Handbook of Epidemiology

Wolfgang Ahrens
Iris Pigeot

Editors

Handbook of Epidemiology

With 165 Figures and 180 Tables

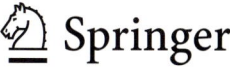 Springer

Editors
Prof. Dr. rer. nat. Wolfgang Ahrens
Prof. Dr. rer. nat. Iris Pigeot

Division of Epidemiological Methods and Ethiologic Research
and
Division of Biometrie and Data Management
Bremen Institute for Prevention Research and Social Medicine (BIPS)
Linzer Str. 8–10
28359 Bremen
Germany

Library of Congress Control Number: 2004106521

ISBN 3-540-00566-8 Springer Berlin Heidelberg New York

Springer is a part of Springer Science+Business Media

springeronline.com

© Springer-Verlag Berlin Heidelberg 2005
Printed in Germany

Typesetting and Production: LE-TEX Jelonek, Schmidt & Vöckler GbR, Leipzig
Cover design and production: deblik, Berlin
Printed on acid-free paper   40/3142/YL   5 4 3 2 1 0

Foreword

When I was learning epidemiology nearly 50 years ago, there was barely one suitable textbook and a handful of specialized monographs to guide me. Information and ideas in journals were pretty sparse too. That all began to change about 25 years ago and soon we had a plethora of books to consider when deciding on something to recommend to students at every level from beginners to advanced postgraduates. This one is different from all the others. There has never been a single source of detailed descriptive accounts and informed discussions of all the essential aspects of practical epidemiology, written by experts and intended as a desk reference for mature epidemiologists who are in practice, probably already specializing in a particular field, but in need of current information and ideas about every aspect of the state of the art and science. Without a work like this, it is difficult to stay abreast of the times. A comprehensive current overview like this where each chapter is written by acknowledged experts chosen from a rich international pool of talent and expertise makes the task considerably easier.

It had been a rare privilege to receive and read the chapters as they have been written and sent to me through cyberspace. Each added to my enthusiasm for the project. I know and have a high regard for the authors of many of the chapters, and reading the chapters by those I did not know has given me a high regard for them too. The book has a logical framework and structure, proceeding from sections on concepts and methods and statistical methods to applications and fields of current research. I have learned a great deal from all of it, and furthermore I have enjoyed reading these accounts. I am confident that many others will do so too.

John M. Last
Emeritus professor of epidemiology
University of Ottawa, Canada

Preface

The objective of this book is to provide a comprehensive overview of the field of epidemiology, bridging the gap between standard textbooks of epidemiology and publications for specialists with a narrow focus on specific areas. It reviews the key issues, methodological approaches and statistical concepts pertinent to the field for which the reader seeks a detailed overview. It thus serves both as a first orientation for the interested reader and a starting point for an in-depth study of a specific area, as well as a quick reference and a summarizing overview for the expert.

The handbook is intended as a reference source for professionals involved in health research, health reporting, health promotion, and health system administration and related experts. It covers the major aspects of epidemiology and may be consulted as a thorough guide for specific topics. It is therefore of interest for public health researchers, physicians, biostatisticians, epidemiologists, and executives in health services.

The broad scope of the book is reflected by four major parts that facilitate an integration of epidemiological concepts and methods, statistical tools, applications, and epidemiological practice. The various facets are presented in 39 chapters and a general introduction to epidemiology. The latter provides the framework in which all other chapters are embedded and gives an overall picture of the whole handbook. It also highlights specific aspects and reveals the interwoven nature of the various research fields and disciplines related to epidemiology. The book covers topics that are usually missing from standard textbooks and that are only marginally represented in the specific literature, such as ethical aspects, practical fieldwork, health services research, epidemiology in developing countries, quality control, and good epidemiological practice. It also covers innovative areas, e.g., molecular and genetic epidemiology, modern study designs, and recent methodological developments.

Each chapter of the handbook serves as an introduction that allows one to enter a new field by addressing basic concepts, but without being too elementary. It also conveys more advanced knowledge and may thus be used as a reference source for the reader who is familiar with the given topic by reflecting the state of the art and future prospects. Of course, some basic understanding of the concepts of probability, sampling distribution, estimation, and hypothesis testing will help the reader to profit from the statistical concepts primarily presented in Part II and from the comprehensive discussion of empirical methods in the other parts. Each chapter is intended to stand on its own, giving an overview of the topic and the most important problems and approaches, which are supported by examples, practical applications, and illustrations. The basic concepts and knowledge, standard procedures and methods are presented, as well as recent advances and new perspectives. The handbook provides references both to introductory texts and to publications for the advanced reader.

The editors dedicate this handbook to Professor Eberhard Greiser, one of the pioneers of epidemiology in Germany. He is the founder of the Bremen Institute for Prevention Research and Social Medicine (BIPS), which is devoted to research into the causes and the prevention of disease. This institute, which started as a small enterprise dedicated to cardiovascular prevention, has grown to become one of the most highly regarded research institutes for epidemiology and public health in Germany. For almost 25 years Eberhard Greiser has been a leader in the field of epidemiology, committing his professional career to a critical appraisal of health practices for the benefit of us all. His major interests have been in pharmaceutical care and social medicine. In recognition of his contributions as a researcher and as a policy advisor to the advancement of the evolving field of epidemiology and public health in Germany we take his 65th birthday in November 2003 as an opportunity to acknowledge his efforts by editing this handbook.

The editors are indebted to knowledgeable experts for their valuable contributions and their enthusiastic support in producing this handbook. We thank all the colleagues who critically reviewed the chapters: Klaus Giersiepen, Cornelia Heitmann, Katrin Janhsen, Jürgen Kübler, Hermann Pohlabeln, Walter Schill, Jürgen Timm, and especially Klaus Krickeberg for his never-ending efforts. We also thank Heidi Asendorf, Thomas Behrens, Claudia Brünings-Kuppe, Andrea Eberle, Ronja Foraita, Andrea Gottlieb, Frauke Günther, Carola Lehmann, Anette Lübke, Ines Pelz, Jenny Peplies, Ursel Prote, Achim Reineke, Anke Suderburg, Nina Wawro, and Astrid Zierer for their technical support. Without the continuous and outstanding engagement of Regine Albrecht – her patience with us and the contributors and her remarkable autonomy – this volume would not have been possible. She has devoted many hours to our handbook over and above her other responsibilities as administrative assistant of the BIPS. Last but not least we are deeply grateful to Clemens Heine of Springer for his initiative, support, and advice in realizing this project and for his confidence in us.

Bremen
June 2004

Wolfgang Ahrens
Iris Pigeot

Table of Contents

II. Statistical Methods in Epidemiology

III. Applications of Epidemiology

IV. Research Areas in Epidemiology

An Introduction to Epidemiology

Wolfgang Ahrens, Klaus Krickeberg, Iris Pigeot

Epidemiology and Related Areas

Various disciplines contribute to the investigation of determinants of human health and disease, to the improvement of health care, and to the prevention of illness. These contributing disciplines stem from three major scientific areas, first from basic biomedical sciences such as biology, physiology, biochemistry, molecular genetics, and pathology, second from clinical sciences such as oncology, gynecology, orthopedics, obstetrics, cardiology, internal medicine, urology, radiology, and pharmacology, and third from public health sciences with epidemiology as their core.

Definition and Purpose of Epidemiology

One of the most frequently used definitions of epidemiology was given by MacMahon and Pugh (1970):

> Epidemiology is the study of the distribution and determinants of disease frequency in man.

The three components of this definition, i.e. frequency, distribution, and determinants embrace the basic principles and approaches in epidemiological research. The measurement of disease *frequency* relates to the quantification of disease occurrence in human populations. Such data are needed for further investigations of patterns of disease in subgroups of the population. This involves "… describing the *distribution* of health status in terms of age, sex, race, geography, etc., …" (MacMahon and Pugh 1970). The methods used to describe the distribution of diseases may be considered as a prerequisite to identify the *determinants* of human health and disease.

This definition is based on two fundamental assumptions: First, the occurrence of diseases in populations is not a purely random process, and second, it is determined by causal and preventive factors (Hennekens and Buring 1987). As mentioned above, these factors have to be searched for systematically in populations defined by place, time, or otherwise. Different ecological models have been used to describe the interrelationship of these factors, which relate to host, agent, and environment. Changing any of these three forces, which constitute the so-called epidemiological triangle (Fig. 1.1), will influence the balance among them and thereby increase or decrease the disease frequency (Mausner and Bahn 1974).

Thus, the search for etiological factors in the development of ill health is one of the main concerns of epidemiology. Complementary to the epidemiological triangle the triad of time, place, and person is often used by epidemiologists to describe the distribution of diseases and their determinants. Determinants that influence health may consist of behavioral, cultural, social, psychological, biological, or physical factors. The determinants by time may relate to increase/decrease

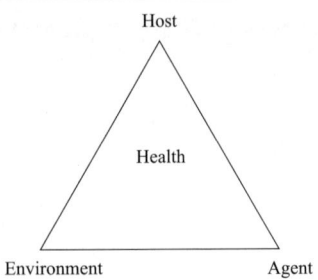

Figure 1.1. The epidemiological triangle

over the years, seasonal variations, or sudden changes of disease occurrence. Determinants by place can be characterized by country, climate zone, residence, and more general, by geographic region. Personal determinants include age, sex, ethnic group, genetic traits, and individual behavior. Studying the interplay between time, place, and person helps to identify the etiologic agent and the environmental factors as well as to describe the natural history of the disease, which then enables the epidemiologist to define targets for intervention with the purpose of disease prevention (Detels 2002). This widened perspective is reflected in a more comprehensive definition of epidemiology as given by Last (2001):

> The study of the distribution and determinants of health-related states or events in specified populations, and the application of this study to control of health problems.

In this broader sense, health-related states or events include "diseases, causes of death, behaviors such as use of tobacco, reactions to preventive regimens, and provision and use of health services" (Last 2001). According to this definition, the final aim of epidemiology is to promote, protect, and restore health. Hence, the major goals of epidemiology may be defined from two overlapping perspectives. The first is a biomedical perspective looking primarily at the etiology of diseases and the disease process itself. This includes

— the description of the disease spectrum, the syndromes of the disease and the disease entities to learn about the various outcomes that may be caused by particular pathogens,

— the description of the natural history, i.e. the course of the disease to improve the diagnostic accuracy which is a major issue in clinical epidemiology,

— the investigation of physiological or genetic variables in relation to influencing factors and disease outcomes to decide whether they are potential risk factors, disease markers or indicators of early stages of disease,

— the identification of factors that are responsible for the increase or decrease of disease risks in order to obtain the knowledge necessary for primary prevention,

— the prediction of disease trends to facilitate the adaptation of the health services to future needs and to identify research priorities,

— the clarification of disease transmission to control the spread of contagious diseases e.g. by targeted vaccination programs.

Achievement of these aims is the prerequisite for the second perspective, which defines the scope of epidemiology from a public health point of view. Especially in this respect, the statement as given in Box 1 was issued by the IEA (International Epidemiological Association) Conference already in 1975.

Box 1. Statement by IEA Conference in 1975 (White and Henderson 1976)

"The discipline of epidemiology, together with the applied fields of economics, management sciences, and the social sciences, provide the essential quantitative and analytical methods, principles of logical inquiry, and rules for evidence for:

— ...;
— diagnosing, measuring, and projecting the health needs of community and populations;
— determining health goals, objectives and priorities;
— allocating and managing health care resources;
— assessing intervention strategies and evaluating the impact of health services."

This list may be complemented by the provision of tools for investigating consequences of disease as unemployment, social deprivation, disablement, and death.

Epidemiology in Relation to Other Disciplines 1.2

Biomedical, clinical and other related disciplines sometimes claim that epidemiology belongs to their particular research area. It is therefore not surprising that biometricians think of epidemiology as a part of biometry and physicians define epidemiology as a medical science. Biometricians have in mind that epidemiology uses statistical methods to investigate the distribution of health-related entities in populations as opposed to handling single cases. This perspective on distributions of events, conditions, etc. is statistics by its very nature. On the other hand, physicians view epidemiology primarily from a substantive angle on diseases and their treatment. In doing so, each of them may disregard central elements that constitute epidemiology.

Moreover, as described at the beginning, epidemiology overlaps with various other domains that provide their methods and knowledge to answer epidemiological questions. For example, measurement scales and instruments to assess subjective well-being developed by psychologists can be applied by epidemiologists to investigate the psychological effects of medical treatments in addition to classical clinical outcome parameters. Social sciences provide indicators and methods of field work that are useful in describing social inequality in health, in investigating social determinants of health, and in designing population-based prevention strategies. Other examples are methods and approaches from demography that are used to provide health reports, from population genetics to identify hereditary factors, and from molecular biology to search for precursors of diseases and factors of susceptibility.

Of course, epidemiology does not only borrow methods from other sciences but has also its own methodological core. This pertains in particular to the development and adaptation of study designs. It is also true for statistical methods. In most cases they can directly be applied to epidemiological data, but sometimes peculiarities in the data structure may call for the derivation of special methods to cope with these requirements. This is in particular currently the case in genetic epidemiology when e.g. modeling gene-environment interactions is needed.

The borderline between epidemiology and related disciplines is often blurred. Let us take clinical medicine as an example. In clinical practice, a physician decides case-by-case to diagnose and treat individual patients. To achieve the optimal treatment for a given subject, he or she will classify this patient and then make use of knowledge on the group to which the person belongs. This knowledge may come from randomized clinical trials but also from (clinical) epidemiological studies. A randomized clinical trial is a special type of a randomized controlled trial (RCT). In a broad sense, a RCT is an epidemiological experiment in which subjects in a population are randomly allocated into groups, i.e. a study group where intervention takes place and a control group without intervention. This indicates an overlap between clinical and epidemiological studies, where the latter focus on populations while clinical trials address highly selected groups of patients. Thus, it may be controversial whether randomized clinical trials for drug approval (i.e. phase III trials) are to be considered part of epidemiology, but it is clear that a follow-up concerned with safety aspects of drug utilization (so-called phase IV studies) needs pharmacoepidemiological approaches.

When discussing the delimitation of epidemiology the complex area of public health plays an essential role. According to Last's definition (Last 2001) public health has to do with the health needs of the population as a whole, in particular the prevention and treatment of disease. More explicitly, "Public health is one of the efforts organized by society to protect, promote, and restore the people's health. It is the combination of sciences, skills, and beliefs that is directed to the maintenance and improvement of the health of all the people through collective or social actions. (...) Public health ... goals remain the same: to reduce the amount of disease, premature death, and disease-produced discomfort and disability in the population. Public health is thus a social institution, a discipline, and a practice." (Last 2001). The practice of public health is based on scientific knowledge of factors influencing health and disease, where epidemiology is, according to Detels and Breslow (2002), "the core science of public health and preventive medicine" that is complemented by biostatistics and "knowledge and strategies derived from biological, physical, social, and demographic sciences".

In conclusion, epidemiology cannot be reduced to a sub-division of one of the contributing sciences but it should be considered as a multidisciplinary science giving input to the applied field of public health.

Overview 1.3

The present handbook intends to reflect all facets of epidemiology, ranging from basic principles (Part I) through statistical methods typically applied in epidemiological studies (Part II) to the majority of important applications (Part III) and to special fields of research (Part IV). Within these four parts, its structure is to a large extent determined by various natural subdivisions of the domain of epidemiology. These correspond mostly to the elements of the definition of epidemiology as given by Last and quoted above, namely study, distribution, determinants (factors, exposures, explanatory variables), health-related states or events (outcomes), populations, applications.

For instance, the concepts of a study and of determinants lead to the distinction of observational epidemiology on the one hand and experimental epidemiology on the other. In the first area, we study situations as they present themselves without intervening. In particular, we are interested in existing determinants within given populations. A typical example would be the investigation of the influence of a risk factor like air pollution on a health-related event like asthma. In experimental epidemiology, however, determinants are introduced and controlled by the investigator in populations which he or she defines by himself or herself, often by random allocation; in fact, experimental epidemiology is often simply identified with RCTs. Clinical trials to study the efficacy of the determinant "treatment" are a special type within this category. They are to be distinguished from trials of preventive interventions, another part of experimental epidemiology.

The idea of the purpose of a study gives rise to another, less clearly defined, subdivision, i.e. explanatory vs. descriptive epidemiology. The objective of an explanatory study is to contribute to the search of causes for health-related events, in particular by isolating the effects of specific factors. This causal element is lacking or at least not prominent in purely descriptive studies. In practice this distinction often amounts to different, and contrasting, sources of data: In descriptive epidemiology they are routinely registered for various reasons whereas in explanatory or analytic epidemiology they are collected for specific purposes. The expression "descriptive epidemiology" used to have a more restrictive, "classical" meaning that is also rendered by the term "health statistics" where as a rule the determinants are time, place of residence, age, gender, and socio-economic status.

"Exposure-oriented" and "outcome-oriented" epidemiology represent the two sides of the same coin. Insofar this distinction is more systematic rather than substantive. If the research question emphasizes disease determinants, e.g. environmental or genetic factors, the corresponding studies usually are classified as exposure-oriented. If, in contrast, a disease or another health-related event like lung cancer or osteoarthritis is the focus, we speak of "outcome-oriented" studies, in which risk factors for the specific disease are searched for. Finally, some subfields of epidemiology are defined by a particular type of application such as prevention, screening, and clinical epidemiology.

Let us now have a short look at the chapters of the handbook. Part I contains general concepts and methodological approaches in epidemiology: After introducing the philosophical background and the conceptual building blocks of epidemiology such as models for causation and statistical ideas (Chap. I.1), Chap. I.2 deepens the latter aspect by giving an overview of various risk measures usually asked for in epidemiological studies. These measures depend heavily on the study type chosen for obtaining the data required to answer the research question. Various designs can be thought of to collect the necessary information. These are described in Chaps. I.3 to I.8. Descriptive studies and disease registries provide the basic information for health reporting. Experimental studies like cohort and case-control studies, modern study designs, and intervention trials serve to examine associations and hypothesized causal relationships. Chapter I.9 discusses in detail the two concepts of interaction and confounding, which are, on the one hand, very technical, but on the other hand fundamental for the analysis of any epidemiological study that involves several determinants. They allow us to describe the synergy of several factors and to isolate the effect of any of them. Chapters I.10 to I.13 concern practical problems to be handled when conducting an epidemiological study: field data collection in Chap. I.10, difficulties specific to exposure assessment in Chap. I.11, some key aspects of the planning of studies in general in Chap. I.12, and quality control and related aspects in Chap. I.13.

Due to the large variety of epidemiological issues, methodological approaches, and types of data, the arsenal of statistical concepts and methods to be found in epidemiology is also very broad. Chapter II.1 treats the question of how many units (people, communities) to recruit into a study in order to obtain a desired statistical precision. Chapter II.2 focuses on the analysis of studies where exposures and/or outcomes are described by continuous variables. Since the relationships between exposures and outcomes, which are the essence of epidemiology, are mostly represented by regression models it is not surprising that Chap. II.3 that is devoted to them is one of the longest of the whole handbook. Chapter II.4 discusses in detail the models used when the outcome variables are in the form of a waiting time until a specific event, e.g. death, occurs. Given that in practice data are often erroneous or missing, methods to handle the ensuing problems are presented in Chaps. II.5 and II.6. Meta-analysis is the art of drawing joint conclusions from the results of several studies together in order to put these conclusions on firmer ground, in particular, technically speaking, to increase their statistical power. It is the subject of Chap. II.7. The last chapter on statistical methodology, Chap. II.8, concerns the analysis of spatial data where the values of the principal explanatory variable are geographic locations. The topic of this chapter is closely related to the fields of application in Part III.

Although each epidemiological study contains its own peculiarities and specific problems related to its design and conduct, depending on the field of application, common features may be identified. Many important, partly classical, partly recent applications of epidemiology of general interest to public health are defined by specific exposures, and hence Part III starts with the presentation of the main exposure-oriented fields: social (III.1), occupational (III.2), environmental (III.3), nutritional (III.4), and reproductive epidemiology (III.5), but also more recent applications such as molecular (III.6) and genetic (III.7). Clinical epidemiology

(III.8) and pharmacoepidemiology (III.9) are large areas where knowledge about the interplay between many types of exposures, e.g. therapies, and many types of outcomes, usually diseases, is being exploited. A similar remark applies to the classical domains of screening in view of early detection of chronic diseases (Chap. III.10) and community-based health promotion, which mostly aims at prevention (Chap. III.11). These fields extend to public health research and build the bridge to the final part of this handbook.

Intensive research is going on in all of the foregoing areas, hence the selection of the topics for Part IV might appear a bit arbitrary, but in our opinion these seem to be currently the subject of particular efforts and widespread interest. The first four are outcome-oriented and deal with diseases of high public health relevance: infectious diseases (Chap. IV.1), cardiovascular diseases (Chap. IV.2), cancer (Chap. IV.3), and muscoloskeletal disorders (Chap. IV.4). The public health perspective is not restricted to these outcome-oriented research areas. The results of epidemiological studies may have a strong impact on political decisions and the health system, an area that is described for developed countries in Chap. IV.5. The particular problems related to health systems in developing countries and the resulting special demands for epidemiological research are addressed in Chap. IV.6. The handbook closes with the very important issue of human rights and responsibilities that have to be carefully considered at the different stages of an epidemiological study. These are discussed in Chap. IV.7 on ethical aspects.

Development of Epidemiology 2

Historical Background 2.1

The word "epidemic", i.e. something that falls upon people (ἐπί upon; δῆμος people), which was in use in ancient Greece, already reflected one of the basic ideas of modern epidemiology, namely to look at diseases on the level of *populations*, or *herds* as they also have been called, especially in the epidemiology of infectious diseases. The link with the search for *causes* of illness was present in early writings of the Egyptians, Jews, Greeks, and Romans (Bulloch 1938). Both Hippocrates (ca. 460–ca. 375 BC) and Galen (129 or 230–200 or 201) advanced etiological theories. The first stressed atmospheric conditions and "miasmata" but considered nutrition and lifestyle as well (Hippocrates 400 BC). The second distinguished three causes of an "epidemic constitution" in a population: an atmospheric one, susceptibility, and lifestyle. The basic book by Coxe (1846) contains a classification of Galen's writings by subject including the subject "etiology". For a survey on the various editions of Galen's work and a biography see the essay by Siegel (1968).

Regarding more specific observations, the influence of dust in quarries on chronic lung diseases was mentioned in a Roman text of the first century. Paracelsus in 1534 published the first treatise on *occupational diseases*, entitled "Von der Bergsucht" (On miners' diseases); see his biography in English by Pagel (1982).

Ramazzini (1713) conjectured that the relatively high incidence of breast cancer among nuns was due to celibacy. Sixty-two years later, Percival Pott (1775) was among the first ones to phrase a comparative observation in quantitative terms. He reported that scrotal cancer was very frequent among London chimney sweeps, and that their death rate due to this disease was more than 200 times higher than that of other workers.

The most celebrated early observational epidemiological study is that of John Snow on cholera in London in 1853. He was able to record the mortality by this disease in various places of residence under different conditions of water supply. And by comparison he concluded that deficient quality of water was indeed the cause of cholera (Snow 1855).

Parallel to this emergence of observational epidemiology, three more currents of epidemiological thinking have been growing during the centuries and interacted among them and with the former, namely the debate on *contagion* and *living causal agents*, *descriptive* epidemiology in the classical sense of health statistics, and *clinical trials*.

A contagion can be suspected from recording cases and their location in time, space, families, and the like. The possibility of its involvement in epidemics has therefore no doubt been considered since time immemorial; it was alluded to in the early writings mentioned at the beginning. Nevertheless, Hippocrates and Galen did not admit it. It played an important role in the thinking about *variolation*, and later on *vaccination* as introduced by Jenner in 1796 (Jenner 1798). The essay by Daniel Bernoulli on the impact of variolation (Bernoulli 1766) was the beginning of the theory of *mathematical modeling* of the spread of diseases.

By contrast to a contagion itself, the existence of *living* pathogens cannot be deduced from purely epidemiological observations, but the discussion around it has often been intermingled with that about contagion, and has contributed much to epidemiological thinking. Fracastoro (1521) wrote about a *contagium animatum*. In the sequel the idea came up again and again in various forms, e.g. in the writings of Snow. It culminated in the identification of specific parasites, fungi, bacteria, and viruses as agents in the period from, roughly, 1840 when Henle, after Arabian predecessors dating back to the ninth century, definitely showed that mites cause scabies, until 1984 when the HIV was identified.

As far as we know, the term "epidemiology" first appeared in Madrid in 1802. From the late 19th century to about the middle of the 20th, it was restricted to *epidemical infectious* diseases until it took its present meaning (see Sect. 2.2 and Greenwood 1932).

Descriptive epidemiology had various precursors, mainly in the form of church and military records on one hand (Marshall and Tulloch 1838), life tables on the other (Graunt 1662; Halley 1693). In the late 18th century, local medical statistics started to appear in many European cities and regions. They took a more systematic turn with the work of William Farr (1975). This lasted from 1837 when he was appointed to the General Register Office in London until his retirement in 1879. In particular, he developed classifications of diseases that led to the first International List of Causes of Death, to be adopted in 1893 by the International

Statistical Institute. Farr took also part in the activities of the London Epidemiological Society, founded in 1850 with him and Snow as founding members, and apparently the oldest learned society featuring the word "epidemiological" in its name.

Geographic epidemiology, i.e. the presentation of health statistics in the form of maps, also started in the 19th century (Rupke 2000).

If we mean by a clinical trial a *planned, comparative,* and *quantitative* experiment on humans in order to learn something about the efficacy of a curative or preventive treatment in a clinical setting, James Lind is considered having done the first one. In 1747 he tried out six different supplements to the basic diet of 12 sailors suffering from scurvy, and found that citrus fruits, and only these, cured the patients (Lind 1753). Later he also compared quinine to treat malaria with less well-defined control therapies (Lind 1771).

The first more or less rigorous trial of a preventive measure was performed by Jenner with 23 vaccinated people, but he still used what is now being called "historical controls," i.e. he compared these vaccinated people with unvaccinated ones of the past who had not been specially selected beforehand for the purpose of the trial (Jenner 1798).

In the 19th century some physicians began to think about the general principles of clinical trials and already emphasized probabilistic and statistical methods (Louis 1835; Bernard 1865). Some trials were done, for example on the efficacy of bloodletting to treat pneumonia, but rigorous methods in the modern sense were established only after World War II (see Sect. 2.2), beginning in 1948 with the pioneer trial on the treatment of pulmonary tuberculosis by streptomycin as described in Hill (1962).

Let us conclude this all too short historical sketch with a few remarks on the history of applications of epidemiology.

Clinical trials have always been tied, by their very nature, to immediate applications as in the above mentioned examples; hence we will not dwell on this anymore.

Observational epidemiology, including classical descriptive epidemiology, has led to hygienic measures. In fact, coming back to a concept of Galen (1951), one might define *hygiene* in a modern and general sense as applied observational epidemiology, its task being to diminish or to eliminate causal factors of any kind. For example, the results of Snow's study on cholera found rapid applications in London but not in places like Hamburg where 8600 people died in the cholera epidemic of 1892.

Hygiene was a matter of much debate and activity during the entire 19th century, although, before the identification of living pathogens, most measures taken were necessarily not directed against a known specific agent, with the exception of *meat inspection* for trichinae. This was made compulsory in Prussia in 1875 as proposed by Rudolf Virchow, one of the pioneers of modern hygiene and also an active politician (Ackerknecht 1953).

Hygienic activities generally had their epidemiological roots in the descriptive health statistics mentioned above. These statistics usually involved only factors like time, place of residence, sex, and age, but Virchow, for example, analyzed during the years 1854–1871 the mortality statistics for the city of Berlin and tried to link those factors with social factors like poverty, crowded dwellings, and dangerous professions, thus becoming a forerunner of *social epidemiology*.

As a result of such reflections as well as of political pressure, large *sewage systems* were built in Europe and North America, the *refuse disposal* was reorganized and the *water supply* improved. Other hygienic measures concerned the structure and functioning of *hospitals*, from reducing the number of patients per room and dispersing wards in the form of pavilions to antiseptic rules. The latter had mainly been inspired by more or less precise epidemiological observations on infections after the treatment of wounds and amputations (Tenon 1788; Simpson 1868–1869, 1869–1870; Ackerknecht 1967), and on puerperal fever (Gordon 1795; Holmes 1842–1843; Semmelweis 1861).

2.2   Milestones in Epidemiological Research

The initiation of numerous epidemiological studies after the Second World War accelerated the research in this field and led to a systematic development of study designs and methods. In the following some exemplary studies are introduced that served as role models for the design and analysis of many subsequent investigations. It is not our intention to provide an exhaustive list of all major studies since that time, if at all feasible, but to exhibit some cornerstones marking the most important steps in the evolution of this science. Each of them had its own peculiarities with a high impact both on methods and epidemiological reasoning as well as on health policies.

The usefulness of descriptive study designs has been convincingly demonstrated by migrant studies comparing the incidence or mortality of a disease within a certain population between the country of origin and the new host country. Such observations offer an exceptional opportunity to distinguish between potential contributions of genetics and environment to the development of disease and thus make it possible to distinguish between the effects of nature and nurture. The most prominent examples are provided by investigations on Japanese migrants to Hawaii and California. For instance, the mortality from stomach cancer is much higher in Japan than among US inhabitants whereas for colon cancer the relationship is reversed. Japanese migrants living in California have a mortality pattern that lies between those two populations. It was thus concluded that dietary and other lifestyle factors have a stronger impact than hereditary factors, which is further supported by the fact that the sons of Japanese immigrants in California have an even lower risk for stomach cancer and a still higher risk for cancer of the colon than their fathers (Buell and Dunn 1965).

One of the milestones in the development of epidemiology was the case-control design, which facilitates the investigation of risk factors for chronic diseases with long induction periods. The most famous study of this type, although not the first, is the study on smoking and lung cancer by Doll and Hill (1950). As early as 1943, the German pathologist Schairer published together with Schöniger from the Scientific Institute for Research into the Hazards of Tobacco, Jena, a case-control study comparing 109 men and women deceased from lung cancer with 270 healthy male controls as well as with 318 men and women who died from other cancers with regard to their smoking habits (Schairer and Schöniger 1943). Judged by modern epidemiological standards this study had several weaknesses, still, it showed a clear association of tobacco use and lung cancer. The case-control study by Doll and Hill was much more sophisticated in methodological terms. Over the whole period of investigation from 1948 to 1952 they recruited 1357 male and 108 female patients with lung cancer from several hospitals in London and matched them with respect to age and sex to the same number of patients hospitalized for non-malignant conditions. For each patient, detailed data on smoking history was collected. Without going into detail here, these data came up with a strong indication for a positive association between smoking and lung cancer. Despite the methodological concerns regarding case-control studies, Doll and Hill themselves believed that smoking was responsible for the development of lung cancer. The study became a landmark that inspired future generations of epidemiologists to use this methodology (cf. Chap. I.6 of this handbook). It remains to this day a model for the design and conduct of case-control studies, with excellent suggestions on how to reduce or eliminate selection, interview, and recall bias (cf. Chaps. I.9, I.10, I.12, I.13).

Because of the strong evidence they started a cohort study of 20,000 male British physicians in 1951, known as the British Doctors' Study. These were followed to further investigate the association between smoking and lung cancer. The authors compared mortality from lung cancer among those who never smoked with that among all smokers and with those who smoked various numbers of cigarettes per day (Doll and Hill 1954, 1964; Doll and Peto 1978).

Another, probably even more important cohort study was the Framingham Heart Study that was based on the population of Framingham, a small community in Massachusetts. The study was initiated in 1949 to yield insights into causes of cardiovascular diseases (CVD) (see Chap. IV.2 of this handbook). For this purpose, 5127 participants free from coronary heart disease (CHD), 30 to 59 years of age, were examined and then followed for nearly 50 years to determine the rate of occurrence of new cases among persons free of disease at first observation (Dawber et al. 1951; Dawber 1980). The intensive biennial examination schedule, long-term continuity of follow-up and investigator involvement, and incorporation of new design components over its decades-long history have made this a uniquely rich source of data on individual risks of CVD events. The study served as a reference and good example for many subsequent cohort studies in this field adopting its methodology. In particular, analysis of these data led to the development of the perhaps most important modeling technique in epidemiology, the multiple logistic regression (Truett et al. 1967; see Chap. II.3).

Two other leading examples of cohort studies conducted within a single population or for comparison of multiple populations to assess risk factors for cardiovascular events are the Whitehall Study of British civil servants (Rose and Shipley 1986; see also Chap. III.1) and the Seven Countries Study of factors accounting for differences in CHD rates between populations of Europe, Japan, and North America (Keys 1980; Kromhout et al. 1995; see Chap. IV.2).

In contrast to the above cohort studies that focused on cardiovascular diseases the U.S. Nurses' Health Study is an impressive example of a multipurpose cohort study. It recruited over 120,000 married female nurses, 30 to 55 years of age, in a mail survey in 1976. In this survey, information on demographic, reproductive, medical and lifestyle factors was obtained. Nurses were contacted every two years to assess outcomes that occurred during that interval and to update and to supplement the exposure information collected at baseline. Various exposure factors like use of oral contraceptives, post-menopausal hormone therapy, and fat consumption were related to different outcomes such as cancer and cardiovascular disease (Lipnick et al. 1986; Willett et al. 1987; Stampfer et al. 1985). The most recent results have had an essential impact on the risk-benefit assessment of post-menopausal hormone therapy speaking against its use over extended periods (Chen et al. 2002).

Final proof of a causal relationship is provided by experimental studies, namely intervention trials. The most famous and largest intervention trial was the so-called Salk vaccine field trial in 1954 where nearly one million school children were randomly assigned to one of two groups, a vaccination group that received the active vaccine and a comparison group receiving placebo. A 50 percent reduction of the incidence of paralytic poliomyelitis was observed in the vaccination group as compared to the placebo group. This gave the basis for the large-scale worldwide implementation of poliomyelitis vaccination programs for disease prevention.

In recent years, the accelerated developments in molecular biology were taken up by epidemiologists to measure markers of exposure, early biological effects, and host characteristics that influence response (susceptibility) in human cells, blood, tissue and other material. These techniques augment the standard tools of epidemiology in the investigation of low-level risks, risks imposed by complex exposures, and the modification of risks by genetic factors. The use of such biomarkers of exposure and effect has led to a boom of the so-called molecular epidemiology (Schulte and Perera 1998; Toniolo et al. 1997; Chap. III.6 of this handbook), a methodological approach with early origins. These developments were accompanied by the sequencing of the human genome and the advances in high-throughput genetic technologies that led to the rapid progress of genetic epidemiology (Khoury et al. 1993; Chap. III.7 of this handbook). The better understanding of genetic factors and their interaction with each other and with environmental factors in disease causation is a major challenge for future research.

2.3   Methodological Limits

The successes of epidemiology in identifying major risk factors of chronic diseases have been contrasted with many more subtle risks that epidemiologists have seemingly discovered. Such risks are difficult to determine and false alarms may result from chance findings. Thus it is not surprising that in recent years many studies showed conflicting evidence, i.e. some studies seem to reveal a significant association while others do not. The uncritical publication of such contradictory results in the lay press leads to opposing advice and thus to an increasing anxiety in the public. This has given rise to a critical debate about the methodological weaknesses of epidemiology that culminated in the article "Epidemiology faces its limits" by Taubes (1995) and the discussions that it prompted.

In investigating low relative risks, say, below 2 or even below 1.5, the methodological shortcomings inherent in observational designs become more serious. Such studies are more prone to yield false positive or false negative findings due to the distorting effects of misclassification, bias, and confounding (see Chaps. I.9 and II.5 of this handbook). For instance, the potential effect of environmental tobacco smoke (ETS) on lung cancer was denied because misclassification of only a few active smokers as non-smokers would result in relative risks that might explain all or most of the observed association between ETS and the risk of lung cancer in non-smokers (Lee and Forey 1996). Validation studies showed that this explanation was unlikely (Riboli et al. 1990; Wells et al. 1998). Thus, the numerous positive findings and the obvious biological plausibility of the exposure-disease relationship support the conclusion of a harmful effect of ETS (Boffetta et al. 1998; Chan-Yeung and Dimich-Ward 2003; IARC Monograph on ETS 2004). This example also illustrates that the investigation of low relative risks is not an academic exercise but may be of high public health relevance if a large segment of the population is exposed.

It is often believed that large-scale studies are needed to identify small risks since such studies result in narrower confidence intervals. However, a narrow confidence interval does not necessarily mean that the overwhelming effects of misclassification, bias and confounding are adequately controlled by simply increasing the size of a study. Even sophisticated statistical analyses will never overcome serious deficiencies of the data base. The fundamental quality of the data collected or provided for epidemiological purposes is therefore the cornerstone of any study and needs to be prioritized throughout its planning and conduct (see Chap. I.13). In addition, refinement of methods and measures involving all steps from design over exposure and outcome assessment to the final data analysis, incorporating e.g. molecular markers, may help to push the edge of what can be achieved with epidemiology a little bit further.

Nevertheless a persistent problem is "The pressures to publish inconclusive results and the eagerness of the press to publicize them ..." (Taubes 1995). This pressure to publish positive findings that are questionable imposes a particular demand on researchers not only to report and interpret study results carefully in peer reviewed journals but also to communicate potential risks also to the lay press in a comprehensible manner that accounts for potential limitations. Both authors and editors have to take care that the pressure to publish does not lead to a publication bias favoring positive findings and dismissing negative results.

Concepts and Methodological
3   # Approaches in Epidemiology

Extending the basic ideas of epidemiology presented above together with its definition, its scope and approaches will now be described further.

3.1   Concepts

Epidemiology may be considered as minor to physical sciences because it does not investigate the biological mechanism leading from exposure to disease as, e.g., toxicology does. However, the ability of identifying modifiable conditions that contribute to health outcome without also identifying the biological mechanism or the agent(s) that lead to this outcome is a strength of epidemiology: It is not always necessary to wait until this mechanism is completely understood in order to facilitate preventive action. This is illustrated by the historical examples of the improvements of environmental hygiene that led to a reduction of infectious diseases like cholera, that was possible before the identification of vibrio cholerae.

What distinguishes epidemiology is its perspective on groups or populations rather than individuals. It is this demographic focus where statistical methods enter the field and provide the tools needed to compare different characteristics relating to disease occurrence between populations. Epidemiology is a comparative discipline that contrasts diseases and characteristics relative to different time periods, different places or different groups of persons. The comparison of groups is a central feature of epidemiology, be it the comparison of morbidity or mortality in populations with and without a certain exposure or the comparison of exposure between diseased subjects and a control group. Inclusion of an appropriate reference group (non-exposed or non-diseased) for comparison with the group of interest is a condition for causal inference.

In experimental studies efficient means are available to minimize the potential for bias. Due to the observational nature of the vast majority of epidemiological studies bias and confounding are the major problems that may restrict the interpretation of the findings if not adequately taken into account (see Chaps. I.9 and I.12 of this handbook). Although possible associations are analyzed and reported on a group level it is important to note that only data that provide the necessary information on an individual level allow the adequate consideration of confounding factors (see Chap. I.3).

Most epidemiological studies deal with mixed populations. On the one hand, the corresponding heterogeneity of covariables may threaten the internal validity of a study, because the inability to randomize in observational studies may impair the comparability between study subjects and referents due to confounding. On the other hand the observation of "natural experiments" in a complex mixture of individuals enables epidemiologists to make statements about the real world and thus contributes to the external validity of the results. This population perspective focuses epidemiology on the judgment of effectiveness rather than efficacy, e.g. in the evaluation of interventions.

Due to practical limitations, in a given study it may not be feasible to obtain a representative sample of the whole population of interest. It may even be desired to investigate only defined subgroups of a population. Whatever the reason, a restriction on subgroups may not necessarily impair the meaning of the obtained results; it may still increase the internal validity of a study. Thus, it is a misconception that the cases always need to be representative of all persons with the disease and that the reference group always should be representative of the general non-diseased population. What is important is a precise definition of the population base, i.e., in a case-control study, cases and controls need to originate from the same source population and the same inclusion/exclusion criteria need to be applied to both groups. This means that any interpretation that extends beyond the source population has to be aware of a restricted generalizability of the findings.

Rarely a single positive study will provide sufficient evidence to justify an intervention. Limitations inherent in most observational studies require the consideration of alternative explanations of the findings and confirmation by independent evidence from other studies in different populations before preventive action is recommended with sufficient certainty. The interpretation of negative studies deserves the same scrutiny as the interpretation of positive studies. Negative results should not hastily be interpreted to prove an absence of the association under investigation (Doll and Wald 1994). Besides chance, false negative results may easily be due to a weak design and conduct of a given study.

Study Designs 3.2

Epidemiological reasoning consists of three major steps. First, a statistical association between an explanatory characteristic (exposure) and the outcome of interest (disease) is established. Then, from the pattern of the association a hypothetical (biological) inference about the disease mechanism is formulated that can be refuted or confirmed by subsequent studies. Finally, when a plausible conjecture about the causal factor(s) leading to the outcome has been acknowledged, alteration or reduction of the putative cause and observation of the resulting disease frequency provide the verification or refutation of the presumed association.

In practice these three major steps are interwoven in an iterative process of hypothesis generation by descriptive and exploratory studies, statistical confirmation of the presumed association by analytical studies and, if feasible, implementation and evaluation of intervention activities, i.e. experimental studies. An overview of the different types of study and some common alternative names are given in Table 1.1.

A first observation of a presumed relationship between exposure and disease is often done at the group level by correlating one group characteristic with an outcome, i.e. in an attempt to relate differences in morbidity or mortality of population groups to differences in their local environment, living habits or other factors. Such correlational studies that are usually based on existing data (see

Table 1.1. Types of epidemiological studies

Type of study	Alternative name	Unit of study
Observational		
Ecological	Correlational	Populations
Cross-sectional	Prevalence; survey	Individuals
Case-control	Case-referent	Individuals
Cohort	Follow-up	Individuals
Experimental	*Intervention studies*	
Community trials	Community intervention studies	Communities
Field trials		Healthy individuals
Randomized controlled trials	RCT	Individuals
Clinical trials	Therapeutic studies[a]	Individual patients

[a] Clinical trials are included here since conceptually they are linked to epidemiology, although they are often not considered as epidemiological studies. Clinical trials have developed into a vast field of its own because of methodological reasons and their commercial importance.

Chap. I.4) are prone to the so-called "ecological fallacy" since the compared populations may also differ in many other uncontrolled factors that are related to the disease. Nevertheless, ecological studies can provide clues to etiological hypotheses and may serve as a gateway towards more detailed investigations. In such studies the investigator determines whether the relationship in question is also present among individuals, either by asking whether persons with the disease have the characteristic more frequently than those without the disease, or by asking whether persons with the characteristic develop the disease more frequently than those not having it. The investigation of an association at the individual level is considered to be less vulnerable to be mixed up with the effect of a third common factor. For a detailed discussion of this issue we refer to Sect. 4.2.5 of Chap. I.3 of this handbook.

Studies that are primarily designed to describe the distribution of existing variables that can be used for the generation of broad hypotheses are often classified as descriptive studies (cf. Chap. I.3 of this handbook). Analytical studies examine an association, i.e. the relationship between a risk factor and a disease in detail and conduct a statistical test of the corresponding hypothesis. Typically the two main types of epidemiological studies, i.e. case-control and cohort, belong to this category (see Chaps. I.5 and I.6 of this handbook). However, a clear-cut distinction between analytical and descriptive study designs is not possible. A case-control study may be designed to explore associations of multiple exposures with a disease. Such "fishing expeditions" may better be characterized as descriptive rather than analytical studies. A cross-sectional study is descriptive when it surveys a community to determine the health status of its members. It is analytic when the association of an acute health event with a recent exposure is analyzed.

Cross-sectional studies provide descriptive data on prevalence of diseases useful for health care planning. Prevalence data on risk factors from descriptive studies also help in planning an analytical study, e.g. for sample size calculations. The design is particularly useful for investigating acute effects but has significant drawbacks in comparison to longitudinal designs because the temporal sequence between exposure and disease usually cannot be assessed with certainty, except for invariant characteristics like blood type. In addition, it cannot assess incident cases of a chronic disease (see Chap. I.3). Both case-control and cohort studies are in some sense longitudinal because they incorporate the temporal dimension by relating exposure information to time periods that are prior to disease occurrence. These two study types – in particular when data are collected prospectively – are therefore usually more informative with respect to causal hypotheses than cross-sectional studies because they are less prone to the danger of "reverse causality" that may emerge when information on exposure and outcome relates to the same point in time. The best means to avoid this danger are prospective designs where the exposure data are collected prior to disease. Typically these are cohort studies, either concurrent or historical, as opposed to retrospective studies, i.e. case-control studies where information on previous exposure is collected from diseased or non-diseased subjects. For further details of the strengths and weaknesses of the main observational designs see Chap. I.12 of this handbook.

The different types of studies are arranged in Table 1.2 in ascending order according to their ability to corroborate the causality of a supposed association. The criteria summarized by Hill (1965) have gained wide acceptance among epidemiologists as a checklist to assess the strength of the evidence for a causal relationship. However, an uncritical accumulation of items from such a list cannot replace the critical appraisal of the quality, strengths and weaknesses of each study. The weight of evidence for a causal association depends in the first place – at least in part – on the type of study, with intervention studies on the top of the list (Table 1.2) (see Chap. I.8). The assessment of causality has then to be based on a critical judgment of evidence by conjecture and refutation (see Chap. I.1 for a discussion of this issue).

Table 1.2. Reasoning in different types of epidemiological study

Study type	Reasoning
Ecological	Descriptive; association on group level may be used for development of broad hypotheses
Cross-sectional	Descriptive; individual association may be used for development and specification of hypotheses
Case-control	Increased prevalence of risk factor among diseased may indicate a causal relationship
Cohort	Increased risk of disease among exposed indicates a causal relationship
Intervention	Modification (reduction) of the incidence rate of the disease confirms a causal relationship

Data Collection

Data are the foundation of any empirical study. To avoid any sort of systematic bias in the planning and conduct of an epidemiological study is a fundamental issue, be it information or selection bias. Errors that have been introduced during data collection can in most cases not be corrected later on. Exceptions from this rule are for example measurement instruments yielding distorted measurements where the systematic error becomes apparent so that the individual measurement values can be adjusted accordingly. In other instances statistical methods are offered to cope with measurement error (see Chap. II.5). However, such later efforts are second choice and an optimal quality of the original data must be the primary goal. Selection bias may be even worse as it cannot be controlled for and may affect both the internal and the external validity of a study. Standardized procedures to ensure the quality of the original data to be collected for a given study are therefore crucial (see Chap. I.13).

Original data will usually be collected by questionnaires, the main measurement instrument in epidemiology. Epidemiologists have neglected for a long time the potential in improving the methods for interviewing subjects in a highly standardized way and thus improving the validity and reliability of this central measurement tool. Only in the last decade it has been recognized that major improvements in this area are not only necessary but also possible, e.g. by adopting methodological developments from the social sciences (Olsen et al. 1998). Chapter I.10 of this handbook is devoted to the basic principles and approaches in this field. Prior to the increased awareness related to data collection methods, the area of exposure assessment has developed into a flourishing research field that provided advanced tools and guidance for researchers (Armstrong et al. 1992; Kromhout 1994; Ahrens 1999; Nieuwenhuijsen 2003; Chap. I.11 of this handbook). Recent advances in molecular epidemiology have introduced new possibilities for exposure measurement that are now being used in addition to the classical questionnaires. However, since the suitability of biological markers for the retrospective assessment of exposure is limited due to the short half-life of most agents that can be examined in biological specimens, the use of interviews will retain its importance but will change its face. Computer-aided data collection with built-in plausibility-checks – that is more and more being conducted in the form of telephone interviews or even using the internet – will partially replace the traditional paper and pencil approach.

Often it may not be feasible to collect primary data for the study purpose due to limited resources or because of the specific research question. In such cases, the epidemiologist can sometimes exploit existing data bases such as registries (see Chap. I.4). Here, he or she usually has to face the problem that such "secondary data" may have been collected for administrative or other purposes. Looking at the data from a research perspective often reveals inconsistencies that had not been noticed before. Since such data are collected on a routine basis without the claim for subsequent systematic analyses they may be of limited quality. The degree of standardization that can be achieved in collection, documentation, and storage is particularly low if personnel of varying skills and levels of training is involved. Moreover, changes in procedures over time may introduce additional systematic variation. Measures for assessing the usefulness and quality of the data and for careful data cleaning are then of special importance.

The scrutiny, time and effort that need to be devoted to any data, be it routine data or newly collected data, before it can be used for data analysis are rarely addressed in standard textbooks of epidemiology and often neglected in study plans. This is also true for the coding of variables like diseases, pharmaceuticals or job titles. They deserve special care with regard to training and quality assurance. Regardless of all efforts to ensure an optimal quality during data collection, a substantial input is needed to guarantee standardized and well documented coding, processing, and storing of data. Residual errors that remain after all preceding steps need to be scrutinized and, if possible, corrected (see Chap. I.13). Sufficient time has to be allocated for this workpackage that precedes the statistical analysis and publication of the study results. Finally, all data and study materials have to be stored and documented in a fashion that allows future use and/or sharing of the data or auditing of the study. Materials to be archived should not only include the electronic files of raw data and files for the analyses, but also the study protocol, computer programs, the documentation of data processing and data correction, measurement protocols, and the final report. Both, during the conduct of the study as well as after its completion, materials and data have to be stored in a physically safe place with limited access to ensure safety and confidentiality even if the data have been anonymized.

Statistical Methods in Epidemiology 4

The statistical analysis of an empirical study relates to all its phases. It starts at the planning phase where ideally all details of the subsequent analysis should be fixed (see Chap. I.12 of this handbook). This concerns defining the variables to be collected and their scale, the methods how they should be summarized e.g. via means, rates or odds, the appropriate statistical models to be used to capture the relationship between exposures and outcomes, the formulation of the research questions as statistical hypotheses, the calculation of the necessary sample size based on a given power or vice versa the power of the study based on a fixed sample size, and appropriate techniques to check for robustness and sensitivity. It is crucial to have in mind that the study should be planned and carried out in such a way that its statistical analysis is able to answer the research questions we are interested in. If the analysis is not already adequately accounted for in the planning phase or if only a secondary analysis of already existing data can be done, the results will probably be of limited validity and interpretability.

Principles of Data Analysis

Having collected the data, the first step of a statistical analysis is devoted to the cleaning of the data set. Questions to be answered are: "Are the data free of measurement or coding errors?" "Are there differences between centers?" "Are the data biased, already edited or modified in any way?" "Have data points been removed from the data set?" "Are there outliers or internal inconsistencies in the data set?" A sound and thorough descriptive analysis enables the investigator to inspect the data. Cross-checks based e.g. on the range of plausible values of the variables and cross-tabulations of two or more variables have to be carried out to find internal inconsistencies and implausible data. Graphical representations such as scatter plots, box plots, and stem-and-leaf diagrams help to detect outliers and irregularities. Calculating various summary statistics such as mean compared to median, standard deviation compared to median absolute deviation from the median is also reasonable to reveal deficiencies in the data. Special care has to be taken to deal with measurement errors and missing values. In both cases, statistical techniques are available to cope with such data (see Chaps. II.5 and II.6 of this handbook).

After having cleaned the data set, descriptive measures such as correlation coefficients or graphical representations will help the epidemiologist to understand the structure of the data. Such summary statistics need, however, to be interpreted carefully. They are descriptive by their very nature and are not to be used to formulate statistical hypotheses that are subsequently investigated by a statistical significance test based on the same data set.

In the next step parameters of interest such as relative risks or incidences should be estimated. The calculated point estimates should always be supplemented by their empirical measures of dispersion like standard deviations and by confidence intervals to get an idea about their stability or variation, respectively. In any case, confidence intervals are more informative than the corresponding significance tests. Whereas the latter just lead to a binary decision, a confidence interval also allows the assessment of the uncertainty of an observed measure and of its relevance for epidemiological practice. Nevertheless, if p-values are used for exploratory purposes, they can be considered as an objective measure to "decide" on the meaning of an observed association without declaring it as "statistically significant" or "non-significant". In conclusion, Rothman and Greenland (1998, p. 6) put it as follows: "The notion of statistical significance has come to pervade epidemiological thinking, as well as that of other disciplines. Unfortunately, statistical hypothesis testing is a mode of analysis that offers less insight into epidemiological data than alternative methods that emphasize estimation of interpretable measures."

Despite the justified condemnation of the uncritical use of statistical hypothesis tests, they are widely used in the close to final step of an analysis to confirm or reject postulated research hypotheses (cf. the next section). More sophisticated techniques such as multivariate regression models are applied in order to describe the functional relationship between exposures and outcome (see Chaps. II.2

and II.3). Such techniques are an important tool to analyze complex data but as it is the case with statistical tests their application might lead to erroneous results if carried out without accounting for the epidemiological context appropriately. This, of course, holds for any statistical method. Its blind use may be misleading with possibly serious consequences in practice. Therefore, each statistical analysis should be accompanied by sensitivity analyses and checks for model robustness. Graphical tools such as residual plots, for instance, to test for the appropriateness of a certain statistical model should also routinely be used.

The final step concerns the adequate reporting of the results and their careful interpretation. The latter has to be done with the necessary background information and substantive knowledge about the investigated epidemiological research field.

Statistical Thinking   4.2

According to the definitions quoted in Sect. 1.1, epidemiology deals with the distribution and determinants of health-related phenomena in *populations* as opposed to looking at *individual* persons or cases. Studying distributions and their determinants in populations in a quantitative way is the very essence of statistics. In this sense, epidemiology means statistical thinking in the context of health including the emphasis on causal analysis as described in Chap. I.1 and the manifold applications to be found all-over in this handbook. However, this conception of epidemiology has started to permeate the field relatively late, and, at the beginning, often unconsciously.

The traditional separation of statistics into its descriptive and its inferential component has existed in epidemiology until the two merged conceptually though not organizationally. The *descriptive* activities, initiated by people like Farr (see Sect. 2.1) continue in the form of *health statistics, health yearbooks* and similar publications by major hospitals, some research organizations, and various health administrations like national Ministries of Health and the World Health Organization, often illustrated by graphics. The visual representation of the geographic distribution of diseases has recently taken an upsurge with the advent of *geographical information systems* (Chap. II.8).

Forerunners of the use of *inferential* statistics in various parts of epidemiology are also mentioned in Sect. 2.1. Thus, in the area of *clinical trials*, the efficacy of citrus fruit to cure scurvy was established by purely statistical reasoning. In the realm of *causal factors* for diseases the discovery of water contamination as a factor for cholera still relied on quite rudimentary statistical arguments whereas the influence of the presence of a doctor at child birth on maternal mortality was confirmed by a quantitative argument coming close to a modern test of significance. The basic idea of statistics that one needs to *compare frequencies* in populations with different levels of the factors (or "determinants") to be studied was already present in all of these early investigations. The same is true for statistics in the domain of *diagnosis* where statistical thinking expresses itself by concepts like *sensitivity* or *specificity* of a medical test although it seems that this was only recently conceived of as a branch of epidemiology on par with the others, indispensable in particular for developing areas like computer-aided diagnosis or tele-diagnosis.

The big "breakthrough" of statistical thinking in epidemiology came after the elaboration of the theory of *hypothesis testing* by Neyman and Pearson. No self-respecting physician wrote any more a paper on health in a population without testing some hypotheses on the significance level 5% or without giving a p-value. Most of these hypotheses were about the efficacy of a curative treatment or, to a lesser degree, the etiology of an ailment, but the efficacy of preventive treatments and diagnostic problems were also concerned.

However, the underlying statistical thinking was often deficient. Non-acceptance of the alternative hypothesis was frequently regarded as acceptance of the null hypothesis. The meaning of an arbitrarily chosen significance level or of a p-value was not understood, and in particular several simultaneous trials or trials on several hypotheses at a time were not handled correctly by confusing the significance level of each part of the study with the overall significance level. Other statistical procedures that usually provide more useful insights like *confidence bounds* were neglected. Above all, *causal interpretations* were often not clear or outright wrong and hence erroneous practical conclusions were drawn. A statistical result in the form of a hypothesis accepted either by a test or by a correlation coefficient far from 0 was regarded as final evidence and not as one element that should lead to further investigations, usually of a biological nature.

Current statistical thinking expresses itself mainly in the study of the effect of several factors on a health phenomenon, be it a causal effect in etiologic research (Chap. I.1), a curative or preventive effect in clinical or intervention trials (Chaps. I.8, III.8, III.9, and IV.1), or the effect of a judgment, e.g. a medical test or a selection of people in diagnosis and screening (Chaps. III.8 and III.10). Such effects are represented in quantitative, statistical terms, and relations between the action of several factors as described by the concepts of interaction and confounding play a prominent role (Chap. I.9). The use of modern statistical ideas and tools has thus allowed a conceptual and practical *unification* of the many parts of epidemiology. The *same* statistical models and methods of analysis (Chaps. II.1 to II.8) are being used in all of them. Let us conclude with a final example of this global view. The concept of the etiological fraction (Chap. I.2) may represent very different things in different contexts: In causal analysis it is the fraction of all cases of a disease *due* to a particular factor whereas in the theory of prevention it means the fraction of all cases prevented by a particular measure, the most prominent application being the *efficacy of a vaccination* in a given population.

4.3   Multivariate Analysis

An epidemiological study typically involves a huge number of variables to be collected from the study participants, which implies a high-dimensional data set that has to be appropriately analyzed to extract the essential information. This curse of dimensionality becomes especially serious in genetic or molecular epidemiological studies due to genetic and familial information obtained from the study subjects. In such situations, statistical methods are called for to reduce the dimensionality of the data and to reveal the "true" underlying association structure. Various multivariate techniques are at hand depending on the structure of the data and the research aim. They can roughly be divided into two main groups. The first group contains methods to structure the data set without distinguishing response and explanatory variables, whereas the second group provides techniques to model and test for postulated dependencies. Although these multivariate techniques seem to be quite appealing at first glance they are not a statistical panacea. Their major drawback is that they cannot be easily followed by the investigator which typically leads to a less deep understanding of the data. This "black box" phenomenon also implies that the communication of the results is not as straightforward as it is when just showing some well-known risk measures supplemented by frequency tables. In addition, the various techniques will usually not lead to a unique solution where each of those obtained from the statistical analysis might be compatible with the observed data. Thus, a final decision on the underlying data structure should not be made without critically reflecting the results based on the epidemiological context, on additional substantive knowledge, and on simpler statistical analyses such as stratified analyses perhaps restricted to some key variables that hopefully support the results obtained from the multivariate analysis.

Multivariate analyses with the aim to structure the data set comprise factor analysis and cluster and discriminant analysis. Factor analysis tries to collapse a large number of observed variables into a smaller number of possibly unobservable, i.e. latent variables, so-called factors, e.g. in the development of scoring systems. These factors represent correlated subgroups of the original set. They serve in addition to estimate the fundamental dimensions underlying the observed data set. Cluster analysis simply aims at detecting highly interrelated subgroups of the data set, e.g. in the routine surveillance of a disease. Having detected certain subgroups of, say, patients, their common characteristics might be helpful e.g. to identify risk factors, prevention strategies or therapeutic concepts. This is distinct to discriminant analysis, which pertains to a known number of groups and aims to assign a subject to one of these groups (populations) based on certain characteristics of this subject while minimizing the probability of misclassification. As an example, a patient with a diagnosis of myocardial infarction has to be assigned to one of two groups, one consisting of survivors of such an event and the other consisting of non-survivors. The physician may then measure his/her systolic and diastolic blood pressure, heart rate, stroke index, and mean arterial pressure. With these data the physician will be able to predict whether or not the patient will survive. A more detailed discussion of these techniques would be beyond the scope of this handbook. We refer instead to classical text books in this field such as Dillon and Goldstein (1984), Everitt and Dunn (2001), and Giri (2004).

However, in line with the idea of epidemiology, epidemiologists are mostly not so much interested in detecting a structure in the data set but in explaining the occurrence of some health outcome depending on potentially explanatory variables. Here, it is rarely sufficient to investigate the influence of a single variable on the disease as most diseases are the result of the complex interplay of many different exposure variables including socio-demographic ones. Although it is very helpful to look first at simple stratified 2×2 tables to account for confounders such techniques become impractical for an increasing number of variables to be accounted for and a restricted number of subjects. In such situations, techniques are needed that allow the examination of the effect of several variables simultaneously for adjustment, but also for prediction purposes.

This is realized by regression models that offer a wide variety of methods to capture the functional relationship between response and explanatory variables (see Chap. II.3 of this handbook). Models with more than one explanatory variable are usually referred to as multiple regression models, multivariable or multivariate models where the latter might also involve more than one outcome. Using such techniques one needs to keep in mind that a statistical model rests on assumptions like normality, variance homogeneity, independence, and linearity that have all to be checked carefully in a given data situation. The validity of the model depends on these assumptions which might not be fulfilled by the data. Various models are therefore available from which an adequate one has to be selected. This choice is partly based on the research question and the a priori epidemiological knowledge on the relevant variables and their measurement. Depending on the scale, continuous or discrete, linear or logistic regressions might then be used for modeling purposes. Even more complex techniques such as generalized linear models can be applied where the functional relationship is no longer assumed to be linear (see Chaps. II.2 and II.3). Once the type of regression model is determined one has to decide which and how many variables should be included in the model where in case that variables are strongly correlated with each other only one of them should be included. Many software packages offer automatic selection strategies such as forward or backward selection, which usually lead to different models that are all consistent with the data at hand. An additional problem may occur due to the fact that the type of regression model will have an impact on the variables to be selected and vice versa. The resulting model may also have failed to recognize effect modification or may have been heavily affected by peculiarities of this particular data set that are of no general relevance. Thus, each model obtained as part of the statistical analysis should be independently validated.

Further extensions of simple regression models are e.g. time-series models that allow for time-dependent variation and correlation, Cox-type models to be applied in survival analysis (see Chap. II.4) and so-called graphical chain models which try to capture even more complex association structures. One of their features is that they allow in addition for indirect influences by incorporating so-called intermediate variables that simultaneously serve as explanatory and response variables. The interested reader is referred to Lauritzen and Wermuth (1989), Wermuth and Lauritzen (1990), Whittaker (1990), Lauritzen (1996), and Cox and Wermuth (1996).

Handling of Data Problems 4.4

Data are the basic elements of epidemiological investigation and information. In the form of values of predictor variables they represent levels of factors (risk factors and covariates), which are the *determinants* of health-related states or events in the sense of the definition of epidemiology quoted in Sect. 1.1. As values of response (outcome) variables they describe the health-related phenomena themselves. Measuring these values precisely is obviously fundamental in any epidemiological study and for the conclusions to be drawn from it. The practical problems that arise when trying to do this are outlined in Chaps. I.10 to I.13. However, even when taking great care and applying a rigorous quality control, some data as registered may still be erroneous and others may be missing. The question of how to handle these problems is the subject of Chaps. II.5 and II.6.

Intuitively, it is clear that in both cases the approach to be taken depends on the particular situation, more precisely, on the type of *additional information* that may be available. We use this information either to correct or to supplement certain data individually or to correct the final results of the study.

Sometimes a naïve approach looks sensible. Here are two examples of the two types of correction. First, if we know that the data at hand represent the size of a tumor in consecutive months, we may be tempted to replace a missing or obviously out-of-range value by an interpolated one. Second, when monitoring maternal mortality in a developing country by studies done routinely on the basis of death registers, we may multiply the figures obtained by a factor that reflects the fact that many deaths in childbed are not recorded in these registers. This factor was estimated beforehand by special studies where all such deaths were searched for, e.g. by visits to the homes of diseased women and retrospective interviews. For example, in Guatemala the correcting factor 1.58 is being used.

Even with such elementary procedures, though, the problem of estimating the influence of their use on the *statistical quality* of the study, be it the power of a test or the width of a confidence interval, is not only at the core of the matter but also difficult. It should therefore not be surprising that the Chaps. II.5 and II.6 are more mathematical.

The basic idea underlying the rigorous handling of measurement errors looks like this. We represent the *true* predictor variables whose values we cannot observe exactly because of errors, via so-called *surrogate* predictor variables that can be measured error free and that are being used for "correcting the errors" or as surrogates for the true predictors. The way a surrogate and a predictor are assumed to be related and the corresponding distributional assumptions form the so-called *measurement error model*. Several types of such models have been suggested and explored, the goal always being to get an idea about the magnitude of the effect on the statistical quality of the study if we correct the final results as directed by the model. Based on these theoretical results, when planning a study, a decision about the model to be used must be taken beforehand, subject to the demand that it be realistic and can be handled mathematically.

The general ideas underlying methods for dealing with missing values are similar although the technical details are of course quite different. The first step consists in jointly modeling the predictor and response variables and the missing value mechanism. This mechanism may or may not consist in filling in missing data individually (data imputation). Next, the influence of correcting under various models is investigated, and finally concrete studies are evaluated using one or several appropriate models.

4.5   Meta-Analysis

The use of meta-analyses to synthesize the evidence from epidemiological studies has become more and more popular. They can be considered as the quantitative parts of systematic reviews. The main objective of a meta-analysis is usually the statistical combination of results from several studies that individually are not powerful enough to demonstrate a small but important effect. However, whereas it is always reasonable to review the literature and the published results on a certain topic systematically, the statistical combination of results from separate epidemiological studies may yield misleading results. Purely observational studies are in contrast to randomized clinical trials where differences in treatment effects between studies can mainly be attributed to random variation. Observational studies, however, may lead to different estimates of the same effect that can no longer be explained by chance alone, but that may be due to confounding and bias potentially inherent in each of them. Thus, the calculation of a combined measure of association based on heterogeneous estimates arising from different studies may lead to a biased estimate with spurious precision. Although it is possible to allow for heterogeneity in the statistical analysis by so-called random-effects models their interpretation is often difficult. Inspecting the sources of heterogeneity and trying to explain it would therefore be a more sensible approach in most instances.

Nevertheless, a meta-analysis may be a reasonable way to integrate findings from different studies and to reveal an overall trend of the results, if existing at all. A meta-analysis from several studies to obtain an overall estimate of association, for instance, can be performed by pooling the original data or by calculating a combined measure of association based on the single estimates. In both cases, it is important to retain the study as unit of analysis. Ignoring this fact would lead to biased results since the variation between the different studies and their different within-variabilities and sample sizes would otherwise not be adequately accounted for in the statistical analysis.

Since the probably first application of formal methods to pool several studies by Pearson (1904) numerous sophisticated statistical methods have been developed that are reviewed in Chap. II.7 of this handbook.

Applications of Epidemiological Methods and Research Areas in Epidemiology

5

Epidemiology pursues three major targets: (1) to describe the spectrum of diseases and their determinants, (2) to identify the causal factors of diseases, and (3) to apply this knowledge for prevention and public health practice.

Description of the Spectrum of Diseases

5.1

Describing the distribution of disease is an integral part of the planning and evaluation of health care services. Often, information on possible exposures and disease outcomes has not been gathered with any specific hypothesis in mind but stems from routinely collected data. These descriptions serve two main purposes. First, they help in generating etiological hypotheses that may be investigated in detail by analytical studies. Second, descriptive data form the basis of health reports that provide important information for the planning of health systems, e.g. by estimating the prevalence of diseases and by projecting temporal trends. The approaches in descriptive epidemiology are presented in Chap. I.3 of this handbook.

Complementary descriptive information relates to the revelation of the natural history of diseases – one of the subjects of clinical epidemiology – that helps to improve diagnostic accuracy and therapeutic processes in the clinical setting. The understanding of a disease process and its intermediate stages also gives important input for the definition of outcome variables, be it disease outcomes that are used in classical epidemiology or precursors of disease and pre-clinical stages that are relevant for screening or in molecular epidemiology studies.

Identification of Causes of Disease

5.2

Current research in epidemiology is still tied to a considerable extent to the general methodological issues summarized in Sects. 3 and 4. These concern *any* kind of exposures (risk factors) and *any* kind of outcomes (health defects). However, the basic ideas having been shaped and the main procedures elaborated, the emphasis is now on more specific questions determined by a particular type of exposure (e.g. Chaps. III.1–III.4, III.7, III.9) or a special kind of outcome (e.g. Chaps. IV.1) or both (e.g. Chap. III.6).

Exposure-oriented Research

The search for extraneous factors that cause a disease is a central feature of epidemiology. This is nicely illustrated by the famous investigation into the causes of cholera by John Snow, who identified the association of ill social and hygienic conditions, especially of the supply with contaminated water, with the disease and thus provided the basis for preventive action. Since that time, the investigation of hygienic conditions has been diversified by examining infective agents

(Chap. IV.1), nutrition (Chap. III.4), pharmaceuticals (Chap. III.9), social conditions (Chap. III.1) as well as physical and chemical agents in the environment (Chap. III.3) or at the workplace (Chap. III.2). A peculiarity is the investigation of genetic determinants by themselves and their interaction with the extraneous exposures mentioned above (Chap. III.7).

Nutrition belongs to the most frequently studied exposures and may serve as a model for the methodological problems of exposure-oriented research and its potential for public health. There are few health outcomes for which nutrition does not play either a direct or an indirect role in causation, and therefore a solid evidence-base is required to guide action aiming at disease prevention and improvement of public health. Poor nutrition has direct effects on growth and normal development, as well as on the process of healthy ageing. For example, 40 to 70% of cancer deaths were estimated to be attributable to poor nutrition. The effect of poor diet on chronic diseases is complex, such as, for example, the role of micronutrients in maintaining optimal cell function and reducing the risk of cancer and cardiovascular disease. Foods contain more than nutrients, and the way foods are prepared may enhance or reduce their harmful or beneficial effects on health. Because diet and behavior are complex and interrelated, it is important, both in the design and the interpretation of studies, to understand how this complexity may affect the results. The major specific concern is how to define and assess with required accuracy the relevant measure of exposure, free from bias.

The latter is a general problem that exposure-oriented epidemiology is faced with, especially in retrospective studies (see Chap. I.11). The use of biological markers of exposure and early effect has been proposed to reduce exposure misclassification. In a few cases, biomarker-based studies have led to important advances, as for example illustrated by the assessment of exposure to aflatoxins, enhanced sensitivity and specificity of assessment of past viral infection, and detection of protein and DNA adducts in workers exposed to reactive chemicals such as ethylene oxide. In other cases, however, initial, promising results have not been confirmed by more sophisticated investigations. They include in particular the search for susceptibility to environmental carcinogens by looking at polymorphism for metabolic enzymes (Chap. III.6). The new opportunities offered by biomarkers to overcome some of the limitations of traditional approaches in epidemiology need to be assessed systematically. The measurement of biomarkers should be quality-controlled and their results should be validated. Sources of bias and confounding in molecular epidemiology studies have to be assessed with the same stringency as in other types of epidemiological studies.

Modern molecular techniques have made it possible to investigate exposure to genetic factors in the development or the course of diseases on a large scale. A familial aggregation has been shown for many diseases. Although some of the aggregation can be explained by shared risk factors among family members, it is plausible that a true genetic component exists for most human cancers and for the susceptibility to many infectious diseases. The knowledge of low-penetrance genes responsible for such susceptibility is still very limited, although research has currently focused on genes encoding for metabolic enzymes, DNA repair, cell-cycle control, and hormone receptors. In many studies only indirect evidence can be used since the suspected disease-related gene (candidate gene) is not directly observable. To locate or to identify susceptibility genes, genetic markers are used either in a so-called whole genome scan or in the investigation of candidate genes (Chap. III.7). The latter can be performed through linkage studies, where the common segregation of a marker and a disease is investigated in pedigrees; and through association studies, where it is investigated whether certain marker alleles of affected individuals will be more or less frequent than in a randomly selected individual from the population. Both, population-based and family designs are complementary and play a central role in genetic epidemiological studies. In the case of low-penetrance genes, association studies have been successful in identifying genetic susceptibility factors. Given the lack of dependence of genetic markers from time of disease development, the case-control approach is particularly suitable for this type of investigation because their assessment is not prone to recall bias. More pronounced than in classic epidemiology, the three main complications in genetic epidemiology are dependencies, use of indirect evidence and complex data sets.

Outcome-oriented Research

Epidemiology in industrialized countries is nowadays dominated by research on chronic diseases, among them cardiovascular diseases (Chap. IV.2), cancer (Chap. IV.3) and musculoskeletal disorders (Chap. IV.4). Their epidemiology – especially the one of cancer – is characterized more than any other outcome-defined epidemiology by the abundance of observational studies to find risk factors of all kind.

Cardiovascular diseases have a multi-factorial etiology and confounding effects are especially intriguing. For example, clustering of coronary heart diseases in families could be due both to genetic factors and to common dietary habits. High blood pressure plays both the role of an outcome variable and of a risk factor. Typical features of the epidemiology of cardiovascular diseases are the existence of many long term prospective studies, of intervention programmes like those described in Chap. III.11, and of a decline of morbidity and mortality in some areas and population groups whose causes are manifold, too, including for example control of blood pressure and blood cholesterol.

In many respects cancer epidemiology exemplifies the strengths and the weaknesses of the discipline at large. Although it is a relatively young discipline, it has been the key tool to demonstrate the causal role of important cancer risk factors, like smoking, human papilloma virus infections in cervical cancer, solar radiation in skin cancer, and obesity in many neoplasms. Cancer epidemiology is an area in which innovative methodological approaches are developed as illustrated by the increasing use of biological and genetic markers pertaining to causal factors and early outcomes.

By comparison, the epidemiology of musculoskeletal disorders is less developed. Already the definition of the various disorders and the distinction between them are still subject to debate. Case ascertainment is often tricky. In spite of the high prevalence of for example back pain or osteoarthritis and their enormous negative impact on quality of life, mortality caused by them is significantly lower than that by cancer or cardiovascular diseases. Even simple estimates of prevalence leave wide margins. Regarding established risk factors, we find for instance for osteoarthritis and depending on its location, genetic factors, gender, obesity, heavy physical workload, and estrogen use, but not much more seems to be known although certain nutritional factors have been mentioned like red meat and alcohol.

The investigation of infectious diseases is the most important historical root of epidemiology and is still of primary importance in developing countries. If a person suffers from a particular outcome like tuberculosis, the exposure "infection by the relevant micro-organism", i.e. by mycobacterium tuberculosis, must have been present by the very definition of the disease. However, it is not a sufficient condition for overt disease, and many analytical studies examine the influence of co-factors like social conditions, nutrition, and co-morbidities regarded as risk factors for opportunistic infections. Purely descriptive health statistics, too, play a very important role in controlling infectious diseases. Related activities are general *epidemic surveillance*, *outbreak studies* by tracing possible carriers, and the search for infectious sources like salmonella as sources of food poisoning or the various origins of *nosocomial* illness. The most specific features of the epidemiology of infectious diseases are *mathematical modeling* and *prevention by immunization*. Modeling is to be understood in the sense of population dynamics. What is being modeled is typically the time evolution of the incidence or prevalence of the disease in question. The model, be it deterministic or stochastic, describes the mechanism of the infection and depends on specific parameters like contact frequencies between infected and susceptible subjects and healing rates. It is interesting to note that the discoverer of the infectious cycle of malaria, Ronald Ross, also designed and analyzed a mathematical model for it that led him to conceive of the *threshold principle* (Bailey 1975; Diekmann and Heesterbeek 2000). Prevention of infectious diseases can in principle be done in three ways: by acting on co-factors of the type mentioned above; by interfering with the infectious process via hygiene, separation of susceptible persons from carriers or vectors, and elimination of vectors; or by raising the immunity of susceptible people by various measures like preventive drug treatment, the main method of immunization being a vaccination, though. The effect of a vaccination in a population can be modeled in its turn, which leads in particular to the basic epidemiological concept of *herd immunity*.

5.3   Application of Epidemiological Knowledge

Epidemiological knowledge concerns *populations*. There are two ways to use this knowledge. The first is *group-oriented*: It consists in applying knowledge about a specific population directly to this population itself. This is part of *Public Health*. The conceptually simplest applications of this kind concern the planning of the health system (Chap. IV.5) and of health strategies. For instance, epidemiological studies have shown that people exposed to inhaling asbestos fibers are prone to develop asbestosis and its sequels like cor pulmonale. We apply this knowledge to the entire population by prohibiting the use of asbestos.

The second path is taken when we are confronted with an individual person, typically in a clinical setting: We can then regard this person as a member of an appropriate specific population for which relevant epidemiological knowledge is available, and deal with her or him accordingly. As an example, a physician confronted with a child suffering from medium dehydration due to acute diarrhea, knows from clinical trials that oral rehydration (see Chap. IV.6) will normally be a very efficient treatment. Hence she/he will apply it in this particular case.

Clinical epidemiology plays a major role for the second path, where epidemiological knowledge is applied in all phases of clinical decision making, i.e. in daily clinical practice, starting with diagnosis, passing to therapy, and culminating in prognosis and advice to the patient – including individual preventive measures.

Prevention

The first of the two preceding examples belongs to *population-based prevention* (see Chaps. I.8, III.11 and IV.6). The underlying idea is to diminish the influence of risk factors identified by previous observational epidemiological studies. These factors may be geographic, environmental, social, occupational, behavioral, nutritional, or genetic. Risks of transmission of infectious diseases have long played a particular role in Public Health: Their influence was reduced by public hygiene in the classical sense. Applying observational epidemiology in order to diminish or eliminate risk factors has therefore been termed *hygiene* in a modern, general sense. Preventive measures in this context are sometimes themselves subject to an a posteriori evaluation which may bear on one hand on the way they have been implemented and on the other hand on their effectiveness.

Population-based preventive measures can also be derived from results of experimental epidemiology. The most important applications of this kind are *vaccinations* performed systematically within a given population. They have to be subjected to rigorous efficacy trials before implementation. *Preventive drug treatments*, e.g. against malaria or cardiovascular events, fall into the same category.

In many cases the target population itself is determined by a previous epidemiological study. For instance, dietary recommendations to reduce cardiovascular problems, and vaccinations against hepatitis B, yellow fever or influenza, are usually given only to people that were identified as being of *high risk* to contract the disease in question.

Screening

Population-based *treatments* as a measure of Public Health are conceivable but hardly ever implemented. There exists, however, a population-based application of epidemiology in the realm of *diagnosis*, viz. screening (see Chap. III.10). Its purpose is to find yet unrecognized diseases or health defects by appropriate tests that can be rapidly executed within large population groups. The ultimate aim is mostly to allow a treatment at an early stage. Occasionally, screening was also performed in order to isolate infected people, e.g. lepers. Classical examples of screening include mass X-ray examination to detect cases of pulmonary tuberculosis or breast cancer, and cytological tests to identify cancer of the cervix uteri. Screening programs may concentrate on *high risk groups* if it would be unfeasible, too expensive, or too dangerous to examine the entire original population. A striking example is the screening for pulmonary tuberculosis in Norway where most of the prevalent cases were found at an early stage by systematic X-ray examinations of only a small fraction of the population.

Case Management

The concept of the *individual* risk of a person (see Chaps. I.2 and I.5) that underlies the definition of risk groups represents a particular case of the second way of applications of epidemiology, viz. dealing with an individual person on the basis of epidemiological knowledge about populations to which she or he is deemed to belong. The most important application of this idea, however, is *clinical epidemiology* which was also called *statistics in clinical medicine*. It is the art of case-management in the most general sense: diagnosis using the epidemiological characteristics of medical tests like sensitivity and specificity, treatment using the results of clinical trials, prognosis for a specific case based again on relevant epidemiological studies. Chapter III.3 describes in detail fairly sophisticated procedures involving all aspects of case-management including the opinion of the patient or his/her relatives and considerations of cost, secondary effects, and quality of life as elements entering the therapeutic decision.

Health Services

Health services research (HSR) is a vast and multiform field. It has no concise and generally accepted definition but still there is a more or less general agreement about its essential ideas. Its purpose is to lay the *general, scientific* foundations for health policy in order to improve the health of people as much as possible under the constraints of society and nature. The subjects of HSR are, in the first place, the underlying *structures*, i.e. the basic elements concerned by questions of health and the relations between them, in the second place the *processes* of health care delivery, and in the third place the *effects* of health services on the health of the public.

On the methodological side, HSR means *analysis* and *evaluation* of all of these aspects. The tools are mainly coming from mathematics and statistics, economics, and sociology together with knowledge from clinical medicine and basic sciences like biology. Epidemiology plays a particularly important role.

Evaluation implies *comparison*: comparison of different existing health care systems, and comparison of an existing one with theoretical, ideal systems in order to design a better one. Comparison of health care systems of different countries has been a favorite subject. One of the main "factors" that distinguishes them is the way medical services are being paid for and the form of health insurance.

The basic elements are physicians, nurses and other personnel, hospitals, equipment, and money, but also the population getting into contact with the health system and its health status. Relations between these elements comprise *health needs* and *access to services*, but also the *organization* of the health system.

Processes of health care delivery may of course mean the usual clinical curative treatment of patients but also person- or community-based preventive actions including environmental measures, health education, or health strategies like the one that led to the eradication of smallpox.

Finally, the effects of health services, i.e. the *output*, can be measured in many ways, e.g. by morbidity and mortality, life expectancy, quality of life preserved or restored, and economic losses due to illness. Questions of *effectiveness*, i.e. the value of outputs relative to (usually monetary) inputs, are in the limelight.

Epidemiology as a method serves two purposes. On the one hand, the results of epidemiological investigations enter the field as basic parameters. Some experimental epidemiological studies like intervention trials are even considered as *belonging* to health services research. On the other hand, many methods used in health services research that stem from mathematical statistics and whose goal is to study the influence of various factors on outcomes, are formally the same as those employed in epidemiology.

Given the enormity and complexity of the subject many different "approaches" and "models" have been proposed and tried out. Earlier ones were still fairly descriptive and static, focusing on the functioning of the health services or on health policy with a strong emphasis on the economic aspects. The input-output model where the effects of changes of essential inputs on the various outcomes of interest are studied, if possible in a quantitative way, is more recent. More than others it allows to a large extent a "modular" approach, separating from each other the investigation of different parts or levels of the health services.

Ethical Aspects 5.4

The protection of human rights is one of the most crucial aspects of all studies on humans. Although there are substantial differences between experimental and observational studies they both have to face the challenging task to protect the privacy of all individuals taking part in a study. This also implies as a basic principle that study subjects are asked for their informed consent.

Another ethical angle of epidemiological research concerns the study quality. Poorly conducted research may lead to unsubstantiated and wrong decisions in clinical practice or policy making in public health and may thus cause harm to individuals, but also to society as a whole. Therefore, guidelines have been prepared to maintain high study quality and to preserve human rights such as the "Good Epidemiological Practice" provided by the International Epidemiological Association in 1998.

Of course, the four general principles of the Declaration of Helsinki (World Medical Association 2000) have to be followed, i.e. autonomy (respect for individuals), beneficence (do good), non-maleficence (do no harm), and justice. These principles are of particular relevance in randomized controlled trials, where the intervention (or non-intervention) may involve negative consequences for participants.

Various recent developments in epidemiological research constitute a new challenge regarding ethical aspects. First, automated record linkage databases are now at least partly available that capture both exposure and outcome data on an individual level. Such databases have raised questions about confidentiality of patient's medical records, authorizing access to person-specific information, and their potential misuse. Second, the inclusion of molecular markers in epidemiological studies has led to a controversial debate on the potential benefit or harm of results gained by genetic and molecular epidemiological studies. This raises the following questions: Can knowledge on genetic markers be used in primary prevention programs? How should this knowledge be communicated to the study subjects who may be forced into the conflict between their individual "right to know" and their "right not to know"? A third driver of ethical questioning has been the discussion about integrity and conflict of interests, in particular in cases of sponsored epidemiological studies or when the results are contradictory.

As a consequence, an increasing awareness that ethical conduct is essential to epidemiological research can be observed among epidemiologists. Thus, it is not surprising that now basic principles of integrity, honesty, truthfulness, fairness and equity, respect for people's autonomy, distributive justice, doing good and not harm have become an integral part in the planning and conduct of epidemiological studies. Chapter IV.7 of this handbook is devoted to all of these aspects.

References

Ackerknecht EH (1953) Rudolf Virchow. Doctor – statesman – anthropologist. University of Wisconsin Press, Madison

Ackerknecht EH (1967) Medicine at the Paris hospital, 1794–1848. Johns Hopkins, Baltimore

Ahrens W (1999) Retrospective assessment of occupational exposure in case-control studies. ecomed Verlagsgesellschaft, Landsberg

Armstrong BK, White E, Saracci R (1992) Principles of exposure measurement in epidemiology. Oxford University Press, Oxford, New York, Tokio

Bailey NTJ (1975) The mathematical theory of infectious diseases and its applications. Griffin, London

Bernard C (1865) Introduction à l'étude de la médecine expérimentale. J.B. Baillière et Fils, Paris

Bernoulli D (1766) Essai d'une nouvelle analyse de la mortalité causée par la petite vérole, & desavantages de l'inoculation pour la prévenir. Mém Math Phys Acad Roy Sci, Paris

Boffetta P, Agudo A, Ahrens W, Benhamou E, Benhamou S, Darby SC, Ferro G, Fortes C, Gonzalez CA, Jöckel KH, Krauss M, Kreienbrock L, Kreuzer M, Mendes A, Merletti F, Nyberg F, Pershagen G, Pohlabeln H, Riboli E, Schmid G, Simonato L, Tredaniel J, Whitley E, Wichmann HE, Saracci R (1998) Multicenter case-control study of exposure to environmental tobacco smoke and lung cancer in Europe. J Natl Cancer Inst 90:1440–1450

Buell P, Dunn JE (1965) Cancer mortality among Japanese Issei and Nisei of California. Cancer 18:656–664

Bulloch W (1938) The history of bacteriology. Oxford University Press, London

Chan-Yeung M, Dimich-Ward H (2003) Respiratory health effects of exposure to environmental tobacco smoke. Respirology 8:131–139

Chen WY, Colditz GA, Rosner B, Hankinson SE, Hunter DJ, Manson JE, Stampfer MJ, Willett WC, Speizer FE (2002) Use of postmenopausal hormones, alcohol, and risk for invasive breast cancer. Ann Intern Med 137:798–804

Cox D, Wermuth N (1996) Multivariate dependencies – models, analysis and interpretation. Chapman and Hall, London

Coxe JR (1846) The writings of Hippocrates and Galen. Lindsay and Blackiston, Philadelpia

Dawber TR (1980) The Framingham study: The epidemiology of atherosclerotic disease. Harvard University Press, Cambridge Mass.

Dawber TR, Meadors GF, Moore FE Jr (1951) Epidemiological approaches to heart disease: the Framingham Study. Am J Public Health 41:279–286

Detels R (2002) Epidemiology: The foundation of public health. In: Detels R, McEwen J, Beaglehole R, Tanaka H (eds) Oxford textbook of public health. Vol 2: The methods of public health, 4th edn. Oxford University Press, Oxford, New York, pp 485–491

Detels R, Breslow L (2002) Current scope and concerns in public health. In: Detels R, McEwen J, Beaglehole R, Tanaka H (eds) Oxford textbook of public health. Vol 1: The scope of public health, 4th edn. Oxford University Press, Oxford, New York, pp 3–20

Diekmann O, Heesterbeek JAP (2000) Mathematical epidemiology of infectious diseases. Wiley, Chichester

Dillon W, Goldstein M (1984) Multivariate analysis, methods and applications. Wiley, New York

Doll R, Hill AB (1950) Smoking and carcinoma of the lung: Preliminary report. Brit Med J 2:739–748

Doll R, Hill AB (1954) The mortality of doctors in relation to their smoking habits: A preliminary report. Brit Med J 1:1451–1455

Doll R, Hill AB (1964) Mortality in relation to smoking: Ten years' observation of British doctors. Brit Med J 1:1399–1410; 1460–1467

Doll R, Peto R (1978) Cigarette smoking and bronchial carcinoma: Dose and time relationships among regular smokers and lifelong non-smokers. J Epidemiol Comm Health 32:303–313

Doll R, Wald NJ (1994) Interpretation of Negative Epidemiological Evidence for Carcinogenicity. IARC Scientific Publications vol 65. International Agency for Research on Cancer (IARC), Lyon

Everitt B, Dunn G (2001) Applied multivariate data analysis, 2nd edn. Edward Arnold, London

Farr W (1975) Vital statistics: a memorial volume of selections from the reports and writings of William Farr. New York Academy of Sciences. Scarecrow Press, Metuchen NJ

Fracastoro G (1521) De contagione et contagiosis morbis et eorum curatione. English translation by Wright WC (1930). G P Putnam's Sons, New York

Galen (1951) De sanitate tuenda, English translation by Green R. C C Thomas, Springfield Ill

Giri NC (2004) Multivariate statistical analysis, 2nd edn. Marcel Dekker, New York

Gordon A (1795) A treatise on the epidemic puerperal fever of Aberdeen. London

Graunt J (1662) Natural and political observations mentioned in a following index, and made upon the Bills of mortality ... with reference to the government, religion, trade, growth, ayre, diseases, and the several changes of the said city ... Martin, Allestry, and Dicas, London

Greenwood M (1932) Epidemiology, historical and experimental. Johns Hopkins, Baltimore

Halley E (1693) An estimate of the degrees of the mortality of mankind, drawn from curious tables of the births and funerals at the city of Breslau; with an attempt to ascertain the price of annuities upon lives. Philos Trans Roy Soc London 17:596–610, 654–656

Hennekens CH, Buring JE (1987) Epidemiology in medicine. Little, Brown and Company, Boston, Toronto

Hill AB (1962) Statistical methods in clinical and preventive medicine. Livingstone, Edinburgh

Hill AB (1965) The environment and disease: association or causation? Proc R Soc Med 58:295–300

Hippocrates (400 BC, approximately) On airs, waters, and place. There exist several editions in English, among others in: (1846) Coxe, see above; (1939) The genuine works of Hippocrates. Williams and Wilkins, Baltimore; (1983) Lloyd (ed) Hippocratic writings. Penguin Classics, Harmondsworth (http://classics.mit.edu/Hippocrates/airwatpl.html) Accessed May 24, 2004

Holmes OW (1842–43) The contagiousness of puerperal fever. N Engl Quart J Med Surg 1:503–540

IARC (2004) Tobacco smoke and involuntary smoking. IARC Monographs vol 83. International Agency for Research on Cancer (IARC), Lyon

Jenner E (1798) An inquiry into the causes and effects of the variolae vaccinae, a disease known by the name of Cow Pox. Published by the author, London

Keys A (1980) Seven Countries: a multivariate analysis of death and coronary heart disease. Harvard University Press, Cambridge

Khoury MJ, Beaty TH, Cohen BH (1993) Fundamentals of genetic epidemiology. Oxford University Press, New York

Kromhout D, Menotti A, Bloemberg B, Aravanis C, Blackburn H, Buzina R, Dontas AS, Fidanza F, Giampaoli S, Jansen A, Karvonen M, Katan M, Nissinen A, Nedeljkovic S, Pekkanen J, Pekkarinen M, Punsar S, Räsänen L, Simic B, Toshima H (1995) Dietary saturated and trans fatty acids and cholesterol and 25-year mortality from coronary heart disease: the Seven Countries Study. Prev Med 24:308–315

Kromhout H (1994) From eyeballing to statistical modelling. Methods for assessment of occupational exposure. 1–210. 1994. Landbouwuniversiteit de Wageningen

Last JM (ed) (2001) A dictionary of epidemiology, 4th edn. Oxford University Press, New York, Oxford, Toronto

Lauritzen SL, Wermuth N (1989) Graphical models for associations between variables, some of which are qualitative and some quantitative. Ann Statist 17:31–57

Lauritzen SL (1996) Graphical models. Oxford University Press, Oxford

Lee PN, Forey BA (1996) Misclassification of smoking habits as a source of bias in the study of environmental tobacco smoke and lung cancer. Stat Med 15:581–605

Lind J (1753) A treatise on the scurvy. Sands, Murray, and Cochran, Edinburgh

Lind J (1771) An essay on diseases incidental to Europeans in hot climates with the method of preventing their fatal consequences, 2nd edn. T Becket and PA De Hondt, London

Lipnick RJ, Buring JE, Hennekens CH, Rosner B, Willett W, Bain C, Stampfer MJ, Colditz GA, Peto R, Speizer FE (1986) Oral contraceptives and breast cancer. A prospective cohort study. JAMA 255:58–61

Louis PCA (1835) Recherches sur les effets de la saignée dans quelques maladies inflammatoires et sur l'action de l'émétique et les vésicatoires dans la pneumonie. Baillière, Paris

MacMahon B, Pugh TF (1970) Epidemiology: principles and methods. Little, Brown and Company, Boston, Massachusetts

Marshall H, Tulloch AM (1838) Statistical report on the sickness, mortality and invaliding in The West Indies. Prepared from the records of the Army Medical Department and War Office returns. Clowes & Sons, London

Mausner JS, Bahn AK (1974) Epidemiology: An introductory text. W.B. Saunders Company, Philadelphia, London, Toronto

Nieuwenhuijsen JM (ed) (2003) Exposure assessment in occuppational and environmental epidemiology. Oxford University Press, Oxford

Olsen J, Ahrens W, Björner J, Grönvold M, Jöckel KH, Keiding L, Lauritsen JM, Levy-Desroches S, Manderson L, Olesen F (1998) Epidemiology deserves better questionnaires. Int J Epidemiol 27:935 (http://ije.oupjounals.org/cgi/reprint/27/6/935.pdf) Accessed May 24, 2004

Pagel W (1982) Paracelsus, 2nd edn. Karger, Basel

Pearson K (1904) Report on certain enteric fever inoculation statistics. Brit Med J 3:1243–1246

Pott P (1775) Chirurgical observations relative to the cataract, the polypus of the nose, the cancer of the scrotum, the different kinds of ruptures, and the mortification of the toes and feet. Hawes, Clarke and Collins, London

Ramazzini B (1713) De morbis artificum diatriba. Baptistam Conzattum, Padua

Riboli E, Preston-Martin S, Saracci R, Haley NJ, Trichopoulos D, Becher H, Burch JD, Fontham ETH, Gao YT, Jindal SK, Koo LC, Marchand LL, Segnan N, Shimizu H, Stanta G, Wu-Williams AH, Zatonski W (1990) Exposure of nonsmoking women to environmental tobacco smoke: a 10-country collaborative study. Cancer Causes Control 1:243–252

Rose G, Shipley M (1986) Plasma cholesterol concentration and death from coronary heart disease: 10 year results of the Whitehall Study. BMJ 293:306–307

Rothman KJ, Greenland S (1998) Modern epidemiology, 2nd edn. Lippincott-Raven, Philadelphia

Rupke N (ed) (2000) Medical geography in historical perspective. Medical History, Supplement No 20. The Wellcome Trust Centre for the History of Medicine at UCL, London

Schairer E, Schöniger E (1943) Lungenkrebs und Tabakverbrauch. Z Krebsforsch 54:261–269 (English translation: Schairer E, Schöniger E (2001) Lung cancer and tobacco consumption. Int J Epidemiol 30:24–27)

Schulte P, Perera FP (eds) (1998) Molecular epidemiology: Principles and practices, 2nd edn. Academic Press, New York

Semmelweis IP (1861) Die Aetiologie, der Begriff und die Prophylaxe des Kindbettfiebers. Hartleben, Pest, Wien, Leipzig

Siegel RE (1968) Galen's system of physiology and medicine. Karger, Basel

Simpson JY (1868–1869, 1869–1870) Our existing system of hospitalism and its effects. Edinburgh Mon J Med Sci 14:816–830, 1084–1115; 15:523–532

Snow J (1855) On the mode of communication of cholera, 2nd edn. Churchill, London

Stampfer MJ, Willett WC, Colditz GA, Rosner B, Speizer FE, Hennekens CH (1985) A prospective study of postmenopausal estrogene therapy and coronary heart disease. N Engl J Med 331:1044–1049

Taubes G (1995) Epidemiology faces its limits. Science 269:164–169

Tenon JR (1788) Mémoires sur les hôpitaux de Paris. Pierres, Paris

Toniolo P, Boffetta P, Shuker D, Rothman N, Hulka B, Pearce N (1997) Application of biomarkers to cancer epidemiology. IARC Scientific Publications No 142. International Agency for Research on Cancer, Lyon

Truett J, Cornfield J, Kannel E (1967) Multivariate analysis of the risk of coronary heart disease in Framingham. J Chronic Disease 20:511–524

Wells AJ, English PB, Posner SF, Wagenknecht LE, Perez-Stable EJ (1998) Misclassification rates for current smokers misclassified as smokers. Am J Public Health 88:1503–1509

Wermuth N, Lauritzen SL (1990) On substantive research hypotheses, conditional independence, graphs and graphical chain models. J Roy Statist Soc Series B 52:21–50

White KL, Henderson MM (1976) Epidemiology as a fundamental science. Its uses in health services planning, administration, and evaluation. Oxford University Press, New York

Whittaker J (1990) Graphical models in applied multivariate statistics. Wiley, Chichester

Willett WC, Stampfer MJ, Colditz GA, Rosner BA, Hennekens CH, Speizer FE (1987) Dietary fat and the risk of breast cancer. N Engl J Med 316:22–28

World Medical Association (2000) The revised Declaration of Helsinki. Interpreting and implementing ethical principles in biomedical research. Edinburgh: 52nd WMA General Assembly. JAMA 284:3043–3045

Part I

Concepts and Methodological Approaches in Epidemiology

Basic Concepts*

Kenneth J. Rothman, Sander Greenland

* This chapter is adapted from Rothman KJ and Greenland S (eds) (1998) Modern epidemiology, 2nd edn. Lippinroth Williams Wilkins & Publishers, Philadelphia

Introduction

Epidemiology is the science that focuses on the occurrence of disease in its broadest sense, with the fundamental aim to understand and to control its causes. This chapter deals with the conceptual building blocks of epidemiology. First we offer a model for causation, from which a variety of insights relevant to epidemiologic understanding emerge. We then discuss the basis by which we attempt to infer that an identified factor is indeed a cause of disease; the guidelines lead us through a rapid review of modern scientific philosophy. The remainder of the chapter deals with epidemiologic fundamentals of measurement, including the measurement of disease and the measurement of causal effects.

Causation and Causal Inference

A General Model of Causation

In *The Magic Years*, Selma Fraiberg (1959) characterizes every toddler as a scientist, busily fulfilling an earnest mission to develop a logical structure for the strange objects and events that make up the world that he or she inhabits. To survive successfully requires a useful theoretical scheme to relate the myriad events that are encountered. As a youngster, each person develops and tests an inventory of causal explanations that brings meaning to the events that are perceived and ultimately leads to increasing power to control those events.

If everyone begins life as a scientist, creating his or her own inventory of causal explanations for the empirical world, everyone also begins life as a pragmatic philosopher, developing a general causal theory that some events or states of nature are causes with specific effects or effects with specific causes. Without a general theory of causation, there would be no skeleton on which to hang the substance of the many specific causal theories that one needs to survive. Unfortunately, the concepts of causation that are established early in life are too rudimentary to serve well as the basis for scientific theories. We need to develop a more refined set of concepts that can serve as a common starting point in discussions of causal theories.

Concept of Sufficient Cause and Component Causes

To begin, we need to define *cause*. For our purposes, we can define a cause of a specific disease event as an antecedent event, condition, or characteristic that was necessary for the occurrence of a specific instance of the disease at the moment it occurred, given that other conditions are fixed. In other words, a cause of a disease event is an event, condition or characteristic that preceded the disease event and without which the disease event either would not have occurred at all or would not have occurred until some later time. With this definition it may be that no specific event, condition, or characteristic is sufficient by itself to produce disease. This definition, then, does not define a complete causal mechanism, but only a component of it.

A common characteristic of the concept of causation that we develop early in life is the assumption of a one-to-one correspondence between the observed cause and effect. Each cause is seen as necessary *and* sufficient in itself to produce the effect. Thus, the flick of a light switch appears to be the singular cause that makes the lights go on. There are less evident causes, however, that also operate to produce the effect: the need for an unspent bulb in the light fixture, wiring from the switch to the bulb, and voltage to produce a current when the circuit is closed. To achieve the effect of turning on the light, each of these is equally as important as moving the switch, because absence of any of these components of the causal constellation will prevent the effect.

For many people, the roots of early causal thinking persist and become manifest in attempts to find single causes as explanations for observed phenomena. But experience and reflection should easily persuade us that the cause of any effect must consist of a constellation of components that act in concert (Mill 1843). A "sufficient cause", which means a complete causal mechanism, can be defined as a set of minimal conditions and events that inevitably produce disease; "minimal" implies that all of the conditions or events are necessary. In disease etiology, the completion of a sufficient cause may be considered equivalent to the onset of disease. (Onset here refers to the onset of the earliest stage of the disease process, rather than the onset of signs or symptoms.) For biologic effects, most and sometimes all of the components of a sufficient cause are unknown (Rothman 1976).

For example, tobacco smoking is a cause of lung cancer, but by itself it is not a sufficient cause. First, the term *smoking* is too imprecise to be used in a causal description. One must specify the type of smoke (e.g., cigarette, cigar, pipe), whether it is filtered or unfiltered, the manner and frequency of inhalation, and the onset and duration of smoking. More important, smoking, even defined explicitly, will not cause cancer in everyone. So who are those who are "susceptible" to the effects of smoking? Or, to put it in other terms, what are the other components of the causal constellation that act with smoking to produce lung cancer?

When causal components remain unknown, we are inclined to assign an equal risk to all individuals whose causal status for some components is known and identical. Thus, men who are heavy cigarette smokers are said to have approximately a 10% lifetime risk of developing lung cancer. Some interpret this statement to mean that all men would be subject to a 10% probability of lung cancer if they were to become heavy smokers, as if the outcome, aside from smoking, were purely a matter of chance. In contrast, we view the assignment of equal risks as reflecting nothing more than assigning to everyone within a specific category, in this case male heavy smokers, the average of the individual risks for people in that category. In the classical view, these risks are either one or zero, according to whether the individual will or will not get lung cancer.

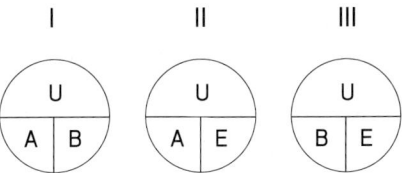

Figure 1.1. Three Sufficient Causes of a Disease

We cannot measure the individual risks, and assigning the average value to everyone in the category reflects nothing more than our ignorance about the determinants of lung cancer that interact with cigarette smoke. It is apparent from epidemiologic data that some people can engage in chain smoking for many decades without developing lung cancer. Others are or will become "primed" by unknown circumstances and need only to add cigarette smoke to the nearly sufficient constellation of causes to initiate lung cancer. In our ignorance of these hidden causal components, the best we can do in assessing risk is to classify people according to measured causal risk indicators, and then assign the average risk observed within a class to persons within the class. As knowledge expands, the risk estimates assigned to people will depart from average according to the presence or absence of other factors that affect the risk.

For example, we now know that smokers with substantial asbestos exposure are at higher risk of lung cancer than those who lack asbestos exposure. Consequently, with adequate data we could assign different risks to heavy smokers based on their asbestos exposure. Within categories of asbestos exposure, the average risks would be assigned to all heavy smokers until other risk factors are identified.

Figure 1.1 provides a schematic diagram of sufficient causes in a hypothetical individual. Each constellation of component causes represented in Fig. 1.1 is minimally sufficient to produce the disease; that is, there is no redundant or extraneous component cause – each one is a necessary part of that specific causal mechanism. A specific component cause may play a role in one, two or all three of the causal mechanisms pictured.

Figure 1.1 does not depict aspects of the causal process such as prevention, sequence or timing of action of the component causes, dose, and other complexities. These aspects of the causal process must be accommodated in the model by an appropriate definition of each causal component. Thus, if the disease is lung cancer and the factor E represents cigarette smoking, it might be defined more explicitly as smoking at least 2 packs a day of unfiltered cigarettes for at least 20 years. If the outcome is smallpox, which is completely prevented by immunization, U could represent "unimmunized". More generally, preventive effects of a factor C can be represented by placing its complement "no C" within sufficient causes.

Strength of Effects   1.2.3

We will call the set of conditions necessary and sufficient for a factor to produce disease the *causal complement* of the factor. Thus, the condition "(A and U) or

(B and U)" is the causal complement of E in the above example. The strength of a factor's effect on a population depends on the relative prevalence of its causal complement. This dependence of the effects of a specific component cause on the prevalence of its causal complement has nothing to do with the biologic mechanism of the component's action, since the component is an equal partner in each mechanism in which it appears. Nevertheless, a factor will appear to have a strong effect if its causal complement is common. Conversely, a factor with a rare causal complement will appear to have a weak effect.

In epidemiology, the strength of a factor's effect is usually measured by the change in disease frequency produced by introducing the factor into a population. This change may be measured in absolute or relative terms. In either case, the strength of an effect may have tremendous public health significance, but it may have little biologic significance. The reason is that given a specific causal mechanism, *any* of the component causes can have strong or weak effects. The actual identity of the constituent components of the cause amount to the biology of causation, whereas the strength of a factor's effect depends on the time-specific distribution of its causal complements in the population. Over a span of time, the strength of the effect of a given factor on the occurrence of a given disease may change, because the prevalence of its causal complements in various mechanisms may also change. The causal mechanisms in which the factor and its complements act could remain unchanged, however.

1.2.4   Interaction Among Causes

Two component causes acting in the same sufficient cause may be thought of as interacting biologically to produce disease. Indeed, one may define biological interaction as the participation of two component causes in the same sufficient cause. Such interaction is also known as causal co-action or joint action. The joint action of the two component causes does not have to be simultaneous action: one component cause could act many years before the other, but it would have to leave some effect that interacts with the later component.

For example, suppose a traumatic injury to the head leads to a permanent disturbance in equilibrium. Many years later, the faulty equilibrium may lead to a fall while walking on an icy path, causing a broken hip. The causal mechanism for the broken hip includes the traumatic injury to the head as a component cause, along with its consequence of a disturbed equilibrium. The causal mechanism also includes the walk along the icy path. These two component causes have interacted with one another, although their time of action is many years apart. They also would interact with the other component causes, such as the type of footwear, the absence of a handhold, and any other conditions that were necessary to the causal mechanism of the fall and the broken hip that resulted.

The degree of observable interaction between two specific component causes depends on how many different sufficient causes produce disease, and the proportion of cases that occur through sufficient causes in which the two component

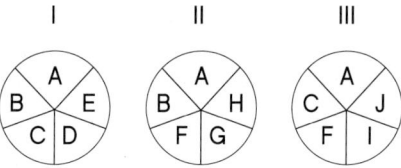

Figure 1.2. Another Example of Three Sufficient Causes of a Disease

causes both play some role. For example, in Fig. 1.2, suppose that G were only a hypothetical substance that did not actually exist. Consequently, no disease would occur from Sufficient Cause II, because it depends on an action by G, and factors B and F would act only through the distinct mechanisms represented by sufficient causes I and III. Thus, B and F would be biologically independent. Now suppose G is present; then B and F would interact biologically. Furthermore, if C is completely absent, then cases will occur only when factors B and F act together in the mechanism represented by Sufficient Cause II. Thus, the extent or apparent strength of biologic interaction between two factors is dependent on the prevalence of other factors.

Proportion of Disease Due to Specific Causes 1.2.5

In Fig. 1.1, assuming that the three sufficient causes in the diagram are the only ones operating, what fraction of disease is caused by U? The answer is all of it; without U, there is no disease. U is considered a "necessary cause". What fraction is due to E? E causes disease through two mechanisms, I and II, and all disease arising through either of these two mechanisms is due to E. This is not to say that all disease is due to U alone, or that a fraction of disease is due to E alone; no component cause acts alone. Rather, these factors interact with their complementary factors to produce disease.

There is a tendency to think that the sum of the fractions of disease attributable to each of the causes of the disease should be 100%. For example, in their widely cited work, *The Causes of Cancer*, Doll and Peto created a table giving their estimates of the fraction of all cancers caused by various agents; the total for the fractions was nearly 100% (Doll and Peto 1981, Table 20). Although they acknowledged that any case could be caused by more than one agent, which would mean that the attributable fractions would not sum to 100%, they referred to this situation as a "difficulty" and an "anomaly". It is, however, neither a difficulty nor an anomaly, but simply a consequence of allowing for the fact that no event has a single agent as the cause. The fraction of disease that can be attributed to each of the causes of disease in all the causal mechanisms actually has no upper limit: for cancer, or any disease, the upper limit for the total of the fraction of disease attributable to all the component causes of all the causal mechanisms that produce it is not 100% but infinity. Only the fraction of disease attributable to a single component cause cannot exceed 100%.

Induction Period and Latent Period

The diagram of causes in Fig. 1.2 also provides a model for conceptualizing the *induction period*, which may be defined as the period of time from causal action until disease occurrence. If, in Sufficient Cause I, the sequence of action of the causes is A, B, C, D, and E, and we are studying the effect of B, which, let us assume, acts at a narrowly defined point in time, disease does not occur immediately after B acts. It occurs only after the sequence is completed, so there will be a delay while C, D, and finally E act. When E acts, disease occurs. The interval between the action of B and the disease occurrence is the induction time for the effect of B.

In the example given earlier of an equilibrium disorder leading to a later fall and hip injury, the induction time between the occurrence of the equilibrium disorder and the later hip injury might be very long. In an individual instance, we would not know the exact length of an induction period, since we cannot be sure of the causal mechanism that produces disease in an individual instance, nor when all the relevant component causes acted. We can characterize the induction period relating the action of a component cause to the occurrence of disease in general, however, by accumulating data for many individuals. A clear example of a lengthy induction time is the cause-effect relation between exposure of a female fetus to diethylstilbestrol (DES) and the subsequent development of clear cell adenocarcinoma of the vagina. The cancer usually occurs between the ages of 15 and 30. Since the causal exposure to DES occurs early in pregnancy, there is an induction time of about 15–30 years for the carcinogenic action of DES. During this time, other causes presumably are operating; some evidence suggests that hormonal action during adolescence may be part of the mechanism (Rothman 1981).

It is incorrect to characterize a disease itself as having a lengthy or brief induction time. The induction time can be conceptualized only in relation to a specific component cause. Thus, we say that the induction time relating DES to clear cell carcinoma of the vagina is 15–30 years, but we cannot say that 15–30 years is the induction time for clear cell carcinoma in general. Since each component cause in any causal mechanism can act at a time different from the other component causes, each can have its own induction time. For the component cause that acts last, the induction time equals zero. If another component cause of clear cell carcinoma of the vagina that acts during adolescence were identified, it would have a much shorter induction time for its carcinogenic action than DES. Thus, induction time characterizes a specific cause-effect pair rather than just the effect.

Disease, once initiated, will not necessarily be apparent. The time interval between disease occurrence and detection has been termed the *latent* period (Rothman 1981), although others have used this term interchangeably with induction period. The latent period can be reduced by improved methods of disease detection. The induction period, on the other hand, cannot be reduced by early detection of disease, since disease occurrence marks the end of the induction period. Earlier detection of disease, however, may reduce the apparent induction period (the time between causal action and disease detection), since the time when disease is detected, as a practical matter, is usually used to mark the time of disease occurrence. Thus, diseases such as slow-growing cancers may appear to have long induction periods with respect to many causes because they have long latent periods. The latent period, unlike the induction period, is a characteristic of the disease and the detection effort applied to the person with the disease.

Although it is not possible to reduce the induction period proper by earlier detection of disease, it may be possible to observe intermediate stages of a causal mechanism. The increased interest in biomarkers such as DNA adducts is an example of attempting to focus on causes more proximal to the disease occurrence. Such biomarkers may reflect the effects of earlier acting agents on the organism.

Some agents may have a causal action by shortening the induction time of other agents. Suppose that exposure to factor A leads to epilepsy after an interval of 10 years, on the average. It may be that exposure to a drug, B, would shorten this interval to 2 years. Is B acting as a catalyst or as a cause of epilepsy? The answer is both: a catalyst *is* a cause. Without B the occurrence of epilepsy comes eight years later than it comes with B, so we can say that B causes the onset of the early epilepsy. It is not sufficient to argue that the epilepsy would have occurred anyway. First, it would not have occurred at that time, and the time of occurrence is part of our definition of an event. Second, epilepsy will occur later only if the individual survives an additional eight years, which is not certain. Agent B not only determines when the epilepsy occurs, it can determine whether it occurs. Thus, we should call any agent that acts as a catalyst of a causal mechanism, speeding up an induction period for other agents, as a cause in its own right. Similarly, any agent that postpones the onset of an event, drawing out the induction period for another agent, is a preventive. It should not be too surprising to equate postponement to prevention: we routinely use such an equation when we employ the euphemism that we prevent death, which actually can only be postponed. What we prevent is death at a given time, in favor of death at a later time.

Philosophy of Scientific Inference

1.2.7

Modern science began to emerge around the 16th and 17th centuries, when the knowledge demands of emerging technologies (such as artillery and transoceanic navigation) stimulated inquiry into the origins of knowledge. An early codification of the scientific method was Francis Bacon's *Novum Organum*, published in 1620, which presented an *inductivist* view of science. In this philosophy, scientific reasoning is said to depend on making generalizations, or inductions, from observations to general laws of nature; the observations are said to induce the formulation of a natural law in the mind of the scientist. Thus, an inductivist would have said that Jenner's observation of lack of smallpox among milkmaids induced in Jenner's mind the theory that cowpox (common among milkmaids) conferred immunity to smallpox. Inductivist philosophy reached a pinnacle of sorts in the canons of John Stuart Mill (1843), which evolved into inferential criteria that are still in use today.

Inductivist philosophy was a great step forward from the medieval scholasticism that preceded it, for at least it demanded that a scientist make careful observations of people and nature, rather than appeal to faith, ancient texts, or authorities. Nonetheless, by the 18th century, the Scottish philosopher David Hume had described a disturbing deficiency in inductivism: An inductive argument carried no logical force; instead, such an argument represented nothing more than an *assumption* that certain events would in the future follow in the same pattern as they had in the past. Thus, to argue that cowpox caused immunity to smallpox because no one got smallpox after having cowpox corresponded to an unjustified assumption that the pattern observed so far (no smallpox after cowpox) will continue into the future. Hume pointed out that, even for the most reasonable-sounding of such assumptions, there was no logic or force of necessity behind the inductive argument.

Causal inference based on mere coincidence of events constitutes a logical fallacy known as *post hoc ergo propter hoc* (Latin for "after this therefore on-account-of this"). This fallacy is exemplified by the inference that the crowing of a rooster is necessary for the sun to rise because sunrise is always preceded by the crowing. The *post hoc* fallacy is a special case of a more general logical fallacy known as the *fallacy of affirming the consequent*. This fallacy of confirmation takes the following general form: "We know that if H is true, B must be true; and we know that B is true; therefore H must be true". This fallacy is used routinely by scientists in interpreting data. It is used, for example, when one argues as follows: "if sewer service causes heart disease, then heart disease rates should be highest where sewer service is available; heart disease rates are indeed highest where sewer service is available; therefore, sewer service causes heart disease". Here, H is the hypothesis "sewer service causes heart disease" and B is the observation "heart disease rates are highest where sewer service is available". The argument is of course logically unsound, as demonstrated by the fact that we can imagine many ways in which the premises could be true but the conclusion false; for example, economic development could lead to both sewer service and elevated heart disease rates, without any effect of the latter on the former.

1.2.8   Refutationism

Many philosophers and scientists from Hume's time forward attempted to set out a firm logical basis for scientific reasoning. Perhaps none has attracted more attention from epidemiologists than the philosopher Karl Popper.

Popper (1968) addressed Hume's problem by asserting that scientific hypotheses can never be proven or established as true in any logical sense. Instead, Popper observed that scientific statements can simply be found to be consistent with observation. Since it is possible for an observation to be consistent with several hypotheses that themselves may be mutually inconsistent, consistency between a hypothesis and observation is no proof of the hypothesis. In contrast, a valid observation that is inconsistent with a hypothesis implies that the hypothesis as stated is false, and so refutes the hypothesis. If you wring the rooster's neck before it crows and the sun still rises, you have disproved that the rooster's crowing is a necessary cause of sunrise. Or consider a hypothetical research program to learn the boiling point of water (Magee 1985). A scientist who boils water in an open flask and repeatedly measures the boiling point at 100 °C will never, no matter how many confirmatory repetitions are involved, prove that 100 °C is always the boiling point. On the other hand, merely one attempt to boil the water in a closed flask or at high altitude will refute the proposition that water always boils at 100 °C.

According to Popper, science advances by a process of elimination that he called conjecture and refutation. Scientists form hypotheses based on intuition, conjecture, and previous experience. Good scientists use deductive logic to infer predictions from the hypothesis, and then compare observations with the predictions. Hypotheses whose predictions agree with observations are confirmed only in the sense that they can continue to be used as explanations of natural phenomena. At any time, however, they may be refuted by further observations, and replaced by other hypotheses that better explain the observations. This view of scientific inference is sometimes called *refutationism* or *falsificationism*.

Refutationists consider induction to be a psychological crutch: repeated observations did not in fact induce the formulation of a natural law, but only the belief that such a law has been found. For a refutationist, only the psychological comfort that induction provides explains why it still has its advocates. One way to rescue the concept of induction from the stigma of pure delusion is to resurrect it as a psychological phenomenon, as Hume and Popper claimed it was, but one that plays a legitimate role in hypothesis formation. The philosophy of conjecture and refutation places no constraints on the origin of conjectures. Even delusions are permitted as hypotheses, and therefore inductively inspired hypotheses, however psychological, are valid starting points for scientific evaluation. This concession does not admit a logical role for induction in confirming scientific hypotheses, but it allows the process of induction to play a part, along with imagination, in the scientific cycle of conjecture and refutation.

The philosophy of conjecture and refutation has profound implications for the methodology of science. The popular concept of a scientist doggedly assembling evidence to support a favorite thesis is objectionable from the standpoint of refutationist philosophy, because it encourages scientists to consider their own pet theories as their intellectual property, to be confirmed, proven, and when all the evidence is in, cast in stone and defended as natural law. Such attitudes hinder critical evaluation, interchange, and progress. The approach of conjecture and refutation, in contrast, encourages scientists to consider multiple hypotheses and to seek crucial tests that decide between competing hypotheses by falsifying one of them. Since falsification of one or more theories is the goal, there is incentive to depersonalize the theories. Criticism leveled at a theory need not be seen as criticism of its proposer. It has been suggested that the reason why certain fields of science advance rapidly while others languish is that the rapidly advancing fields are propelled by scientists who are busy constructing and testing competing hypotheses; the other fields, in contrast, "are sick by comparison, because they have forgotten the necessity for alternative hypotheses and disproof" (Platt 1964).

1.2.9   Bayesianism

There is another philosophy of inference that, like refutationism, holds an objective view of scientific truth and a view of knowledge as tentative or uncertain, but which focuses on evaluation of knowledge rather than truth. Like refutationism, the modern form of this philosophy evolved from the writings of 18th century British philosophers, but the focal arguments first appeared in a pivotal essay by Thomas Bayes (1763), and hence the philosophy is usually referred to as Bayesianism (Howson and Urbach 1993). Like refutationism, it did not reach a complete expression until after World War I, most notably in the writings of Ramsey (1931) and DeFinetti (1937), and, like refutationism, it did not begin to appear in epidemiology until the 1970s (see, for example, Cornfield 1976).

The central problem addressed by Bayesianism is the following: In classical logic, a deductive argument can provide you no information about the truth or falsity of a scientific hypothesis unless you can be 100% certain about the truth of the premises of the argument. Consider the logical argument called *modus tollens*: "If H implies B, and B is false, then H must be false". This argument is logically valid, but the conclusion follows only on the assumptions that the premises "H implies B" and "B is false" are true statements. If these premises are statements about the physical world, we cannot possibly know them to be correct with 100% certainty, since all observations are subject to error. Furthermore, the claim that "H implies B" will often depend on its own chain of deductions, each with its own premises of which we cannot be certain.

For example, if H is "television viewing causes homicides" and B is "homicide rates are highest where televisions are most common", the first premise used in modus tollens to test the hypothesis that television viewing causes homicides will be "If television viewing causes homicides, homicide rates are highest where televisions are most common". The validity of this premise is doubtful – after all, even if television does cause homicides, homicide rates may be low where televisions are common because of socioeconomic advantages in those areas.

Continuing to reason in this fashion, we could arrive at a more pessimistic state than even Hume imagined: not only is induction without logical foundation, but *deduction* has no scientific utility because we cannot ensure the validity of all the premises. The Bayesian answer to this problem is partial, in that it makes a severe demand on the scientist and puts a severe limitation on the results. It says roughly this: If you can assign a degree of certainty, or personal probability, to the premises of your valid argument, you may use any and all the rules of probability theory to derive a certainty for the conclusion, and this certainty will be a logically valid consequence of your original certainties. The catch is that your concluding certainty, or *posterior probability*, may heavily depend on what you used as initial certainties, or *prior probabilities*. And, if those initial certainties are not those of a colleague, that colleague may very well assign a different certainty to the conclusion than you derived.

Because the posterior probabilities emanating from a Bayesian inference depend on the person supplying the initial certainties, and so may vary across individuals, the inferences are said to be *subjective*. This subjectivity of Bayesian inference is often mistaken for a subjective treatment of truth. Not only is such a view of Bayesianism incorrect, but it is diametrically opposed to Bayesian philosophy. The Bayesian approach represents a constructive attempt to deal with the dilemma that scientific laws and facts should not be treated as known with certainty, whereas classical deductive logic yields conclusions only when some law, fact, or connection is asserted with 100% certainty.

A common criticism of Bayesian philosophy is that it diverts attention away from the classical goals of science, such as the discovery of how the world works, towards psychological states of mind called "certainties", "subjective probabilities", or "degrees of belief" (Popper 1968). This criticism fails, however, to recognize the importance of a scientist's state of mind in determining what theories to test and what tests to apply.

Most epidemiologists desire some interval estimate or evaluation of the likely range for an effect in light of available data. This estimate must inevitably be derived in the face of considerable uncertainty about methodologic details and various events that led to the available data, and can be extremely sensitive to the reasoning used in its derivation. Psychological investigations have found that most people, including scientists, reason poorly in general and especially poorly in the face of uncertainty (Kahneman et al. 1982). Bayesian philosophy provides a methodology for such reasoning, and in particular provides many warnings against being overly certain about one's conclusions.

Such warnings are echoed in refutationist philosophy. As Peter Medawar put it,

> I cannot give any scientist of any age better advice than this: the intensity of the conviction that a hypothesis is true has no bearing on whether it is true or not. (Medawar 1979)

We would only add that intensity of conviction that a hypothesis is false has no bearing on whether it is false or not.

Impossibility of Proof 1.2.10

Vigorous debate is a characteristic of modern scientific philosophy, no less in epidemiology than in other areas (Rothman 1988). Perhaps the most important common thread that emerges from the debated philosophies is Hume's legacy that proof is impossible in empirical science. This simple fact is especially important to epidemiologists, who often face the criticism that proof is impossible in epidemiology, with the implication that it is possible in other scientific disciplines. Such criticism may stem from a view that experiments are the definitive source of scientific knowledge. Such a view is mistaken on at least two counts. First, the nonexperimental nature of a science does not preclude impressive scientific discoveries; the myriad examples include plate tectonics, the evolution of species, planets orbiting other stars, and the effects of cigarette smoking on human health. Even when they are possible, experiments (including randomized trials) do not provide anything approaching proof, and in fact may be controversial, contradictory, or irreproducible. The cold-fusion debacle demonstrates well that neither physical nor experimental science is immune to such problems (Taubes 1993).

Some experimental scientists hold that epidemiologic relations are only suggestive, and believe that detailed laboratory study of mechanisms within single individuals can reveal cause-effect relations with certainty. This view overlooks the fact that *all* relations are suggestive in exactly the manner discussed by Hume: Even the most careful and detailed mechanistic dissection of individual events cannot provide more than associations, albeit at a finer level. Laboratory studies often involve a degree of observer control that cannot be approached in epidemiology; it is only this control, not the level of observation, that can strengthen the inferences from laboratory studies. And again, such control is no guarantee against error.

All of the fruits of scientific work, in epidemiology or other disciplines, are at best only tentative formulations of a description of nature, even when the work itself is carried out without mistakes. The tentativeness of our knowledge does not prevent practical applications, but it should keep us skeptical and critical, not only of everyone else's work, but of our own as well.

1.2.11   Causal Inference in Epidemiology

Biologic knowledge about epidemiologic hypotheses is often scant, making the hypotheses themselves at times little more than vague statements of causal association between exposure and disease, such as "smoking causes cardiovascular disease". These vague hypotheses have only vague consequences that can be difficult to test. To cope with this vagueness, epidemiologists usually focus on testing the negation of the causal hypothesis, that is, the null hypothesis that the exposure does *not* have a causal relation to disease. Then, any observed association can potentially refute the hypothesis, subject to the assumption (auxiliary hypothesis) that biases are absent.

If the causal mechanism is stated specifically enough, epidemiologic observations can provide crucial tests of competing non-null causal hypotheses. For example, when toxic shock syndrome was first studied, there were two competing hypotheses about the origin of the toxin. Under one hypothesis, the toxin was a chemical in the tampon, so that women using tampons were exposed to the toxin directly from the tampon. Under the other hypothesis, the tampon acted as a culture medium for staphylococci that produced the toxin. Both hypotheses explained the relation of toxic shock occurrence to tampon use. The two hypotheses, however, lead to opposite predictions about the relation between the frequency of changing tampons and the risk of toxic shock. Under the hypothesis of a chemical intoxication, more frequent changing of the tampon would lead to more exposure to the toxin and possible absorption of a greater overall dose. This hypothesis predicted that women who changed tampons more frequently would have a higher risk than women who changed tampons infrequently. The culture-medium hypothesis predicts that the women who change tampons frequently would have a lower risk than those who leave the tampon in for longer periods, because a short duration of use for each tampon would prevent the staphylococci from multiplying enough to produce a damaging dose of toxin. Thus, epidemiologic research, which showed that infrequent changing of tampons was associated with the risk of toxic shock, refuted the chemical theory.

Another example of a theory easily tested by epidemiologic data related to the finding that women who took replacement estrogen therapy were at a considerably higher risk for endometrial cancer. Horwitz and Feinstein (1978) conjectured a competing theory to explain the association: they proposed that women taking estrogen experienced symptoms such as bleeding that induced them to consult a physician. The resulting diagnostic workup led to the detection of endometrial cancer at an earlier stage in these women, as compared with women not taking estrogens. Many epidemiologic observations could have been and were used to evaluate these competing hypotheses. The causal theory predicted that the risk of endometrial cancer would tend to increase with increasing use (dose, frequency and duration) of estrogens, as for other carcinogenic exposures. The detection bias theory, on the other hand, predicted that women who had used estrogens only for a short while would have the greatest risk, since the symptoms related to estrogen use that led to the medical consultation tend to appear soon after use begins. Because the association of recent estrogen use and endometrial cancer was the same in both long-term and short-term estrogen users, the detection bias theory was refuted as an explanation for all but a small fraction of endometrial cancer cases occurring after estrogen use. (Refutation of the detection bias theory also depended on many other observations. Especially important was the theory's implication that there must be a large reservoir of undetected endometrial cancer in the typical population of women to account for the much greater rate observed in estrogen users.)

The endometrial cancer example illustrates a critical point in understanding the process of causal inference in epidemiologic studies: Many of the hypotheses being evaluated in the interpretation of epidemiologic studies are non-causal hypotheses, in the sense of involving no causal connection between the study exposure and the disease. For example, hypotheses that amount to explanations of how specific types of bias could have led to an association between exposure and disease are the usual alternatives to the primary study hypothesis that the epidemiologist needs to consider in drawing inferences. Much of the interpretation of epidemiologic studies amounts to the testing of such non-causal explanations for observed associations.

Causal Criteria

1.2.12

In practice, how do epidemiologists separate out the causal from the non-causal explanations? Despite philosophic criticisms of inductive inference, inductively-oriented causal criteria have commonly been used to make such inferences. If a set of necessary and sufficient causal criteria could be used to distinguish causal from non-causal relations in epidemiologic studies, the job of the scientist would be eased considerably. With such criteria, all the concerns about the logic or lack thereof in causal inference could be forgotten: it would only be necessary to consult the checklist of criteria to see if a relation were causal. We know from philosophy that a set of sufficient criteria does not exist. Nevertheless, lists of causal criteria have become popular, possibly because they seem to provide a road map through complicated territory. A commonly used set of criteria was proposed by Hill (1965); it was an expansion of a set of criteria offered previously in the landmark Surgeon General's report on Smoking and Health (1964), which in turn were anticipated by the inductive canons of Mill (1843) and the rules given by Hume. Hill suggested that the following aspects of an association be considered in attempting to distinguish causal from noncausal associations: (1) strength, (2) consistency, (3) specificity, (4) temporality, (5) biologic gradient, (6) plausibility, (7) coherence, (8) experimental evidence, and (9) analogy.

Despite the popular view that these criteria should be used for causal inference, there is no necessary or sufficient criterion for determining whether an observed association is causal. This conclusion accords with the views of Hume, Popper, and others that causal inferences cannot attain the certainty of logical deductions. Although some scientists continue to promulgate causal criteria as aids to inference (Susser 1991), others argue that it is actually detrimental to cloud the inferential process by considering checklist criteria (Lanes and Poole 1984). An intermediate, refutationist approach seeks to transform the criteria into deductive tests of causal hypotheses (Maclure 1985; Weed 1986). Such an approach avoids the temptation to use causal criteria simply to buttress pet theories at hand, and instead allows epidemiologists to focus on evaluating competing causal theories using crucial observations.

1.3   Measures of Disease Frequency

A central task in epidemiologic research is to quantify the occurrence of disease in populations. We discuss here four basic measures of disease occurrence. *Incidence times* are simply the times at which new disease occurs among population members. *Incidence rate* measures the occurrence of new disease per unit of person-time. *Incidence proportion* measures the proportion of people who develop new disease during a specified period of time. *Prevalence*, a measure of status rather than of newly occurring disease, measures the proportion of people who have disease at a specific time.

1.3.1   Incidence Time

In attempting to measure the frequency of disease occurrence in a population, it is insufficient merely to record the number of people or even the proportion of the population that is affected. It is also necessary to take into account the time elapsed before disease occurs, as well as the period of time during which events are counted. Consider the frequency of death. Since all people are eventually affected, the time from birth to death becomes the determining factor in the rate of occurrence of death. If, on average, death comes earlier to the members of one population than to members of another population, it is natural to say that the first population has a higher death rate than the second.

In an epidemiologic study, we may measure the time of events in an individual's life relative to any one of several reference events. Using age, for example, the reference event is birth, but we might instead use the start of a treatment or the start of an exposure as the reference event. The reference event may be unique to each person, as it is with birth, or it may be identical for all persons, as with calendar time. The time of the reference event determines the time origin or *zero time* for measuring time of events.

Given an outcome event or "incident" of interest, a person's *incidence time* for this outcome is defined as the time span from zero time to the time at which the event occurs if it occurs. A man who experienced his first MI in 1990 at age 50 has an incidence time of 1990 in (Western) calendar time, and an incidence time of 50 in age time. A person's incidence time is undefined if that person never experiences the event. (There is a useful convention that classifies such a person as having an unspecified incidence time that is known to exceed the last time the person could have experienced the event. Under this convention, a woman who had a hysterectomy in 1990 without ever having had endometrial cancer is classified as having an endometrial cancer incidence time greater than 1990.)

Incidence Rate

Epidemiologists often study events that are not inevitable, or that may not occur during the period of observation. In such situations, the set of incidence times for a specific event in a population will not all be defined or observed, and another incidence measure must be sought. Ideally, such a measure would take into account the number of individuals in a population that become ill as well as the length of time contributed by all persons during the period they were in the population and events are counted.

Consider any population, and a risk period over which we want to measure incidence in this population. Every member of the population experiences a specific amount of time in the population over the risk period; the sum of these times over all population members is called the total *person-time* at risk over the period. Person-time should be distinguished from clock time in that it is a summation of time that occurs simultaneously for many people, whereas clock time is not. Person-time represents the observational experience in which disease onsets can be observed. The number of new cases of disease divided by the person-time is the *incidence rate* of the population over the period:

$$\text{Incidence rate} = \frac{\text{no. disease onsets}}{\sum_{\text{persons}} \text{time at risk for getting disease}}$$

When the risk period is of fixed length Δt, the total person-time at risk over the period is equal to the average size of the population over the period, $\overline{N}$, times the length of the period, Δt. If we denote the incident number by A, it follows that the person-time rate equals $A/(\overline{N} \times \Delta t)$. This formulation makes clear that the incidence rate has units of inverse time (per year, per month, per day, etc.). The units attached to an incidence rate can be written as year^{-1}, month^{-1}, or day^{-1}.

It is an important principle that the only events eligible to be counted in the numerator of an incidence rate are those that occur to persons who are contributing time to the denominator of the incidence rate at the time that the disease onset occurs. Likewise, only time contributed by persons eligible to be counted in the numerator if they suffer an event should be counted in the denominator. The time contributed by each person to the denominator is sometimes known as the "time at risk", that is, time at risk of an event occurring. Analogously, the people who contribute time to the denominator of an incidence rate are referred to as the "population at risk".

Incidence rates often include only the first occurrence of disease onset as an eligible event for the numerator of the rate. For the many diseases that are irreversible states, such as diabetes, multiple sclerosis, cirrhosis or death, there is at most only one onset that a person can experience. For some diseases that do recur, such as rhinitis, we may simply wish to measure the incidence of "first" occurrence, even though the disease can occur repeatedly. For other diseases, such as cancer or heart disease, the first occurrence is often of greater interest for study than subsequent occurrences in the same individual. Therefore, it is typical that the events in the numerator of an incidence rate correspond to the first occurrence of a particular disease, even in those instances in which it is possible for an individual to have more than one occurrence.

When the events tallied in the numerator of an incidence rate are first occurrences of disease, then the time contributed by each individual who develops the disease should terminate with the onset of disease. The reason is that the individual is no longer eligible to experience the event (the first occurrence can only occur once per individual), so there is no more information to obtain from continued observation of that individual. Thus, each individual who experiences the event should contribute time to the denominator up until the occurrence of the event, but not afterwards. Furthermore, for the study of first occurrences, the number of disease onsets in the numerator of the incidence rate is also a count of people experiencing the event, since only one event can occur per person.

An epidemiologist who wishes to study both first and subsequent occurrences of disease may decide not to distinguish between first and later occurrences, and simply count all the events that occur among the population under observation. If so, then the time accumulated in the denominator of the rate would not cease with the occurrence of the event, since an additional event might occur in the same individual. Usually, however, there is enough of a biologic distinction between first and subsequent occurrences to warrant measuring them separately. One approach is to define the "population at risk" differently for each occurrence of the event: the population at risk for the first event would consist of individuals who have not experienced the disease before; the population at risk for the second event, or first recurrence, would be limited to those who have experienced the event once and only once, etc. A given individual should contribute time to the denominator of the incidence rate for first events only until the time that the disease first occurs. At that point, the individual should cease contributing time to the denominator of that rate, and should now begin to contribute time to the denominator of the rate measuring the second occurrence. If and when there is a second event, the individual should stop contributing time to the rate measuring the second occurrence, and begin to contribute to the denominator of the rate measuring the third occurrence, and so forth.

Closed and Open Populations

Conceptually we can imagine the person-time experience of two distinct types of populations, the *closed population* and the *open population*. A closed population adds no new members over time, and loses members only to death, whereas an open population may gain members over time, through immigration or birth, or lose members who are still alive through emigration. (Some demographers and ecologists use a broader definition of closed population in which births (but not immigration or emigration) are allowed.) Suppose we graph the survival experience of a closed population of 1000 people. Since death eventually claims everyone, after a period of sufficient time the original 1000 will have dwindled to zero. A graph of the size of the population with time might approximate that in Fig. 1.3.

The curve slopes downward because as the 1000 individuals in the population die, the population at risk of death is reduced. The population is closed in the sense that we consider the fate of only the 1000 individuals present at time zero. The person-time experience of these 1000 individuals is represented by the area under the curve in the diagram. As each individual dies, the curve notches downward;

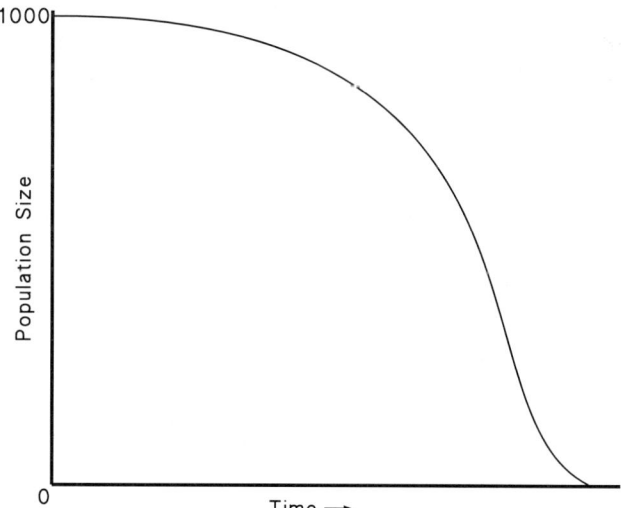

Figure 1.3. Size of a closed population of 1000 people, by time

that individual no longer contributes to the person-time denominator of the death (mortality) rate. Each individual's contribution is exactly equal to the length of time that individual is followed from start to finish; in this example, since the entire population is followed until death, the finish is the individual's death. In other instances, the contribution to the person-time experience would continue until either the onset of disease or some arbitrary cutoff time for observation, whichever came sooner.

Suppose we added up the total person-time experience of this closed population of 1000 and obtained a total of 75,000 person-years. The death rate would be $(1000/75,000) \times \text{year}^{-1}$ since the 75,000 person-years represent the experience of all 1000 people until their deaths. Furthermore, if time is measured from start of follow-up, the average death time in this closed population would be 75,000 person-years/1000 persons = 75 years, which is the inverse of the death rate.

A closed population facing a constant death rate would decline in size exponentially (which is what is meant by the term "exponential decay"). In practice, however, death rates for a closed population change with time, since the population is aging as time progresses. Consequently, the decay curve of a closed human population is never exponential. *Life-table* methodology is a procedure by which the death rate (or disease rate) of a closed population is evaluated within successive small age or time intervals, so that the age or time dependence of mortality can be elucidated. Even with such methods, it can be difficult to distinguish any age-related effects from those related to other time axes, since each individual's age increases directly with an increase along any other time axis. For example, a person's age increases with increasing duration of employment, increasing calendar time, and increasing time from start of follow-up.

An open population differs from a closed population in that individual contributions need not begin at the same time. Instead, the population at risk is open to new members who become eligible with passing time. People can enter a population open in calendar time through various mechanisms. Some are born into it; others migrate into it. For a population of people of a specific age, individuals can become eligible to enter the population by aging into it. Similarly, individuals can exit from the person-time observational experience defining a given incidence rate by dying, aging out of a defined age group, emigrating, or by becoming diseased (the latter method of exiting applies only if first bouts of a disease are being studied).

1.3.4   Steady State

If the number of people entering a population is balanced by the number exiting the population in any period of time within levels of age, sex, and other determinants of risk, the population is said to be *stationary*, or in a *steady state*. Steady state is a property that can occur only in open populations, not closed populations. It is, however, possible to have a population in steady state in which no immigration or emigration is occurring; this situation would occur if births perfectly balanced deaths in the population. The graph of the size of an open population in steady

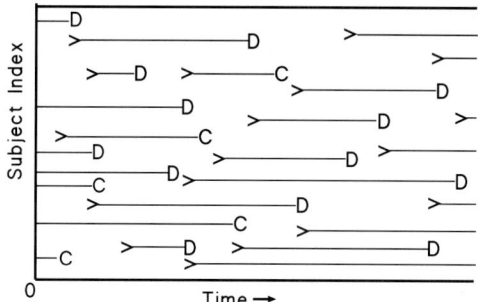

Figure 1.4. Composition of an open population in approximate steady state, by time. > indicates entry into the population, *D* indicates disease onset, and *C* indicates exit from the population without disease

state is simply a horizontal line. People are continually entering and leaving the population in a way that might be diagrammed as shown in Fig. 1.4.

In the diagram, the symbol > represents a person entering the population, a line segment represents their person-time experience, and the termination of a line segment represents the end of their experience. A terminal *D* indicates that the experience ended because of disease onset, and a terminal *C* indicates that the experience ended for other reasons. In theory, any time interval will provide a good estimate of the incidence rate in a stationary population. The value of incidence will be the ratio of the number of cases of disease onset, indicated by *D*, to the area depicting the product of population × time. Because this ratio is equivalent to the density of disease onsets in the observational area, the incidence rate has also been referred to as *incidence density* (Miettinen 1976). The measure has also been called the *person-time rate, force of morbidity* (or *force of mortality* in reference to deaths), *hazard rate*, and *disease intensity*, although the latter three terms are more commonly used to refer to the theoretical limit approached by an incidence rate as the time interval is narrowed toward zero.

Interpretation of an Incidence Rate

The numerical portion of an incidence rate has a lower bound of zero, but has no upper bound; it has the mathematical range for the ratio of two non-negative quantities, in this case the number of events in the numerator and the person-time in the denominator. At first it may seem surprising that an incidence rate can exceed the value of 1.0, which would seem to indicate that more than 100% of a population is affected. It is true that at most only 100% of persons in a population can get a disease, but the incidence rate does not measure the proportion of a population with illness, and in fact is not a proportion at all. Recall that incidence rate is measured in units of the reciprocal of time. Among 100 people, no more than 100 deaths can occur, but those 100 deaths can occur in 10,000 person-years, in 1000 person-years, in 100 person-years, or even in 1 person-year (if the 100 deaths occur after an average of 3.65 days each). An incidence rate of 100 cases (or deaths) per 1 person-year might be expressed as

$$100 \frac{\text{cases}}{\text{person-year}}.$$

It might also be expressed as

$$10,000 \frac{\text{cases}}{\text{person-century}}$$

or

$$8.33 \frac{\text{cases}}{\text{person-month}}$$

or

$$1.92 \frac{\text{cases}}{\text{person-week}}$$

or

$$0.27 \frac{\text{cases}}{\text{person-day}}.$$

The numerical value of an incidence rate in itself has no interpretability because it depends on the arbitrary selection of the time unit. It is thus essential in presenting incidence rates to give the appropriate time units, either as in the examples given above or as in 8.33 month^{-1} or 1.92 week^{-1}. Although the measure of time in the denominator of an incidence rate is often taken in terms of years, one can have units of years in the denominator regardless of whether the observations were collected over one year of time, over one week of time, or over ten years of time.

The reciprocal of time is an awkward concept that does not provide an intuitive grasp of an incidence rate. The measure does, however, have a close connection to more interpretable measures of occurrence in closed populations. Referring back to Fig. 1.3, one can see that the area under the curve is equal to $N \times T$, where N is the number of people starting out in the closed population and T is the average time until death. Equivalently, the area under the curve in Fig. 1.3 is equal to the area of a rectangle with height N and width T. Since T is the average time until death for the N people, the total person-time experience is $N \times T$. The time-averaged death rate when the follow-up for the closed population is complete is $N/(N \times T) = 1/T$; that is, the death rate equals the reciprocal of the average time until death.

More generally, in a stationary population with no migration, the crude incidence rate of an inevitable outcome such as death will equal the reciprocal of the average time until the outcome. The time until the outcome is sometimes referred to as the "waiting time" until the event occurs (Morrison 1979). Thus, in a stationary population with no migration, a death rate of 0.04 years^{-1} would translate to an average time until death of 25 years.

If the outcome of interest is not death but either disease onset or death from a specific cause, the waiting time interpretation must be modified slightly: The waiting time is the average time until disease onset, assuming that a person is not at risk of other causes of death, or other events that remove one from risk of the outcome of interest. That is, the waiting time must be redefined to account for *competing risks*, that is, events that "compete" with the outcome of interest to remove persons from the population at risk.

Unfortunately, the interpretation of incidence rates as the inverse of the average "waiting time" will usually not be valid unless the incidence rate is calculated for a stationary population with no migration (no immigration or emigration) or a closed population with complete follow-up. For example, the death rate for the United States in 1977 was 0.0088 year^{-1}; in a steady state this rate would correspond to a mean life-span, or expectation of life, of 114 years. Other analyses, however, indicate that the actual expectation of life in 1977 was 73 years (Alho 1992). The discrepancy is due to immigration and to the lack of a steady state. Note that the no-migration assumption cannot hold within specific age groups, for people are always "migrating" in and out of age groups as they age.

While the notion of incidence is a central one in epidemiology, it cannot capture all aspects of disease occurrence. Consider that a rate of 1 case/(100 years) = 0.01 years^{-1} could be obtained by following 100 people for an average of 1 year and observing 1 case, but could also be obtained by following two people for 50 years and observing 1 case, a very different scenario. To distinguish these situations, concepts that directly incorporate the notion of follow-up time and risk are needed.

Incidence Proportions and Survival Proportions 1.3.6

For a given interval of time, we can divide the number of new cases of disease occurring during that interval by the population size. If we measure the population size at the start of the interval and no one enters the population (immigrates) or leaves alive (emigrates) after the start of the interval, such a measure becomes the proportion of people who become cases during the time interval among those who were in the population at the start of the interval. We call this quantity the incidence *proportion*, which may also be defined as the proportion of a closed population at risk that becomes diseased within a given period of time. This quantity is often called the "cumulative incidence" (Miettinen 1976), but the term "cumulative incidence" is also used for another quantity we will discuss below. A more traditional term for incidence proportion is "attack rate", but we reserve the term "rate" for person-time incidence rates.

If *risk* is defined as the probability of an individual developing disease in a specified time interval, then incidence proportion is a measure, or estimate, of average risk. Although this concept of risk applies only to individuals and incidence proportion to populations, incidence proportion is sometimes called "risk". "Average risk" is a more accurate synonym, one that we will sometimes use.

Like any proportion, the value of an incidence proportion ranges from zero to one and is dimensionless. It is uninterpretable, however, without specification of the time period to which it applies. An incidence proportion of death of 3% means something very different when it refers to a 40-year period than when it refers to a 40-day period.

A useful complementary measure to the incidence proportion is the *survival proportion*, which may be defined as the proportion of a closed population at risk that does *not* become diseased within a given period of time. If R and S denote the incidence and survival proportions, we have that $S = 1 - R$ and $R = 1 - S$. Another measure that is commonly used is the *incidence odds*, defined as $R/S = R/(1-R)$, the ratio of the proportion getting the disease to the proportion not getting the disease. If R is small, $S \doteq 1$ and $R/S \doteq R$; that is, the incidence odds will approximate the incidence proportion when both quantities are small. Otherwise, because $S < 1$, the incidence odds will be greater than the incidence proportion.

Under certain conditions there is a very simple relation between the incidence proportion and the incidence rate of a nonrecurrent event. Consider a closed population over an interval t_0 to t_1, and let $\Delta t = t_1 - t_0$ be the length of the interval. If N is the size of the population at t_0, and A is the number of disease onsets over the interval, then the incidence and survival proportions over the interval are $R = A/N$ and $S = (N - A)/N$. Now suppose the size of the population at risk declines only slightly over the interval. Then $N - A \doteq N$, $S \doteq 1$, and so $R/S \doteq R$. Furthermore, the average size of the population at risk will be approximately N, and so the total person-time at risk over the interval will be approximately $N\Delta t$. Thus, the incidence rate (I) over the interval will be approximately $A/N\Delta t$, and we obtain

$$R = A/N = (A/N\Delta t)\Delta t \doteq I\Delta t \doteq R/S.$$

In words, the incidence proportion, incidence odds, and the quantity $I\Delta t$ will all approximate one another if the population at risk declines only slightly over the interval. We can make this approximation hold to within an accuracy of $1/N$ by making Δt so short that no more than one person leaves the population at risk over the interval. Thus, given a sufficiently short time interval, one can simply multiply the incidence rate by the time period to approximate the incidence proportion. This approximation offers another interpretation for the incidence rate: it can be viewed as the limiting value of the ratio of the average risk to the time period for the risk as the duration of the time period approaches zero.

A specific type of incidence proportion is the *case fatality rate*, or *case fatality ratio*, which is the incidence proportion of death among those who develop an illness (it is therefore not a rate in our sense but a proportion). The time period for measuring the case fatality rate is often unstated, but it is always better to specify it.

1.3.7   Prevalence

Unlike incidence measures, which focus on events, *prevalence* focuses on disease status. Prevalence may be defined as the proportion of a population that has disease at a specific point in time. The terms *point prevalence*, *prevalence proportion*, and *prevalence rate* are sometimes used to mean the same thing. The *prevalence pool* is the subset of the population with the disease. An individual who dies with or from disease is removed from the prevalence pool; consequently, death from an illness decreases prevalence. Diseases with large incidence rates may have low prevalences if they are rapidly fatal. People may also exit the prevalence pool by recovering from disease or emigrating from the population.

Recall that a stationary population has an equal number of people entering and exiting during any unit of time. Suppose that both the population at risk and the prevalence pool are stationary, and that everyone is either at risk or has the disease. Then the number of people entering the prevalence pool in any time period will be balanced by the number exiting from it:

$$\text{Inflow (to prevalence pool)} = \text{outflow (from prevalence pool)}.$$

People can enter the prevalence pool from the nondiseased population and by immigration from another population. Suppose there is no immigration into or emigration from the prevalence pool, so that no one enters or leaves the pool except by disease onset, death, or recovery. If the size of the population is N and the size of the prevalence pool is P, then the size of the population at risk that "feeds" the prevalence pool will be $N - P$. Also, during any time interval of length Δt, the number of people who enter the prevalence pool will be

$$I(N - P)\Delta t,$$

where I is the incidence rate, and the outflow from the prevalence pool will be

$$I'P\Delta t,$$

where I' represents the incidence rate of exiting from the prevalence pool, that is, the number who exit divided by the person-time experience of those in the prevalence pool.

Prevalence, Incidence and Mean Duration

Earlier we mentioned that, in the absence of migration, the reciprocal of an incidence rate in a stationary population equals the mean time spent in the population before the incident event. Therefore, in the absence of migration and in a stationary population, the reciprocal of I' will be the mean duration of the disease, $\overline{D}$, which is the mean time until death or recovery. It follows that

$$\text{inflow} = I(N - P)\Delta t = \text{outflow} = \left(1/\overline{D}\right)P\Delta t$$

which yields

$$\frac{P}{N - P} = I \times \overline{D},$$

$P/(N - P)$ is the ratio of diseased to nondiseased people in the population, or equivalently, the ratio of the prevalence proportion to its complement (1 − prevalence proportion). (We could call those who are nondiseased healthy except that we mean they do not have a specific illness, which doesn't imply an absence of all illness.) The ratio $P/(N - P)$ is called the *prevalence odds*; it is the odds of having a disease relative to not having the disease. As shown above, the prevalence odds equals the incidence rate times the mean duration of illness. If the prevalence is small, say less than 0.1, then

$$\text{Prevalence proportion} \doteq I \times \overline{D}$$

since the prevalence proportion will approximate the prevalence odds for small values of prevalence. More generally (Freeman and Hutchison 1980), under the assumption of stationarity and no migration in or out of the prevalence pool,

$$\text{Prevalence proportion} = \frac{I \times \overline{D}}{1 + I \times \overline{D}}$$

which can be obtained from the above expression for the prevalence odds, $P/(N-P)$.

Like the incidence proportion, the prevalence proportion is dimensionless, with a range of zero to one. The above equations are in accord with these requirements, because in each of them the incidence rate, with a dimensionality of the reciprocal of time, is multiplied by the mean duration of illness, which has the dimensionality of time, giving a dimensionless product.

Furthermore, the product $I \times \overline{D}$ has the range of zero to infinity, which corresponds to the range of prevalence odds, whereas the expression

$$\frac{I \times \overline{D}}{1 + I \times \overline{D}}$$

is always in the range zero to one, corresponding to the range of a proportion.

Unfortunately, the above formulas have limited practical utility because of the no-migration assumption, and because they do not apply to age-specific prevalence (Miettinen 1976). If we consider the prevalence pool of, say, diabetics age 60–64, we can see that this pool experiences considerable immigration from younger diabetics aging into the pool, and considerable emigration from members aging out of the pool. Under such conditions we require more elaborate formulas that give prevalence as a function of age-specific incidence, duration, and other population parameters (Preston 1987; Keiding 1991; Alho 1992).

1.3.9   Utility of Prevalence in Etiologic Research

Seldom is prevalence of direct interest in etiologic applications of epidemiologic research. Since prevalence reflects both the incidence rate and the probability of surviving with disease, studies of prevalence, or studies based on prevalent cases, yield associations that reflect the determinants of survival with disease just as much as the causes of disease. The study of prevalence can be misleading in the paradoxical situation in which better survival from a disease and therefore a higher prevalence follows from the action of preventive agents that mitigate the disease once it occurs. In such a situation, the preventive agent may be positively associated with the prevalence of disease, and so be misconstrued as a causative agent.

Nevertheless, for one class of diseases, namely, congenital malformations, prevalence is usually employed. The proportion of babies born with some malformation is a prevalence proportion, not an incidence rate. The incidence of malformations refers to the occurrence of the malformations among the susceptible populations of embryos. Many malformations lead to early embryonic or fetal death that is classified, if recognized, as a miscarriage rather than a birth. Thus, malformed babies at birth represent only those individuals who survived long enough with their malformations to be recorded as a birth. This is indeed a prevalence measure, the reference point in time being the moment of birth. The measure classifies the population of newborns as to their disease status, malformed or not, at the time of birth. This example illustrates that the time reference for a prevalence need not be a common point in calendar time: it can be a point on another time scale, such as an individual's life span.

It would be more useful and desirable to study the incidence than the prevalence of congenital malformations; as already noted, studying prevalence makes it impossible to distinguish the effects of agents that increase the incidence rate from the effects of agents that increase survival with the disease once the disease occurs. Unfortunately, it is seldom possible to measure the incidence rate of malformations, since the population at risk, young embryos, is difficult to ascertain, and learning the occurrence and timing of the malformations among the embryos is equally problematic. Consequently, in this area of research, incident cases are not usually studied, with most investigators settling for the theoretically less desirable but much more practical study of prevalence at birth.

Prevalence is sometimes used to measure the occurrence of nonlethal degenerative diseases with no clear moment of onset. It is also used in seroprevalence studies of the incidence of infection, especially when the infection has a long asymptomatic (silent) phase that can only be detected by serum testing (such as HIV infection). In these and other situations, prevalence is measured simply for convenience, and inferences are made about incidence by using assumptions about the duration of illness. Of course, in epidemiologic applications outside of etiologic research, such as planning for and managing health resources and facilities, health economics, and other public-health activities, prevalence may be a more relevant measure than incidence.

Measures of Effect   1.4

Epidemiologists use the term *effect* in two senses. In one sense, any case of a given disease may be the effect of a given cause. *Effect* is used in this way to mean the endpoint of a causal mechanism, identifying the type of outcome that a cause produces. For example, we may say that HIV infection is an effect of sharing needles for drug use. This use of the term *effect* merely identifies HIV infection as one consequence of the activity of sharing needles. Other effects of the exposure, such as hepatitis B infection, are also possible.

In a more particular and quantitative sense, an *effect* is also the amount of change in a population's disease frequency caused by a specific factor. If disease frequency is measured in terms of incidence rate or proportion, then the effect is the change in incidence rate or proportion brought about by a particular factor. We might say that for drug users, the effect of sharing needles, compared with not sharing needles, is to increase the average risk of HIV infection from 0.001 in one year to 0.01 in one year. Although it is customary to use the definite article in referring to this second type of effect ("the" effect of sharing needles), it is not meant to imply that this is a unique effect of sharing needles. An increase in risk for hepatitis or other diseases remains possible, and the increase in risk of HIV infection may differ across populations and time.

In epidemiology it is customary to refer to potential causal characteristics as *exposures*. Thus, "exposure" can refer to a behavior (such as needle sharing), a treatment (such as an educational program about hazards of needle sharing), a trait (such as genotype), or an exposure in the ordinary sense (such as injection of contaminated blood).

Population effects are most commonly expressed as effects on incidence rates or incidence proportions, but other measures based on the incidence times or prevalences may also be used. Epidemiologic analyses that focus on survival time until death or recurrence of disease are examples of analyses that measure effects on incidence times. *Absolute effects* are differences in incidence rates, incidence proportions, prevalences or incidence times. *Relative effects* involve ratios of these measures.

1.4.1   Simple Effect Measures

Consider a cohort followed over a specific time interval – say 1996 to 2000, or age 50 to 69. If we can imagine the experience of this cohort over the same interval under two different conditions – say, "exposed" and "unexposed" – then we can ask what the incidence rate of any outcome would be under the two conditions. Thus, we might consider a cohort of smokers and an exposure that consisted of mailing to each cohort member a brochure of current smoking cessation programs in their county of residence. We could then ask what the lung-cancer incidence rate would be in this cohort if we carry out this treatment, and what it would be if we did not carry out this treatment. The difference between the two rates we call the absolute effect of our mailing program on the incidence rate, or the *causal rate difference*. To be brief we might refer to the causal rate difference as the excess rate due to the program (which would be negative if the program prevented some lung cancers).

In a parallel manner, we may ask what the incidence proportion would be if we carry out this treatment, and what it would be if we do not carry out this treatment. The difference of the two proportions we call the absolute effect of our treatment on the incidence proportions, or *causal risk difference* or excess risk for short. Also in a parallel fashion, the difference in the average lung-cancer-free years of life lived over the interval under the treated and untreated conditions is another absolute effect of treatment.

To illustrate the above measures in symbolic form, suppose we have a closed cohort of size N at the start of a fixed time interval, and that anyone alive without the disease is at risk of the disease. Further, suppose that if every member of the cohort gets exposed throughout the interval, A_1 cases will occur and the total time at risk will be T_1, but if no member of the same cohort is exposed during the interval, A_0 cases will occur and the total time at risk will be T_0. Then the causal rate difference will be

$$\frac{A_1}{T_1} - \frac{A_0}{T_0},$$

the causal risk difference will be

$$\frac{A_1}{N} - \frac{A_0}{N},$$

and the causal difference in average disease-free time will be

$$\frac{T_1}{N} - \frac{T_0}{N}.$$

Each of these measures compares disease occurrence by taking differences, and so are called difference measures, or absolute measures.

More commonly, effect measures are defined by taking ratios. Examples of such ratio (or relative) measures are the *causal rate ratio*

$$\frac{A_1/T_1}{A_0/T_0} = \frac{I_1}{I_0},$$

where $I_j = A_j/T_j$ is the incidence rate under condition j (1 = exposed, 0 = unexposed); the *causal risk ratio*

$$\frac{A_1/N}{A_0/N} = \frac{A_1}{A_0} = \frac{R_1}{R_0},$$

where $R_j = A_j/N$ is the incidence proportion (average risk) under condition j; and the *causal ratio of disease-free time,*

$$\frac{T_1/N}{T_0/N} = \frac{T_1}{T_0}.$$

The rate ratio and risk ratio are often called relative risk measures. The three ratio measures are related by the simple formula

$$\frac{R_1}{R_0} = \frac{R_1 N}{R_0 N} = \frac{A_1}{A_0} = \frac{I_1 T_1}{I_0 T_0},$$

which follows from the fact that the number of cases equals the disease rate times the time-at-risk. A fourth relative risk measure can be constructed from the incidence odds. If we write $S_1 = 1 - R_1$ and $S_0 = 1 - R_0$, the *causal odds ratio* is then

$$\frac{R_1/S_1}{R_0/S_0} = \frac{A_1/(N - A_1)}{A_0/(N - A_0)}.$$

The definitions of effect just given are sometimes called *counterfactual*, or potential-outcome definitions. Such definitions may be traced back to the writings of Hume, but received little attention from scientists until the 20th century (see Lewis (1973) and Rubin (1990) for early references in philosophy and statistics, respectively). They are called counterfactual because at least one of the two circumstances in the definitions must be contrary to fact: The cohort may be exposed or "treated" (e.g., every member sent a mailing) or untreated (no one sent a mailing); if the cohort is treated, then the untreated condition will be counterfactual, and if it is untreated, then the treated condition will be counterfactual. Both conditions may be counterfactual: If only part of the cohort is sent the mailing, both conditions in the definitions will be contrary to this fact. Although some authors have objected to counterfactual causal concepts on philosophical grounds, it turns out that such concepts directly parallel concepts found in graphical and structural-equation models of causality (Pearl 2000; Greenland and Brumback 2002).

An important feature of counterfactual definitions of effect is that they involve two distinct conditions: an index condition, which usually involves some exposure or treatment, and a reference condition against which this exposure of treatment will be evaluated – such as no treatment. To ask for "the" effect of exposure is meaningless without reference to some other condition. In the above example, the effect of one mailing is only defined in reference to no mailings. We could have instead asked about the effect of one mailing relative to four mailings; this is a very different comparison than one versus no mailing.

1.4.2   Effect Measure Modification

Suppose we divide our cohort into two or more distinct categories, or strata. In each stratum, we can construct an effect measure of our choosing. These stratum-specific effect measures may or may not equal one another. Rarely would we have any reason to suppose that they do equal one another. If indeed they are not equal, we say that the effect measure is *heterogeneous* or *modified* across strata. If they are equal, we say that the measure is *homogeneous*, *constant* or *uniform* across strata.

A major point about effect measure modification is that, if effects are present, it will usually be the case that only one or none of the effect measures discussed above will be uniform across strata. In fact, if the exposure has any effect on an occurrence measure at most one of the ratio or difference measures of effect can be uniform across strata. As an example, suppose among males the average risk would be 0.50 if exposure was present, but would be 0.20 if exposure was absent, whereas among females the average risk would be 0.10 if exposure was present but would be 0.04 if exposure was absent. Then the causal risk difference for males is

0.50 − 0.20 = 0.30, five times the female difference of 0.10 − 0.04 = 0.06. In contrast, for both sexes the causal risk ratio is 0.50/0.20 = 0.10/0.04 = 2.5. Now suppose we change this example to make the differences uniform, say by making the exposed male risk 0.26 instead of 0.50. Then both differences would be 0.06, but the male risk ratio would be 0.26/0.20 = 1.3, much less than the female risk ratio of 2.5.

Relative versus Absolute Measures

1.4.3

As mentioned above, we refer to differences in incidence rates, incidence proportions, prevalences or incidence times as absolute measures. Relative effect measures are based on the ratio of an absolute effect measure to a baseline measure of occurrence. Analogous measures are used routinely whenever change or growth is measured. For example, suppose that an investment of a sum of money has yielded a gain of $ 1000 in 1 year. Knowing the gain might be useful in itself for some purposes, but the absolute increase in value does not reveal by itself how effective the investment was. If the initial investment was $ 5000 and grew to $ 6000 in 1 year, then we could judge the investment by relating the absolute gain, $ 6000 − $ 5000, to the initial amount. That is, we take the $ 1000 gain and divide it by the $ 5000 of the original principal, obtaining 20% as the relative gain. The relative gain puts the absolute gain into a perspective that reveals how effective the investment was.

Because the magnitude of the relative effect depends on the magnitude of the baseline occurrence, the same absolute effect in two populations can correspond to greatly differing relative effects (Peacock 1971). Conversely, the same relative effects for two populations could correspond to greatly differing absolute effects.

Attributable Fractions

1.4.4

Although the counterfactual approach to effects has provided the foundation for extensive statistical and philosophical developments in causal analysis, it takes no account of the mechanisms that produce effects. Suppose that all sufficient causes of a particular disease were divided into two sets, those that contain a specific cause (exposure) and those that do not, and that the exposure is never preventive. This situation is summarized in Fig. 1.5.

C and C' may represent many different combinations of causal components. Each of the two sets of sufficient causes represents a theoretically large variety of causal mechanisms for disease, perhaps as many as one distinct mechanism for

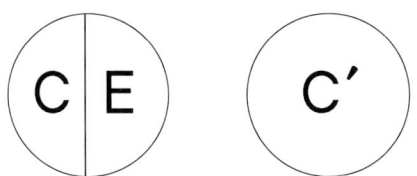

Figure 1.5. Two Types of Sufficient Causes of a Disease

every case that occurs. Disease can occur either with or without E, the exposure of interest. The causal mechanisms are grouped in the diagram according to whether or not they contain the exposure. We say that the exposure E causes disease if a sufficient cause that contains E gets completed. Thus, we say that exposure can cause disease if exposure will cause disease under at least some set of conditions C.

Perhaps the most straightforward way to quantify the effect of the exposure would be to estimate the numbers of cases that were caused by E. This number is not estimable from ordinary incidence data, because the observation of an exposed case does not reveal the mechanism that caused the case. In particular, people who have the exposure can develop the disease from a mechanism that does not include the exposure. For example, a smoker may develop lung cancer through some mechanism that does not involve smoking (for example, one involving asbestos or radiation exposure). For such lung cancer cases, their smoking was incidental; it did not contribute to the cancer causation. There is currently no way to tell which exposures are responsible for a given case. Therefore, exposed cases include some cases of disease caused by the exposure, if the exposure is indeed a cause, and some cases of disease that occur through mechanisms that do not involve the exposure.

The observed incidence rate or proportion among the exposed reflects the incidence of cases in both sets of sufficient causes represented in Fig. 1.5. The incidence of sufficient causes containing E could be found by subtracting the incidence of the sufficient causes that lack E. Unfortunately, the latter incidence cannot be estimated if we cannot distinguish cases for which exposure played an etiologic role from cases for which exposure was irrelevant (Greenland and Robins 1988). Thus, if I_1 is the incidence rate of disease in a population when exposure is present, and I_0 is the rate in that population when exposure is absent, the rate difference $I_1 - I_0$ does not necessarily equal the rate of disease with the exposure as a component cause.

To see the source of this difficulty, imagine a cohort in which, for every member, the causal complement of exposure, C, will be completed before the sufficient cause C' is completed. If the cohort is unexposed, every case of disease must be attributable to the cause C'. But, if the cohort is exposed from start of follow-up, every case of disease occurs when C is completed (E being already present), so every case of disease must be attributable to the sufficient cause containing C and E. Thus, the incidence rate of cases caused by exposure is I_1 when exposure is present, not $I_1 - I_0$.

Several other measures have often been incorrectly interpreted as the fraction of cases,

$$\frac{I_1 - I_0}{I_1} = \frac{I_1/I_0 - 1}{I_1/I_0} = \frac{IR - 1}{IR},$$

caused by exposure, or etiologic fraction. One such measure is the *rate fraction* also known as the *relative excess rate*, in which IR denotes the incidence rate ratio. The preceding example shows that the rate fraction is generally *not* equal to the fraction of cases in which exposure played a role in the disease etiology, for in the example the latter fraction is 100%. Another fractional measure is $(A_1 - A_0)/A_1$, the excess caseload due to exposure, which has been called the *excess fraction* (Greenland and Robins 1988). The preceding example shows that this measure may be far less than the etiologic fraction, for in the example the latter fraction is 100%, regardless of A_0.

There has been much confusion in the epidemiologic literature over the definition and interpretation of terms related to the above concepts. The term "attributable risk" has, at one time or another, been used to refer to the risk difference, the rate fraction, the etiologic fraction, and the excess fraction. The terms "etiologic fraction", "attributable fraction", and "attributable proportion" have each been used to refer to the etiologic fraction at one time, the excess fraction at others, and the rate fraction at still other times.

In a closed cohort, the fraction of the exposed incidence proportion $R_1 = A_1/N$ that is attributable to exposure is exactly equal to the excess fraction:

$$\frac{R_1 - R_0}{R_1} = \frac{A_1/N - A_0/N}{A_1/N} = \frac{A_1 - A_0}{A_1},$$

where $R_0 = A_0/N$ is what the incidence proportion would be with no exposure. An equivalent formula for the excess fraction is

$$\frac{R_1 - R_0}{R_1} = \frac{R_1/R_0 - 1}{R_1/R_0} = \frac{RR - 1}{RR},$$

where RR is the causal risk ratio. The rate fraction is often mistakenly equated with either the etiologic fraction or the excess fraction. To see that it is not equal to the excess fraction, let T_1 and T_0 represent the total time at risk that would be experienced by the cohort under exposure and nonexposure during the interval of interest. The rate fraction $(I_1 - I_0)/I_1$ then equals

$$\frac{A_1/T_1 - A_0/T_0}{A_1/T_1}.$$

If exposure has any effect, and if the disease removes people from further risk (as when the disease is irreversible), then T_1 will be less than T_0. The last expression cannot equal the excess fraction $(A_1 - A_0)/A_1$ if $T_1 \neq T_0$, although if the exposure effect on total time at risk is small, T_1 will be close to T_0 and so the rate fraction will approximate the excess fraction. Although the excess fraction and rate fraction for an uncommon disease will usually be close to one another, for reasons outlined above both may be much less than the etiologic fraction (Greenland and Robins 1988). This discrepancy leads to some serious issues in policy and legal settings, in which the etiologic fraction corresponds to the probability of causation (PC), i.e., the probability that the disease of a randomly selected case had exposure as a component cause. In these settings an estimate of the excess fraction or rate fraction in the exposed is often presented as an estimate of PC. Unfortunately, the excess fraction and rate fraction can be considerably different from the PC, even if the disease is rare; hence, such presentations are misleading (Greenland and Robins 2000).

For convenience, we refer to the family of fractional measures, including the etiologic, excess, and rate fractions as "attributable fractions", a term originally introduced by Ouellet et al. (1979) and Deubner et al. (1980). They are also often called "attributable risk percent" (Cole and MacMahon 1971) or "attributable risk" (Walter 1976), although the latter term is also used to denote the risk difference (MacMahon and Pugh 1970). These measures were intended for use with exposures that have a net causal effect; they become negative and hence difficult to interpret with a net preventive effect. One simple approach for dealing with preventive exposures is to interchange the exposed and unexposed quantities in the above formulas, interchanging I_1 with I_0, P_1 with P_0, A_1 with A_0, and T_1 with T_0. The resulting measures have been called *preventable fractions*, and are easily interpreted. For example, $(A_0 - A_1)/A_0 = (R_0 - R_1)/R_0 = 1 - R_1/R_0 = 1 - RR$ is the fraction of the caseload under nonexposure that could be prevented by exposure.

1.4.5 Population Attributable Fractions and Impact Fractions

One often sees in the literature a definition of "population attributable risk" or "population attributable fraction" as the reduction in incidence that would be achieved if the population had been entirely unexposed, compared with its current (actual) exposure pattern. One should recognize that this concept, due to Levin (1953), is just a special case of the definition of attributable fraction based on exposure pattern. In particular, it is a comparison of the incidence (either rate or number of cases, which must be kept distinct) under the observed pattern of exposure, and the incidence under a counterfactual pattern in which exposure or treatment is entirely absent from the population. A more general concept is the "impact fraction" (Morgenstern and Bursic 1982), which is a comparison of incidence under the observed exposure pattern, and incidence under a counterfactual pattern in which exposure is only partially removed from the population. Again, this is a special case of our definition of attributable fraction based on exposure pattern.

1.4.6 Estimation of Effects

Effects are defined in reference to a *single*, enumerable population, under two distinct conditions. Such definitions require that one can meaningfully describe each condition for the one population. Consider, for example, the "effect" of sex (male versus female) on heart disease. For these words to have content, we must be able to imagine a cohort of men, their heart-disease incidence, and what their incidence would have been had the very same men been women instead. The apparent ludicrousness of this demand reveals the vague meaning of sex effect. To reach a reasonable level of scientific precision, sex effect could be replaced by more precise mechanistic concepts, such as hormonal effects and effects of other sex-associated factors. With such concepts, we can imagine what it means for the men to have their exposure changed: hormone treatments, sex-change operations, and so on.

The single population in an effect definition can only be observed under one of the two conditions in the definition (and sometimes neither). This leads to the problem of effect *estimation*, which is to predict accurately what the magnitude of disease occurrence would have been in the single population under conditions that did not in fact occur (counterfactual conditions). For example, we may have observed $I_1 = 50$ deaths/100,000 person-years in a target cohort of smokers over a 10 year follow-up, and ask what rate reduction would have been achieved had these smokers quit at the start of follow-up. Here, we observed a rate I_1 and are asking about I_0, the rate that would have occurred under complete smoking cessation.

Since I_0 is not observed, we must predict what it would have been. To do so, we would want to refer to outside data such as data from a cohort that was not part of the target cohort. From these data, we would construct a prediction of I_0. The point we wish to emphasize here is that neither the outside cohort nor the prediction derived from it are part of the effect measure: they are only ingredients in our estimation process. This point is overlooked by effect definitions that refer to two separate "exposed" and "unexposed" populations. Such definitions confuse the concept of effect with the concept of *association*.

Measures of Association

1.4.7

Consider a situation in which we contrast a measure of occurrence in *two* different populations. For example, we could take the ratio of cancer incidence rates among males and females in Canada. This cancer rate ratio comparing the male and female subpopulations is *not* an effect measure, because its two component rates refer to different groups of people. In this situation, we say that the rate ratio is only a *measure of association*; in this example, it is a measure of the association of gender with cancer incidence in Canada.

As another example, we could contrast the incidence rate of dental caries in a community in the year before and in the third year after the introduction of fluoridation of the water supply. If we take the difference of the rates in these before and after periods, this difference is *not* an effect measure, because its two component rates refer to two different subpopulations, one before fluoridation and one after. There may be considerable or even complete overlap in the persons present in the before and after periods; nonetheless, the experiences compared refer to different time periods. In this situation, we say that the rate difference is only a measure of association; in this example, it is a measure of the association of fluoridation with dental caries incidence in the community.

1.5   **Confounding**

In the preceding example of dental caries, it is tempting to ascribe any and all of a decline in incidence following fluoridation to the act of fluoridation itself. Let us analyze what such an inference translates into in terms of measures of effect and association. The *effect* we wish to measure is that which fluoridation had on the rate; to measure this effect, we must contrast the actual rate under fluoridation with the rate that would have occurred *in the same time period* had fluoridation *not* been introduced. We cannot observe the latter rate, for it is counterfactual. Thus, we substitute in its place, or exchange, the rate in the time period before fluoridation. In doing so, we substitute a measure of association (the rate difference before and after fluoridation) for what we are really interested in (the causal rate difference between rates without and with fluoridation in the post-fluoridation time period).

This substitution will be misleading to the extent that the rate before fluoridation does not equal and so should not be exchanged with the counterfactual rate (i.e., the rate that would have occurred in the post-fluoridation period if fluoridation had not been introduced). If the two are not equal, then the measure of association we are using will not equal the measure of effect we are substituting it for. In such a circumstance, we say that our measure of association is *confounded* (for our desired measure of effect). Other ways of expressing the same idea is that the before-after rate difference is confounded for the causal rate difference, or that *confounding* is present in the before-after difference (Greenland and Robins 1986). On the other hand, if the rate before fluoridation does equal the counterfactual rate, so that the measure of association equals our desired measure of effect, we say that the before-after difference is unconfounded, or that no confounding is present in this difference.

The preceding definitions apply to ratios as well as differences. Because ratios and differences contrast the same underlying quantities, confounding of a ratio measure implies confounding of the corresponding difference measure and vice versa: If the value substituted for the counterfactual rate or risk does not equal that rate or risk, both the ratio and difference will be confounded.

The above definitions also extend immediately to situations in which the contrasted quantities are average risks, incidence times, or prevalences. For example, one could wish to estimate the impact of fluoridation on caries prevalence three years after fluoridation began. Here, the needed but unobserved counterfactual is what the caries prevalence would have been three years after fluoridation began had fluoridation not begun; for it, we might substitute the prevalence of caries at the time fluoridation began. It is possible (though perhaps rare in practice) for there to be confounding for one effect measure and not another if the two effect measures derive from different underlying occurrence measures. For example, there could in theory be confounding of the rate ratio but not the risk ratio.

One point of confusion in the literature is the failure to recognize that odds are risk-based measures, and hence odds ratios will be confounded under exactly the same circumstances as risk ratios (Miettinen and Cook 1981; Greenland and Robins 1986; Greenland 1987). The confusion arises because of the peculiarity that the causal odds ratio for a whole cohort can be closer to the null than any stratum-specific causal odds ratio. Such noncollapsibility of the causal odds ratio is usually confused with confounding, even though it has nothing to do with the latter phenomenon (Greenland et al. 1999).

Consider again the fluoridation example. Suppose that, within the year after fluoridation began, dental-hygiene education programs were implemented in some of the schools in the community. If these programs were effective, then (other things being equal) some reduction in caries incidence would have occurred as a consequence of the programs. Thus, even if fluoridation had not begun, the caries incidence would have declined in the post-fluoridation time period. In other words, the programs alone would have caused the counterfactual rate in our effect measure to be lower than the pre-fluoridation rate that substitutes for it. As a result, the measure of association (which is the before-after rate difference) must be larger than the desired measure of effect (the causal rate difference). In this situation, we say the programs *confounded* the measure of association, or that the program effects are confounded with the fluoridation effect in the measure of association. We also say that the programs are *confounders* of the association, and that the association is confounded by the programs.

Confounders are factors (exposures, interventions, treatments, etc.) that explain or produce confounding. In the present example, the programs explain why the before-after association overstates the fluoridation effect: The before-after risk difference or ratio includes the effects of programs, as well as the effects of fluoridation. More generally, a confounder explains a discrepancy between the desired (but unobservable) counterfactual risk or rate (which the exposed would have had, had they been unexposed) and the unexposed risk or rate that was its substitute. In order for a factor to explain some of this discrepancy, and thus confound, it must be capable of affecting or at least predicting the risk or rate in the unexposed (reference) group. In the above example, we assumed that the presence of the dental-hygiene programs in the years after fluoridation accounted for some of the discrepancy between the before-fluoridation rate and the (counterfactual) rate that would have occurred 3 years after fluoridation if fluoridation had not been introduced.

A large portion of epidemiologic methods are concerned with avoiding or adjusting (controlling) for confounding. Such methods inevitably rely on the gathering and proper use of confounder measurements. The most fundamental adjustment methods rely on the notion of *stratification* on confounders. If we make our comparisons within specific levels of a confounder, those comparisons cannot be confounded by that confounder. For example, we could limit our before-after fluoridation comparisons to schools in states in which no dental-hygiene program was introduced. In such schools, program introductions could not have had an effect (because no program was present), and so any decline following fluoridation could not be explained by effects of programs in those schools.

1.6 Selection Bias

Selection biases are distortions that result from procedures used to select subjects, and from factors that influence study participation. The common element of such biases is that the relation between exposure and disease is different for those who participate and those who should be theoretically eligible for study, including those who do not participate. The result is that associations observed in the study represent a mix of forces determining participation, as well as forces determining disease.

1.6.1 Self-Selection Bias

One form of such bias is self-selection bias. When the Centers for Disease Control (CDC) investigated subsequent leukemia incidence among troops who had been present at the Smoky Atomic Test in Nevada (Caldwell et al. 1980), 76% of the troops identified as members of that cohort had known outcomes. Of this 76%, 82% were traced by the investigators, but the other 18% contacted the investigators on their own initiative in response to publicity about the investigation. This self-referral of subjects is ordinarily considered a threat to validity, since the reasons for self-referral may be associated with the outcome under study (Criqui et al. 1979). In the Smoky study, there were four leukemia cases among the $0.18 \times 0.76 = 15\%$ of cohort members who referred themselves and four among the $0.82 \times 0.76 = 62\%$ of cohort members traced by the investigators, for a total of eight cases among the 76% of the cohort with known outcomes. These data indicate that self-selection bias was a small but real problem in the Smoky study. If the 24% of the cohort with unknown outcomes had a leukemia incidence like that of the subjects traced by the investigators, we should expect that only $4(24/62) = 1.5$ or about 1 or 2 cases occurred among this 24%, for a total of only 9 or 10 cases in the entire cohort. If, however, we assumed that the 24% with unknown outcomes had a leukemia incidence like that of subjects with known outcomes, we would calculate that $8(24/76) = 2.5$ or about 2 or 3 cases occurred among this 24%, for a total of 10 or 11 cases in the entire cohort.

Self-selection can also occur before subjects are identified for study. For example, it is routine to find that the mortality of active workers is less than that of the population as a whole (McMichael 1976; Fox and Collier 1976). This "healthy-worker effect" presumably derives from a screening process, perhaps largely self-selection, that allows relatively healthy people to become or remain workers, whereas those who remain unemployed, retired, disabled, or otherwise out of the active worker population are as a group less healthy (Wang and Miettinen 1982).

1.6.2 Diagnostic Bias

Another type of selection bias occurring before subjects are identified for study is diagnostic bias (Sackett 1979). When the relation between oral contraceptives and venous thromboembolism was first investigated with case-control studies of hospitalized patients, there was concern that some of the women had been hospitalized with a diagnosis of venous thromboembolism because their physicians suspected a relation between this disease and oral contraceptives and had known about oral contraceptive use in patients who presented with suggestive symptoms (Sartwell et al. 1969). A study of hospitalized patients with thromboembolism could lead to an exaggerated estimate of the effect of oral contraceptives on thromboembolism if the hospitalization and determination of the diagnosis were influenced by the history of oral-contraceptive use.

Information Bias 1.7

Once the subjects to be compared have been identified, the information to be compared must be obtained. Bias in evaluating an effect can occur from errors in obtaining the needed information. Information bias can occur whenever there are errors in the measurement of subjects, but the consequences of the errors are different depending on whether the distribution of errors for one variable (for example, exposure or disease) depends on the actual value of other variables.

For discrete variables (variables with only a countable number of possible values, such as indicators for sex), measurement error is usually called classification error or misclassification. Classification error that depends on the values of other variables is referred to as *differential misclassification*. Classification error that does not depend on the values of other variables is referred to as *nondifferential misclassification*.

Differential Misclassification 1.7.1

Suppose a cohort study were undertaken to compare incidence rates of emphysema among smokers and nonsmokers. Emphysema is a disease that may go undiagnosed without unusual medical attention. If smokers, because of concern about health-related effects of smoking or as a consequence of other health effects of smoking (such as bronchitis), seek medical attention to a greater degree than nonsmokers, then emphysema might be diagnosed more frequently among smokers than among nonsmokers simply as a consequence of the greater medical attention. Unless steps were taken to ensure comparable follow-up, an information bias would result: A spurious excess of emphysema incidence would be found among smokers compared with nonsmokers that is unrelated to any biologic effect of smoking. This is an example of differential misclassification, since the underdiagnosis of emphysema, a classification error, occurs more frequently for nonsmokers than for smokers. Sackett (1979) has described it as a diagnostic bias, but unlike the diagnostic bias in the studies of oral contraceptives and thromboembolism described earlier, it is not a selection bias, since it occurs among subjects already included in the study. Nevertheless, the similarities between some selection biases and differential misclassification biases are worth noting.

In case-control studies of congenital malformations, the etiologic information may be obtained at interview from mothers. The case mothers have recently given birth to a malformed baby, whereas the vast majority of control mothers have recently given birth to an apparently healthy baby. Another variety of differential misclassification, referred to as recall bias, can result if the mothers of malformed infants recall exposures more thoroughly than mothers of healthy infants. It is supposed that the birth of a malformed infant serves as a stimulus to a mother to recall all events that might have played some role in the unfortunate outcome. Presumably such women will remember exposures such as infectious disease, trauma, and drugs more accurately than mothers of healthy infants, who have not had a comparable stimulus. Consequently, information on such exposures will be ascertained more frequently from mothers of malformed babies, and an apparent effect, unrelated to any biologic effect, will result from this recall bias. Recall bias is a possibility in any case-control study that uses an anamnestic response, since the cases and controls by definition are people who differ with respect to their disease experience, and this difference may affect recall. Klemetti and Saxen (1967) found that the amount of time lapsed between the exposure and the recall was an important indicator of the accuracy of recall; studies in which the average time since exposure was different for interviewed cases and controls could thus suffer a differential misclassification.

The bias that is caused by differential misclassification can either exaggerate or underestimate an effect. In each of the examples above, the misclassification serves to exaggerate the effects under study, but examples to the contrary can also be found. Because of the relatively unpredictable effects of differential misclassification, some investigators go through elaborate procedures to insure that the misclassification will be nondifferential, such as blinding of exposure evaluations with respect to outcome status. Unfortunately, even in situations when blinding is accomplished or in cohort studies in which disease outcomes have not yet occurred, collapsing continuous or categorical exposure data into fewer categories can induce differential misclassification (Wacholder 1991; Flegal et al. 1991).

1.7.2   Nondifferential Misclassification

Nondifferential exposure or disease misclassification occurs when the proportion of subjects misclassified on exposure does not depend on disease status, or when the proportion of subjects misclassified on disease does not depend on exposure. Under certain conditions, any bias introduced by such nondifferential misclassification of a binary exposure or disease is predictable in direction, namely toward the null value (Newell 1962; Keys and Kihlberg 1963; Gullen et al. 1968; Copeland et al. 1977). Contrary to popular misconceptions, however, nondifferential exposure or disease misclassification can sometimes produce bias away from the null (Walker and Blettner 1985; Dosemeci et al. 1990; Chavance et al. 1992; Kristensen 1992). In particular, when both exposure and disease are nondifferentially misclassified but the classification errors are dependent, it is possible to obtain bias away from the null (Chavance et al. 1992; Kristensen 1992), and the simple bias relations just given will no longer apply. Dependent errors can arise easily in many situations, such as in studies in which exposure and disease status are both determined from interviews.

Because the bias from independent nondifferential misclassification of a dichotomous exposure is always in the direction of the null value, historically it has not been a great source of concern to epidemiologists, who have generally considered it more acceptable to underestimate effects than to overestimate effects. Nevertheless, such misclassification is a serious problem: The bias it introduces may account for certain discrepancies among epidemiologic studies. Many studies ascertain information in a way that guarantees substantial misclassification, and many studies use classification schemes that can mask effects in a manner identical to nondifferential misclassification.

Suppose aspirin transiently reduces risk of myocardial infarction. The word transiently implies a brief induction period. Any study that considered as exposure aspirin use outside of a narrow time interval before the occurrence of a myocardial infarction would be misclassifying aspirin use: There is relevant use of aspirin, and there is use of aspirin that is irrelevant because it does not allow the exposure to act causally under the causal hypothesis with its specified induction period. Many studies ask about "ever use" (use at any time during an individual's life) of drugs or other exposures. Such cumulative indices over an individual's lifetime inevitably augment possibly relevant exposure with irrelevant exposure, and can thus introduce a bias toward the null value through nondifferential misclassification.

In cohort studies in which there are disease categories with few subjects, investigators are occasionally tempted to combine outcome categories to increase the number of subjects in each analysis, thereby gaining precision. This collapsing of categories can obscure effects on more narrowly defined disease categories. For example, Smithells and Shepard (1978) investigated the teratogenicity of the drug Bendectin, a drug indicated for nausea of pregnancy. Because only 35 babies in their cohort study were born with a malformation, their analysis was focused on the single outcome, "malformation". But no teratogen causes all malformations; if such an analysis fails to find an effect, the failure may simply be the result of the grouping of many malformations not related to Bendectin with those that are. In fact, despite the authors' claim that "their study provides substantial evidence that Bendectin is not teratogenic in man", their data indicated a strong (though imprecise) relation between Bendectin and cardiac malformations. Unwarranted assurances of a lack of effect can easily emerge from studies in which a wide range of etiologically unrelated outcomes are grouped.

Nondifferential exposure and disease misclassification is a greater concern in interpreting studies that seem to indicate the absence of an effect. Consequently, in studies that indicate little or no effect, it is crucial for the researchers to consider the problem of nondifferential misclassification to determine to what extent a real effect might have been obscured. On the other hand, in studies that describe a strong nonzero effect, preoccupation with nondifferential exposure and disease misclassification is rarely warranted, provided that the errors are independent. Occasionally, critics of a study will argue that poor exposure data or a poor disease classification invalidate the results. This argument is incorrect, however, if the results indicate a nonzero effect and one can be sure that the classification errors produced bias towards the null, since the bias will be in the direction of underestimating the effect.

The importance of appreciating the likely direction of bias was illustrated by the interpretation of a study on spermicides and birth defects (Jick et al. 1981a, b). This study reported an increased prevalence of several types of congenital disorder among women who were identified as having filled a prescription for spermicides during a specified interval before the birth. The exposure information was only a rough correlate of the actual use of spermicides during a theoretically relevant time period, but the misclassification that resulted was in all probability nondifferential and independent of errors in outcome ascertainment, because prescription information was recorded on a computer log before the outcome was known. One of the criticisms raised about the study was that inaccuracies in the exposure information cast doubt on the validity of the findings (Felarca et al. 1981; Oakley 1982). Whatever bias was present on this account, however, would not likely have led to an underestimation of any real effect, so this criticism is inappropriate (Jick et al. 1981b).

Generally speaking, it is incorrect to dismiss a study reporting an effect simply because there is substantial nondifferential misclassification of exposure, since an estimate of effect without the misclassification could be even greater, provided that the misclassification probabilities apply uniformly to all subjects. Thus, the implications of nondifferential misclassification depend heavily on whether the study is perceived as "positive" or "negative". Emphasis on measurement instead of on a qualitative description of study results lessens the likelihood for misinterpretation, but even so it is important to bear in mind the direction and likely magnitude of a bias.

1.7.3   Misclassification of Confounders

If a confounding variable is misclassified, the ability to control confounding in the analysis is hampered (Greenland 1980; Brenner 1993; Marshall and Hastrup 1996). While independent nondifferential misclassification of exposure or disease usually biases study results in the direction of the null hypothesis, independent nondifferential misclassification of a confounding variable will usually reduce the degree to which confounding can be controlled and thus can cause a bias in either direction, depending on the direction of the confounding. For this reason, misclassification of confounding factors can be a serious problem.

If the confounding is strong and the exposure-disease relation is weak or zero, misclassification of the confounding factor can lead to extremely misleading results. For example, a strong causal relation between smoking and bladder cancer, coupled with a strong association between smoking and coffee drinking, makes smoking a strong confounder of any possible relation between coffee drinking and bladder cancer. Since the control of confounding by smoking depends on accurate smoking information, and since some misclassification of the relevant smoking information is inevitable no matter how smoking is measured, some residual confounding is inevitable (Morrison et al. 1982). The problem of residual confounding would be even worse if the only available information on smoking were a simple dichotomy such as "ever smoked" versus "never smoked", since the lack of detailed specification of smoking prohibits adequate control of confounding. The resulting confounding is especially troublesome because to many investigators and readers it may appear that confounding by smoking has been controlled.

Conclusions 1.8

Epidemiology is concerned with making inferences about the distribution and causes of disease and health in human populations. One should bear in mind that these inferences, like any scientific inference, can never be drawn with complete certainty, and will often be highly tentative in light of unresolved validity issues, such as uncontrolled confounding. The uncertainties stemming from validity issues cannot always be addressed by statistical methods; hence the process of epidemiologic inference is a more complicated process than statistical inference. Epidemiologic inference is further complicated by subtleties that arise when quantifying and measuring population effects, such as the distinction between number of individuals harmed by an exposure and the excess caseload produced by an exposure. These subtleties also cannot be addressed using ordinary statistical theory, and yet they can be of crucial importance in attempts to employ epidemiologic results in decision-making contexts. The proper conduct and interpretation of epidemiologic research and its application in public health requires mastery of epidemiologic concepts and methods that are outlined in this chapter and elucidated further in the subsequent chapters of this handbook.

References

Alho JM (1992) On prevalence, incidence and duration in stable populations. Biometrics 48:578–592

Bayes T (1763) Essay towards solving a problem in the doctrine of chances. Philosophical Transactions of the Royal Society 53:370–418

Brenner H (1993) Bias due to non–differential misclassification of polytomous confounders. J Clin Epidemiol 46:57–63

Caldwell GG, Kelley DB, Heath Jr CW (1980) Leukemia among participants in military maneuvers at a nuclear bomb test: A preliminary report. JAMA 244:1575–1578

Chavance M, Dellatolas G, Lellouch J (1992) Correlated nondifferential misclassifications of disease and exposure. Int J Epidemiol 21:537–546

Cole P, MacMahon B (1971) Attributable risk percent in case-control studies. Br J Prev Soc Med. 25:242–244

Copeland KT, Checkoway H, Holbrook RH, McMichael AJ (1977) Bias due to misclassification in the estimate of relative risk. Am J Epidemiol 105:488–495

Cornfield J (1976) Recent methodological contributions to clinical trials. Am J Epidemiol 104:408–424

Criqui MH, Austin M, Barrett–Connor E (1979) The effect of non–response on risk ratios in a cardiovascular disease study. J Chron Dis 32:633–638

DeFinetti B (1937) Foresight: its logical laws, its subjective sources. Reprinted in: Kyburg HE, Smokler HE (eds) Studies in subjective probability. Wiley, New York, 1964

Deubner DC, Wilkinson WE, Helms MJ, Tyroler HA, Hanes CG (1980) Logistic model estimation of death attributable to risk factors for cardiovascular disease in Evans County, Georgia. Am J Epidemiol 112:135–143

Doll R, Peto R (1981) The causes of cancer. Oxford University Press, New York

Dosemeci M, Wacholder S, Lubin J (1990) Does nondifferential misclassification of exposure always bias a true effect toward the null value? Am J Epidemiol 132:746–749

Felarca LC, Wardell DM, Rowles B (1981) Vaginal spermicides and congenital disorders. JAMA 246:2677

Flegal KM, Keyl PM, Nieto FJ (1991) Differential misclassification arising from nondifferential errors in exposure measurement. Am J Epidemiol 134:1233–1244

Fox AJ, Collier PF (1976) Low mortality rates in industrial cohort studies due to selection for work and survival in the industry. Br J Prev Soc Med 30:225–230

Fraiberg S (1959) The magic years. Scribner's, New York

Greenland S (1980) The effect of misclassification in the presence of covariates. Am J Epidemiol 112:564–569

Greenland S (1987) Interpretation and choice of effect measures in epidemiologic analysis. Am J Epidemiol 125:761–768

Greenland S, Brumback BA (2002) An overview of relations among causal modelling methods. International Journal of Epidemiology 31:1030–1037

Greenland S, Robins JM (1986) Identifiability, exchangeability and epidemiological confounding. Int J Epidemiol 15:413–419

Greenland S, Robins JM (1988) Conceptual problems in the definition and interpretation of attributable fractions. Am J Epidemiol 128:1185–1197

Greenland S, Robins JM, Pearl J (1999) Confounding and collapsibility in causal inference. Statistical Science 14:19–46

Greenland S, Robins JM (2000) Epidemiology, justice, and the probability of causation. Jurimetrics 40:321–340

Gullen WH, Berman JE, Johnson EA (1968) Effects of misclassification in epidemiologic studies. Public Health Rep 53:1956–1965

Hill AB (1965) The environment and disease: Association or causation? Proc R Soc Med 58:295–300

Horwitz RI, Feinstein AR (1978) Alternative analytic methods for case–control studies of estrogens and endometrial cancer. N Engl J Med 299:1089–1094

Howson C, Urbach P (1993) Scientific reasoning: The Bayesian approach, 2nd edn. Open Court, LaSalle, Illinois

Jick H, Walker AM, Rothman KJ, Hunter JR, Holmes LB, Watkins RN, D'Ewart DC, Danford A, Madsen S (1981a) Vaginal spermicides and congenital disorders. JAMA 245:1329–1332

Jick H, Walker AM, Rothman KJ, et al. (1981b) Vaginal spermicides and congenital disorders (letter). JAMA 246:2677–2678

Kahnemann D, Slovic P, Tversky A (1982) Judgment under uncertainty; heuristics and biases. Cambridge University Press, New York

Keiding N (1991) Age-specific incidence and prevalence: a statistical perspective. J Royal Statist Soc A 154:371–412

Keys A, Kihlberg JK (1963) The effect of misclassification on the estimated relative prevalence of a characteristic. Am J Public Health 53:1656–1665

Klemetti A, Saxen L (1967) Prospective versus retrospective approach in the search for environmental causes of malformations. Am J Public Health 57:2071–2075

Kristensen P (1992) Bias from nondifferential but dependent misclassification of exposure and outcome. Epidemiology 3:210–215

Lanes SF, Poole C (1984) "Truth in packaging?" The unwrapping of epidemiologic research. J Occup Med 26:571–574

Levin ML (1953) The occurrence of lung cancer in man. Acta Unio Int Contra Cancrum 9:531–541

Lewis D (1973) Causation. J Philos 70:556–567 (Reprinted with postscript in: Lewis D (1986) Philosophical papers. Oxford, New York)

Maclure M (1985) Popperian refutation in epidemiology. Am J Epidemiol 121:343–350

MacMahon B, Pugh TF (1970) Epidemiology: Principles and methods. Little, Brown and Co., Boston, pp 137–198, 175–184

Magee B (1985) Philosophy and the real world. An introduction to Karl Popper. Open Court, La Salle, Illinois

Marshall JR, Hastrup JL (1996) Mismeasurement and the resonance of strong confounders: Uncorrelated errors. Am J Epidemiol 143:1069–1078

McMichael AJ (1976) Standardized mortality ratios and the "healthy worker effect": Scratching beneath the surface. J Occup Med 18:165–168

Medawar PB (1979) Advice to a young scientist. Basic Books, New York

Miettinen OS, Cook EF (1981) Confounding: essence and detection. Am J Epidemiol 114:593–603

Miettinen OS (1976) Estimability and estimation in case-referent studies. Am J Epidemiol 103:226–235

Mill JS (1843) A system of logic, ratiocinative and inductive, 5th edn. Parker, Son and Bowin, London

Morgenstern H, Bursic ES (1982) A method for using epidemiologic data to estimate the potential impact of an intervention on the health status of a target population. J Comm Health 7:292–309

Morrison AS (1979) Sequential pathogenic components of rates. Am J Epidemiol 109:709–718

Morrison AS, Buring JE, Verhoek WG, Aoki K, Leck I, Ohno Y, Obata K (1982) Coffee drinking and cancer of the lower urinary tract. J Nat Cancer Inst 68:91–94

Newell DJ (1962) Errors in interpretation of errors in epidemiology. Am J Public Health 52:1925–1928

Oakley G Jr (1982) Spermicides and birth defects. JAMA 247:2405

Ouellet BL, Ræmeder J-M, Lance J-M (1979) Premature mortality attributable to smoking and hazardous drinking in Canada. Am J Epidemiol 109:451–463

Peacock PB (1971) The non–comparability of relative risks from different studies. Biometrics 27:903–907

Pearl J (2000) Causality. Cambridge University Press, Cambridge

Platt JR (1964) Strong inference. Science 146:347–353

Popper KR (1968) The logic of scientific discovery. Harper & Row, New York

Preston SH (1987) Relations among standard epidemiologic measures in a population. Am J Epidemiol 126:336–345

Ramsey FP (1931) Truth and probability. Reprinted in: Kyburg HE, Smokler HE (eds) Studies in subjective probability. Wiley, New York, 1964

Rothman KJ (1976) Causes. Am J Epidemiol 104:587–592

Rothman KJ (1981) Induction and latent periods. Am J Epidemiol 114:253–259

Rothman KJ (ed) (1988) Causal inference. Epidemiology Resources, Inc., Boston

Rubin DB (1990) Comment: Neyman (1923) and causal inference in experiments and observational studies. Stat Science 5:472–480

Sackett DL (1979) Bias in analytic research. J Chron Dis 32:51–63

Sartwell PE, Masi AT, Arthes FG, Greene GR, Smith HE (1969) Thromboembolism and oral contraceptives: An epidemiologic case-control study. Am J Epidemiol 90:365–380

Smithells RW, Shepard S (1978) Teratogenicity testing in humans: a method demonstrating the safety of Bendectin. Teratology 17:31–36

Susser M (1991) What is a cause and how do we know one? A grammar for pragmatic epidemiology. Am J Epidemiol 133:635–648

Taubes G (1993) Bad science. The short life and weird times of cold fusion. Random House, New York

U.S. Department of Health, Education and Welfare. Smoking and Health (1964) Report of the Advisory Committee to the Surgeon General of the Public Health Service. Public Health Service Publication No. 1103. Government Printing Office, Washington, D.C.

Wacholder S (1991) Practical considerations in choosing between the case–cohort and nested case–control design. Epidemiol 2:155–158

Walker AM, Blettner M (1985) Comparing imperfect measures of exposure. Am J Epidemiol 121:783–790

Walter SD (1976) The estimation and interpretation of attributable risk in health research. Biometrics 32:829–849

Wang J, Miettinen OS (1982) Occupational mortality studies: principles of validity. Scand J Work Environ Health 8:153–158

Weed D (1986) On the logic of causal inference. Am J Epidemiol 123:965–979

Rates, Risks, Measures of Association and Impact

I.2

Jacques Benichou, Mari Palta

Introduction

A major aim of epidemiologic research is to measure disease occurrence in relation to various characteristics such as exposure to environmental, occupational, or lifestyle risk factors, genetic traits or other features. In this chapter, various measures will be considered that quantify disease occurrence, associations between disease occurrence and these characteristics as well as their consequences in terms both of disease risk and impact at the population level. As is common practice, the generic term exposure will be used throughout the chapter to denote such characteristics. Emphasis will be placed on measures based on occurrence of new disease cases, referred to as disease incidence. Measures based on disease prevalence, i.e., considering newly occurring and previously existing disease cases as a whole will be considered more briefly.

We will first define the basic measure of disease incidence, namely the incidence rate, from which other measures considered in this chapter can be derived. These other measures, namely measures of disease risk, measures of association between exposure and disease risk (e.g., relative risk), and measures of impact of exposure-disease associations (e.g., attributable risk) will be considered successively. Additional points will be made regarding standardized incidence rates and measures based on prevalence.

Incidence and Hazard Rates

Definition

The incidence rate of a given disease is the number of persons who develop the disease (number of incident cases) among subjects at risk of developing the disease in the source population over a defined period of time or age. Incidence rates are not interpretable as probabilities. While they have a lower bound of zero, they have no upper bound. Units of incidence rates are reciprocal of person-time, such as reciprocals of person-years or multiples of person-years (e.g., 100,000 person-years). For instance, if 10 cases develop from the follow-up of 20 subjects and for a total follow-up time of five years, the incidence rate is $10/100 = 0.1$ cases per person-year (assuming an instantaneous event with immediate recovery and all 20 subjects being at risk until the end of the observation period).

Usually, incidence rates are assessed over relatively short time periods compared with the time scale for disease development, e.g., intervals of five-years for chronic diseases with an extended period of susceptibility such as many cancers.

Synonyms for incidence rate are average incidence rate, force of morbidity, person-time rate, or incidence density (Miettinen 1976), the last term reflecting the interpretation of an incidence rate as the density of incident case occurrences in an accumulated amount of person-time (Morgenstern et al. 1980).

Mortality rates (overall or cause-specific) can be regarded as a special case of incidence rates, the outcome considered being death rather than disease occurrence.

Incidence rates can be regarded as estimates of a limiting theoretical quantity, namely the hazard rate, $h(t)$, also called the incidence intensity or force of morbidity. The hazard rate at time t, $h(t)$, is the instantaneous rate of developing the disease of interest in an arbitrarily short interval Δ around time t, provided the subject is still at risk at time t (i.e., has not fallen ill before time t). Technically, it has the following mathematical definition:

$$h(t) = \text{limit}_{\Delta \downarrow 0} \Delta^{-1} \Pr(t \leq T < t + \Delta | t \leq T) , \tag{2.1}$$

where T is the time period for the development of the disease considered and Pr denotes probability. Indeed, for time intervals in which the hazard rate can be assumed constant, the incidence rate as defined above represents a valid estimate of the hazard rate. Thus, this result applies when piecewise constant hazards are assumed, which can be regarded as realistic in many applications, especially when reasonably short time intervals are used, and leads to convenient estimating procedures, e.g., based on the Poisson model.

Strictly speaking, incidence and hazard rates do not coincide. Hazard rates are formally defined as theoretical functions of time whereas incidence rates are defined directly as estimates and constitute valid estimates of hazard rates under certain assumptions (see above). For the sake of simplicity however, we will use the terms incidence rates and hazard rates as synonyms in the remainder of this chapter unless a clear distinction is needed.

2.2.2   Estimability and Basic Principles of Estimation

From the definitions above, it ensues that individual follow-up data are needed to obtain incidence rates or estimate hazard rates. Alternatively, in the absence of individual follow-up data, person-time at risk can be estimated as the time period width times the population size at midpoint. Such estimation makes the assumption that individuals who disappear from being at risk, either because they succumb, or because they move in or out, do so evenly across the time interval. Thus, population data such as registry data can be used to estimate incidence rates as long as an exhaustive census of incident cases can be obtained.

Among the main designs considered in Part I of this handbook, the cohort design (cf. Chap. I.5) is the ideal design to obtain incidence or hazard rates for various levels or profiles of exposure, i.e., exposure-specific incidence or hazard rates. This is because follow-up is available on subjects with various profiles of exposure. In many applications, obtaining exposure-specific incidence rates is not trivial however. Indeed, several exposures are often considered, some with several exposed levels and some continuous. Moreover, it may be necessary to account for confounders or effect-modifiers. Hence, estimation often requires modeling.

Methods of inference based on regression models are considered in detail in Part II of this handbook, particularly Chaps. II.3 and II.4.

Case-control data (cf. Chap. I.6) pose a more difficult problem than cohort data because case-control data alone are not sufficient to yield incidence or hazard rates. Indeed, they provide data on the distributions of exposure respectively in diseased subjects (cases) and non-diseased subjects (controls) for the disease under study, which can be used to estimate odds ratios (see Sect. 2.4.3) but are not sufficient to estimate exposure-specific incidence rates. However, it is possible to arrive at exposure-specific incidence rates from case-control data if case-control data are complemented by either follow-up or population data, which happens for nested or population-based case-control studies. In a nested case-control study, the cases and controls are selected from a follow-up study. In a population-based case-control study, they are selected from a specified population in which an effort is made to identify all incident cases diagnosed during a fixed time interval, usually in a grouped form (e.g., number of cases and number of subjects by age group). In both situations, full information on exposure is obtained only for cases and controls. Additionally, complementary information on composite incidence (i.e., counts of events and person-time) can be sought from the follow-up or population data. By combining this information with odds ratio estimates, exposure-specific incidence rates can be obtained. This has long been recognized (Cornfield 1951, 1956; MacMahon 1962; Miettinien 1974, 1976; Neutra and Drolette 1978) and is a consequence of the relation (Miettinen 1974; Gail et al. 1989):

$$h_0 = h^*(1 - \text{AR}) , \qquad (2.2)$$

where AR is the attributable risk in the population for all exposures considered, a quantity estimable from case-control data (see Sect. 2.5.1), h_0 is the baseline incidence rate, i.e., the incidence rate for subjects at the reference (unexposed) level of all exposures considered and h^* is the composite or average incidence rate in the population that includes unexposed subjects and subjects at various levels of all exposures (i.e., with various profiles of exposure). The composite incidence rate h^* can be estimated from the complementary follow-up or population data. Equation (2.2) simply states that the incidence rate for unexposed subjects is equal to the proportion of the average incidence rate in the population that is not associated with any of the exposures considered. Equation (2.2) can be specialized to various subgroups or strata defined by categories of age, sex or geographic location such as region or center, on which incidence rates are assumed constant. From the baseline rate h_0, incidence rates for all levels or profiles of exposure can be derived using odds ratio estimates, provided odds ratio estimates are reasonable estimates of incidence rate ratios as in the case of a rare disease (see Sect. 2.4). Consequently, exposure-specific incidence rates can be obtained from case-control data as long as they are complemented by follow-up or population data that can be used to estimate average incidence rates.

Example 1.   Exposure-specific incidence rates of breast cancer were obtained based on age as well as family history in first-degree relatives, reproductive history (i.e., age at menarche and age at first live birth), and history of benign disease from the Breast Cancer Detection and Demonstration Project (BCDDP). The BCDDP combined the prospective follow-up of 284,780 women over five years, and a nested case-control study (Gail et al. 1989) with about 3000 cases and 3000 controls. For each five-year age group from ages 35 to 79 years, composite incidence rates were obtained from the follow-up data. In age groups 40–44 and 45–49 years, 162 and 249 new cases of breast cancer developed from the follow-up of 79,526.4 and 88,660.7 person-years, yielding composite incidence rates of 203.7 and 280.8 per 10^5 person-years, respectively. For all women less than 50 years of age, the attributable risk for family history, reproductive history and history of benign breast disease was estimated at 0.4771 from the nested case-control data (see Sect. 2.5.1). By applying (2.2), baseline incidence rates for women at the reference level of all these factors were $203.7 \times (1 - 0.4771) = 106.5$ and $280.8 \times (1 - 0.4771) = 146.8$ per 10^5 person-years, respectively. For a nulliparous woman of age 40, with menarche at age 12, one previous biopsy for benign breast disease, and no history of breast-cancer in her first-degree relatives, the corresponding odds ratio was estimated at 2.89 from logistic regression analysis of the nested case-control data (see Sect. 2.4.6), yielding an exposure-specific incidence rate of $106.5 \times 2.89 = 307.8$ per 10^5 person-years. For a 45-year old woman with the same exposure profile, the corresponding exposure-specific incidence rate was $146.8 \times 2.89 = 424.3$ per 10^5 person-years.   ◆

Finally, cross-sectional data cannot provide any assessment of incidence rates but instead will yield estimates of disease prevalence proportions as discussed in Sect. 2.6 of this chapter.

2.2.3   Relation with Other Measures

The reason why exposure-specific incidence or hazard rates are central quantities is that, once they are available, most other quantities described in this chapter can be obtained from them, namely measures of disease risk, measures of association between exposure and disease risk, and measures of exposure impact in terms of new disease burden at the population level. However, it should be noted that measures of impact as well as some measures of association (i.e., odds ratios) can be estimated from case-control data alone without relying on exposure-specific incidence rates (see Sects. 2.3 and 2.4). Moreover, cross-sectional data can yield estimates of measures of association and impact with respect to disease prevalence (see Sect. 2.6.2).

Measures of Disease Risk

2.3

Definition

2.3.1

Disease risk is defined as the probability that an individual who is initially disease-free will develop a given disease over a specified time or age interval (e.g., one year or lifetime). Of all incidence and risk measures, this measure is probably the one most familiar and interpretable to most consumers of health data.

If the interval starting at time a_1 and ending just before time a_2, i.e., $[a_1, a_2)$, is considered, disease risk can be written formally as:

$$\pi(a_1, a_2) = \int_{a_1}^{a_2} h(a)\{S(a)/S(a_1)\}\,da \ . \tag{2.3}$$

In (2.3), $h(a)$ denotes the disease hazard at time or age a (see Sect. 2.2). The function $S(\cdot)$, with $(\cdot)$ an arbitrary argument, is the survival function, so that $S(a)$ denotes the probability of still being disease-free at time at age a, and $S(a)/S(a_1)$ denotes the conditional probability of staying disease-free up to time or age a for an individual who is free of disease at the beginning of the interval $[a_1, a_2)$. Equation (2.3) integrates over the interval $[a_1, a_2)$ the instantaneous incidence rate of developing disease at time or age a for subjects still at risk of developing the disease (i.e., subjects still disease-free). Because the survival function $S(\cdot)$ can be written as a function of disease hazard through:

$$S(a_2)/S(a_1) = \exp\left\{-\int_{a_1}^{a_2} h(a)\,da\right\} , \tag{2.4}$$

disease risk is also a function of disease hazard.

By specializing the meaning of functions $h(\cdot)$ and $S(\cdot)$, various quantities can be obtained that measure disease risk in different contexts. First, the time scale on which these functions as well as disease risk are defined corresponds to two specific uses of risk. In most applications, the relevant time scale is age, since disease incidence is influenced by age in most applications. Note that by considering the age interval $[0, a_2)$, one obtains lifetime disease risk up to age a_2. However, in clinical epidemiology settings, risk refers to the occurrence of an event, such as relapse or death in subjects already presenting with the disease of interest. In this context, the relevant time scale becomes time from disease diagnosis or, possibly, time from some other disease-related event, such as a surgical resection of a tumor or occurrence of a first myocardial infarction.

Second, risk definition may account or not for individual exposure profiles. If no risk factors are considered to estimate disease hazard, the corresponding measure of disease risk defines the average or composite risk over the entire population that includes subjects with various exposure profiles. This measure, also called cumulative incidence (Miettinen 1976), may be of value at the population level.

However, the main usefulness of risk is in quantifying an individual's predicted probability of developing disease depending on the individual's exposure profile. Thus, estimates of exposure-specific disease hazard have to be available for such exposure-specific risk (also called individualized or absolute risk) to be estimated.

Third, the consideration of competing risks and the corresponding definition of the survival function $S(\cdot)$ yields two separate definitions of risk. Indeed, although risk is defined with respect to the occurrence of a given disease, subjects can die from other causes (i.e., competing risks), which obviously precludes disease occurrence. The first option is to define $S(a)$ as the theoretical probability of being disease-free at time or age a if other causes of death (competing risks) were eliminated yielding a measure of disease risk in a setting with no competing risks. This measure may not be of much practical value. Moreover, unless unverifiable assumptions regarding incidence of the disease of interest and deaths from other causes can be made, for instance assuming that they occur independently, the function $S(\cdot)$ will not be estimable. For these reasons, it is more feasible to define $S(a)$ as the probability that an individual will be alive and disease-free at age a as the second option, yielding a more practical definition of disease risk as the probability of developing disease in the presence of competing causes of death (see Sect. 2.3.5).

From the definition of disease risk above, it appears that disease risk depends on the incidence rate of disease in the population considered and can also be influenced by the strength of the relationship between exposures and disease if individual risk is considered. One consequence is that risk estimates may not be portable from one population to another, as incidence rates may vary widely among populations that are separated in time and location or even among subgroups of populations, possibly because of differing genetic patterns or differing exposure to unknown risk factors. Additionally, competing causes of death (competing risks) may also have different patterns among different populations, which might also influence values of disease risk.

2.3.2   Range

Disease risk is a probability and therefore lies between 0 and 1, and is dimensionless. A value of 0 while theoretically possible would correspond to very special cases such as a purely genetic disease for an individual not carrying the disease gene. A value of 1 would be even more unusual and might again correspond to a genetic disease with a penetrance of 1 for a gene carrier but, even in this case, the value should be less than 1 if competing risks are accounted for.

2.3.3   Synonyms

Beside the term "disease risk", "absolute risk" or "absolute cause-specific risk" have been used by several authors (Dupont 1989; Benichou and Gail 1990a, 1995; Benichou 2000a; Langholz and Borgan 1997). Alternative terms include "individualized risk" (Gail et al. 1989), "individual risk" (Spiegelman et al. 1994), "crude probability" (Chiang 1968), "crude incidence" (Korn and Dorey 1992), "cumulative incidence" (Gray 1988; Miettinen 1976), "cumulative incidence risk" (Miettinen 1974) and "absolute incidence risk" (Miettinen 1976).

The term "cumulative risk" refers to the quantity $\int_{a_1}^{a_2} h(a)\,da$ and approximates disease risk closely in the case where disease is rare.

The term "attack rate" defines the risk of developing a communicable disease during a local outbreak and for the duration of the epidemic or the time during which primary cases occur (MacMahon and Pugh 1970, Chap. 5; Rothman and Greenland 1998, Chap. 27).

The term "floating absolute risk", introduced by Easton et al. (1991), refers to a different concept from disease risk. It was derived to remedy the standard problem that measures of association such as ratios of rates, risks or odds are estimated in reference to a baseline group, which causes their estimates for different levels of exposure to be correlated and may lead to lack of precision if the baseline group is small. The authors proposed a procedure to obtain estimates unaffected by these problems and used the term "floating absolute risk" to indicate that standard errors were not estimated in reference to an arbitrary baseline group.

Interpretation and Usefulness   2.3.4

If exposure profiles are not taken into account, the resulting average risk has little usefulness in disease prediction. Average risk estimates may be useful only for diseases for which no risk factors have been identified. Otherwise, they only provide overall results such as "one in nine women will develop breast cancer at sometime during her life" (American Cancer Society 1992), which are of no direct use in quantifying the risk of women with given exposure profiles and no direct help in deciding on preventive treatment or surveillance measures.

Upon taking individual exposure profiles into account, resulting individual disease risk estimates become useful in providing an individual measure of the probability of disease occurrence, and can therefore be useful in counseling. They are well suited to predicting risk for an individual, unlike measures of association that quantify the increase in the probability of disease occurrence relative to subjects at the baseline level of exposure, but do not quantify that probability itself.

Individual risk has been used as a tool for individual counseling in breast cancer (Benichou et al. 1996; Gail and Benichou 1994; Hoskins et al. 1995). Indeed, a woman's decision to take a preventive treatment such as Tamoxifen (Fisher et al. 1998; Wu and Brown 2003) or even undergo prophylactic mastectomy (Hartman et al. 2001; Lynch et al. 2001) depends on her awareness of the medical options, on personal preferences, and on individual risk. A woman may have several risk factors, but if her individual risk of developing breast cancer over the next 10 years is small, she may be reassured and she may be well advised simply to embark on a program of surveillance. Conversely, she may be very concerned about her absolute risk over a longer time period, such as 30 years, and she may decide to use prophylactic medical treatment or even undergo prophylactic mastectomy if her absolute risk is very high.

Estimates of individual risk of breast cancer are available based on age, family history, reproductive history and history of benign disease (Gail et al. 1989; Costantino et al. 1999) and were originally derived from the BCDDP that combined a follow-up study and a nested case-control study (Gail et al. 1989). This example illustrates that not only exposures or risk factors per se (such as family history) may be used to obtain individual risk estimates but also markers of risk such as benign breast disease which are known to be associated with an increase in disease risk and may reflect some premalignant stage. In the same fashion, it has been suggested to improve existing individual risk estimates of breast cancer by incorporating mammographic density, a risk marker known to be associated with increased breast cancer risk (Benichou et al. 1997). In the cardiovascular field, individual risk estimates of developing myocardial infarction, developing coronary heart disease, dying from coronary heart disease, developing stroke, developing cardiovascular disease, and dying from cardiovascular disease were derived from the Framingham heart and Framingham offspring cohort studies. These estimates are based on age, sex, HDL, LDL and total cholesterol levels, smoking status, blood pressure and diabetes history (Anderson et al. 1991).

Individual risk is also useful in designing and interpreting trials of interventions to prevent the occurrence of a disease. At the design stage, disease risk may be used for sample size calculations because the sample sizes required for these studies depend importantly on the risk of developing the disease during the period of study and the expected distribution of exposure profiles in the study sample (Anderson et al. 1992). Disease risk has also been used to define eligibility criteria in such studies. For example, women were enrolled in a preventive trial to decide whether the drug Tamoxifen can reduce the risk of developing breast cancer (Fisher et al. 1998). Because Tamoxifen is a potentially toxic drug and because it was to be administered to a healthy population, it was decided to restrict eligibility to women with somewhat elevated absolute risks of breast cancer. All women over age 59 as well as younger women whose absolute risks were estimated to equal or exceed that of a typical 60-year old woman were eligible to participate (Fisher et al. 1998). Individual risk has been used to interpret results of this trial through a risk-benefit analysis in order to help define which women are more likely to benefit from using Tamoxifen. Women were identified, who had a decrease in breast cancer risk and other events such as hip fracture from using Tamoxifen surpassing the Tamoxifen-induced increase in other events such as endometrial cancer, pulmonary embolism or deep vein thrombosis (Gail et al. 1999).

Disease risk can also be important in decisions affecting public health. For example, in order to estimate the absolute reduction in lung cancer incidence that might result from measures to reduce exposure to radon, one could categorize a general population into subgroups based on age, sex, smoking status and current radon exposure levels and then estimate the absolute reduction in lung cancer incidence that would result from lowering radon levels in each subgroup (Benichou and Gail 1990a; Gail 1975). Such an analysis would complement estimation of population attributable risk or generalized impact fractions (see Sect. 2.5).

The concept of risk is also useful in clinical epidemiology as a measure of the individualized probability of an adverse event, such as a recurrence or death in diseased subjects. In that context, risk depends on factors that are predictive of recurrence or death, rather than on factors influencing the risk of incident disease, and the time-scale of interest is usually time from diagnosis or from surgery rather than age. It can serve as a useful tool to help define individual patient management and, for instance, the absolute risk of recurrence in the next three years might be an important element in deciding whether to prescribe an aggressive and potentially toxic treatment regimen (Benichou and Gail 1990a; Korn and Dorey 1992).

Properties   2.3.5

Two main points need to be emphasized. First, as is evident from its definition, disease risk can only be estimated and interpreted in reference to a specified age or time interval. One might be interested in short time spans (e.g., five years), or long time spans (e.g., 30 years). Of course, disease risk increases as the time span increases. Sometimes, the time span is variable such as in lifetime risk.

Disease risk can be influenced strongly by the intensity of competing risks (typically competing causes of death, see above). Disease risk varies inversely as a function of death rates from other causes.

Estimability   2.3.6

It follows from its definition that disease risk is estimable as long as hazard rates for the disease (or event) of interest are estimable. Therefore, disease risk is directly estimable from cohort data, but case-control data have to be complemented with follow-up or population data in order to obtain the necessary complementary information on incidence rates (see Sect. 2.2.2).

It has been argued above (see Sect. 2.3.1) that disease risk is a more useful measure when it takes into account competing risks, that is the possibility for an individual to die of an unrelated disease before developing the disease (or disease-related event) of interest. In this setting, disease risk is defined as the probability of disease occurrence *in the presence* of competing risks, which is more relevant for individual predictions and other applications discussed above than the underlying (or "net" or "latent") probability of disease occurrence *in the absence* of competing risks. Moreover, disease risk is identifiable without any unverifiable competing risk assumptions in this setting, such as the assumption that competing risks act independently of the cause of interest because, as Prentice et al. (1978) emphasize, all functions of the disease hazard rates are estimable. Death rates from other causes can be estimated either internally from the study data or from external sources such as vital statistics.

Example 1. *(continued)*

In order to obtain estimates of breast cancer risk in the presence of competing risks, Gail et al. (1989) used 1979 United States (US) mortality rates from year 1979 for all causes except breast cancer to estimate the competing risks with more precision than from the BCDDP follow-up data. In age groups 40–44 and 45–49 years, these death rates were 153.0 and 248.6 per 10^5 person-years, respectively, hence of the same order of magnitude as breast cancer incidence rates. In older age groups, these death rates were much higher than breast cancer incidence rates, thus strongly influencing breast cancer risk estimates for age intervals including these age groups. For instance, death rates from causes other than breast cancer were 1017.7 and 2419.8 per 10^5 person-years in age groups 65–69 and 70–74 years, respectively, whereas average incidence rates of breast cancer were 356.1 and 307.8 per 10^5 person-years in these age groups, respectively.   ◆

2.3.7   Estimation from Cohort Studies

Estimation of disease risk rests on estimating disease incidence and hazard rates, a topic also addressed in Part II of this handbook. Several approaches have been worked out fully for disease risk estimation. A brief review of these approaches is given here starting with average risk estimates that do not take exposure profiles into account and continuing with exposure-specific estimates.

Estimates of Average Disease Risk

The density or exponential method (Miettinen 1976; Kleinbaum et al. 1982, Chap. 6; Rothman and Greenland 1998, Chap. 3) relies on subdividing the time or age scale in successive time or age intervals $I_1, \ldots, I_i, \ldots, I_I$ (e.g., one- or five-year intervals) on which the rate of disease incidence is assumed constant (i.e., piecewise constant). Disease risk over time or age interval $[a_1, a_2)$, that is the probability for an individual to experience disease occurrence over interval $[a_1, a_2)$ is taken as one minus the probability of staying disease-free through the successive intervals included in $[a_1, a_2)$. Assuming that disease is rare on each of the successive intervals considered, disease risk can be estimated as:

$$\widehat{\pi}(a_1, a_2) = 1 - \exp\left(-\sum_i \widehat{h}_i \Delta_i\right) . \tag{2.5}$$

The sum is taken over all intervals included in $[a_1, a_2)$. Notation Δ_i denotes the width of interval i, whereas $\widehat{h}_i$ denotes the incidence rate in interval i, obtained as the ratio of the number of incident cases over the person-time accumulated during follow-up in that interval.

While (2.5) is simple to apply, its validity depends on several assumptions. The assumption that disease incidence is constant over each time or age interval considered makes it a parametric approach. However, if intervals are small enough, this will not amount to a strong assumption. Moreover, it relies on the assumption that disease incidence is small on each interval. If this is not the case, a more complicated formula will be needed. Finally, this approach ignores competing risks.

Benichou and Gail (1990a) generalized this approach by lifting the condition on small incidence on each interval and allowing competing risks to be taken into account. They derived a generalized expression for the estimate of disease risk over time or age interval $[a_1, a_2)$ as:

$$\widehat{\pi}(a_1, a_2) = \sum_i \frac{\widehat{h}_{1i}}{\widehat{h}_{1i} + \widehat{h}_{2i}} \left[1 - \exp\left\{-\left(\widehat{h}_{1i} + \widehat{h}_{2i}\right)\Delta_i\right\}\right] A(i), \qquad (2.6)$$

$$\text{with} \quad A(i) = \prod_{j<i} \exp\left\{-\left(\widehat{h}_{1j} + \widehat{h}_{2j}\right)\Delta_j\right\} .$$

In (2.6), the sum is taken over all intervals included in $[a_1, a_2)$, Δ_i denotes the width of interval i, $\widehat{h}_{1i}$ denotes the disease incidence rate in interval i, $\widehat{h}_{2i}$ the death rate from other causes in interval i, and the product in $A(i)$ is taken over time intervals in $[a_1, a_2)$ from the first one to the one just preceding interval i. Death rates can be obtained in a similar fashion as disease incidence rates. It should be noted that disease risk can be estimated for a much longer duration than the actual follow-up of individuals in the study if age is the time scale (open cohort) provided there is no secular trend in disease incidence.

Variance estimates were derived by Benichou and Gail (1990a). Moreover, based on simulations of a closed cohort, they found that resulting confidence intervals have satisfactory coverage, especially with the log transformation, and observed little or no bias on risk estimates with a sufficient number of intervals even when disease incidence varied sharply with time.

The actuarial method or life table method (Cutler and Ederer 1958; Elveback 1958; Fleiss et al. 1976; Kleinbaum et al. 1982, Chap. 6; Rothman and Greenland 1998, Chap. 3) shares similarities with the density method, although it was derived from a less parametric viewpoint. As with the density method, time is split into intervals. In each time interval i, the probability for an individual who is disease-free at the beginning of the interval to stay disease-free throughout the interval is estimated. Disease risk is obtained as one minus the estimated probability of staying disease-free throughout the successive time intervals included in $[a_1, a_2)$ as:

$$\widehat{\pi}(a_1, a_2) = 1 - \prod_i \frac{(n_i - w_i/2 - d_i)}{(n_i - w_i/2)}, \qquad (2.7)$$

where the product is taken over all intervals included in $[a_1, a_2)$, n_i denotes the number of disease-free subjects at the beginning of interval i, d_i the number of incident cases occurring in interval i, and w_i the number of subjects either lost to follow-up or dying from other causes (competing risks) in interval i. The actuarial approach is most appropriate when grouped data are available and the actual follow-up of each individual in each interval is not known. The person-years of follow-up for subjects lost to follow-up or affected with competing risks in interval i is not used directly but, if one assumes that the mean withdrawal time occurs at the midpoint of the interval, then the denominator in each product term of (2.7) can be regarded as the effective number of persons at risk of developing the disease in the corresponding interval. Namely, it represents the number of disease-free persons that would be expected to produce d_i incident cases if all persons could be followed for the entire interval (Elandt-Johnson 1977; Kleinbaum et al. 1982, Chap. 6; Littell 1952). The actuarial method can be regarded as a refinement of the simple cumulative method (Kleinbaum et al. 1982, Chap. 6) that ignores quantity w_i and simply estimates disease risk as the number of individuals who contract the disease, divided by the total number in the cohort, or exposure subgroup of interest. The actuarial method is preferable to this direct method because, in practice, it is rare that a large enough cohort can be followed over a long enough time to reliably estimate the risk of disease by this simple method. Moreover, the simple cumulative method cannot handle the case when subjects are followed for varying lengths of time, which often occurs because subjects can be enrolled at different times whereas the follow-up ends at the same time for all subjects.

As shown by several authors (Cutler and Ederer 1958; Fleiss et al. 1976), the actuarial method results in biased estimates of risk even in the unlikely and most favorable event (in terms of bias) of all withdrawals occurring at the interval midpoints. Alternative approaches based on different choices of the quantity to subtract from n_i (i.e., choices different from $w_i/2$) are not subject to less bias, however (Elandt-Johnson 1977). The problem can be best handled by using narrow intervals but this is done at the expense of a larger random error (i.e., less precise estimates of risk).

Compared to the density method ((2.5) and (2.6)), the actuarial method has the advantage of not requiring knowledge of individual follow-up times in each interval but only knowledge of the number at risk at the beginning of the interval and the number of withdrawals. The density method could be used however without knowledge of follow-up time by assigning a follow-up time of half the interval width to subjects who are lost to follow-up, develop disease or die from other causes, in an analogous fashion as with the actuarial method (Benichou and Gail 1990a). The actuarial method requires neither the assumption of constant incidence rate nor rarity of disease incidence on all time intervals. However, bias is less of a problem with the density than the actuarial method and the density method applies naturally to open cohorts and extends easily to risk estimates that take exposure profiles into account (see below).

When individual follow-up times are all known, a fully nonparametric risk estimate can be obtained in the spirit of the Kaplan–Meier estimate of survival (Kaplan and Meier 1958; see also Chap. II.4 of this handbook). Disease risk is estimated through summation on all distinct times in $[a_1, a_2)$ at which new disease cases occur (Aalen and Johansen 1978; Kay and Schumacher 1983; Gray 1988; Matthews 1988; Keiding and Andersen 1989; Benichou and Gail 1990a; Korn and Dorey 1992). Corresponding variance estimates were derived (Aalen 1978; Aalen and Johansen 1978; Keiding and Andersen 1989; Benichou and Gail 1990a; Korn and Dorey 1992) from which confidence intervals can be obtained, based on the log transformation as suggested by Benichou and Gail (1990a) and Keiding and Andersen (1989), or based on the approach of Dorey and Korn (1987).

Upon comparing the generalized density method (see (2.6)) and the nonparametric method, Benichou and Gail (1990a) showed that the loss of efficiency of the nonparametric method is small compared to the density method. Moreover, the nonparametric method yields little bias in risk estimates as well nearly nominal coverage for confidence intervals of risk with the log transformation. Nominal coverage refers to the theoretical probability of a confidence interval to cover the true parameter and may be assessed using simulations (i.e., a 95% confidence interval will be said to have nominal coverage if it does include the true parameter value in 95% of the cases). Hence, properties of the generalized density and nonparametric methods agree closely. However, the generalized density method has the advantage of simplicity of computation and is better suited to open cohorts.

Estimates of Exposure-specific Disease Risk

In order to obtain risk estimates that depend on exposure profiles, the cohort could be subdivided into subcohorts based on exposure levels and the methods above applied to these subcohorts. However, this approach would be impractical because it would yield risk estimates with very low precision. In order to remedy this problem, a natural approach to incorporate exposures is to model incidence rates through regression models.

Benichou and Gail (1990a) proposed a direct extension of the generalized density method (2.6). This extension is based on assuming that the disease hazard rate on each time or age interval i is the product of a constant baseline hazard rate for subjects at the reference level of exposure in interval i and a function of the various exposures. The corresponding parameters, i.e., baseline hazard rates and hazard ratio parameters for exposure can be jointly estimated by maximizing the piecewise exponential likelihood, which is equivalent to the usual Poisson likelihood for the analysis of cohort data (Holford 1980; Laird and Oliver 1981). Corresponding variance estimates are available (Benichou and Gail 1990a). In simulations, risk estimates appeared subject to little bias, variance estimates were also little biased and coverage of confidence intervals was nearly nominal, except for the exposure profiles with very few subjects (Benichou and Gail 1990a). Other parametric approaches were considered to obtain risk estimates of cardiovascular events from the Framingham studies (Anderson et al. 1991). Semi-parametric estimators of risk were also derived (Benichou and Gail 1990a). In contrast with the previous approach where a piecewise exponential or Poisson distribution is assumed, the baseline disease hazard rate is expressed as an unspecified function of time or age rather than a constant, which corresponds to the semi-parametric Cox regression model (Cox 1972). Risk estimates are obtained as functions of the partial likelihood estimates (Cox 1975) of hazard ratio parameters and related Nelson-Aalen estimates of cumulative baseline hazards (Borgan 1998). From results in Tsiatis (1981) and Andersen and Gill (1982) on the joint distribution of these parameter estimates, Benichou and Gail (1990a) derived an asymptotic variance estimator.

Regression based methods appear well suited for estimating exposure-specific disease risk and are therefore useful for the purpose of individual prediction. Compared to the semi-parametric approach, the generalized density method appears easier to implement while providing a good compromise between bias and precision.

2.3.8   Estimation from Population-based or Nested Case-Control Studies

As discussed above, whereas disease risk is directly estimable from cohort data, case-control data have to be complemented with follow-up or population data in order to obtain the necessary information on incidence rates. If such complementary data are available, exposure-specific incidence rates and exposure-specific disease risk can be estimated. All approaches proposed in the literature rely on regression methods.

The Hybrid Approach

This approach relies on the assumption of piecewise constant incidence rates and on (2.2) to obtain baseline incidence rates in strata defined by factors such as age, sex, race or geographic area (see Sect. 2.2.2). Odds ratio estimates are then combined with baseline incidence rates to arrive at exposure-specific incidence rates (see Sect. 2.2.2). Applying (2.6) to these rates and death rates from competing causes, disease risk estimates can be obtained for desired time intervals. This approach has been used in practice to obtain individual risks of breast cancer by Gail et al. (1989) (see Example 1 below). Resulting disease risk estimates can be termed estimates of individual breast cancer risk since they depend on age and individual exposure profile (216 profiles were considered overall). The approach can be seen as a multivariate extension of earlier work by Miettinen (1974). It has been termed a hybrid approach (Benichou 2000a) since it relies on two models, namely the piecewise exponential model that underlies the density method (i.e., constant incidence by age group) and the logistic model used to obtain odds ratio estimates from the nested case-control data (see Sect. 2.4.6). It can be applied to population-based case-control data with no individual follow-up of subjects in a similar manner as to nested case-control data, as discussed and illustrated for bladder cancer by Benichou and Wacholder (1994) (see Example 2 below).

Variance estimators for risk estimates are complex since exposure-specific incidence rate estimates involve odds ratio parameters obtained through logistic regression from the case-control data and counts of incident cases from the follow-up or population data. Estimators of variances and covariances of age- and exposure-specific incidence rates that take into account all sources of variability have been fully worked out for various sampling schemes regarding control selection in the general case (Benichou and Gail 1990a) and specifically to account for the special features of the BCDDP data (Benichou and Gail 1995). Simulations tailored to the BCDDP data showed a small upward bias in risk estimates due to the small upward bias incurred by using odds ratios to estimate hazard ratios when the rare-disease assumption appeared questionable. Variance estimates had very little bias and yielded confidence intervals with near nominal coverage. Coverage was improved with the logit transformation.

Example 1. *(continued)*
Applying (2.6) to exposure-specific incidence rates of breast cancer estimated from the BCDDP data (see Sect. 2.2.2) and death rates from other causes estimated from US mortality data (see Sect. 2.3.6), risk estimates of breast cancer can be obtained. For instance, the 10-year risk of developing breast cancer between ages 40 and 50 years for a woman initially free of breast cancer at age 40 years and with the exposure profile considered in Sect. 2.2.2 (i.e., nulliparous woman with menarche at age 12 years, one previous biopsy for benign breast disease, and no history of breast cancer in her first-degree relatives) is obtained as a sum of two terms. The first term $\widehat{\pi}_1$, corresponding to age interval 40–44, is obtained from (2.6) as:

$$\widehat{\pi}_1 = \frac{307.8 \times 10^{-5}}{307.8 \times 10^{-5} + 153.0 \times 10^{-5}} \left[1 - \exp\left\{ -5\left(307.8 \times 10^{-5} + 153.0 \times 10^{-5}\right)\right\}\right]$$

$$= 0.0152 \, .$$

The second term $\widehat{\pi}_2$, corresponding to age interval 45–49, is obtained from (2.6) as the product of the probability of developing breast cancer in age interval 45–49 times the probability of having stayed free of breast cancer and not died from other causes in age interval 40–44:

$$\widehat{\pi}_2 = \frac{424.3 \times 10^{-5}}{424.3 \times 10^{-5} + 248.6 \times 10^{-5}} \left[1 - \exp\left\{ -5\left(424.3 \times 10^{-5} + 248.6 \times 10^{-5}\right)\right\}\right]$$

$$\times \exp\left\{ -5\left(307.8 \times 10^{-5} + 153.0 \times 10^{-5}\right)\right\} = 0.0204 \, .$$

Thus, the 10-year risk of developing breast cancer is obtained as the sum 0.0152 + 0.0204 = 0.0356, or 3.6%. The corresponding 95% confidence interval based on taking all sources of variability into account can be estimated as 3.0% to 4.2% through computations described in Benichou and Gail (1995). Breast cancer risk estimates can be obtained for all age intervals in the range 20–80 years and all 216 exposure profiles including the profile considered above. This whole approach to individual breast cancer risk estimation is known as the "Gail model" and has enjoyed widespread use in individual counseling, designing and interpreting prevention trials. Practical implementation has been greatly facilitated by the development of graphs (Benichou et al. 1996) as well as a computer program (Benichou 1993a) and its modified version that is available on the US National Cancer Institute web site at http://bcra.nci.nih.gov/brc/. ◆

Example 2. In the year 1978, incident cases of bladder cancer were identified through 10 cancer registries in the United States. For instance, 32 incident cases were identified among white males aged 45–64 years whose population numbered 97,420 individuals. Assuming that this population remained constant throughout the year 1978, these data yielded an average incidence rate of 32.8 per 10^5 person-years. The National Bladder Cancer Study was a population-based case-control study conducted at the ten cancer registries. Incident cases aged 21–84 years were selected from the registries. Controls aged 21–84 years were selected from telephone sampling or Health Care Financing Administration rosters and frequency-matched to cases on geographic area, age and sex. Based on case-control data from two states (Utah and New Jersey) and one large city (Atlanta), odds ratios were estimated for smoking status (never smoker, ex-smoker, current light smoker, current heavy smoker) and occupational exposure to carcinogens (yes, no) using logistic regression (see Sect. 2.4.6). Moreover, the attributable risk for smoking and occupational exposure was estimated for white males in each of the nine strata resulting from the three areas and three age groups (i.e., 21–44, 45–64 and 65+ years) (see Sect. 2.5.1). Among white males aged 45–64 years in Utah, it was estimated at 54.0%, yielding a baseline incidence rate of $32.8 \times (1 - 0.540) = 15.1$ per 10^5 person-years. The odds ratios for current heavy smokers (≥ 20 cigarettes per day) and occupational exposure were estimated at 2.9 and 1.6. Hence, among white males aged 45–64 years in Utah, exposure-specific incidence rates were estimated at $15.1 \times 1.6 = 24.1$ per 10^5 person-years for never smokers with a history of occupational exposure, and $15.1 \times 2.9 \times 1.6 = 69.8$ per 10^5 person-years for current heavy smokers with a history of occupational exposure assuming a multiplicative effect of smoking and occupational exposure (and allowing for rounding error). From these exposure-specific incidence rates, estimates of the risk of bladder cancer over specified age intervals could be derived, using (2.6). ◆

Other Parametric Approaches

A pseudo-likelihood approach also relying on the assumption on piecewise constant incidence (i.e., piecewise exponential model) has been proposed as an alternative to the hybrid approach (Benichou and Wacholder 1994). In each stratum separately, observed distributions of exposure in the cases and controls are applied to counts of incident cases and person-time to obtain respective expected numbers of incident cases and of person-time per stratum and exposure level. Then, baseline incidence rates and hazard ratios are jointly estimated from these expected quantities under a piecewise exponential model. Joint estimation proceeds from maximizing the likelihood corresponding to this model. Since this likelihood includes expected rather than observed counts, it is termed a pseudo-likelihood. Thus, the procedure includes two steps. In the first step, expected numbers of incident cases and person-time per exposure and stratum are calculated. Then, the parameters of interest (i.e., stratum-specific baseline incidence rates and hazard ratios) are estimated from these expected counts through maximizing a pseudo-likelihood. This approach is easy to implement, as was illustrated on population-based case-control data of bladder cancer.

Example 2. *(continued)*
    Among white males aged 45–64 years and in all other strata separately, observed proportions of cases (respectively controls) with given joint level of smoking and occupational exposure among the eight (four times two) joint levels considered were applied to counts of incident cases (respectively person-time) to obtain expected counts by stratum and joint exposure level. Namely, the products of the counts by the observed proportions were formed. Using these expected counts, a pseudo-likelihood based on the piecewise exponential model was maximized yielding estimates of relative hazards and stratum-specific baseline incidence rates. For instance, the baseline incidence rate for white males aged 45–64 years in Utah was estimated at 13.7 per 10^5 person-years and relative hazards for current heavy smoking and occupational exposure were estimated at 2.9 and 1.5, respectively. Hence, among white males aged 45–64 years in Utah, exposure-specific incidence rates were estimated at $13.7 \times 1.5 = 20.6$ per 10^5 person-years for never smokers with a history of occupational exposure, and $13.7 \times 2.9 \times 1.5 = 61.9$ per 10^5 person-years for current heavy smokers with a history of occupational exposure still assuming a multiplicative effect of smoking and occupational exposure (and allowing for rounding error). ◆

A full likelihood approach has also been proposed based on the piecewise exponential model (Benichou and Wacholder 1994). All parameters (i.e., baseline rates, hazard ratios and conditional probabilities for the distribution of exposure in the cases and controls) are estimated jointly through maximizing a likelihood involving all parameters. This approach may prove intractable in practice except in simple situations with few exposure levels considered. A full likelihood approach based on the logistic model (Greenland 1981) appears much easier to implement. Baseline incidence rates are obtained by simply adding to the stratum parameter estimates from the logistic model a term corresponding to the logarithm of the ratio of sampling fractions among cases and controls in the stratum (Greenland 1981; Prentice and Pyke 1979; also similar to discussion of (2.8) in Sect. 2.4.6).

Example 2. *(continued)*
    Although it required the estimation of 60 additional parameters relative to the pseudo-likelihood approach, the full likelihood approach based on the piecewise exponential model could be implemented. The 60 additional parameters described the conditional probabilities of exposure (smoking and occupational exposure) in the cases and controls for all nine strata. For instance, the baseline incidence rate for white males aged 45–64 years in Utah was estimated at 13.9 per 10^5 person-years and relative hazards for current heavy smoking and occupational exposure were estimated at 2.9 and 1.6, respectively. Hence, among white

males aged 45–64 years in Utah, exposure-specific incidence rates were estimated at $13.9 \times 1.6 = 22.2$ per 10^5 person-years for never smokers with a history of occupational exposure, and $13.9 \times 2.9 \times 1.6 = 64.1$ per 10^5 person-years for current heavy smokers with a history of occupational exposure still assuming a multiplicative effect of smoking and occupational exposure (and allowing for rounding error). ◆

Upon comparing the pseudo-likelihood, full likelihood and hybrid approach on population-based case-control data of bladder cancer, Benichou and Wacholder (1994) noted that the hybrid approach seemed to be less efficient for incidence rate estimation than the other two approaches, which were themselves equally efficient. They discussed other advantages of the pseudo-likelihood and full likelihood approaches. Namely, these approaches allow direct estimation of hazard ratios rather than odds ratios. Furthermore, the pseudo-likelihood approach and the full likelihood approach (in its version relying on the piecewise exponential model) can be applied to more general regression models, e.g., models with an additive form using hazard rate difference parameters rather than hazard ratio parameters (see Sects. 2.4.4 and 2.4.6). Finally, all three approaches require that cases and controls be selected completely at random and that incident cases or at least a known proportion of them (i.e., known sampling fraction) be fully identified.

Semi-parametric Approach

In nested case-control studies, controls are usually individually matched to cases on time. Namely, for each case, one (or several) control(s) is (are) selected among subjects with the same age and length of follow-up in the cohort as the case (Breslow et al. 1983; Liddell et al 1977; Mantel 1973; see also Chap. I.7 of this handbook). The three parametric approaches described above do not apply readily to this context of individual time matching of controls to cases. Langholz and Borgan (1997) developed a semi-parametric approach to handle this case. Their approach can be regarded as an extension of the semi-parametric approach for cohort studies described above (see Sect. 2.3.7). Incidence rates are expressed as the product of baseline incidence rates of an unspecified form times a function of the covariates representing the hazard ratio (Cox 1972). Hazard ratio parameter estimates are obtained from maximizing the partial likelihood of the Cox model for nested case-control data (Oakes 1981; Prentice and Breslow 1978). Risk estimates are obtained by combining partial likelihood hazard ratio parameter estimates and corresponding cumulative hazard estimates.

A direct comparison of the semi-parametric approach with the parametric approaches presented above is not possible because the semi-parametric approach applies only to time-matched data, which the parametric approaches cannot handle. The semi-parametric approach requires observation of individual follow-up time of each subject in the original cohort in order to form the risk sets for each failure time and enable control selection. It is therefore potentially less widely applicable than the parametric approaches.

Final Notes and Additional References 2.3.9

General problems of definition of disease risk, interpretation and usefulness, properties, estimation and special problems have been reviewed in detail (Benichou 2000a). Special problems include accounting for continuous or time-dependent exposure, estimation of disease risk from two-stage case-control data, and validation procedures for disease risk estimates. Finally, an important challenge is to increase awareness of the proper interpretation and use of disease risk in practice and develop general software for easier implementation.

Measures of Association 2.4

Definitions and General Points 2.4.1

Measures of association have a long history and have been reviewed in many textbooks. They assess the strength of associations between one or several exposures and the risk of developing a given disease. Thus, they are useful in etiologic research to assess and quantify associations between potential risk (or protective) factors and disease risk. The question addressed is whether and to what degree a given exposure is associated with occurrence of the disease of interest. In fact, this is the primary question that most epidemiologic studies are trying to answer.

Depending on the available data, measures of association may be based on disease rates, disease risks, or even disease odds, i.e., $\pi/(1 - \pi)$, with π denoting disease risk. They contrast rates, risks or odds for subjects with various levels of exposure, e.g., risks or rates of developing breast cancer for 40-year old women with or without a personal history of benign breast disease. They can be expressed in terms of ratios or differences of risks or rates among subjects exposed and non-exposed to given factors or among subjects with various levels of exposure.

Measures of association can be defined for categorical or continuous exposures. For categorical exposures, any two exposure levels can be contrasted using the measures of association defined below. However, it is convenient to define a reference level to which any exposure level can be contrasted. This choice is sometimes natural (e.g., non-smokers in assessing the association of smoking with disease occurrence) but can be more problematic if the exposure considered is of continuous nature, where a range of low exposures may be considered potentially inconsequential. The choice of a reference range is important for interpreting results. It should be wide enough for estimates of measures of association to be reasonably precise. However, it should not be so wide that it compromises meaningful interpretation of the results, which depend critically on the homogeneity of the reference level. For continuous exposures, measures of association can also be expressed per unit of exposure, e.g., for each additional gram of daily alcohol consumption. The reference level may then be a precise value such as no daily alcohol consumption or a range of values such as less than 10 grams of daily alcohol consumption.

2.4.2   Usefulness and Interpretation

When computing a measure of association, it is usually assumed that the relationship being captured has the potential to be causal, and efforts are taken to remove the impact of confounders from the quantity. Section 2.4.6 provides a summary of techniques for adjustment for confounders. Nonetheless, except for the special case of randomized studies, most investigators retain the word "association" rather than "effect" when describing the relationship between exposure and outcome to emphasize the possibility that unknown confounders may still influence the relationship.

Rothman and Greenland (Chap. I.4 of this handbook) take efforts to differentiate the concepts of effect and association, and adopt the framework of *counterfactuals*, popular in the field of economics (Wooldridge 2001), to define the term *effect size*. They then define "measure of association" as computed to compare two actual populations. Hence, the distinction is one of a true causal concept versus one that may be subject to the confounding of the true effect arising from the population mix of characteristics at hand. These definitions are more precise and serve as reminders of the true nature of causality. We will retain the less precise, but more common terminology where "measure of association" refers to either or both concepts. We also note that the discussion here is limited to measures of association with a *binary* (i.e. coded as 1 = present, 0 = absent) or event *count* (number of events) outcome. In many situations, classification into disease versus no disease is not clear-cut. For example, the definition of an abnormal lipid profile has undergone frequent change. In such cases, using measures based on continuous outcomes may be a better choice. We comment on relationships between measures of association for continuous and categorical outcomes in Sect. 2.4.6.

When choosing a measure of association, the primary goal is interpretability and familiarity to consumers of the information. Another guideline is that the measure of association should allow as simple a description of the association as possible. For example, it has been empirically observed that risk ratios are more likely than risk differences to remain constant across subpopulations with different risk levels (Breslow and Day 1980, Chap. 2), hence simplifying description of the association of the exposure with the outcome. Breslow and Day (1980, Chap. 2) also point out that ratios can be converted to differences by taking the logarithm of the risk or rate.

Definitions and properties of measures of association as well as relations among them are reviewed below for measures based on ratios and measures based on differences. Then, estimability of these measures from cohort and case-control designs and general points regarding estimation of these measures are considered, including an overview of techniques to adjust for confounders. More details regarding inference, namely estimating these measures and assessing the statistical significance of apparent associations, will be presented in Part II of this handbook.

The below Table 2.1 provides an overview of measures of association discussed in this chapter:

Table 2.1. Measures of association discussed in this chapter (GLM = generalized linear model; see Sect. 2.4.6)

Measure	Lower limit	Upper limit	Null value	Definition	Link function in GLM
Rate ratio (HR)	0	$+\infty$	1	$h_E/h_{\bar{E}}$	Log
Risk ratio (RR)	0	$+\infty$	1	$\pi_E/\pi_{\bar{E}}$	Log
Odds ratio (OR)	0	$+\infty$	1	$[\pi_E/(1-\pi_E)]/$ $[\pi_{\bar{E}}/(1-\pi_{\bar{E}})]$	Logit
Rate difference	$-\infty$	$+\infty$	0	$h_E - h_{\bar{E}}$	Identity
Risk difference	-1	$+1$	0	$\pi_E - \pi_{\bar{E}}$	Identity

Measures Based on Ratios

2.4.3

General Properties

Ratio based measures of association are particularly appropriate when the effect of the exposure is multiplicative, which means there is a similar percent increase or decrease associated with exposure in rate, risk or odds across exposure subgroups. As noted above, effects have often been observed to be multiplicative, leading to ratios providing a simple description of the association (e.g., see Breslow and Day 1980, Chap. 2). Ratio measures are dimensionless and range from zero to infinity, with one designating no association of the exposure with the outcome. When the outcome is death or disease, and the ratio has the rate, risk or odds of the outcome with the exposed group in the numerator, a value less than one indicates a protective effect of exposure. The exposure is then referred to as a protective factor. When the ratio in this set-up is greater than one, there is greater disease occurrence with exposure, and the exposure is then referred to as a risk factor.

It can be shown that numerically, the odds ratio falls the furthest from the null, and the risk ratio the closest, with the rate ratio in between. For example, from the below Table 2.2, based on a fictitious data from a cohort study for a disease that is not rare, we would obtain a risk ratio $\widehat{RR} = 0.3/0.1 = 3.00$ and an odds ratio $\widehat{OR} = [(30)(90)]/[(10)(70)] = 3.86$. If we assume a constant hazard, so that the risk for each group is $1 - \exp(-hT)$, with T being the follow-up time for each subject, we have the rate ratio $\widehat{HR} = \ln(1-0.3)/\ln(1-0.1) = 3.39$ (see Sects. 2.3.1 and 2.4.6). Hence $1 < \widehat{RR} < \widehat{HR} < \widehat{OR}$.

Table 2.2. Data from fictitious cohort study

	Exposed	Unexposed
Diseased	30	10
Non-diseased	70	90

The difference in magnitude between the above ratio measures is important to keep in mind when interpreting them for diseases or outcomes that are not rare. For rare outcomes the values of the three ratio measures tend to be close. Ratios become differences on the logarithmic scale, and estimation and inference often take place on the log scale, where zero indicates no association.

Rate Ratios

As the name implies, the rate ratio is the ratio between the rate of disease among those exposed and those not exposed or $h_E/h_{\bar{E}}$. Conceptually, the rate ratio is identical to a hazard ratio HR. The latter term tends to be used when time dependence of the rate is emphasized, as the hazard is a function that may depend on time. The situation of a constant rate ratio over time is referred to as *proportional hazards*. The proportional hazards assumption is often made in the analysis of rates (see below). Theoretically, the hazard ratio at a given time point is the limiting value of the rate ratio as the time interval around the point becomes very short, just as the hazard is the limiting quantity for incidence rate (see Sect. 2.2.1). The rate ratio has also been called the *Incidence Density Ratio* (Kleinbaum et al. 1982, Chap. 8). It may be noted that the rate ratio is attenuated by less than perfect specificity of the outcome criteria, but relatively unaffected by less than perfect sensitivity, especially when the rate is low, as long as the sensitivity is unaffected by exposure. In other words, if cases are equally missed in the exposed and unexposed groups, the rate ratio is relatively unaffected. However, if non-cases are considered cases, the ratio will be lower than if diagnostic criteria identified only true cases. Even in the fictitious example above with high incidence rates, 80% sensitivity leads to a slightly attenuated rate ratio of 3.29 from

$$\widehat{HR} = \ln\left[1 - (0.80)(0.3)\right]/\ln\left[1 - (0.80)(0.1)\right] = 3.29$$

(as compared to the correct rate ratio of 3.39 from Table 2.2), while 80% specificity leads to a severely biased rate ratio of

$$\widehat{HR} = \ln\left[0.80(1 - 0.3)\right]/\ln\left[0.80(1 - 0.1)\right] = 1.77 .$$

Rate ratios are extremely useful because of the ease of estimating them in many contexts. They refer to population dynamics, and are not as easily interpretable on the individual level. It has been argued, however, that rate ratios make more sense than risk ratios (see below) when the period subjects are at risk is longer than the observation period (Kleinbaum et al. 1982, Chap. 8). Numerically, the rate ratio is further from the null than the risk ratio. When rates are low, the similarity of risk and rate leads to rate ratios being close to risk ratios, as discussed below. Some investigators tend to refer to rate ratios as relative risks, creating some confusion in terminology. Further considerations of how the rate ratio relates to other ratio based measures of association are offered by Rothman and Greenland (1998, p 50).

Risk Ratios

The risk ratio, relative risk or ratio of risks of disease among those exposed π_E and those not exposed $\pi_{\bar{E}}$, RR $= \pi_E/\pi_{\bar{E}}$, has been viewed as the gold standard among measures of association for many years. It is eminently interpretable on the individual level as a given-fold increase in risk of disease. Like other ratio-based measures, it tends to be more stable than the risk difference across population groups at widely different risk. However, similar to rate ratios and odds ratios (introduced in Sect. 2.4.3), the risk ratio can be viewed as misleading in the public eye when the risk among both the unexposed and the exposed is very low, yet many-fold increased by exposure. Another disadvantage of the risk ratio is its asymmetry with respect to the definition of an event, so that the risk ratio for not having an event, $(1 - \pi_E)/(1 - \pi_{\bar{E}})$, cannot be directly computed from the risk ratio for having an event. For example, knowing that the risk ratio for an event RR $= 3.00$, the scenario $\pi_E = 0.3$, $\pi_{\bar{E}} = 0.1$ results in $(1 - \pi_E)/(1 - \pi_{\bar{E}}) = 0.7/0.9 = 0.78$, while the scenario $\pi_E = 0.6$, $\pi_{\bar{E}} = 0.2$, which represents the same risk ratio of 3.00, results in $(1 - \pi_E)/(1 - \pi_{\bar{E}}) = 0.4/0.8 = 0.50$. The risk ratio depends on the length of the time interval considered because risk itself refers to a specific interval (see Sect. 2.3.1). In the literature, the term relative risk is often used to denote the rate ratio as well as the risk ratio, creating some confusion. Therefore, we will avoid the term "relative risk" in the following. Numerically the risk ratio is closer to the null than the rate ratio for the same data (see above).

Cornfield et al. (1959), in the smoking versus lung cancer debate, derived several theoretical properties of the risk ratio, which have further supported its use. In this debate, Cornfield, along with Doll and Hill, argued against strong opposition from R.A. Fisher and Joseph Berkson that the association was causal, and not likely due to unmeasured confounders, such as a genetic predisposition to both smoke and contract lung cancer. First of all, Cornfield et al. (1959) turned attenuation of the risk ratio due to lack of specificity of the outcome into an advantage, by noting that the ratio will become stronger as the disease subtype affected by the exposure is honed. Second, Cornfield et al. demonstrated that if a confounder is to explain the outcome with exposure risk ratio RR > 1, that confounder has to have risk ratio at least RR, and in addition the prevalence of the confounder must be at least RR times greater among the exposed than among the unexposed. Lin et al. (1998) presented more general formulas that confirm Cornfield et al.'s assertions under assumptions of no interaction between the confounder and exposure. These theoretical results have led investigators to reason that high risk ratios (say above 1.4; Siemiatycki et al. 1988) are not likely to be explained by uncontrolled confounding.

Odds Ratios

For several reasons, the odds ratio has emerged as the most popular measure of association. The odds ratio is the ratio of odds, OR $= [\pi_E/(1 - \pi_E)]/[\pi_{\bar{E}}/(1 - \pi_{\bar{E}})]$. Historically, the odds ratio was considered an approximation to the risk ratio obtainable from case-control studies. The reason for this is that the probabilities of being sampled into case and control groups cancel in the calculation of the odds ratio, as long as sampling is independent of exposure status. Furthermore, when π_E and $\pi_{\bar{E}}$ are small, the ratio $(1 - \pi_{\bar{E}})/(1 - \pi_E)$ has little influence on the odds ratio, making it approximately equal to the risk ratio $\pi_E/\pi_{\bar{E}}$. The assumption of small π_E and $\pi_{\bar{E}}$ is referred to as the *rare-disease assumption*. Kleinbaum et al. (1982) have pointed out that in a case-control study of a stable population with incident cases and controls being representative of non-cases, the odds ratio is the rate ratio. Numerically, the odds ratio is the furthest from the null of the three ratio measures considered here.

More recently, the odds ratio has gained status as an association measure in its own right, and is often applied in cohort studies and clinical trials, as well as in case-control studies. This is due to many desirable properties of the odds ratio. First of all, focusing on risk rather than odds may be a matter of convention rather than a preference based on fundamental principles, and using the same measure across settings has the advantage of consistency and makes comparisons and meta-analyses easy. In contrast to the risk ratio, the odds ratio is symmetric so that the odds ratio for disease is the inverse of the odds ratio for no disease. Furthermore, the odds ratio based on exposure probabilities equals the odds ratio based on disease probabilities, a fact that follows from Bayes' theorem (e.g., Cornfield 1951; Miettinen 1974; Neutra and Drolette 1978) or directly from consideration of how cases and controls are sampled. The disease and exposure odds ratios are sometimes referred to as *prospective* and *retrospective odds ratios*, respectively. Finally, odds ratios from both case-control and cohort studies are estimable by logistic regression, which has become the most popular approach to regression analysis with binary outcomes (see Sect. 2.4.6).

Some investigators feel that the risk ratio is more directly interpretable than the odds ratio, and have developed methods for converting odds ratios into risk ratios for situations when risks are not low (Zhang and Yu 1998).

2.4.4   Measures Based on Differences

General Properties

Difference based measures are appropriate when effects are additive (e.g., see Breslow and Day 1980, Chap. 2), which means that the exposure leads to a similar absolute increase or decrease in rate or risk across subgroups. The difference in odds is very rarely used, and not addressed here. As noted above, additive relationships are less common in practice, except on the logarithmic scale, when they are equivalent to ratio measures. However, difference measures may be more understandable to the public when the outcome is rare, and relate directly to measures of impact discussed below (see Sect. 2.5).

The numerical ranges of difference measures depend on their component parts. The rate difference ranges from minus to plus infinity, while the risk difference is bounded between minus and plus one. The situation of no association is reflected by a difference measure of zero. When the measure is formed as the rate or risk among the exposed minus that among the non-exposed, a positive value indicates that the exposure is a risk factor, while a negative value indicates that it is a protective factor. It can be shown that the risk difference falls numerically nearer to the null than does the rate difference. For example, Table 2.2 yields a risk difference of $0.30 - 0.10 = 0.20$, while the rate difference is $\ln(0.70) + \ln(0.90) = 0.25$. However, they will be close for rare outcomes. In contrast to ratio measures, difference measures are always attenuated by less than perfect sensitivity (i.e., missed cases), but the rate difference is unaffected by less than perfect specificity. The risk difference is also relatively unaffected when risk is low. In the fictitious example above, if the sensitivity of the test used to detect disease is 80%, the rate difference is $-\ln[1 - (0.80)(0.3)] + \ln[1 - (0.80)(0.1)] = 0.19$, but if the specificity is 80%, the rate difference remains at 0.25.

Rate Differences

The rate difference is defined as $h_E - h_{\bar{E}}$, and has been commonly employed to compare mortality rates and other demographic rates between countries, time periods and/or regions. In such comparisons, the two rates being compared are often *directly standardized* (see Sect. 2.6) to the age and sex distribution of a standard population chosen, e.g., as the population of a given country in a given census year.

For the special case of a dichotomous exposure, the rate difference, i.e., the difference between the incidence rates in the exposed and unexposed subjects has been termed "excess incidence" (Berkson 1958; MacMahon and Pugh 1970; Mausner and Bahn 1974), "excess risk" (Schlesselman 1982), "Berkson's simple difference" (Walter 1976), "incidence density difference" (Miettinen 1976), or even "attributable risk" (Markush 1977; Schlesselman 1982), which may have caused some confusion.

Risk Differences

The risk difference $\pi_E - \pi_{\bar{E}}$ is parallel to the rate difference discussed above, and similar considerations apply. Due to the upper and lower limits of plus, minus one on risk, but not on rate, risk differences are more difficult to model than rate differences.

Estimability   2.4.5

Because exposure-specific incidence rates and risks can be obtained from cohort data, all measures of association considered (based on ratios or differences) can be obtained as well. This is also true of case-control data complemented by follow-up or population data (see Sects. 2.2 and 2.3). Case-control data alone allow estimation of odds ratios thanks to the identity between disease and exposure odds ratios (see Sect. 2.4.3) that extends to the logistic regression framework. Prentice and Pyke (1979) showed that the unconditional logistic model (see also Breslow and Day 1980, Chap. 6) applies to case-control data as long as the intercept is disregarded (see Sect. 2.4.6). Interestingly, time-matched case-control studies allow estimation of hazard rates (e.g., see Miettinen 1976; Greenland and Thomas 1982; Prentice and Breslow 1978).

Estimation

The most popular measures of association have a long history of methods for estimation and statistical inference. Some traditional approaches have the advantage of being applicable in small samples. Traditional methods adjust for confounders by *direct standardization* (see Sect. 2.6.1) of the rates or risks involved, prior to computation of the measure of association, or by *stratification*, where association measures are computed separately for subgroups and then combined. For measures based on the difference of rates or risks, direct standardization and stratification can be identical, if the same weights are chosen (Kahn and Sempos 1989). Generally, however, direct standardization uses predetermined weights chosen for external validity, while *optimal* or *efficient* weights are chosen with stratification. Efficient weights make the standard error of the combined estimator as small as possible. *Regression adjustment* is a form of stratification, which provides more flexibility, but most often relies on large sample size for inference.

In modern epidemiology, measures of association are most often estimated from regression analysis. Such methods tend to require large sample sizes, in particular when based on *generalized linear models* (often abbreviated *GLM*). In this context, the ratio, difference or other association measures arise from the regression coefficient of the exposure indicator, and different measures of association result depending on the transformation applied to the mean of the outcome variable. Note that the mean of an event count over a unit time interval is the rate, and the mean of a binary outcome is the risk. For example a model may use the logarithm of the rate ($\ln(h)$) or risk ($\ln(\pi)$) as the outcome to be able to estimate ratio measures of association.

The function applied to the rate or risk in a regression analysis is referred to as the *link function* in the framework of generalized linear models underlying such analyses (see McCullagh and Nelder (1989) and Palta (2003) for theory and practical application). For example, linear regression would regress the risk or rate directly on exposure without any transformation, which is referred to as using the *identity link*. When the exposure is the only predictor in such a model, all link functions fit equally well and simply represent different ways to characterize the association. However, when several exposures or confounders are involved, or if the exposure is measured as a continuous or ordinal variable, some link functions and not others may require interaction or non-linear terms to improve the fit. The considerations in choosing the link function parallel those for choosing a measure of association as multiplicative or additive and as computed from rates, risks or odds, discussed above (see Table 2.1).

Both traditional and regression estimation is briefly overviewed below, with more details provided in Chap. II.3 and Chap. II.4 of this handbook.

Estimation and Adjustment for Confounding of Rate Ratios

Estimation of the rate or hazard ratio between exposed and non-exposed individuals can be based on either event counts (overall or in subgroups and/or subintervals of time), or on the time to event for each individual, where the time for subjects without events are entered as time to end of follow-up, and are referred to as being *censored* (see Chap. II.4).

In the first case, estimation can proceed directly by forming ratios of interest, or by modeling the number of events on exposure by a generalized linear model. When ratios are formed directly as the ratio of the number of cases D_E divided by the person time at risk t_E, i.e. D_E/t_E, in those exposed and $D_{\bar{E}}/t_{\bar{E}}$ in those unexposed, the 95% confidence interval of the resulting rate ratio $HR = D_E/t_E/D_{\bar{E}}/t_{\bar{E}}$ is obtained as (Rothman and Greenland 1996)

$$\left[\exp\left(\ln(\widehat{HR}) - 1.96(1/D_E + 1/D_{\bar{E}})^{1/2} \right), \exp\left(\ln(\widehat{HR}) + 1.96(1/D_E + 1/D_{\bar{E}})^{1/2} \right) \right] .$$

In either case, it is often necessary to adjust for confounding factors, including age and sex. When rate ratios are formed directly, the rates are generally adjusted by direct standardization (see Sect. 2.6.1) or by use of the *standardized mortality (or morbidity or incidence) ratio SMR or SIR* (see Sect. 2.6.1). The SMR and SIR have found wide application in investigations of the potential health effects of occupational exposures.

A common regression approach to estimating rate ratios requires information on event count and person time at risk for each subgroup, time interval and exposure level of interest. To obtain rate ratios from the regression requires that the logarithm of the mean number of events be modeled. This is referred to in the generalized linear model framework as using a *log link* function. The resulting regression equation is

$$\ln(h_i) = -\ln(t_i) + \beta_0 + \beta_E E_i + \beta_1 X_{1i} + \beta_2 X_{2i} + \dots ,$$

where the subscript i indicates subject, $i = 1, \dots, n$, E_i is an indicator that equals 0 for the unexposed and 1 for the exposed. In this equation, β_0 is the logarithm of the rate per time unit for the unexposed with confounder values, $X_1, X_2, \dots = 0$. Care should be taken to center confounders so that this intercept is meaningful. The quantity $\ln(t_i)$ is referred to as the offset, and allows event counts over different size denominators to be used as the outcome variable. In the case when disease rates in a population are modeled, t_i are population sizes. The rate ratio for exposure adjusted for confounders $X_1, X_2, \dots$ is obtained as $\exp(\beta_E)$. Differences in rate ratios across levels of X can easily be accommodated by the inclusion of interaction terms in the model. Inferences on the rate ratio follow from the standard error of the estimate $\widehat{\beta}_E$ of β_E, which is approximately normally distributed with reasonable large sample sizes, so that a 95% confidence interval for the rate ratio is

$$\left[\exp\left(\widehat{\beta}_E - 1.96 se\left(\widehat{\beta}_E \right) \right), \exp\left(\widehat{\beta}_E + 1.96 se\left(\widehat{\beta}_E \right) \right) \right] .$$

The standard errors $se(\widehat{\beta}_E)$ can be obtained from maximum likelihood theory, assuming that the counts follow a *Poisson* or *negative binomial distribution*. The variance of the Poisson distribution equals the rate, while the negative binomial distribution allows for possible clustering of events leading to the variance being larger than the rate.

There are also several approaches available in most statistical software packages to adjust standard errors for so called *overdispersion*. Overdispersion refers to variability in rates being larger than expected from a Poisson count process. For example, events may cluster in time, or there may be unmeasured characteristics of the population influencing the rate, so that the overall count arises from a mixture of different rates. An example of overdispersion (Palta 2003) arises in overall cancer rates because different cancers predominate for different ages and genders. One of the approaches to adjusting for overdispersion, is to use a *robust* or *sandwich* estimator of the standard error of $\hat{\beta}_E$ available in software packages, such as PROC GENMOD in SAS (1999) that fit *generalized estimating equations* (Liang and Zeger 1986).

When the data consist of times to event for individuals, the rate ratio, or hazard ratio can be estimated by techniques designed for *survival analysis* (e.g., see Hosmer and Lemeshow 1999 and Chap. II.4 of this handbook). Most parametrically specified survival distributions (i.e., distributions $S(t) = 1 - F(t)$, where F is the distribution of time to event) lead to hazard ratios $h_E(t)/h_{\bar{E}}(t)$ that vary over time. When the hazard ratio remains constant, this is referred to as proportional hazards. This property holds when the time to event follows the *exponential distribution*, so that the probability of avoiding an event up to time t is given by $S(t) = \exp(-ht)$ where h is a constant hazard, and for the *Weibull distribution* $S(t) = \exp[(-ht)^y]$ as long as y is the same for the exposed and non-exposed groups. Models are sometimes fit that assume that the exponential distribution holds over short intervals, i.e., piecewise constant hazard. In these models, the hazard ratio is constant across short intervals, but can be allowed to change over time. An exponential distribution for time to event leads to the Poisson distribution for number of events in a given time period.

In the situation of proportional hazards, estimation of the hazard ratio can proceed without specifying the actual survival distribution via the *Cox model*, where estimation is based on so called *partial likelihood* (Cox 1972). The reason this works is that the actual level of the hazard cancels out; similarly to how the offset becomes part of the intercept in the regression model given by (2.8) above.

Estimation and Adjustment for Confounding for Risk Ratios

In a cohort study with a fixed follow-up time, the risk ratio can be estimated in a straightforward manner. From a 2×2 table (see Table 2.3) with cells a, b, c, d, where a is the number diseased and exposed, b is the number diseased and unexposed, c the number non-diseased and exposed and d the number non-diseased and unexposed, the risk ratio is estimated by $\widehat{RR} = \{a/(a + c)\}/\{b/(b + d)\}$.

Table 2.3. Notation for a generic 2×2 table from cohort or case-control study

	Exposed	Unexposed
Diseased	a	b
Non-diseased	c	d

Statistical inference can be based on the approximate standard error (Katz et al. 1978) which can be estimated as $se(\ln(\widehat{RR})) = \{a/(a+c)+d/b(b+d)\}^{1/2}$. In cases where follow-up time is not fixed, the risk ratio can be calculated from the individual risks estimated from the rate or hazard function. However, this is rarely done, as investigators tend to prefer the rate or hazard ratio as the measure of association in such situations. The risk ratio can be estimated from case-control studies only when the ratio of sampling probabilities of cases and controls is known, or by using the odds ratio (see above) as an approximation.

Although standardization can be used either as direct standardization to adjust risks before forming ratios or as indirect standardization to compute the SMR (see Sect. 2.6.1) from risks in a reference population, it is often more appropriate to apply stratified analyses to adjust the risk ratio for confounders (see also Sect. 2.6.1). For example, a study of cancer risk in individuals exposed or not exposed to a risk factor may be stratified into age groups, or a study investigating outcomes in neonates may be stratified by birth weight. Stratum-specific risk ratio estimates can be calculated and then be combined for instance by the popular Mantel–Haenszel estimator that is known to have good properties. It is given by

$$\widehat{RR}_{MH} = \sum \left(a_i \left(b_i + d_i \right) / n_i \right) \Big/ \sum \left(b_i \left(a_i + c_i \right) / n_i \right) ,$$

where the sums are across strata and n_i is the number of subjects in stratum i. This estimator is stable in small samples, but has a larger standard error than the corresponding estimator from regression modeling. Formulas for the standard error are provided by Breslow and Day (1987) and by Rothman and Greenland (1998).

From regression analysis, the risk ratio can be obtained as $\exp(\beta_E)$ from fitting the binary or *binomial* (grouped binary events) outcome to the model:

$$\ln(\pi_i) = \beta_0 + \beta_E E_i + \beta_1 X_{1i} + \dots .$$

This is a generalized linear model with error distribution reflecting each binary outcome being independent with variance $\pi_i(1 - \pi_i)$ and log link. Clearly, the log link is not ideal, as $\pi_i > 1$ can result from some exposure-confounder combinations. Nonetheless, this model tends to be reasonable with low risks. Maximum likelihood or generalized estimating equation fitting automatically provides large sample inference, with or without adjustment for deviations from the binomial error structure by robust standard errors. Deviations from binomial structure may result from clustering or correlation between events within subgroups, or from multiple events per person (e.g., cavities in teeth when teeth are individually counted).

Another option for the link function when modeling the risk by a generalized linear model is the so-called *complementary log-log link* resulting in the model:

$$\ln(-\ln(1 - \pi_i)) = \beta_0 + \beta_E E_i + \beta_1 X_{1i} + \dots .$$

This model has the advantage of always estimating risks to be in the range 0 to 1. However, $\exp(\beta_E)$ is the rate ratio rather than the risk ratio.

Estimation and Adjustment for Confounding for Odds Ratios

In the traditional setting, the odds ratio in an unmatched case-control or cohort study is estimated from a 2×2 table (see Table 2.3) as $\widehat{OR} = ad/bc$. Inference can be based on exact methods, which historically were difficult to implement, but are now available in most statistical software packages, such as the SAS procedure PROC FREQ. With the exact approach, the confidence interval for the odds ratio is obtained from the *non-central hypergeometric distribution*. Over the years, many approximations to this interval have been developed, the most accurate of which is the *Cornfield approximation* (Cornfield 1956). Another, less accurate method is based on the approximate standard error of $\ln(\widehat{OR})$ known as the Woolf (1955) or *logit method*, where $se(\ln(\widehat{OR}))$ is calculated as $(1/a + 1/b + 1/c + 1/d)^{1/2}$. The logit method takes its name from being related to an approximation used for fitting logistic regression. Although the approximation has limited use for reporting final study results, it is useful to have an explicit approximation of the standard error for study planning purposes.

Stratified methods for estimating the odds ratio either build on taking a weighted average of the stratum specific log odds ratios, using the inverses of the logit method standard errors for each stratum as the weights, or using the Mantel–Haenszel stratified odds ratio estimator (Mantel and Haenszel 1959),

$$\widehat{OR}_{MH} = \left(\sum a_i c_i / n_i \right) / \left(\sum b_i d_i / n_i \right) ,$$

where the sums are across strata with tables as depicted in Table 2.3 for each stratum and n_i is the number of subjects in stratum i. This odds ratio estimator has been shown to have excellent properties even when strata are very small (Birch 1964; Breslow 1981; Breslow and Day 1980, Chaps. 4–5; Landis et al. 1978, 2000; Greenland 1987; Robins and Greenland 1989). The confidence interval for a stratified odds ratio can be obtained by exact methods or by the approximation of Miettinen (1976) where $se(\ln(\widehat{OR}))$ is calculated as $\ln(\widehat{OR}_{MH})/\chi_{MH}$. Here χ_{MH} is the square root of the *Mantel–Haenszel stratified chi-square test* used to test the null hypothesis that the odds ratio equals one (Mantel and Haenszel 1959). This test statistic is computed as

$$\chi^2_{MH} = \sum \left[a_i - (a_i + b_i)(a_i + c_i)/n_i \right]^2 /$$
$$\left[(a_i + b_i)(a_i + c_i)(d_i + b_i)(d_i + c_i)/ \left(n_i^2 (n_i - 1) \right) \right] .$$

The 95% confidence interval for the odds ratio is then given by

$$\left[\exp \left(\ln \left(\widehat{OR} \right) - 1.96 \left(\ln \left(\widehat{OR}_{MH} \right) / \chi_{MH} \right) \right), \exp \left(\ln \left(\widehat{OR} \right) + 1.96 \left(\ln \left(\widehat{OR}_{MH} \right) / \chi_{MH} \right) \right) \right] .$$

A special case of stratification occurs when data are pair matched, such that each case is matched to a control, e.g., based on kinship or neighborhood. In this case, the Mantel–Haenszel odds ratio estimator becomes m_{++}/m_{--}, where m_{++} is the number of pairs (matched sets) where both the case and the control are exposed, and m_{--} is the number of pairs where neither is exposed. Breslow and Day (1980,

Chap. 7) provide additional formulas for the situation when several controls are matched to each case. Confidence intervals can again be obtained by exact formulas (Breslow and Day 1980, Chap. 7). It is well known that although matched studies are not technically confounded by the factors matched on because cases and controls are balanced on these, odds ratios based on the matched formula are larger than odds ratios not taking the matching into account. We discuss this phenomenon further in the logistic model framework below.

Increasingly, logistic regression is used for the estimation of odds ratios from clinical trials, cohort and case control studies. Logistic regression fits the equation:

$$\ln\left(\pi_i/(1 - \pi_i)\right) = \beta_0 + \beta_E E_i + \beta_1 X_{1i} + \ldots , \qquad (2.8)$$

with E_i denoting the exposure status and $X_{1i}, X_{2i}, \ldots$ the confounder variables of individual i. For a cohort study β_0 is $\ln(\pi_i/(1 - \pi_i))$ for an unexposed individual with all *confounders equal* to 0. For such a person, then, the risk of disease $\pi_i = \exp(\beta_0)/[1+\exp(\beta_0)]$. In a case-control study, the intercept in (2.11) is $\beta_0 = \beta_{0,\text{cohort}} + \ln(P_1/P_0)$, with P_1 and P_0 the probabilities for being sampled into the study for cases and controls, respectively. We see again that risk can be estimated from a case-control study only when the sampling scheme of cases and controls is known. The odds ratio for exposure, adjusted for confounders is $\exp(\beta_E)$.

In the generalized linear model framework, (2.8) is said to use the *logit link*, where the logit function is defined as $g(\pi) = \ln(\pi/(1 - \pi))$. The logit link is the one that follows most naturally from the mathematical formulation of the binomial distribution (McCullagh and Nelder 1989), and is referred to as the *canonical link*, whereas the log is the canonical link for rates. Just as for other generalized linear models, maximum likelihood based and robust standard errors are available, with the latter taking into account clustering of events. It should be noted, however, that generalizations of logistic regression to the longitudinal or clustered setting by generalized estimating equations do not work for case-control studies (Neuhaus and Jewell 1990).

Matched data can be analyzed by *conditional logistic regression* that fits the model:

$$\ln(\pi_{ji}/(1 - \pi_{ji})) = \beta_{0j} + \beta_E E_{ji} + \beta_1 X_{1ji} + \ldots \qquad (2.9)$$

for individual i in the matched set j. Estimation of β_E and $\beta_1, \ldots$ is based on algorithms that compare individuals only within and not between matched sets. For example, for matched pairs, estimation is based on differences in exposure and confounders. These algorithms do not actually estimate the matched set specific intercepts β_{0j} that cancel out. All variables that do not vary within matched sets are automatically absorbed into β_{0j} although interactions of such variables with those that vary within set can be included in the model. For example, in SAS, PROC PHREG can be tricked into fitting this model (e.g., see Palta 2003). While the conditional logistic regression model is usually fit by large sample methods, such as maximum likelihood, exact procedures have also become available (e.g., Mehta et al. 2000). Again, taking matching into account in the analysis results in larger coefficients than those of the unmatched model (2.11). When all matching variables are explicit (such as age and sex) they can be directly entered as covariates in (2.11).

It is useful to know that, when an outcome is originally normally distributed, but dichotomized and analyzed by logistic regression, the resulting coefficients in the unconditional model (2.11) are approximately 1.7 times as large as the coefficients that would have resulted from ordinary regression of the original continuous outcome, "standardized" by being divided by its residual standard deviation. (Note that the word *standardized* here is used to denote a conversion to standard deviation units, rather than in the sense of direct standardization discussed in Sect. 2.6.1.) This result emerges from the relationship between the variances of the logistic and normal distributions (Johnson and Kotz 1970). While the logit link is related to the logistic distribution, another link function, the *probit* can be shown to arise directly when a continuous outcome from ordinary regression with normally distributed errors is dichotomized (Palta 2003). The probit link is defined as $g(\pi) = \Phi^{-1}(\pi)$ where Φ^{-1} is the inverse of the cumulative normal distribution. This link yields the same coefficients as the "standardized" ones from ordinary regression of the continuous outcome. Apart from this difference, the logit and probit provide a very similar fit. In both cases, of course, dichotomizing the outcome results in loss of information and thus in loss of statistical efficiency, which yields larger standard errors relative to the size of the regression coefficients.

The idea of logistic regression providing coefficients that are related by "standardization" to those that would arise from regression analysis of an underlying continuous variable (e.g., blood pressure being dichotomized into hypertension or not) also provides a framework for understanding the difference between a matched and an unmatched analysis. In an unmatched analysis, the coefficients are for the outcome "standardized" to the scale of the overall residual standard deviation across the population. This means that the original continuous regression coefficient is divided by that standard deviation. In a matched analysis, the coefficients are "standardized" to the residual standard deviation within each matched set. This happens by explicitly including a matched set specific intercept in the model (see (2.12)). Hence, the standard deviation within matched sets does not contain the variation arising from different matched sets having a different level of the outcome, and hence matched coefficients are larger (Palta et al. 1997; Palta and Lin 1999).

Estimation and Adjustment for Confounding for Rate Differences

Regression estimation of the rate difference with and without adjustment for confounders can be done in the generalized linear model framework by specifying the identity link function, resulting in linear regression of the rates with variance arising from the Poisson distribution. Overdispersion can be handled the same way as for ratios. However, unequal time intervals cannot be as easily accommodated with the identity link. Instead, weighted ordinary regression of observed rates can be employed, where inverse variance weights automatically account for the interval length (Breslow and Day 1987, Chap. 4).

Measures of Impact

Measures of impact are used to assess the contribution of one or several exposures to the occurrence of incident cases at the population level. Thus, they are useful in public health to weigh the impact of exposure on the burden of disease occurrence and assess potential prevention programs aimed at reducing or eliminating exposure in the population. They are sometimes referred to as measures of *potential* impact to convey the notion that the true impact at the population level may be different from that reflected by these measures except under very specific conditions (see Sect. 2.5.1). The most commonly used measure of impact is the attributable risk. This measure is presented in some detail below. Then, other measures are briefly described. Table 2.4 provides an overview of measures of impact discussed in this chapter.

Attributable Risk

Definition

The term "attributable risk" (AR) was initially introduced by Levin in 1953 (Levin 1953) as a measure to quantify the impact of smoking on lung cancer occurrence. Gradually, it has become a widely used measure to assess the consequences of an association between an exposure and a disease at the population level. It is defined as the following ratio:

$$AR = \left\{ \Pr(D) - \Pr\left(D|\overline{E}\right) \right\} / \Pr(D) . \tag{2.10}$$

The numerator contrasts the probability of disease, $\Pr(D)$, in the population, which may have some exposed, E, and some unexposed, $\overline{E}$, individuals, with the hypothetical probability of disease in the same population but with all exposure eliminated $\Pr(D|\overline{E})$. Thus, it measures the additional probability of disease in the population that is associated with the presence of an exposure in the population, and AR measures the corresponding proportion. Probabilities in (2.10) will usually refer to disease risk although, depending on the context, they may be replaced with incidence rates.

Unlike measures of association (see Sect. 2.4), AR depends both on the strength of the association between exposure and disease and the prevalence of exposure in the population p_E. This can be seen for instance through rewriting AR from (2.10). Upon expressing $\Pr(D)$ as

$$\Pr(D|E)p_E + \Pr\left(D|\overline{E}\right) p_{\overline{E}} \quad \text{with} \quad p_{\overline{E}} = 1 - p_E ,$$

both in the numerator and the denominator, and noting that

$$\Pr(D|E) = RR \times \Pr\left(D|\overline{E}\right) ,$$

the term $\Pr(D|\overline{E})$ cancels out and AR is obtained as (Cole and MacMahon 1971; Miettinen 1974):

$$AR = \left\{ p_E(RR - 1) \right\} / \left\{ 1 + p_E(RR - 1) \right\} , \tag{2.11}$$

Table 2.4. Measures of impact discussed in this chapter

Measures	Definition[a]	Range	Usual interpretation(s)[b]
Attributable risk (AR)	1) $\{\Pr(D) - \Pr(D\mid\bar{E})\}/\Pr(D)$ 2) $\{p_E(RR - 1)\}/\{1 + p_E(RR - 1)\}$ 3) $p_{E\mid D}(RR - 1)/RR$	$-\infty$ to 1 0 to 1 for risk factor	Proportion of disease cases in the population attributable to exposure. Proportion of disease cases in the population potentially preventable by eliminating exposure
Attributable risk among the exposed (AR$_E$)	1) $\{\Pr(D\mid E) - \Pr(D\mid\bar{E})\}/\Pr(D\mid E)$ 2) $(RR - 1)/RR$	$-\infty$ to 1 0 to 1 for risk factor	Proportion of disease cases among the exposed attributable to exposure
Sequential attributable risk	Contributions of a given exposure to the joint attributable risk to several exposures for a given order of exposures	0 to 1 for risk factor	Proportion of disease cases in the population potentially preventable by eliminating a given exposure when several exposures are removed in a given sequence
Partial attributable risk	Average contribution of a given exposure to the joint attributable risk to several exposures over all possible exposure orders	0 to 1 for risk factor	Average proportion of disease cases in the population potentially preventable by eliminating a given exposure when several exposures are removed in sequence over all possible orders of removal
Prevented (preventable) fraction (PF)	1) $\{\Pr(D\mid\bar{E}) - \Pr(D)\}/\Pr(D\mid\bar{E})$ 2) $p_E(1 - RR)$	$-\infty$ to 1 0 to 1 for protective factor	Proportion of disease cases averted ("prevented fraction") in relation to the presence of a protective exposure or intervention in the population. Proportion of cases that could be potentially averted ("preventable fraction") if a protective exposure or intervention were introduced *de novo* in the population

Measures	Range	Definition[a]	Usual interpretation(s)[b]
Generalized impact fraction	$-\infty$ to 1 for risk factor and modified distribution with lowering of exposure	$[\Pr(D) - \Pr^*(D)]/\Pr(D)$	Proportion of disease cases potentially averted (fractional reduction of disease occurrence) from changing the current distribution of exposure in the population to some modified distribution
Person-years of life lost (PYLL)	≥ 0 for risk factor (person-years)	Difference between current life expectancy and life expectancy with exposure removed at the population level	Person-time of life lost at the population level attributable to exposure
Average potential years of life lost (PYLL)	≥ 0 for risk factor (years)	Average difference per exposed person between current life expectancy and life expectancy with exposure removed	Average loss of life expectancy per person attributable to exposure

[a] $\Pr(D)$, $\Pr(D|\bar{E})$, $\Pr(D|E)$ and $\Pr^*(D)$ denote probabilities of disease (disease risks), namely the overall probability of disease in the population, the probability of disease in the population with all exposure eliminated, the probability of disease among exposed individuals, and the overall probability of disease under a modified distribution of exposure, respectively. Alternatively, they may refer to disease rates depending on the context. The terms p_E and $p_{E|D}$ respectively refer to the overall exposure prevalence in the population and the exposure prevalence in the diseased individuals. The term RR refers to risk or rate ratios for exposed relative to unexposed individuals.
[b] Interpretations subject to conditions (see text)

a function of both the prevalence of exposure in the population, p_E, and the rate ratio or relative risk, RR.

An alternative formulation underscores this joint dependency in yet another manner. Again, upon expressing $\Pr(D)$ as

$$\Pr(D|E)p_E + \Pr\left(D|\overline{E}\right)p_{\overline{E}} \quad \text{with} \quad p_{\overline{E}} = 1 - p_E$$

and noting that

$$\Pr(D|E) = RR \times \Pr\left(D|\overline{E}\right) ,$$

the numerator in (2.10) can be rewritten as

$$p_E\Pr(D|E) - p_E\Pr(D|E)/RR .$$

From using Bayes' theorem to express $\Pr(D|E)$ as $\Pr(E|D)\Pr(D)/p_E$, it then becomes equal to

$$\Pr(D)p_{E|D}(1 - 1/RR) ,$$

after simple algebra. This yields (Miettinen 1974):

$$AR = p_{E|D}(RR - 1)/RR , \qquad (2.12)$$

a function of the prevalence of exposure in diseased individuals, $p_{E|D}$, and the rate ratio or relative risk, RR.

A high relative risk can correspond to a low or high AR depending on the prevalence of exposure, which leads to widely different public health consequences. One implication is that, portability is not a usual property of AR, as the prevalence of exposure may vary widely among populations that are separated in time or location. This is in contrast with measures of association such as the relative risk or rate ratio which are more portable from one population to another, as the strength of the association between disease and exposure might vary little among populations (unless strong interactions with environmental or genetic factors are present). However, portability of RR can be questioned as well in the case of imperfect specificity of exposure assessment, since misclassification of non-exposed subjects as exposed will bias RR towards unity, which will affect differentially RR estimates in various populations depending on their exposure prevalence. This is not a problem with AR, which is not affected by imperfect specificity of exposure assessment.

Range

When the exposure considered is a risk factor (RR > 1), it follows from the above definition that AR lies between 0 and 1. Therefore, it is very often expressed as a percentage. AR increases both with the strength of the association between exposure and disease measured by RR, and with the prevalence of exposure in the population. A prevalence of 1 (or 100%) yields a value of AR equal to the attributable risk among the exposed, that is $(RR-1)/RR$ (see Sect. 2.5.2). AR approaches 1 for an infinitely high RR provided the exposure is present in the population (i.e., non-null prevalence of exposure).

AR takes a null value when either there is no association between exposure and disease ($RR = 1$) or there are no exposed subjects in the population. Negative AR values are obtained for a protective exposure ($RR < 1$). In this case, AR varies between 0 and $-\infty$, a scale on which AR lacks a meaningful interpretation. One solution is to reverse the coding of exposure (i.e., interchange exposed and unexposed categories) to go back to the situation of a positive AR, sometimes called the preventable fraction in this case (Benichou 2000c; Greenland 1987; Last 1983). Alternatively, one must consider a different parameter, namely the prevented fraction (see Sect. 2.5.4).

Synonyms

Some confusion in the terminology arises from the reported use of as many as 16 different terms in the literature to denote attributable risk (Gefeller 1990, 1995). However, a literature search by Uter and Pfahlberg (Uter and Pfahlberg 1999) found some consistency in terminology usage, with "attributable risk" and "population attributable risk" (MacMahon and Pugh 1970) the most commonly used terms by far followed by "etiologic fraction" (Miettinen 1974). Other popular terms include "attributable risk percentage" (Cole and MacMahon 1971), "fraction of etiology" (Miettinen 1974), and "attributable fraction" (Greenland and Robins 1988; Last 1983; Ouellet et al. 1979; Rothman and Greenland 1998, Chap. 4).

Moreover, additional confusion may originate in the use by some authors (MacMahon and Pugh 1970; Markush 1977; Schlesselman 1982) of the term "attributable risk" to denote a measure of association, the excess incidence, that is the difference between the incidence rates in exposed and unexposed subjects (see Sect. 2.4.4). Context will usually help the readers detect this less common use.

Interpretation and Usefulness

While measures of association such as the rate ratio and relative risk are used to establish an association in etiologic research, AR has a public health interpretation as a measure of the disease burden attributable or at least related to one or several exposures. Consequently, AR is used to assess the potential impact of prevention programs aimed at eliminating exposure from the population. It is often thought of as the fraction of disease that could be eliminated if exposure could be totally removed from the population.

However, this interpretation can be misleading because, for it to be strictly correct, the three following conditions have to be met (Walter 1976). First, estimation of AR has to be unbiased (see below). Second, exposure has to be causal rather than merely associated with the disease. Third, elimination of exposure has to be without any effect on the distribution of other risk factors. Indeed, as it might be difficult to alter the level of exposure to one factor independently of other risk factors, the resulting change in disease load might be different from the AR estimate.

For these reasons, various authors elect to use weaker definitions of AR, such as the proportion of disease that can be related or linked, rather than attributable, to exposure (Miettinen 1974).

A fundamental problem regarding causality has been discussed by Greenland and Robins (1988) and Robins and Greenland (1989) who considered the proportion of disease cases for which exposure played an etiologic role, i.e., cases for which exposure was a component cause of disease occurrence. They termed this quantity the etiologic fraction and argued that it was a more relevant measure of impact than AR. Rothman and Greenland (1998, Chap. 4) argued that AR and the etiologic fractions are different quantities using logical reasoning regarding causality and the fact that disease occurrence may require several component causal factors rather than one. The main problem with the etiologic fraction is that it is usually impossible to distinguish exposed cases for whom exposure played an etiologic role from those where exposure was irrelevant. As a consequence, estimating the etiologic fraction will typically require non-identifiable biologic assumptions about exposure actions and interactions to be estimable (Cox 1984, 1985; Robins and Greenland 1989; Seiler 1986). Thus, despite its limitations, AR remains a useful measure to assess the potential impact of exposure at the population level and can serve as a suitable guide in practice to assess and compare various prevention strategies.

Several authors have considered an interpretation of AR in terms of etiologic research. The argument is that if an AR estimate is available for several risk factors jointly, then its complement to 1, $1 - AR$, must represent a gauge of the proportion of disease cases not explained by the risk factors used in estimating AR. Hence, $1 - AR$ would represent the proportion of cases attributable to other (possibly unknown) risk factors. For instance, it was estimated that the AR of breast cancer was 41% for late age at first birth, nulliparity, family history of breast cancer and higher socioeconomic status, which suggested that at least 59% of cases had to be attributable to other risk factors (Madigan et al. 1995). A similar type of reasoning was used in several well-known reports of estimated percentages of cancer death or incidence attributable to various established cancer risk factors (e.g., smoking, diet, occupational exposure to carcinogens ...). Some of these reports conveyed the impression that little remained unexplained by factors other than the main established preventable risk factors and that cancer was a mostly preventable illness (Colditz et al. 1996, 1997; Doll and Peto 1981; Henderson et al. 1991; Ames et al. 1995). Such interpretation has to be taken with great care since ARs for different risk factors may add to more than 100% because multiple exposures are usually possible (e.g., smoking and occupational exposure to asbestos). Moreover, this interpretation can be refuted on the basis of logical arguments regarding the fact that disease occurrence may require more than one causal factor (see Rothman and Greenland 1998, Chap. 2). Furthermore, one can note that once a new risk factor is considered, the joint unexposed reference category changes from lack of exposure to all previously considered risk factors to lack of exposure to those risk factors *and* the new risk factor (Begg 2001). Because of this change in the reference category, the AR for the new risk factor may surpass the quantity $1 - AR$

for previously considered risk factors. Thus, while it is useful to know that only 41% of breast cancer cases can be attributed to four established risk factors in the above example, it is entirely conceivable that new risk factors of breast cancer may be elicited which yield an AR of more than 59% by themselves in the above example.

Properties

AR has two main properties. First, AR values greatly depend on the definition of the reference level for exposure (unexposed or baseline level). A more stringent definition of the reference level corresponds to a larger proportion of subjects exposed and, as one keeps depleting the reference category from subjects with higher levels of risk, AR values and estimates keep rising. This property has a major impact on AR estimates as was illustrated by Benichou (1991) and Wacholder et al. (1994). For instance, Benichou (1991) found that the AR estimate of esophageal cancer for an alcohol consumption greater or equal to 80 g/day (reference level of 0–79 g/day) was 38% in the Ille-et-Vilaine district of France, and increased dramatically to 70% for an alcohol consumption greater or equal to 40 g/day (i.e., using the more restrictive reference level 0–39 g|day) (see Example 3 below). This property plays a role whenever studying a continuous exposure with a continuous gradient of risk and when there is no obvious choice of threshold. Therefore, AR estimates must be reported with reference to a clearly defined baseline level in order to be validly interpreted.

Example 3. A case-control study of esophageal cancer conducted in the Ille-et-Vilaine district of France included 200 cases and 775 controls selected by simple random sampling from electoral lists (Tuyns, Pequignot and Jensen 1977). The assessment of associations between alcohol consumption and smoking with esophageal cancer has been the focus of detailed illustration by Breslow and Day (1980) who presented various approaches to odds ratio estimation with or without adjustment for age. As in previous work (Benichou, 1991), four levels of alcohol consumption (0–39, 40–79, 80–119 and 120+ g/day) are considered here as well as three levels of smoking (0–9, 10–29, 30+ g/day) and three age groups (25–44, 45–54, 55+ years). There were 29, 75, 51 and 45 cases with respective alcohol consumptions of 0–39, 40–79, 80–119 and 120+ g/day. Corresponding numbers of controls were 386, 280, 87 and 22, respectively. The first reference level considered, 0–79 g/day, included 104 cases and 666 controls, leaving 96 cases and 109 controls in the exposed (i.e., 80+ g/day) category (see Table 2.5). The corresponding crude (unadjusted) odds ratio was estimated as $(96 \times 666)/(104 \times 109) = 5.6$ (see Sect. 2.4.6). Using methods described below, the crude AR estimate was 39.5% for alcohol consumption and the age- and smoking-adjusted AR estimates were close to 38%. The second reference level considered, 0–39 g/day, was more restrictive and included only 29 cases and 286 controls, leaving 171 cases and 489 controls in the exposed (i.e., 40+ g/day) category (see Table 2.5). The corresponding crude odds ratio was estimated as $(171 \times 386)/(29 \times 389) = 5.9$ (see Sect. 2.4.6). Using

Table 2.5. Numbers of cases and controls in the reference and exposed categories of daily alcohol consumption according to two definitions of the reference category – Data from a case-control study of esophageal cancer (from Tuyns, Pequignot and Jensen 1977)

| | More restrictive definition of reference category (0–39 g/day) | | |
	Reference category (0–39 g/day)	Exposed category (40+ g/day)	Total
Cases	29	171	200
Controls	386	389	775
Total	315	660	975

| | Less restrictive definition of reference category (0–79 g/day) | | |
	Reference category (0–79 g/day)	Exposed category (80+ g/day)	Total
Cases	104	96	200
Controls	666	109	775
Total	770	205	975

methods described below, the crude AR estimate was 70.9% and adjusted AR estimates were in the range 70% to 72%. The marked increase mainly resulted from the much higher proportion of subjects exposed with the more restrictive definition of the reference category (63% instead of 14% of exposed controls). ♦

The second main property is distributivity. If several exposed categories are considered instead of just one, then the sum of the category-specific ARs equals the overall AR calculated from combining those exposed categories into a single one, regardless of the number and the divisions of the original categories (Benichou 1991; Wacholder et al. 1994; Walter 1976), provided the reference category remains the same. This property applies strictly to crude AR estimates and to adjusted AR estimates calculated on the basis of a saturated model including all possible interactions (Benichou 1991). It applies approximately to adjusted estimates not based on a saturated model (Wacholder et al. 1994). Thus, if an overall AR estimate is the focus of interest, there is no need to break the exposed category into several mutually exclusive categories, even in the presence of a gradient of risk with increasing level of exposure. Of course, if the impact of a partial removal of exposure is the question of interest, retaining detailed information on the exposed categories will be necessary (Greenland 2001).

Example 3. *(continued)*
For the more restrictive definition of the reference category of daily alcohol consumption (0–39 g/day), the crude AR was estimated at 70.9%. The sep-

arate contributions of categories 40–79, 80-119 and 120+ g/day were 27.0%, 22.2% and 21.7%, summing to the same value 70.9%. Similarly, for the less restrictive definition of the reference category (0–79 g/day), the crude AR was estimated at 39.5% and the separate contributions of categories 80–119 g/day and 120+ g/day were 18.7% and 20.8%, summing to the same value 39.5%.   ♦

Estimability and Basic Principles of Estimation

AR can be estimated from cohort studies since all quantities in (2.10), (2.11) and (2.12) are directly estimable from cohort studies. AR estimates can differ depending on whether rate ratios, risk ratios or odds ratios are used but will be numerically close for rare diseases. For case-control studies, exposure-specific incidence rates or risks are not available unless data are complemented with follow-up or population-based data (see Sect. 2.2.2). Thus, one has to rely on odds ratio estimates, use (2.11) and estimate p_E from the proportion exposed in the controls, making the rare-disease assumption also involved in estimating odds ratios rather than relative risks. For crude AR estimation, the estimate of the odds ratio is taken as ad/bc and that of p_E as $c/(c + d)$, where, as in Table 2.3, a, b, c and d respectively denote the numbers of exposed cases, unexposed cases, exposed controls and un-exposed controls. Alternatively, one can use (2.12), in which the quantity $p_{E|D}$ can be directly estimated from the diseased individuals (cases) as $a/(a + b)$ and RR can be estimated from the odds ratio again as ad/bc. Using either equation, the resulting point estimate is given by $(ad - bc)/\{d(a + b)\}$.

Variance estimates of crude AR estimates are based on applying the delta-method (Rao 1965). For instance, an estimate of the variance for case-control data is given by the quantity

$$\text{var}\left(\widehat{AR}\right) = b(c + d)\{ad(c + d) + bc(a + b)\}/\{d^3(a + b)^3\} \ .$$

Various $(1 - \alpha)\%$ confidence intervals for AR have been proposed that can be applied to all epidemiologic designs once point and variance estimates are obtained. They include standard confidence intervals for AR based on the untransformed AR point estimate, namely

$$\widehat{AR} \pm z_{1-\alpha/2} se\left(\widehat{AR}\right) \ ;$$

AR confidence intervals based on the log-transformed variable $\ln(1 - AR)$, namely

$$1 - \left(1 - \widehat{AR}\right)\left[\exp\left\{\pm z_{1-\alpha/2} se\left(\widehat{AR}\right)/\left(1 - \widehat{AR}\right)\right\}\right] \quad \text{(Walter 1975)} \ ;$$

as well as confidence intervals based on the logit-transformed variable $\ln\{AR/(1 - AR)\}$, namely

$$\left\{1 + \left\{\left(1 - \widehat{AR}\right)/\widehat{AR}\right\}\left(\exp\left[\pm z_{1-\alpha/2} se\left(\widehat{AR}\right)/\left\{\widehat{AR}\left(1 - \widehat{AR}\right)\right\}\right]\right)\right\}^{-1}$$

(Leung and Kupper 1981).

In the previous formulae, $z_{1-\alpha/2}$ denotes the $(1-\alpha/2)$th percentile of the standard normal distribution, $\widehat{AR}$ denotes the AR point estimate and $se(\widehat{AR})$ its corresponding standard error estimate. Whittemore (1982) noted that the log-transformation yields a wider interval than the standard interval for AR > 0. Leung and Kupper (1981) showed that the interval based on the logit transform is narrower than the standard interval for values of AR strictly between 0.21 and 0.79, whereas the reverse holds outside this range for positive values of AR. While the coverage probabilities of these intervals have been studied in some specific situations and partial comparisons have been made, no general studies have been performed to determine their relative merits in terms of coverage probability.

Detailed reviews of estimability and basic estimation of AR for various epidemiologic designs can be found in Walter (1976) and Benichou (2000b, 2001) who provide explicit formulae for $\widehat{AR}$ and $se(\widehat{AR})$ for cohort and case-control designs.

Example 3. *(continued)*

For the more restrictive definition of the reference category of daily alcohol consumption (0–79 g/day), the crude AR estimate was obtained as:

$$(171 \times 386 - 29 \times 389)/(386 \times 200) = 0.709 ,$$

or 70.9%. Its variance was estimated as:

$$29 \times 775 \times (171 \times 386 \times 775 + 29 \times 389 \times 200)/\left(386^3 \times 200^3\right) = 0.00261 ,$$

yielding a standard error estimate of 0.051, or 5.1%. The corresponding 95% confidence intervals for AR are given by 60.9% to 80.9% (no transformation), 58.9% to 79.4% (log transformation), and 60.0% to 79.8% (logit transformation), very similar to each other in this example.   ♦

Adjusted Estimation

As is the case for measures of association, unadjusted (or crude or marginal) AR estimates may be inconsistent (Miettinen 1974; Walter 1976, 1980, 1983). The precise conditions under which adjusted AR estimates that take into account the distribution and effect of other factors will differ from unadjusted AR estimates that fail to do so were worked out by Walter (1980). If E and X are two dichotomous factors taking levels 0 and 1, and if one is interested in estimating the AR for exposure E, then the following applies. The adjusted and unadjusted AR estimates coincide (i.e., the crude AR estimate is unbiased) if and only if (a) E and X are such that $\Pr(E = 0, X = 0)\Pr(E = 1, X = 1) = \Pr(E = 0, X = 1)\Pr(E = 1, X = 0)$, which amounts to the independence of their distributions, or (b) exposure to X alone does not increase disease risk, namely $\Pr(D|E = 0, X = 1) = \Pr(D|E = 0, X = 0)$. When considering one (or several) polychotomous factor(s) X forming J levels $(J > 2)$, conditions (a) and (b) can be extended to a set of analogous sufficient conditions. Condition (a) translates into a set of $J(J-1)/2$ conditions for all pairs of levels j and j' of X, amounting to an independent distribution of E and all factors in X. Condition (b) translates into a set of $J-1$ conditions stating that in the absence of exposure to E, exposure to any of the other factors in X, alone or in combination, does not increase disease risk.

The extent of bias varies according to the severity of the departure from conditions (a) and (b) above. Although no systematic numerical study of the bias of unadjusted AR estimates has been performed, Walter (1980) provided a revealing example of a case-control study assessing the association between alcohol, smoking and oral cancer. In that study, severe positive bias was observed for crude AR estimates, with a very large difference between crude and adjusted AR estimates both for smoking (51.3% vs. 30.6%, a 20.7 difference in percentage points and 68% relative difference in AR estimates) and alcohol (52.2% vs. 37.0%, a 15.2% absolute difference and 48% relative difference). Thus, the prudent approach must be to adjust for factors that are suspected or known to act as confounders in a similar fashion as for estimating measures of associations.

Two simple adjusted estimation approaches discussed in the literature are inconsistent. The first approach was presented by Walter (1976) and is based on a factorization of the crude risk ratio into two components similar to those in Miettinen's earlier derivation (Miettinen 1972). In this approach, a crude AR estimate is obtained under the assumption of no association between exposure and disease (i.e., values of RR or the odds ratio are taken equal to 1 separately for each level of confounding). This term reflects the AR only due to confounding factors since it is obtained under the assumption that disease and exposure are not associated. By subtracting this term from the crude AR estimate that ignores confounding factors and thus reflects the impact of both exposure and confounding factors, what remains is an estimate of the AR for exposure adjusted for confounding (Walter 1976). The second approach is based on using (2.11) and plugging in a common adjusted RR estimate (odds ratio estimate in case-control studies), along with an estimate of p_E (Cole and MacMahon 1971; Morgenstern 1982). Both approaches, while intuitively appealing, were shown to be inconsistent (Ejigou 1979; Greenland and Morgenstern 1983; Morgenstern 1982) and, accordingly, very severe bias was exhibited in simulations of cross-sectional and cohort designs (Gefeller 1995).

By contrast, two adjusted approaches based on stratification yield valid estimates. The Mantel Haenszel approach consists in plugging-in an estimate of the common adjusted RR (odds ratio in case-control studies) and an estimate of the prevalence of exposure in diseased individuals, $p_{E|D}$, in (2.12) in order to obtain an adjusted estimate of AR (Greenland 1984, 1987; Kuritz and Landis 1987, 1988a,b). In doing so, it is possible to adjust for one or more polychotomous factors forming J levels or strata. While several choices are available for a common adjusted RR or odds ratio estimator, a usual choice is to use a Mantel–Haenszel estimator of RR in cohort studies (Kleinbaum et al. 1982, Chaps. 9 and 17; Landis et al. 2000; Rothman and Greenland 1998, Chaps. 15–16; Tarone 1981) or odds ratio in case-control studies (Breslow and Day 1980, Chaps. 4–5; Kleinbaum et al. 1982, Chaps. 9, 17; Landis et al.,

2000; Mantel and Haenszel 1959; Rothman and Greenland 1998, Chaps. 15–16) (see Sect. 2.4.6). For this reason, the term "Mantel–Haenszel approach" has been proposed to denote this approach to adjusted AR estimation (Benichou 1991). When there is no interaction between exposure and factors adjusted for, Mantel–Haenszel type estimators of RR or odds ratio have favorable properties, as they combine lack of (or very small) bias even for sparse data (e.g., individually matched case-control data) and good efficiency except in extreme circumstances (Birch 1964; Breslow 1981; Breslow and Day 1980, Chaps. 4–5; Landis et al. 1978; Landis et al., 2000). Moreover, variance estimators are consistent even for sparse data ("dually-consistent" variance estimators) (Greenland 1987; Robins and Greenland 1989). Simulation studies of cohort and case-control designs (Gefeller 1992; Greenland 1987; Kuritz and Landis 1988a,b) showed that adjusted AR estimates are little affected by small-sample bias when there is no interaction between exposure and adjustment factors, but can be misleading if such interaction is present.

Example 3.   *(continued)*

In order to control for age and smoking, nine strata (joint categories) of smoking × age have to be considered. The Mantel–Haenszel odds ratio estimate can be calculated from quantities a_j, b_j, c_j and d_j that respectively denote the numbers of exposed cases, unexposed cases, exposed controls and unexposed controls in stratum j, using the methods in Sect. 2.4.6. With the more restrictive definition of the reference category for daily alcohol consumption, the Mantel–Haenszel odds ratio was estimated at 6.2, thus slightly higher than the crude odds ratio of 5.9. Combined with an observed proportion of exposed cases of $171/200 = 0.855$, this resulted in an adjusted AR estimate of $0.855 \times (6.2 - 1)/6.2 = 0.716$ or 71.6% using (2.12) (allowing for rounding error), slightly higher than the crude AR estimate of 70.9%. The corresponding estimate of the standard error was 5.1%. ◆

The weighted-sum approach also allows adjustment for one or more polychotomous factors forming J levels or strata. The AR is written as a weighted sum over all strata of stratum-specific ARs, i.e., $\sum_{j=1}^{J} w_j AR_j$ (Walter 1976; Whittemore 1982, 1983). Using crude estimates of AR_j separately within each stratum j and setting weights w_j as proportions of diseased individuals (cases) yields an asymptotically unbiased estimator of AR, which can be seen to be a maximum-likelihood estimator (Whittemore 1982). This choice of weights defines the "case-load method". The weighted-sum approach does not require the assumption of a common relative risk or odds ratio. Instead, the relative risks or odds ratios are estimated separately for each adjustment level with no restrictions placed on them, corresponding to a fully saturated model for exposure and adjustment factors (i.e., a model with all interaction terms present). From these separate relative risk or odds ratio estimates, separate AR estimates are obtained for each level of adjustment. Thus, the weighted-sum approach not only accounts for confounding but also for interaction. Simulation studies of cohort and case-control designs (Gefeller 1992; Kuritz and Landis 1988a,b; Whittemore 1982) show that the weighted-sum approach can be affected by small sample bias, sometimes severely. It should be avoided when analyzing sparse data, and should not be used altogether for analyzing individually matched case-control data.

Example 3. *(continued)*

As with the Mantel–Haenszel approach, nine strata (joint categories) of smoking × age have to be considered in order to control for age and smoking. In each stratum separately, an AR estimate is calculated using the methods for crude AR estimation (see above). For instance, among heavy smokers (30+ g/day) in age group 65+ years, there were 15 exposed cases, five unexposed cases, four exposed controls, and six unexposed controls, yielding an odds ratio estimate of 4.5 and an AR estimate of 58.3%. The corresponding weight was $20/200 = 0.1$, so that the contribution of this stratum to the overall adjusted AR was 5.8%. Summing the contributions of all nine strata yielded an adjusted AR estimate of 70.0%, thus lower than both the crude and Mantel–Haenszel adjusted AR estimates. The corresponding standard error estimate was 5.8%, higher than the standard error estimate from the Mantel–Haenszel approach because fewer assumptions were made. Namely, the odds ratio was not assumed common to all strata, so that nine separate odds ratios had to be estimated (one for each stratum) rather than a single common odds ratio from all strata. To circumvent the problem of empty cells, the standard error estimate was obtained after assigning the value 0.5 to all zero cells. ◆

A natural alternative to generalize these approaches is to use adjustment procedures based on regression models, in order to take advantage of their flexible and unified approach to efficient parameter estimation and hypothesis testing. Regression models allow one to take into account adjustment factors as well as interaction of exposures with some or all adjustment factors. This approach was first used by Walter (1976), Sturmans et al. (1977) and Fleiss (1979) followed by Deubner et al. (1980) and Greenland (1987). The full generality and flexibility of the regression approach was exploited by Bruzzi et al. (1985) who developed a general AR estimate based on rewriting AR as

$$ 1 - \sum_{j=1}^{J} \sum_{i=0}^{I} \varrho_{ij} RR_{i|j}^{-1} \, . $$

Quantities ϱ_{ij} represent the proportion of diseased individuals with level i of exposure ($i = 0$ at the reference level, $i = 1, \ldots, I$ for exposed levels) and j of confounding and can be estimated from cohort or case-control data (or cross-sectional survey data) using the observed proportions. The quantity $RR_{i|j}^{-1}$ represents the inverse of the rate ratio, risk ratio or odds ratio depending on the context, for level i of exposure at level j of confounding. It can be estimated from regression models (see Sect. 2.4.6), both for cohort and case-control data (as well as cross-sectional data), which allows confounding and interactions to be accounted for. Hence, this regression-based approach to AR estimation allows control for confounding and interaction and can be used for the main epidemiologic designs. Depending on the design, conditional or unconditional logistic, log-linear or Poisson models can be used. Variance estimators were developed based on an extension of the delta-method to implicitly related random variables in order to take into account the variability in estimates of terms ϱ_{ij} and $RR_{i|j}^{-1}$ as well as their correlations (Basu and Landis 1995; Benichou and Gail 1989, 1990b). This regression approach includes the crude and two stratification approaches as special cases and offers additional options (Benichou 1991). The unadjusted approach corresponds to models for $RR_{i|j}^{-1}$ with exposure only. The Mantel–Haenszel approach corresponds to models with exposure and confounding factors, but no interaction terms between exposure and adjustment factors. The weighted-sum approach corresponds to fully saturated models with all interaction terms between exposure and confounding factors. Intermediate models are possible, for instance models allowing for interaction between exposure and only one confounder, or models in which the main effects of some confounders are not modeled in a saturated way.

Example 3. *(continued)*
Still considering the more restrictive definition of the reference category for daily alcohol consumption, an unconditional logistic model (see Sect. 2.4.6) with two parameters, one general intercept and one parameter for elevated alcohol consumption, was fit, ignoring smoking and age. The resulting unadjusted odds ratio estimate was 5.9 as above. The formula above for $1 - AR$ reduced to a single sum with two terms ($i = 0, 1$) corresponding to unexposed and exposed categories, respectively. The resulting unadjusted AR estimate was 70.9% (standard error estimate of 5.1), identical to the crude AR estimate above. Adding eight terms for smoking and age in the logistic model increased the fit significantly ($p < 0.001$, likelihood ratio test) and yielded an adjusted odds ratio estimate of 6.3, slightly higher than the Mantel–Haenszel odds ratio estimate of 6.2 (see above). This resulted in an adjusted AR estimate of 71.9%, slightly higher than the corresponding Mantel–Haenszel AR estimate of 71.6%, and with a slightly lower standard error estimate of 5.0%. Adding two terms for interactions of smoking with alcohol consumption (thus allowing for different odds ratio estimates depending on smoking level) resulted in a decreased AR estimate of 70.3% (with a higher standard error estimate of 5.4% because of the additional parameters estimated). Adding six more terms allowed for all two-by-two interactions between alcohol consumption and joint age × smoking level and yielded a fully saturated model. Thus nine odds ratios for alcohol consumption were estimated (one for each stratum) as with the weighted-sum approach. This resulted in little change as regards AR, with an AR estimate of 70.0%, identical to the AR estimate with the weighted sum approach, which precisely corresponds to a fully saturated model. The corresponding standard error estimate was increased to 5.6% due to the estimation of additional parameters. ◆

A modification of Bruzzi et al.'s approach was developed by Greenland and Drescher (1993) in order to obtain full maximum likelihood estimates of AR. The modification consists in estimating the quantities ϱ_{ij} from the regression model rather than simply relying on the observed proportions of cases. The two model-based approaches seem to differ very little numerically (Greenland and Drescher 1993). Greenland and Drescher's approach might be more efficient in small samples although no difference was observed in simulations of the case-control design even for samples of 100 cases and 100 controls (Greenland and Drescher 1993). It might be less robust to model misspecification, however, as it relies more heavily on the RR or odds ratio model used. Finally, it does not apply to the conditional logistic model, and if that model is to be used (notably, in case-control studies with individual matching), the original approach of Bruzzi et al. is the only possible choice.

Detailed reviews of adjusted AR estimation (Benichou 1991, 2001; Coughlin et al. 1994; Gefeller 1992) are available. Alternative methods to obtain estimates of variance and confidence intervals for AR have been developed either based on resampling techniques (Gefeller 1992; Greenland 1992; Kahn et al. 1998; Kooperberg and Petitti 1991; Llorca and Delgado-Rodriguez 2000; Uter and Pfahlberg 1999) or on quadratic equations (Lui 2001a,b, 2003).

Final Notes and Additional References

General problems of AR definition, interpretation and usefulness as well as properties have been reviewed in detail (Benichou 2000b; Gefeller 1992; Miettinen 1974; Rockhill et al. 1998a,b; Walter 1976). Special issues were reviewed by Benichou (2000b, 2001). They include estimation of AR for risk factors with multiple levels of exposure or with a continuous form, multiple risk factors, recurrent disease events, and disease classification with more than two categories. They also include assessing the consequences of exposure misclassification on AR estimates. Specific software for attributable risk estimation (Kahn et al. 1998; Mezzetti et al. 1996) as well as a simplified approach to confidence interval estimation (Daly 1998) have been developed to facilitate implementation of methods for attributable risk estimation. Finally, much remains to be done to promote proper use and interpretation of AR as illustrated in a recent literature review (Uter and Pfahlberg 2001).

Attributable Risk Among the Exposed   2.5.2

The attributable risk in the exposed (AR_E) or attributable fraction in the exposed is defined as the following ratio (Cole and MacMahon 1971; Levin 1953; MacMahon and Pugh 1970; Miettinen 1974):

$$AR_E = \left\{ \Pr(D|E) - \Pr\left(D|\overline{E}\right) \right\} / \Pr(D|E), \tag{2.13}$$

where $\Pr(D|E)$ is the probability of disease in the exposed individuals (E) and $\Pr(D|\overline{E})$ is the hypothetical probability of disease in the same subjects but with all exposure eliminated. Depending on the context, these probabilities will refer to disease risk or may be replaced with incidence rates (see Sect. 2.5.1). AR_E can be rewritten as:

$$AR_E = (RR - 1)/RR \,, \qquad (2.14)$$

where RR denotes the risk or rate ratio. Following Greenland and Robins (1988), Rothman and Greenland (1998, Chap. 4) proposed to use the terms "excess fraction" for the definition of AR_E based on risks or risk ratios and "rate fraction" for the definition of AR_E based on rates or rate ratios.

Like AR, AR_E lies between 0 and 1 when exposures considered are risk factors (RR > 1) with a maximal limiting value of 1, is equal to zero in the absence of association between exposure and disease (RR = 1), and is negative for protective exposures (RR < 1).

As for AR, AR_E has an interpretation as a measure of the disease burden attributable or at least related to one or several exposures among the exposed subjects. Consequently, AR_E could be used to assess the potential impact of prevention programs aimed at eliminating exposure from the population. These interpretations are subject to the same limitations as corresponding interpretations for AR however (see Sect. 2.5.1). Moreover, AR_E does not have a clear public health interpretation because it does not depend on the exposure prevalence but only on the risk or rate ratio of which it is merely a one-to-one transformation. For the assessment of the relative impact of several exposures, AR_E will not be an appropriate measure since AR_E for different exposures refer to different groups of subjects in the population (i.e., subjects exposed to each given exposure).

AR_E being a one-to-one function of RR, issues of estimability and estimation for AR_E are similar to those for RR. They depend on whether rates or risks are considered. For case-control studies, odds ratios can be used. Greenland (1987) specifically derived adjusted point estimates and confidence intervals for AR_E based on the Mantel–Haenszel approach.

2.5.3   Sequential and Partial Attributable Risks

Upon considering multiple exposures, separate ARs can be estimated for each exposure as well as the overall AR for all exposures jointly. Except in very special circumstances worked out by Walter (1983) (i.e., lack of joint exposure or additive effects of exposures on disease risk or rate), the sum of separate AR estimates over all exposures considered will not equal the overall AR estimate.

Because this property is somewhat counter-intuitive and generates misinterpretations, three alternative approaches have been suggested, one based on considering variance decomposition methods (Begg et al. 1998) rather than estimating AR, one based on estimating assigned share or probability of causation of a given exposure with relevance in litigation procedures for individuals with multiple exposures (Cox 1984, 1985; Lagakos and Mosteller 1986; Seiler 1986; Seiler and Scott 1987; Benichou 1993b; McElduff et al. 2002), and one based on an extension of the concept of AR (Eide and Gefeller 1995; Land et al. 2001). This last approach relies on partitioning techniques (Gefeller et al. 1998; Land and Gefeller 1997) and keeps with the framework of AR estimation by introducing the sequential AR that generalizes the concept of AR. The principle is to define an order among the exposures considered. Then, the contribution of each exposure is assessed sequentially according to that order. The contribution of the first exposure considered is calculated as the standard AR for that exposure separately. The contribution of the second exposure is obtained as the difference between the joint AR estimate for the first two exposures and the separate AR estimate for the first exposure, the contribution of the third exposure is obtained as the difference between the joint AR estimates for the first three and first two exposures, etc .... Thus, a multidimensional vector consisting of contributions of each separate exposure is obtained.

These contributions are meaningful in terms of potential prevention programs that consider successive rather than simultaneous elimination of exposures from the population. Indeed, each step yields the additional contribution of the elimination of a given exposure once higher-ranked exposures are eliminated. At some point, additional contributions may become very small, indicating that there is not much point in considering extra steps. By construction, these contributions sum to the overall AR for all exposures jointly, which constitutes an appealing property. Of course, separate vectors of contributions are obtained for different orders. Meaningful orders depend on practical possibilities in implementing potential prevention programs in a given population. Average contributions can be calculated for each given exposure by calculating the mean of contributions corresponding to that exposure over all possible orders. These average contributions have been termed partial attributable risks (Eide and Gefeller 1995) and represent another potentially useful measure. Methods for visualizing sequential and partial ARs are provided by Eide and Heuch (2001). An illustration is given by Fig. 2.1. A detailed review of properties, interpretation, and variants of sequential and partial ARs was provided by Land et al. (2001).

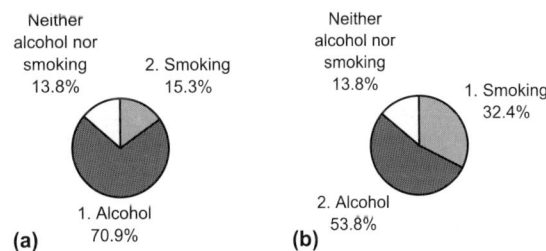

Figure 2.1. Sequential attributable risk estimates for elevated alcohol consumption (80+ g/day) and heavy smoking (10+ g/day) for two different orders of removal (a: alcohol, then smoking; b: smoking, then alcohol) – Case-control data on esophageal cancer (Tuyns, Pequignot and Jensen 1977; cf. Example 3)

Example 3. *(continued)*
Smoking is also a known risk factor of esophageal cancer so that it is important to estimate the impact of smoking and the joint impact of smoking

and alcohol consumption on esophageal cancer in addition to that of alcohol consumption alone. Using the first category (i.e., 0–9 g/day) as the reference level of smoking, there were 78 cases in the reference level of smoking, 122 cases in the exposed level (i.e., 10+ g/day), 447 controls in the reference level and 328 controls in the exposed level. From these data, the crude odds ratio estimate for smoking at least 10 g/day was 2.1 and the crude AR estimate for smoking at least 10 g/day was 32.4%. Moreover, there were nine cases and 252 controls in the joint reference level of alcohol consumption and smoking (i.e., 0–39 g/day of alcohol and 0–9 g/day of tobacco), which yielded a crude joint odds ratio estimate of 10.2 and a crude joint AR estimate for drinking at least 40 g/day of alcohol or smoking at least 10 g/day of tobacco of 86.2%.

Furthermore, the crude AR estimate for alcohol consumption of at least 40 g/day was estimated at 70.9% in Sect. 2.5.1. Hence, considering the first order of risk factor removal (i.e., eliminating alcohol consumption above 39 g/day followed by eliminating smoking above 9 g/day) yields sequential AR estimates of 70.9% for elevated daily alcohol consumption and 86.2% − 70.9% = 15.3 percentage points for heavy smoking so that, once elevated alcohol consumption is eliminated, the additional impact of eliminating heavy smoking appears rather limited (Fig. 2.1a). Considering the second order (i.e., eliminating heavy smoking first) yields sequential AR estimates of 32.4% for heavy smoking and 86.2% − 32.4% = 53.8 percentage points for elevated alcohol consumption so that, once heavy smoking is eliminated, the additional impact of eliminating elevated alcohol consumption remains major (Fig. 2.1b). A summary of these results is provided by partial ARs for elevated alcohol consumption and heavy smoking, with estimated values of 62.4% and 23.9%, respectively, again reflecting the higher impact of elevated alcohol consumption on esophageal cancer.

◆

2.5.4   Preventable and Prevented Fractions

When considering a protective exposure or intervention, an appropriate alternative to AR is the preventable or prevented fraction (PF) defined as the ratio (Miettinen 1974):

$$\text{PF} = \left\{ \Pr\left(D|\bar{E}\right) - \Pr(D) \right\} / \Pr(D|\bar{E}) , \tag{2.15}$$

where $\Pr(D)$ is the probability of disease in the population, which may have some exposed (E) and some unexposed ($\bar{E}$) individuals, and $\Pr(D|\bar{E})$ is the hypothetical probability of disease in the same population but with all (protective) exposure eliminated. Depending on the context, these probabilities will refer to disease risk or may be replaced with incidence rates (see sections above). PF can be rewritten as:

$$\text{PF} = p_E(1 - \text{RR}) , \tag{2.16}$$

a function of both the prevalence of exposure, p_E, and the risk or rate ratio, RR. Thus, a strong association between exposure and disease may correspond to a high or low value of PF depending on the prevalence of exposure, as for AR. Moreover, portability is not a typical property of PF, as for AR. As for AR again, it may be useful to compare PF estimates among population subgroups to target prevention efforts to specific subgroups with a potentially high impact (as measured by the PF).

For a protective factor (RR < 1), PF lies between 0 and 1 and increases with the prevalence of exposure and the strength of the association between exposure and disease.

PF measures the impact of an association between a protective exposure and disease at the population level. It has a public health interpretation as the proportion of disease cases averted ("prevented fraction") in relation to the presence of a protective exposure or intervention in the population, among the totality of cases that would have developed in the absence of that factor or intervention in the population. In this case, it is useful to assess prevention programs *a posteriori*. Alternatively, it can be used to assess prevention programs *a priori* by measuring the proportion of cases that could be potentially averted ("preventable fraction") if a protective exposure or intervention were introduced *de novo* in the population (Gargiullo et al. 1995). These interpretations are subject to the same limitations as corresponding interpretations for AR however (see Sect. 2.5.1).

PF and AR are mathematically related through (Walter 1976):

$$1 - PF = 1/(1 - AR) . \tag{2.17}$$

From (2.17), it appears that, for a protective factor, PF estimates will usually differ from AR estimates obtained by reversing the coding of exposure. This follows from the respective definitions of AR and PF. While AR, with reverse coding, measures the potential reduction in disease occurrence that could be achieved if all subjects in the current population became exposed, PF measures the reduction in disease occurrence obtained from introducing exposure at the current prevalence in a formally unexposed population (Benichou 2000c).

In view of (2.17), estimability and estimation issues are similar for AR and PF. Specific PF adjusted point and confidence interval estimates were derived using the Mantel–Haenszel approach (Greenland 1987) and weighted-sum approaches (Gargiullo et al. 1995).

Generalized Impact Fraction

2.5.5

The generalized impact fraction (GIF) or generalized attributable fraction was introduced by Walter (1980), and Morgenstern and Bursic (1982) as the ratio:

$$GIF = \{Pr(D) - Pr^*(D)\}/Pr(D) , \tag{2.18}$$

where $Pr(D)$ and $Pr^*(D)$ respectively denote the probability of disease under the current distribution of exposure and under a modified distribution of exposure.

As for AR and PF, these probabilities denote risks or can be replaced by incidence rates depending on the context.

The generalized impact fraction not only depends on the association between exposure and disease as well as the current distribution (rather than just the prevalence) of exposure, but also on the target distribution of exposure considered that will yield $\Pr^*(D)$. It is a general measure of impact that includes AR and PF as special cases. AR contrasts the current distribution of exposure with a modified distribution defined by the absence of exposure. Conversely, PF contrasts a distribution defined by the absence of exposure with the current distribution of exposure (prevented fraction) or target distribution of exposure (preventable fraction).

The generalized impact fraction can be interpreted as the fractional reduction of disease occurrence that would result from changing the current distribution of exposure in the population to some modified distribution. Thus, it can be used to assess prevention programs or interventions, targeting all subjects or subjects at specified levels, and aimed at modifying or shifting the exposure distribution (reducing exposure), but not necessarily eliminating exposure. For instance, heavy smokers could be specifically targeted by interventions rather than all smokers. The special AR case corresponds to the complete elimination of exposure by considering a modified distribution putting unit mass on the lowest risk configuration and can be used to assess interventions aimed at eliminating (rather than reducing) exposure. Alternatively, the general impact fraction could be used to assess the increase in disease occurrence as a result of exposure changes in the population, such as the increase in breast cancer incidence as a result of delayed childbearing (Kleinbaum et al. 1982, Chap. 9). Such interpretations are subject to the same limitations as for AR and PF (see Sect. 2.5.1).

The generalized impact fraction has been used for instance by Lubin and Boice (1989) who considered the impact on lung cancer of a modification in the distribution of radon exposure consisting in truncating the current distribution at various thresholds and by Wahrendorf (1987) who examined the impact of various changes in dietary habits on colo-rectal and stomach cancers.

Issues of estimability are similar to those for AR and PF. Methods to estimate the generalized impact fraction are similar to methods for estimating AR and PF. However, unlike for AR or PF, it might be useful to retain the continuous nature of exposures to define the modification of the distribution considered (for instance a shift in the distribution), and extensions of methods for estimating AR for continuous factors (Benichou and Gail 1990b) are relevant in this context. Drescher and Becher (1997) proposed extending model-based approaches of Bruzzi et al. (1985) and Greenland and Drescher (1993) to estimate the generalized impact fraction in case-control studies and considered continuous as well as categorical exposures.

2.5.6   Person-Years of Life Lost

Person-years of life lost (or potential years of life lost, PYLL) for a given cause of death is a measure defined as the difference between current life expectancy of the population and potential life expectancy with the cause of death eliminated (Smith 1998). For instance, one may be interested in PYLL due to prostate cancer in men, breast cancer in women, or cancer as a whole (all sites) in men and women. Methods for estimating PYLL rely on calculating cause-deleted life tables. Total PYLL at the population level or average PYLL per person may be estimated. As an example, a recent report from the Surveillance, Epidemiology and End Results (SEER) estimated that 8.4 million years of life overall were lost due to cancer in the US population (both sexes, all races) in the year 2001, with an average value of potential years of life lost per person of 15.1 years. Corresponding numbers were 779,900 years overall and 18.8 years on average for breast cancer in women, and 275,200 years overall and 9.0 years on average for prostate cancer in men (Ries et al. 2004).

PYLL represents an assessment of the impact of a given disease. Thus, it is not directly interpretable as a measure of exposure impact, except perhaps for diseases with a dominating risk factor, such as asbestos exposure for mesothelioma or human papilloma virus for cervical cancer.

However, it is possible to obtain a corresponding measure of the impact of a given exposure by converting PYLL due to a particular cause of death to PYLL due to a particular exposure. Estimation of an exposure-specific PYLL is obtained through applying an AR estimate for that exposure to the disease-specific PYLL, namely calculating the product PYLL times AR, which yields the fraction of PYLL attributable to exposure. In this process, several causes of deaths may have to be considered. For instance, the fractions of PYLL for mesothelioma and lung cancer would need to be added in order to obtain the overall PYLL for asbestos exposure. In contrast with AR that provides a measure of exposure impact as a fraction of disease incidence (or death), such calculations of PYLL will provide a measure of exposure impact on the life expectancy scale. As for AR, the impact of a given exposure on the PYLL scale will depend on the prevalence of exposure in the population and strength of association between exposure and disease(s). Moreover, it will depend critically on the age-distribution of exposure-associated diseases and their severity, i.e. case fatality.

Other Topics

2.6

Standardization of Risks and Rates

2.6.1

Risks and rates can usually not be directly compared between countries, regions or time periods because of differences in age structure. For example, an older population may appear to have higher rates of certain cancers, not because of the presence of risk factors, but because of the higher age itself. This is a form of confounding. In the tradition of demography, so called standardization is applied to reported rates and risks to adjust for differences in age and possibly other confounders. Direct standardization is the most commonly used technique. It proceeds by forming a weighted average of age specific rates or risks, where the weights reflect a known population structure. This structure is typically chosen as that of a country in a given census year, the so-called *standard population*. A directly standardized rate can be written:

$$\text{SR} = \sum n_j^S h_j / \sum n_j^S = \sum w_j^S h_j , \qquad (2.19)$$

where n_j^S is the number of individuals in age group j in the standard population, h_j are age specific rates in the population under study, and w_j^S are weights such that $\sum w_j^S = 1$. A standardized risk can be computed in the same manner. Since the weights are fixed and not estimated, the variance of the estimated standardized rate is

$$\text{var}\left(\sum w_j^S h_j\right) = \sum \left(w_j^S\right)^2 h_j , \qquad (2.20)$$

based on the Poisson assumption for the age specific rates. For risks, the binomial assumption may be used for the age specific risks.

When age-specific rates or risks are not available in the population under study, *indirect standardization* may be used. This technique is less common, but requires knowledge only of the age distribution, and not the age-specific rates, in the population under study. The indirectly standardized rate is obtained by (SMR)(CR^0), where SMR is the *standardized mortality or morbidity ratio* (see below), and CR^0 is the *crude* (i.e., original overall) rate in a reference population that provides stratum-specific rates.

The standardized mortality or morbidity ratio is a ratio between observed and expected event counts, where the expected count is based on age specific rates or risks in a reference population, which is a non-exposed or general population group. Then the standardized mortality (or morbidity or incidence) ratio

$$\text{SMR or SIR} = D_E/E_0 = \sum n_j h_j / \sum n_j h_{0j} ,$$

where D_E is the number of events in the exposed and E_0 is the expected number of events obtained from the rates h_{0j} in the unexposed applied to the sample composition of the exposed. The SMR can also be re-written as a weighted average of sex- and age-specific (say) rate ratios h_j/h_{0j} with weights $w_j = n_j h_{0j}$. It can be shown that these weights minimize the standard error of the weighted average (Breslow and Day 1987, Chap. 2) as long as the rates in the reference population are assumed to be known rather than estimated. Stratified analyses as discussed above, on the other hand, choose weights that minimize the standard errors when the rates are estimated among both the exposed and the unexposed. The SMR has the advantage that age- and sex-specific rates are not needed for the exposed group.

The denominator of the SMR is generally obtained from age- and sex-specific rates in the entire regional population. This allows the random variation of the denominator to be considered to be none, and confidence intervals can be based on the estimate $1/D_E^{1/2}$ for the standard error of ln(SMR). This standard error computation also assumes that the events among the exposed are uncorrelated (do not cluster), or more specifically, that the event count follows a Poisson distribution.

It may be noted that directly standardized rates are based on a choice of standard population to generate weights. While the weights used for the SMR result from the composition of the comparison group and do not involve a true standard population, the weights used in direct standardization are external as they result from information outside the samples being compared. In principle, the latter weights are similar to survey weights applied in for examples the National Health and Nutrition Examination Survey (NHANES), where the sample must be standardized to the US population to account for the methodology used in drawing it. While improving external validity, weights from direct standardization and survey weights always result in loss of statistical efficiency, i.e., standard errors will be larger than for crude, or non-weighted rates and risks. In contrast, many of the methods to adjust for confounding discussed in Sect. 2.4 are internal to the specific comparison and designed to optimize statistical efficiency.

Measures Based on Prevalence   2.6.2

Prevalence is the number of cases either at a given point in time (point prevalence) or over a time period (period prevalence) divided by the population size. Prevalence can be easier to obtain than incidence. For example, a population survey can determine how many individuals in a population suffer from a given illness or health condition at a point in time.

Measures of association based on prevalence parallel those for risk (for point prevalence) or incidence rates (for period prevalence). For example, one can form prevalence ratios, prevalence differences and prevalence odds ratios. Measures of impact based on prevalence can also be obtained.

Prevalence and the measures of association based on it are useful entities for health policy planning and for determining the level of services needed for individuals with a given health condition in the population. It is usually considered less useful for studying the etiology of a disease. The reason for this is that under certain assumptions prevalence of a disease equals its incidence multiplied by its duration (Kleinbaum et al. 1982, Chap. 8). These assumptions are that the population is stable, and that both the incidence and prevalence remain constant. Under more general conditions, prevalence still reflects both incidence and duration, but in a more complex manner. For a potentially fatal or incurable disease, duration means survival, and the exposures that increase incidence may reduce or increase survival and hence the association of an exposure with prevalence may be very different than its association with incidence. On the other hand, when a disease or condition can be of limited duration due to recovery or cure, and its duration is maintained by the same exposures that caused it, prevalence can be more meaningful than incidence. For example, it is conceivable that weight gain in a person may have caused hypertension, and when the person loses the same amount of weight she/he moves out of being hypertensive. In this latter case, the prevalence ratio between the percentages with hypertension in those exposed and unexposed to the risk factor captures the increase in the risk of living with the condition caused by the exposure, while the incidence ratio captures only part of the etiologic association.

2.7   Conclusions

Disease frequency is measured through the computation of incidence rates or estimation of disease risk. Both measures are directly accessible from cohort data. They can be obtained from case-control data only if they are complemented by follow-up or population data. Using regression techniques, methods are available to derive incidence rates or risk estimates specific to a given exposure profile. Exposure-specific risk estimates are useful in individual prediction.

A wide variety of options and techniques are available for measuring association. The odds ratio is presently the most often used measure of association for both cohort and case control studies. Adjustment for confounding is key in all analyses of observational studies, and can be pursued by standardization, stratification and by regression techniques. The flexibility of the latter, especially in the generalized linear model framework, and availability of computer software, has made it widely applied in the last several years.

Several measures are available to assess the impact of an exposure in terms of the occurrence of new disease cases at the population level, among which the attributable risk is the most commonly used. Several approaches have been developed to derive adjusted estimates of the attributable risk from case-control as well as cohort data, either based on stratification or on more flexible regression techniques. The concept of attributable risk has been extended to handle preventive exposures, multiple exposures, as well as assessing the impact of various modifications of the exposure distribution rather than the mere elimination of exposure.

References

Aalen O (1978) Nonparametric estimation of partial transition probabilities in multiple decrement models. Annals of Statistics 6:534–545

Aalen O, Johansen S (1978) An empirical transition matrix for nonhomogeneous Markov chains based on censored observations. Scandinavian Journal of Statistics 5:141–150

American Cancer Society (1992) Cancer facts and figures. American Cancer Society, Atlanta, Georgia

Ames BN, Gold LS, Willett WC (1995) The causes and prevention of cancer. Proceedings of the National Academy of Sciences of the United States of America 254:1131–1138

Andersen PK, Gill RD (1982) Cox's regression models for counting processes: A large-sample study. Annals of Statistics 4:1100–1120

Anderson KM, Wilson PW, Odell PM, Kannel WB (1991) Cardiovascular disease risk profiles. A statement for health professionals. Circulation 83:356–362

Anderson SJ, Ahnn S, Duff K (1992) NSABP Breast Cancer Prevention Trial Risk Assessment Program, Version 2. University of Pittsburgh Department of Bio-statistics, Pittsburgh, PA

Basu S, Landis JR (1995) Model-based estimation of population attributable risk under cross-sectional sampling. American Journal of Epidemiology 142:1338–1343

Begg CB (2001) The search for cancer risk factors: When can we stop looking? American Journal of Public Health 91:360–364

Begg CB, Satagopan JM, Berwick M (1998) A new strategy for evaluating the impact of epidemiologic risk factors for cancer with applications to melanoma. Journal of the American Statistical Association 93: 415–426

Benichou J (1991) Methods of adjustment for estimating the attributable risk in case-control studies: A review. Statistics in Medicine 10:1753–1773

Benichou J (1993a) A computer program for estimating individualized probabilities of breast cancer. Computers and Biomedical Research 26:373–382

Benichou J (1993b) Re: "Methods of adjustment for estimating the attributable risk in case-control studies: A review" (letter). Statistics in Medicine 12:94–96

Benichou J (2000a) Absolute risk. In: Gail MH, Benichou J (eds) Encyclopedia of epidemiologic methods. Wiley, Chichester, pp 1–17

Benichou J (2000b) Attributable risk. In: Gail MH, Benichou J (eds) Encyclopedia of epidemiologic methods. Wiley, Chichester, pp 50–63

Benichou J (2000c) Preventable fraction. In: Gail MH, Benichou J (eds) Encyclopedia of epidemiologic methods. Wiley, Chichester, pp 736–737

Benichou J (2001) A review of adjusted estimators of the attributable risk. Statistical Methods in Medical Research 10:195–216

Benichou J, Gail MH (1989) A delta-method for implicitly defined random variables. American Statistician 43:41–44

Benichou J, Gail MH (1990a) Estimates of absolute cause-specific risk in cohort studies. Biometrics 46:813–826

Benichou J, Gail MH (1990b) Variance calculations and confidence intervals for estimates of the attributable risk based on logistic models. Biometrics 46:991–1003

Benichou J, Gail MH (1995) Methods of inference for estimates of absolute risk derived from population-based case-control studies. Biometrics 51:182–194

Benichou J, Wacholder S (1994) A comparison of three approaches to estimate exposure-specific incidence rates from population-based case-control data. Statistics in Medicine 13:651–661

Benichou J, Gail MH, Mulvihill JJ (1996) Graphs to estimate an individualized risk of breast cancer. Journal of Clinical Oncology 14:103–110

Benichou J, Byrne C, Gail MH (1997) An approach to estimating exposure-specific rates of breast cancer from a two-stage case-control study within a cohort. Statistics in Medicine 16:133–151

Berkson J (1958) Smoking and lung cancer. Some observations on two recent reports. Journal of the American Statistical Association 53:28–38

Birch MW (1964) The detection of partial associations, I: The 2×2 case. Journal of the Royal Statistical Society, Series B 27:313–324

Borgan Ø (1998) Nelson-Aalen estimator. In: Armitage P, Colton T (eds) Encyclopedia of epidemiologic methods. Wiley, Chichester, pp 2967–2972

Breslow NE (1981) Odds ratio estimators when the data are sparse. Biometrika 68:73–84

Breslow NE, Day NE (1980) Statistical methods in cancer research vol I: The analysis of case-control studies. International Agency for Research on Cancer Scientific Publications No. 32, Lyon

Breslow NE, Day NE (1987) Statistical methods in cancer research vol II: The design and analysis of cohort studies. International Agency for Research on Cancer Scientific Publications No. 82, Lyon

Breslow NE, Lubin JH, Marek P, Langholz B (1983) Multiplicative models and cohort analysis. Journal of the American Statistical Association 78:1–12

Bruzzi P, Green SB, Byar DP, Brinton LA, Schairer C (1985) Estimating the population attributable risk for multiple risk factors using case-control data. American Journal of Epidemiology 122:904–914

Chiang CL (1968) Introduction to stochastic processes in biostatistics. Wiley, New York

Colditz G, DeJong W, Hunter D, Trichopoulos D, Willett W (eds) (1996) Harvard report on cancer prevention, vol 1. Cancer Causes and Control 7(suppl.):S3–S59

Colditz G, DeJong W, Hunter D, Trichopoulos D, Willett W (eds) (1997) Harvard report on cancer prevention, vol 2. Cancer Causes and Control 8(suppl.):S1–S50

Cole P, MacMahon B (1971) Attributable risk percent in case-control studies. British Journal of Preventive and Social Medicine 25:242–244

Cornfield J (1951) A method for estimating comparative rates from clinical data: Applications to cancer of the lung, breast and cervix. Journal of the National Cancer Institute 11:1269–1275

Cornfield J (1956) A statistical problem arising from retrospective studies. In: Neyman J (ed) Proceedings of the Third Berkeley Symposium, vol IV. University of California Press, Monterey, pp 133–148

Cornfield J, Haenszel W, Hammond EC, Lilienfeld AM, Shimkin MB, Wynder EI (1959) Smoking and lung cancer: recent evidence and a discussion of some questions. Journal of the National Cancer Institute 22:173–203

Costantino JP, Gail MH, Pee D, Anderson S, Redmond CK, Benichou J, Wieand HS (1999) Validation studies for models projecting the risk of invasive and total breast cancer incidence. Journal of the National Cancer Institute 91:1541–1548

Coughlin SS, Benichou J, Weed DL (1994) Attributable risk estimation in case-control studies. Epidemiologic Reviews 16:51–64

Cox DR (1972) Regression models and lifetables (with discussion). Journal of the Royal Statistical Society, Series B 34:187–220

Cox DR (1975) Partial likelihood. Biometrika 62:269–276

Cox LA (1984) Probability of causation and the attributable proportion of risk. Risk Analysis 4:221–230

Cox LA (1985) A new measure of attributable risk for public health applications. Management Science 7:800–813

Cutler SJ, Ederer F (1958) Maximum utilization of the life table method in analyzing survival. Journal of Chronic Diseases 8:699–712

Daly LE (1998) Confidence limits made easy: interval estimation using a substitution method. American Journal of Epidemiology 147:783–790

Deubner DC, Wilkinson WE, Helms MJ, Tyroler HA, Hames CG (1980) Logistic model estimation of death attributable to risk factors for cardiovascular disease in Evans County, Georgia. American Journal of Epidemiology 112:135–143

Doll R, Peto R (1981) The causes of cancer. Oxford University Press, New York

Dorey FJ, Korn EL (1987) Effective sample sizes for confidence intervals for survival probabilities. Statistics in Medicine 6:679–687

Drescher K, Becher H (1997) Estimating the generalized attributable fraction from case-control data. Biometrics 53:1170–1176

Dupont DW (1989) Converting relative risks to absolute risks: A graphical approach. Statistics in Medicine 8:641–651

Easton DF, Peto J, Babiker AG (1991) Floating absolute risk: An alternative to relative risk in survival and case-control analysis avoiding an arbitrary reference group. Statistics in Medicine 10:1025–1035

Eide GE, Gefeller O (1995) Sequential and average attributable fractions as aids in the selection of preventive strategies. Journal of Clinical Epidemiology 48:645–655

Eide GE, Heuch I (2001) Attributable fractions: fundamental concepts and their vizualization. Statistical Methods in Medical Research 10:159–193

Ejigou A (1979) Estimation of attributable risk in the presence of confounding. Biometrical Journal 21:155–165

Elandt-Johnson RC (1977) Various estimators of conditional probabilities of death in follow-up studies. Summary of results. Journal of Chronic Diseases 30:247–256

Elveback L (1958) Estimation of survivorship in chronic disease: The "actuarial" method. Journal of the American Statistical Association 53:420–440

Fleiss JL (1979) Inference about population attributable risk from cross-sectional studies. American Journal of Epidemiology 110:103–104

Fleiss JL, Dunner DL, Stallone F, Fieve RR (1976) The life table: A method for analyzing longitudinal studies. Archives of General Psychiatry 33:107–112

Fisher B, Costantino JP, Wickerham L, Redmond CK, Kavanah M, Cronin WM, Vogel V, Robidoux A, Dimitrov N, Atkins J, Daly M, Wieand S, Tan-Chiu E, Ford L, Womark N, other National Surgical Adjuvant Breast and Bowel project Investigators (1998) Tamoxifen for prevention of breast cancer: Report of the National Surgical Adjuvant Breast and Bowel Project P-1 Study. Journal of the National Cancer Institute 90:1371–1388

Gail MH (1975) Measuring the benefit of reduced exposure to environmental carcinogens. Journal of Chronic Diseases 28:135–147

Gail MH, Benichou J (1994) Validation studies on a model for breast cancer risk (editorial). Journal of the National Cancer Institute 86:573–575

Gail MH, Brinton LA, Byar DP, Corle DK, Green SB, Schairer C, Mulvihill JJ (1989) Projecting individualized probabilities of developing breast cancer for white females who are being examined annually. Journal of the National Cancer Institute 81:1879–1886

Gail MH, Costantino JP, Bruant J, Croyle R, Freedman L, Helzsouer K, Vogel V (1999) Weighing the risks and benefits of Tamoxifen treatment for preventing breast cancer. Journal of the National Cancer Institute 91:1829–1846

Gargiullo PM, Rothenberg R, Wilson HG (1995) Confidence intervals, hypothesis tests, and sample sizes for the prevented fraction in cross-sectional studies. Statistics in Medicine 14:51–72

Gefeller O (1990) Theory and application of attributable risk estimation in cross-sectional studies. Statistica Applicata 2:323–331

Gefeller O (1992) The bootstrap method for standard errors and confidence intervals of the adjusted attributable risk [letter]. Epidemiology 3:271–272

Gefeller O (1995) Definitions of attributable risk-revisited. Public Health Reviews 23:343–355

Gefeller O, Land M, Eide GE (1998) Averaging attributable fractions in the multifactorial situation: Assumptions and interpretation. Journal of Clinical Epidemiology 51:437–451

Gray RJ (1988) A class of k-sample tests for comparing the cumulative incidence of a competing risk. Annals of Statistics 16:1141–1151

Greenland S (1981) Multivariate estimation of exposure-specific incidence from case-control studies. Journal of Chronic Diseases 34:445–453

Greenland S (1984) Bias in methods for deriving standardized mortality ratio and attributable fraction estimates. Statistics in Medicine 3:131–141

Greenland S (1987) Variance estimators for attributable fraction estimates, consistent in both large strata and sparse data. Statistics in Medicine 6:701–708

Greenland S (1992) The bootstrap method for standard errors and confidence intervals of the adjusted attributable risk [letter]. Epidemiology 3:271

Greenland S (2001) Attributable fractions: bias from broad definition of exposure. Epidemiology 12:518–520

Greenland S, Drescher K (1993) Maximum-likelihood estimation of the attributable fraction from logistic models. Biometrics 49:865–872

Greenland S, Morgenstern H (1983) Morgenstern corrects a conceptual error [letter]. American Journal of Public Health 73:703–704

Greenland S, Robins JM (1988) Conceptual problems in the definition and interpretation of attributable fractions. American Journal of Epidemiology 128:1185–1197

Greenland S, Thomas DC (1982) On the need for the rare disease assumption. American Journal of Epidemiology 116:547–553

Hartman LC, Sellers TA, Schaid DJ, Franks TS, Soderberg CL, Sitta DL, Frost MH, Grant CS, Donohue JH, Woods JE, McDonnell SK, Vockley CW, Deffenbaugh A, Couch FJ, Jenkins RB (2001) Efficacy of bilateral prophylactic mastectomy in BRCA1 and BRCA2 gene mutation carriers. Journal of the National Cancer Institute 93:1633–1637

Henderson BE, Ross RK, Pike MC (1991) Toward the primary prevention of cancer. Science 254:1131–1138

Holford TR (1980) The analysis of rates and of survivorship using log-linear models. Biometrics 36:299–305

Hosmer D, Lemeshow S (1999) Applied survival analysis: Regression modeling of time to event data. John Wiley & Sons, Hoboken, New Jersey

Hoskins KF, Stopfer JE, Calzone K, Merajver SD, Rebbeck TR, Garber JE, Weber BL (1995) Assessment and counseling for women with a family history of breast cancer. A guide for clinicians. Journal of the American Medical Association 273:577–585

Johnson NL, Kotz S (1970) Distributions in statistics, vol 2. Houghton-Mifflin, Boston

Kahn HA, Sempos CT (1989) Statistical methods in epidemiology. Monographs in epidemiology and biostatistics, vol 12, Oxford University Press, Oxford, New York

Kahn MJ, O'Fallon WM, Sicks JD (1998) Generalized population attributable risk estimation. Technical Report #54, Mayo Foundation, Rochester, Minnesota

Kaplan EL, Meier P (1958) Nonparametric estimation from incomplete observations. Journal of the American Statistical Association 53:457–481

Katz D, Baptista J, Azen SP, Pike MC (1978) Obtaining confidence intervals for the risk ratio in a cohort study. Biometrics 34:469–474

Kay R, Schumacher M (1983) Unbiased assessment of treatment effects on disease recurrence and survival in clinical trials. Statistics in Medicine 2:41–58

Keiding N, Andersen PK (1989) Nonparametric estimation of transition intensities and transition probabilities: A case study of a two-state Markov process. Applied Statistics 38:319–329

Kleinbaum DG, Kupper LL, Morgenstern H (1982) Epidemiologic research: Principles and quantitative methods. Lifetime Learning Publications, Belmont

Kooperberg C, Petitti DB (1991) Using logistic regression to estimate the adjusted attributable risk of low birthweight in an unmatched case-control study. Epidemiology 2:363–366

Korn EL, Dorey FJ (1992) Applications of crude incidence curves. Statistics in Medicine 11:813–829

Kuritz SJ, Landis JR (1987) Attributable risk estimation from matched-pairs case-control data. American Journal of Epidemiology 125:324–328

Kuritz SJ, Landis JR (1988a) Summary attributable risk estimation from unmatched case-control data. Statistics in Medicine 7:507–517

Kuritz SJ, Landis JR (1988b) Attributable risk estimation from matched case-control data. Biometrics 44:355–367

Lagakos SW, Mosteller F (1986) Assigned shares in compensation for radiation-related cancers (with discussion). Risk Analysis 6:345–380

Laird N, Oliver D (1981) Covariance analysis of censored survival data using log-linear analysis techniques. Journal of the American Statistical Association 76:231–240

Land M, Gefeller O (1997) A game-theoretic approach to partitioning attributable risks in epidemiology. Biometrical Journal 39:777–792

Land M, Vogel C, Gefeller O (2001) Partitioning methods for multifactorial risk attribution. Statistical Methods in Medical Research 10:217–230

Landis JR, Heyman ER, Koch GG (1978) Average partial association in three-way contingency tables: A review and discussion of alternative tests. International Statistical Review 46:237–254

Landis JR, Sharp TJ, Kuritz SJ, Koch G (2000) Mantel–Haenszel methods. In: Gail MH, Benichou J (eds) Encyclopedia of epidemiologic methods, Wiley, Chichester, pp 499–512

Langholz B, Borgan Ø (1997) Estimation of absolute risk from nested case-control data. Biometrics 53:767–774

Last JM (1983) A dictionary of epidemiology. Oxford University Press, New York

Leung HM, Kupper LL (1981) Comparison of confidence intervals for attributable risk. Biometrics 37:293–302

Levin ML (1953) The occurrence of lung cancer in man. Acta Unio Internationalis contra Cancrum 9:531–541

Liang KY, Zeger SL (1986) Longitudinal data analysis using generalized linear models. Biometrika 73:13–22

Liddell JC, McDonald JC, Thomas DC (1977) Methods of cohort analysis: Appraisal by application to asbestos mining (with discussion). Journal of the Royal Statistical Society, Series A 140:469–491

Lin DY, Psaty BM, Kronmal RA (1998) Assessing the sensitivity of regression results to unmeasured confounders in observational studies. Biometrics 54:948–963

Littell AS (1952) Estimation of the t-year survival rate from follow-up studies over a limited period of time. Human Biology 24:87–116

Llorca J, Delgado-Rodriguez M (2000) A comparison of several procedures to estimate the confidence interval for attributable risk in case-control studies. Statistics in Medicine 19:1089–1099

Lubin JH, Boice JD Jr (1989) Estimating Rn-induced lung cancer in the United States. Health Physics 57:417–427

Lui KJ (2001a) Interval estimation of the attributable risk in case-control studies with matched pairs. Journal of Epidemiology and Community Health 55:885–890

Lui KJ (2001b) Notes on interval estimation of the attributable risk in cross-sectional sampling. Statistics in Medicine 20:1797–1809

Lui KJ (2003) Interval estimation of the attributable risk for multiple exposure levels in case-control studies with confounders. Statistics in Medicine 22:2443–2557

Lynch HT, Lynch JF, Rubinstein WS (2001) Prophylactic mastectomy: obstacles and benefits (editorial). Journal of the National Cancer Institute 93:1586–1587

MacMahon B (1962) Prenatal X-ray exposure and childhood cancer. Journal of the National Cancer Institute 28:1173–1191

MacMahon B, Pugh TF (1970) Epidemiology: Principles and methods. Little, Brown and Co, Boston

Madigan MP, Ziegler RG, Benichou J, Byrne C, Hoover RN (1995) Proportion of breast cancer cases in the United States explained by well-established risk factors. Journal of the National Cancer Institute 87:1681–1685

Mantel N (1973) Synthetic retrospective studies and related topics. Biometrics 29:479–486

Mantel N, Haenszel W (1959) Statistical aspects of the analysis of data from retrospective studies of disease. Journal of the National Cancer Institute 22:719–748

Markush RE (1977) Levin's attributable risk statistic for analytic studies and vital statistics. American Journal of Epidemiology 105:401–406

Matthews DE (1988) Likelihood-based confidence intervals for functions of many parameters. Biometrika 75:139–144

Mausner JS, Bahn AK (1974) Epidemiology: An introductory text. W.B. Saunders, Philadelphia

McCullagh P, Nelder JA (1989) Generalized linear models, 2nd edn. CRC Press, Boca Raton

McElduff P, Attia J, Ewald B, Cockburn J, Heller R (2002) Estimating the contribution of individual risk factors to disease in a person with more than one risk factor. Journal of Clinical Epidemiology 55:588–592

Mehta CR, Patel R, Senchaudhuri P (2000) Efficient Monte Carlo methods for conditional logistic regression. Journal of the American Statistical Association 95:99–108

Mezzetti M, Ferraroni M, Decarli A, La Vecchia C, Benichou J (1996) Software for attributable risk and confidence interval estimation in case-control studies. Computers and Biomedical Research 29:63–75

Miettinen OS (1972) Components of the crude risk ratio. American Journal of Epidemiology 96:168–172

Miettinen OS (1974) Proportion of disease caused or prevented by a given exposure, trait or intervention. American Journal of Epidemiology 99:325–332

Miettinen OS (1976) Estimability and estimation in case-referent studies. American Journal of Epidemiology 103:226–235

Morgenstern H (1982) Uses of ecologic analysis in epidemiological research. American Journal of Public Health 72:1336–1344

Morgenstern H, Bursic ES (1982) A method for using epidemiologic data to estimate the potential impact of an intervention on the health status of a target population. Journal of Community Health 7:292–309

Morgenstern H, Kleinbaum D, Kupper LL (1980) Measures of disease incidence used in epidemiologic research. International Journal of Epidemiology 9:97–104

Neuhaus JM, Jewell NP (1990) The effect of retrospective sampling on binary regression models for clustered data. Biometrics 46:977–990

Neutra RR, Drolette ME (1978) Estimating exposure-specific disease rates from case-control studies using Bayes' theorem. American Journal of Epidemiology 108:214–222

Oakes D (1981) Survival times: Aspects of partial likelihood (with discussion). International Statistical Review 49:235–264

Ouellet BL, Romeder JM, Lance JM (1979) Premature mortality attributable to smoking and hazardous drinking in Canada. American Journal of Epidemiology 109:451–463

Palta M, Lin C-Y, Chao W (1997) Effect of confounding and other misspecification in models for longitudinal data. In: Modeling longitudinal and spatially correlated data. Lecture Notes in Statistics Series 122. Proceeding of the Nantucket Conference on Longitudinal and Correlated Data. Springer-Verlag, Heidelberg, New York, pp 77–88

Palta M, Lin C-Y (1999) Latent variables, measurement error and methods for analyzing longitudinal binary and ordinal data. Statistics in Medicine 18:385–396

Palta M (2003) Quantitative methods in population health: Extensions of ordinary regression. John Wiley & Sons, Hoboken, New Jersey

Prentice RL, Breslow NE (1978) Retrospective studies and failure time models. Biometrika 65:153–158

Prentice RL, Kalbfleisch JD, Peterson AV, Flournoy N, Farewell VT, Breslow NE (1978) The analysis of failure times in the presence of competing risks. Biometrics 34:541–554

Prentice RL, Pyke R (1979) Logistic disease incidence models and case-control studies. Biometrika 66:403–411

Rao CR (1965) Linear statistical inference and its application. John Wiley, New York, pp 319–322

Ries LAG, Eisner MP, Kosary CL, Hankey BF, Miller BA, Clegg L, Mariotto A, Feuer EJ, Edwards BK (eds) (2004) SEER Cancer Statistics Review, 1975–2001, National Cancer Institute. Bethesda, MD. (http://seer.cancer.gov/csr/1975_2001) Accessed May 21, 2004

Robins JM, Greenland S (1989) Estimability and estimation of excess and etiologic fractions. Statistics in Medicine 8:845–859

Rockhill B, Newman B, Weinberg C (1998) Use and misuse of population attributable fractions. American Journal of Public Health 88:15–21

Rockhill B, Weinberg C, Newman B (1998) Population attributable fraction estimation for established breast cancer risk factors: considering the issues of high prevalence and unmodifyability. American Journal of Epidemiology 147:826–833

Rothman KJ, Greenland S (1998) Modern epidemiology. Lippincott-Raven, Philadelphia.

SAS Institute Inc. (1999) SAS/STAT user's guide. Version 8. SAS Institute Inc, Cary, NC

Schlesselman JJ (1982) Case-control studies. Design, conduct and analysis. Oxford University Press, New York

Seiler FA (1986) Attributable risk, probability of causation, assigned shares, and uncertainty. Environment International 12:635–641

Seiler FA, Scott BR (1986) Attributable risk, probability of causation, assigned shares, and uncertainty. Environment International 12:635–641

Siemiatycki J, Wacholder S, Dewar R, Cardis E, Greenwood C, Richardson L (1988) Degree of confounding bias related to smoking, ethnic group and SES in estimates of the associations between occupation and cancer. J Occup Med 30:617–625

Smith L (1998) Person-years of life lost. In: Armitage P, Colton T (eds) Encyclopedia of biostatistics. Wiley, Chichester, pp 3324–3325

Spiegelman D, Colditz GA, Hunter D, Hetrzmark E (1994) Validation of the Gail et al model for predicting individual breast cancer risk. Journal of the National Cancer Institute 86:600–607

Sturmans F, Mulder PGH, Walkenburg HA (1977) Estimation of the possible effect of interventive measures in the area of ischemic heart diseases by the attributable risk percentage. American Journal of Epidemiology 105:281–289

Tarone RE (1981) On summary estimators of relative risk. Journal of Chronic Diseases 34:463–468

Tsiatis AA (1981) A large-sample study of Cox's regression model. Annals of Statistics 9:93–108

Tuyns AJ, Pequignot G, Jensen OM (1977) Le cancer de l'œsophage en Ille-et-Vilaine en fonction des niveaux de consommation d'alcool et de tabac. Bulletin of Cancer 64:45–60

US National Cancer Institute (2004) Breast cancer risk assessment tool. An interactive tool to measure a woman's risk of invasive breast cancer. (http://bcra.nci.nih.gov/brc) Accessed May 12, 2004

Uter W, Pfahlberg A (1999) The concept of attributable risk in epidemiological practice. Biometrical Journal 41:985–999

Uter W, Pfahlberg A (2001) The application of methods to quantify attributable risk in medical practice. Statistical Methods in Medical Research 10:231–237

Wacholder S, Benichou J, Heineman EF, Hartge P, Hoover RN (1994) Attributable risk: Advantages of a broad definition of exposure. American Journal of Epidemiology 140:303–309

Wahrendorf J (1987) An estimate of the proportion of colo-rectal and stomach cancers which might be prevented by certain changes in dietary habits. International Journal of Cancer 40:625–628

Walter SD (1975) The distribution of Levin's measure of attributable risk. Biometrika 62:371–374

Walter SD (1976) The estimation and interpretation of attributable risk in health research. Biometrics 32:829–849

Walter SD (1980) Prevention for multifactorial diseases. American Journal of Epidemiology 112:409–416

Walter SD (1983) Effects of interaction, confounding and observational error on attributable risk estimation. American Journal of Epidemiology 117:598–604

Whittemore AS (1982) Statistical methods for estimating attributable risk from retrospective data. Statistics in Medicine 1:229–243

Whittemore AS (1983) Estimating attributable risk from case-control studies. American Journal of Epidemiology 117:76–85

Wooldridge JM (2001) Econometric analysis of cross section and panel data. MIT Press, Boston

Woolf B (1955) On estimating the relationship between blood group and disease. Annals of Human Genetics 19:251–253

Wu K, Brown P (2003) Is low-dose Tamoxifen useful for the treatment and prevention of breast cancer (editorial)? Journal of the National Cancer Institute 95:766–767

Zhang J, Yu KF (1998) What's the relative risk? A method of correcting the odds ratio in cohort studies of common outcomes. JAMA 280:1690–1691

Descriptive Studies

D. Maxwell Parkin, Freddie I. Bray

3.1   **Introduction**

We begin by setting out some definitions in descriptive epidemiology, the sources of data from which such studies arise and provide a brief outline of the sections that comprise this chapter.

3.1.1   **Definitions**

A distinction has traditionally be drawn between "descriptive" and "analytic" epidemiology, and their characteristics as 'hypothesis generating' or 'hypothesis testing', respectively, have been taught to generations of students. This distinction may perhaps reflect the dichotomy between distribution and of causes of disease, in the dictionary definition of Epidemiology (Last 2001): "The study of the distribution and determinants of health-related states or events in specified populations, and the application of this study to control of health problems".

Describing the distribution of disease is an integral part of the planning and evaluation of health care services, but, in the context of investigative epidemiology, the distinction is an arbitrary one. There are no real differences in the concepts, methods, or deductive processes between descriptive and analytic epidemiology, for example, between the information conveyed by the observations of an *association* between the risk of liver cancer and being engaged in a specific occupation, or having markers of infection by a certain virus. Both *may* tell us something about the *cause* of liver cancer. Only the *sources* of information differ. In the former case, it has derived from some routine source (a dataset or register maintained for general disease surveillance purposes, or even for unrelated administrative reasons). These sources include information on possible exposures or disease outcomes *that have not been collected with the testing of any specific hypothesis in mind*. It is this use of routinely collected data that characterises descriptive studies.

Descriptive epidemiology is certainly not synonymous with ecological studies of groups, as suggested by some authors (Estève et al. 1994), since most "descriptive" studies have information on distribution and levels of several exposure variables for individual members of the population studied. In their classic textbook, MacMahon and Trichopoulos (1996) liken this phase of epidemiological investigation to the early questions in the parlour game "20 questions" – using generally available information to focus down the field of enquiry to one that may need expensive ad hoc study. But the variables available in routine data sources are no less "exposures" from the point of view of methodology, or deductive reasoning, than are those measured by questionnaire, physical examination, or biochemical tests. The fact that some "exposures" may be remote from the molecular mechanisms involved in disease aetiology is a familiar one when considering "cause" of disease, especially from a public health perspective of devising appropriate methods of prevention. "Cause" is a relative concept, that only has meaning in epidemiology terms of its removal being associated with a diminished risk of the disease, and, in this context, it is just as relevant to improve educational levels in a population as a means of reducing infection by HIV as it is to identify the mechanisms by which the virus enters the host cell.

"Exposures" in descriptive epidemiology are those characteristics of individuals that are present in the pre-existing data sets available for study. The most commonly available are personal characteristics, the so-called "demographic" variables, systematically collected by vital statistics and health care institutions. They include birth date (or age), sex, address (current place of residence), birthplace, race/ethnic group, marital status, religion, occupation, and education. From sources within the health sector, there may be much more detail on diagnostic and therapeutic interventions, while community surveys may include information on health determinants, such as tobacco and alcohol use, weight, height, blood pressure, and so forth.

Disease outcomes may be in terms of incident cases (from disease registers), deaths (vital statistics), episodes of morbidity (utilisation statistics from health services), or prevalence of, especially, chronic conditions from population surveys.

Information on "exposure" and "outcome" for the same individual may be taken from a single source (e.g. a disease register, or population survey), or it may be necessary to perform record linkage between different sources to obtain exposure and outcome information on individuals in the population under study.

Sources of Data   3.1.2

There is a wide variety of sources of information that can be drawn upon for information on exposure and disease outcome. They are of two broad types: systems based on populations, containing data collected through personal interviews or examinations; and systems based on records, containing data collected from vital and medical records. They include:

- Census data, or population registers
- Vital statistics (especially death certificate data)
- Disease registers, recording new cases of specific diseases in defined populations (the best known example being cancer registries)
- Notification systems (especially for infectious diseases)
- Hospital activity statistics, especially on admissions/discharges from hospital, including diagnosis
- Primary care contacts
- Diagnostic services (pathology, etc)
- Community surveys (e.g., those carried out by the NCHS in the USA (Freid et al. 2003).

Some of these are described in Chap. I.4 of this handbook.

Outline of the Chapter   3.1.3

The chapter comprises four sections, beginning with an introduction of the most important measurements in descriptive epidemiology. Since these are primarily concerned with risk or burden of disease in a single population, appropriate methods for comparisons between populations – the hallmark of epidemiology – are required. Section 3.4 illustrates how these tools can be applied in the study designs familiar to epidemiologists, with a special emphasis on ecological studies. Section 3.5 provides a series of examples, illustrating the principles of descriptive studies.

3.2   Measurement

3.2.1   Incidence

Incidence is the number of new cases occurring. It can be expressed as an absolute number of cases or in relation to the size of the population at risk, and time during which the cases occur, as an incidence rate (cf. Chaps. I.2 and I.5 of this handbook). Incidence requires definition of the moment at which the disease "begins", when an individual becomes a new "case". This may be straightforward for many infectious diseases. However, for most, time of onset is less clear cut, and is by convention considered to be the time of diagnosis, although this is a somewhat arbitrary point in time, and dependant upon local circumstances. Incidence may refer to the number of new disease events, or to the number of individuals affected. The distinction is important where the same individual may have more than one event of the same disease, during the period of observation (e.g. common infections, accidents, etc).

Incidence data are available from disease registers, including notification systems for infectious diseases. Disease registers are part of surveillance systems for various diseases. When they are based on notification of disease events, their success depends upon the patient seeking medical advice, the correct diagnosis being made, and notification of it being made to the public health authorities. Completeness is very variable, but probably higher for serious or highly contagious diseases. Registers have been more important, and successful, for cancer than for any other condition. This is because of the serious nature of most cancers, which means that, except in a few societies without access to medical care and concepts, those affected will almost always present for diagnosis (and treatment, if available). As a result, enumeration of incident cases of cancer is relatively easy in comparison with other diseases, and this has permitted the establishment of a worldwide network of cancer registries, providing data on defined populations (Jensen et al. 1991). Incidence data from cancer registries worldwide that meet defined criteria regarding completeness and validity are published at five-year intervals in the Cancer Incidence in Five Continents series. The latest volume (8th) contains comparable incidence information from 186 registries in 57 countries, mainly over the period 1993–1997 (Parkin et al. 2002).

Other sources of information on incidence include:

1.   Retrospective or prospective surveys for incident cases of a particular disease. The approach is similar to ongoing registers, except that it is limited in time.

2. Community surveys. General morbidity surveys record all cases of disease appearing in a sample of the community, e.g. at primary care level, during a period of time. They are most efficient for relatively common conditions.

3. Hospital activity statistics. These summarise hospital admissions. Such statistics are usually *event*-based, so there may be multiple admissions for the same disease event. The numbers of hospitalisations is also affected by the facilities available, admissions policies, and social factors. It may be difficult to define the population at risk, unless national-level data can be compiled.

Incidence rates are of particular value in the study of disease aetiology, since they are informative about the risk of developing the disease in different population groups.

Prevalence

3.2.2

Prevalence is the number, or more usually, the proportion of a population that has the disease at a given point in time (Rothman and Greenland 1998; cf. Chap. I.2 of this handbook). For many diseases (e.g., hypertension, diabetes), prevalence usefully describes the number of individuals requiring care, and may be useful in planning health services. Prevalence is proportional to the incidence of the disease, and its duration (and when both are constant, then Prevalence = Incidence × Duration). In the absence of useful data on incidence or mortality, prevalence may be used to compare the risk of disease between populations, although this has clear drawbacks, not least because prevalence is related also to the mean duration of the disease. The mean duration may simply reflect the availability of effective treatment, allowing prolonged survival. For some chronic diseases, what to consider as the moment of cure (after which an individual is no longer a "case") is a problem when trying to calculate comparable indices of prevalence between populations (Pisani et al. 2002). Population surveys are a common source of information on prevalence of the more common conditions or complaints, including those that may exist in asymptomatic form, and therefore remain unrecognised in a clinical setting.

A less commonly used measure is *period prevalence*, which is the sum of all cases of the disease that have existed during a given period, divided by the average population at risk during the period. It has been used for studying mental illness, where the exact time of onset is difficult to define, and when it may be difficult to know whether the condition was present at a particular point in time.

Case Fatality/Survival

3.2.3

Case fatality is a measure of the severity of a disease. It is the proportion of cases of a particular disease that are fatal within a specified time. *Survival* is proportion of cases that do not die in a given interval after diagnosis (and is equal to 1-*fatality*). The survival time is defined as the time that elapsed between diagnosis and death. Computation of survival depends upon follow-up of diagnosed patients for deaths or withdrawal from observation. There are two related approaches to the estimation of survival: the Kaplan–Meier and actuarial, or life-table, methods. The former (Kaplan and Meier 1958) is particularly useful when exact survival times are available, since smooth estimates of survival as a function of time since diagnosis can be obtained. The actuarial method requires a life-table with survival times grouped usually into intervals that permit the calculation of the cumulative probability of survival at time t_i from the conditional probabilities of survival during consecutive intervals of follow-up time up to and including t_i (Cutler and Ederer 1958; Ederer et al. 1961). Information from all cases is used in the estimation of survival, including those withdrawn due their follow-up ending owing to closure of study, and those who are lost to follow-up before the termination. In both cases follow-up is censored before the time of the outcome event, usually the death of the patient. "Observed survival" is influenced not only by mortality from the disease of interest, but also by deaths from other causes. If these deaths can be identified, they can be treated as withdrawals, and the "corrected survival" (also referred to as "net survival") calculated. Alternatively, allowance for deaths due to causes other than the disease under study is made by calculation of "relative survival" (Ederer et al. 1961). This makes use of an appropriate population life-table to estimate expected numbers of deaths. The issue of competing risks is discussed in detail in Chap. I.2 of this handbook. For comparisons between different populations, age standardisation of survival is necessary (see Sect. 3.3.1).

For a more detailed description of survival analysis, see Chap. II.4 of this handbook.

3.2.4   Mortality

Mortality is the number of deaths occurring in a population, and is the product of the incidence and the fatality of the disease.

Mortality statistics derive from the information on death certificates, collected by civil registration systems recording vital events (births, marriages, deaths). The responsible authority varies between countries, but usually the first level of data collection and processing is the municipality or province, with collation of national statistics being the responsibility of the Ministry of Health, or the Interior Ministry. Death certificates record information on the person dying, and the cause of death, as certified, usually by a medical practitioner. The International Classification of Diseases (ICD) provides a uniform system of nomenclature and coding, and a recommended format for the death certificate (WHO 1992). Mortality statistics are produced according to the underlying cause of death; this may not equate with the presence of a particular disease. Although the ICD contains a set of rules and guidelines that allow the underlying cause to be selected in a uniform manner, interpretation of the concept probably varies considerably e.g. when death occurs from pneumonia in a person previously diagnosed as having cancer. Comprehensive mortality statistics thus require that diagnostic data is available on decedents, which are transferred in a logical, standardised fashion to death certificates, which are then accurately and consistently coded, compiled and analysed.

It is well known that mortality data may be deficient both in completeness of ascertainment, and in the validity of the recorded cause of death (Alderson 1981). A huge number of studies of the validity of cause of death statements in vital statistics data have been carried out. These compare cause of death entered on the death certificate with a reference diagnosis, which may be derived from autopsy reports (e.g. Heasman and Lipworth 1966), detailed clinical records (Puffer and Wynne-Griffith 1967), or cancer registry data (Percy et al. 1981). They reveal that the degree of accuracy of the stated cause of death declines as the degree of precision in the diagnosis increases. Despite the problems, mortality data remain the most valuable source of information on disease burden, and a useful proxy for risk of disease in many circumstances. A major advantage is in their widespread availability. About 30% of the world population is covered by national vital registration systems producing mortality statistics, including all of the developed countries, and many of the developing countries. National level statistics are collated and made available by the WHO (2004, http://www3.who.int/whosis). Nevertheless, some knowledge of the likely accuracy of the data available is a prerequisite to their intelligent use. Thus, the fact of publication by national and international authorities is not a guarantee of data quality. For some countries, or time periods, coverage of the population is manifestly incomplete, and the so-called mortality rates produced are implausibly low. The WHO Statistical Information System publishes tables of estimated coverage and completeness of mortality statistics in their database. As well as deficiencies in these, quality of cause of death information may be poor. This can sometimes be predicted when a substantial proportion of certificates are completed by non-medical practitioners. (WHO formerly published a useful table in 'World Health Statistics Annual' (WHO 1998) giving – for a few countries at least – the relevant percentage). Otherwise, quality of data must be judged from indicators such as the proportion of deaths coded to *Senility and Ill Defined Conditions*.

The mortality rate – the number of deaths in relation to the population at risk, in a specified period of time – provides an indicator of the average risk to the *population* of dying from a given cause (while fatality represents the probability that an *individual* with the disease will die from it). Mortality rates are the most useful measure of the impact, or burden of disease in a population. They are probably equally often used as a convenient proxy measure of the risk of acquiring the disease (incidence) when comparing different groups, because of their availability, although such use introduces the assumption of equal survival/fatality in the populations being compared.

The *infant mortality rate* is a widely used indicator of the level of health and development. It is calculated as the number of deaths in children aged less than one, during a given year, divided by the number of live births in the same year. Other similar indicators include the fetal death rate, stillbirth or late fetal death rate, perinatal mortality rate, neonatal mortality rate, and post neonatal mortality rate. These data may be collected by household survey, rather than the vital statistics system, especially in developing countries (United Nations 1984).

3.2.5 Person-Years of Life Lost (PYLL)

The concept of person-years of life lost (PYLL) was introduced over 50 years ago (Dempsey 1947) in order to refine the traditional mortality rates, by providing a weighting for deaths occurring at different ages. These methods started to become more widely used from the late 1970's in health services planning (Murray and Axtell 1974). There are many variations in the calculations used (summarised by Murray 1994). There are four variants of 'normal' lifespan against which to compare premature death. The simplest is to choose a fixed value for the potential limit where ages ranging from 60 to 85 have been used. *Potential years of life lost* are calculated as

$$\sum_{x=0}^{L} d_x(L-x) \, ,$$

where d_x is the number of deaths at age x, and L is the potential limit to life. This method gives no importance to deaths over the upper limit. To avoid this, calculating the *expected years of life lost*, using the expectation of life at the age of death (e_x), derived from an appropriate life-table, seems a better solution:

$$\sum_{x=0}^{l} d_x e_x \, ,$$

where l is the last age group and e_x is the expectation of life at each age. The expectation of life (e_x) may be taken from a period life-table, or more appropriately, be cohort-specific. This method is not suitable, however, for comparing between populations with different expectations of life. For this purpose, a standard expectation of life (e_x^*), taken from some ideal standard population, should be used. The calculated indicator then becomes the *standard expected years of life lost*. Another variation is to give different weights to years of life lost at different ages. The rationale is that the economic, or social, "value" of individuals varies with their age. In addition, discounting may be used, to give decreasing weights to the life years saved over time, admitting that life years in the future are valued less highly than at present (Das Gupta et al. 1972; Layard and Glaister 1994).

The approach has been taken a step further, with the development of indices that take into account non-fatal health outcomes of disease, such as "*Quality Adjusted Life Years (lost)*" (QALYs) or "*Disability Adjusted Life Years (lost)*" (DALYs) (Murray 1994; Morrow and Bryant 1995). Essentially, these admit that, between onset of a disease, and death or recovery, there is a spectrum of morbidity, which can be quantified in terms of its duration and severity. Three elements are needed in calculating these indices, therefore- the incidence of the disease, its mean duration or, equivalently, survival probability, and a measure of life "quality" in between onset and end of disease. The problem in using these indices lies in ascribing values to quality of life, or level of disability, since both are subjective, and will vary with time since diagnosis, and in different cultural and socio-economic settings. Nevertheless, the estimation of DALYs for different conditions worldwide has been widely used by the World Health Organization (WHO) as a means of establishing priorities for health care programmes (WHO 2000). The calculation involves summing the standard expected years of life lost (using a standard model life-table with expectation at life at birth being 82.5 for females and 80 for males), with the time lived between onset and death in different disability classes having a severity weighting between 0 and 1 (Table 3.1). Both an age weighting function, and a discount rate (of 3% per year) are applied (Murray and Lopez 1996).

Table 3.1. Definitions of disability weighting (Murray 1994)

	Description	Weight
Class 1	Limited ability to perform at least one activity in one of the following areas: recreation, education, procreation or occupation.	0.096
Class 2	Limited ability to perform most activities in one of the following areas: recreation, education, procreation or occupation.	0.220
Class 3	Limited ability to perform activities in two or more of the following areas: recreation, education, procreation or occupation.	0.400
Class 4	Limited ability to perform most activities in all of the following areas: recreation, education, procreation or occupation.	0.600
Class 5	Needs assistance with instrumental activities of daily living such as meal preparation, shopping or housework.	0.810
Class 6	Needs assistance with activities of daily living such as eating, personal hygiene or toilet use.	0.920

Rates of Disease 3.2.6

Although the dimensions of a health problem may be expressed by the absolute numbers of events (for example, the numbers of cases of infectious diseases, including AIDS, reported through WHO's surveillance data (WHO 2004, http://www3.who.int/whosis)), comparisons between population groups require that the number of events is related to the size of the population in which they occur, by the calculation of rates or proportions. "Rate", as the name implies, incorporates a time dimension – the number of events occurring in a defined population during a defined time period. The term rate is often used interchangeably with *risk*, although, the risk of disease is a probability, or proportion, and describes the accumulation of the effect of rates over a given period of time. Ideally, we would estimate a rate by ascertaining, for every individual in the population, the risk of being diagnosed or dying at a given age and specific point in time. This *instantaneous rate* requires that the designated period of time is infinitely small, approaching zero. In practice, the average rate of occurrence of new cases or deaths in a sufficiently large population is calculated for a sufficiently long time period. In this formulation, the denominator is the underlying *person-time at risk* in which the cases or deaths in the numerator arose. Prevalence, and survival, as defined above, are proportions (or percentages), not rates, as there is no time dimension, although the term "rate" is frequently appended.

3.2.7   Population at Risk

For the denominators of proportions, such as prevalence and survival, the population at risk comprises the number of individuals at a point in time. When rates are calculated, the time period of observation also needs to be specified. The denominator is calculated as units of person-time (Last 2001), whereby each person in the study population contributes one person-year for each year of observation before disease develops, or the person is lost to follow-up. In prospective cohort studies, the individuals can be followed up until the end of the study, and summation of the varying lengths of individual follow-up accurately represents the person-time at risk of disease. However, in descriptive epidemiology, information on the population-at-risk is not usually available at the individual level, unless there is an accurate population register. It is usually necessary to approximate person-years at risk using cross-sectional population data from national statistical organisations. The estimation of the denominator, a summation of the mid-year estimates for each of the years under consideration, is thus dependent on both the availability and completeness of demographic information on the population under study. In most developing and developed countries, 10-yearly population censuses provide basic population estimates by age, sex and census year, and statistical offices often produce estimates for intercensal years, based on rates of birth, death and migration. The approximation assumes there is stability in the underlying population, as individuals traverse the age-time plane represented by the well-known Lexis diagram (Fig. 3.1). The German demographer Lexis (1875) described this graphical representation of the life history of subjects according to birth cohort (the abscissa) and age (the ordinate). The modern interpretation of the Lexis diagram displays subjects arranged by calendar year of event and age at time of event on the same unit scale, with each cell corresponding to a year of birth, the diagonal tracing the experience of subjects born in the same year, who are under observation until either the end of follow-up, the event of interest occurs, or they are lost to follow-up. In the commonly tabulated system used for vital rates, a synthetic birth cohort over a 10-year range is derived from the combined experience of a 5-year age group over 5 years of occurrence. Approximate cohorts are identified by their central year of birth, and overlap each other by exactly five years. Given a steady state of demographic gains and losses, where the number of individuals in a designated period entering an age group equals the number that leave, the method can be considered to provide adequate estimates of the person-time at risk in most circumstances. For diseases that are relatively rare (of low prevalence), the estimate is not unduly biased by the fact that the numerator is a subset of the denominator.

It should be recalled that the number of units of person-time does not represent a number of independent observations. 100 person-years of observation may

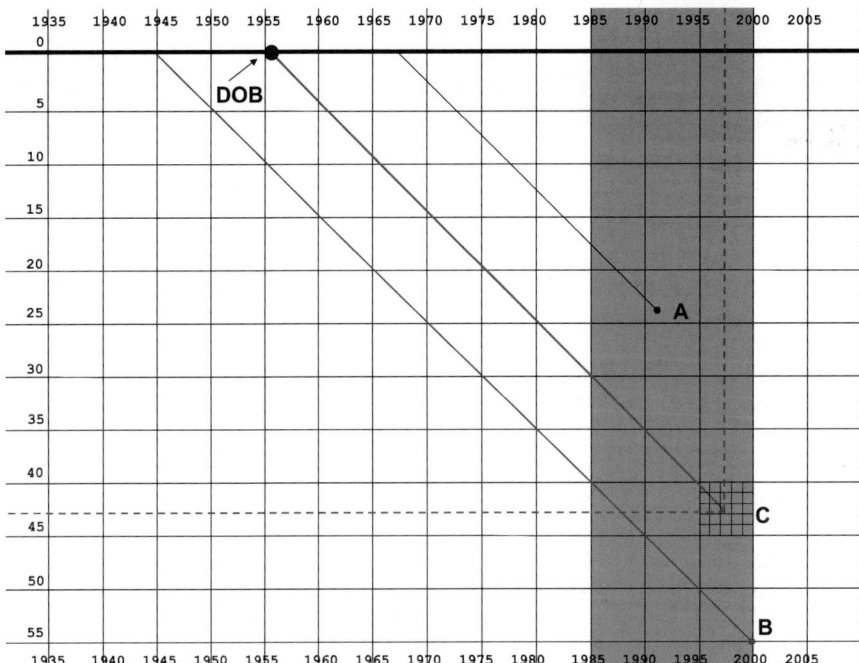

Figure 3.1. The modern Lexis diagram depicting three subjects under observation between 1985–2000. Individual A is lost to follow up aged 24 in 1991, B is alive at the end of follow-up (end of 2000) and C has the outcome of interest at the age of 42 in 1997 – the year of birth (DOB) can be ascertained for C by period – age = 1955, and his "life journey" represented by the diagonal line from DOB to 1997

result from 100 persons being followed for 1 year each, or from 20 people under observation for 5 years.

Population at risk should, ideally, only include those persons who are potentially susceptible to the disease being studied. Sometimes, this is taken into account in the denominator, for example in studying occupational diseases (where only those in the relevant occupation are at risk), and in infectious disease epidemiology, where a large proportion of the population is immune.

Comparisons Between Populations   3.3

In descriptive studies, comparisons between two or more populations are usually based on rates that account for the person-time at risk in each group using mid-year population estimates. The summary measure is estimated by stratifying on some well-known factor to remove its effect as a potential confounder. Comparisons of disease risk as a rule must take into account the effects of age, given its influence on both the disease process and the exposure of interest across groups.

The graphical representation of age-specific rates in a particular population describes how risk evolves with age. In comparing age disease curves in two (or more) populations it is a useful point of departure, often alerting the researcher to anomalies in the data, or to certain hypotheses that warrant further investigation. Standard methods exist for comparing rates in two or more populations. The simple techniques include the comparison of rates based on age standardisation, and stratification methods that pool the age-specific rates to obtain a weighted ratio (Mantel and Haenszel 1959). In the presence of heterogeneity in the age-specific rates, pooling or standardisation may not provide a satisfactory measure of relative risk, and visual inspections together with statistical tests that look for departures from the assumption of proportionality (homogeneity) should be investigated (Estève et al. 1994).

Greater flexibility and a more unified framework is a prerequisite when dealing with a series of population comparisons and, given most diseases are multifactorial, the analysis must consider the association between numerous factors on disease risk whilst adjusting for several potential confounders. Statistical models offer quantitative and comparable estimates of disease risk according to level of exposure based on objective criteria for choosing the best description of the data and whether variations observed are real or due to chance. Some methods for the analysis of two groups, and multiple groups are briefly described below.

3.3.1   Comparisons Between Two Groups

Standardisation

The Direct Method.   Crude rates can be thought of as a weighted sum of age-specific rates that render *biased* comparisons between populations, if the weights that represent the size of each age-stratum are different in each population compared. The age-standardised rate is the summary rate that would have been observed, given the schedule of age-specific rates, in a population with the age composition of some reference population, called the *standard*. The calculation of the standardised rate is an example of *direct standardisation*, whereby the observed age-specific rates in each group are applied to the *same* standard, i.e. the same age-specific weights. Age groups are indexed by the subscript i, d_i is the number of cases, y_i is the number of person-time at risk (frequently obtained by multiplying population estimates based on those at risk by the length of the observation period) and w_i is the proportion of persons or *weight* of age group i in the chosen standard population. The age-standardised rate (ASR) is given by:

$$\text{ASR} = \sum_i d_i w_i / y_i \, .$$

The main criticism of the technique stems from the need to select an arbitrary standard population. The most widely used reference for global comparisons is the world standard, as proposed by Segi (1960) on the basis of the pooled population of 46 countries, and modified for the first volume of *Cancer Incidence in Five Continents* by Doll et al. (1966). Although this does not really resemble the age structure of the current population of the world (so that ASR's will rarely be similar to crude rates), this is of little importance, since it is the *ratio* of ASR's (the standardised rate ratio), an estimate of relative risk between populations, that is the focus of interest. This has been shown to be quite insensitive to the choice of standard (Bray et al. 2002; Gillum 2002).

Another form of direct standardisation involves the cumulative risk, defined as the probability that an individual will develop the disease in question during a certain age span, in the absence of other competing causes of death. The age span over which the risk is accumulated must be specified. The age ranges 0–64 and 0–74 are generally used, and attempt to give two representations of the lifetime risk of developing the disease. Other age ranges may be more appropriate for more specific needs, such as investigating childhood diseases. If the cumulative risk using the above age ranges is less than 10%, as is the case for relatively rare diseases, it can be approximated very well by the cumulative rate (cf. Chap. I.2).

The cumulative rate is the summation of the age-specific rates over each year of age from birth to a defined upper age limit. As age-specific incidence rates are typically computed for five-year age intervals, the cumulative rate is then five times the sum of the age-specific rates calculated over the five-year age groups, assuming the age-specific rates are the same for all ages within the five-year age stratum. The cumulative rate from 0 to 74 is given by:

$$5 \sum_{i=1}^{15} d_i/y_i \, .$$

The precise mathematical relationship between the cumulative rate and the cumulative risk (Day 1992) is:

$$\text{cumulative risk} = 1 - \exp(-\text{cumulative rate}) \, .$$

The cumulative rate has several advantages over age-standardised rates. Firstly, the predicament of choosing an arbitrary reference population is irrelevant. Secondly, as an approximation to the cumulative risk, it has a greater intuitive appeal, and is more directly interpretable as a measurement of lifetime risk, assuming no other causes of death are in operation.

The Indirect Method. An alternative form of age standardisation, known as the *indirect method*, involves calculating the ratio of the total number of cases *observed* in the population of interest, $O = \sum_i d_i$, to the number of cases which would be *expected*, E, if the age-specific risks of some reference population applied. The expected number of cases in a study population is given by

$$E = \sum_i m_i y_i \, ,$$

where the m_i are age-specific rates for the reference population, and y_i the number of persons in age class i in the population of interest. The ratio is termed the standardised mortality ratio (SMR) when deaths and mortality rates are used; the terms "standardised incidence ratio" (SIR) or "standardised morbidity ratio" are used for incidence data. Expressed as a percentage, the calculation is:

$$\text{SMR (or SIR)} = \frac{O}{E} \times 100 \ .$$

There are two ways in which the reference population can be chosen. If the aim is to compare several populations with a specific reference population, then it would be sensible to choose a reference population with relatively large numbers of observed cases, since this increases the precision of the reference rates. A second strategy would be to create a pooled population from those to be compared; this has the advantage of increasing the precision of the reference rates and is analogous to comparing the observed rate in each population with that expected if the true age-specific risks were identical in all of the populations. Whichever approach is taken, it is important to realise that the SMRs of the individual populations can only be compared with the reference population. In addition, the SMR for population A compared with population B is *not* the inverse of the SMR for B compared with A.

Both direct and indirect standardisation can give a reasonable summary of a multiplicative effect, and are normally close in practice. Indirect standardisation however requires a further assumption of uniformity of the effect – the SMR has optimal statistical properties only if the force of incidence in the population of interest is *proportional* to that of the reference.

Direct standardisation is preferred for statistical reasons, given that a ratio of SMRs for two comparison groups may in some instances misrepresent the underlying stratum-specific ratios (Breslow and Day 1987). The risk ratio of two directly standardised rates (based on the same standard) has an associated confidence interval based on either exact variance calculations (Rothman and Greenland 1998) or a close approximation given by Smith (1987). As already mentioned, heterogeneity in the age-specific rates may render the relative risk estimate invalid.

Stratification: The Mantel–Haenszel (MH) Estimate

The standardised rate ratio is not a very efficient estimator of relative risk, since the weightings for the age strata are entirely arbitrary. More efficient summary measures assume uniformity across strata. The common rate ratio ϱ for population 1 compared with population 0 is $\varrho = \lambda_{1i}/\lambda_{0i}$. This relation can be written as $\lambda_{1i} = \lambda_{0i}\varrho$ or, in the form of a *log-linear model*, as:

$$\ln\left(\lambda_{1i}\right) = \ln\left(\lambda_{0i}\right) + \ln\left(\varrho\right) \ .$$

This is sometimes called the *multiplicative model*.

The Mantel–Haenszel (MH) estimate of the common rate ratio ϱ is simply the weighted average of the ratio of the age-specific rates

$$\hat{\varrho} = \frac{\sum\limits_{i} \dfrac{d_{1i} y_{0i}}{y_{\cdot i}}}{\sum\limits_{i} \dfrac{d_{0i} y_{1i}}{y_{\cdot i}}} ,$$

where $\cdot$ denotes summation over the index it replaces.

The Cochran–Mantel–Haenszel (CMH) tests the hypothesis $\varrho \neq 1$ against the null hypothesis $\varrho = 1$ (Cochran 1954), e.g. whether the force of incidence is identical in the two populations being compared ($\varrho = 1$). However the CMH test is valid only if the age-specific rate ratios are approximately proportional, i.e. $\varrho_i \approx \varrho$. Therefore, it is important to check this assumption. Several such tests are described by Breslow (1984); one method involves comparing the numbers of cases observed and expected under the assumption of proportionality, while another tests the same null hypothesis against the specific alternative of a trend (increasing or decreasing) in the age-specific rate ratios. The different hypotheses which can be tested and their corresponding alternative hypotheses are shown in Table 3.2 and Fig. 3.2. More details and the required formulae can be found in Estève et al. (1994).

Table 3.2. Null hypotheses and corresponding alternatives for the common rate ratio ϱ

H_0 (null hypothesis)	H_a (alternative hypothesis)
$\varrho = 1$	$\varrho \neq 1$, test for a common rate ratio (i.e. assumes proportionality)
$\varrho_i = \varrho$	ϱ_i unrestricted, test for heterogeneity in the ϱ_i
$\varrho_i = \varrho$	$\varrho_i = \varrho \times f(i)$, test for trend in the ϱ_i with the age values i

Comparisons Between Multiple Groups   3.3.2

In practice, when comparing multiple populations the simple methods above offer some serious limitations. Generally, a series of pairwise comparisons may yield spurious significant results due to multiple testing, and is therefore not appropriate. In indirect standardisation the choosing of the age-specific risks of one population as a reference over several others is inconsistent: the *ratio* of population 1 relative to population 0 is not the inverse of the *ratio* of the population 0 relative to population 1.

In most studies, there are a number of confounders that require examination and possible adjustment, other than age. The Mantel–Haenszel estimates may be extended to adjust simultaneously for several confounders but we may not have sufficient data to simultaneously consider many strata. In addition, it is not possible to classify an explanatory variable as an exposure or a confounder using

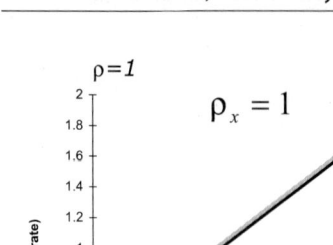

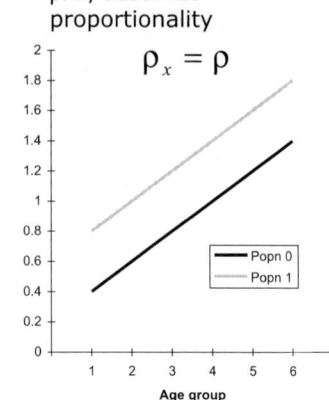

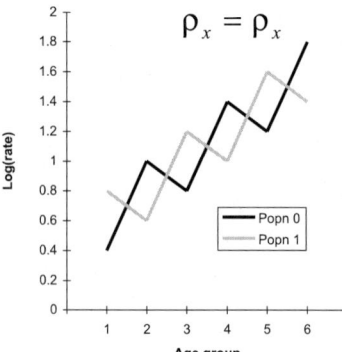

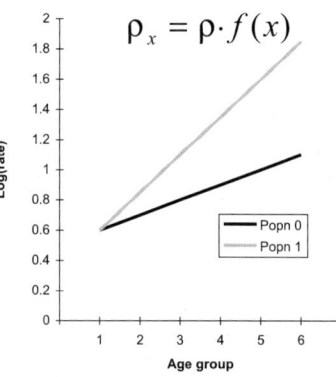

Figure 3.2. Graphical representation of the null hypotheses and alternatives described in Table 3.2

this method, and a separate analysis is required to obtain rate ratios for each exposure adjusted for the confounders.

A regression model provides a uniform framework for estimating the magnitude of the effect of interest, testing whether the effect is uniform across subgroups of the populations (effect modification), whether the effects of potential confounders may account for the effect, and whether a particular model given a parsimonious but adequate description of the observed data.

Further details on appropriate regression models as well as the techniques and strategies required in statistical modelling are described in Chaps. II.3 and II.4 of this handbook. A particular model that attempts to quantify trends in rates over time as a function of age, period of event, and year of birth is described in detail in Sect. 3.5.3.

Study Designs
in Descriptive Epidemiology

Data on Individuals

Investigation of observed associations between exposure variables, and disease outcome in individuals, may be investigated using cohort (prospective) (cf. Chap. I.5 of this handbook), case-control (retrospective) (cf. Chap. I.6) and cross-sectional-study designs.

Cohort Designs

The basic descriptive epidemiological study involves a comparison of disease rates in individuals categorized according to exposure variables that have been obtained from "routine" data sources, and relate to personal (demographic) characteristics, place (of residence, birth, diagnosis), and time (of birth, of diagnosis). The focus is on the risk in one exposure group, relative to another. Relative risks may be approximated by the ratio of disease rates, with person-years at risk estimated from census data (or population registers, if available). The simplest way to adjust for the major confounders (especially age) is by standardisation of the rates used for the rate ratios (Sect. 3.3.1). The idea of comparing summary rates for two populations seems appealing since we would hope to describe the differences between the two as a simple ratio. However, this simple description would only be appropriate if the proportional differences in age specific rates were constant across all age groups, i.e. – if the assumption of proportionality holds (see Sect. 3.3.1). The multiplicative model presented in Sect. 3.3.1 is important in descriptive cancer epidemiology, since the aim is generally to estimate ϱ and its statistical significance (Breslow 1984; Estève et al. 1994).

Alternatives to the rate ratios of age standardised rates are the Mantel–Haenszel estimate (MH) introduced in Sect. 3.3.1, which has been shown to be particularly robust, and the internal standardisation method of maximum likelihood (ML), which has optimal statistical properties (Breslow and Day 1975). Providing the assumption of proportionality of the ratio of the age-specific rates in the two groups is valid, the values obtained from the three methods should be close.

An alternative method of comparison is to calculate the standardised incidence ratio (SIR) for the populations being compared to a reference population (Sect. 3.3.1). This indirect standardisation is often preferred to direct standardisation to increase statistical precision for rare diseases or small populations. As already mentioned in Sect. 3.3.2, when more than one confounding variable (age) is present, the adjustment methods discussed above are not suitable, and it is more efficient to use standard log-linear modelling methods (Kaldor et al. 1990). When the population-at-risk in each cell of the cross-classification is available, it is assumed that the number of cases or deaths per cell has a Poisson distribution, with mean value proportional to the number of person-years at risk, and that the logarithm of the rate is a linear function of the classification variables. Poisson regression provides adjusted relative risk estimates for each population group, with reference to an appropriate standard. Even when age is the only confounding variable, statistical modelling has advantages over standardisation and related techniques in relative risk estimates with greater numerical stability (Breslow and Day 1987).

Case-Control Comparisons

Very often, in descriptive studies, the information on the cases/deaths is more detailed, in terms of variables of interest, than that on the population at risk. For example, the case file may include information on occupation, socio-economic status, or details about date of immigration, while the population-at-risk cannot be categorized in such detail. Analysis has to rely entirely on the numerator data, that is, on proportionate incidence or mortality data. Comparison of proportions between different case series via the proportionate mortality ratio (PMR) or proportionate incidence ratio (PIR) is generally, implicitly at least, an attempt to approximate the relative risk or ratio of rates. Confounding by age (as a result of different age structures of the case series being compared) can be removed by indirect standardisation techniques, with the fraction of deaths or of cases due to specific causes in the reference series as the standard (Breslow and Day 1987). Proportionate methods are, however, relative measures, and the PMR for a specific disease (age standardized) is close in value to the ratio of the SMR for the disease, to the SMR for all causes (Kupper et al. 1978).

Odds ratios provide a better estimate of relative risk than the ratio of proportions, in most circumstances (Miettinen and Wang 1981). Odds ratios are estimated by case-control comparisons, comparing exposure status among the cases of the disease of interest, and cases/deaths of other (control) diseases. Unconditional logistic regression or stratified analyses are performed to obtain maximum likelihood estimates of the odds ratios (Breslow and Day 1980). The odds ratio values based on logistic regression are heavily dependent on the choice of the controls: if the risk for the subjects used as controls is unrelated to exposure, the estimates from the logistic model for the effects of exposure closely approximate those which would be obtained using Poisson regression with denominator populations.

These methods have been widely used in the study of disease risk by social status and occupation (Logan 1982), and in migrant populations (Marmot et al. 1984; Kaldor et al. 1990).

Cross-Sectional Studies

In contrast to longitudinal studies, for which observations of cause and effect represent different points in time, cross-sectional studies *simultaneously* observe exposure status and outcome status at a single point in time, or over a short period in the life of members of a sample population. The analysis proceeds by determining the prevalence "rates" in exposed and non-exposed persons, or according to level of exposure, commonly using data from complete population surveys to correlate putative aetiological factors with outcome.

Cross-sectional studies are relevant to public health planning, in that they may provide information on the care requirements of a population at a given point in time. In the context of investigative enquiries, they can be considered advantageous to more complex designs in measuring the association between diseases of slow inception and long duration, where the time of onset is difficult to establish, such as osteoarthritis or certain mental disorders, and exposures that endure over a prolonged time period e.g. HLA antigens or air pollution levels. They are simpler, quicker and more economical than cohort (longitudinal studies), as no follow-up of individuals is required. In addition, the sample may be more representative of the target population as they are based on a sample of the general population.

There are however two major drawbacks to cross-sectional studies. Firstly, it is difficult to establish whether the temporal sequence is from that of exposure to outcome or vice versa. Are individuals, for instance, in lower socio-economic groups more likely to develop mental disorders, or is it that mental illness triggers a series of events that relegates persons from a wide-spectrum of socio-economic groups to a lower status at the time of measurement? Thus it is important to consider the possibility of reverse causation – whereby exposure status is in part a consequence of disease – the association obtained in a cross-sectional study may be wholly different from that obtained at time of the disease origin. Secondly, as it is usually not possible to determine incidence in cross-sectional studies, the use of prevalence as a proxy of frequency may distort the exposure-disease relationship as, by definition, the prevalence measure will include a larger number of cases with a long duration of disease relative to incidence. Hence persons who die or recover quickly tend to be less likely to be included as a prevalent case than persons with long-lasting disease.

In descriptive studies, measures of exposure and outcome are taken directly from existing survey datasets. These include general purpose datasets, such as that derived from the General Household Survey in the UK (Office for National Statistics 2004), a multi-purpose continuous survey which collects information on a range of topics, including health and the use of health services from people living in private households in Great Britain. Other datasets, more specific to health topics include the National Health Interview Survey (NHIS) and National Health and Nutrition Examination Survey (NHANES) carried out by the National Center for Health Statistics (2004) in the USA.

The analysis proceeds by classifying exposure and outcome status dichotomously in a contingency table. A *prevalence rate ratio* can be calculated as the ratio of the prevalence of the outcome in those exposed to the putative risk factor compared with those not exposed, or where the level of exposure varies by intensity, test for a trend in outcome by exposure category. A case-control approach to the analysis can also be taken, whereby the *odds ratio* is calculated, although it is important to appreciate that the two ratios are not equivalent and only approximate each other when the prevalence and odds are small and the disease is rare (cross-sectional studies however require relatively common outcomes). Confounding is an important bias (cf. Chap. I.9 of this handbook) and multivariate techniques such as logistic regression (estimating odds ratios) and proportional hazards models (estimating prevalence rate ratios) can be used when the outcome is, for example, the presence or absence of disease.

3.4.2   Ecological Studies

Main Characteristics

The characteristic of ecological studies is that *exposure* and *outcome* are measured on *populations/groups*, rather than on individuals. The units of observation may be populations defined by place of residence (counties, regions, districts, etc), by personal characteristics, such as race, religion, or socio-economic status, or by time (birth cohorts). Usually, these studies are descriptive, in that they exploit pre-existing sources of information, rather than data collected to investigate a specific hypothesis. Thus, the outcome (disease) data are the likes of mortality rates, incidence rates, or prevalence data from health surveys. Exposure information may be from sources such as household/community surveys, environmental measurements, or commercial sources (data on production or sales). Exposure is expressed as an aggregate (summary) measure such as population mean, median, proportion etc. based on observations from individuals within the group. Exposure data may also be some environmental measurement (e.g. of air pollution, ambient temperature, etc). The essential difference from most epidemiological study designs is that there is no information on the joint distribution of exposure and outcome in the individuals *within* the populations being studied. Table 3.3 shows two populations (A and B). In studies in which data on individuals are available, the numbers in the individual cells of each table are known, and we may calculate relative risks or odds ratios for each (and combine the results from the two strata). However, in an ecological study, only the values in the margins of each table (with n_{EA} denoting the number of exposed and $n_{\bar{E}A}$ the number of non-exposed subjects in population A and n_{DA} denoting the number of diseased and $n_{\bar{D}A}$ the number of non-diseased subjects in population A, analogously for population B) are known, so that we have simply prevalence of exposure, and disease incidence or prevalence, for populations A and B.

Ecological studies may be used to generate (or test) aetiological hypotheses, and to evaluate interventions at the population level.

The main problem, as described below, is that ecological designs are usually being employed to make such inferences (concerning cause/prevention) about individuals, based upon observations using groups. Such interpretations are prey to a variety of artefact, referred to collectively as "the ecological fallacy" (Piantadosi et al. 1988). However, ecological studies may have particular value when some characteristic of the group (rather than the sum of individuals within it) is important in determining outcome, so that ecological designs are more appropriate than studies of individuals within the groups (see Sect. 3.4.2). Similarly, ecological studies may be used to evaluate the effect of population-level interventions, especially if the interest is in the effect at group rather than individual level. Thus, the relationship between exercise and mortality from cardiovascular disease may be known from individual based studies, but the effectiveness of an educational programme on

Table 3.3. Ecological study: comparison of prevalence of exposure and outcome in two populations A and B

	A		
	Diseased	Non-diseased	Total
Exposed	?	?	n_{EA}
Unexposed	?	?	$n_{\bar{E}A}$
Total	n_{DA}	$n_{\bar{D}A}$	

$$\text{prevalence of exposure in A} = \frac{n_{EA}}{n_{EA} + n_{\bar{E}A}}$$

$$\text{rate of disease in A} = \frac{n_{DA}}{n_{DA} + n_{\bar{D}A}}$$

	B		
	Diseased	Non-diseased	Total
Exposed	?	?	n_{EB}
Unexposed	?	?	$n_{\bar{E}B}$
Total	n_{DB}	$n_{\bar{D}B}$	

$$\text{prevalence of exposure in B} = \frac{n_{EB}}{n_{EB} + n_{\bar{E}B}}$$

$$\text{rate of disease in B} = \frac{n_{DB}}{n_{DB} + n_{\bar{D}B}}$$

the topic in influencing disease rates might choose an ecological design, to capture the combined effect at group and individual level.

Types of Design

Exploratory Ecological Studies.   The term "exploratory ecological study" has sometimes been used to describe the comparison of disease rates between populations defined, for example, by place of residence, ethnic group, birthplace, or birth cohort (Estève et al. 1994; Morgenstern 1982). In fact, it is hard to understand the justification for the use of the term "ecological" for such studies. They compare disease risk among individuals characterised by various exposure variables (such as place of residence, or birthplace, or period of birth), and as such, differ only in the source of information, from cohort studies using questionnaires or biological measurements, comparing disease rates according to exposure type or level (occupational groups, smoking status, etc). Probably, the term should be reserved for comparisons between groups in which "exposure" has not been measured, but is simply assumed from some sort of a priori knowledge or guesswork. This is the basis of many studies carried out with quite sophisticated laboratory methods, where the subjects comprise some sort of sample (usually by no means random) from populations believed to be at high/medium/low exposure of something. Another version would be studies in which exposure is not measured, and may not even be defined, but is assumed to have some underlying spatial or temporal distribution; the purpose of the analysis is to see if disease risk in the population groups studied has, too. This includes studies of geographical clustering and of spatial autocorrelation (cf. Chap. II.8 of this handbook).

Multigroup Comparison Ecological Study. This is the most commonly used study design. For several populations (usually geographical regions), outcome (disease) levels (prevalence, rates) are compared with exposure (means, proportions) to variables of interest. An example is given by the early studies suggesting the importance of blood lipids in the aetiology of ischaemic heart disease. Coronary heart disease rates were compared with plasma cholesterol and dietary fat intake in different populations (McGill 1968). Figure 3.3 shows a well-known example from Doll and Peto (1981), relating lung cancer mortality to consumption of manufactured cigarettes.

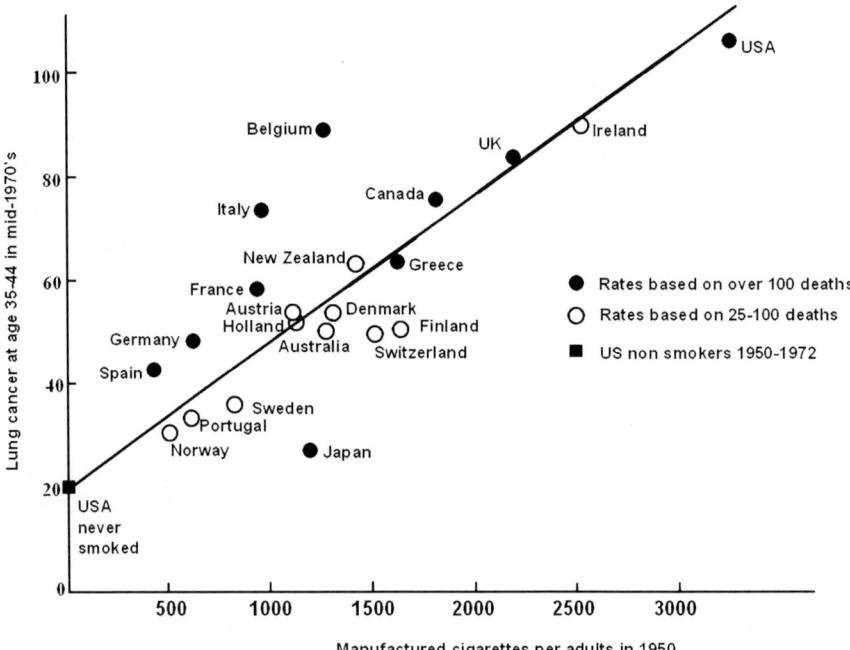

Figure 3.3. International correlation between manufactured cigarette consumption per adult in 1950 while one particular generation was entering adult life (in 1950), and lung cancer rates in that generation as it enters middle age (in the mid-1970s)

Time Trend Ecological Studies. A single population is studied, but is cut up into *groups* corresponding to different time periods. The objective of the study is to determine whether the time trend in outcome (disease rates) corresponds to time trend in exposure.

Multiple Group Time-trend Ecological Studies. These are a mixture of multigroup and time trend designs. Change in exposure and outcome over time is compared for several populations. Dwyer and Hetzel (1980) compared time trends in coronary heart disease mortality in three countries in relation to changes in major risk factors. The advantage of this design is that it is less subject to confounding than with a single population, i.e. the unmeasured factor, related to both exposure and outcome (change in disease) is unlikely in several different populations, but quite possible in one.

Analytic Methods

The simplest level of analysis is to plot the disease rate and indicator of exposure for each population on a scattergram, and to calculate a correlation coefficient. This merely indicates the level (strength and direction) of association between the parameters; it does not necessarily imply that the exposure variables predict outcome, rather that other influencing factors (confounders) are likely to have been well controlled in the ecological grouping. Moreover, the correlation coefficients may be quite biased, especially if the groups for study have been chosen on the basis of their level of exposure.

More usually, interest lies in quantifying the magnitude of the effect to be expected from different levels of exposure, and regression of group-specific disease rates (Y) on group-specific exposure prevalence (x) is the method employed. The simple linear model ($Y = \alpha + \beta x + \varepsilon$ with ε denoting an error term) is typically used. An estimate of the effect of exposure (at the individual level) can be derived from the regression results (Beral et al. 1979). The relative risk is the ratio of the disease rate (Y) in an exposed population ($x = 1$) divided by the rate in an unexposed population ($x = 0$) Assuming the above linear model for Y, this results in

$$RR = \frac{\alpha + \beta \times 1}{\alpha + \beta \times 0} = \frac{\alpha + \beta}{\alpha} = 1 + \frac{\beta}{\alpha} .$$

If a log-linear model is fitted, such that $\ln(Y) = \alpha + \beta x + \varepsilon$, then the estimate of relative risk can be derived as $\exp(\beta)$. For more details on regression models we refer to Chap. II.3 of this handbook.

These equations assume that the groups studied are perfectly homogenous for exposure, and that the relationship modelled (prediction of disease rate) is valid at both extremes of exposure (nil, or total), a situation that is rarely observed in practice. Homogeneity of exposure is unlikely, of course, and the summary statistics (means, medians) have large and unknown error terms. Trying to mitigate the problem by studying small population gives rise to different technical problems (measurement error, migration), and a larger variance of estimated disease rates.

In the situation where the rates in the different populations being compared have different precision (due to varying size), weighted regression is frequently used, to give more emphasis to the larger units. The usual weighting applied is the inverse of the variance, although maximum likelihood methods (taking into account variation in rates that would be expected by chance) may be more appropriate (Pocock et al. 1981)

Time Lagging. It is reasonable to take exposure date from an earlier period than that for the outcome (disease). Varying the interval to obtain the best fit (correlation, for example) has been used to provide information on the possible induction period between exposure and disease. Rose (1982) found that the correlation between serum cholesterol and coronary heart disease mortality in men aged 40–59 in 7 countries was maximal when the interval between the two measures was 15 years.

Advantages of Ecological Studies

There are several advantages to ecological study designs.

- They are very economical, since they use existing data on exposure and outcome, with no costs involved in collection.
- They are very rapid; even compared with case-control studies, where time is needed for recruitment, e.g., for investigating suspect clusters.
- Very large numbers can be studied, so that *small* increases in risk can be investigated. Small risks affecting large numbers of people are important from a public health point of view.
- They may – and ideally do – include populations with a very wide range of exposure level (more than can be found in a single population used for conventional cohort or case-control studies). For example, the range of variation in dietary fat intake in a single population may be too small to demonstrate the differences in risk at different levels (Prentice and Sheppard 1990).
- They may be the only practical analytic approach to investigating the effects of an exposure that is *relatively constant* in a population, but differs *between* populations e.g. exposure to external environment (air, radiation, water).
- In many circumstances, individual measures of exposure are difficult or impossible to obtain. This is often the case in studies of diet and disease, since collection of individual food records is difficult, may not reflect habitual intake, and does not allow for individual variability in metabolic response to a given diet. 24-hour dietary recalls, although of little value in the study of dietary exposures in individuals, may, when averaged for a population, may provide a useful indicator of exposure for ecological analysis. The same principles apply to average exposures to air pollution, trace elements in soil/water, and so on.
- There may be interest in "contextual effects", that is group or community level effects, rather than inferences about individual exposure-outcome. This is particularly important in communicable disease epidemiology, where models of transmission have a group component e.g. transmission of vector borne-diseases will be dependant upon the prevalence of carriers in the population (Koopman and Longini 1994). Ecological studies are relevant in examining the effects of policy, laws, social processes where contextual, as well as individual effects, are relevant to the outcome.

Disadvantages of Ecological Studies

The above advantages have to be contrasted with several disadvantages, not only from a technical perspective.

Technical Disadvantages.

— *Data problems*

The data on exposure are obtained from existing sources, usually not compiled for the purpose for which they are being used, and may in consequence lead to a somewhat inaccurate estimator of the relevant exposure. Thus, data based on production, sales, or food disappearance give only an approximate guide to actual exposure, even at the group level. If the data are from a sample of the population, this may be unrepresentative of the group. The outcome (disease) variables are subject to similar concerns. Data quality may differ between the populations, due, for example, to varying completeness of death registration. Lack of comparability may also result from changes in disease classification or coding over time. A further concern is the accuracy of person-years at risk for group data. This is an issue for all types of descriptive study, where person-years at risk are estimated from cross-sectional counts, rather than longitudinal observation of individuals. Moreover, migration of populations will make comparisons over time difficult since cases of disease may not be exactly from the exposed population. This problem is compounded if migration is related to the presence of the disease studied. A solution commonly adopted is simply to assert that the populations studied are "stable", without having any objective evidence to that effect.

Misclassification of exposure within the groups being studied may have surprising consequences. Even when non-differential (unrelated to outcome) the bias in estimated risk of exposure may be away from the null value – the opposite to the familiar situation in individual-based studies (Brenner et al. 1992).

— *Availability of data*

The number of variables available for the populations studied is quite limited. There is little scope for any adjustment for possible confounding (limited though this is in ecological studies).

— *Problem of induction period*

It is reasonable to assume that there is some delay between exposure and outcome, and that both should not be measured at the same time. It is not difficult to find published studies in which the exposure measures post-date those of outcome. Some time lag should be included (e.g. Fig. 3.3), but this involves assumptions, possibly arbitrary, as to the appropriate mean interval to use. Furthermore, exposure information may not be available for the relatively distant past, and, when it is, the population in the units of analysis will comprise different individuals, if exposure and outcome measures are far apart in time.

— *Ecological fallacy*

It is the main problem when inferences about individual exposure-outcome associations are being inferred from observations at the group level (Piantadosi et al. 1988). In this instance, the assumption being made is that the single

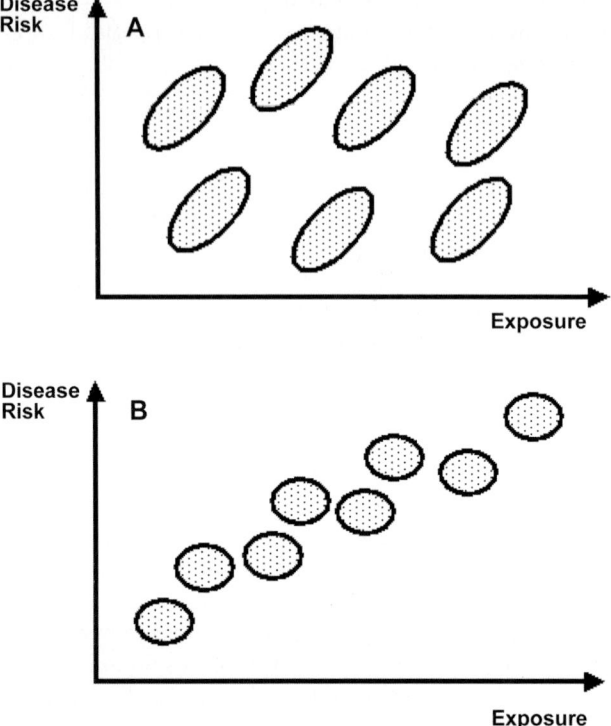

Figure 3.4. Two situations illustrating the difference between ecological and individual associations between exposure and disease (from Walter 1991)

measure of exposure applies to all members of the group. This is rarely so. Often, it is obvious (e.g. exposure variable is a group mean, with its own variance). Else, it is intuitive (e.g. exposure variable is an environmental measure – e.g. solar UV, nitrate in drinking water) but individual behaviours result in varying exposure to it (wearing hats, long holidays or work periods elsewhere, using bottled water, etc.). As a result, there may be a difference between the relationship at the individual level (within groups) and group level (between groups). Ecological associations may be weaker, or stronger, than relevant associations at individual region. Figure 3.4 (from Walter 1991) illustrates two extreme scenarios. In A, there is a strong covariance between exposure and outcome within groups, but a very weak one between groups. An ecological analysis, based on a single aggregate measure of exposure and outcome for each group would show only a weak association. In B, the association within groups is weak, but appears strong when examined between groups.

– *Ecological bias*
Due to the failure of the expected ecological effect estimates to reflect the biological effect at the individual level, two forms of bias are said to exist (Mor-

genstern 1982). Aggregation bias: data are aggregated, ignoring the information from the subgroups from which the individual observations came. Specification bias: a problem of using groups that in some way are related to the disease (irrespective of the exposure under study). It may result from extraneous risk factors being differentially distributed by group, or from property of the group itself (contextual effects). The sum of these two components provides "the ecological bias" (cross level bias) which is present. Table 3.4 gives an example.

Table 3.4. An example of ecological (cross level) bias

Population	Prevalence of exposure	Exposed		
		n_E	N_E	R_E
A	0.25	1200	1×10^6	1.2
B	0.50	3330	2×10^6	1.67
C	0.75	6000	3×10^6	2.0
All	(0.50)	10,530	6×10^6	1.76

Population	Non-exposed			Total		
	$n_{\bar{E}}$	$N_{\bar{E}}$	$R_{\bar{E}}$	n_T	N_T	R_T
A	1800	3×10^6	0.6	3000	4×10^6	0.75
B	1670	2×10^6	0.84	5000	4×10^6	1.25
C	1000	1×10^6	1.0	7000	4×10^6	1.75
All	4470	6×10^6	0.75	15,000	12×10^6	1.25

The relative risk of exposure in each of the three populations, A, B and C, is 2.0 ($R_E/R_{\bar{E}}$ with R_E and $R_{\bar{E}}$ denoting the disease rates in the exposed and non-exposed subjects, respectively), i.e., there is no difference in the effect of exposure within the different groups. Although the overall (crude) relative risk, summing the cases and populations at risk for the three groups is 2.35 = 1.76/0.75, the relative risk, standardized for group, can be estimated by

$$\widehat{RR} = \frac{\sum n_E}{\sum (n_{\bar{E}} N_E)/N_{\bar{E}}},$$

where the summation is across groups, with n_E denoting the number of diseased subjects among the exposed and N_E denoting the total number of exposed subjects in the population (analogously for the non-exposed and the total population). In the example shown, therefore

$$\widehat{RR} = \frac{1200 + 3330 + 6000}{(1800*1)/3 + (1670*2)/2 + (1000*3)/1} = 2.0 .$$

The difference between the unadjusted and adjusted estimates (2.35 and 2.0) shows that there is confounding by other risk factors, which are different between the groups (as shown by different risks in the non-exposed) indicating a specification bias. Figure 3.5 shows the linear regression of the rate of disease (R_T) on the prevalence of exposure, and the ecological estimate of relative risk (Sect. 3.4.2). The large difference between the estimates based on ecologic and crude individual data (9.0 and 2.35) is the result of aggregation bias since the extraneous factor that increases the risk among the non-exposed is most prevalent in the most exposed population (C).

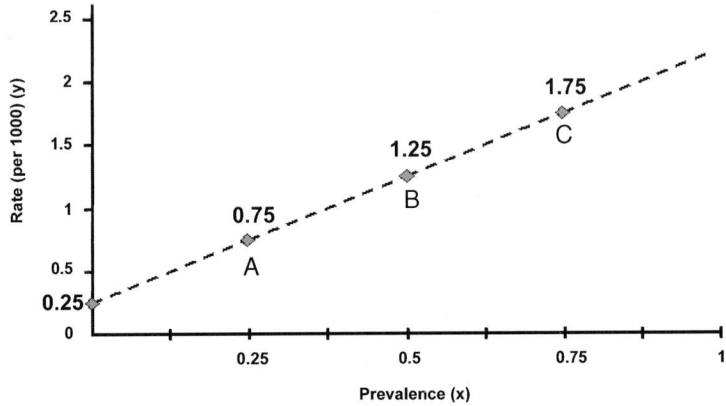

Figure 3.5. Ecological analysis (linear regression: $y = \alpha + \beta x$) of the hypothetical data summarised in Table 3.4: $\alpha = 0.25$, $\beta = y - \alpha/x = 2.0$, $RR = 1 + \beta/\alpha = 9.0$

Confounding and Effect Modification in Ecological Studies. Confounding in epidemiological studies arises when two exposure variables are statistically associated (correlated), and at least one of them is also an independent risk factor for the disease under study, so that both will appear to be so if examined separately. In individual-based studies, with many subjects, it is feasible to separate their effects (by stratification, or multivariate methods), because perfect correlation between variables is very unlikely. When groups are studied, however, there may be perfect correlation between variables, particularly if the populations studied are few in number (e.g. the hi-lo two group studies beloved of laboratory workers), and large in size.

Furthermore, risk factors that are independent of exposure at the individual level may be correlated with it, and thus be confounders, when aggregated at the population level. Conversely, a confounding variable at the individual level may not be so at the ecological level; for example, although the risk of most cancers is quite different in males and females, sex, as an ecological variable, will not be associated with disease rates in geographical areas because the ratio of males to females is broadly similar in all.

Effect modification (or interaction) refers to variation in the magnitude of the effect of an exposure across the levels of a third (covariate). Effect modification can be present in an ecological association, even when not evident at the individual level. Greenland and Morgenstern (1989) give an example of a cofactor (e.g. nutritional deficiency) with different prevalence in the populations (regions) studied, which is not a risk factor in the absence of the study factor (smoking). Thus, the non-smoker rates would be the same in all regions (and region would not, therefore, be a confounder in an individual based study of smoking and disease), but the effect of smoking would differ by region.

Descriptive Studies

Personal Characteristics

Routine sources of information on morbidity and mortality include information on the so-called "demographic" variables (age, sex, marital status, religion, race, education, occupation etc) of the cases, and the corresponding data on population-at-risk may likewise be available. This allows investigations of how characteristics of the individual relate to the risk of disease. Since they may often have striking effects on disease intensity, a number of these variables (particularly age) can be considered as amongst the foremost risk factors for many diseases. Exploration of the relationship between personal characteristics and disease have generated and confirmed many hypotheses, and importantly, elucidated particular mechanisms concerning other putative factors, by taking account of the strong confounding effects of routine variables that may otherwise have distorted the relationship between outcome and the exposure of interest.

Age

The increases with age in morbidity of, and mortality from, disease are more apparent than for any other variable. Excluding accidental and violent deaths, there is a 500-fold variation in the death rate from all causes between the ages of 20 and 80 (Peto and Doll 1997). For epithelial cancers, as well as for cardiovascular disease and chronic respiratory disease, there is more than a 1000-fold difference. The age-specific patterns also differ between and within diseases; Fig. 3.6 compares the age-specific incidence of several types of cancer. The effects of age are most commonly ascribed to an individual's cumulative exposure to environmental insults (e.g. socio-cultural or behavioural factors) over a life span, or in the case of, for example, breast cancer, to the effects of hormonal changes. While the process of ageing is commonly put forward as a possible mechanism in its own right e.g. through declining immunological defences, or an increasing number of mutations in certain somatic cells (Lilienfeld and Lilienfeld 1980), others suggest that while ageing is clearly related to disease, there is no evidence that ageing itself is a biological process that causes disease (Peto and Doll 1997).

The fundamental importance of age as a major confounder in almost all epidemiological studies is exemplified by age standardisation or stratification to control for its effects (see Sect. 3.3.1).

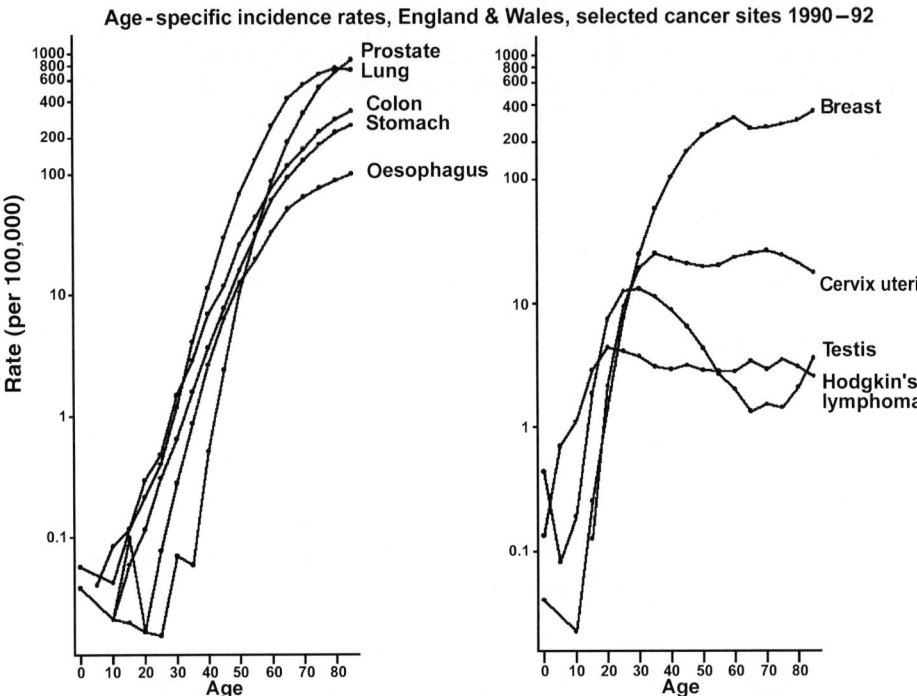

Figure 3.6. Age-specific incidence rates. England and Wales, selected cancer sites, 1990–1992

Interesting forms of the distribution of disease risk by age have motivated a series of hypotheses as to the biological mechanisms underlying particular diseases. The bimodality of Hodgkin lymphoma (Fig. 3.6) suggested that it comprised at least two distinct forms of the cancer, and the likelihood of differing aetiologies. Early investigations seeking biological explanations for particular age-disease patterns led to hypotheses concerning the importance of early development to disease later in life. More recently, a life course approach to chronic and infectious disease has been conceptualised, which considers the long-terms effects of factors during gestation, childhood and adolescence on subsequent adult morbidity or mortality (Kuh and Ben-Shlomo 1997).

The importance of period of birth (birth cohort) is clear when investigating changes in disease risk over time (see Sect. 3.5.3); it was through the study of age-curves that the influence of generation effects on disease were first realised, however. In examining the age-specific mortality rates from tuberculosis in different calendar periods of time, Frost (1939) after Andvord (1930) showed that the peak in more recent cross-sectional age-mortality curves (in 1930) at later ages (50–60) compared to peaks in young children (0–4) previously (in 1880) and at the ages 20–40 (in 1910) was an illusion – an examination of the same age curves by cohort indicated subjects comprising the 1930 age curve passed through greater risks in previous decades – the class of individuals whom were children in 1880 and who were aged 50–60 (if still alive) by 1930 (Fig. 3.7). In concluding, he noted that contemporary peaks of mortality in later life did not signify a postponement of maximum risk, but rather were the residuals of higher rates in early life.

Korteweg (1951) similarly demonstrated that a cross-sectional view of age curves of lung cancer mortality led to an erroneous interpretation as the age curves were artificially pushed down by the increase in lung cancer in younger age groups – the consistent pattern of declining rates at relatively early ages (65 and over) for five consecutive periods between 1911 and 1945 was therefore not an observation that required a biological explanation. The mechanisms that promoted lung cancer, he observed, acted particularly (but not exclusively) in younger people.

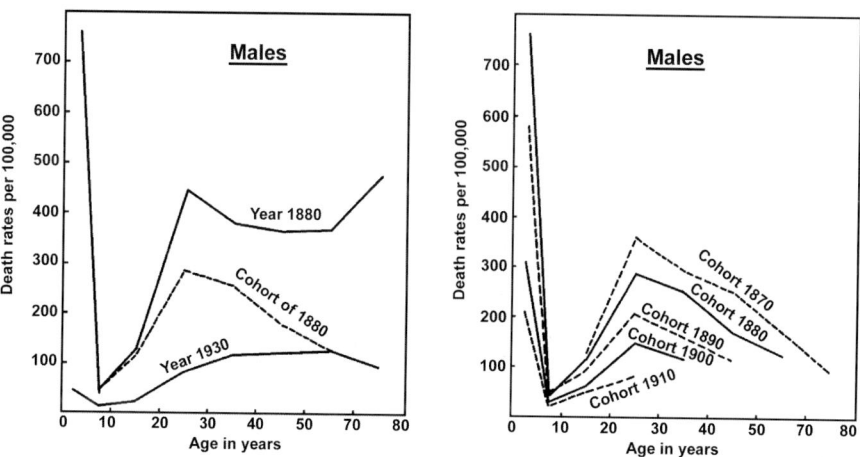

Figure 3.7. Age-specific mortality rates from tuberculosis in Massachusetts, by period (a) and by birth cohort (b) (Frost 1939)

Several well-known biases may distort the underlying age disease relationship. The quality of mortality statistics in the very elderly is particularly affected by the precision and coding of the death certificate, as well as the decision as to the underlying cause of death. For incidence data, case ascertainment is less effective in the very old, in part due to inaccuracy in the abstraction and coding of diagnostic information, in part due to competing causes of death.

Sex

There are, for certain diseases, substantial differentials in the rates in men compared to women (sex ratio), that may represent fundamental differences in exposure to environmental risk factors, and/or response to them. Mortality rates from several common causes of death, such as ischaemic heart disease, malignant neoplasms, and HIV-AIDS (in western countries), have sex ratios substantially greater than one. The disparity is perhaps not surprising given the contrasting social, cultural and behavioural practices of men and women, and the strong lifestyle component of such diseases. Other than environmental exposures, endogenous factors, such as the sex hormones, may contribute to differences in risk between the sexes, acting as promoters of disease pathogenesis or as protective factors, while our understanding of the putative impact of sex-specific genetic predisposing factors is in its infancy.

The marked differences between the sexes in the incidence of some common cancers are shown in Fig. 3.8; for many of these neoplasms much of the variation can be explained by contrasting levels of exposure to well-established carcinogens in men relative to women. Hence, the high male:female (M:F ratio) for mesothelioma is largely a consequence of historical exposure to asbestos in men through certain occupations, while lung cancer largely replicates the past history of tobacco smoking in men relative to women. Based on site-specific M:F ratios of age-standardised rates in developed countries, the majority of the cancers of the head and neck, as well as of the bladder and oesophagus are also much more common in men reflecting the heavier alcohol consumption acting independently and multiplicatively with tobacco smoking.

For M:F ratios lower than one, the most outstanding example is for breast cancer for which there is a 500-fold difference in risk in women relative men, which might be attributable to the mammary gland mass, as a correlate of the number of cells susceptible to transformation, as well as hormonal milieu. Differences in gallbladder cancer are probably attributable to a higher prevalence of gallstones in women relative to men. A corresponding distribution of sex-ratios is observed for cancer mortality, but additionally, differences in survival, (through gender rather than biological differences e.g. stage of presentation) modifies the differentials.

Ethnic Group

Variations in the risk of disease and differences in the health experience of individuals from different ethnic groups have been the subject of many studies (Macbeth and Shetty 2001). Studies within multi-ethnic societies are more valuable than international comparisons, if the primary variable of interest is ethnicity or racial group, since at least some of the environmental differences present in international comparisons are reduced or eliminated. There are plenty of examples of such studies from multi-ethnic populations in all parts of the world.

Interpretation of ethnic differences in risk should first consider the possibility of data artefact. Even within a single country, it is possible that differential access to health care and diagnostic services by ethnic group may influence reporting rates of disease, for example, access to and acceptance of screening programmes has been shown to differ by ethnic group in several countries (Parker et al. 1998; Seow et al. 1997). Differences in access to treatment certainly can affect outcome, so that survival rates from cancer are well known to vary by race/ethnicity (Baquet and Ringen 1986); since mortality rates are determined by both incidence of disease and survival, this is a major consideration if mortality is being used, as it often is, to provide information on cancer risk.

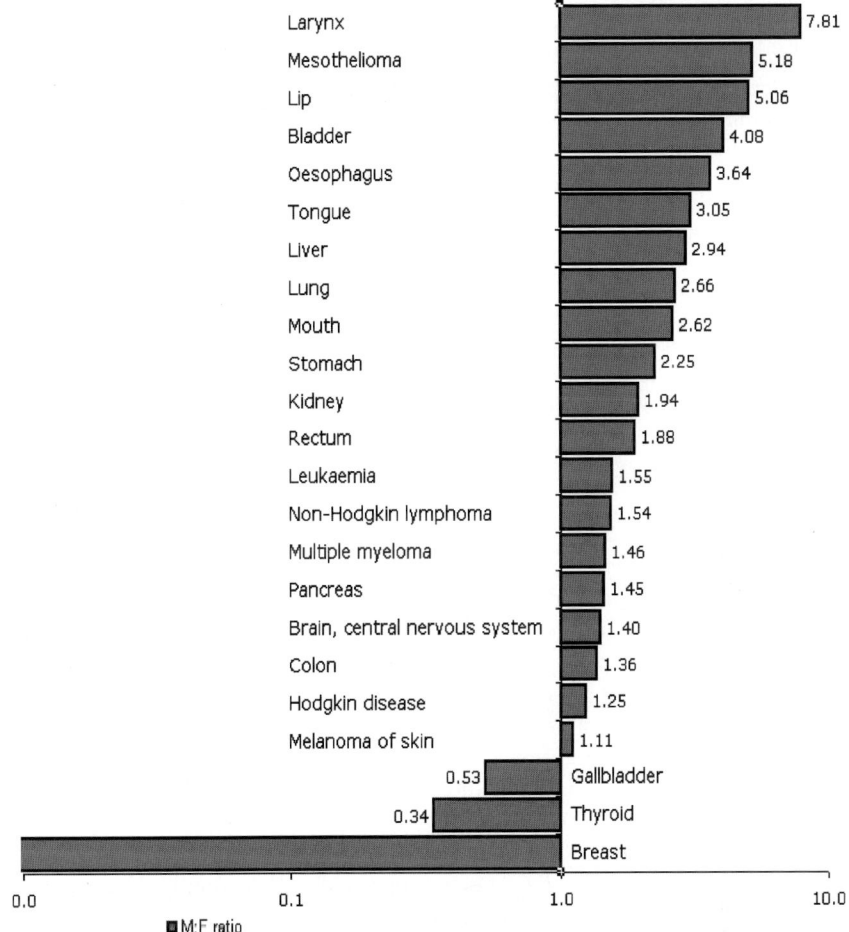

Figure 3.8. M:F ratios of age-standardised rates for the common cancers in developed areas worldwide (Parkin et al. 2002)

Artefact aside, the principal question posed by observed inter-ethnic differences in risk is how much is due to variation in exposure (to "carcinogens" or "risk factors"), and how much is the result of inherent differences in susceptibility to such exposures (and hence genetically determined).

From an epidemiological point of view, the variable 'ethnicity' or 'race' defines a constellation of genetic factors, which relate to susceptibility to a given disease. Of course, there is considerable variation *within* a given ethnic or racial group (however this is defined), but there are often sufficiently large differences between them to yield distinctive patterns of risk. If "ethnicity" is the variable of interest, the first consideration is to eliminate the effect of confounding variables, associated with the risk of disease and differentially distributed by ethnic group. The relevant exposure variable are quite likely to be exposures such as tobacco, alcohol, diet, infection etc, but in descriptive studies, there will generally only be information on so-called demographic variables such as social class (or occupation, educational level), place of residence, marital status and so on, that are proxies for these.

A striking illustration of the likely influence of genetic factors on risk of disease is provided by certain cancers of childhood. For bone tumours (Fig. 3.9), there are very marked differences in incidence between ethnic groups for which no plausible environmental "exposure" can be imagined. Any such exposure would have to be very carcinogenic (to act so early in life), very tissue specific, and be very unevenly distributed by ethnic group.

The most fruitful approach using routine data sources is through the study of migrants (see Sect. 3.5.4), that attempt to separate the "genetic" and "environmental" components of differences by studying disease risk in a given migrant population in comparison with that in the host population (similar environment, different genetics) and in the population living in place of origin (similar genetics, different environment).

Socio-economic Status

Socio-economic status is an extremely important but rather vague term for a whole host of factors that require individual consideration and action, such as income, occupation, living conditions, education and access to services. For many diseases, such as cardiovascular disease (Rose and Marmot 1981) and cancer (Smith et al. 1991; Kogevinas et al. 1997), a clear gradient by social class is observed, with the highest disease rates or the poorest outcome often observed within the lowest socio-economic grouping. The influence of social status has a marked effect on disease outcomes in adults and in both prenatal development and infant mortality.

While the magnitude of gradients of many disease outcomes tend to vary additionally with time reflecting in part changing social and economic circumstances (Marmot 1999), the impact of general improvements in health often fail to reach the most disadvantaged: Since the 1920s, for instance, improving infant survival rates over half a century in the U.K. was not observed amongst those considered least advantaged (with the consistently highest infant mortality rates) (Rosen 1993). A recent advance has been the linking of "deprivation" scores, an index that combines a number of social variables from censuses according to area of residence, to data records from routine data sources (e.g. cancer registries) at the small area level (Carstairs 1995).

In measuring socio-economic status, a number of potential surrogates may provide a reproducible definition, such as affluence (income), living conditions or occupation. From a perspective of routine systems based on populations, some of the most illustrative stem from the pioneering series of reports published by the Office for National Statistics, formerly the Registrar General for England and Wales. The Registrar General's social classes were derived from a classification of occupations according to status and level of responsibility (and for married women, on the basis of their husband's employment). Figure 3.10 demonstrates

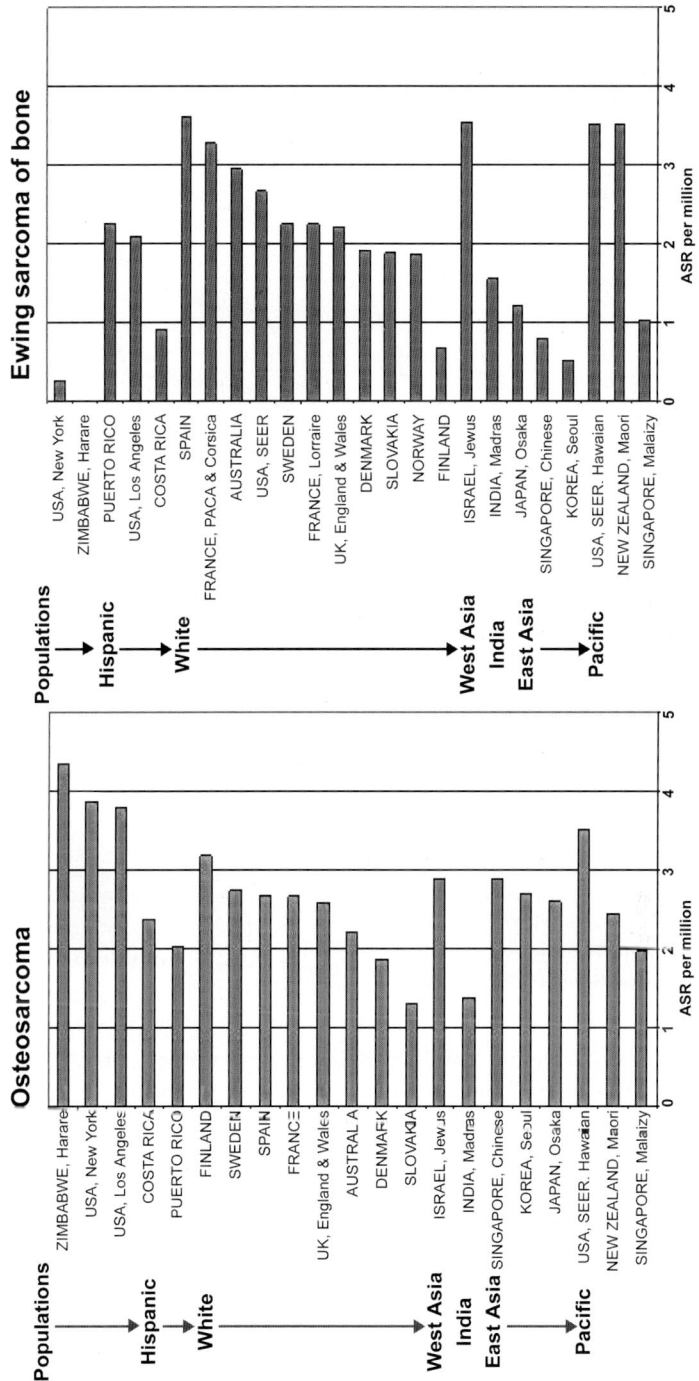

Figure 3.9. Incidence of osteosacoma and Ewing's sarcoma in childhood (Parkin et al. 1998)

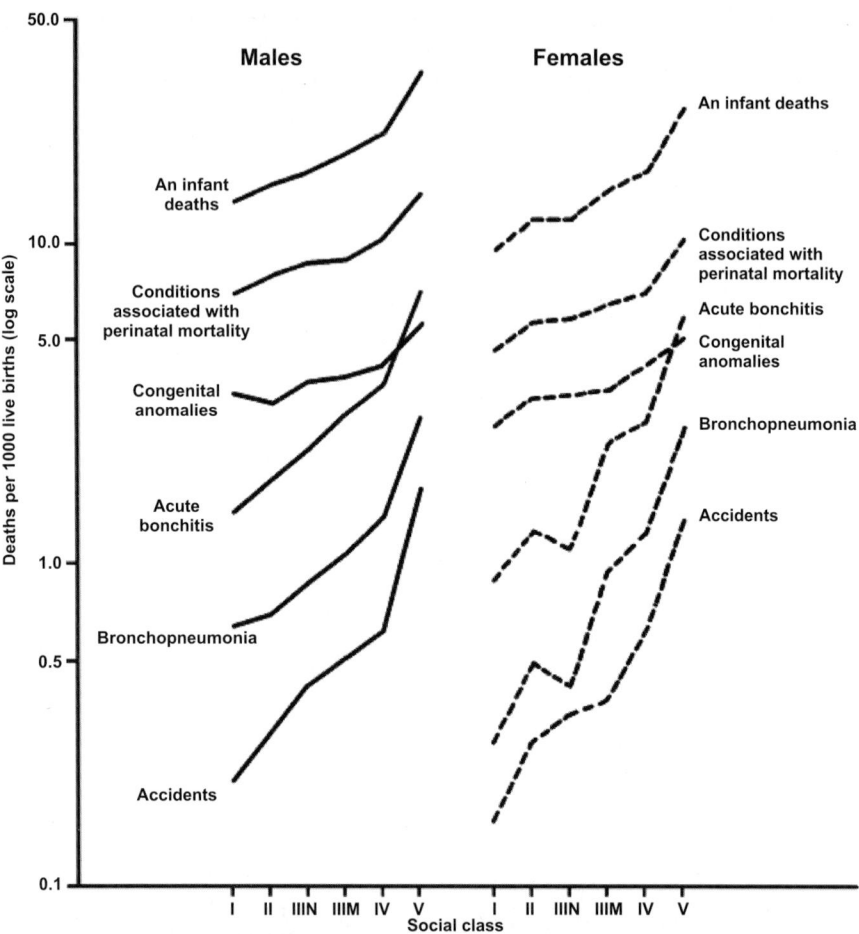

Figure 3.10. Infant mortality by sex, occupational class and cause of death (Occupational Mortality 1970–1972; Registrar General's Office for England and Wales 1978, p 158)

the uniform socio-economic gradients of infant mortality by cause, with the most abrupt increases observed for accidents and respiratory disease.

There are interpretational difficulties with socio-economic data from routine sources. Although selection bias should be minimal if the comparison of health events with survey data is made from the same population at the same time, measurement bias is of particular concern. In occupational studies, the respondent is asked for only one occupation, even though they may have had a history of different professions (see Sect. 3.5.1).

The consistent findings of poorer disease outcomes amongst the more disadvantaged social groups have political as well as public health implications. In addition to pinpointing the need for health promotion and disease prevention strategies targeted at low socio-economic groups, health inequality also demonstrates a need for change at the societal level: improving health by improving incomes, basic housing, and working conditions. However, the practical importance of the variable as an independent risk factor in epidemiological studies is perhaps overstated. Health-deprivation gradients are now well established in most disease domains, and specific public health actions are difficult to formulate and implement given social class acts as a surrogate for a vast and complex array of social and environmental processes, congenital characteristics and early life experiences.

Marital Status

A number of epidemiological studies have examined marital status in relation to disease risk. While it is apparent that there are major differences in disease rates according to this variable – married persons often have lower death rates than single persons – there are commonly difficulties inferring the true nature of the association. The main difficulty arises in determining whether being married per se offers health advantages, or if there are certain characteristics of good health or long life that favour an individual's predisposition to marriage. The variable has, however, proved useful in determining certain surrogate populations – such as never-married males as proxies for homosexual men (Biggar et al. 1987). In this context, the variable was used to establish increases from the mid-1970 s in AIDS-related cancers such as Kaposi's sarcoma in single men aged 20 to 49 years old (Biggar et al. 1987).

Occupation

Descriptive studies have made an important contribution to occupational epidemiology, through the analysis of routine record sources. In some countries, occupations are recorded on death certificates or in disease registers. Such routine record data sets can be used to calculate cancer risks in different occupations. If the comparisons are to involve rates (of mortality, or incidence), then suitable population-at-risk data must be available from the census or population register, with occupations classified in the same way; failing this, proportionate methods may be used (Sect. 3.4.1). Routine record studies are relatively inexpensive and often entail very large numbers of subjects. Occupation is specified in terms of job titles. A limiting factor of such analyses is the validity of the job title information collected. With an interviewer-administered questionnaire, quite valid job histories can be obtained, but the validity of occupations recorded on routine records such as death certificates or tumour registers is typically mediocre (Wigle et al. 1982; Steenland and Beaumont 1984; Armstrong et al. 1994). In addition, routine records typically contain only one of the subject's jobs, usually the most recent which may include "retired". In a large sample of Montreal workers, it was estimated that, on average, about 62% of working years were spent in the job of longest duration, and about 50% in the last job (Siemiatycki 1996). Some of the defects of the limited information on occupation available in routine records can be reduced by linkage with more valid sources of occupational data. Examples are in Canada (Howe and Lindsay 1983) where a government-run labour force survey was linked to mortality records, and especially in the Nordic countries where census data has been linked to the cancer registry (Lynge and Thygesen 1990; Andersen et al. 1999). Despite these limitations, analyses using job titles are useful. Several associations with cancer have been discovered by means of analyses based on job titles. Table 3.5 shows results from the Decennial Occupational Mortality analysis (Registrar General 1978) based on deaths occurring in England and Wales in 1970–1972, and cancer registrations in 1968–1969. Analyses such as these are most valid and valuable when the workers have a relatively homogeneous exposure profile – for example miners, motor vehicle drivers, butchers and cabinetmakers. However, job titles are limited as descriptors of occupational exposures (Siemiatycki et al. 1981). On the one hand, many job titles cover workers with very diverse exposure profiles, while on the other, multiple exposures are found to occur in many occupation categories. Several approaches have been used to better define actual exposures. One such is the Job Exposure Matrix (JEM). A JEM is simply an automatic set of indicators showing which exposures may occur in which occupations (Hoar et al. 1980; Siemiatycki 1996; Chap. I.11 of this handbook).

3.5.2   Place of Residence

Place of residence is an important variable in descriptive epidemiology. It is almost always available in routine sources of events of disease (registers, surveys, death certificates), and population-at-risk is very often available for small geographic units too. "Geographic pathology"-comparisons of disease rates or risk of individuals living in different areas has been one of the longest established and productive types of descriptive study for more than a century (Hirsch 1883). National populations have often been the unit of study. The reason is that this dimension is the one for which statistics – especially mortality – are collected and published. Differences in disease between countries may indeed be striking. Sometimes, the reasons are obvious, and correspond to the known distribution of causal agents – as for some infectious diseases. But for some diseases, the clear international variations in incidence or mortality have prompted research to better understand the reasons behind them.

Valid comparisons of data deriving from routine data sources in international studies require that there is fair comparability in diagnostic criteria, and in recording and coding the events concerned. Variation in quality and completeness of death registration has been mentioned as a source of bias in epidemiological studies, and it is easy to find examples of uncritical use of such data (Carroll 1975). For diseases where there are differences in diagnostic criteria internationally, special studies of disease incidence/prevalence may be undertaken, using similar definitions and criteria in the different participating centres. Examples are international studies of cardiovascular disease and its determinants (the MONICA project, Tunstall-Pedoe et al. 1988) and of Asthma (ISAAC study, Pearce et al. 1993).

National boundaries have not always been based on levels of exposure to environmental risk factors, nor of the genetic homogeneity of the populations within

Table 3.5. Stomach cancer deaths and registrations by occupation unit and cancer: men aged 15–74 giving units with significantly raised PMRs and PIRs in 1968–1969 ($p < 0.01$) (Registrar General's Office for England and Wales 1978)

Cancer (ICD number) Occupation			Deaths 1970–1972			Registrations 1968–1969	
			Observed	All cancer PMR		All cancer PIR Observed	
Order	Unit	Title	15–74	15–64	65–74	15–74	15–74
Stomach (151)							
II	007	Coal mine – face workers	615	142**	127**	44	182**
II	008	Coal miner – other underground	120	159**	139*	45	214**
II	007	Coal mine-workers above ground	615	142**	127**	34	207**
II	015	Coal miners (so described)	16	122	72	270	146**
IV		Furnacemen, kilnmen, glass and ceramics	262	121*	133**	9	173
VII	054	Other metal making; working; jewellery and electrical production process workers	35	191*	110	96	145**
X	064	Fibre preparers	44	123	122	13	194*
XIV	089	Workers in rubber	256	102	106	27	175**
XV	098	Construction workers nec	121	107	120	127	132**
XVI	102	Boiler firemen	65	103	113	69	143**
XVIII	106	Railway lengthmen	149	109	78	33	156*
XVIII	113	Labourers and unskilled Workers nec, building and contracting	1120	114**	113**	56	143*
XVIII	114	Labourers and unskilled workers nec, other	84	94	109	781	122**
XIX	123	Inspectors, supervisors, transport	664	103	111	50	149**
XX	136	Warehousemen, storekeepers and assistants	109	89	100	314	129**
XXII	144	Shop salesmen and assistants				11	111

* those results significant at the 1% level are denoted ** and those at the 5% level *
nec = not elsewhere classified

them. Thus, study of populations within, and sometimes across, national boundaries has been particularly informative. The geographic units of study can be as small as compatible with a sufficient number of events to generate stable disease rates within them, and availability of information on the population-at-risk. Issues of comparability, that may be a source of bias in international comparisons, are usually less important, because recording procedures are in general more similar within countries than between them.

Mapping

"Spot maps", which show the location of individual cases/deaths have a long history, initially in the investigation of the epidemiology of infectious diseases, more recently as an adjunct to the investigation of clusters of disease (Sect. 3.5.4). For non-communicable diseases, the more familiar method is the chloropleth (thematic) map, which uses distinct shading or colour to geographic units, usually these are administrative or statistical areas. The reasons for presenting data on risk by place of residence as a map rather than a table are not simply aesthetic. As well as conveying the actual value associated with a particular area, a map conveys a sense of the overall geographic pattern of the mapped variable, and allows comparison between the patterns on different maps. This is especially valuable when used to suggest possible causative hypotheses. There are now a large number of disease atlases available, for individual countries (USA, Pickle et al. 1987; UK, Gardner et al. 1984; France, Salem et al. 1999; China, Editorial Committee 1979), or for regions where it is considered that issues of comparability between the participating countries can be overcome (Europe, WHO 1997; Baltic region, Pukkala et al. 2001).

There are a number of specific technical issues to be considered

— Choice of map

As well as the various map projections, the *cartogram* has been used by some authors (see Fig. 3.11) (e.g. Verhasselt and Timmermans 1987; Howe 1977). This allocates to the units of study an area proportional to their population size. The idea is to draw attention to the relative numerical importance of the differences displayed, but the resulting maps generally appear somewhat bizarre.

— Choice of geographic unit

As noted above, the size of the unit for study is a compromise between the need to provide as much geographic detail as possible (so as to show up any pockets of high or low risk), and achieving stable rates (small variance), so that any spatial patterns are not obscured by random variation.

— Choice of parameter

The functions plotted are usually rates or ratios. The basic problem is how to compromise between illustrating the actual value of the rate/ratio (generally age standardised in some way) in the different units, which may be influenced by random variation, and giving more weight to those areas with lower variance in the statistic, that are unlikely to be due to chance. It is often the case that sparsely populated units cover large geographic areas, while densely populated cities are small. Mapping may well result in impressive high or low values for eye-

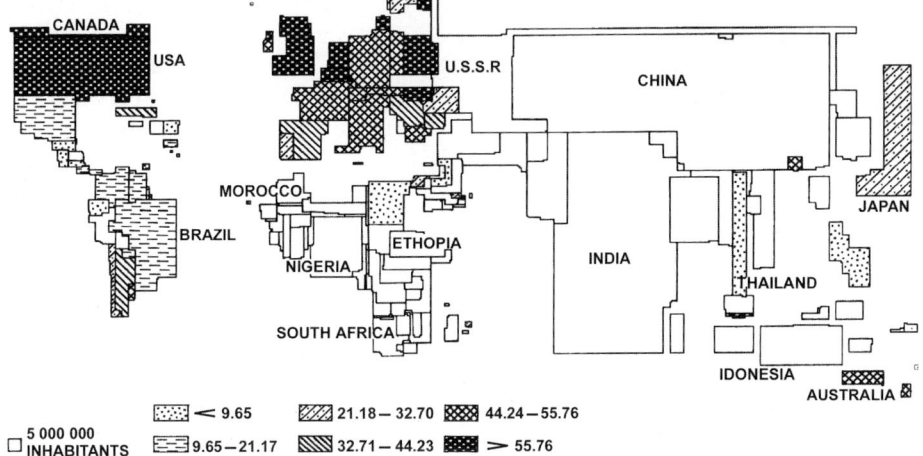

Figure 3.11. Cartogramm of mortality from cancers of the trachea, bronchus and lung (1981–1984) (Howe 1977)

catchingly big areas. Plotting the *p*-values as level of "statistical significance" is not the answer, as this simply highlights differences between the populous units, even when the magnitude of the difference (reflecting its biological significance) is small.

There have been various attempts to circumvent this fundamental problem. The US Atlas of Cancer Mortality used a scale that was a combination of the relative value (e.g., top 10th percentile) and its statistical significance. There is no logical solution to the problem of how to present such maps (is a relative risk of 2 with $p = 0.002$ more or less impressive than an $\widehat{RR}$ of 4 and $p = 0.05$?). A different approach is to try to reduce the random variation of rates in small units by assuming that rates in adjacent units will tend to be similar, under the assumption that there is an underlying geographic pattern. Pukkala et al. (2001) colour their maps by giving a value to each unit that is the weighted (by distance) average of the other units within 200 km (Fig. 3.12). A more formal method is to plot empirical Bayes estimates of the rates, whereby the values for the units (areas) that are imprecise are improved by estimates from other appropriate areas (Clayton and Kaldor 1987).

– Choice of range

The number of classes into which to divide the range of values is a compromise between detail and clarity. Usually, 5–10 classes are used. There are various choices for the class intervals to be used. The simplest is to use constant intervals (equal steps), in which the range of values is divided into a number of categories of equal size; this works well if the distribution of the data between the units is relatively even, but otherwise may be dominated by extreme values, even leaving some classes with no entries at all. If the data set displays an approximately normal frequency distribution, class intervals may be standard

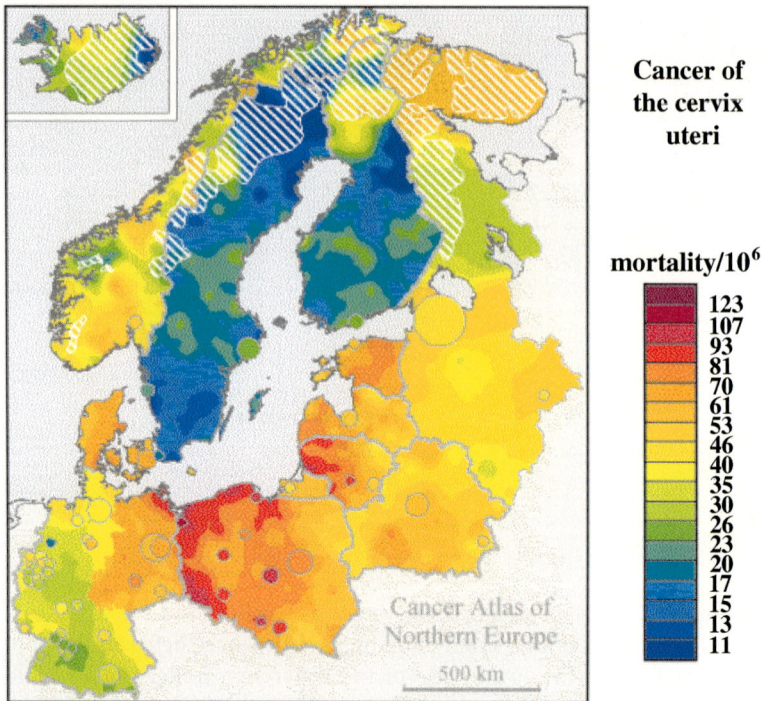

Figure 3.12. Mortality rates from cancer of the cervix uteri in Northern Europe (Pukkala et al. 2001)

deviation values; it is useful if the idea of the map is to illustrate deviations from a mean value. Natural divisions of the scale may be used, based upon low points observed in the actual frequency distribution, or on some prior knowledge or hypothesis of important dividing values. A relative scale, based on percentiles of the units being mapped, results in irregular variable intervals, but a predictable number of values in each class. The percentiles do not need to be even – in the Scottish Cancer Atlas, the percentiles were 5th, 15th, 35th, 65th, 85th, 95th, which draws attention to areas of both high and low incidence (Kemp et al. 1985). The same scheme was used for the atlas of cancer mortality in Europe (Smans et al. 1992; Fig. 3.13). This approach means that there is no arbitrary selection of values to plot, and that the colouring of all maps tends to be about the same. However, it will obscure outlying (very high or very low values).

— Choice of shading/colour

The change of shading or colour should convey as closely as possible the progression of risk. Colour maps are more visually pleasing, and can convey more information than those in monochrome. The choice of colours to illustrate the gradations of the scale of the map is not arbitrary, and ideally should follow a scale based on the sequence of the spectrum, and degree of whiteness (chroma) (Smans and Estève 1992).

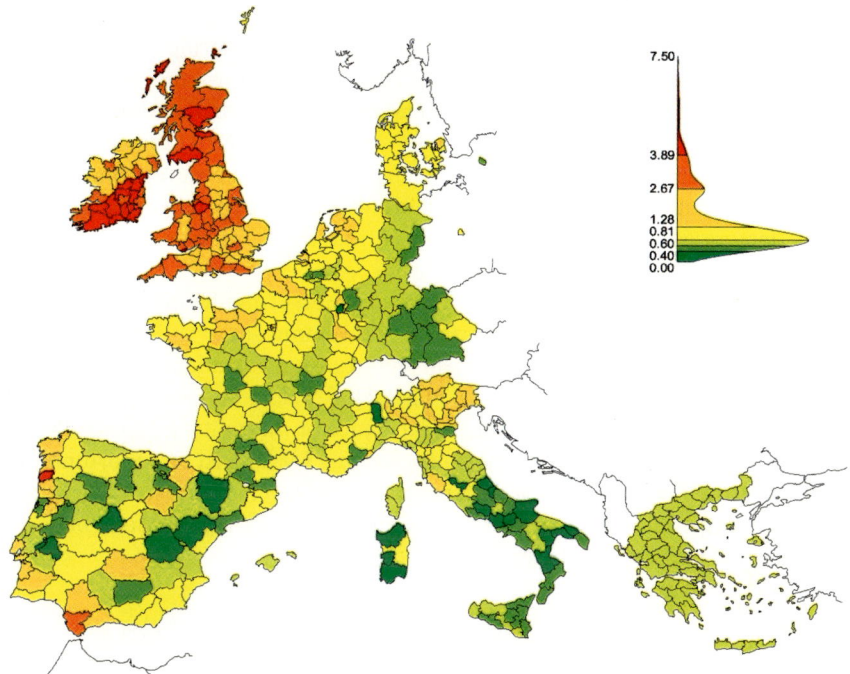

Figure 3.13. Mortality from oesophageal cancer in Europe 1971–1978 (females) (Smans et al. 1992)

Urban-Rural Comparisons

There have been many studies in which individuals have been classified into urban or rural dwellers, on the basis of some characteristic of their place of residence, usually, its administrative designation or otherwise as a town/city, or on the basis of population density of the administrative areas (Nasca et al. 1980; Friis and Storm 1993; Barnett et al. 1996). Although distinct differences in the risk of various diseases may be observed, the reasons underlying them are generally obscure. Often, the interest may be in the effects of air pollution on health, given that most air pollution (due to traffic, domestic smoke, or industry) will be more intense in urban areas. However, urban-rural classifications of place of residence is an inefficient way to approach this topic, given the multiplicity of covariates involved.

Clustering

The topic is briefly introduced in Sect. 3.5.4, where combinations of person, place and time are considered.

Time   3.5.3

Investigations of the occurrence of diseases over time are standard tools in epidemiological science and public health surveillance. In the context of investigative epidemiology, temporal studies may generate novel aetiological hypotheses, or provide confirmatory evidence of existing ones. As well as offering a unique possibility to quantify how risk in populations is changing over time, they offer clues as to the underlying determinants of the observation. Changes in the evolution of incidence rates with time usually imply (in the absence of artefacts) consideration of plausible mechanisms of, and changes in, environmental exposures (time-lagged by an approximation of the induction period). Excepting large migrational effects, genetic factors only have a minor impact on time trends of disease (MacMahon and Pugh 1970).

Time trends are also of major importance in measuring the impact of disease control; in studying the effects of primary prevention interventions, screening programmes, and the efficacy of treatment regimes. The evaluation of implemented programmes (planned or unplanned), may take a 'before and after' approach to assess the impact of the intervention on incidence or mortality at the population level. In determining the effectiveness of screening (organised or opportunistic), trends in incidence or mortality, dependant on the specific disease under study, targeted population before and after implementation, or comparisons between screening and non-screened groups.

Time Trends of Routine Data

The strengths and weaknesses of incidence and mortality data in studying time trends is a subject of much debate. There are complexities in examining trends in either measure, and to avoid erroneous conclusions it is usually necessary to consider the possibility that artefactual changes over time may have in some way distorted the observed trend.

If the mortality rate is used as a surrogate measure of the risk of developing the disease, a strong assumption of constancy over time in the fatality ratio is required. As survival for many diseases has been improving for several decades, it may be inappropriate to utilise mortality trends as proxies for risk other than for the most fatal diseases. Ideally, mortality rates are best utilised as measures of outcome, rather than occurrence in time trends studies.

Generally a description that utilises several of these indicators serves to clarify their key properties and aid understanding of the underlying disease processes. There are also a number of temporal datasets on putative or known risk factors collected for particular studies based on, for example, repeated surveys or national surveys, that may be of some utility in elucidating observed trends. Correlation analyses that link such data with trends may clarify particular hypotheses, but are limited by their coverage and quality, as well as various potential ecological biases (Morgenstern 1998, Sect. 3.4.2).

Describing Secular Trends

Time trend data should be analysed according to the problem under investigation, and the structural characteristics of the data. In the field of health monitoring, the goal might be to determine the nature of the recent secular trend. An estimate of the magnitude and direction (the EAPC – estimated annual percentage change) of the trend over a limited period of time (the last 10 years, say) could be obtained using a simple log-linear model. The EAPC is a useful descriptive measure, but should be interpreted with some caution. 95% confidence intervals for the slope should always be given and should help in assessing whether the fitted linear trend may have arisen through chance. If there are elements of curvature in the trend, the EAPC will give incorrect and imprecise estimates of the average unit change. In describing recent trend patterns, the particular choice of time points is often arbitrary and, in the absence of highly stable rates over time, the EAPC may vary according to the period of time nominated. A preferable description might involve some modelling procedure that could identify sudden changes in the long-term trend, and on that basis, estimate the direction and magnitude of the slope for each epoch of time in which rates are relatively stable.

Methods that seek abrupt linear changes in trend have been devised by Chu et al. (1999), and by Kim et al. (2000), the latter technique having been implemented in a specially written (and freely available) statistical software package entitled "JoinPoint". The joinpoint regression model essentially searches the temporal data for a few continuous linear phases. The procedure is motivated by the problem of determining the number of joinpoints, i.e. breaks in time where abrupt linear changes occur, and an estimate of the EAPC between joinpoints. The minimum and maximum number of joinpoints are user-specified in the software package. To determine up to two joinpoints, for example, a model indicating no change is compared against the model containing two joinpoints. If the null hypothesis of no joinpoints is rejected, then the procedure is applied to test the null hypothesis of one joinpoint against the alternative of two joinpoints. Otherwise, the test for the null hypothesis of no change is considered against the alternative of one joinpoint.

Statistical models may also be used to make forecasts of the likely future cancer burden. Prediction models are an important (but hazardous) aspect of public health surveillance, and predictions can help answer both scientific and administrative questions (Hakulinen and Hakama 1991). The choice of statistical model, prediction base, future year of prediction, and the precision of the estimates (Dyba et al. 1997) are important considerations in making predictions of burden that account for risk and demographic effects of ageing and population growth.

Age Period Cohort Analyses

The first use of the term "cohort" is attributed to Frost in a letter written to a colleague in 1935. The note was published posthumously alongside his landmark paper that discussed some insights that could be attained by visually examining age-specific death rates from tuberculosis according to cohorts, members of a community who share the same birth period, rather than simply in the usual cross-sectional way (Frost 1939). The present day usage of cohort obviously extends well beyond the closed or hypothetical sense of the term – *age-period-cohort analysis* is usually employed to describe temporal studies that include birth cohort analyses, to distinguish it from the generic usage of cohorts in prospective studies (Liddell 1988). In general, such an analysis allows one to examine the influence of each of the three time components, and the importance of the particular properties they represent:

— Birth cohort effects may relate to birth itself, or may approximate factors related to birth only by exerting influences that are shared in the same group as they age together. An examination of rates according to birth cohort may thus give some insight into the nature and intensity of disease-correlated exposures that may vary across successive generations, and has played a vital role in corroborating evidence from other types of epidemiological study. Temporal patterns in environmental risk factors tend to affect particular generations of individuals in the same way as they age together, and are more likely to exert particular influence on earlier stages of disease development.

— Period effects, on the other hand, may act as surrogate measures of events that quickly change incidence or mortality with the same order of magnitude regardless of the age group under study. These effects may be the result of planned interventions that act at later stages of the disease process e.g. novel therapies that improve survival in all age groups. More frequently, they are due to artefactual changes over time e.g. changes in ICD revisions or improvements in diagnostic procedures.

— Age is without doubt a powerful determinant of cancer risk, since it parallels the cumulative exposure to carcinogens over time, and the accumulation of the series of mutations necessary for the unregulated cell proliferation that leads to cancer.

A graphical representation of the age-specific rates by period and birth cohort is an essential element of the analysis. Time-specific rates by age though common representations (as in Fig. 3.14), are sometimes not helpful in elucidating the importance of each of the time components – without transformation of the *y*-axis, the rates can be too closely packed to clearly display the changes, while additionally for cohort trends, they are difficult to interpret, in view of the obvious fact that each generation-specific rate is only observed for a maximum of a few age groups, and at the extremes, only for one age band. Much more informative is the depiction of the age-specific rates with period and cohort representing the *x* coordinates of the two graphs respectively (Fig. 3.15). Time effects of either origin are therefore apparent when the age-specific trends are changing in consecutive periods or cohorts in the same way across all age groups.

The effects of the components are sometimes evident to the extent that further investigation may seem unnecessary, given the limited number of variables that require attention. The interpretation of the majority of temporal analyses is however usually more complicated. Rates may fluctuate over time according to the level of random error inherent in the data, dependent on the magnitude of the person-time and the rarity of the disease under investigation. In most situations, the random

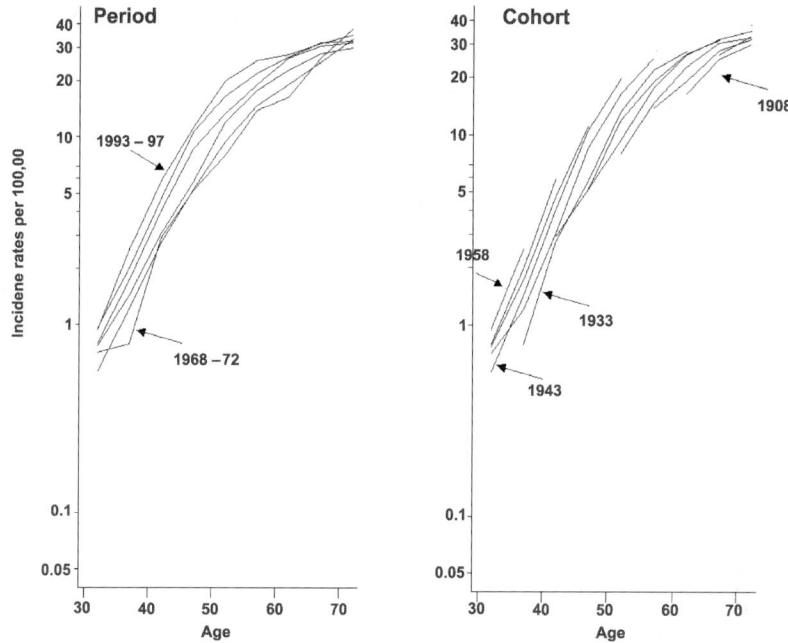

Figure 3.14. Cohort-specific incidence rates by age, England, oral cavity cancer, males, 1968–1997. *Arrows* indicate the midpoint of the period of disease events and year of birth in the left and right figure, respectively

variation is particularly high in younger persons in recent cohorts. The attribution of changes in the trend to period or cohort effects on the basis of visual means is therefore often not straightforward nor satisfactory, and a comparison of the two-dimensional age-period versus age-cohort graphs can lead to arbitrary opinions as to which component more adequately describes the data. It is in these situations that our understanding of the evolution of cancer risk can be greatly enhanced by the use of more formal statistical procedures. Models offer quantitative and comparable estimates of trend based on objective criteria for choosing the best description of the data, and statistical tests to decide whether the trends are real or random (Estève 1990). The consequences of subjective judgments based exclusively on graphical descriptions are thus avoided. Statistical models of this nature do not provide definitive answers, but offer some guidance as to the importance of each component.

The Age-Period-Cohort Model

The emerging importance of birth cohort analyses is in part due to the extensive theoretical and applied research into the age-period-cohort (APC) model in recent times, and importantly, knowledge of its inherent mathematical limitations (Holford 1983; Clayton and Schifflers 1987a,b). The accumulation of available data, advances in statistical theory, including development of the generalised lin-

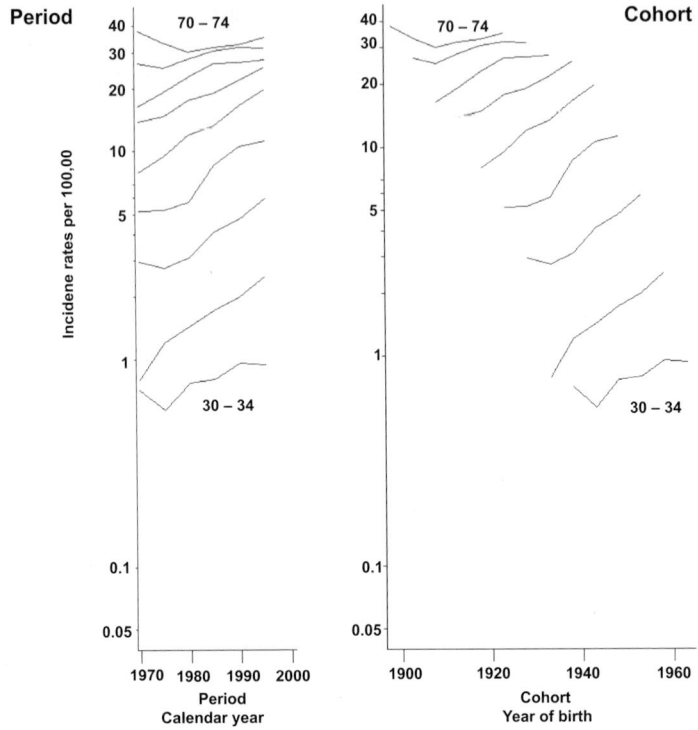

Figure 3.15. Age-specific incidence rates by birth cohort, England, oral cavity cancer, males, 1968–1997. The youngest and oldest age groups are indicated in the figures

ear model (Nelder and Wedderburn 1972) alongside an increasing availability of software dedicated to fitting such models also contribute to the development.

As birth cohort is related to a linear function of calendar period and age, the full APC model cannot, given a default set of model constraints, identify all of the parameters of the three components, nor – on introduction of a further constraint – provide a unique set of estimates. While the APC model is used extensively in applied temporal analyses of disease, the statistical methodologies used to circumvent this problem are numerous and diverse, an indicator of an enduring lack of consensus as to how best to provide satisfactory inferences.

In parallel with advances in statistical theory and computing power, theoretical and applied research on the APC model began to flourish in the late 1970's. During the next couple decades, a number of solutions were offered as how should one present the joint components (e.g. Glenn 1976; Moolgavkar et al. 1979; Day and Charnay 1982; Osmond and Gardner 1982; Holford 1983; Fienberg and Mason 1985; Kupper et al. 1985; Clayton and Schifflers 1987a,b; Tarone and Chu 1992, 1996). A number of reviews and critique of APC models has also been published (e.g. Holford 1998).

The Lexis diagram (see Sect. 3.2.7) considers the location of incident cases on one plane, with three time coordinates used to classify events, the date of diagnosis, age at diagnosis, and the date of birth of the individual(s) affected. The third axis, denoted by the diagonal bands crossing the plane from top left to bottom right, represents the date of birth. The APC regression model involves additive contributions of the three time effects on the rate, and is given by:

$$E\left[\ln r_{ij}\right] = \mu + a_i + p_j + c_k \, ,$$

where $r_{ij} = Y_{ij}/n_{ij}$ is the incidence (or mortality) rate with n_{ij} is the number of person-time in age group i and period j, assumed fixed and known. a_i is the fixed effect of age group i ($i = 1, 2, \ldots, I$), p_j the fixed effect of period j ($j = 1, 2, \ldots, J$), and c_k the fixed effect of birth cohort with $k = 1, 2, \ldots, K$ where $k = I - i + j$. The number of cancer cases, y_{ij} are assumed to be distributed as a Poisson random variable with mean λ_{ij}. The model can be estimated readily using maximum likelihood techniques. The numbers of events are fitted via a generalised linear model assuming Poisson errors and a log-link function relating the mean to the linear component. The logarithm of the corresponding person-time is declared as an *offset*, an added constant set to unity for which estimation is not required. The goodness-of-fit is determined as usual by the deviance.

The Identifiability Problem.   Intrinsic to recognising the inherent limitations of the APC model is the fact that knowledge of any two factors implies knowledge of the third, making one of the factors redundant. As mentioned above, the index of cohort is defined by the corresponding indexes of age and period, and hence the three factors are exactly linearly dependant on each other. One further linear constraint must be imposed to ensure the parameter estimates are unique, but the crux of the problem is that this choice of constraint is completely arbitrary in the absence of compelling external information that one can bring to bear in making the selection.

Period and cohort can be considered as weak proxies for our own ignorance regarding the real determinants of time trends (Hobcraft et al. 1985), and it is important that the APC model should be considered as an exploratory tool for investigating the underlying reasons for significant period and cohort effects, adjusted for age. Despite their limitations, such models can render informative results capable of augmenting interpretations based on purely visual approaches.

Classifying Solutions to the Identifiability Problem.   A number of methods have been proposed that introduce particular constraints on the above APC parameterisation so that the identifiability problem appears to be at once resolved, thus yielding unique trend estimates. Such methods often make assumptions founded, necessarily, on mathematical rather than biological principles, that, if inconsistent with reality, induce a bias in all trends, leading to erroneous interpretation. Therefore, such solutions must be carefully scrutinised alongside our present knowledge of the aetiology of the cancer under study. Amongst the methods proposed, a distinction can be drawn that classifies ways of dealing with the analysis and presentation of results from the APC model.

As Holford (1998) points out, that a number of quantifies can be derived that are estimable and may fulfil the investigative objectives of a temporal study. Such *estimable functions* avoid any imposition of mathematical statements. Rather they are specific reparameterisations that offer summaries of the trends that are identical for any particular set of APC parameters. These conservative but (statistically) correct strategies will be compared with methods that incorporate external data or provide a certain mathematical solution for the cancer outlined, in order to ascertain the level of insight obtained, and the similarities and differences between the methods.

Several authors, notably, Holford (1983) and Clayton and Schifflers (1987b) have noted that certain reparameterisations of the parameters are unique regardless of the constraints imposed, ensuring identifiability, without making any further biological, epidemiological or mathematical assumptions. Holford (1983) suggested, given the large number of parameters included in the full APC model, for simplicity it is sensible to highlight the non-identifiability in terms of two parameters, one representing a linear function of the three (non-identifiable) slopes and the other, the identifiable curvature of each effect. Clayton and Schifflers (1987a) introduced the term *drift* or *net drift* in describing a model for which the two-factor models, age-period and age-cohort, fit the data equally well.

Drift or δ can be thought of as the average annual change in the rates over time, the passage of time that is common to both axes, calendar period *and* birth cohort, a quantity that cannot be disentangled between the time axes of calendar period and birth cohort. It has become an integral part of the APC modelling strategy, drift being utilised as an estimate of the rate of change of the regular trend, and a partitioner of first order and curvature effects. The age-drift model implies the same linear change in the logarithm of the rates over time in each age group. Given the linear component over time is identifiable but cannot be allocated in any way to period or cohort, δ can be estimated by either specifying period or cohort as a continuous covariate, and the resulting EAPC estimated as $e^\delta - 1$, expressed in the unit of origin.

Perhaps the easiest way to avoid the issue is to ignore the possibility of a three-factor model. However, if such a preference is founded simply on the basis of adequacy of model fit, such an approach may be biased if one of the three effects follows a purely linear pattern (Kupper et al. 1985). In addition, the age-period and age-cohort models are not nested within each other and are therefore not directly comparable. Given its simplicity relative to methods dealing with the three-factor model, however, two-factors models are commonly applied, often when there are, *a priori* beliefs in the nature of the temporal pattern.

Combinations

Space Time Clustering

Clustering results from the aggregation of cases (or deaths) in terms of disease group, time and space, where the number of cases is substantially greater than we would expect when the natural history of the disease and chance fluctuations are taken into account. Investigation of observed clusters, or search for clustering of different diseases is probably one of the most frequent types of study in descriptive epidemiology. There are, in general, two aims: to identify a possible aetiological role for infectious agents in non-communicable diseases, and to identify health hazards of sources of environmental contamination, the most popular suspects being sources of pollution (toxic waste dumps, industrial plants) or radiation (nuclear power, electro magnetic fields). Cancer and congenital malformations are the usual subjects of study. It is doubtful if the aetiological insights gained are commensurate with the huge volume of research effort (Rothman 1990), although explanations for some clusters of disease have been forthcoming (mesothelioma and sources of asbestos (Baris et al. 1987; Driscoll et al. 1988), mercury and Minimata disease in Japan (Tsuchiya 1992) and dental caries and fluoride in water (Dean 1938)).

Studies of clustering are either a priori or ad hoc. A priori investigation is the search for evidence of clustering in space and/or time in data sets where none is known to exist beforehand, but where the investigator may have some prior hypothesis about its existence. Post hoc clusters are observed groupings of events in neighbourhoods, schools, occupational units, households or families, that are considered by someone to be unusual. In both cases, the existence of a point source, responsible for the observed excess, may be suspected.

There are some important considerations in all cluster investigations. The boundaries or units of investigation need to be clearly defined, without reference to the actual observations. The definition should include the disease entity studied, including the diagnostic criteria of a case, the age and sex groups of subjects to be included, and the geographic and temporal boundaries within which the disease event will be counted. Ideally, these are based on biological criteria, or on the a priori hypothesis that is being tested. The boundaries should not be defined by the nature of the observations themselves. Demonstrating a clustering effect means that the observed spatial/temporal patterns of disease are significantly different from the expected result, based on an appropriate reference area. Any diligent investigator should be able to achieve this, if sufficient sub-analyses are performed, on varying combinations of diseases, areas, and timescales. Less ideally, post hoc clusters are, by definition, combinations of place, time, and disease that accidentally appeared to be significantly unusual.

A large number of methodological approaches are available for examining datasets for evidence of clustering (see Smith 1982; Marshall 1991; Alexander and Cuzick 1992; Bithell 1992; Alexander and Boyle 1996). Guidelines have been prepared to aid epidemiologists working in public health departments to investigate local post hoc clusters brought to their attention (Centers for Disease Control 1990; Leukaemia Research Fund 1997).

Migrant Studies

Migrant studies provide a useful insight into the relative importance of environment and genetic make-up in disease aetiology. Disease risk is compared between populations of similar genetic background living in different physical and social environments. Figure 3.16 illustrates the principles; comparison is usually between the rate of disease in migrants (R_{m1}), and the population from which they originated (R_0), or between the rates in migrants and those of the new host country in which they have settled (R_{m1} vs. R_h). The most informative migrant studies are those that permit study of the rate of change of risk following migration. This may be by partitioning migrant rates (R_{m1}) according to age at migration or duration of residence, or by comparison of risk in first generation migrants (R_{m1}) and their offspring (R_{m2}).

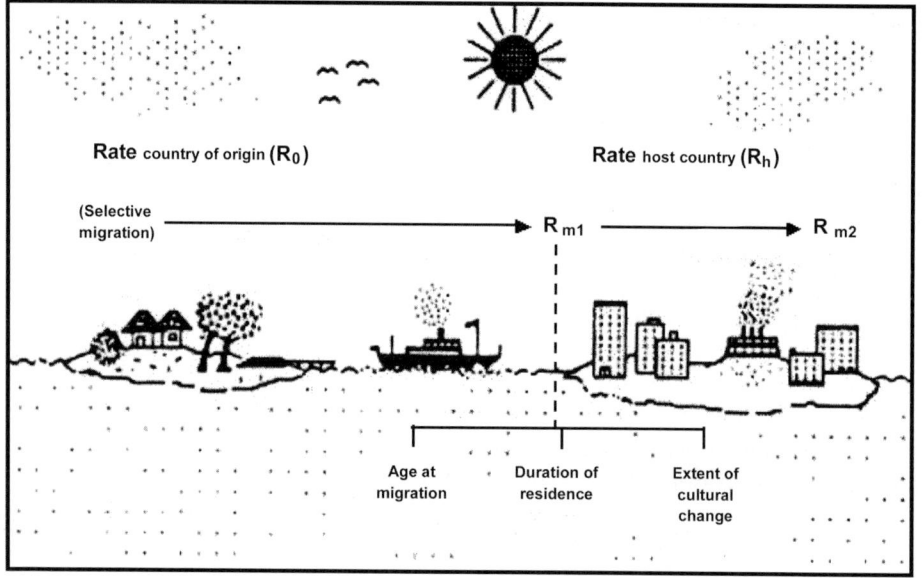

Figure 3.16. Principles of migrant studies (McMichael and Giles 1988)

Studies of disease risk in migrants may involve interview/examination of subjects, in which case information is available not only on the variables of place of origin/place of residence- the focus of migrant studies- but also on covariates. Descriptive studies rely upon data from routine sources (Sect. 3.1.2), and all environmental exposures are subsumed by the variables birthplace and place of residence. Although these may be highly reproducible and subject to little misclassification, in an aetiological sense they are themselves related to numerous more proximate unmeasured 'exposures', not only in the external environment (air, soil, water), but also through socio-cultural factors (diet, fertility, smoking, etc.), as well as genetic predispositions to them. Adjustment for confounding factors related to birthplace is generally limited, since the variables available are usually few (sex, age, place of residence, occupation etc.). Nevertheless, as well as the simplicity and convenience that characterise descriptive studies in general, such studies are population based and often of large size, (for example, 120,000 subjects in one study of migrants to Israel; Steinitz et al. 1989). The prospective (cohort) design of most permits risk for several different diseases to be examined.

Migrant studies can only provide useful information when there is a difference in risk between the country of origin (specifically, the population from which the migrants came) and the host population. In the particular instance of the host population comprising the offspring of earlier migrants, there might well be less difference than were it genotypically quite different. Migrants from Spain and Italy might have considerable genetic similarity to the inhabitants of Argentina and Uruguay, for example, countries with populations largely of southern European descent.

Descriptive studies in which "exposure" is investigated in terms of birthplace and residence are not very useful for diseases for which there are obvious causes, with a high population attributable fraction. For example, tobacco smoking is responsible for such a large proportion of cases of lung cancer that risk in migrants will be almost entirely determined by past smoking habits, and the contributions of other environmental factors, for example air pollution, will be quite impossible to evaluate in the absence of detailed knowledge of exposure to tobacco smoke. Conversely, the changes of risk experienced by migrants for cancers of the breast, large bowel, pancreas and prostate have been far more useful pointers to the relative importance of environmental factors in aetiology, and to the stage of carcinogenesis at which they may act.

The definition of migrant status is dependent upon the data sources used in a particular study. The most common classification is by place of birth, a relatively well-defined, unchanging attribute, likely to be comparable between the data sources being used (census, vital statistics, registration). Place of birth can also be used in the study of migrants within one country (internal migration). Citizenship or nationality is often recorded on death certificates; it is less useful than place of birth, since migrants will become naturalised to varying degrees, and there are more problems of definition (e.g. dual nationality, stateless persons). Other variables, particularly ethnic group (but also language or religion), have been widely used in comparative studies of populations of different genetic background living in similar environments (or vice versa), in a manner analogous to studies of risk by birthplace (Sect. 3.5.1). Studies that employ a combination of ethnic group and birthplace to distinguish first-generation migrants and their offspring are much more informative than either one alone.

The term "environment" embraces, of course, more than the physical surroundings of an individual; it also encompasses all elements of lifestyle that influence disease risk. Thus, while certain aspects of the physical environment (e.g. air and its pollutants, water and trace elements, irradiation-solar and other forms) change abruptly on migration, other aspects of lifestyle which are related to socio-cultural norms will be retained to a greater or lesser degree in the new place of residence. Examples are patterns of diet, childbearing, alcohol and tobacco consumption, sexual habits, and so on. Socio-cultural factors also influence the degree of exposure to external environmental agents; thus, given that potential exposure to ultraviolet radiation from the sun is determined by geographical locality, the actual exposures will be modified by culturally defined behaviour. As a result, although migrants to countries with sunny climates, such as Israel or Australia, clearly have the same potential for exposure to ultraviolet radiation as the local population, they may be culturally more or less inclined to avoid the sun than the locally born.

The study of disease risk in relation to duration of residence in the new country, or, alternatively, according to the age at the time of migration, is feasible when information is available on the date of migration of the individuals. Provided migrants settle permanently in the host country, age at diagnosis or death is the summation of age at arrival and duration of stay, and it is not possible to evaluate the effect of one of these variables independently of the other. As age is such a strong determinant of risk, and an essential component of any analysis, there is no variability left in duration of stay after controlling for age at arrival, or vice versa; these two variables are therefore inextricably linked. This problem constitutes an extension of the non-identifiability property of age/period/cohort models in the study of time trends (see Sect. 3.5.3). A pragmatic solution is to examine each variable in turn (age/duration of residence, or age/age at arrival) to see which provides the most plausible pattern of change of risk. "Duration of residence" can be interpreted in terms of dose, i.e. assuming that longer periods spent in the new location imply a greater change in cumulative exposure to the relevant aetiological factors. It might equally be interpreted in terms of the stage of the disease process at which particular environmental exposures may act. Thus, a rapid change in risk following migration implies change in exposure to a relevant factor, and a short period between exposure and disease. Alternatively, the pattern of change may suggest that prolonged exposure is needed before risk is altered, or that the agent is only important with respect to exposures early in life. Analysis of risk by "age at migration" may show a clear distinction, in this case, between migrants arriving as children or as adults.

The importance of genetic susceptibility in determining risk is suggested by the persistence of characteristic rates between generations, since the offspring of migrants have been exposed to the environment of the host country for their entire lifespan. However, it is quite likely that they retain some aspects of their parents' lifestyle (as well as their genetic makeup). Some insight into the effect of this can be gained if the rates in the second generation (R_{m2}) can be partitioned according to birthplace of parents (neither, one, or both in the country of origin). These studies require that the data source used contains information on birthplace of parent(s), or ethnicity (if the migrants comprise a distinct ethnic group), or both.

Descriptive studies using routine sources for disease incidence, mortality or prevalence will have no information on levels of exposure (diet, tobacco, fertility, etc.). However, other data sources may be able to provide population-level data on prevalence or intensity of exposures, and permit ecological analyses of risk versus exposure according to birthplace (see Sect. 3.4.2). The opportunities for such studies are, unfortunately, limited. Although population surveys may be available, based on interviews (smoking, drinking, dietary habits, reproductive history) or physical examinations (height/weight, blood pressure, blood sugar, etc.), either place of birth is not recorded or, if it is, the samples are usually too small for meaningful results to emerge for any particular group of migrants, who usually comprise only a small fraction of the general population. Occasionally, there have been special ad hoc surveys of migrant populations-and sometimes data from control groups in case-control studies where ethnicity or place of birth has been a major variable of interest (e.g., in studies of diet and cancer in Hawaii (Kolonel et al. 1980; Hankin et al. 1983)). These may provide information on, for example, dietary habits in different migrant groups for comparison with those of the locally-born population.

Biases in Migrant Studies.

— *Use of mortality data*

Mortality data are normally used as a proxy for incidence (risk of disease), a perfectly valid procedure providing the ratio between mortality and incidence is constant for the groups being compared. This may not be true for international comparisons, since there are known differences in survival between countries (Berrino et al. 1999; Sankaranarayanan et al. 1998). It is less clear whether there are differences in survival by birthplace within a country, although ethnic-specific differences are well documented in the USA (Miller et al. 1996).

— *Data quality*

Variation in the quality of data from different sources is particularly troublesome when mortality rates in one country (locally-born and migrants) are compared with those from another (country of origin). International variation in completeness and accuracy of death certificate data has been discussed above (Sect. 3.2.4). It may introduce spurious differences in mortality rates. Thus, if the migrant population under study moves from a country with poor certification (of all causes, or a specific cause of death) to one with more accurate recording, there will be an apparent increase in the observed rate. Better ascertainment of cause of death, especially for diseases that present diagnostic difficulties, may account for some of the examples of "overshoot" (rates in migrants higher than host country, but country of origin rates lower), reported in several studies (Lilienfeld et al. 1972; McMichael et al. 1980).

Incidence rates from cancer registries are probably more comparable between countries than mortality data. Nevertheless, incidence can be influenced by the detection of asymptomatic cancers during screening, surgery, or autopsy, and is thus related to the extent and nature of such practices. Systematic histological examination of material removed at transurethral prostectomy was responsible for the detection of many 'incidental' (non-symptomatic) cancers of the prostate in the USA, and it has been suggested (Shimizu et al. 1991) that the incidence in Japan would have been three to four times higher in the same circumstances. This would explain the apparent rapid increase in the risk of prostate cancer in Japanese migrants to the USA.

— *Mismatching numerator/denominator*

In descriptive studies, person-years at risk are estimated from census data (or from population registers), typically broken down by rather few variables including, in addition to birthplace, age, sex and place of residence. It is essential that the definition of migrant status is the same in the census and case/death data, but even with the same definition, individuals may be classified in a different way in the two sources. Lilienfeld et al. (1972) present unpublished data on differences between country-of-birth statements on death certificates and census returns for the USA in 1960 – this varied from a 10.8% deficit on death certificates for UK birth to 16.7% excess for Ireland. A source of bias more difficult to detect results from migration that is related to the disease event itself-for example, when migrants return to their country of origin soon before death (so that mortality rates of migrants in the host country are underestimated).

A more practical difficulty in using population-at-risk data results from the fact that censuses are rather infrequent, and interpolations are needed to derive person-years at risk. This can be quite prone to error when several variables are involved, and active migration is still occurring during the study period.

— *Selection bias*

Migrant populations are a non-random (self-selected) sample of the population of their country of origin. Very often they come from quite limited geographical areas. For example, migrants to the United States of Italian origin come mainly from the south of that country (Geddes et al. 1993) and a large proportion of US Chinese originate from Guangdong province (King et al. 1985). Alternatively, the migrants may be special social or religious groups with quite distinctive disease patterns. For example, Jews comprised a large proportion of the migrants from Central Europe in the late 1930 s and 1940 s. Whenever possible, disease rates appropriate to the source population of the migrants should be used for comparisons, rather than the national country of origin rates.

Migrants are often assumed to be healthier than the average population (the 'healthy migrant effect'); this may be because the fact of seeking a new life overseas implies a population that is resourceful and energetic (or at least not chronically ill), or because the sick and disabled are excluded by the immigration authorities of the host country. Conversely, it has been suggested (Steinitz et al. 1989) that permission for Jews to migrate to Israel from countries of the Soviet block was more easily obtained for those in ill health, giving rise to an 'unhealthy migrant effect'. It is possible to check for the 'healthy/unhealthy migrant effect' if risk according to duration of stay in the new country can be estimated. A significant change in rates from those in the host country in recent migrants should suggest this form of bias. Swerdlow (1991) found no sign of any such effect in Vietnamese refugees to England and Wales, and Steinitz et al. (1989) found that exclusion of cancer cases diagnosed within a year of arrival in Israel made no difference to relative risks for short stay (less than 10 years) migrants.

– *Confounding*

Several demographic variables recorded in the sources of disease information (death certificates, disease registers, etc.) can be considered as confounders – influencing disease risk and associated with exposure (migrant status) – in a study aiming to investigate the effect of birthplace on disease risk. These include date of diagnosis/death, marital status, place of residence, and possibly ethnic group, occupation, socio-economic status (such as employment status, income, educational level, etc.).

Migrants are in the first place rarely distributed homogeneously in their new host country: they tend to settle in certain areas, generally in urban areas, and the establishment of a migrant 'colony' in a place tends to attract later migrants to settle there. It may well be inappropriate therefore to compare disease rates in migrants with the entire population of the host country. Table 3.6 illustrates an example of confounding by place of residence. Polish migrants to Argentina live mainly in Buenos Aires (81.2%, compared with 48% of the local-born), where mortality rates from colon and breast cancer are higher than elsewhere. Adjustment for place of residence reduces the relative risk of both cancers, and for colon cancer the difference from the local-born is no longer statistically significant.

Table 3.6. Confounding by place of residence in a study of cancer mortality in Polish migrants to Argentina (95% confidence intervals in brackets)

Cancer mortality and place of residence	Buenos Aires	Elsewhere in Argentina
Relative risk of colon cancer (M)	1.9	1.0
Relative risk of breast cancer (F)	1.4	1.0
Place of residence and birthplace	Buenos Aires	Elsewhere in Argentina
Born in Poland	81.2%	18.8%
Born in Argentina	47.9%	52.1%
Cancer mortality and birthplace [Relative risk in Poland-born vs. Argentina-born (1.0)]	Crude	Adjusted for place of residence
Colon cancer (M)	1.34 (1.06–1.68)	1.16 (0.95–1.43)
Breast cancer (F)	0.90 (0.75–1.08)	0.82 (0.63–1.05)

Social class and occupation are also known to be strong determinants of disease risk, and it is often clear from census data that migrants are over-represented in specific occupational categories, and are atypical of the general population in their socio-economic profile. Meaningful comparisons should therefore take the social dimension into account.

Temporal trends in incidence or mortality of disease may also be different in the migrant population and in the host country. When data from a long time period are used, the relative risk between them may differ according to time period. This is particularly troublesome when the effect of duration of stay is being studied, since, in general, data from more recent time periods will contain more migrants with long periods of residence than those from earlier years: an adjustment for time period is thus necessary.

Examples of Migrant Studies

— *Single-comparison studies* are the least informative, showing differences in risk between migrants and the locally born, but providing no information on the populations from which the migrants came. This may be the consequence of absence of appropriate sources of data (for example, no accurate mortality statistics), or that rates of disease are unavailable for the appropriate population subgroups from which the migrants came.

Figure 3.17 (Marmot et al. 1984) shows data on mortality from hypertensive disease (ICD-8 A82) and from coronary heart disease (A83) in men of different migrant groups in England and Wales. There is very large variation in the former (five fold), and a rather poor correlation of death rates from these two causes between the populations. For most of the countries of origin of the migrants there are no available data on mortality.

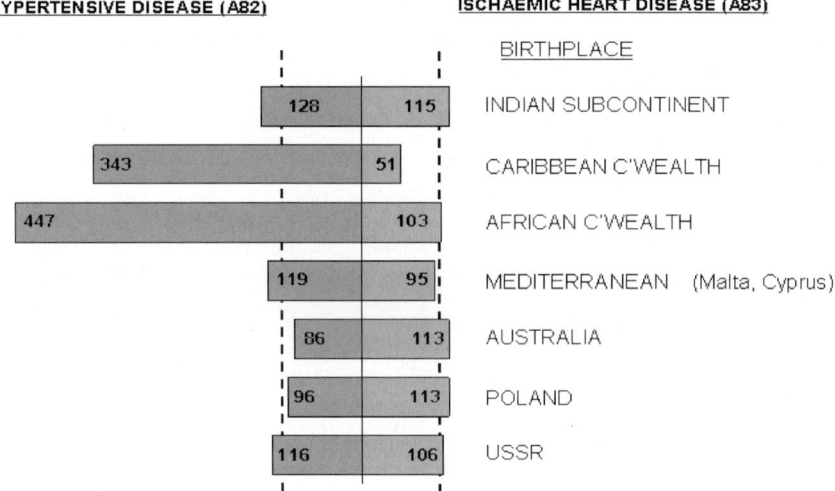

Figure 3.17. Mortality in migrants to England and Wales, age 20+, 1970–1972 SMR (relative to England and Wales = 100) (Marmot et al. 1984)

— *Two-comparison studies* are the most common type of study reported. They aim to demonstrate the degree to which the risk of a given disease changes in the migrant population away from that in the country of origin and towards that of natives in the new host country. Examples are the several studies that examine mortality rates in populations of pre-dominantly European origin moving to the United States (Haenszel 1961; Lillienfeld et al. 1972), Australia (Armstrong et al. 1983; McCredie 1998), England & Wales (Marmot et al. 1984; Grulich et al. 1992) and South America (Matos et al. 1991; de Stefani et al. 1990). The fact that the data for the two comparisons came from different sources must always be borne in mind, and bias in the first (country of origin) probably explains some of the findings in published studies.

Figure 3.18 shows results from a study of migrant mortality in the United States (Lilienfeld et al. 1972), comparing age-specific rates in migrants, with those in US born whites, and in the countries of origin of the migrants. One of the most impressive differences between migrants and country of origin is for Italians. It is probably in part the result of selection bias: Italian migrants originated mainly from southern Italy, where stomach cancer rates are much lower than in the north (or for the country as a whole) (Geddes et al. 1993).

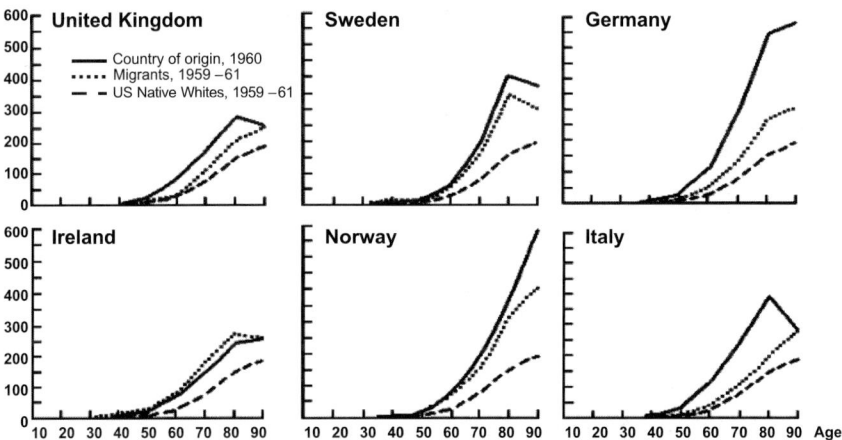

Figure 3.18. Mortality from cancer of stomach (rate per 10^5) in migrants to United States (Lilienfeld et al. 1972)

— *Studies with a time dimension* are studies of the effect of duration of residence or age at migration. Relatively few published studies have been able to study cancer rates in first-generation migrants by duration of stay (or age at arrival) in the host country. The routine recording in Australian death certificates of date of migration has permitted several studies of mortality in relation to duration of residence in Australia; the findings in relation to gastro-intestinal cancers (McMichael et al. 1980) and to malignant melanoma (Khlat et al. 1992) are of particular interest. Figure 3.19 (Khlat et al. 1992) shows the risk of death from melanoma of six migrant populations in relation to either duration of stay or age at arrival, using the Australia-born as the reference group. Since these two variables are completely interdependent (long durations of stay are associated with early ages at arrival), it is impossible to separate their effects. The figure gives the impression that arrival in childhood is associated with relatively high risks, but that in age groups 15–24 years, and 25 years and above, risk remains significantly lower than that of the Australia-born. The irregular increase in risk with duration of stay, with a relatively sharp increase after 30 years for many of the groups makes little biological sense, and could well reflect the excess of childhood immigrants in the long stay category.

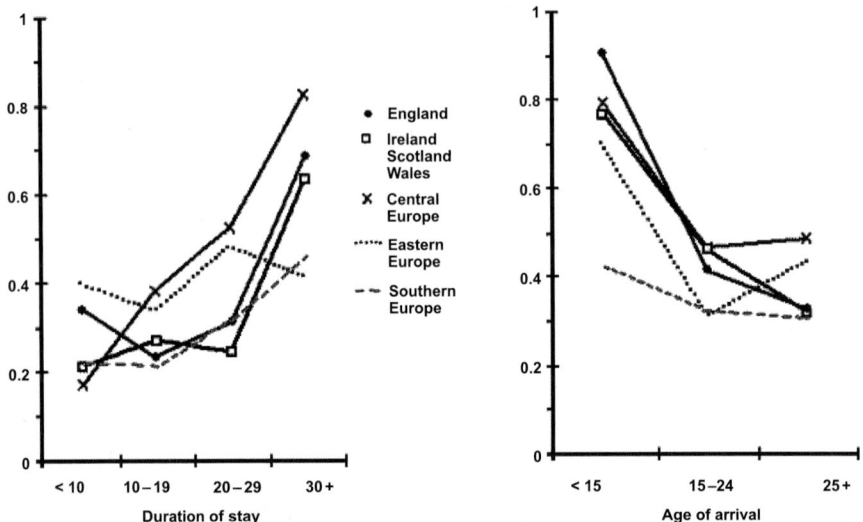

Figure 3.19. Estimated relative risks of melanoma in male immigrants to Australia, by region of birth and according to duration of stay and age at arrival (both in years), compared with the Australian-born and adjusted for age, period, cohort, and state: Australia, 1964–1985 (Khlat et al. 1992)

The Israel Cancer Registry records date of migration for all cases of cancer. This has allowed the risk of cancer to be examined for different populations of migrants in relation to their duration of residence in Israel (Steinitz et al. 1989; Parkin and Iscovich 1997). Figure 3.20 illustrates the risk of cervical cancer in migrants to Israel, relative to the local-born, in relation to duration of stay. The data derive from a long time period (1961–1981) during which there were marked temporal trends in the risk of cervical cancer, and in particular a striking increase in incidence (2.5 times) in the Israel-born, but little change or even slight declines in risk for the migrant groups. Because most migration took place before the data collection period, duration of stay is strongly confounded by time period (short duration-of-stay cases come mainly from earlier periods, and vice versa), and adjustment for time period has a very striking effect on relative risks (Fig. 3.20). These observations may be explicable in terms of cumulative exposure to Pap smear testing following migration, since the high risk of cervical cancer in these populations is well known to clinicians.

— *Studies of second and subsequent generations of migrants.* The best known studies are those of Japanese in the USA (Haenszel & Kurihara, 1968; Locke & King, 1980) and Hawaii (Kolonel et al. 1980; Hankin et al. 1983), and of Chinese in

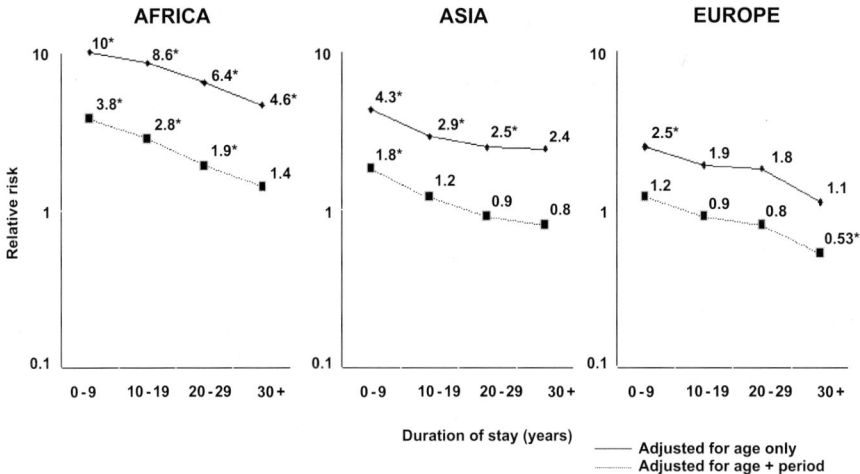

Figure 3.20. Risk of cervix cancer in migrants (relative to local born) (Parkin et al. 1990)

the USA (King et al. 1985), distinguishing the foreign-born (first-generation migrants) from the USA-born (their offspring).

Figure 3.21 shows incidence rates of stomach cancer in two ethnic groups in Hawaii-Japanese and Caucasian (white) in relation to place of birth, and provides rates for the populations of the countries of origin, Japan and USA. Incidence rates in Japanese migrants to Hawaii are lower than in Japan, and in Hawaii-born Japanese they are lower still, but still higher than in the white population. Conversely, in the white population of Hawaii, there is an increase in stomach cancer risk in the locally born compared to US whites (or migrants from the USA).

Birthplace of parents, which is sometimes recorded on death certificates or cancer registries, has been little used to study cancer risk in offspring of migrants. Balzi et al. (1995) used mortality data from Canada to study cancer risks in Italian migrants and Canadian-born individuals of Italian parentage. The latter group was separated into either those with two parents born in Italy, or only one. Figure 3.22 shows results for the two most common cancers, stomach and lung. The risk of stomach cancer, which in migrants is 2–3 times that in the reference population (Canada-born of Canadian parents), is no longer significantly raised in their offspring, while trends in the opposite direction are seen for lung cancer. Parkin and Iscovich (1997), using data from the Israel Cancer Registry, presented odds ratios for migrants and the Israel-born population according to parents' birthplace. Individuals with parents from North Africa retained the increased risk of nasopharynx cancer seen in migrants from that area, while the risk of melanoma remained low in migrants from this area and their offspring.

— *Studies that include information on exposures* at population-level data for the migrants and the population of the host country, and sometimes for country of origin, are examples of ecological studies (Sect. 3.4.2).

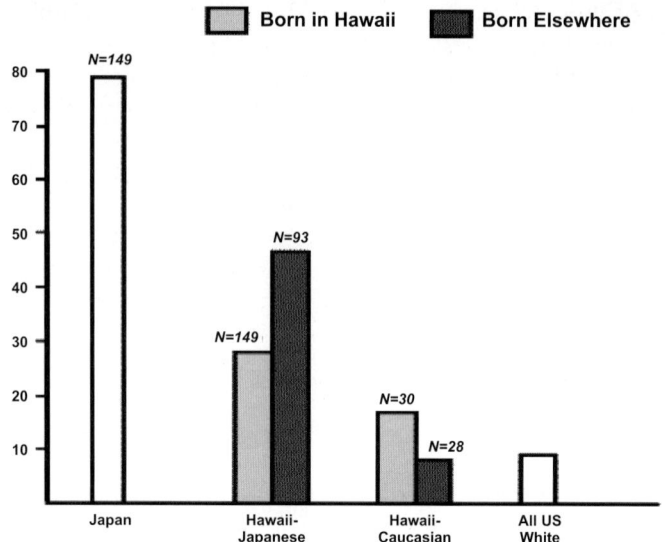

Figure 3.21. Age-adjusted stomach cancer incidence in Hawaii-Japanese and Caucasians by place of birth, 1973 to 1977 (Kolonel et al. 1981)

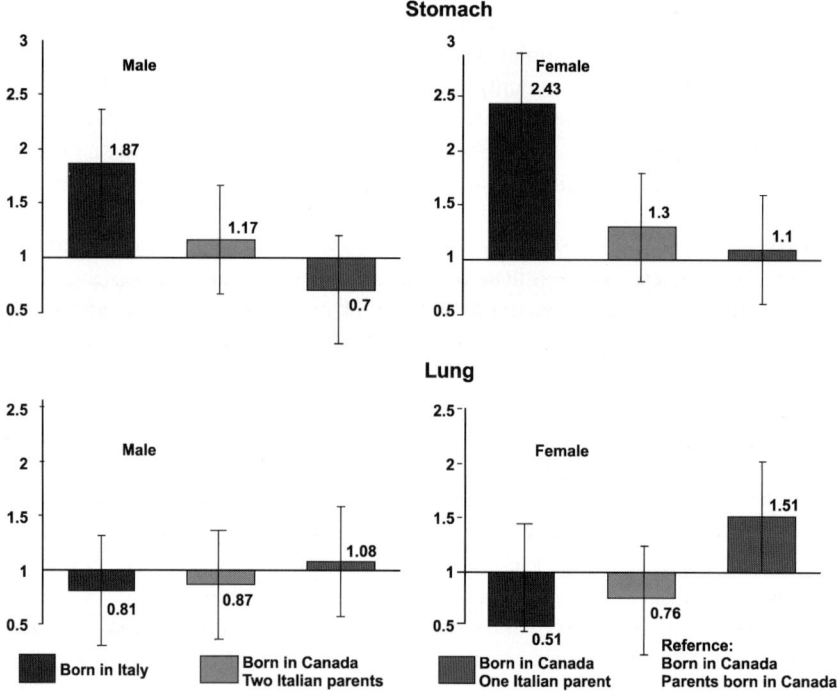

Figure 3.22. Risks and 95% confidence intervals of stomach and lung cancer in Italian migrants and Canadian-born individuals of Italian parentage (reference population: Canada-born of Canadian parents, Balzi et al. 1995)

McMichael and colleagues (1980) related mortality rates from gastro-intestinal cancers in European migrants to Australia with per capita food consumption data from a period 10 years earlier in Australia and the countries of origin; results from a national dietary survey were included later (McMichael and Giles 1988).

For the Japanese population of Hawaii, the dietary intake of a range of nutrients can be estimated from the control subjects in case-control studies and from special surveys (Kolonel et al. 1980; Hankin et al. 1983), and the Japanese population (as well as Hawaii whites) can be separated into those born in Hawaii or elsewhere. The Japan-Hawaii heart study also provides a large amount of information on dietary patterns in Japan and Hawaii (Kagan et al. 1974). These data have been used to help in the interpretation of the changes in risk of stomach cancer in Japanese migrant populations (Fig. 3.21). Thus, second-generation Japanese eat less pickled vegetables and dried salted fish than Japanese migrants (born in Japan), whereas the whites who were born in Hawaii seem to eat these foods more frequently than whites born elsewhere. Both of these items have been associated with an increase in the risk of stomach cancer in case-control studies. The observations were similar for consumption of rice (and total carbohydrate intake), also suggested as aetiologically important in some studies.

Conclusions 3.6

Studies of disease patterns using registers of vital events are often cited as the foundations of modern epidemiology – the work of Graunt on "Bills of Mortality" (Graunt 1662) foreshadowing the enormous contribution of Farr, as statistician to the Registrar General, in analyzing the material on cause of death, provided by the routine registration of vital events in England and Wales. Descriptive epidemiology is a continuation of this theme. The increasing availability of databases related to the health of individuals, or to their possible exposure to causes of disease, has enormously increased the scope for investigations providing clues to aetiological associations. As we describe in this chapter, the information on individuals that is contained in personalized databases is rarely closely related to pathogenetic mechanisms, so that observed associations will generally be suggestive only of causative pathways, and a stimulus to more focused investigations. Thus, differences in the risk of disease according to locality (place of residence, or of birth, or both) may be quite suggestive of an underlying cause (for example, in contaminants of water, background radiation, soil mineral deficiencies, etc.), but the hypotheses will require testing, if possible, by studies that involve collection of information from individual subjects, on variables that are related to the hypothesized more proximal causes.

This chapter provides some background on the tools available in descriptive epidemiology: The sources of routine data on health status, and the basics of measurement and comparison. It illustrates how these can be applied in the study designs familiar to epidemiologists. The second section provides a series of examples, illustrating the principles of descriptive studies.

In an era of genomics, proteomics, metabolomics, etc., the study of disease risk according to demographic characteristics of individuals, or their place of birth, or residence, and the evolution of risk over time, may seem mundane, with little relevance to unraveling the secrets of life. However, the relative simplicity of descriptive studies, in which large populations can be investigated, at relatively little expense, means that they will continue to be widely used. The ecological study, for all its defects, is probably the most popular study design in epidemiology (and much beloved of other disciplines too, for example in economics). Even within the framework of aetiological research, some of the most basic observations remain a challenge to biological explanation (the striking sex ratios for some cancers, for example).

Descriptive epidemiology has, of course, a wide application beyond the realm of the academic epidemiologist focused on investigating the causation of disease. Epidemiology, is, after all, concerned with "The *application* of this study [of the distribution and determinants of health-related states or events in specified populations] to control of health problems" (Sect. 3.1.1). Planning and evaluation of health care requires a knowledge of the magnitude of different problems – their distribution in subgroups within the community, their past and likely future evolution, their amenability to different interventions – and monitoring of the effectiveness of interventions, be they in prevention, early diagnosis, or therapy. Epidemiology is the keystone of Public Health, and attention to the well-being of the health of the populace requires a sound knowledge of the principles of descriptive epidemiology, rather than a detailed knowledge of the proteomics of gene interactions. It is the basic toolkit of the community orientated health specialist.

References

Alderson M (1981) International mortality statistics. McMillan, London

Alexander FE, Boyle P (eds) (1996) Methods for investigating localised clustering of disease. IARC Scientific Publications No 135. International Agency for Research on Cancer, Lyon

Alexander FE, Cuzick J (1992) Methods for the assessment of disease clusters. In: Elliot P, Cuzick J, English D, Stern R (eds) Geographical and environmental epidemiology: Methods for small-area studies. Oxford University Press, Oxford, pp 238–250

Andersen A, Barlow L, Engeland A, Kjaerheim K, Lynge E, Pukkala E (1999) Work-related cancer in the Nordic countries. Scand J Work Environ Health 25 Suppl 2:1–116

Andvord KF (1930) What can we learn from studying tuberculosis by generations? Norsk Mag Loegevidensk 91:642–60

Armstrong BK, White E, Saracci R (1994) Principles of exposure measurement in epidemiology. Oxford University Press, Oxford

Armstrong BK, Woodings TL, Stenhouse NS, McCall MG (1983) Mortality from cancer in migrants to Australia – 1962 to 1971. Nedlands, University of Western Australia, p 138

Balzi D, Geddes M, Brancker A, Parkin DM (1995) Cancer mortality in Italian migrants and their offspring in Canada. Cancer Causes Control 6:68–74

Baquet CR, Ringen K (1986) Cancer among blacks and other minorities: Statistical profiles. National Cancer Institute, USDHHS, National Institute of Health Publication 86–2785, Washington DC

Baris I, Simonato L, Artvinli M, Pooley F, Saracci R, Skidmore J, Wagner C (1987) Epidemiological and environmental evidence of the health effects of exposure to erionite fibres: A four-year study in the Cappadocian region of Turkey. Int J Cancer 39:10–17

Barnett E, Strogatz D, Armstrong D, Wing S (1996) Urbanisation and coronary heart disease mortality among African Americans in the US South. J Epidemiol Community Health 50:252–257

Beral V, Chilvers C, Fraser P (1979) On the estimation of relative risk from vital statistical data. J Epidemiol Community Health 33:159–162

Berrino F, Capocaccia R, Estève J, Gatta G, Micheli A, Hakulinen T, Sant M, Verdecchia A (1999) Survival of cancer patients in Europe: The EUROCARE-2 study. IARC Scientific Publication No 151. International Agency for Research on Cancer, Lyon

Biggar RJ, Horm J, Goedert JJ, Melbye M (1987) Cancer in a group at risk of acquired immunodeficiency syndrome (AIDS) through 1984. Am J Epidemiol 126:578–586

Bithell J (1992) Statistical methods for analysing point source exposures. In: Elliot P, Cuzick J, English D, Stern R (eds) Geographical and environmental epidemiology: Methods for small-area studies. Oxford University Press, Oxford, pp 221–230

Bray F, Guilloux A, Sankila R, Parkin DM (2002) Practical implications of imposing a new World standard population. Cancer Causes Control 13:175–182

Brenner H, Savitz DA, Jockel KH, Greenland S (1992) Effects of nondifferential exposure misclassification in ecologic studies. Am J Epidemiol 135:85–95

Breslow NE (1984) Elementary methods of cohort analysis. Int J Epidemiol 13:112–115

Breslow NE, Day NE (1975) Indirect standardization and multiplicative models for rates, with reference to the age adjustment of cancer incidence and relative frequency data. J Chronic Dis 28:289–303

Breslow NE, Day NE (1980) Statistical methods in cancer research, vol I: The analysis of case-control studies. IARC Scientific Publications No 32. International Agency for Research on Cancer, Lyon

Breslow NE, Day NE (1987) Statistical methods in cancer research, vol II: The design and analysis of case-control studies. IARC Scientific Publications No 82. International Agency for Research on Cancer, Lyon

Carroll KK (1975) Experimental evidence of dietary factors and hormone-dependent cancers. Cancer Res 35:3374–3383

Carstairs V (1995) Deprivation indices: Their interpretation and use in relation to health. J Epidemiol Community Health 49 Suppl 2:S3–8

Centers for Disease Control (1990) Guidelines for investigating clusters of health events. Morbidity & Mortality Weekly Report 39 (No. RR-11):1–23

Chu KC, Baker SG, Tarone RE (1999) A method for identifying abrupt changes in U.S. cancer mortality trends. Cancer 86:157–169

Clayton D, Kaldor J (1987) Empirical Bayes estimates of age-standardised relative risks for use in diease mapping. Biometrics 43:671–681

Clayton D, Schifflers E (1987a) Models for temporal variation in cancer rates. I: Age-period and age-cohort models. Stat Med 6:449–467

Clayton D, Schifflers E (1987b) Models for temporal variation in cancer rates. II: Age-period-cohort models. Stat Med 6:469–481

Cochran WG (1954) Some methods for strengthening the common χ^2 tests. Biometrics 10:417–451

Cutler SJ, Ederer F (1958) Maximum utilization of the life table method in analyzing survival. J Chronic Dis 8:699–712

Das Gupta P, Sen A, Marglin S (1972) Guidelines for project evaluation. United Nations, New York

Day NE (1992) Cumulative rate and cumulative risk. In: Parkin DM, Muir CS, Whelan SL, Gao Y-T, Ferlay J, Powell J (eds) Cancer incidence in five continents, vol VI. IARC Scientific Publications No 120. International Agency for Research on Cancer, Lyon

Day NE, Charnay B (1982) Time trends, cohort effects and aging as influence on cancer incidence. In: Magnus K (ed) Trends in cancer incidence – causes and practical implications. Hemisphere Publication Corporation, Washington, pp 51–65

De Stefani E, Parkin DM, Khlat M, Vassalo A, Abella M (1990) Cancer in migrants to Uruguay. Int J Cancer 46:233–237

Dean HT (1938) Endemic fluorosis and its relation to dental caries. Public Health Reports 53:1443–1452

Dempsey M (1947) Decline in tuberculosis: the death rate fails to tell the entire story. American Review of Tuberculosis 86:157–164

Doll R, Payne P, Waterhouse J (eds) (1966) Cancer incidence in five continents: A technical report. Springer, New York

Doll R, Peto R (1981) The causes of cancer. Oxford University Press, Oxford

Driscoll RJ, Mulligan WJ, Schultz D, Candelaria A (1988) Malignant mesothelioma. A cluster in a Native American pueblo. New Engl J Med 318:1437–1438

Dwyer T, Hetzel BS (1980) A comparison of trends of coronary heart disease mortality in Australia, USA and England & Wales with reference to three major risk factors – hypertension, cigarette smoking and diet. Int J Epidemiol 9:67–71

Dyba T, Hakulinen T, Paivarinta L (1997) A simple non-linear model in incidence prediction. Stat Med 16:2297–2309

Ederer F, Axtell LM, Cutler SJ (1961) The relative survival rate: A statistical methodology. Natl Cancer Inst Monogr 6:101–121

Editorial Committee for the Atlas of Cancer Mortality (1979) Atlas of cancer mortality in the People's Republic of China. China map press

Estève J (1990) International study of time trends. Some methodological considerations. Ann N Y Acad Sci USA 609:77–84

Estève J, Benhamou E, Raymond L (1994) Statistical methods in cancer research, vol IV. Descriptive epidemiology. IARC Scientific Publications No 128. International Agency for Research on Cancer, Lyon

Fienberg SE, Mason WM (1985) Specification and implementation of age, period, and cohort models. In: Mason WM, Fienberg SE (eds) Cohort Analysis in Social Research: Beyond the Identification Problem. Springer-Verlag, New York, pp 44–88

Freid VM, Prager K, MacKay AP, Xia H (2003) Chartbook on trends in the health of Americans. Health, United States, 2003. National Center for Health Statistics, Hyattsville, Maryland

Friis S, Storm H (1993) Urban-rural variation in cancer incidence in Denmark 1943–1987. Eur J Cancer A 29:538–544

Frost WH (1939) The age selection of mortality from tuberculosis in successive decades. Am J Hyg 30:91–96

Gardner MJ, Winter PD, Taylor CP, Acheson ED (1984) Atlas of cancer mortality in England & Wales, 1968–1978. Wiley, Chichester

Geddes M, Parkin DM, Khlat M, Balzi D, Buiatti E (eds) (1993) Cancer in Italian migrant populations. IARC Scientific Publication No 123. International Agency for Research on Cancer, Lyon

Gillum RF (2002) New considerations in analyzing stroke and heart disease mortality trends: The year 2000 age standard and the international statistical classification of diseases and related health problems, 10th revision. Stroke 33:1717–1721

Glenn NK (1976) Cohort analysts' futile quest: Statistical attempts to separate age, period and cohort effects. Am Sociol Rev 41:900–904

Graunt J (1662) Natural and political observations mentioned in a following index, and made upon the bills of mortality. London

Greenland S, Morgenstern H (1989) Ecological bias, confounding and effect modification. Int J Epidemiol 18:269–274

Grulich AE, Swerdlow AJ, Head J, Marmot MG (1992) Cancer mortality in African and Caribbean migrants to England and Wales. Br J Cancer 66:905–911

Haenszel W (1961) Cancer mortality among the foreign born in the United States. J Natl Cancer Inst 26:37–132

Haenszel W, Kurihara M (1968) Studies of Japanese migrants. I. Mortality from cancer and other diseases among Japanese in the United States. J Natl Cancer Inst 40:43–68

Hakulinen T, Hakama M (1991) Predictions of epidemiology and the evaluation of cancer control measures and the setting of policy priorities. Soc Sci Med 33:1379–1383

Hankin JR, Kolonel LN, Yano K, Heilbrun L, Nomura AMY (1983) Epidemiology of diet related diseases in the Japanese migrant population of Hawaii. Proc Nutr Soc Austr 8:22–40

Heasman MA, Lipworth L (1966) Accuracy of certification of cause of death. Studies in Medical and Population Subjects 20. HMSO, London

Hirsch A (1883) Handbook of geographical and historical pathology, vols I–III. Translated from the Second German Edition by Creighton C. The New Syden-ham Society, London

Hoar SK, Morrison AS, Cole P, Silverman DT (1980) An occupation and exposure linkage system for the study of occupational carcinogenesis. J Occup Med 22:722–726

Hobcraft J (1985) Age, period, and cohort effects in demography: A review. In: Mason W M FSE, editor. Cohort Analysis in Social Research: Beyond the Iden-tification Problem. Springer-Verlag, New York, pp 89–135

Holford TR (1983) The estimation of age, period and cohort effects for vital rates. Biometrics 39:311–324

Holford TR (1998) Age-period cohort analysis. In: Armitage P, Colton T (eds). Encyclopaedia of Biostatistics. John Wiley & Sons, Chichester, pp 82–99

Howe GM (1977) A world geography of human diseases. Academic Press, London, New York, San Francisco

Howe GR, Lindsay JP (1983) A follow-up study of a ten-percent sample of the Canadian labor force. I. Cancer mortality in males, 1965–1973. J Natl Cancer Inst 70:37–44

Jensen OM, Parkin DM, MacLennan R, Muir CS, Skeet RG (eds) (1991) Cancer registration: Principles and methods. International Agency for Research on Cancer, Lyon

Kagan A, Harris BR, Winkelstein W, Johnson KG, Kato H, Syne SL, Rhoads GG, Gay ML, Nichaman MZ, Hamilton HB, Tillotson J (1974) Epidemiologic studies of coronary heart disease and stroke in Japanese men living in Japan, Hawaii and California: Demographic, physical, dietary and biochemical characteristics. J Chron Dis 27:345–364

Kaldor J, Khlat M, Parkin DM, Shiboski S, Steinitz R (1990) Log linear models for cancer risk among migrants. Int J Epidemiol 19:233–239

Kaplan EL, Meier P (1958) Nonparametric estimation from incomplete observa-tions. J Am Stat Assoc 53:457–481

Kemp I, Boyle P, Smans M, Muir C (eds) (1985) Atlas of cancer in Scotland 1975–1980. IARC Scientific Publications No 72. International Agency for Research on Cancer, Lyon

Khlat M, Vail A, Parkin DM, Green A (1992) Mortality from melanoma in migrants to Australia: variation by age at arrival and duration of stay. Am J Epidemiol 135:1103–1113

Kim HJ, Fay MP, Feuer EJ, Midthune DN (2000) Permutation tests for joinpoint regression with applications to cancer rates. Stat Med 19:335–351

King H, Li JY, Locke FB, Pollack ES, Tu JJ (1985) Patterns of site-specific displacement in cancer mortality among migrants: The Chinese in the United States. Am J Public Health 75:237–242

Kogevinas M. Pearce N, Susser M, Boffetta P (eds) (1997) Social inequalities and cancer. IARC Scientific Publications No 138. International Agency for Research on Cancer, Lyon

Kolonel LN, Hinds MW, Hankin JR (1980) Cancer patterns among migrant and native-born Japanese in Hawaii in relation to smoking, drinking and dietary habits. In: Gelboin LJV, MacMahon B, Matsushima T, Sugimura T, Takayama S, Takebe H (eds) Genetic and environmental factors in experimental and human cancer. Japan Scientific Societies Press, Tokyo, pp 327–340

Koopman JS, Longini IM Jr. (1994) The ecological effects of individual exposures and non-linear disease dynamics in populations. Am J Public Health 84:836–842

Korteweg R (1951) The age curve of lung cancer. Br J Cancer 5:21–27

Kuh DL, Ben-Shlomo Y (1997) A life course approach to chronic disease epidemiology; tracing the origins of ill-health from early to adult life. Oxford University Press, Oxford

Kupper LL, Janis JM, Karmous A, Greenberg BG (1985) Statistical age-period-cohort analysis: a review and critique. J Chron Dis 38:811–830

Kupper LL, McMichael AJ, Symon MJ, Most BM (1978) On the utility of proportional mortality analysis. J Chron Dis 31:15–22

Last JM (ed) (2001). A dictionary of epidemiology, 4th edn. Oxford University Press, New York

Layard R, Glaister S (1994). Cost-benefit analysis, 2nd edn. Cambridge University Press, Cambridge

Leukaemia Research Fund Centre for Clinical Epidemiology (1997) Handbook and guide to the investigation of clusters of diseases. University of Leeds, UK

Lexis W (1875) Einleitung in die Theorie der Bevölkerungsstatistik. Karl J. Trübner, Strassburg

Liddell FD (1988) The development of cohort studies in epidemiology: A review. J Clin Epidemiol 41:1217–1237

Lilienfeld AM, Lilienfeld, DE (1980) Foundations of Epidemiology. Oxford University Press, New York

Lilienfeld AM, Levin ML, Kessler II (1972) Mortality among the foreign born and in their countries of origin. In: Lee HP, Lilienfeld AM, Levin ML, Kessler II (eds) Cancers in the United States. Harvard University Press, Cambridge, Massachusetts, pp 233–278

Locke FB, King H (1980) Cancer mortality among Japanese in the United States. J Natl Cancer Inst 65:1149–1156

Logan WPD (1982) Cancer mortality by occupation and social class, 1851–1971. IARC Scientific Publications No 36 & Studies on Medical and Population Subjects

No 44. International Agency for Research on Cancer, Lyon, Her Majesty's Stationery Office, London

Lynge E, Thygesen L (1990) Occupational cancer in Denmark. Cancer incidence in the 1970 census population. Scand J Work Environ Health 16 Suppl 2:3–35

Macbeth H, Shetty P (eds) (2001) Health and ethnicity. Taylor & Francis; London, New York

MacMahon B, Pugh H (1970) Epidemiology: Principles and methods. Little Brown and Company, Boston

MacMahon B, Trichopoulos D (1996) Epidemiology: Principles and methods, 2nd edn. Little Brown and Company, Boston

Mantel N, Haenszel W (1959) Statistical aspects of the analysis of data from retrospective studies of disease. J Natl Cancer Inst 22:719–748

Marmot M (1999) Epidemiology of socioeconomic status and health: Are determinants within countries the same as between countries? Ann NY Acad Sci 896:16–29

Marmot MG, Adelstein AM, Bulusu L (1984) Immigrant mortality in England and Wales 1970–1978: Causes of death by country of birth. Studies on Medical and Population Subjects No 47. Her Majesty's Stationery Office, London, p 144

Marshall RJ (1991) A review of methods for the statistical analysis of spatial patterns of disease. In: J R Stat Soc Ser A 154:S421–441

Matos E, Khlat M, Loria DI, Vilensky M, Parkin DM (1991) Cancer in migrants to Argentina. Int J Cancer 49:805–811

McCredie M (1998) Cancer epidemiology in migrant populations. Recent results. Cancer Res 154:298–305

McGill HC (ed) (1968) Geographic pathology of atherosclerosis. Williams & Williams, Baltimore, MD

McMichael AJ, Giles GG (1988) Cancer in migrants to Australia: Extending the descriptive epidemiological data. Cancer Res 48:751–756

McMichael AJ, McCall MG, Hartshorne JM, Woodings TL (1980) Patterns of gastrointestinal cancer in European migrants to Australia: The role of dietary change. Int J Cancer 25:431–437

Miettinen OS, Wang JD (1981) An alternative to the proportionate mortality ratio. Am J Epidemiol 114:144–148

Miller BA, Kolonel LN, Bernstein L, Young JL, Swanson GM, West D, Key CR, Liff JM, Glover CS, Alexander GA (eds) (1996) Racial/ethnic patterns of cancer in the United States 1988–1992. National Cancer Institute, NIH Publication No. 96–4104, Bethesda, MD

Moolgavkar SH, Stevens RG, Lee JA (1979) Effect of age on incidence of breast cancer in females. J Natl Cancer Inst 62:493–501

Morgenstern H (1998) Ecologic studies. In: Rothman KJ, Greenland S (eds) Modern epidemiology, 2nd edn. Lippincott-Raven, Philadelphia

Morgenstern H (1982) Uses of ecologic analysis in epidemiologic research. Am J Public Health 72:1336–1344

Morrow RH, Bryant JH (1995) Health policy approaches to measuring and valuing human life: Conceptual and ethical issues. Am J Public Health 85:1356–1360

Murray CJL, Lopez AD (eds) (1996) The global burden of disease: a comprehensive assessment of mortality and disability from diseases, injuries, and risk factors in 1990 and projected to 2020. Harvard University Press, Cambridge

Murray CJL (1994) Quantifying the burden of disease: the technical basis for disability-adjusted life years. Bull World Health Org 72:429–445

Murray JL, Axtell LM (1974) Editorial: Impact of Cancer: years of life lost due to cancer mortality. J Natl Cancer Inst 52:3–7

Nasca PC, Burnett WS, Greenwald P, Brennan K, Wolfgang P, Carlton K (1980) Population density as an indicator of urban-rural differences in cancer incidence, upstate New York, 1968–1972. Am J Epidemiol 112:362–375

National Center for Health Statistics (2004) Surveys and data collection systems. (http://www.cdc.gov/nchs/express.htm) Accessed May 23, 2004

Nelder JA, Wedderburn RWM (1972) Generalized linear models. Journal of the Royal Statistical Society (Series A) 135:370–384

Office of National Statistics, UK (2004) General household survey. (http://www.statistics.gov.uk/ssd/surveys/general_household_survey.asp) Accessed May 23, 2004

Osmond C, Gardner MJ (1982) Age, period and cohort models applied to cancer mortality rates. Stat Med 1:245–59

Parker SL, Davis KJ, Wingo PA, Ries LA, Heath-CW J (1998) Cancer statistics by race and ethnicity. CA Cancer J Clin 48:31–48

Parkin DM, Iscovich JA (1997) The risk of cancer in migrants and their descendants in Israel: II Carcinomas and germ cell tumours. Int J Cancer 70:654–660

Parkin DM, Steinitz R, Khlat M, Kaldor J, Katz L, Young J (1990) Cancer in Jewish migrants to Israel. Int J Cancer 45:614–621

Parkin DM, Kramarova E, Draper GJ, Masuyer E, Michaelis J, Neglia J, Qureshi S, Stiller CA (1998) International incidence of childhood cancer, vol II. IARC Scientific Publications No 144. International Agency for Research on Cancer, Lyon

Parkin DM, Whelan SL, Ferlay J, Teppo L, Thomas DB (eds) (2002) Cancer incidence in five continents, vol. VIII. IARC Scientific Publications No 155. International Agency for Research on Cancer, Lyon

Pearce N, Weiland S, Keil U, Langridge P, Anderson HR, Strachan D, Bauman A, Young L, Gluyas P, Ruffin D, Crane J, Beasley R (1993) Self-reported prevalence of asthma symptoms in children in Australia, England, Germany and New Zealand: An international comparison using the ISAAC protocol. Eur Resp J 6:1455–1461

Percy C, Stanek E, Gloeckner L (1981) Accuracy of cancer death certificates and its effect on cancer mortality statistics. Amer J Publ Hlth 71:242–250

Peto R, Doll R (1997) There is no such thing as aging. BMJ 315:1030–1032

Piantadosi S, Byar DP, Green SB (1988) The ecological fallacy. Am J Epidemiol 127:893–904

Pickle LM, Mason TJ, Howard N, Hoover R & Fraumeni JF Jr. (1987) Atlas of US cancer mortality among whites, 1950–1980. DHEW Publ No (NIH) 87-2900, Washington DC

Pisani P, Bray F, Parkin DM (2002) Estimates of the world-wide prevalence of cancer for 25 sites in the adult population. Int J Cancer 97:72–81

Pocock SJ, Cook DG, Beresford SAA (1981) Regression of area mortality rates on explanatory variables; what weighting is appropriate? Appl Stat 30:286–295

Prentice RL, Sheppard L (1990) Dietary fat and cancer; consisitency of the epidemiological data, and disease prevention that may follow from a practical reduction in dietary fat consumption. Cancer Causes & Control 1:81–97

Puffer RR, Wynne-Griffith G (1967) Patterns of urban mortality, Pan American Health Organization Scientific Publication 151, Washington

Pukkala E, Söderman B, Okeanov A, Storm H, Rahu M, Hakulinen T, Becker N, Stabenow R, Bjarnadottir K, Stengrevics A, Gurevicius R, Glattre E, Zatonski W, Men T, Barlow L (2001) Cancer atlas of northern Europe. Cancer Society of Finland, Publ. No 62, Helsinki

Registrar General's Office for England and Wales (1978) Occupational mortality: The Registrar General's Decennial Supplement for England and Wales, 1970–72, XVIII. Series D S 1. HMSO No. [O 11 69064483]. Her Majesty's Stationery Office, London

Rose G (1982) Incubation period of coronary heart disease. Brit Med J 284:1600–1601

Rose G, Marmot M (1981) Social class and coronary heart disease. Br.Heart J 45:13–19

Rosen G (1993) A history of public health. Johns Hopkins University Press, Baltimore

Rothman KJ (1990) A sobering start for the cluster busters conference. Amer J Epidemiol 132:6–11

Rothman KJ, Greenland S (eds) (1998) Modern epidemiology, 2nd edn. Lippincott-Raven, Philadelphia

Salem G, Rican S, Jougla E (1999) Atlas de la Sante en France. John Libbey Eurotext, Paris

Sankaranarayanan R, Black RJ, Parkin DM (eds) (1998) Cancer survival in developing countries. IARC Scientific Publications No 145. International Agency for Research on Cancer, Lyon

Segi M (1960) Cancer mortality for selected sites in 24 countries (1950–57). Tohoku University of Medicine, Sendai, Japan

Seow A, Straughan PT, Ng EH, Emmanuel SC, Tan CH, Lee HP (1997) Factors determining acceptability of mammography in an Asian population: A study among women in Singapore. Cancer Causes & Control 8:771–779

Shimizu H, Ross RK, Bernstein L, Yatoni R, Henderson BE, Mack TM (1991) Cancers of the prostate and breast among Japanese and white immigrants in Los Angeles County. Br J Cancer 63:963–966

Siemiatycki J (1996) Exposure assessment in community-based studies of occupational cancer. Occup Hyg 3:41–58

Siemiatycki J, Day NE, Fabry J, Cooper JA (1981) Discovering carcinogens in the occupational environment: a novel epidemiologic approach. J Natl Cancer Inst 66:217–225

Smans M, Estève J (1992) Practical approaches to disease mapping. In: Elliott P, Cuzick J, English D, Stern R (eds) Geographical and environmental epidemiology: Methods for small-area studies. Oxford University Press, Oxford, pp 141–150

Smans M, Muir CS, Boyle P (1992) Atlas of cancer mortality in the European Economic Community. IARC Scientific Publications No 107. International Agency for Research on Cancer, Lyon

Smith GD, Leon D, Shipley MJ, Rose G (1991) Socioeconomic differentials in cancer among men. Int J Epidemiol 20:339–344

Smith P (1987) Comparison between registries: age-standardized rates. In: Muir C, Waterhouse J, Mack T, Powell J, Whelan S (eds) Cancer incidence in five continents, vol V. IARC Scientific Publications No 88. International Agency for Research on Cancer, Lyon

Smith PG (1982) Spatial and temporal clustering In: Schottenfeld D, Fraumeni JF (eds) Cancer epidemiology and prevention. WB Saunders Comp, Philadelphia, Chap. 21

Steenland K, Beaumont J (1984) The accuracy of occupation and industry data on death certificates. J Occup Med 26:288–296

Steinitz R, Parkin DM, Young JL, Bieber CA, Katz L (1989) Cancer incidence in Jewish migrants to Israel 1961–1981. IARC Scientific Publications No 98. International Agency for Research on Cancer, Lyon

Swerdlow A (1991) Mortality and cancer incidence in Vietnamese refugees in England and Wales: A follow-up study. Int J Epidemiol 20:13–19

Tarone RE, Chu KC (1992) Implications of birth cohort patterns in interpreting trends in breast cancer rates. JNCI 84:1402–1410

Tarone RE, Chu KC (1996) Evaluation of birth cohort patterns in population disease rates. Am J Epidemiol 143:85–91

Tsuchiya K (1992) The discovery of the causal agent of Minamata disease. Amer J Ind Med 21:275–280

Tunstall-Pedoe H for WHO MONICA Project Principal Investigators (1988) The World Health Organisation MONICA Project (Monitoring Trends and Determinants in Cardiovascular Disease): A major international collaboration. J Clin Epidemiol 41:105–114

United Nations (1984) Handbook of household surveys. United Nations, New York

Verhasselt Y, Timmermans A (1987) World maps of cancer mortality. Geografisch Instituut VUB, Brussels

Walter SD (1991) The ecologic method in the study of environmental health. II Methodologic issues and feasibility. Env Health Persp 94:67–73

WHO (1992) International statistical classification of diseases and related health problems, 10th revision. World Health Organization, Geneva

WHO (1997) Atlas of mortality in Europe: Subnational patterns 1980/1981 and 1990/1991. WHO Regional Publications; European Series No 75, World Health Organization, Geneva

WHO (1998) Reported information on mortality statistics. World Health Statistics Annual 1996. World Health Organization, Geneva, pp xvi–xxi

WHO (2000) The World Health Report 2000 Health Systems: Improving Performance, WHO, Geneva

WHO (2004) WHO Statistical Information System (WHOSIS). (http://www3.who.int/whosis) Accessed May 28, 2004

Wigle DT, Mao Y, Howe G, Lindsay J (1982) Comparison of occupation on survey and death records in Canada. Can J Public Health 73:242–247

Use of Disease Registers

Måns Rosén, Timo Hakulinen

4.1 # Introduction

Routine data are data collected continuously or at least repeatedly with some time intervals. They could be collected in various ways, e.g. registration by the health services or by interviews with patients or population groups. For epidemiological purposes, it is necessary that the disease cases collected can be related to a specified population base, thus providing the ability to calculate different epidemiological measures as incidence, prevalence etc. The data could then be stored and administered in registers. Health data or disease registers are restricted to persons with diseases or health-related events. The coverage can vary from a total registration to a sample of the population and from national to regional coverage. Data can be routinely collected for various reasons, from economic and administrative purposes to more strict epidemiological purposes.

We have mainly limited our review to registers with data on individuals, i.e. where each individual can be followed-up. The reason is that anonymous data and statistics in registers have limited value for epidemiological purposes. With anonymous data it is, for example, not possible to know whether one individual has been treated 10 times or if ten individuals have been treated once. It is also impossible to add data for follow up without data on individuals to observe the sequence of events. However, some comments on the usefulness of routine anonymous data for descriptive epidemiology will be made.

This chapter is outlined in the following way. First, a presentation of registers will be made including types of registers, organisation, contents and variables in the registers as well as the quality of registers. Second, analytical options for register-based studies will be presented followed by examples of the usefulness and discussions on potentials and limitations of different designs. The ethical questions of autonomy and confidentiality will also briefly be discussed.

4.2 # Types of Registers

The most widespread and well-known registers are the cause of death- and cancer registers. Most countries in the world have cause of death registers, mostly based on total registration and in some cases on a sample of deaths. The coverage of cause of death is usually very high since it is usually not allowed to bury a person before you have a death certificate. Cancer registers are also frequently used around the world. In several countries it is mandatory for the physician to report all patients they have diagnosed with malignant neoplasms.

Medical birth registers are also disease registers common in many countries, though not as widespread as the cause of death and cancer registers. This kind of registers usually has medical data on the new-born child and sometimes also information on the mother. In some countries, registers on congenital malformations are in operation. Several of these registers started as a consequence of the thalidomide catastrophe in the 1960s (Ericson et al. 1977).

A fourth type of register is the hospital discharge register with data on hospitalised patients. Mainly they contain data on diagnoses and treatments of the patient. Hospital discharge registers are not always population-based or nationwide and data are, from an epidemiological point of view, more difficult to interpret since they do not cover the whole chain of care. Different care strategies can heavily affect whether patients with the same disease are hospitalised or treated in out-patient settings.

These four types of registers are the most common ones. There are also a lot of local research registers covering other disease groups like cardiovascular and psychiatric diseases. They usually follow a cohort for a long time and are administered by research groups. However, we have excluded research registers since they cannot usually be considered as routinely collected. In countries where disease registers are lacking, data from health insurance systems can be a basis for epidemiological research. They can be routinely collected data on sickness absence of employees or health outcomes of the insured population. One problem is that insurance systems and insured populations usually vary in many aspects, which may create biases and lack of comparability. Validity may also be impaired due to the fact that these data are generated for administrative purposes. Diagnoses and treatments may be influenced by aspects related to payments and accounting. Another problem is that the insurance registers are not always accessible because of confidentiality.

A more recent phenomenon is the development of quality registers. In Sweden, there are about 50 national quality registers covering treatment procedures and outcomes for different disease groups or medical interventions (NBHW 2000). There are quality registers for hip replacement, hernia operations, diabetes, cataract, cardiac intensive care etc. New data sets or registers have also been created by record-linkages, the most common ones being linkages between the population censuses and the cause of death and cancer registers. The purposes and epidemiological applications for these linkages will be presented later on in this section. In a few countries like Denmark there are individual-based registers for drugs and abortions. In the following, we have restricted our presentation to the four most common registers, i.e. cause of death, cancer, medical birth and hospital discharge registers.

Organisation of Registries 4.3

According to the IEA dictionary of epidemiology (Last 1988) the term "register" is applied to the file of data that can be related to a population base, i.e. the actual document, while the registry is the system of ongoing registrations. The organisation of registries and collection of data differ from country to country, but they have always some basic governmental or other public funding. In most countries, the registries are organised within a governmental body like national statistical offices or national boards of health and welfare. Many cancer registries have more or less close links to cancer societies from where they also typically get their funding.

The Nordic countries have a long tradition of collecting data on deaths and diseases. They employ epidemiological registers of high quality covering the whole population. The cause of death has been registered in Sweden since 1751 (computerised from 1952) onwards while the oldest cancer register is the Danish one dating back to 1943. The register of congenital malformations was established in Sweden in 1964 as an early warning system and as a direct response to the thalidomide catastrophe. The medical birth register founded in the 1970s includes information on mothers and children, e.g. diagnoses, birth weight and height, operations, maternal tobacco and drug use during pregnancy etc. In Denmark in-patient care is recorded since 1977 and ambulatory care since 1995. The National Hospital Discharge Register covers all publicly run in-patient care in Sweden from 1987, including information on diagnoses, surgical procedures etc. From 2001, the Government has empowered the National Board also to collect information on hospital out-patient care. The value of these registers grows continuously as time passes.

The routine registers may not always be in an optimal shape for reliable statistics and research. It has proven useful to dedicate scientifically qualified staff to run the register (Jensen and Whelan 1991). This personnel has a research interest in the data. When the register data are good enough for scientific research they normally also are guaranteed to be very good for routine statistics production. Moreover, the dedicated personnel is very useful in helping other researchers with the data use by knowing the strengths and weaknesses and the most relevant method issues. Of course, there is a risk that researchers give priority to their own research instead of giving service to outside researchers. This potential problem is best dealt with by careful instruction and legislation concerning equal access to data.

In many countries, e.g. in Finland, the existence of such personnel has been guaranteed by creating a cancer registry (Finnish Cancer Registry 2002). The Finnish Cancer Registry is a research organisation specialised in statistics and studies making use of the nation-wide cancer register in Finland. In Sweden, the Centre for Epidemiology is an organisation responsible for several other diseases and health registers in addition to the cancer register in Sweden (EpC 2003a; www.sos.se/epc). These research organisations have a multidisciplinary scientific staff consisting of epidemiologists, statisticians, physicians, social scientists, computer scientists etc.

It is necessary to have legislation on the registration and its supporting scientific organisation. Both in Finland and in Sweden, the existence of the health registers and the way they are run with responsibilities, rights and obligations is based on laws. It is also important to have secured funding and the core scientific staff, in addition to the clerical staff, on permanent funding. The knowledge required cannot possibly be maintained by scientists on short-term project funding contracts only.

Contents and Variables in the Registers

A necessity in registers with data on individuals is a unique identity, usually in forms of a person identification number (PIN) or a social security number. In some countries it is necessary to rely on names and addresses as the identifier which creates some biases and practical problems as for follow-up.

Using the unique personal identification number, it is possible to link data from other sources about exposure or treatment to outcomes in these health data registers. This Nordic system has created large data banks that are invaluable to the research community, since data do not have to be collected from scratch. Thousands of scientific articles have been published based on data from these registers.

Variables usually collected in all these registers are PIN, sex, age and residential area of the individual (Table 4.1). The cause of death register usually includes data on underlying and contributory causes of death, place and date of death and basis of cause certification. For the cancer registers, data on tumours, date of diagnosis, histological type, reporting department, hospital and pathology/cytology department etc. are available. Medical birth registers generally include data on sex, weight, length, size of head, analgesia, birth conditions and operations of the children, but also data on the mother's previous gestation, smoking habits and in Sweden also drugs taken during pregnancy. Hospital discharge registers include data on main and secondary diagnoses, external cause of injury and poisoning, surgical procedures, date of admittance and discharge, length of stay, hospital and clinical department. Except operations, there are in general few or no data on type of interventions during hospital stay.

Table 4.1. Common variables in health data registers in the Nordic countries

Register	Variables
Cause of death register	PIN (personal identification number), age, sex, place of residence, date and place of death, underlying cause of death, nature of the injury, contributing causes of death, autopsy (clinical or forensic), place of death
Cancer register	Name, PIN, age, sex, place of residence, site of tumour, histological type, basis of diagnosis, date of diagnosis, reporting hospital and department and reporting pathology/cytology department
Medical birth register	Infants date of birth (PIN), sex, weight, length, head circumference, gestational age and diagnoses. Mothers PIN, age, smoking habits, medication, diagnoses, place of residence, operations, type of analgesia, type of delivery, reporting hospital
Hospital discharge register/ patient register	PIN, sex, age, place of residence, date of admission, date of discharge, acute/planned admission, main and secondary diagnoses, external cause of injury and poisoning, surgical procedures and hospital/department These registers are in some countries enlarged to also include out-patient visits at hospitals.

The Quality of Data in Registers

The quality and validity of routinely collected data can hardly be as consistent as for those obtained in clinical trials where pre-defined criteria for diagnosis have been chosen. However, many studies have been conducted showing relatively good quality and validity of diagnoses in these registers. In general, cancer diagnoses have good quality as well as causes of death based on autopsies. The quality is in general better for younger than for older people who often have several diseases.

Cancer registration in the Nordic countries is based on compulsory reports from all physicians and all pathologists, in both public and private administration. One Swedish study from the 1980s estimated the deficit in cancer registration to be 4.5% and less than 2% when the diagnosis had been histologically verified (Mattsson 1984). A Finnish study showed good coverage for solid tumours, but a roughly 10% underregistration for benign neoplasms of the central nervous system, chronic lymphatic leukaemia and multiple myeloma (Teppo et al. 1994). Technical quality control procedures are usually applied by cancer registries, e.g. the computers are programmed to detect invalid codes, inconsistent combinations of codes, duplicate registrations and illogical time sequences. Examples of inconsistent combination of codes are testis cancer in a female and distant metastasis associated with carcinoma in situ. This kind of quality control reduces some types of errors, but cannot deal with missing data or false primary diagnoses. In the Finnish Cancer Register, some 2% of all cancers are coded to "primary site unknown" (Teppo et al. 1994). Some cancers will never be diagnosed during the life-time of individuals, but may occur on the death certificate after an autopsy. Thus, changes and differences in autopsy rates between time periods and regions may affect the validity of cancer registration. The increase in incidence of prostate cancer during the last decade is to a large extent due to extensive PSA tests rather than a real increase in incidence (Tretli et al. 1996; Walsh 2002).

The quality of cause of death registers varies considerable depending on the age of the deceased, underlying and contributing diseases and depending on practise variations among physicians and coders. In general, fatal diseases where the deceased has been treated for some time before death have good quality, e.g. most cancers and ischaemic heart disease. The autopsy rates are usually higher for younger people and accidents, which makes this group of diagnoses quite reliable. Diabetes is a more troublesome diagnosis and is usually underreported, mainly as a contributing cause of death. In one quality study, the hospital discharge records were compared with death certificates (Johansson and Westerling 2002). The conclusion was that most differences between underlying cause of death and final main diagnosis in hospitals can be explained by differences in ICD (International Classification of Diseases) selection procedures. An international death certificate study showed variations in classification procedures by country (Percy and Muir 1989) and also regional variations within a country should be interpreted with caution due to potential practise variations.

A general problem in many cause of death registers are the declining autopsy rates (Lindström et al. 1997). In Sweden the overall autopsy rate was about 41% in 1980 and about 15% in 2000.

The quality of data in hospital discharge registers varies considerably mainly due to type of diagnosis and age of the patients. In the Swedish hospital register, estimations of underreporting are hard to make for psychiatric and geriatric care, but the underreporting has been estimated to be less than 2% for somatic short-term care. In 2001, personal identification numbers were missing in 0.4% of number of stays and the main diagnosis was missing in 0.9% of the stays reported from Swedish hospitals. Two types of diagnostic errors can occur, false positives and false negatives. In a Swedish validity study of acute myocardial infarction in the hospital discharge register, about 6% of those with an infarction in the register were considered false while 3% of those with other diagnoses in the hospital discharge register ought to have had an acute myocardial infarction as the main diagnosis (Rosén et al. 2000). This bias must be considered minor in epidemiological studies, especially considering the high coverage and large number of cases. At present the register contains more than 500,000 cases of acute myocardial infarction. Another validity study of 875 discharges in the hospital patient register in 1990 showed inconsistencies in main diagnoses of about 3% for ICD-chapters, 12% for 3-digit codes and 14% for 4-digit codes (www.sos.se/epc/par).

The Swedish Medical Birth Register completely misses about 0.5%–3.9% of all records for infants (EpC 2003b). Single items of information may also be missing to a varying degree. Missing data significantly affect estimates of incidence, but has only a slight effect on risk estimates. In most cases, variables are fairly valid, but for studies of extreme outcomes caution must be exercised. Omissions with regard to severely ill neonatals are selective due to several reasons including referals of babies between hospitals. However, since only 1%–2% of those records are missing, the problem is manageable. With regard to exposure data, information on smoking in early pregnancy is good, while information on maternal drug use is incomplete (EpC 2003b). For some drugs, it is likely that the woman or the reporting midwife does not regard them as significant and therefore does not record them. However, since all exposure data are obtained prospectively, this will have little effect on risk estimates.

Study Designs in Register-based Studies   4.6

Disease and mortality registers could be used to measure incidence, prevalence, mortality and survival of different diseases over time and for different geographical areas and population groups. This is an important task for descriptive epidemiology (cf. Chap. I.3 of this handbook), but the main advantage of registers for analytical purposes is that data from other sources can be connected to the outcome data in registers. Record linkage of two or more national registers is one option. An early application of record linkage conducted already in the 1960s was to link the population censuses with the cancer and cause of death registers. The primary aim was to identify occupational groups with excess risks in order to prevent occupational hazards. Record linkage of the cancer and cause of death register facilitates survival analysis of cancer patients.

One common application is that researchers use their own collected cohort as a baseline and then make follow-up in the national health data registers. The "Study of men born in 1913" is one such example of a cohort study where subjects with local registration of risk factors for cardiovascular disease were followed-up for decades in health data registers like the cause of death register (Tibblin et al. 1975).

In case-control studies, you identify cases in the disease registers and choose a control group from the general population or from a group of patients with other diseases and then add information on exposure to some risk factors or to treatment.

In the Nordic tradition it is from a practical point of view quite easy to make record-linkage by using the personal identification number. Of course, you have to consider confidentiality and national legislation.

4.7 Potentials and Limitations of Register-based Studies

In general, the advantages of routine collected and register-based studies are that data are already collected and in an objective way with regard to specific studies, the number of observations is large and data are often nation-wide and cover a whole population. Register-based studies have the limitations of having a restricted number of variables collected, which are not specified in advance for the research question in focus. Quality of data can differ, but as described above, they are usually manageable for epidemiological research.

For analytical purposes, the big difference is whether data are individual-based or aggregated. Due to concerns about integrity, some routine collected data include aggregated data only and do not have observations on individual subjects. Analyses restricted to studies of aggregated data are usually called ecological studies. Thus, the group rather than the individual is the unit of observation and analysis. The groups may be defined according to occupation, place of residence, socio-economic positions etc.

The limitation of ecological studies is that causal inference on individuals is not possible to conduct. In 1950, Robinson showed that data describing group level conditions cannot be inferred to the behaviour of individuals, a problem he called "ecological fallacy" (Robinson 1950). Ecological fallacy can be illustrated in different ways. One such often quoted example is the high correlation in trends between a decreasing number of breeding storks and a similar decrease in birth-rate among the Danish population. The problem of ecological fallacy has also

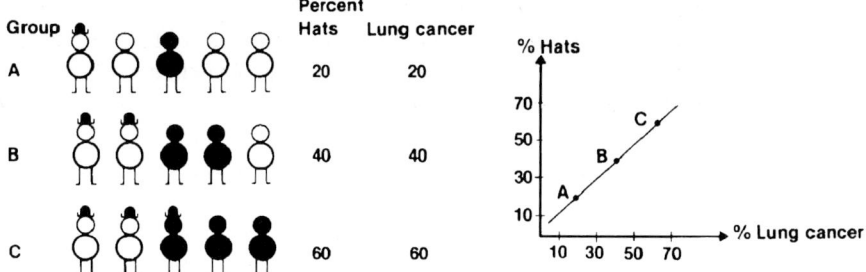

Figure 4.1. An example of ecological correlation (Rosén et al. 1985)

been illustrated in an article (Rosén et al. 1985) by imaging three groups: *A*, *B* and *C* (Fig. 4.1). These may denote counties, municipalities or occupations. Group *A* consists of 5 individuals, one of whom wears a hat and one has lung cancer (black figure). This means that one out of 5 – i.e. 20% – wear hat and 20% have lung cancer in group *A*. Group *B* and *C* are then computed accordingly. Simple correlation analysis will give a correlation coefficient (r) of 1.0 on the group level. However, if each individual is studied separately, those who wear hats and those who develop lung cancer are generally not one and the same.

In spite of this limitation, high correlation coefficients between group data are indications of associations and have been frequently used to generate valuable hypotheses. High correlation between fat intake and ischaemic heart disease (Keys 1953) or between fibre intake and colorectal cancer (Bingham et al. 1979) have generated dietary hypotheses followed up by studies with analytical designs.

Without doubt, accessibility to individual-based data in register research has a tremendous advantage when it comes to causal inferences. In the following some examples of the usefulness of register-based studies will be demonstrated, mainly when individual data are a necessity.

Examples of the Usefulness   4.8

Many registers in the Nordic countries are nation-wide and cover the whole population. It may, however, be questioned, particularly in larger countries, whether it is not sufficient to do periodic surveys or registration in geographically limited areas for the assessment of the occurrence of disease in a country. The answer may depend on the disease and on the desired goals of the registration or study. For rare diseases, it is important to have large samples in order to come to conclusive answers. In environmental studies, it is an advantage to have data covering many different areas of a country. This will be illustrated later in this chapter. If epidemiological data are used for planning purposes like identifying needs of preventive actions, studies of equity in access to care or allocating health care resources, it is also important to have data from all parts of a country.

Many thousands of scientific articles have been published based on data from national registers around the world and particularly from the Nordic countries. In many cases the studies have added a piece of knowledge to the existing state of the art or later been replicated with other kinds of epidemiological studies, in others it has been nearly impossible for economic reasons to conduct studies without the use of registers. In general, register-based studies are very cost-effective due to the fact that data have already been collected for a long time period. Illustrations of the usefulness of register-based studies will be presented under four headings, environmental studies, occupational studies and social epidemiology, survival analysis and surveillance of drug effects.

4.8.1   Environmental Studies

If the goal is to give answers related to environmental exposures, it is useful to have the registration in the whole country and over a longer period of time. In Finland, the Chernobyl accident in 1986 resulted in a radioactive fallout with rain (Auvinen et al. 1994). The exposure level varied strongly between areas that were quite irregular in shape and did not coincide with health districts. The cancer registry had been in existence by that date for 33 years. Thus, it was possible to reconstruct historical trends in childhood leukaemia incidence in each of these different irregular areas and to study whether any changes in these trends could be related to the exposure level in the area. The answer was negative for the periods of 1986–1988 and 1989–1992 (Auvinen et al. 1994).

More than 500,000 cleanup workers from the former Soviet Union were forced to clean the accident site in Chernobyl and its environment. The number from Estonia was almost 5000 (Rahu et al. 1997). Since there had been a reliable cancer registration in Estonia since 1978 that continued also after the accident and the return of the cleanup workers it was possible to estimate whether or not the cancer risk of the workers had been affected. The result has been negative for the period of 1986–1993 (Rahu et al. 1997). However, in the former workers an increased risk of dying through suicide has been shown by the Cause of Death Register. Biologic dosimetry done on the workers has also indicted that the range of doses the workers received was not likely to cause markedly increased cancer risks (Bigbee et al. 1997).

On the other hand, the majority of the 500,000 cleanup workers came from areas in the former USSR where there was no reliable cancer registration (IPHECA 1996). Had there been a reliable cancer registration it would have been possible to give much more accurate estimates of possible excess risks.

Cancer registration also revealed excess cancer risks related to the Chernobyl accident: children having lived in the nearby areas of Chernobyl experienced an epidemic of thyroid cancer (Kazakov et al. 1992). This was totally unexpected given the scientific knowledge available at the time of the accident.

Another example on routine register use is provided by a much smaller local exposure. In 1987, increased concentrations of chlorophenol were detected in the drinking water source of Järvelä, the center of Kärkölä municipality in Southern Finland (Lampi et al. 1992). According to the International Agency for Research on Cancer, exposure was related to possible increased risks at eight sites of cancer. The cancer registration in Finland covered Kärkölä, the other municipalities in the same local health care district and all the municipalities in the corresponding cancer control region. It was therefore very easy to quantify whether the population in the exposed municipality had faced any increased risks since 1953 related to the suspected eight forms of cancer or related to any other cancer. The results showed an increased risk of non-Hodgkin lymphoma and of soft-tissue tumours during the most recent 15 years but not before that time. Subsequent case-control studies in the local health care district based on the material from the cancer registry confirmed that only these two cancers were concerned and the excess risk could be related to chloropherol exposure. The exposure had come from a sawmill in Järvelä and was related to anti-fungal treatment of timber. Subsequent sediment analyses revealed that the exposure had been there for decades.

The cancer registry receives very often concerns about possible local increases in cancer risk. Then it is necessary to count the expected numbers of cases on the basis of suitable reference populations (e.g. neighbours or the cancer control region) and to evaluate the historical development in the area itself and in the other comparable areas. Moreover, it is useful to evaluate the development with all the other cancers, as well. All these evaluations can be done really quickly when the historical database and the software are in an appropriate condition. In Finland, it is indeed easy to follow the guidelines in this situation (Centers for Disease Control 1990).

The cancer register has been an important source e.g. for analysing the association between residential radon exposure and lung cancer in Sweden (Pershagen et al. 1994) and the potential effects of magnetic fields (Feychting and Ahlbom 1993). The Swedish medical birth register was used to show that there was no significant adverse pregnancy outcome in Sweden after the Chernobyl accident (Ericson and Källén 1994). For a more detailed discussion of environmental epidemiology in general we refer to Chap. III.3 of this handbook.

Occupational Studies and Social Epidemiology   4.8.2

Occupations at high risk for cancer and premature mortality have been followed and analysed using record linkages of population censuses with the cancer register or the cause of death register (Andersen et al. 1999; EpC 1999; Pollán and Gustavsson 1999). By linking two population censuses, 1960 and 1970, with the cancer register, risks of long-term occupational exposure could be studied. Based on analysis of this data set, some research results were confirmed, while other hypotheses were rejected (EpC 1999). Excess risks for lip cancers among farmers and fishermen, and excess lung cancer risks among miners and chimneysweeps were confirmed. On the other hand, earlier found associations between bladder cancer and dental technicians or between brain tumours and engine-drivers could not be found in this study of long-term occupational exposure. Overall, work environment nowadays plays a less important role in causing cancer. Rather psycho-social factors are in the focus of occupational research and one study based on a record-linkage between a population census and the Swedish hospital discharge register showed an increased risk of myocardial infarction among men and women working in a stressful and monotonous environment (Alfredsson et al.1985) (for more details on occupational epidemiology see Chap. III.2 of this handbook).

The national registers have been used continuously to study social inequalities in health by record-linking health data registers with population censuses (Persson et al.(eds) 2001; Hallqvist et al. 1998) and disease risks for vulnerable groups, e.g. psychiatric patients, immigrants and single mothers (Ringbäck et al. 1998, 2000). In these cases national registers have been the only source. Other aspects related to social epidemiology are discussed in Chap. III.1 of this handbook.

Many studies of the health and social outcomes of single parents and their children have been conducted by linking several registers, i.e. population census, total enumeration income survey, hospital discharge register and the cause of death register. The studies show increased premature mortality and morbidity both for single parents and their children even after adjustments for socio-economic factors and previous somatic and psychiatric inpatient history (Ringbäck et al. 2000, 2003). Socio-economic factors, especially a lack of economic resources explained some of the disadvantages. Still, the results indicated an independent excess risk for single parents irrespective of socio-economic factors and health selection into single parenthood. The credibility of the studies was considered to be very high, mainly due to the complete coverage and long follow up. These studies covered more than 90,000 lone mothers, more than 622,000 cohabitant mothers, about 65,000 children with single parents and more than 921,000 children with two parents.

4.8.3 Survival Analysis

Survival analysis of cancer patients is a common application where registers have been used as extensive sources. Linking date of cancer incidence in cancer registers to date of death in the cause of death register create opportunities for survival analysis. Many large survival analyses have been published based on registers (Berrino et al. (eds) 1995, 1999; Stenbeck and Rosén (eds) 1995; Dickman et al. 1999; Adami et al. 1989). The EUROCARE-2 Study included follow-up of nearly 1.3 million cancer cases (Berrino et al. 1999). One methodological problem in survival analysis is that survival analysis by definition must be based on historical data, thus, assessing the effects of old treatment strategies. This problem is universal irrespective if the study is based on registers or not. However, one way to reduce this problem is to conduct period analysis using the latest information available (Brenner and Hakulinen 2002). Further methodological aspects are discussed in Chap. II.4 of this handbook. The social dimension of cancer survival has also been investigated in some studies by linking population census and cancer register (Vågerö and Persson 1987; Dickman et al. 1997).

It has also been possible to create databases of the incidence of acute myocardial infarction (AMI) in Sweden, Denmark and Finland by linking the hospital discharge register and the cause of death register (Rosén et al. 2000; Abildström et al. 2003; Salomaa et al. 1992). The validity of this AMI register is, as presented in an earlier section, quite high. The Swedish database was established in 1995 and includes in 2003 more than 500,000 patients with acute myocardial infarction. The register is used for many research purposes and for following trends in the incidence, mortality and case fatality of myocardial infarction. In 1987, 47% of those with an AMI died within 28 days. In 2000 less than 37% died within 28 days. Sex differences in case fatality after AMI have been analysed by using this type of database (Rosengren et al. 2001; Rosén et al. 1999).

Surveillance of Drug Effects   4.8.4

The study of vitamin K and childhood cancer well illustrates the advantages of large national health registers. A case-control study by Golding et al. (1992) published in the BMJ indicated that intramuscular vitamin K administration doubled the risk of childhood cancer compared to oral administration. Since intramuscular administration was recommended by the National Board of Health and Welfare, this result created much concern in Sweden, but also in other countries. In Sweden, a study based on the medical birth and cancer registers was initiated. However, the Swedish study, also published in the BMJ, showed no increased risk of childhood cancer (Ekelund et al. 1993). Later studies have confirmed the Swedish results. There were several differences between the British case-control study and the Swedish register-based study. One was sample size: the case-control study included 195 cases and 558 controls while the register-based study included more than 2300 childhood cancers and 1.3 million controls. In the register-based study, data were already available in the registers and data from the medical birth and cancer register were record-linked. Supplemented with data on maternity hospital routines for vitamin K administration, the study was complete within a few months. This example well illustrates both the reliability advantages of using large national registers as well as the cost-effectiveness of such an approach. For more details on pharmacoepidemiologic studies please refer to Chap. III.9 of this handbook.

Since 1994, data on drug use during pregnancy have been collected in the Swedish medical birth register to monitor potential side-effects of drugs. To our knowledge, this is the only register in the world prospectively collecting data both on drug use during pregnancy and on perinatal outcomes. Several studies have already been published (Ericson et al. 1999; Källén 1998; Källén et al. 1999; Källén and Otterblad Olausson 2003; Gerhardsson de Verdier and Norjavaara 2001). Two studies showed no excess risk of using inhaled budesonide during pregnancy (Källén et al. 1999; Gerhardsson de Verdier and Norjavaara 2001). The Food and Drug Administration in the United States changed their safety classification based on these studies. Data from the Swedish medical birth register have been used in one study to find an association between maternal use of the anti-allergic drug loratadine and congenital hypospadias (Källén and Otterblad Olausson 2002). A biological mechanism explaining the association is still unknown. The study was first discussed with the Swedish Medical Products Agency and is now followed by the European Agency for the Evaluation of Medical Products (EMEA).

4.8.5   **Other Examples of Etiological Research**

Epidemiological registers have often been used in etiological research, i.e. search-ing for risk factors to different diseases and health outcomes. The study of men born 1913 in Gothenburg is one such study displaying risk factors for cardiovascular disease.

The medical birth register has been used extensively, e.g. to analyse the risk of smoking during pregnancy (Ericson et al. 1991; Cnattingius and Haglund 1997), teenage pregnancy outcomes (Otterblad Olausson et al. 1999) and effects on chil-dren born after in-vitro fertilisation (Bergh et al. 1999).

A family-cancer database has been constructed in Sweden by linking population registers and the national cancer register in order to study familial cancer risks (Hemminki and Vaittinen 1998). The database includes approximately 6 million persons and more than 30,000 cancers in offspring diagnosed at ages 15–51 years and their parents. Numerous studies have been published based only on this database (Hemminki and Vaittinen 1998; Hemminki and Li 2001).

Risk factors for breast cancer have been studied with cancer registers as the main data base (Lambe et al. 1994, 1996). The long-term effects of oestrogen and oestrogen-progestin-replacement therapies on breast cancer and hip fracture have been analysed by register data (Magnusson et al. 1999, Naessén et al. 1990). Most of the randomised controlled studies of mammography screening for breast cancer have been conducted in Sweden (Nyström et al. 2002). Also the effects of service screening have been extensively followed (Duffy et al. 2002, Jonsson et al. 2001). In all these assessments, the cause of death register has been the main source for follow-up of mortality.

This short summary of conducted studies shows clearly both the present and the future benefits of register-based epidemiological research.

4.8.6   **Quality Control in Medical Care Using Registers**

There is a general trend world-wide to improve systems for quality control in medical care (OECD 2002). Outcomes of care have often been assessed by mortality analysis. One famous example is the coronary bypass mortality study in New York State (Hannan et al. 1994, 1995) where they gathered clinical data whereby results could be adjusted for risks or patient mix. Frequent discussions and analyses of mortality after bypass surgery took place. During the study period mortality declined by 41% while it went down by only 18% in the rest of the country. The improvement was claimed to partly be due to the fact that less successful teams abandoned the market and partly to quality improvements by the other teams (OECD 2002).

Another approach is to routinely collect data on treatment procedures and outcomes of care in clinical or quality registers. An early example is the registry for total hip replacement surgery in Sweden which started in 1979 (NBHW 2000). Serious complications have served as a measure of the quality improvement of prosthetic techniques over time. Nowadays more than 50 quality registers are in operation in Sweden (NBHW 2000). Besides many orthopaedic and surgical registers, there are quality registers for cardiac intensive care, stroke, cataract, several cancer sites etc. The Federation of County Councils and the National Board of Health and Welfare collaborate at the national level in providing financial and other kinds of support for creation and development of the national quality registers. Similar developments can be seen internationally, both in the Nordic and in other European countries. The Hip Fracture Register in Sweden started in 1988, but has now expanded to a European Commission Concerted Action Project where data are compared and analysed between almost all EU's Member States (Parker et al. 1998).

Ethics, Confidentiality and Legislation 4.9

The principles of autonomy, doing good, doing no harm, justice and solidarity must guide decisions on how to administer national registers. The decision is a trade-off between benefits and risks (Allebeck 2002). The registers and their use are governed by national legislation.

There is one main difference between research based on these types of disease registers and other research projects where it is necessary to collect data on individuals. In the latter there is a need for informed consent from all participants. This is not possible for routinely collected national disease registers. For this kind of routinely collected national data bank it would be practically and economically impossible to apply the informed-consent rule. To do so would substantially hamper clinical work and take resources from other important health service tasks. One may say that parliament and the government have given informed consent on behalf of the population by national legislation. This exception from the rule of informed consent is based on the judgement that the benefits far outweigh the negative consequences. Here principles of doing good and justice or solidarity outweigh that of autonomy.

Another important topic is the risk of violating individual integrity. This risk of doing harm may be twofold: the risk of unlawful trespass/encroachment of data on individual diseases, and the perceived uneasiness/discomfort at just being registered. No system could guarantee 100% security, but after more than four decades of administer health data registers in the Nordic countries, there is no known case of misuse or data leakage to unauthorised persons. The risk of data trespass is very small.

That some people feel discomfort at just being registered is a negative aspect we must consider seriously. Public confidence in health data registers is influenced by mass media debate and knowledge of how the registers are being handled. This confidence could vary from country to country. In surveys, about 9% of the Swedish population feel registration is a threat to personal integrity. Dissemination of the purposes and the usefulness, and the careful administration, of these registers are therefore important and never-ending responsibilities for administrators and users.

It may well be concluded that it is worth having routine registers and registries also for giving a good basis for scientific research. Thus, scientific research should not primarily be seen as a utilizer of registers created mainly for other purposes. The only justification of registration is that the registered data are used. The use has to be guaranteed by securing the manpower and resources and by finding a correct balance between the individual's right to privacy protection and the right of the individual and the mankind to benefit from research knowledge based on data registers (International Association of Cancer Registries 1992). For a broad discussion of ethical aspects in epidemiologic research please refer to Chap. IV.7 of this handbook.

4.10   Conclusions

The quality of health data registers is crucial for their usefulness for research. Many validity studies of the registers have been conducted, indicating variations in diagnostic procedures. However, the studies indicate mostly good data quality provided the registers are run by scientific staff and the data is analysed with care.

Many studies, not least in the field of cardiovascular epidemiology, are criticised for focusing on men, or on a limited age-group or a specific geographical area, etc. This kind of limitation can be disregarded when using national registers, since they include both sexes, all age groups and all parts of a country: an important advantage when assessing health services.

The small selection of studies using routine data and disease registers presented here could also have been conducted by collecting new data sets. In that case, however, one would have to accept the use of much greater resources and more time before answers to the research questions were available. In some cases, it is not even feasible to conduct a study without national registers.

There are, of course, also disadvantages with national health data registers. For example, data are collected without specifying diagnostic criteria in advance. Focus is on outcomes and the number of variables collected is also strictly limited. Consequently, it is harder to control for confounders and patient characteristics. Some of these disadvantages can be handled in cohort and case-control studies by combining data collection from specific research projects with national health data registers. Many of the examples presented in this chapter have used this approach.

In the next couple of years, it is important that hospital discharge registers will be transformed to hospital patient registers where all visits to hospitals are included. Otherwise, the value of such registers will diminish as more and more patients are treated in out-patient settings.

In a future perspective, the most promising development would be if nation-wide drug registers to monitor negative side effects could be in operation for research. In Denmark, a national drug register is already in operation, but has so far not been used extensively for research. In Sweden, a governmental investigation has made a proposal for a nation-wide drug register for research purposes. Today, we know very little about the long-range benefits and risks of taking medication for chronic diseases. By linking drug data to outcome data in the hospital discharge, the cancer and the cause of death register tremendous opportunities would arise, all for the benefit of public health.

References

Abildström SZ, Rasmusussen S, Rosén M, Madsen M (2003) Trends in incidence and case fatality rate of acute myocardial infarction in Denmark and Sweden. Heart 89:507–511

Adami HO, Sparén P, Bergström R, Holmberg L, Krusemo UB, Pontén J (1989) Increasing survival trend after cancer diagnosis in Sweden: 1960–1984. J Natl Cancer Inst 81:1640–1647

Alfredsson L, Spetz C-L, Theorell T (1985) Type of occupation and near-future hospitalization for myocardial infarction and some other diagnoses. Int J Epidemiol 14:378–388

Allebeck P (2002) The revised Helsinki declaration: Good for patients? Good for public health? Scand J Public Health 30:1–4

Andersen A, Barlow L, Engeland A, Kjaerheim K, Lynge E, Pukkala E (1999) Work-related cancer in the Nordic countries. Scand J Work Environment Health 25 (suppl. 2):1–116

Auvinen A, Hakama M, Arvela H, Hakulinen T, Rahola T, Suomela M, Söderman B, Rytömaa T (1994) Fallout from Chernobyl and incidence of childhood leukemia in Finland, 1976–92. Brit Med J 309:151–154

Bergh T, Ericson A, Hillensjö T, Nygren K-G, Wennerholm UB (1999) Deliveries and children born after in-vitro fertilization in Sweden 1982–1995: a retrospective cohort study. Lancet 354:1579–1585

Berrino F, Sant M, Verdecchia A, Capocaccia R, Hakulinen T, Esteve J (eds) (1995) Survival of cancer patients in Europe: the EUROCARE study. International Agency for Research on Cancer IARC Scientific Publications No. 132, Lyon

Berrino F, Capocaccia R, Estève J, Gatta G, Hakulinen T, Micheli A, Sant M, Verdecchia A (1999) Survival of cancer patients in Europe: the EUROCARE-2 study. International Agency for Research on Cancer IARC Scientific Publications No. 151, Lyon

Bigbee WL, Jensen RH, Veidebaum T, Tekkel M, Rahu M, Stengrevics A, Auvinen A, Hakulinen T, Servomaa K, Rytömaa T, Obrams GI, Boice JD Jr (1997) Biodosimetry of Chernobyl cleanup workers from Estonia and Latvia using the glycophorin A in vivo somatic cell mutation assay. Radiat Res 147:215–224

Bingham S, Williams DRR, Cole TJ, James WPT (1979) Dietary fibre and regional large-bowel cancer mortality in Britain. Br J Cancer 40:456–463

Brenner H, Hakulinen T (2002) Up-to-date long-term survival curves of patients with cancer by period analysis. J Clin Oncol 20:826–832

Centers for Disease Control (1990) Guidelines for investigating clusters of health events. CDC Morbidity and Mortality Weekly Report 1990; 39: July 27, 1990

Cnattingius S, Haglund B (1997) Decreasing smoking prevalence during pregnancy in Sweden: The effect for small-for-gestational-age birth. Am J Public Health 87:410–413

Dickman PW, Gibberd RW, Hakulinen T (1997) Estimating potential savings in cancer deaths by eliminating regional and social class variation in cancer survival in the Nordic countries. J Epidemiol Comm Health 51:289–298

Dickman PW, Hakulinen T, Luostarinen T, Pukkala E, Sankila R, Söderman B, Teppo L (1999) Survival of cancer patients in Finland 1955–1994. Acta Oncologica 38:suppl. 12

Duffy SW, Tabár L, Chen H-H, Holmqvist M, Yen M-F, Abdsalah S, Epstein B, Frodis E, Ljungberg E, Hedborg-Melander C, Sundbom A, Tholin M, Wiege M, Åkerlund A, Wu H-M, Tung T-S, Chiu Y-H, Chiu C-P, Huang C-C, Smith RA, Rosén M, Stenbeck M, Holmberg L (2002) The impact of organized mammography service screening on breast carcinoma mortality in seven Swedish counties. A collaborative evaluation. Cancer 95:458–469

Ekelund H, Finnström O, Gunnarskog J, Källén B, Larsson Y (1993) Administration of vitamin K to newborn infants and childhood cancer. BMJ 307:89–91

EpC, Centre for Epidemiology, National Board of Health and Welfare (1999) Cancer and occupation in Sweden 1971–1989. EpC rappor :1, Stockholm

EpC, Centre for Epidemiology, National Board of Health and Welfare (2003a) A finger on the pulse. Monitoring public health and social conditions in Sweden 1992–2002. EpC, Stockholm

EpC, Centre for Epidemiology, National Board of Health and Welfare (2003b) The Swedish Medical Birth Register – A summary of content and quality. Research report from EpC, Stockholm

Ericson A, Källén B (1994) Pregnancy outcome in Sweden after the Chernobyl accident. Environmental Research 67:149–159

Ericson A, Källén B, Winberg J (1977) Surveillance of malformations at birth: a comparison of two record systems run in parallel. Int J Epidemiol 6:35–41

Ericson A, Gunnarskog J, Källén B, Otterblad Olausson P (1991) Surveillance of smoking during pregnancy in Sweden, 1983–1987. Acta Obstet Gynaecol Scand 70:111–117

Ericson A, Källén B, Wiholm B-E (1999) Delivery outcomes after the use of antidepressants in early pregnancy. Eur J Clin Pharmacol 55:503–508

Feychting M, Ahlbom A (1993) Magnetic fields and cancer in children residing near Swedish high voltage power lines. Am J Epidemiol 138:467–481

Finnish Cancer Registry – Institute for Statistical and Epidemiological Cancer Research (2002) Cancer incidence in Finland 1998 and 1999. Cancer Society of Finland Publication No. 63, Helsinki

Gerhardsson de Verdier M, Norjavaara E (2001) Normal birth weight and length of babies whose mother used inhaled budesonide during pregnancy. Respiratory and Critical Care Medicine 163:A376

Golding J, Greenwood R, Birmingham K, Mott M (1992) Childhood cancer, intramuscular vitamin K, and pethidine given during labour. BMJ 305:341–346

Hallqvist J, Lundberg M, Diderichsen F, Ahlbom A (1998) Socioeconomic differences in risk of myocardial infarction 1971–1994 in Sweden: time trends, relative risks and population attributable risks. Int J Epidemiol 27:410–415

Hannan EL, Kilburn JF, Racz M, Shields E, Chassin MR (1994) Improving the outcomes of coronary artery bypass surgery in New York State. JAMA 271:761–766

Hannan EL, Siu AL, Kumar D, Kilburn H Jr, Chassin MR (1995) The decline in coronary bypass surgery mortality in New York State. The role of surgeon volume. JAMA 273:209–213

Hemminki K, Li X (2001) Familial colorectal adenocarcinoma from the Swedish Family-Cancer database. Int J Cancer 94:743–748

Hemminki K, Vaittinen P (1998) National database of familial cancer in Sweden. Genet Epidemiol 15:225–236

International Association for Cancer Registries (1992) Guidelines on Confidentiality in the Cancer Registry. International Agency for Research on Cancer IARC Internal Report No. 92/003, Lyon

IPHECA (International Programme on the Health Effects of the Chernobyl Accident (1996) Health consequences of the Chernobyl accident. Results of the IPHECA pilot projects and related national programmes. World Health Organization, Geneva

Jensen OM, Whelan S (1991) Chap 4: Planning a cancer registry. In: Jensen OM, Parkin DM, Maclennan R, Muir CS, Skeet RG (eds) Cancer registration: principles and methods. IARC Scientific Publications No. 95, Lyon, pp 22–28

Johansson LA, Westerling R (2002) Comparing hospital discharge records with death certificates – can the differences be explained? J Epidemiol Comm Health 56:301–308

Jonsson H, Nyström L, Törnberg S, Lenner P (2001) Service screening with mammography of women aged 50–69 years in Sweden: effects on mortality from breast cancer. J Med Screen 8:152–160

Kazakov VS, Demidchik EP, Astakhova LN (1992) Thyroid cancer after Chernobyl. Nature 359:21

Keys A (1953) Atherosclerosis – a problem in newer public health. J Mount Sinai Hosp 20:118–139

Källén B (1998) The teratogenicity of antirheumatic drugs – what is the evidence? Scand J Rheumatol 27 suppl. 107:119–124

Källén B, Otterblad Olausson P (2002) Monitoring of maternal drug use and infant congenital malformations. Does loratadine cause hypospadias? Int J Risk Safety Med 14:115–119

Källén B, Otterblad Olausson P (2003) Maternal drug use in early pregnancy and infant cardiovascular defect. Reproductive Toxicology 17:255–261

Källén B, Rydhström H, Åberg A (1999) Congenital malformations after the use of inhaled budesonide in early pregnancy. Obstet Gynecol 93:392–395

Lambe M, Hsieh C-C, Chan H-W, Ekbom A, Trichopoulos D, Adami HO (1996) Parity, age at first and last birth and risk of breast cancer. A population based study in Sweden. Breast Cancer Res and Treat 38:305–311

Lambe M, Hsieh C-C, Trichopoulos D, Ekbom A, Paiva M, Adami H-O (1994) Transient increase in the risk of breast cancer after giving birth. New Engl J Med 331:5–9

Lampi P, Hakulinen T, Luostarinen T, Pukkala E, Teppo L (1992) Cancer incidence following chlorophenol exposure in a community in Southern Finland. Arch Environ Health 47:167–175

Last JM (1988) A dictionary of epidemiology. International Epidemiological Association. 2nd edn. Oxford University Press, New York, Oxford, Toronto

Lindström P, Janzon L, Sternby NH (1997) Declining autopsy rate in Sweden: a study of causes and consequences in Malmö, Sweden. J Intern Med 50:367–375

Magnusson C, Baron JA, Correia N, Bergström R, Adami HO, Persson I (1999) Breast-cancer risk following long-term oestrogen- and oestrogen-progestin-replacement therapy. Int J Cancer 81:339–344

Mattsson B (1984) Cancer registration in Sweden. Studies on completeness and validity of incidence and mortality registers. Thesis. Karolinska Institutet, Stockholm

Naessén T, Persson I, Adami HO, Bergström R, Bergkvist L (1990) Hormone replacement therapy and the risk for first hip fracture; a prospective population-based cohort study. Ann Intern Med 113:95–103

NBHW, National Board of Health and Welfare (2000) National health care quality registries in Sweden 1999. National Board of Health and Welfare and the Federation of County Councils, Stockholm

Nyström L, Andersson I, Bjurstam N, Frisell J, Nordenskjöld B, Rutqvist LE (2002) Long-term effects of mammography screening: updated overview of the Swedish randomised trials. Lancet 359:909–919

OECD, Organisation for Economic Co-operation and Development (2002) Measuring up. Improving health system pperformance in OECD countries, Paris

Otterblad Olausson P, Cnattingius S, Haglund B (1999) Teenage pregnancies and risk of late fetal death and infant mortality. Br J Obstet Gynaecol 106:116–121

Parker MJ, Currie CT, Mountain JA, Thorngren K-G (1998) Standardised audit of hip fracture in Europe (SAHFE). Hip International 8:10–15

Percy C, Muir C (1989) The international comparability of cancer mortality data. Results of an international certificate study. Am J Epidemiol 129:934–946

Pershagen G, Åkerblom G, Axelson O, Clavensjö B, Damber L, Desai G, Enflo A, Lagarde F, Mellander H, Svartengren M, Swedjemark GA (1994) Residential radon exposure and lung cancer in Sweden. New Engl J Med 330:159–164

Persson G, Boström G, Diderichsen F, Lindberg G, Pettersson B, Rosén M, Stenbeck M, Wall S (eds) (2001) Health in Sweden. The National Public Health Report 2001. Scand J Public Health suppl 58:1–239

Pollán M, Gustavsson P (1999) Cancer and occupation in Sweden 1971–89. EpC Report:1

Rahu M, Tekkel M, Veidebaum T, Pukkala E, Hakulinen T, Auvinen A, Rytömaa T, Inskip PD, Boice JD Jr (1997) The Estonian study of Chernobyl cleanup workers: II. Incidence of cancer and mortality. Radiat Res 147:653–657

Ringbäck Weitoft G, Gullberg A, Rosén M (1998) Avoidable mortality among psychiatric patients. Soc Psychiatry Psychiatr Epidemiol 33:430–437

Ringbäck Weitoft G, Haglund B, Rosén M (2000) Mortality among lone mothers in Sweden: a population study. Lancet 355:1215–1219

Ringbäck Weitoft G, Hjern A, Haglund B, Rosén M (2003) Mortality, severe morbidity and injury in children living with single parents in Sweden: a population-based study. Lancet 361:289–295

Robinson WS (1950) Ecological correlations and the behavior of individuals. Am Sociol Rev 15:51–57

Rosén M, Nyström L, Wall S (1985) Guidelines for regional mortality analysis: An epidemiological approach to health planning. Int J Epidemiol 14:293–299

Rosén M, Spetz C-L, Hammar N (1999) Coronary artery disease in men and women. New Engl J Med 341:1931–1932

Rosén M, Alfredsson L, Hammar N, Kahan T, Spetz CL, Ysberg AS (2000) Attack rate, mortality and case fatality for acute myocardial infarction in Sweden 1987–1995. Results from the Swedish Myocardial Infarction Register. J Internal Med 248:159–164

Rosengren A, Spetz C-L, Köster M, Hammar N, Alfredsson L, Rosén M (2001) Sex differences in survival after myocardial infarction in Sweden. Eur Heart J 22:314–322

Salomaa V, Arstila M, Kaarsalo E, Ketonen M, Kuulasmaa K, Lehto S, Miettinen H, Mustaniemi H, Niemelä M, Palomäki P (1992) Trends in the incidence of and mortality from coronary heart disease in Finland 1983–88. Am J Epidemiol 136:1303–1315

Stenbeck M, Rosén M (eds) (1995) Cancer survival in Sweden in 1961–1991. Acta Oncologica suppl. 4:1–124

Teppo L, Pukkala E, Lehtonen M (1994) Data quality and quality control of a population-based cancer registry. Acta Oncologica 33:365–369

Tibblin G, Wilhelmsen L, Werkö L (1975) Risk factors for myocardial infarction and death due to ischaemic disease and other causes. Am J Cardiol 35:514–522

Tretli S, Engeland A, Haldorsen T, Hakulinen T, Hörte LG, Luostarinen T, Schou G, Sigvaldason H, Storm HH, Tulinius H, Vaittinen P (1996) Prostate cancer – Look to Denmark? J Natl Cancer Inst 88:128

Walsh PC (2002) Overdiagnosis due to prostate antigen screening: lessons from U.S. prostate cancer incidence trends. J Natl Cancer Inst 94:981–990

Vågerö D, Persson G (1987) Cancer survival and social class in Sweden. J Epidemiol Comm Health 41:204–209

Cohort Studies

I.5

Anthony B. Miller, David C. Goff Jr., Karin Bammann, Pascal Wild

5.1   Introduction

This chapter summarises our basic understanding of cohort studies, a type of observational epidemiology study that some have also called longitudinal, or prospective. A cohort study evaluates the risk of disease or disease-related outcome in a population that is characterised in terms of relevant risk factors or exposures, placed under observation, and followed for some time until disease develops or not. In contrast to its classical counterpart, the case-control study (cf. Chap. I.6 of this handbook), cohort studies can relate multiple diseases to the exposure or exposures identified. On the other hand, cohort studies are frequently restricted to a limited number of exposures and potential confounders that can be included in the study, if historical data is used.

The chapter is organised as follows: First, a brief historical perspective on cohort studies is given, showing the importance of this study design by giving examples from the past and from today. Second, conceptual features of cohort studies are presented, where the two basic types of cohort studies, concurrent and non-concurrent historical cohort studies are summarised, and the basic concepts of data analysis in cohort studies are described. These concepts include the description of outcome events in the cohort, the comparison with external data and the analysis of effects of exposure. The chapter then deals with key concerns of cohort studies, like selection of the study population, and on the important question of how to determine exposure and outcome events in the framework of a cohort study. A review on ethical issues, mainly raised through the potential future use of specimens, is given.

5.2   A Brief Historical Perspective on Cohort Studies

Cohort studies have been used for over a century to study determinants of disease. Since the early days of epidemiology, they have been used as a powerful tool to study a broad range of exposures like infections, nutritional factors, occupational exposures, and lifestyle factors as the following examples illustrate.

The classical study on the London cholera epidemic of 1849 conducted by John Snow is an example of a cohort study on infectious diseases (Snow 1855; Sutherland 2002). Previous reports from the Registrar General had drawn attention to the possibility that differences in water supply were associated with differences in cholera rates across sections of London. Two different water companies (the Lambeth and the Southwark & Vauxhall) supplied households within various regions of London, and frequently these two water companies supplied adjacent households. The companies differed in one important feature, the location of the water intake. The Lambeth had moved their water intake upstream from the sewage discharge point in 1849; whereas, the Southwark & Vauxhall continued to obtain water downstream of the sewage discharge point. Dr. Snow classified households according to their exposure to the two water sources and showed a substantial difference in cholera mortality, 315 versus 37 cholera deaths per 10,000 households served by the Lambeth and Southwark & Vauxhall companies, respectively.

Cohort studies continue to be an important tool in the investigation of infectious diseases. For example, McCray (1986) used a cohort design to quantify the risk of developing the acquired immunodeficiency disorder (AIDS) among healthcare workers exposed to blood and body fluids of AIDS patients.

Joseph Goldberger employed a variety of epidemiological approaches, including cohort methods, to study pellagra, a systemic disease endemic in the southeast of the United States in the late 19th and early 20th century (Terris 1964). In one investigation, Goldberger examined the dietary exposures of households in relation to the occurrence of pellagra and demonstrated that a cornmeal subsistence diet was associated with pellagra. Subsequent trials showed that pellagra could not be transmitted from person to person, as might be expected for an infectious disease, but could be prevented by the "pellagra preventive factor" later determined to be niacin. More recently, Oomen and colleagues studied the association of trans-fatty acids, a hydrogenation product of oils containing polyunsaturated fatty acids, and heart disease among men in the Netherlands (Oomen et al. 2001). They found a relative risk of 1.28 of heart disease for an increase of 2% of energy from trans-fatty acids intake at baseline.

Occupational epidemiology is another classical field of application of cohort studies. Typically workers exposed to a putative harmful substance are compared to other workers in the industry or to the general population. Occupational cohorts were used to study, for example, the association between exposure to dyes and urinary bladder cancer (Case et al. 1954), exposure to mustard gas and respiratory cancer (Wada et al. 1968), and exposure to benzene and leukaemia (Rinsky et al. 1987). The health effects for workers exposed to asbestos continue to be examined. Ulvestad and colleagues (2004) conducted a cohort study of members of the Norwegian Trade Union of Insulation Workers hired between 1930 and 1975 and followed through 2002, demonstrating relative increases in risk of mesothelioma and lung cancer when compared with the experience of the general population.

In addition to diet, other lifestyle exposures have attracted the attention of epidemiologists, including physical activity, tobacco and alcohol use. Morris and colleagues (1953a, b) demonstrated that British bus drivers had approximately twice the risk of heart disease in comparison to the more active conductors (who went up and down the stairs to collect tickets). This result was confirmed in a comparison of postmen with telephonists and clerks (Morris et al. 1953a,b). In 1951, Doll and Hill (1954) initiated a cohort study of British physicians by collecting data on tobacco use via questionnaire. By collecting death certificate data, they were able to demonstrate a 10-fold increased risk of lung cancer death for smokers compared to non-smokers (Doll and Peto 1976). Doll and colleagues also reported on the association of alcohol consumption with mortality among British doctors (Doll et al. 1994a) demonstrating a u-shaped relationship, with greater mortality among abstainers and heavy drinkers and the lowest mortality among moderate drinkers, defined as 1–2 drinks per day on average. Concerns persist that the increased risk described in abstainers may be falsely elevated by the experience of former drinkers who may have quit drinking due to health decline. This concern has been addressed by Eigenbrodt and colleagues using cohort methodology within the Atherosclerosis Risk in Communities (ARIC) study (Eigenbrodt et al. 2001). Eigenbrodt and colleagues measured perceived health status and alcohol consumption behaviour longitudinally and were able to identify changes in health status that preceded changes in drinking behaviour. They demonstrated that perceived health decline predicted cessation of drinking, thereby providing evidence that the risk among abstainers may have been inflated in studies that failed to distinguish between lifelong abstainers and former drinkers.

Despite disadvantages regarding cost and complexity, cohort studies remain until today of substantial public health importance as indicated by several of the previously cited examples and by such evidence as was recently provided by the National Institutes of Health (NIH). The NIH is considering the establishment of a 500,000-person cohort study to examine genetic and environmental influences on common diseases in the United States (National Institutes of Health 2004). The large sample size under consideration for this study would enable the examination of gene-gene- and gene-environment interaction in the general population and in subgroups of interest. Therefore, a sound understanding of cohort methodology is of substantial importance to the modern epidemiologist.

5.3   Conceptual Foundations

5.3.1   Types of Cohort Studies: Concurrent and Non-concurrent Approaches

The central feature of a cohort study is the collection of exposure data in a defined population and the subsequent surveillance of possible outcome events regarding health, morbidity, and mortality. For this purpose, healthy members of a defined population (the cohort) are classified according to their exposure status (e.g. exposed vs. unexposed) and followed over a longer period with respect to their health status. Then, the question can be answered if incidence of outcome events is associated with former presence or absence of exposure, which would indicate a possible causal relationship.

Within this framework, cohort studies can be classified in two major categories depending on the timing of follow-up period relative to the time of study conduct. In *concurrent cohort studies*, sometimes referred to as prospective cohorts (Fig. 5.1), a defined population is assembled and possibly screened to eliminate persons with disease. Then, information on exposure, possible confounders, and other important factors is gathered. The cohort members are subsequently followed for a specified period into the future recording outcome events of interest. In *non-concurrent* or *historical cohort studies* (Fig. 5.1), a population is assembled

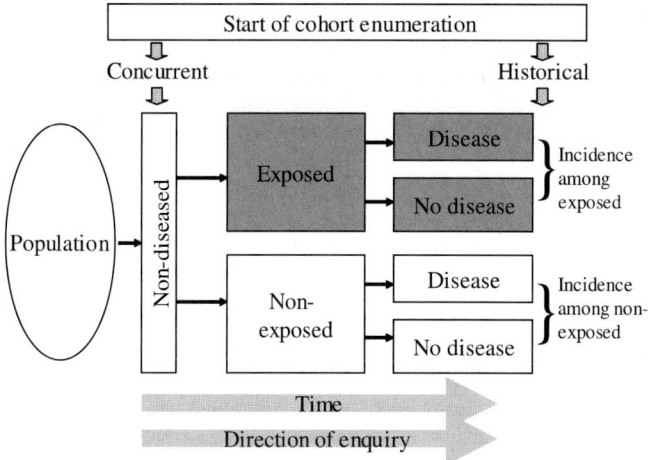

Figure 5.1. Design of a cohort study

from available data records, for example from company files. Exclusion of persons with disease and assessment of exposure and other factors is based on the available data from the past. Cohort members are monitored for outcome events through existing documents and data systems (e.g. vital statistics files or disease registries) to some point in the past. As in concurrent studies, outcome rates may be compared across exposure categories within the cohort, or, if all members of the cohort are assumed to be exposed, outcome rates may be compared between the cohort and the general population, assumed to be unexposed. A combined approach is also possible, with the cohort assembled and followed initially through historical documents or other data sources such as data from registries and subsequently followed using concurrent methods. The distinction between these two major categories of cohort studies has important implications regarding data collection.

In concurrent studies, the methods for cohort assembly and data collection can more easily be controlled; whereas, in non-concurrent studies, the investigators must rely on data recorded in historical records almost always for reasons other than medical research. This notable disadvantage of the non-concurrent approach is compensated by the ability to study exposures, such as occupational exposures, that meet one or more of the following key conditions: (1) the exposure can be attributed to selected employed populations based on individual records of job descriptions or other employment data, (2) the exposure is relatively rare in the general population outside the occupations of interest, (3) the induction period is long, and (4) the health concern is substantial, making the continued exposure required for a concurrent study undesirable from a public health perspective.

Because many of the non-infectious diseases tend to be multi-factorial in causation, a crucial point in the validity of cohort studies is the inclusion of data on possible confounders at baseline. This is a problem in historical cohort studies, that will be discussed in the section on determining exposures below.

Two modern extensions of cohort studies that try to integrate the advantages of cohort and case-control studies are designed to have nearly all the power of classic cohort studies, but utilise relatively economically detailed exposure information from questionnaires, biomarkers or other biological measurements determined from the collection of biological specimens at the time the study is initiated. These analytic designs, i.e. nested case-control studies and case-cohort studies, are discussed in detail in Chap. I.7 of this handbook and will not further be considered here.

<table>
<tr><td>5.3.2</td><td></td></tr>
</table>

Description of Outcome Events in the Cohort

In contrast to case-control studies, cohort studies with their straightforward design allow direct comparisons of exposed and unexposed persons and can provide measures of effects for various outcome events, like e.g. different endpoints (morbidity, mortality, pre-morbidity) and/or different diseases. Nevertheless, analysis of cohort data requires reasonable care especially in the steps of data preprocessing for description and analysis. The often necessary change of perspective from persons at risk to person-time at risk needs special attention to ensure that unbiased results can be obtained. This subsection will refer mainly to disease incidence; however other measures can principally be treated in the same manner.

The results from a cohort study can be presented as shown in Table 5.1.

Table 5.1. 2×2 table summarising the results of a cohort study

		Second observe		Total
		Disease contracted	No disease	
First	Exposed	a	b	$a + b = n_E$
select	Non-exposed	c	d	$c + d = n_{\bar{E}}$
Total		$a + c$	$b + d$	$a + b + c + d = N$

The easiest way to describe outcome events in a cohort is by counting the number of persons experiencing the event of interest and to relate this number to the crude number of persons at risk in the cohort. Disease incidence, for example, can be described by the cumulative incidence or risk, which is calculated by dividing the number of incident cases by the number of persons at risk at baseline:

$$\widehat{\text{Risk}} = \text{number of incident cases/number of persons at risk}, \quad (5.1)$$

that can be calculated as

$$\widehat{\text{Risk}} = (a + c)/N \quad (5.2)$$

and accordingly for the exposed and unexposed study populations as

$$\widehat{Risk}_E = a/(a + b) = a/n_E$$

$$\widehat{Risk}_{\bar{E}} = c/(c + d) = c/n_{\bar{E}}.$$

The cumulative incidence or risk is unit-free and represents an individual risk of developing the disease. It is a proportion, not a rate and it does not account for possible different periods of disease-free follow-up time of cohort members, but assumes a fixed cohort. In cohort studies on acute diseases with short induction periods and a short time of follow-up, like outbreaks, the risk of disease can be estimated directly using the cumulative incidence, given a fixed cohort with fixed period of follow-up and a low fraction of drop-outs. In cohort studies on chronic diseases with their long follow-up periods, however, the use of the cumulative incidence is not appropriate because usually disease-free follow-up periods differ strongly among cohort members. In this case, outcome events are preferably described by rates, that represent the number of outcome events divided by the cumulated duration of event-free follow-up periods of all cohort members at risk. For further analysis, all rates presented in the following can be used to determine rate ratios and rate differences as described in Chap. I.2 of this handbook. Disease incidence can be expressed as incidence rate (I):

$$\widehat{I} = \text{number of incident cases/person-time at risk}, \tag{5.3}$$

where each cohort member is contributing the time from entry into the study to either development of disease or end of follow-up to the denominator of the incidence rate, thus accounting for different times at risk of the cohort members to develop the disease. The incidence rate is sometimes called incidence density and should not be confused with the above mentioned cumulative incidence. Assuming total person-time of follow-up of t, with t_E and $t_{\bar{E}}$ follow-up of exposed (E) and unexposed ($\bar{E}$) populations, (5.3) results in

$$\widehat{I} = (a + c)/(N \times t), \tag{5.4}$$

where $N \times t$ denotes the person-time at risk. Calculating the incidence rates separately for the exposed and unexposed study populations gives

$$\widehat{I}_E = a/[(a + b) \times t_E] = a/(n_E \times t_E)$$

$$\widehat{I}_{\bar{E}} = c/[(c + d) \times t_{\bar{E}}] = c/(n_{\bar{E}} \times t_{\bar{E}}).$$

Measures of risk and incidence of disease may provide important information regarding the public health burden of the outcome or disease of interest.

Since incidence rates often vary considerably by e.g. age, sex, calendar year, and race, the calculation of specific incidence rates instead of crude incidence rates may be desirable. For this purpose, different strata (for one group variable) or cells (for two or more group variables) have to be defined over the group variables' range.

The individual contributions of the cohort members to numerator and denominator of the incidence rate have to be assigned to the respective stratum or cell. Usually, each cohort member will contribute to more than one stratum or cell as he/she moves through the cohort during follow-up. Age- and calendar-specific incidence rates can be approximated well enough on the base of calendar year data if more precise information on months and days is not available (see Breslow and Day 1987).

A simple example demonstrates the principle steps for the calculation of specific incidence rates for the age groups 30–39 years, 40–49 years, and 50–59 years. Table 5.2 shows the data of a fictitious cohort, for which we will calculate age-specific incidence rates. Since exact dates in terms of months and days are not available in our example, age and follow-up time will be approximated by full and half years. The contribution of the year at entry into the study and the year of diagnosis is approximated as half a year (see Fig. 5.2).

The cohort consists of 10 persons who were followed for 20 years resulting in a total of 155 person-years of follow-up, deaths and drop-outs accounted for the lacking 45 person-years. Three cases of the disease of interest occurred in the cohort during follow-up, resulting in a crude incidence rate of $3/135 = 0.022$ cases/person-year. The difference between the total of 155 observed person-years and the 135 person-years in the denominator of the incidence rate results from 20 years of cumulated follow-up time after diagnosis in the three cases. A useful general way in which to think of cohort data is to separate person-time at risk and person-time under observation.

A subject is "at risk" at a given moment if the event of interest can happen. Thus if a subject gets a thyroid surgery, she/he is no longer at risk of getting a thyroid cancer. If on the other hand the event of interest were a pregnancy, a woman would not be "at risk" of becoming pregnant if she already is pregnant or during spells of abstinence. In this case, however, the woman is "at risk" again from the moment on she desires another child. In the example above, a subject is no longer

Table 5.2. Data from a fictitious cohort

No.	Age at entry	Years of follow-up	Age at end of follow-up	Age at diagnosis	Person-years at risk
1	34	15	49		15
2	39	20	59	54	15
3	31	12	43		12
4	36	17	53	41	5
5	38	9	47		9
6	38	16	54	51	13
7	41	11	52		11
8	32	20	52		20
9	39	18	57		18
10	42	17	59		17
Total		155			135

considered "at risk", after diagnosis of the disease. Of course no subject is "at risk" from the moment of his/her death. Being at risk depends only on the endpoint studied.

On the contrary, being under observation, (i.e. being followed up), depends on the precise definition of the cohort and the method of follow-up considered in the epidemiological study. A subject is under observation at a time t, if, were the event of interest to occur at this moment, it would be recorded. Thus for example if the cohort definition were "all subjects employed in a given factory with at least one year of employment", the follow-up would start only at the moment the subject satisfies this criterion. In this case, all the person-time in the first year must be ignored. If the event of interest occurred in this year, it would not satisfy the inclusion category. Similarly a subject would be dropped from the follow-up at a time t if no information as to his/her disease status could be retrieved from time t on (e.g. the subject moves abroad), the subject is then considered "lost to follow-up". A subject contributes person-time to the study at any moment t if and only if at this moment he/she is "at risk" and "under observation".

Coming back to the example, each incident case is assigned to the age group he/she belonged to until diagnosis. In the same manner, the disease-free time of follow-up of each cohort member is allocated to the three age groups yielding the age-specific incidence rates presented in Table 5.3.

Incidence rates are commonly re-scaled e.g. to cases per 100,000 person-years underlining their reference to populations rather than to individuals. The crude

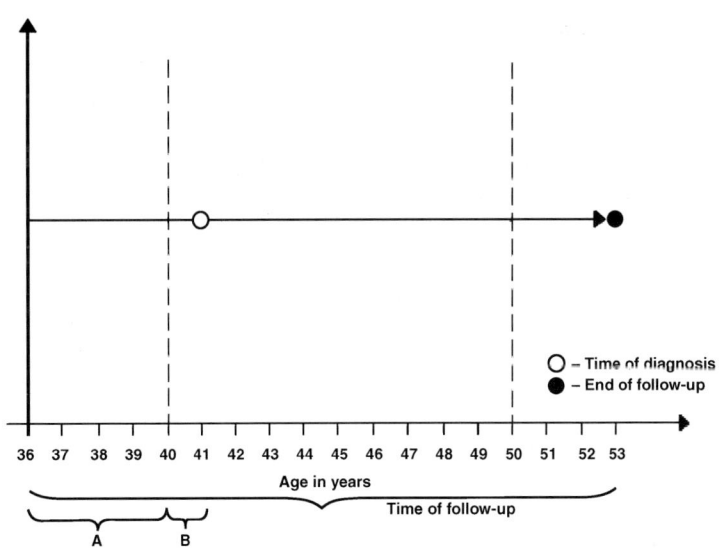

A - Span contributing to incidence rate: 30–39 years
B - Span contributing to incidence rate: 40–49 years

Figure 5.2. Follow-up time of cohort member No. 4 of the fictitious cohort

Table 5.3. Age-specific incidence rates for fictitious cohort data

Age group	Incident cases	Disease-free follow-up time	Age-specific incidence rate
30–39	0	5.5+0.5+8.5+3.5+1.5+1.5+0+7.5+0.5+0 = 29	0/29 = 0
40–49	1	9.5+10+3.5+**1.5**+7.5+10+8.5+10+10+7.5 = 78	1/78 = 0.013
50–59	2	0+**4.5**+0+**0**+0+**1.5**+2.5+2.5+7.5+9.5 = 28	2/28 = 0.071

incidence rate of 0.022 cases/person-year of the fictitious cohort, for example, would then be expressed as 2222/100,000 person-years.

In Fig. 5.2 the follow-up time of cohort member No. 4 is depicted schematically with respect to age. The first three and a half years, denoted with A, of the five years of disease-free follow-up time (41 years at time of diagnosis – 36 years at entry into the study) are contributing to the denominator of the incidence rate of the first age group (30–39 years), the next one and a half year, denoted with B, contribute to the numerator of the incidence rate of the second age group (40–49 years).

To quantify the frequency of exposure in the population under study the prevalence of exposure may be considered:

$$\widehat{P}_E = (a + b)/N = n_E/N. \tag{5.5}$$

The various quantities presented here can be used to derive measures of association accordingly (see Sect. 5.3.4).

5.3.3   External Comparisons

One important task in cohort studies is the comparison of the cohort with external data, preferably from the general population. Irrespective of the existence of internal comparison groups, external comparisons always give valuable insights by putting the cohort data in a broader context. For external comparisons either age-, sex- and calendar year-specific incidence or mortality rates or cumulative measures can be used. Standardised incidence rates can be calculated from specific incidence rates by weighting them with the age-, sex- and calendar year-distribution of the external comparison data (direct standardisation). However, cumulative measures have to be interpreted cautiously since they can mask underlying differences in specific disease patterns, like e.g. an unusually high incidence rate among younger persons in the cohort. With d_i denoting the number of cases in the age group i, n_i denoting the disease-free person-years accumulated in the age group i and w_i denoting the proportion of persons in the age group i in the standard population, the directly age-standardised incidence rate $\widehat{I}_W$ calculates as:

$$\widehat{I}_W = \sum_{i=1}^{I} w_i d_i/n_i, \tag{5.6}$$

Indirectly standardised measures requiring morbidity or mortality rates of the standard population are the standardised morbidity or incidence ratio (SIR) and the standardised mortality ratio (SMR). Since morbidity data is not routinely available in most countries the standardised mortality ratio is used much more frequently. The SMR compares the observed numbers of deaths in the cohort with the expected numbers, given the age structure of the cohort and the age-specific mortality rates λ_i of a reference population. With d_i denoting the number of deaths in the age group and n_i denoting the person-years accumulated in the age group, the SMR is estimated as

$$\widehat{SMR} = \sum_{i=1}^{I} d_i / \sum_{i=1}^{I} n_i \lambda_i , \qquad (5.7)$$

where $\sum_{i=1}^{I} d_i$ represents the total number of observed deaths in the cohort under investigation and $\sum_{i=1}^{I} n_i \lambda_i$ the expected number of deaths that are obtained by applying age-specific incidence rates of the reference population to the cohort under investigation. A SMR above 1 indicates a larger mortality in the cohort, a SMR below 1 a smaller mortality in the cohort compared to that of the reference population. Statistical testing of a single SMR can be done with a simple χ^2-test (observed vs. expected) with one degree of freedom. Assuming that the number of observed cases $D = \sum_{i=1}^{I} d_i$ follows a Poisson distribution with expectation $\gamma = E(D)$, confidence limits for the SMR ($\widehat{SMR}_L$, $\widehat{SMR}_U$) can be obtained by finding confidence limits $\hat{\gamma}_L$, $\hat{\gamma}_U$ for the number of observed cases:

$$\widehat{SMR}_L = \hat{\gamma}_L / \sum_{i-1}^{I} n_i \lambda_i \quad \text{and} \quad \widehat{SMR}_U = \hat{\gamma}_U / \sum_{i=1}^{I} n_i \lambda_i . \qquad (5.8)$$

The confidence limits for γ can be determined as:

$$\hat{\gamma}_L = (1/2)\chi^2_{2D,\alpha/2} \quad \text{and} \quad \hat{\gamma}_U = (1/2)\chi^2_{2(D+1),1-\alpha/2} , \qquad (5.9)$$

where $\chi^2_{2D,\alpha/2}$ denotes the $100(\alpha/2)$th percentile of the χ^2-distribution with $2D$ degrees of freedom, and $\chi^2_{2(D+1),1-\alpha/2}$ denotes the $100(1 - \alpha/2)$th percentile of the χ^2-distribution with $2(D + 1)$ degrees of freedom (see e.g. Sahai and Khurshid 1996).

If the age-specific rates of the standard population are just estimations of the exact rates, as is often the case with morbidity data, calculation of confidence intervals for the SMR can be performed by the method described in Silcocks (1994). A method for estimating the SMR where information on vital status is complete but information on cause of death is partly missing as may be the case in historical cohort studies can be found in Rittgen and Becker (2000).

Comparison of rates by direct standardisation has poor statistical properties, especially due to large variances of age-specific rates in small cohorts. Therefore, indirect standardisation is usually preferred (see Chap. I.2 of this handbook).

5.3.4   Summary Effects of Exposure

The main goal of cohort studies is to compare morbidity and/or mortality in exposed and non-exposed subjects or between different exposure groups of the cohort, and to investigate dose-effect relationships between exposure and disease. If the exposure is constant and can be determined at entry into the cohort, internal comparisons can be performed by calculating specific incidence rates for each exposure category separately as if each group were a separate cohort. Cumulative rates can be used, again provided the subgroups do not differ in important determinants of disease, like e.g. age.

In the simple case of a single dichotomous exposure several measures of association of exposure with disease can be estimated from results provided by a cohort study (see Table 5.1). In the following, the most important ones will be briefly introduced. A detailed discussion of their properties and examples for their calculation can be found in Chap. I.2 of this handbook.

The perhaps most popular measure of association is the risk ratio (RR), also known as relative risk, that compares the experience of exposed and unexposed populations. With the notation given in Table 5.1 and the risks for the exposed and unexposed subjects calculated according to (5.2) it can be estimated as

$$\widehat{RR} = \widehat{Risk}_E / \widehat{Risk}_{\bar{E}} = [a/(a+b)]\,/\,[c/(c+d)] = (a/n_E)/(c/n_{\bar{E}})\,. \qquad (5.10)$$

The incidence ratio (IR) compares the incidence rates in the exposed and unexposed study populations. According to (5.4) its estimator is given as

$$\widehat{IR} = \widehat{I}_E / \widehat{I}_{\bar{E}} = \left\{ a/\left[(a+b) \times t_E\right] \right\} / \left\{ c/\left[(c+d) \times t_{\bar{E}}\right] \right\} = [a/(n_E \times t_E)]\,/\,[c/(n_{\bar{E}} \times t_{\bar{E}})] \qquad (5.11)$$

The RR and IR provide estimates of the relative strength of the association between the exposure of interest and the outcome or disease of interest.

The absolute difference in risk (AR) between the exposed and unexposed groups provides an estimate of the impact of the exposure on the risk of disease in absolute terms. This measure is not to be confused with the absolute risk, which is the absolute probability that a disease-free individual will develop a given disease over a specific time-interval (Benichou 1998). Using the above formulas for the risks among exposed and unexposed it can be obtained from a cohort study as

$$\widehat{AR} = \widehat{Risk}_E - \widehat{Risk}_{\bar{E}} = [a/(a+b)] - [c/(c+d)] = a/n_E - c/n_{\bar{E}}\,. \qquad (5.12)$$

Based on the attributable risk several other measures can be derived. The so-called attributable fraction (AF) can be interpreted as the proportion of risk due to exposure in exposed individuals. It may be useful for quantifying the degree to which risk can be reduced at the individual level if the exposure (and its effects) can be eliminated. It may, therefore, be a sensible measure for counselling individuals:

$$\widehat{AF} = \widehat{AR}/\widehat{Risk}_E = \left\{[a/(a+b)] - [c/(c+d)]\right\}/[a/(a+b)] = \left(a/n_E - c/n_{\overline{E}}\right)/\left(a/n_E\right). \tag{5.13}$$

The population attributable risk (PAR) reflects the absolute level of risk of the outcome in the population due to the exposure. It can be used to estimate the public health impact, in absolute terms, of elimination of the exposure, at least with respect to the outcome of interest. Based on the attributable risk and the prevalence of exposure (see (5.5)) it is given as

$$\widehat{PAR} = \widehat{AR}/\widehat{P}_E = \left\{[a/(a+b)] - [c/(c+d)]\right\}/[(a+b)/N] = (a/n_E - c/n_{\overline{E}})/(n_E/N). \tag{5.14}$$

The last measure to be mentioned here may be used to estimate the proportion of all events of interest that could be prevented in the overall population if the exposure (and its effects) can be eliminated. The population attributable fraction (PAF) is defined as the proportion of all events of interest that occur in the population due to the exposure:

$$\widehat{PAF} = \widehat{PAR}/\widehat{Risk} = (a/n_E - c/n_{\overline{E}})/\left\{(n_E/N)\,[(a+c)/N]\right\}. \tag{5.15}$$

Internal Modelling of the Effects of Exposure $\qquad$ 5.3.5

The situation is more complicated, if cohort members continuously add exposure over follow-up time. Simple categorisation on the basis of cumulative exposure would lead to biased results. Person-years accumulated shortly after entry into the study of cohort members with high cumulative exposure would wrongly be allocated to a high exposure category, although the cumulative exposure at that time-point was still low for these cohort members, resulting in underestimation of high exposures and overestimation of low exposures. Therefore, the disease-free person-time of each subject has to be subdivided and assigned to the respective age- and sex-specific exposure category the cohort member belongs to as he or she moves through the cohort, meaning that most cohort members contribute to different age-exposure-categories. In the same manner, the incident cases have to be assigned to the categories where they occurred.

In Fig. 5.3 the follow-up time of cohort member No. 4 is again depicted schematically, this time with respect to age and cumulative exposure assuming that the exposure starts at the beginning of the follow-up and that it is constant over time. For age- and exposure-specific incidence rates, the disease-free follow up time is assigned to the groups according to the squares in the figure that are defined by the categorisation of the group variables, resulting in a contribution of cohort member No. 4 of two and a half year to the denominator of the incidence rate of category A $\times$ C (30–39 years of age and < 3 units of cumulative exposure), one year to the denominator of the incidence rate of category A $\times$ D (30–39 years of age and 3

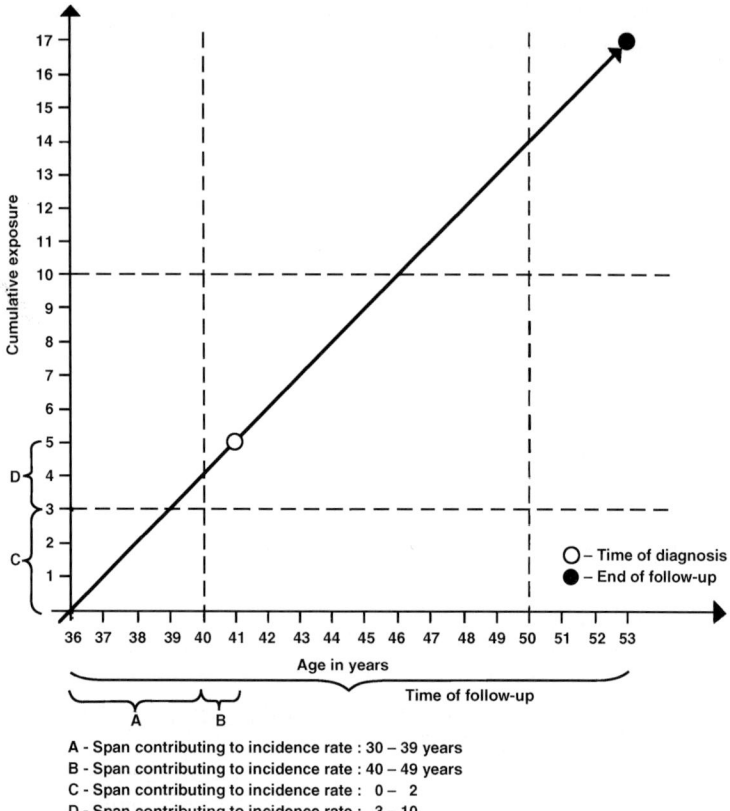

A - Span contributing to incidence rate : 30 – 39 years
B - Span contributing to incidence rate : 40 – 49 years
C - Span contributing to incidence rate : 0 – 2
D - Span contributing to incidence rate : 3 – 10

Figure 5.3. Follow-up time of cohort member No. 4 of the fictitious cohort

to smaller than 10 units of cumulative exposure), and one and a half year to the denominator of the incidence rate of category B × D (40–49 years of age and 3–< 10 units of cumulative exposure). The case itself contributes to the nominator of the incidence rate of category B × D, since this is the category in which he/she was diagnosed.

This procedure can be extended in several ways. The exposure may have started before beginning of follow-up or may start later. It can vary over time, it can even vary from individual to individual or can be lagged to account for induction time. Several measures of exposure (e.g. time since first exposure and and/or confounders) can be considered simultaneously and possible confounders can be included in the analyses as additional variables. Figures 5.4, 5.5 and 5.6 illustrate some of these features. For simplicity no half-years are considered in these examples.

In Fig. 5.4, a subject is followed up from age 23 but has been exposed from age 19 on, he/she is exposed until age 27 followed by an unexposed 5 year period. He/she is again exposed until age 39 at which time his/her person-time at risk ceases either

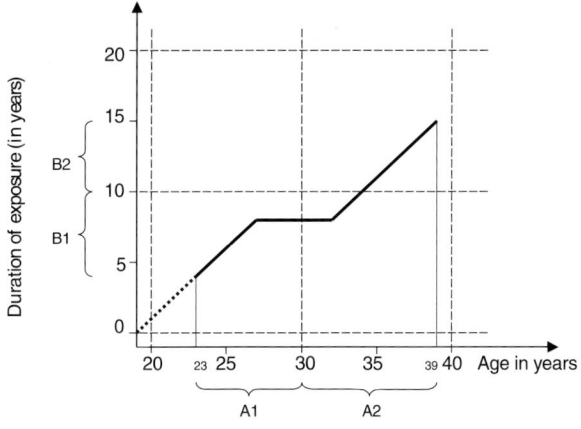

A1 - Span contributing to incidence rate 20 − 29 years
A2 - Span contributing to incidence rate 30 − 39 years
B1 - Span contributing to incidence rate 0 − 9 years of exposure
B2 - Span contributing to incidence rate 10 − 19 years of exposure

Figure 5.4. Person-time classification with varying duration of exposure

because of disease diagnosis or because of end of follow-up. This subject would contribute 7 years (from age 23 to age 30) to the A1 × B1 group (20–29 years of age, 0–10 years exposure) 4 years (from age 30 to 34) to the A2 × B1 (30–39 years of age, 0–10 years of exposure), 5 years (from age 34 to 39) to A2 × B2 ((30–39 years of age, 10–19 years of exposure).

Fig. 5.5 presents the same subject assuming that the first exposure spell was twice as intensive (e.g. 20 ppm of a given chemical) than the second exposure (10 ppm). The unit of cumulative exposure y-axis is now in ppm.years. The subject would contribute 1 year to group A1 × B1, (his cumulative exposure is then 100 ppm.years) then 5 years to group A1 × B2 (at age 30 his cumulative exposure is 160 ppm.years), then 6 years (from age 30 to age 36 at which he reaches 200 ppm.years) in group A2 × B2) and finally 3 years in group A2 × B3.

Fig. 5.6 considers the same subject again but this time the exposure is lagged by 10 years, say, to account for disease induction time. The first period would then be a non-exposed period. The rationale is that, were the disease to occur in these first 10 years, it would not be attributable to exposure. Applying the same rationale as before, the subject would contribute 6 years in group B0 × A1, then 1 year in group B1 × A1, finally 9 years in group B1 × A2, the lagged cumulative exposure at end of follow up (i.e. at age 39) is 160 ppm−years.

Another exposure can occur during the follow-up, e.g. the preceding subject starts smoking at age 25. In this case a further splitting of the time periods would be done separating periods in which the subject was a non-smoker and periods in which he/she smoked.

This splitting of person-time into age and exposure groups must be done for each subject of the cohort and gets more complex with a growing number of group

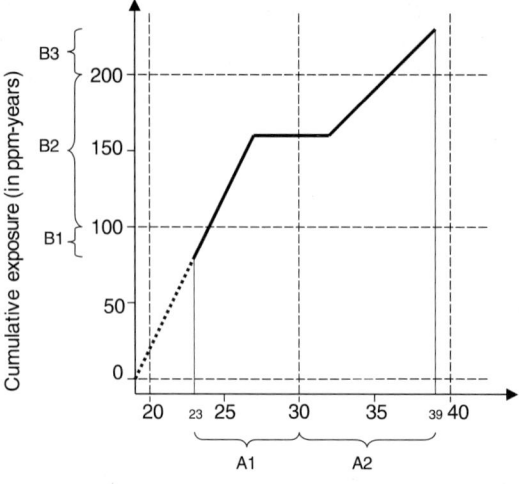

A1 - Span contributing to incidence rate   20 – 29 years
A2 - Span contributing to incidence rate   30 – 39 years
B1 - Span contributing to incidence rate   0 – 99 ppm-years
B2 - Span contributing to incidence rate 100 – 199 ppm-years
B3 - Span contributing to incidence rate 200 + ppm-years

Figure 5.5. Person-time classification with varying cumulative exposure

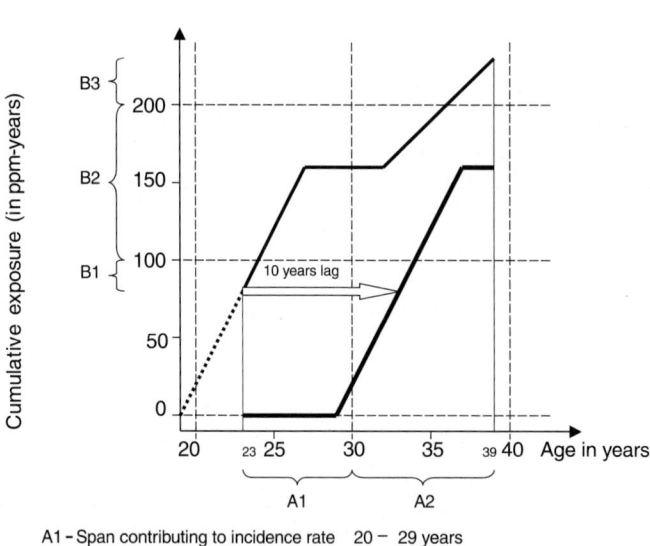

A1 - Span contributing to incidence rate   20 – 29 years
A2 - Span contributing to incidence rate   30 – 39 years
B1 - Span contributing to incidence rate   0 – 99 ppm-years
B2 - Span contributing to incidence rate 100 – 199 ppm-years
B3 - Span contributing to incidence rate 200 + ppm-years

Figure 5.6. Person-time classification with varying lagged cumulative exposure

variables. Specialised software packages exist (e.g. Coleman et al. 1986) to perform these computations but they are usually limited in the complexity they can handle. Interestingly, these restrictions do not apply to some more general packages as Stata (version 7 or later – StataCorp. 2001) or Epicure (Preston et al. 1993) in which the statistical modelling procedures of such data are furthermore included. The end result of the calculations carried out in these packages can then be presented as a data table with each line corresponding to a separate combination of age and exposure classes (other classifications like calendar periods might also be included) and containing the following variables: the value of each age and exposure group, the number of person-years n_i accumulated in this category over the entire cohort and the number d_i of events of interest falling in this category.

In epidemiological cohort studies the standard model for analysing such data is the Poisson model which is a statistical model of the disease rates. Basically the Poisson model assumes that the number of events d_i in each category i (combination of age category j and the kth combination of exposure variables) follows a Poisson distribution with parameter $n_i\lambda_i$. The standard (multiplicative) model would then assume that

$$\ln(\lambda_i) = \alpha_j + \beta_k \qquad (5.16)$$

where λ_i are the unknown true disease rates, the α_j are nuisance parameters specifying the effects of age and (possibly) other stratification variables like calendar periods and β_k the parameters that describe the effects of primary interest. As usual in regression models $\beta_0 = 0$ would be a baseline category. $\exp(\beta_k)$ is then an estimate, adjusted on the nuisance parameters, of the relative risk of the kth exposure category vs. the baseline category assuming absence of interaction between exposure. The full modelling strategy of the Poisson regression is beyond the scope of this chapter but is not different from any regression modeling (see Chaps. II.3 and II.4 of this handbook). A comprehensive account of Poisson modeling is given by Breslow and Day (1987, Chap. 4).

An alternative way of analysing event history data (another denomination of cohort data focussed on events), is by using Cox' proportional hazard model. This model acknowledges that the categorisation of continuous data always implies a loss of information and therefore a loss in statistical power. Moreover, there is no need to explicitly estimate the effects of nuisance parameters if it can be avoided.

The first step in proportional hazard model is the choice of one of the time variables considered. This basic time variable can either be age as was implicit at the beginning of this chapter, but in some settings, this variable can be the calendar time or even the time since the beginning of follow-up. Once this special time variable has been fixed, its effects are estimated nonparametrically.

The key idea of Cox's regression is that no information is lost when considering only the time points t_i at which an event of interest occurs. At each such time point a "risk set" is set up including all members of the cohort contributing person-time (at risk and under observation) at this time point. If one wants to use a Cox model, the first step is thus to identify all risk sets. Then, one must obtain the value at each time t_i of all variables to be included in the model for all members of the corresponding risk set. The statistical analysis is then similar (in fact the same software can be used) to a conditional logistic regression analysis, in which the matching variable is the indicator of the risk set. As in the logistic regression, the exposure at time t_i of the case, i.e. the subject experiencing the event at time t_i, and the exposure at time t_i of the other members of the risk set are compared. Again, the full modelling strategy of the Cox proportional hazard model and its various extensions are beyond the scope of this chapter (see Chaps. II.3 and II.4). A comprehensive account of this model is given by Breslow and Day (1987, Chap. 5). As for Poisson models, both Stata and Epicure provide easy to use software, but once the risk sets and the corresponding exposure variables have been computed for each risk set, any logistic regression package (e.g. Proc PHREG in SAS) can be used.

5.3.6   Internal Versus External Comparisons

In Sect. 5.3.3 the event rate (morbidity or mortality) of a cohort is compared to the rates of an external population. This is done by comparing the observed number of deaths in the cohort with the expected numbers, given the age structure of the cohort and the age-specific mortality rates λ_i of a reference population. The ratio of observed to expected (the SMR) is then interpreted as a rate ratio between the cohort and the general population taken as a reference.

If the cohort is set up for investigating a specific risk factor, as would be the case in an occupational cohort, one can be tempted to interpret the SMR as a risk ratio due to the risk factor under investigation. However, this interpretation would only be valid if the cohort were comparable to the general population for all factors except for the risk factor under investigation. This is obviously only rarely the case. The general population consists of all subjects including the very ill and very poor, which would rarely be included in the same proportion in a cohort. Thus the mortality in the general population is usually higher than in any (unexposed) cohort. In occupational cohorts, this phenomenon has been termed the "*Healthy Worker Effect*" (see e.g. Li and Sung 1999; Goldberg and Luce 2001). Other factors, like regional differences, owing to social, behavioural, nutritional and environmental factors, might cause the mortality of a regionally based cohort to be different from a nationwide general population. In summary, the SMR is a biased estimate of the effect of any risk factor.

This bias can be reduced by choosing a reference population which is as comparable as possible (except for the risk factor of interest) to the cohort under investigation. This implies to carefully select the reference population and in the end to compare the cohort to another reference cohort. In this case, however, the computation of the confidence interval of the SMR is no longer valid as it assumes that, because of the large number of subjects in the reference population, the disease rates and hence the expected numbers are observed without any sampling error. In this case, the only statistically valid methods are those presented in the preceding section, although the confidence intervals of the risk ratio become wider. The choice between an external comparison and an internal comparison is thus the choice between accepting an (often small) bias and accepting a larger variance, which implies a lower power. Such a choice can only be made in the context of each study and, if possible, both approaches should be tried. Finally, methods have been proposed including external reference rates to stabilise internal comparisons (e.g. Breslow and Day 1987, p 151) that might be used as reasonable compromise.

Key Concerns in Cohort Studies   5.4

Selection of the Study Population   5.4.1

Usually, vital statistics data of the general population, or data derived from national disease registries are used as a reference for the calculation of expected cases. However, they can only be regarded as valid for deriving an expectation of mortality and disease rates if the cohort under investigation is a representative sample of the general population. Indeed, many cohorts are convenience samples, derived from a group that happens to be accessible. Representative cohorts can for example be derived from national censuses, utilizing the data collected for the specific census. Obtaining access to census data is generally not easy, since most censuses guarantee confidentiality to participants. Exceptions to that rule are for example, a Swedish occupational census-based sample or a 10% sample of the Canadian labour force, derived from data collected from Canadian having a social insurance number that is required for all who are employed in an active occupation (Howe and Lindsay 1983). These types of population samples are very valuable, because subsets among them chosen for specific analysis can be regarded as comparable to the general population apart from the characteristics that caused them to enter, or be selected for, that subset.

Occupational cohorts (cf. Chap. III.2 of this handbook) are usually identified by company files or sometimes by workers' union files. Access to these cohorts is usually granted, if the company or union is interested in determining whether a suspected increase in disease rates has occurred, or there is concern that exposure to a potential hazard bears an increased risk of disease. Many carcinogens have been confirmed in humans, after first evidence from animal studies, by investigations of specific cohorts (Tomatis et al. 1990). This mechanism is still being used, as exhibited by a tri-utility study of electrical and magnetic field exposures (Theriault et al. 1994), and a study of Motorola employees on the potential risks of exposure to radiofrequency fields (Morgan et al. 2000). It is very helpful, if employment records indicate exposure to specific agents. This is the case when routine measurements are taken for safety reasons, as for most workers exposed to radiation. In their absence estimation of exposures may be required, as discussed further below.

So-called multi-purpose cohorts identified for study, however, have to be recruited by some mechanism that provides the opportunity for potential subjects to volunteer. For example, much has been learnt from an ongoing study of American nurses, who were given the opportunity to volunteer for the study by completing a questionnaire of dietary and other lifestyle factors (Willett et al. 1992). Similar studies were initiated in Canada by providing self-administered questionnaires to women already participating in a mammography screening trial (Howe et al. 1991) and in Sweden by approaching women who participated in a routine mammography screening programme (Wolk et al. 1998). In Europe, a large multi-centre cohort study was initiated in 10 countries using different approaches (Riboli and Kaaks 1997). Some used population registers as the basis for mailing invitations to participate. The response proportions were good in most countries, but still tended to include more health conscious and more highly educated people than the general population as is often the case in volunteer studies (cf. Chap. I.10 of this handbook).

Another recent feature of cohort studies has been the attempt to bring many together and analyse them almost as a multicentre study to enable the investigators to identify risks which none of them individually were capable of demonstrating. The Pooling Project is a case in point, originally funded to evaluate further uncertain associations between diet and breast cancer, it has proven a very useful source of additional knowledge because of the ability of cohort studies to identify multiple endpoints. Thus it has already been extended to lung cancer (Smith-Warner et al. 2003), with findings similar to the EPIC study (Miller et al. 2004), and other diseases will follow.

When a truly representative cohort cannot be obtained, because the mechanism used involves the opportunity to volunteer, and to refuse to participate, comparisons with the general population in terms of mortality and disease rates may not be valid. Thus the cohort may lack external validity. However, provided that the recruitment mechanism is unbiased with regard to the exposure of interest, and the data obtained on exposure enables the investigators to stratify their population into exposed and unexposed subgroups, the estimation of the association between the exposure and the outcome will be valid (internal validity).

Tables 5.4 and 5.5 demonstrate the effects of different participation patterns (selection) on estimates that can be obtained from cohort studies. In the presence of a fair sample, all of the measures of disease occurrence and association will be unbiased (Table 5.4). In the presence of over-representation of exposed persons (Table 5.5), the prevalence of the exposure will be overestimated and the risk of the outcome will be over- or under-estimated depending on whether the exposure is positively or negatively associated with disease. Nevertheless, the estimates of the relative risk and the attributable risk will be unbiased. Since the estimate of the prevalence of exposure is biased, estimates of the public health impact will be biased. Other participation patterns that can theoretically introduce selection bias including over-representation of diseased individuals and participation rates

Table 5.4. Effects of a fair sampling process on the measures of disease occurrence and association

Target Population				Selection Weights		Study Population			
		Disease						Disease	
		Yes	No					Yes	No
At Risk Yes	40	160	200			At Risk Yes	20	80	100
				50	50				
At Risk No	60	740	800			At Risk No	30	370	400
				50	50				
	100	900	1000				50	450	500

Target Population		Study Population
10%	Prevalence of Disease	10%
20%	Prevalence of Risk Factor	20%
2.67	Relative Risk	2.67
3.08	Odds Ratio	3.08
125/1000	Attributable Risk	125/1000

Table 5.5. Effects of oversampling of exposed individuals on the measure of disease occurence and assiociation (positive association between exposure and outcome)

Target Population				Selection Weights		Study Population			
		Disease						Disease	
		Yes	No					Yes	No
At Risk Yes	40	160	200			At Risk Yes	40	160	200
				100	100				
At Risk No	60	740	800			At Risk No	6	74	80
				10	10				
	100	900	1000				46	234	280

Target Population		Study Population
10%	Prevalence of Disease	16%
20%	Prevalence of Risk Factor	71%
2.67	Relative Risk	2.67
3.08	Odds Ratio	3.08
125/1000	Attributable Risk	125/1000

that differ by both, exposure and disease status, are unlikely to affect cohort studies due to the customary exclusion of persons with the outcome of interest at baseline. This assurance is only relative, relying on the degree to which persons with prevalent disease can be excluded from the cohort. In general, selection bias can be minimized by avoiding the use of volunteers (or using volunteers exclusively) and by minimizing non-participation. The potential for selection bias can be assessed by evaluating non-participants for study characteristics, if possible.

5.4.2   Exposure and Confounders in Cohort Studies

As already indicated, some cohorts will have exposure data readily available, especially those derived from occupational groups where exposure was routinely collected for safety monitoring purposes. It is the strength of such cohorts that they offer the possibility to report the exposure before the disease occurs. However, for population-based cohorts, the investigators will have to collect data specifically for the study, or to refine existing data.

Because most cohorts will be very large, the collection of exposure data is not a simple task. If exposure data is to be collected by questionnaires, the scale of the effort required will generally mean that neither personal nor telephone interviews are feasible, as would normally be planned for case-control studies. This means that the exposure data will generally be collected by mailed self-administered questionnaires, often linked to the recruitment mechanism of the cohort, with response to the questionnaire qualifying the individual for inclusion in the study. Inevitably, the amount of data that can be collected by self-administered questionnaire is limited. The degree of detail for a given variable that can be obtained by such instruments is also restricted (cf. Chap. I.11 of this handbook), so that in addition to the problems of the ability of the respondent to recall accurately the exposure he/she has experienced, the data will be potentially subjected to major misclassification.

The extent of misclassification in cohort studies has only recently been appreciated, probably explaining the fact that the results of many cohort studies, especially when diet was the exposure of interest, have been negative (Day and Ferrari 2002). Thus although many of the questionnaires used in cohort studies have been subject of validation studies, and correlation with other assessment methods seemed reasonable, these validation studies have served to reassure the investigators, but probably have not protected them from reporting negative, or very weak results. Even for smoking, the information obtained in cohort studies cannot be regarded as precise as investigators would have wished.

Misclassification of exposure can be differential or non-differential with respect to the outcome of interest; that is, the degree of misclassification of the exposure can differ, or not, by outcome status. In cohort studies, non-differential misclassification is the more typical form of misclassification due to the customary exclusion of persons with prevalent disease at baseline. It is unlikely that the measurement of exposure at baseline will be influenced by the development of an outcome sometime in the future. Differential misclassification is potentially a much greater problem in case-control and cross-sectional studies. Non-differential misclassification always introduces a bias toward a null finding (a finding of no association) if the exposure

Table 5.6. Non-differential misclassification of exposure

		True Cohort (no error)						Observed Cohort (error)		
		MI	No MI					MI	No MI	
Cigarettes	Yes	60	300	360		Cigarettes	Yes	54	270	324
	No	30	330	360			No	36	360	396
		90	630	720				90	630	720

2.00	Rate Ratio	1.83

status is dichotomized; whereas, differential misclassification can introduce a less predictable bias. Table 5.6 shows the impact of a 10% non-differential error rate in classifying smokers. In this example, 90% of exposed individuals were correctly classified regarding exposure and 100% of unexposed individuals were correctly classified. Assuming a true relative risk of 2.0, the observed relative risk would be 1.8. With greater degrees of misclassification, the bias towards the null would increase. This bias can be minimized through the use of standardized and validated procedures for exposure assessment.

Another issue that affects cohort studies differently than case-control studies is the effect of change in exposure with time. In case-control studies detailed exposure biographies that include changes in exposure patterns, e.g. change in intensity of smoking, or cessation of smoking, or even measures taken to affect dietary change, can be retrieved using just one survey, with the problem of uncertainty, and possibly differential error, in recall. The concurrent cohort study with its prospective data collecting does offer the possibility of assessing changes in exposure while they happen. To assess changes in exposure patterns, a mechanism has, however, to be set up specifically e.g. by re-administering the questionnaire on a regular basis. This could be done as part of the follow-up mechanism adopted, though some loss to follow-up will be inevitable. An alternative to incorporating this new information into the analysis is shown in the Nurses Health Study (Willett et al. 1992). The follow-up period with regard to the time from the first exposure information to the second was used as a separate cohort from the follow-up period subsequent to the second exposure information. This is justifiable as blocks of person-time in different periods are statistically independent, regardless of the extent they are derived from the same people (Rothman and Greenland 1998). However, sometimes cohorts are analysed with regard to the exposure determined at baseline, and although that may seem distant from the period when many endpoints are determined, for those with a long induction period from exposure to outcome, as for many cancers, this has not always been regarded as a major disadvantage.

Exposure assessment by questionnaires always depends on subjects' accuracy of recall and their willingness to participate, and many efforts have been made to introduce more objective measures of exposure determination. For radiation exposure, cohorts with occupations that require wearing film badges provide cumulative, and in some instances, peak measurements of exposure. For uranium and other hard rock miners, measures of the radiation exposure in mines were often made for safety reasons to limit the length of exposure of those at risk and these measurements can be assigned to the job history of the individual.

However, in many instances, exposure has to be estimated simply from the type of occupation at a certain time since no further information is available, and misclassification of exposure assessment cannot be avoided. In occupational studies, attempts have been made to refine exposure assessment by developing a job exposure matrix (cf. Chap. I.11). Often using data from hygiene assessments performed in the past, a matrix can be constructed with the different job tasks in the rows, and columns indicating the probability and/or intensity of exposure within that job to the agents (chemical or physical) of interest. The approach was for example used in a study of electrical and magnetic field exposures in electric utility workers in Canada and France (Theriault et al. 1994). Extension of the work upon a sample of workers wearing portable electric and magnetic field exposure meters, and using historical data of electrical usage in the province enabled the investigators to identify strong associations of leukaemia and non-Hodgkin's lymphoma risk with high electric field exposure (Miller et al. 1996; Villeneuve et al. 1998).

Another source of exposure data collected in cohort studies is gained from biological material of the cohort members. Historically, rather simple parameters were under study, like blood pressure or cholesterol levels, derived from blood samples that were collected in the framework of large cohort and intervention studies on cardiovascular disease. Now, there is increasing interest in the study of disease aetiology by biomarkers of exposure and/or of genetic factors, as e.g. in the European Prospective Investigation of Diet and Cancer (EPIC) (Riboli and Kaaks 1997).

The findings of cohort studies regarding the effects of exposure can be strengthened if it is possible to evaluate a dose-response relationship. This requires the assessment of intensity of exposure that can be quantified as peak, average, or cumulative exposure. Sometimes duration of exposure is used as a surrogate for cumulative exposure. However, using duration in this way is problematic if the exposure is associated with an early, perhaps toxic effect. Then it could be anticipated that these workers would tend to change their employment and could not cumulate long durations of exposure. If such workers represented a particularly susceptible subgroup, perhaps for genetic reasons, it is possible that in this subgroup a relatively brief exposure results in the same incidence of disease than in subgroups with a longer duration of exposure that are less susceptible. The absence of a dose-response relationship without appropriate statistical control for the genetic background might then be incorrectly interpreted as indicator that the exposure is not causal for the disease (Blair and Stewart 1992).

The treatment of potential confounding factors is the major challenge of the analysis of cohort studies. This is in part because the basic data set may not contain information on all relevant confounders, particularly not in historical cohort studies, but also because the data available on confounders may not be assessed with sufficient precision to take account of their effect. An example is the possible confounding effect of cigarette smoking with fruit and vegetable consumption and lung cancer. Although two large cohort studies (one multicentre and one the result of a pooled analysis) which fully adjusted for the effects of cigarette smoking in the opinion of the investigators were available (Miller et al. 2004; Smith-Warner et al. 2003) a working group of the International Agency for Research on Cancer (IARC) was not convinced that there was not residual confounding of fruit consumption by smoking with lung cancer, and therefore judged the evidence to be limited rather than sufficient (IARC 2003).

Determining Outcome Events

5.4.3

A limiting factor for cohort studies is that most diseases are relatively rare, with rates determined in the population per 100,000 persons. Therefore to accrue sufficient cases of the disease the size of the cohort has to be large, and/or the follow-up time has to be long. Another factor affecting the length of follow-up relates to the long induction period from the beginning of many exposures to the occurrence of disease. For many cancers, for example, the induction period exceeds ten, often 20 years. One example for the importance of a long enough follow-up period is the British Doctors' Study that showed much higher lung cancer risks of cigarette smoking after 40 years of follow-up than in the ten- and twenty-year reports of this study (Doll et al. 1994b). The reason for this was a dominant effect of duration of smoking compared to intensity of exposure on the risk of lung cancer (see also Flanders et al. 2003). It seems probable that this is not the only example of this phenomenon – it may particularly affect exposures with a long induction period from initiation of exposure to effect. The possibility of such an effect should encourage investigators to maintain the follow-up of well documented cohorts for as long as proves feasible, and granting agencies will agree to provide the necessary funds. If grants are limited it may be useful to store the necessary data and extend the follow-up after a certain time lapse. It is unusual for cohort studies to start from the first exposure and the possible initiation of disease, covering the whole spectrum of exposure in a subject's lifetime. Attempts have to be made to determine or to estimate past exposure, with all the error and potential misclassification of such inquiries. Nevertheless, a major advantage of cohort studies over case-control studies is that exposure is determined prior to the diagnosis of disease, thus avoiding a major bias of concern in case-control studies, the recall bias.

As already indicated, the follow-up of cohorts enables multiple endpoints to be determined, e.g. different types of cardiovascular disease and/or different cancer sites. In determining endpoints in cohort studies, it is essential that ascertainment bias is avoided. Ascertainment bias relates to the possibility that the surveillance of cohort members, by virtue of the fact that they are in a study, may result in greater efforts to make a diagnosis than would occur in the general population. Special surveillance mechanisms in a cohort study are valid if internal comparisons of exposed versus unexposed within the cohort are planned, but would invalidate external comparisons with general population data. Orencia and colleagues (1995) provided an example of this bias in a non-concurrent cohort study examining the association of mitral valve prolapse (MVP) with stroke. Using the database of the Mayo Clinic, they assembled a cohort of persons with MVP, followed them for the occurrence of stroke, and compared the rate of stroke with the rate in the general population of Olmsted County, Minnesota. The overall standardized mortality ratio was 2.1, indicating a risk of stroke twice of that of the general population. However, Orencia noted that MVP can be diagnosed by auscultation or as a serendipitous finding during an echocardiogram conducted for other medical reasons (e.g. following myocardial infarction, chronic heart failure, atrial fibrillation) often associated with risk of stroke. When the cohort was further subdivided according to method of diagnosis, the auscultatory group demonstrated no increase in risk. The increased risk was confined to the group identified serendipitously during a cardiac evaluation motivated by other medical concerns associated with risk of stroke.

In some cohort studies, annual or less frequent contact by mail, generally with the cohort member directly, or sometimes with his or her designated physician, will identify the probable occurrence of a study endpoint, or death from a cause unrelated to the disease of interest. However, these processes are costly, and also pose the risk of losing an increasing proportion of cohort members with time. Further, if the participant has died, family members may not always be willing to collaborate in providing the required information. Hence, in many studies, other mechanisms are used for follow-up, and indeed may have to be used also for subjects lost if the basic mechanism of follow-up is by mail. Losses to follow-up lead to a loss of power due to the resultant loss of sample size and can introduce bias in a manner similar to the selection processes described previously. Losses that do not differ by either exposure or disease status result in a picture similar to that shown in Table 5.4, that is, no bias, but a loss of power. Losses that differ by exposure (but not outcome) status introduce the same bias as that described in Table 5.5. More problematic are losses that differ by outcome status (Table 5.7) and those that differ by both exposure and outcome status (Table 5.8). In these situations, estimates of the relative risk may be biased in unpredictable directions.

Apart from special surveillance mechanisms, including screening for the disease of interest, there are many sources of routinely collected data for endpoints in cohort studies. These include medical records of physicians, health maintenance organizations and hospitals, vital statistics systems and disease registries. The process to determine whether a particular record relates to a cohort member involves some form of record linkage, determining whether the identifying data in the study file of a cohort member corresponds with the identifying data on the medical or other record of endpoint information. In the past, much of this linkage used to be done manually. Increasingly some form of computerised record linkage is performed. Although such linkages are easier if both sets of records contain the same (national) identifying number, computerised record linkage can still be extremely efficient, and less costly than individual-based follow-up. If record linkage is planned to determine endpoints in a cohort study, great care should be taken at the time of recruitment to collect sufficient identifying information for record linkage purposes, this includes full name, full date of birth, place of birth, mothers maiden name, social security number, other identifying number (if available), and current address. Further, the name and address of friends or relatives of the cohort member should also be collected, to facilitate tracing an individual if other means of tracing them have failed, or if record linkage to another data source has resulted in an uncertain linkage.

In many countries, in addition to disease registries, such as cancer registries, there are other data sources that have been developed to facilitate record linkage for cohort studies and large scale trials. These include the National Health Service Central Register in the UK, the Canadian National Mortality Data Base, the National Death Index in the USA, and similar national registers in the Scandinavian countries. Relatively new in this context are the population-wide registries of genetic data, like the registry already established in Iceland or the one planned in Estonia. Record linkage using these national data bases overcomes many of the issues regarding confidentiality of data, as confidentiality procedures are readily available for such systems. In Canada, what is returned to the investigator is generally anonymous (i.e. stripped of personal identifiers), unless the subjects have signed a prior consent form that specifically permitted record linkage. This was

Table 5.7. Effects of losses to follow-up that differ by outcome status on estimates of disease occurence and assiociation

Target Population			Selection Weights		Study Population			
Disease						Disease		
	Yes	No					Yes	No
At Risk Yes	40	160	200	100	10	**At Risk** Yes	40	16	56
No	60	740	800	100	10	No	60	74	134
	100	900	1000				100	90	190

Target Population			Study Population	
	10%	Prevalence of Disease		53%
	20%	Prevalence of Risk Factor		29%
	2.67	Relative Risk		1.60
	3.08	Odds Ratio		3.08
	125/1000	Attributable Risk		260/1000

Table 5.8. Effects of losses to follow-up that differ by both exposure and outcome status on estimates of disease occurence and assiociation

Target Population			Selection Weights		Study Population		
Target Population Disease Yes / No					**Study Population** Disease Yes / No		
At Risk Yes	40	160	200		At Risk Yes	20	160	180
				50	100			
At Risk No	60	740	800		At Risk No	60	740	800
				100	100			
	100	900	1000			80	900	980

Target Population		Study Population
10%	Prevalence of Disease	8%
20%	Prevalence of Risk Factor	18%
2.67	Relative Risk	1.48
3.08	Odds Ratio	1.54
125/1000	Attributable Risk	36/1000

the case, for example in a cohort study that was linked to a large multi-centre trial of breast screening (Howe et al. 1991).

5.5   Ethical Issues

It is now generally accepted that studies on humans should be carried out with informed consent. This principle, originally developed in relation to controlled clinical trials, has generally now been extended to observational epidemiology studies, including cohort studies.

In the past, if a cohort was recruited that involved the subjects participation in providing data, their agreement to supply the data (e.g. respond to a question-naire) was generally regarded as implied consent. However, now, in addition to providing information on questionnaires, for many cohorts, biological specimens (e.g. blood, buccal cells) are requested, and then it becomes mandatory that the respondent provide consent for the future use of such specimens for research purposes. However, at the time the specimens are provided, it is impossible to know the precise use the investigators may wish to apply to this material. An example relates to the fact that the majority of participants in the sub-cohorts of the European Prospective Investigation of Diet and Cancer (EPIC; Riboli and Kaaks 1997) provided blood specimens in the early 1990s; a few without signing a consent form, the majority did so. However, now that genetic studies are com-monplace on such specimens, it has become apparent that some of the consent forms did not specifically mention genetic analyses as potential research usages. This has led to difficulties in obtaining approval for such sub-studies from human experimentation committees, some of which wanted new consent forms to be signed, specific to the genetically-associated sub-study planned. Obtaining new consent, however, will become increasingly difficult as time goes on, and a number of subjects with the endpoint of interest may have died. In the United States, potential restrictions upon studies such as these have caused difficulties. In Europe, especially Scandinavia, there has been a more relaxed view of the ethical acceptability of studies on stored specimens, many such collections having been originally made without a formal informed consent process, but for which studies conducted with full preservation of confidentiality have been deemed to be ethically acceptable.

The issue as to whether respondents whose stored specimens have been tested should be informed of the results of such tests is also controversial. The European view tends to be that as the testing is being conducted as part of research, it may be impossible to interpret the results of tests for individuals, until this particular research track reaches agreed conclusions. Thus, it is not necessary, indeed possibly unethical, to inform the respondent of the results. Some consent forms specifically state this as a policy. In the United States, however, the opposite viewpoint tends to hold, say, it being regarded as ethically inappropriate for investigators to take a decision on whether or not a subject receives information on themselves. The difficulty with a universal application of such a principle is that for some, the test results may come too late for any possibility of benefit, but, especially in the case of genetic-related information, this may not preclude the test result having implications for the relatives of the subject, and such knowledge is not always a blessing. However, all would agree that if a test reveals information of potential benefit to a subject, they should be informed.

The question of consent for historical cohort studies in general does not arise, though again, there may be issues on informing subjects of the findings of the research. In general, as the research is unlikely to harm the individuals, and providing confidentiality is maintained, human experimentation committees will approve such studies.

One further ethical issue has already been mentioned in Sect. 5.4.3, and that relates to the use of record linkage in obtaining outcome data. In general, providing full confidentiality is maintained, this should not cause difficulties in obtaining approval from human experimentation committees. For further discussions of ethical aspects we refer to Chap. IV.7 of this handbook.

Conclusions   5.6

Cohort studies are a critical method for evaluating causality in epidemiology, and may also be used in evaluating screening (see Chap. III.10 of this handbook).

There are, however, several needs if they are to be valid. You need skilled investigators being familiar with the peculiarities of the planning and the conduct of cohort studies, a sensible source for cohort recruitment, evaluable hypotheses to consider, a validated questionnaire for use at enrolment, unbiased mechanisms to administer the questionnaire as well as for follow-up, quality controlled procedures to collect biological material if relevant for the question under research, facilities for data entry and of course the expertise as well as the facilities for analysis and interpretation.

Cohort studies are often rated at a higher level than case-control studies, largely because the latter are susceptible to recall bias. However, both are usually regarded as "level II" evidence (level I are randomised controlled trials) and there are potential deficiencies in cohort studies that may be less intrusive than in case-control studies, especially a greater propensity for measurement error. Both, however, continue to have an important role in disease epidemiology.

References

Blair A, Stewart PA (1992) Do quantitative exposure assessments improve risk estimates in occupational studies of cancer? Am J Ind Med 21:53–63

Benichou J (1998) Absolute risk. In: Armitage P, Colton T (eds) Encyclopedia of biostatistics. Wiley, New York

Breslow NE, Day NE (1987) Statistical methods in cancer research. Volume II: The design and analysis of cohort studies. IARC Scientific Publications No. 82. International Agency for Research on Cancer, Lyon

Case RA, Hosker ME, McDonald DB, Pearson JT (1954) Tumours of the urinary bladder in workmen engaged in the manufacture and use of certain dyestuff intermediates in the British chemical industry. Br J Ind Med 11:75–104

Coleman M, Douglas A, Hermon C, Peto J (1986) Cohort study analysis with a FORTRAN computer program. Int J Epidemiol 15:134–137

Day NE, Ferrari P (2002) Some methodological issues in nutritional epidemiology. In: Riboli E, Lambert A (eds) Nutrition and lifestyle: Opportunities for cancer prevention. IARC Scientific Publications No. 156. International Agency for Research on Cancer, Lyon, pp 5–10

Doll R, Hill AB (1954) The mortality of doctors in relation to their smoking habits: A preliminary report. Br Med J 1:1451–1455

Doll R, Peto R (1976) Mortality in relation to smoking: 20 years' observations on male British doctors. Br Med J 2:1525–1536

Doll R, Peto R, Hall E, Wheatley K, Gray R (1994a) Mortality in relation to consumption of alcohol: 13 years' observations on male British doctors. Br Med J 309:911–918

Doll R, Peto R, Wheatley K, Gray R, Sutherland I (1994b) Mortality in relation to smoking: 40 years' observations on male British doctors. Br Med J 309:901–911

Eigenbrodt ML, Mosley TH, Hutchinson RG, Watson RL, Chambless LE, Szklo M (2001) Alcohol consumption with age: a cross-sectional and longitudinal study of the Atherosclerosis Risk in Communities (ARIC) study, 1987–1995. Am J Epidemiol 153:1102–1111

Flanders WD, Lally CA, Zhu BP, Henley SJ, Thun MJ (2003) Lung cancer mortality in relation to age, duration of smoking, and daily cigarette consumption: Results from Cancer Prevention Study II. Cancer Res 63:6556–6562

Goldberg M, Luce D (2001) Selection effects in epidemiological cohorts: Nature, causes and consequences. Rev Epidemiol Sante Publique 49:477–492

Howe GR, Friedenreich CM, Jain M, Miller AB (1991) A cohort study of fat intake and risk of breast cancer. J Natl Cancer Inst 83:336–340

Howe GR, Lindsay JP (1983) A follow-up of a ten-percent sample of the Canadian labor force. I. Cancer mortality in males, 1965–1973. J Natl Cancer Inst 70:37–44

IARC Working Group (2003) IARC handbooks on cancer prevention, vol 8: Fruits and vegetables. International Agency for Research on Cancer, Lyon

Li CY, Sung FC (1999) A review of the healthy worker effect in occupational epidemiology. Occup Med 49:225–229

McCray E (1986) Occupational risk of the acquired immunodeficiency syndrome among health care workers. N Engl J Med 314:1127–1132

Miller AB, To T, Agnew DA, Wall C, Green LM (1996) Leukemia following occupational exposure to 60-Hz electric and magnetic fields among Ontario electric utility workers. Am J Epidemiol 144:150–160

Miller AB, Altenburg H-P, Bueno de Mesquita, B, Boshuizen HC, Agudo A, Berrino F, Gram IT, Janson L, Linseisen J, Overvad K, Rasmuson T, Vineis P, Lukanova A, Allen N, Amiano P, Barricarte A, Berglund G, Boeing H, Clavel-Chapelon F, Day NE, Hallmans G, Lund E, Martinez C, Navarro C, Palli D, Panico S, Peeters PH, Quiros JR, Tjonneland A, Tumino R, Trichopoulou A, Trichopoulos D, Slimani N, Riboli E (2004) Fruits and vegetables and lung cancer: Findings from the European Prospective Investigation into Cancer and Nutrition. Int J Cancer 108:269–276

Morgan RW, Kelsh MA, Zhao K, Exuzides KA, Heringer S, Negrete W (2000) Radiofrequency exposure and mortality from cancer of the brain and lymphatic/hematopoietic systems. Epidemiology 11:118–127

Morris JN, Heady JA, Raffle PA, Roberts CG, Parks JW (1953a) Coronary heart disease and physical activity of work. Lancet 265:1053–1057

Morris JN, Heady JA, Raffle PA, Roberts CG, Parks JW (1953b) Coronary heart disease and physical activity of work. Lancet 265:1111–1120

National Institutes of Health (2004) Request for information: design and implementation of a large-scale prospective cohort study of genetic and environmental influences on common diseases. (http://grants.nih.gov/grants/guide/notice-files/NOT-OD-04-041.html) Accessed May 11, 2004

Oomen CM, Ocke MC, Feskens EJ, van Erp-Baart MA, Kok FJ, Kromhout D (2001) Association between trans fatty acid intake and 10-year risk of coronary heart disease in the Zutphen Elderly Study: a prospective population-based study. Lancet 357:746–751

Orencia AJ, Petty GW, Khandheria BK, Annegers JF, Ballard DJ, Sicks JD, O'-Fallon WM, Whisnant JP (1995) Risk of stroke with mitral valve prolapse in population-based cohort study. Stroke 26:7–13

Preston DL, Lubin JH, Pierce DA, McConney ME (1993) Epicure user's guide. HiroSoft International Corp, Seattle

Riboli E, Kaaks R (1997) The EPIC project: rationale and study design. European Prospective Investigation into Cancer and Nutrition. Int J Epidemiol 26 Suppl 1:S6–14

Rinsky RA, Smith AB, Hornung R, Filloon TG, Young RJ, Okun AH, Landrigan PJ (1987) Benzene and leukemia. An epidemiologic risk assessment. New Engl J Med 316:1044–1050

Rittgen W, Becker N (2000) SMR analysis of historical follow-up studies with missing death certificates. Biometrics 56:1164–1169

Rothman KJ, Greenland S (1998) Modern epidemiology, 2nd edn. Lippincott Williams & Wilkins, Philadelphia

Sahai H, Khurshid A (1996) Statistics in epidemiology. Methods, techniques, and applications. CRC Press, Boca Raton New York London Tokyo

Silcocks P (1994) Estimating confidence limits on a standardised mortality ratio when the expected number is not error free. J Epidemiol Community Health 48:313–317

Smith-Warner SA, Spiegelman D, Yaun SS, Albanes D, Beeson WL, van den Brandt PA, Feskanich D, Folsom AR, Fraser GE, Freudenheim JL, Giovannucci E, Goldbohm RA, Graham S, Kushi LH, Miller AB, Pietinen P, Rohan TE, Speizer FE, Willett WC, Hunter DJ (2003) Fruits, vegetables and lung cancer: a pooled analysis of cohort studies. Int J Cancer 107:1001–1011

Snow J (1855) On the mode of communication of cholera. Churchill, London

Sutherland J (2002) EXTRACTS from appendix (A) to the Report of the General Board of Health on the Epidemic Cholera of 1848 & 1849. Int J Epidemiol 31:900–907

StataCorp (2001) Stata statistical software: Release 7.0. Stata Corporation, College Station

Terris M (ed) (1964) Goldberger on pellagra. Louisiana State University Press, Baton Rouge

Theriault G, Goldberg M, Miller AB, Armstrong B, Guenel P, Deadman J, Imbernon E, To T, Chevalier A, Cyr D (1994) Cancer risks associated with occupational exposure to magnetic fields among electric utility workers in Ontario and Quebec, Canada, and France: 1970–1989. Am J Epidemiol 139:550–572

Tomatis L, Aitio A, Day NE, Heseltine E, Kalder J, Miller AB, Parkin DM, Riboli E (eds) (1990) Cancer: Causes, occurrence and control. IARC Scientific Publications No. 100. International Agency for Research on Cancer, Lyon

Ulvestad B, Kjaerheim K, Martinsen JI, Mowe G, Andersen A (2004) Cancer incidence among members of the Norwegian trade union of insulation workers. J Occup Environ Med 46:84–89

Villeneuve PJ, Agnew DA, Corey PN, Miller AB (1998) Alternate indices of electric and magnetic field exposures among Ontario electrical utility workers. Bioelectromagnetics 19:140–151

Wada S, Miyanishi M, Nishimoto Y, Kambe S, Miller RW (1968) Mustard gas as a cause of respiratory neoplasia in man. Lancet 1:1161–1163

Willett WC, Hunter DJ, Stampfer MJ, Colditz G, Manson JE, Spiegelman D, Rosner B, Hennekens CH, Speizer FE (1992) Dietary fat and fiber in relation to risk of breast cancer. An 8-year follow-up. J Amer Med Assoc 268:2037–2044

Wolk A, Bergstrom R, Hunter D, Willett W, Ljung H, Holmberg L, Bergkvist L, Bruce A, Adami HO (1998) A prospective study of association of monounsaturated fat and other types of fat with risk of breast cancer. Arch Intern Med 158:41–45

Case-Control Studies

I.6

Norman E. Breslow

6.1   Introduction

6.1.1   A Brief History

The case-control study examines the association between disease and potential risk factors by taking separate samples of diseased cases and of controls at risk of developing disease. Information may be collected for both cases and controls on genetic, social, behavioral, environmental or other determinants of disease risk. The basic study design has a long history, extending back at least to Guy's 1843 comparison of the occupations of men with pulmonary consumption to the occupations of men having other diseases (Lilienfeld and Lilienfeld 1979). Beginning in the 1920's, it was used to link cancer to environmental and hormonal exposures. Broders (1920) discovered an association between pipe smoking and lip cancer; Lane-Claypon (1926), who selected matched hospital controls, investigated the relationship between reproductive experience and female breast cancer; and Lombard and Doering (1928) related pipe smoking to oral cancer. The publication in 1950 of three reports on the association between cigarette smoking and lung cancer generated enormous interest in case-control methodology as well as bitter criticism (Levin et al. 1950; Wynder and Graham 1950; Doll and Hill 1950). The landmark study of Doll and Hill (1950, 1952), in particular, inspired future generations of epidemiologists to use this methodology. It remains to this day a model for the design and conduct of case-control studies, with excellent suggestions on how to reduce or eliminate selection, interview and recall bias.

From the mid-1950's to the mid-1970's the number of case-control studies published in selected medical journals increased four- to sevenfold (Cole 1979). Aird et al. (1953) discovered the association between gastric cancer and the ABO blood groups. The impact of hormonal factors on cancers of female organs was brought to light, starting with confirmation of the association between late first pregnancy and breast cancer (MacMahon et al. 1970). Herbst et al. (1971) investigated an unusual outbreak of vaginal adenocarcinoma in young women, finding that mothers of seven of eight cases had exposed their daughters *in utero* to the fertility drug diethylstilbestrol (DES). None of 32 control mothers had a history of estrogen use during pregnancy. Treatment of menopausal women with exogenous estrogens similarly increased the risk of endometrial cancer (Ziel and Finkle 1975; Smith et al. 1975). Powerful joint effects of alcohol and tobacco consumption on esophageal cancer were demonstrated (Tuyns et al. 1977), as was the strong association between liver cancer and hepatitis B carrier status (Prince et al. 1975). These successes encouraged more investigators to adopt the case-control study as the method of choice for the study of rare chronic diseases, particularly cancer. A survey by Correa et al. (1994) identified 223 population-based case-control studies published in the world literature in 1992. Recent discoveries obtained using case-control methodology have included the role of salted fish in the etiology of nasopharyngeal carcinoma in Chinese populations (Armstrong et al. 1983; Yu et al. 1986), the hazards of prone sleeping position for sudden infant death syndrome (SIDS) (Fleming et al. 1990) and the relationship between use of intrauterine devices (IUDs) and tubal infertility (Daling et al. 1985).

This plethora of case-control studies, stimulated by their relatively low cost and short duration, also had its drawbacks. Not all investigators were as careful as Doll and Hill in following a protocol for selection of cases and controls, in conducting the study to mitigate against bias and in thoughtfully analysing the collected data. Nor did they have the good fortune to study associations as strong as that between lung cancer and cigarette smoking. The increasing availability of high speed computers made it possible to collect more and more data, and to look for all manner of associations with putative risk factors. Investigators eager for research funding were sometimes too quick to publish their findings and draw media attention to them. The inevitable result was an increasingly negative reaction on the part of the public, and from segments of the scientific community, to the false alarms and contradictory results (Taubes 1995). One goal of this chapter, and of others in this handbook, is to describe basic scientific principles whose application should help to improve public confidence in published findings of epidemiologic studies.

Early Methodologic Developments 6.1.2

> The sophisticated use and understanding of case-control studies is the most outstanding methodologic development of modern epidemiology.
> (Rothman 1986, p. 62)

The initial interpretation of the case-control study was the comparison of exposure histories for a group of diseased cases with those for non-diseased controls. Typical analyses involved two group comparisons of exposure distributions using chi-squared and t-tests. The critics argued that such comparisons provided no information about the quantities of true epidemiologic interest, namely the disease rates. Cornfield (1951) corrected this misconception by demonstrating that the exposure odds ratio for cases vs. controls was equal to the disease odds ratio for exposed vs. non-exposed. With $D = 1$ indicating disease, $D = 0$ disease-free and $X = 1/0$ likewise denoting exposed or non-exposed, he showed using Bayes theorem that

$$\frac{\Pr(D = 1|X = 1)\Pr(D = 0|X = 0)}{\Pr(D = 0|X = 1)\Pr(D = 1|X = 0)} = \frac{\Pr(X = 1|D = 1)\Pr(X = 0|D = 0)}{\Pr(X = 0|D = 1)\Pr(X = 1|D = 0)} \quad (6.1)$$

and noted that the disease odds ratio approximated the *relative risk* $\Pr(D = 1|X = 1)/\Pr(D = 1|X = 0)$ provided the disease was rare. He also pointed out that, if the overall disease risk was known from other data sources, this could be combined with the relative risk to estimate *absolute* disease risks for exposed and non-exposed, respectively.

Disease risk as considered by Cornfield (1951) was *prevalence*, the probability that a member of the population was ill at a given point in time. For studies of disease etiology, however, it is preferable to work with disease *incidence*, the probability of developing disease during the study period among subjects who are free of disease initially. Otherwise, one confuses the effect of exposure on causation of disease with its effect on the case fatality rate (Neyman 1955). Controls for a study of the cumulative risk of developing disease during a given period would be persons who were free of disease during the entire period. Although it laid the foundation for what was to follow, this conceptualization of the case-control study in terms of cumulative disease risk was awkward, for two reasons. First, as the study interval lengthened the risk of disease increased for both exposed and non-exposed. The relative risk for a common disease could approach one. Even if it did not, it was undesirable to have the basic effect measure so dependent on study duration, which varies between studies. Second, for a study of long duration, ensuring that the controls were disease-free throughout the study period could be problematic in practice. The modern conception of a case-control study involves sampling of controls who are disease-free at random times during the study period (Sect. 6.2.1). Exposure odds ratios are used to estimate ratios of incidence *rates* rather than ratios of risks. No rare disease assumption is needed in this case.

Mantel and Haenszel (1959) clarified the status of the case-control (or retrospective) study in comparison with the cohort (forward or prospective) study in one of the most highly cited papers in the scientific literature (Breslow 1996). They stated emphatically:

> A primary goal is to reach the same conclusions in a retrospective study as would have been obtained from a forward study, if one had been done.
> (Mantel and Haenszel 1959, p. 722)

This insight underlies the modern conception of the case-control study as involving *sampling*, on the basis of outcome, from an ongoing real or imagined cohort study that has been designed to provide the best possible answer to the basic question. Mantel and Haenszel introduced a new test and a simple, highly efficient estimator for the relative risk after stratification on control factors. Their methods required the epidemiologist to carefully examine the tabular data, and thus to identify strata where there was a lack of information or where there were discrepancies between summary and stratum specific relative risks. They remain valuable today as an adjunct to more elaborate model fitting.

By the end of the 1950s, the case-control study was firmly established as the method of choice for the chronic disease epidemiologist, certainly when the budget was limited. The role of statisticians in bringing the study design to this place of scientific respectability was widely acknowledged (Cole 1979; Armenian and Lilienfeld 1994). Further methodological advances were made during the next two decades, particularly in statistical modeling of case-control data. The development of the proportional hazards regression model for life table data (Sheehe 1962; Cox 1972) provided a sound mathematical basis for methods long used by epidemiologists, and led to refinements and extensions of those methods (Breslow et al. 1983). The nested case-control study, originally conceived as a method to reduce the computational burden of fitting Cox's model to data from large cohorts (Liddell et al. 1977), was recognized as an efficient epidemiologic design for the collection of expensive explanatory data (Langholz and Goldstein 1996). It now serves as a paradigm for all case-control studies. Many of the methodological developments were described in texts by Breslow and Day (1980) and Schlesselman (1982) that led to further appreciation and use of the case-control study.

Chapter Outline   6.1.3

The remainder of this chapter discusses the modern conceptualization of the case-control study, largely from a statistical perspective. Matching of controls to cases at the design stage is viewed as a technique to be used in carefully limited contexts to increase the statistical efficiency of a highly stratified analysis. The implications of these theoretical developments for the practical selection of cases and controls are explored. Major pitfalls include the unique susceptibility of the case-control study to selection bias and, especially when exposures are assessed by interview, to measurement error. The design of any particular study usually involves tradeoffs between potential biases arising from these sources. Following established principles of sound statistical science, including the use of an appropriate protocol for subject selection and exposure assessment, can help reduce the variability in study results that has contributed to the low esteem accorded risk factor epidemiology in some scientific circles (Breslow 2003).

Conceptual Foundations   6.2

Sampling from a Real or Fictitious Cohort   6.2.1

The Mantel and Haenszel (1959) goal, of reaching the same conclusions from a case-control study as from a cohort study if one had been done, provides the key to understanding of case-control methodology. Rather than start the planning process by thinking about how to conduct a case-control study, it often is helpful to first plan the ideal cohort study that would be conducted to investigate the same hypothesis if unlimited resources were available. Planning would include cohort identification, definition of the times of entry into and exit from the cohort, ascertainment of the disease endpoint, measurement of the exposure histories, consideration of potential confounders and methods of statistical analysis. The corresponding case-control study would then be viewed as the random sampling of subjects from this idealized cohort to achieve, so far as possible, the stated goal.

Cohort Definition.   In concept the underlying cohort for a case-control study consists of all subjects who, had they experienced the disease endpoint at a specific time, would have been ascertained as a case at that time. When case-control sampling is carried out in the context of an actual cohort study, to select individuals for genotyping or other expensive measurements, for example, the cohort is completely enumerated by and known to the investigator. More typically, however, the underlying cohort is not fully identified and is effectively defined by the method of case ascertainment. When cases are ascertained from a particular hospital, for example, one considers the cohort to consist of all subjects who, had they developed the disease in question, would have been diagnosed in that hospital.

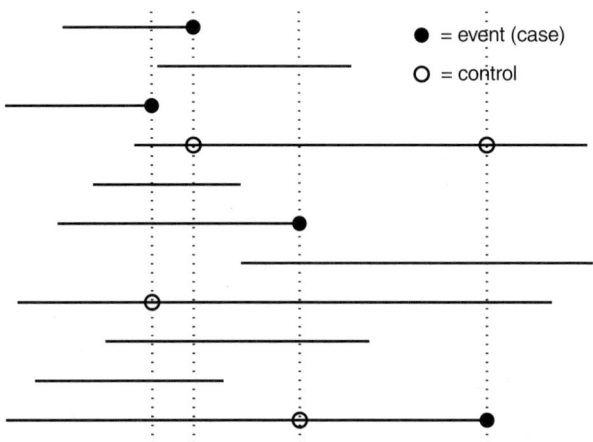

Figure 6.1. Schematic of a (nested) case-control study

Figure 6.1 illustrates the basic idea of case-control sampling. Each of the 11 horizontal lines represents time on study for a member of the cohort. Subjects enter follow-up at the left hand endpoint and exit at the right. They are considered to be *at risk* of becoming a case throughout this period. It is even possible, though not shown here, that a subject could enter the cohort, leave for awhile and then return. Four of the 11 subjects are cases. Their follow-up ends at diagnosis since they are no longer at risk of becoming an incident case thereafter. The vertical dotted lines, plotted at each of the times that a case occurs, intersect the trajectories of those who are at risk at that time, i.e., the trajectories of subjects in the corresponding *risk set*.

Nested Case-Control Sampling.   When the cohort study is a real one, so that times of entry and exit are known for all members, the investigator may completely enumerate each risk set. A nested case-control study is then possible in which controls are selected by finite population random sampling, without replacement, from non-cases in the risk set. The usual assumption is that the sampling of controls from each risk set is completely independent of sampling from all other risk sets. Two consequences are that a subject sampled as a control at one point in time may later become a case, and that the same subject may be sampled more than once as a control. Figure 6.1, which depicts the situation where exactly one control is sampled from each risk set, illustrates each of these possibilities. Robins et al. (1986) describe other sampling schemes, and corresponding methods of analysis, for nested case-control studies.

Density Sampling. These ideas also may be applied, at least in principle, to the more typical situation in which the cohort is not completely enumerated. An essential assumption, which in fact well approximates the design of many studies, is that the cohort is sampled throughout the study period. More specifically, controls are selected at any given time at a rate proportional to the disease incidence rate at that time (Sheehe 1962). Miettinen (1976) termed this *incidence density sampling*. A second assumption is that each subject at risk at a given time has the same probability of being sampled as a control. This implies that, from the standpoint of an individual, the likelihood of being included in the study as a control increases with increasing *time on study*. If the disease incidence rate is constant, someone who is a member of the cohort for twice as long as someone else has twice the chance of being selected as a control. In the statistical literature this is known as *length biased* sampling. One important consequence, under the assumption of constant disease incidence, is that the number of controls sampled is proportional to the *total time at risk*.

Incidence Rate Ratios are Estimable from Odds Ratios 6.2.2

We consider here the simplest situation in which the disease incidence rate is constant and there are two groups of subjects, exposed and non-exposed, that are homogeneous apart from exposure. Confounding is therefore not an issue. Denote by A the total number of incident cases ascertained from the cohort during the study period (t_0, t_1) and suppose that A_0 are determined to be non-exposed whereas $A_1 = A - A_0$ are exposed. Similarly denote by $T = T_0 + T_1$ the total person-time on study, decomposed into its non-exposed (T_0) and exposed (T_1) components. While the numbers of cases A_0 and A_1 are known to the investigator, T_0 and T_1 may not be unless the underlying cohort is a real one. Instead, the case-control study provides information on how many of the total $M = M_0 + M_1$ of controls are non-exposed (M_0) and how many are exposed (M_1). Denoting by M_1/M_0 the observed odds of exposure for controls and likewise by A_1/A_0 the observed odds of exposure for cases, the corresponding exposure odds ratio is $(A_1 M_0)/(A_0 M_1)$.

Let $\pi \tau$ denote the probability that a subject who contributes τ person-years of followup is sampled as a control. With $T = \sum_{i=1}^{N} \tau_i$ denoting the sum of the times-on-study for N cohort members, i.e., the total time at risk, the expected number of controls is $E(M) = \pi T$. In practice π is often selected by the investigator to yield a fixed number of controls, at least as a target value. Its actual value remains unknown unless information is available about T. Nonetheless, provided π is constant for all subjects, both exposed and non-exposed, $E(M_0) = \pi T_0$ and

$E(M_1) = \pi T_1$. Hence the control ratio M_0/M_1 estimates the corresponding ratio T_0/T_1 of person-time. Since the exposure specific incidence rates are estimated by $\hat{\Lambda}_0 = A_0/T_0$ and $\hat{\Lambda}_1 = A_1/T_1$, it follows (see Rothman and Greenland 1998, Chap. 10) that the rate ratio may be estimated by the exposure odds ratio:

$$\frac{\hat{\Lambda}_1}{\hat{\Lambda}_0} = \frac{A_1 T_0}{A_0 T_1} \approx \frac{A_1 M_0}{A_0 M_1}. \tag{6.2}$$

See Sect. 6.3.1 for a numerical example.

6.2.3   Time-dependent Rates and Exposures

Section 6.2.2 assumes that the parameter of interest is the ratio of instantaneous incidence rates, each assumed constant in time, for exposed and non-exposed subjects. A more general conceptualization takes the interest parameter to be the ratio $\psi \equiv \Lambda_1(t)/\Lambda_0(t)$ of instantaneous rates where the ratio, but not necessarily the underlying rates, is assumed constant in t. Let $N(t)$ denote the total number of subjects at risk at time t in the underlying cohort, of which a proportion $p_1(t)$ are exposed and $p_0(t)$ are non-exposed. These proportions could vary with time either because the exposure status for individual subjects changes, or because the exposure composition of the cohort changes through entries and exits. Note that the expected number of exposed cases is given by $\int N(t)p_1(t)\Lambda_1(t)\,dt$ and similarly for the non-exposed cases. The expected number of controls sampled in the interval $(t, t + dt)$ is therefore $M(t)\,dt$ where $M(t) = N(t)[p_0(t)\Lambda_0(t) + p_1(t)\Lambda_1(t)]$. It follows that the unadjusted exposure odds ratio under density sampling estimates

$$\psi^* = \frac{\int N(t)p_1(t)\Lambda_1(t)\,dt \int M(t)p_0(t)\,dt}{\int N(t)p_0(t)\Lambda_0(t)\,dt \int M(t)p_1(t)\,dt}$$

$$= \psi \frac{\int N(t)p_1(t)\Lambda_0(t)\,dt \int M(t)p_0(t)\,dt}{\int N(t)p_0(t)\Lambda_0(t)\,dt \int M(t)p_1(t)\,dt} \tag{6.3}$$

(Greenland and Thomas 1982). Thus the exposure odds ratio estimates the incidence rate ratio, i.e., $\psi^* = \psi$, provided either that the exposure proportions are constant in t or else that $\psi = 1$. Otherwise, time t acts as a *confounder* of the exposure–disease association. In this case, a time-matched analysis using standard methods for matched case-control studies (Breslow and Day 1980, Chap. 7) is needed to estimate ψ unbiasedly. The marginal (unmatched) odds ratio usually provides a slightly *conservative* estimate of this parameter.

6.2.4   Cumulative Risk Ratios and Case-Cohort Sampling

While it is generally agreed that case-control studies of chronic disease are best designed using density sampling to estimate the incidence rate ratio, alternative sampling designs may be superior for other purposes. Vaccine efficacy is usually defined as the proportional reduction, over the study period, in the number of cases among subjects who are vaccinated compared to those who are not. Equivalently, it is 1 minus the ratio of cumulative disease risks for vaccinated vs. non-vaccinated. Suppose the effect of vaccination is to render completely immune a proportion P_I of subjects, while the remainder of those vaccinated have the same disease incidence rates $\lambda_0(t)$ as do non-vaccinated persons (Smith et al. 1984). For simplicity assume that all subjects, both vaccinated and non-vaccinated, are followed from a common starting time t_0 and that there is no loss to follow-up. The cumulative risk of disease by time t_1 for those not vaccinated is $P(t_0, t_1) = 1 - \exp[-\int_{t_0}^{t_1} \lambda_0(t)\,dt]$ and the vaccine efficacy is thus

$$1 - \frac{\text{risk for vaccinated}}{\text{risk for non-vaccinated}} = 1 - \frac{P_I \times 0 + (1 - P_I) \times P(t_0, t_1)}{P(t_0, t_1)} = P_I . \tag{6.4}$$

Here the cumulative risk ratio, not the incidence rate ratio, is independent of study duration $t_1 - t_0$ (Rodrigues and Kirkwood 1990). Suppose now a *subcohort* of M subjects is drawn at random from the combined cohort of vaccinated and non-vaccinated subjects such that each individual has the *same* probability π of inclusion in it, *regardless* of duration of follow-up. If M_0 and M_1 denote the numbers of non-vaccinated and vaccinated in the subcohort, while A_0 and A_1 denote the numbers of disease cases diagnosed by time t_1, then vaccine efficacy is simply estimated as

$$\widehat{P_I} = 1 - \frac{A_1/M_1}{A_0/M_0} . \tag{6.5}$$

More generally, the case-cohort design (Kupper et al. 1975; Miettinen 1982; Prentice 1986) involves random sampling of a subcohort at study entry, without re-

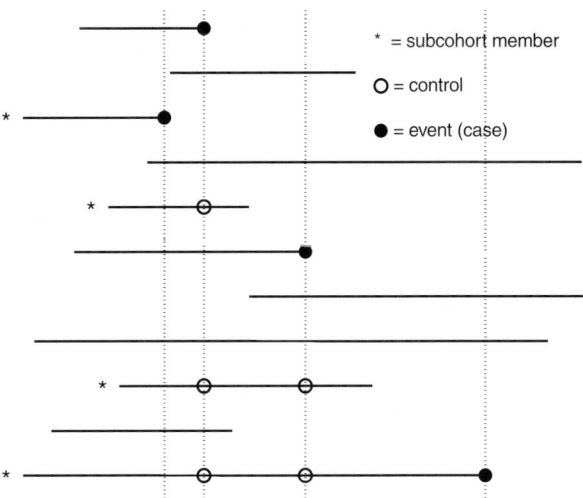

Figure 6.2. Schematic of a case-cohort study

gard to time on study. Figure 6.2 contrasts this design with nested case-control sampling (Fig. 6.1). Incidence rate ratios may be estimated for dynamic (open) cohorts, with staggered entry and loss to follow-up as pictured, just as they are with nested case-control sampling (Prentice 1986; Lin and Ying 1993; Barlow 1994). Subcohort members under observation at the time of disease occurrence serve as the controls for each case in a time-matched analysis. Since the subcohort is a simple random sample from the full cohort, it is suitable for estimation of population genotype or exposure frequencies, whereas the controls from a nested study are not. Furthermore, the same subcohort may be used to provide controls for two or more different types of disease cases. Because of this flexibility, the case-cohort design is increasingly used for sampling from defined cohorts.

6.2.5   Estimation of Absolute Risks

The key feature of case-control sampling in the context of an actual cohort study, where the underlying cohort is completely enumerated and entry and exit times are known for all cohort members, is that the sampling probabilities for cases and controls are known or can be estimated from the available data. The case-control study provides supplementary information on explanatory variables for a randomly selected group of cohort members. Analysis of the combined cohort and case-control data may be approached using standard methods for incomplete data (Little and Rubin 2002). The Horvitz and Thompson (1952) survey sampling approach is often easiest to implement. Here the contribution to estimators or estimating equations from each subject with complete data, i.e., each subject included in the case-control sample, is weighted by (an estimate of) the inverse probability of having been included. Any analysis that could have been carried out were explanatory data available for the entire cohort can also be carried out using the combined data from the cohort and the case-control sample. This principle applies to estimation of absolute as well as relative risks.

Table 6.1. Numbers of lung cancer cases and controls in Greater London among males aged 45–64 years, by average amount smoked in preceding 10 years, with estimated death rates of lung cancer per 1000 persons per year[†]

| | Ave. daily number of cigarettes | | | | | | |
	0	1–4	5–14	15–24	25–49	50+	Total
Controls (n_{0j})	38	87	397	279	119	12	$n_{0+} = 932$
Cases (n_{1j})	2	19	197	171	129	21	$n_{1+} = 539$
Rates ($\hat{\lambda}_j$)	0.14	0.59	1.35	1.67	2.95	4.76*	1.57

[†] Reconstructed from data of Doll and Hill (1952), p. 1278
* Doll and Hill give 4.74 for this entry

A demonstration that absolute risks can be estimated from case-control data that are supplemented with information regarding the underlying population was provided by Doll and Hill (1952). They restricted the analysis to cases and controls drawn from the Greater London area, for which the numbers of persons and the numbers of deaths due to lung cancer were known from government records for each category of age and sex. Table 6.1 shows numbers of male cases n_{1j} and controls n_{0j} aged 45–64 years at the jth of 6 levels of average cigarette consumption during the preceding 10 years ($j = 1, \ldots, 6$). Assuming that the smoking habits of the controls were representative of the habits of the general population in each age-sex category, and likewise that the habits of the cases were reasonably similar to those of persons who died of lung cancer, they were able to estimate the numbers of persons N_j and of deaths D_j at each of the 6 smoking levels. Specifically, knowing that the total male population of Greater London aged 45–64 was $N_+ = 937{,}000$, they estimated the sub-population (in thousands) at the jth smoking level as $\widehat{N}_j = (n_{0j}/932) \times 937$. Similarly, knowing that $D_+ = 1474$ deaths from lung cancer occurred annually in this population, they estimated the numbers of deaths at that level by $\widehat{D}_j = (n_{1j}/539) \times 1474$. Thus the absolute rates per 1000 persons per year at smoking level j were estimated as

$$\hat{\lambda}_j = \frac{\widehat{D}_j}{\widehat{N}_j} = \frac{n_{1j} \cdot n_{0+} \cdot D_+}{n_{0j} \cdot n_{1+} \cdot N_+} \, .$$

See Table 6.1 and Doll and Hill (1952), Table XII. Neutra and Drolette (1978) formally justified this commonly used procedure while Greenland (1987) provided an extension for matched case-control studies.

Langholz and Borgan (1997) developed more specialized methodology for estimation of absolute risks from nested case-control studies under the Cox (1972) model. The absolute risk of disease over the time period (t_0, t_1) for a subject with explanatory variables x who is disease-free at its start is

$$P(t_0, t_1; x) = \int_{t_0}^{t_1} S(t_0, t; x)\lambda(t; x)\,dt \, , \tag{6.6}$$

where $S(t_0, t; x)$ denotes the probability that the subject remains on study and free of disease from t_0 to t and $\lambda(t; x)$ is the disease incidence rate. Increments in the baseline cumulative incidence rate function at each time of disease diagnosis, needed to estimate both S and λ, are obtained from the usual formula for the cohort study applied to *reduced* risk sets consisting of the case and sampled control(s). The denominator term, representing the sum of relative risks for all subjects in the risk set, is weighted by n/m where n denotes the size of the risk set and m the number of subjects, including the case, sampled from it. Benichou and Gail (1995) studied similar methodology for unmatched case-control sampling from an actual cohort when all explanatory variables are discrete. Econometricians also have developed methods for incorporation of external information on background rates into the analyses of data collected in "choice-based" sampling designs, the social science analog of case-control studies (Hsieh et al. 1985).

6.3   **Matching and Stratification**

> While the logical absurdity of attempting to measure an effect for a factor controlled by matching must be obvious, it is surprising how often investigators must be restrained from attempting this. (Mantel and Haenszel 1959, p. 729)

Investigators planning case-control studies used to consider matching of individual controls to cases as a means of making the two groups as comparable as possible, thereby increasing the perceived validity of study results. It is now recognized that such matching, or stratified sampling of controls to make them more like the cases – known as frequency matching, has a much more limited and specific role. This is to improve the efficiency of rate ratio estimators (exposure odds ratios) that are statistically *adjusted* to account for possible confounding effects. Inappropriate matching may have the unintended effect of compromising design efficiency or even of rendering the results completely uninterpretable. Furthermore, since the sampling design must always be considered, matching usually complicates the statistical analysis.

6.3.1   **Consequences of Matching**

The goal of matching in case-control studies is to balance the numbers of cases and controls within strata that will be used for statistical adjustment purposes. If the factor(s) used for stratification are associated with exposure, the matched control sample will generally have an exposure distribution more like that of the cases than would an unmatched control sample.

Some interesting and important consequences of matching are illustrated by the fictitious data shown in Table 6.2, which is adapted from Table 10-5 of Rothman and Greenland (1998). In the underlying cohort the disease rates for exposed and non-exposed are identical for males and females. Consequently, there is no effect modification nor confounding by sex and the crude (marginal) rate ratio equals the sex-specific ratios. The frequency matching of controls to cases by sex, however, has *induced* apparent confounding in the case-control data. The sex specific rate ratios are correctly estimated by the sex-specific odds ratios, in accordance with Equation (6.2), but they are substantially under-estimated by the crude exposure odds ratio. An analysis that accounts for the matching is essential to correctly estimate the interest parameter.

6.3.2   **Efficiency of Matching**

The advantages of a frequency matched sample become evident when one considers extreme situations. In the study of esophageal cancer of Tuyns et al. (1977), for example, 775 controls were sampled at random from electoral rolls for comparison with the 200 cases. Not surprisingly, the lowest age stratum contained only a single

Table 6.2. Distribution of cases and person-years of observation in a fictitious cohort study, and expected distribution of cases and frequency matched controls[†]

	A. Results for underlying cohort study			
	Males		Females	
	Exposed	Non-exposed	Exposed	Non-exposed
Diseased	450	10	50	90
Person-years	90,000	10,000	10,000	90,000
Rate ($\times 10^3$)	5.0	1.0	5.0	1.0
Rate ratio	$\psi_E = 5$		$\psi_E = 5$	
	Crude rate ratio $= \frac{(450+50)/100,000}{(10+90)/100,000} = 5$			

	B. Expected results for the case-control study			
	Males		Females	
	Exposed	Non-exposed	Exposed	Non-exposed
Cases	450	10	50	90
Controls	414	46	14	126
Odds ratio	$\widehat{\psi}_E = 5.0$		$\widehat{\psi}_E = 5.0$	
	Expected crude odds ratio $\approx \widehat{\psi}_E = \frac{(450+50)\times(46+126)}{(10+90)\times(414+14)} = 2$			

[†] Adapted from Table 10-5 of Rothman and Greenland (1998)

case and 115 controls. Since they contributed very little to the age-stratified odds ratio, the time spent interviewing the 115 youngest controls was largely wasted. When the potential for imbalance is less extreme, however, the advantages of matching are not so clear. Some insight is provided by considering the ratio of asymptotic variances of crude and adjusted (stratified) odds ratio estimators for frequency matched and random samples in the simplest of situations, that involving a binary exposure factor, a binary confounding factor and a rare disease. Assuming equal numbers of cases and controls, and that the exposure rate ratio ψ_E is the same at both levels of the confounder, the variances are determined by five quantities: ψ_E; p_E, the population proportion exposed; p_C, the proportion positive for the confounder; ψ_C, the rate ratio for the confounder; and ψ_{CE}, the odds ratio associating confounder and exposure in the population. Table 6.3, adapted from Breslow (1982), shows ratios of variances and biases for different odds ratio estimators when $p_C = 0.5$ and $p_E = 0.3$. Similar results were given by Thomas and Greenland (1983) and by Smith and Day (1984).

A stratified analysis is not needed to control confounding when $\psi_{CE} = 1$ or $\psi_C = 1$. For as shown in rows 1–5, 9 and 13 of Table 6.3, the bias B_R of the pooled estimator using a randomly selected control sample is then zero. Columns labeled V_M/V_R^* show the increase in variance, i.e., the loss in efficiency, if a matched control sample and stratified analysis were used instead. There is no efficiency loss through matching when $\psi_{CE} = 1$ but increasing loss for estimation of large rate

Table 6.3. Variance ratios and biases, in percent, for estimators of ψ_E in case-control studies with matched and random samples[†]

ψ_{CE}	ψ_C	$\psi_E = 1$				$\psi_E = 2$				$\psi_E = 5$				$\psi_E = 10$			
		$\frac{V_M}{V_R}$	$\frac{V_M}{V_{R*}}$	B_R	B_M	$\frac{V_M}{V_R}$	$\frac{V_M}{V_{R*}}$	B_R	B_M	$\frac{V_M}{V_R}$	$\frac{V_M}{V_{R*}}$	B_R	B_M	$\frac{V_M}{V_R}$	$\frac{V_M}{V_{R*}}$	B_R	B_M
1	1	100	100	0	0	100	100	0	0	100	100	0	0	100	100	0	0
	2	97	100	0	0	97	100	0	0	97	100	0	0	97	100	0	0
	5	88	100	0	0	87	100	0	0	87	100	0	0	88	100	0	0
	10	80	100	0	0	79	100	0	0	80	100	0	0	81	100	0	0
2	1	100	103	0	0	100	103	0	-4	100	103	0	-4	104	104	0	-6
	2	95	100	12	0	96	100	12	-4	97	101	12	-4	102	102	12	-5
	5	85	97	24	0	86	97	24	-1	88	98	24	-2	99	99	24	-3
	10	78	96	31	0	78	96	31	-1	81	97	31	-1	98	98	31	-2
5	1	100	113	0	0	99	113	0	-8	101	118	0	-18	105	122	0	-23
	2	93	106	27	0	93	106	27	-7	97	110	27	-14	103	114	27	-18
	5	82	99	58	0	83	99	58	-4	89	102	58	-8	95	105	58	-10
	10	76	95	75	0	77	96	75	-2	82	98	75	-5	88	100	75	-6
10	1	100	126	0	0	98	126	0	-14	100	134	0	-29	107	144	0	-37
	2	91	114	36	0	90	114	36	-11	96	120	36	-23	104	128	36	-28
	5	80	102	82	0	81	102	82	-6	88	107	82	-13	96	111	82	-16
	10	74	97	106	0	76	98	106	-4	82	101	106	-8	90	105	106	-9

† Adapted from Breslow (1982), Table 2 ψ_{CE} = Odds ratio associating exposure and confounder ψ_E = Rate ratio for exposure
ψ_C = Rate ratio for confounder B_R = Bias of pooled estimate of ψ_E, random sample, as percent of ψ_E
B_M = Bias of pooled estimate of ψ_E, matched sample, as percent of ψ_E V_M = Variance of the stratified estimate in the matched sample
V_R = Variance of the stratified estimate in the random sample V_{R*} = Variance of the pooled estimate in the random sample

ratios when the correlation between confounder and exposure is high. Since the "confounder" is not a risk factor for disease ($\psi_C = 1$), it need not be controlled in the analysis. By needlessly matching on it, the exposure distributions for cases and controls have been made more alike, thus reducing the efficiency of estimation of the exposure effect. The negative biases associated with the crude analysis of the matched data reflect the same phenomenon as the example in Table 6.2. This is a case of *overmatching*.

Stratification *is* needed to control confounding when both $\psi_{CE} > 1$ and $\psi_C > 1$. Then, as shown in rows 6–8, 10–12 and 14–16 of the table, the bias B_R using the unadjusted design and analysis is non-zero and becomes increasingly serious as the effect of the confounder and its correlation with the exposure increase. The efficiency of the matched design to the standard design, using in both cases the correct (stratified) analysis, may be read from columns labeled V_M/V_R. Values *under* 100% indicate greater efficiency, meaning a smaller variance, for the matched design. When the potential confounder increases disease risk but exposure does not, matching is always more efficient and its efficiency increases with the degree of confounding. Even in the most extreme situation ($\psi_{CE} = \psi_C = 10$), however, no more than 26% of efficiency is lost by failure to match. A conclusion is that confounder and disease must be strongly associated for matching to produce major gains. Matching may actually *lose* efficiency when ψ_{CE} and ψ_E are both large.

Overmatching 6.3.3

Overmatching refers to matching on a factor that is not a confounder of the disease-exposure association. There are three possibilities.

Factor Related Only to Exposure. This is the situation just considered in Tables 6.2 and 6.3 (rows 5, 9, 13). Matching is not needed to control confounding and leads to a loss of efficiency.

Factor Related Only to Disease. This has been called "the case of futility" because the matching is effectively at random with respect to exposure (Miettinen 1970). Frequency matching has no effect on efficiency, as the variance ratios $V_M/V_{R^*} = 100$ when $\psi_{CE} = 1$ suggest. Were one to "incorrectly" fail to account for the matching in the analysis, however, there would be efficiency loss relative to the frequency matched analysis; note the percentages below 100 in the column labeled V_M/V_R. Individual pair matching in such circumstances could cause a loss of efficiency because of the need to account for this in the analysis and the consequent reduction in degrees of freedom for estimation of the main effect. With binary exposure measurements, for example, only the discordant case-control pairs would contribute to estimation of the exposure odds ratio, and these would become fewer and fewer as the association between the matching factor and disease increased.

"Confounder" an Intermediate in the Causal Pathway. The most serious type of overmatching occurs when one matches on a factor that is both affected by exposure and a cause of disease. If the effect of anti-hypertensive medication on the risk of myocardial infarction was being investigated, for example, yet cases and controls were matched on blood pressure measurements taken after treatment commenced, the data would be completely useless for estimation of treatment effect. Ignoring the matching in the analysis would only compound the error by driving the odds ratio even closer towards unity.

6.3.4 When to Match

In view of the drawbacks of overmatching, and the often modest efficiency gains even when statistical adjustment is indicated, one may well ask whether matching is ever justified. The administrative costs of locating matched controls, and the loss of cases from analysis if none can be found, further argue for careful consideration of matched designs. Individual case-control matching is most appealing when needed to control the effects of a confounder that is not easily measured. The paradigm is use of an identical co-twin to control for genotype (Jablon et al. 1967). Otherwise, stratification of the control sample on gender and broad categories of age to achieve rough comparability with the case distribution, provided that this can be accomplished without great cost, is likely all that is advisable. Greater attention to stratification of the control sample may be needed when the primary goal is to evaluate statistical *interaction*, or effect modification, between exposure and a covariate (Smith and Day 1984).

6.4 Selection of Subjects

The two preceding sections outline the basic ideas of sampling of subjects for a case-control study from a theoretical statistical perspective. While the theory is an important guide to practice, implementation is usually imperfect and requires some compromise to minimize the various types of bias to which case-control studies are particularly susceptible (Sect. 6.5). In this section we consider some of the choices available to the investigator for putting the theory into action.

6.4.1 Selection of Cases

Disease Definition

Careful definition of the disease endpoint to conform to the goals of the study is critical to success. Specific cancers are reasonably well defined by primary site and histologic type. Studies of diabetes, rheumatoid arthritis or psychiatric conditions should follow standard criteria for diagnosis established by professional societies. In the typical study of disease etiology, the investigator may choose to enhance efficiency by including only those cases of disease most likely a priori to have been caused by the particular exposure. Thus, instead of "uterine cancer", studies of hormonal risk factors would best be restricted to adenocarcinoma of the endometrium whereas those investigating sexual practices or viral etiology would focus on squamous cell cancer of the cervix. Of course, in the early stages of an investigation, demonstration that the exposure effect is *specific* to a particular disease subtype can be an important part of the evidence that the association is causal (Hill 1965; Weiss 2002). For case-control studies of the public health impact of exposure, furthermore, a broader definition of disease may be desirable.

As mentioned in Sect. 6.1.2, studies of disease etiology are best restricted to incident cases. This may not always be possible, however. Congenital anomalies are generally ascertained as those that are prevalent at birth, and consideration of possible exposure effects on fetal loss forms an important part of the interpretation. Cohort studies may be preferable for estimating the true effects of exposure on reproductive outcomes (Weinberg and Wilcox 1998).

Sources of Cases

Population Registries.   Population based disease registries, particularly of cancer and birth defects, are often considered the ideal source of cases. This is because the population at risk, whose identification is needed for control selection, is well defined by geographic or administrative boundaries. Practical limitations on their use include the speed with which cases can be identified and interviewed, to avoid selection bias from exclusion of those who may have died, and the feasibility of random sampling of controls.

Health Maintenance Organizations.   Large health maintenance organizations (HMOs) are advantageous as a source of cases, for several reasons. The source population is enumerated and demographic data, as well as some exposure and covariate data, may already be available for everyone. This permits judicious selection of cases and controls using nested case-control, case-cohort or stratified two-phase sampling designs (Sect. 6.6). Relatively objective and inexpensive exposure assessments may be possible using routine medical or pharmacy records, some of which may already exist in electronic form. Similarly, cases are usually easily ascertained from reports of diagnoses within the organization. Of course, some assurance is needed that members of the HMO are unlikely to go elsewhere for diagnosis and treatment.

Hospitals and Clinics.   Historically, many case-control studies have been conducted using either a single or a small group of hospitals or clinics. This facilitates timely access to cases and increases the likelihood of their cooperation, thus limiting selection bias. On the other hand, definition of the source population from which the cases arose may be problematic, not to mention the practicality of obtaining random samples of controls from it.

Exclusion Criteria

In principle, any exclusion criteria may be used for cases so long as they are equally applied to the controls, and vice-versa, since they serve simply to restrict the source population. Thus subjects may be excluded who reside in areas difficult to reach or who are not native speakers of the language of interview. Practical applications of this rule can be more subtle, however. Wacholder (1995) argues, for example, that exclusion of cancer cases who lacked a histologic diagnosis could inadvertently tend to exclude those from smaller, rural hospitals who were more likely to have exposures related to agriculture.

Exposure Opportunity.   Case-control studies are most informative when there is a substantial degree of exposure variability, so that the exposure is neither rare nor ubiquitous (Chase and Klauber 1965). Subjects known a priori to have no opportunity for exposure could be excluded on grounds of efficiency if the exposure was rare, since they would contribute little additional information. Thus, for example, women who were past reproductive age when oral contraceptives became popular should be excluded from a study of OC use and breast cancer (Wacholder et al. 1992a). On the other hand, since they provide valid information on the non-exposed, there is no logical basis for insisting that subjects without the opportunity for exposure should be routinely excluded from cohort and case-control studies (Schlesselman and Stadel 1987; Poole 1987).

6.4.2   Selection of Controls

Principles of Control Selection

Wacholder et al. (1992a) described three basic principles of control selection. The first two correspond roughly to considerations already developed regarding conceptual foundations and the use of matching. The third stems from the desire to minimize the effects of measurement error to which case-control studies are particularly susceptible.

The "study-base" Principle.   This is the principle that controls be randomly se-lected from disease-free members of the underlying cohort, also known as the source population (Kelsey et al. 1996) or study-base (Miettinen 1985), at the times that cases are being ascertained (Sect. 6.2). When controls are in fact selected later, it sometimes mandates the random selection of a reference date for each control so that the distributions of the case diagnosis dates and control reference dates are comparable. Only exposures occurring prior to the reference/diagnosis date would be taken into account. This principle also implies that whatever exclusion criteria have been applied to the cases must also be applied equally to the controls.

The Deconfounding Principle.   This principle underlies the stratified sampling of controls to render possible, or improve the efficiency of, an adjusted analysis designed to control confounding (Sect. 6.3).

The Comparable Accuracy Principle.   This principle, controversial even in the authors' view, suggests that controls be selected so that the errors of measurement of their exposures and covariates are comparable to the measurement errors of the cases. The suggestion that dead controls be selected for dead cases, for example, is sometimes made on the basis of the comparable accuracy principle (Gordis 1982). Unfortunately, there is no guarantee that adherence to the principle will eliminate or even reduce bias (Greenland and Robins 1985). Unless the measurement error can be completely controlled, for example by obtaining error free measurements for a *validation* subsample of cases and controls and appropriately incorporating these data in the analysis, it can seriously compromise study validity even if case and control data are equally error prone (Sect. 6.5.3).

Sources of Controls

The appropriate source population for sampling of controls is determined by the study-base principal. When cases arise from an enumerated source population such as an HMO, controls may be sampled from this cohort using a nested case-control or case-cohort design (Figs. 6.1 and 6.2). One principal advantage of conducting epidemiologic studies in the Nordic countries is their maintenance of national disease and population registers which may be exploited for case and control selection, respectively (see Chap. I.4 of this handbook). Standard survey sampling methods are often used to select controls for "population based" studies in countries that do not maintain population registers. The most difficult and controversial problems of control selection arise with hospital based studies.

Survey Sampling. Methods for scientific sampling of populations have been developed by census bureaus and other government agencies throughout the world. The particular method most advantageous for any given epidemiologic study will likely depend on the local administrative infrastructure. Survey sampling often proceeds in stages, where one first samples a large administrative unit, then a smaller one and finally arrives at an individual household or subject. Such multi-stage "cluster" sampling introduces modest correlations in the responses of individuals sampled from the same primary sampling unit, more marked ones for individuals sampled from the same lower level cluster. Although often ignored by epidemiologists, usually at the cost of some underestimation of the variability in estimated relative risks, these correlations should be accounted for in a rigorous statistical analysis (Graubard et al. 1989). Fortunately, simple methods to accomodate cluster sampling are now routinely incorporated in the standard statistical packages.

Random Digit Dialing. In view of the high costs of census bureau techniques in the United States, methods of survey sampling through the telephone exchanges have been developed (Waksberg 1978; Harlow and Davis 1988). Random digit dialing (RDD) has become increasingly popular for control selection in populations that have high rates of telephone access. Some implementations start with the telephone exchange of each case for sampling of controls that are thereby matched on somewhat ill-defined neighborhood factors (Robison and Daigle 1984). RDD methods may be costly for ascertainment of controls from minority populations, requiring dozens of calls to locate a suitable household (Wacholder et al. 1992b). They are particularly susceptible to bias because of higher selection probabilities for households that have more than one phone line or more than one eligible control and because of high rates of nonresponse (Sect. 6.5.1). The latter problem is likely to become increasingly serious in view of the persistent use of answering machines to screen out unwanted calls. The popularity of cell phones, moreover, eventually may make it infeasible to use RDD to draw a random control sample from a source population defined by geographic or administrative boundaries.

Neighborhood and Friend Controls. Matched controls may also be selected from neighbors or friends of each case. For the former method, a census is taken of all households in the immediate geographic area of the case and these are approached in a random order until a suitable control is found. Care must be taken to ensure that the control was resident at the same time the case was diagnosed. Even with these precautions, neighborhood sampling may yield biased controls for hospital based studies since it will not be guaranteed that the control would have been ascertained as a case if ill, thus violating the study-base principle (Wacholder et al. 1992b). Neighborhood controls are also susceptible to overmatching due to their similarity to the cases on factors associated with exposure that are not risk factors for disease (Sect. 6.3.3). These same difficulties confront the use of friend controls, whereby a random selection is taken from among a census of friends provided by each case. There may be further selection on factors related to popularity since the friend selected as control may well not have listed the case as a friend had the friend become ill (Robins and Pike 1990). The primary advantage of friend controls would be a low level of nonresponse.

Hospital Based Controls. Many studies that ascertain cases through hospitals also select controls from these same hospitals, which is of obvious logistical convenience. Such controls are likely to have the same high response levels as the cases. The fact that they may be interviewed in a hospital setting, as the cases are, is an advantage from the perspective of the comparable accuracy principle (Mantel and Haenszel 1959). The major difficulties stem from the fact that the hypothetical study-base, the *catchment* of persons who would report to the particular hospital if they developed the disease under study, may be different from the catchment population for other diseases. Furthermore, many of the disease categories from which controls could be selected may themselves be associated with the exposure. A large part of the planning of hospital based case-control studies is devoted to the choice of disease categories thought to be independent of exposure and to have a similar catchment. The hope is that controls with such diseases will effectively constitute a random sample, vis-à-vis exposure, from the study-base. Since the independence of exposure and disease diagnosis is rarely known with great certainty, a standard recommendation is to select controls having a variety of diagnoses so that the failure of any one of them to meet the criterion does not compromise the study (Wacholder et al. 1992b; Rothman and Greenland 1998, p. 101). If it is found later that a certain diagnosis is associated with exposure, those controls can be excluded.

How Many Controls per Case?
How Many Control Groups?

Case-Control Ratios. For a fixed number of study subjects, statistical power for testing the null hypothesis is optimized by having equal numbers of cases and controls. When the disease is extremely rare or acquisition of cases particularly expensive, however, it may be important and cost-effective to increase the numbers of controls. In order to have the same statistical power (to reject the null hypothesis of no exposure effect against local alternatives) as a design with equal numbers of cases and controls, a design with M controls per case would need only $(M + 1)/2M$ as many cases. When $M = 2$, for example, this would imply the use of 3/4 as many cases, but twice as many controls, to achieve the same power as a design with equal numbers. For a fixed number of cases, the relative efficiency of a design with M controls per case relative to one that uses an unlimited number of controls is therefore only $M/(M + 1)$. Since 80% of maximum efficiency can thus be obtained with $M = 4$, it is often inadvisable to seek a higher ratio. Exceptions occur when sampling and data collection for controls is substantially cheaper than for cases or if accurate estimation of large rate ratios, rather than a test of the null hypothesis, is the primary statistical objective (Breslow 1982; Breslow et al. 1983).

Multiple Control Groups. Early case-control investigations, including the classic study of Doll and Hill (1952), often utilized two or more control groups. Indeed, multiple control groups were recommended by Dorn (1959) to improve the case-control study so that it would "provide a more valid basis for generalization". As explained by Hill (1971, pp 47–48) "If a whole series of control groups, e.g., of patients with different diseases, gives much the same answer and only the one affected group differs, the evidence is clearly much stronger than if the affected group differs from merely one other group." Similar informal arguments have been put forward in favor of multiple control groups as a means of addressing the possible biases that may be associated with the use of any one of them (Ibrahim and Spitzer 1979). Working from a more formal perspective, Rosenbaum (1987) concluded that a second or third control group was useful *only* if supplemental information was available on whether such use addressed a specific bias. If controls sampled from separate sources have different exposure histories, even after statistical adjustment for potential confounders, this indeed suggests that similar adjustment of the case-control comparison may be inadequate to control confounding. However, failure to detect a difference among control groups may give a false sense of security unless they were deliberately selected to differ with respect to unmeasured potential confounders. Implementation of this last criterion would clearly require some guess as to what those unmeasured confounders might be.

Recent reviews of case-control methods have tended to shy away from the use of multiple control groups (Rothman and Greenland 1998, p. 106; Wacholder et al. 1992b). They argue that there is usually a single "best" control group, and that since the discovery of an adjusted exposure difference with other control groups will force these to be discarded, the effort involved will have been wasted. However, there may not be a "best" control group, or its identification may be controversial. Discovery of a difference between control groups should generally encourage the investigator to seriously suspect that confounding may have compromised study results.

6.5   Pitfalls

Case-control studies are susceptible to the same biases and problems of interpretation that afflict all observational epidemiological studies. These include confounding, selection or sampling bias, measurement error and missing data. Selection bias can be considered an extreme version of bias due to missing data where the entire observational record is missing for subjects who are in the source population but fail to be included in the study. Each of these topics is considered in detail in other chapters of this handbook. Many methods described there for dealing with such issues apply to case-control studies as well as to cohort studies. Attention is confined here to a few of the potential problems to which case-control studies are particularly susceptible.

6.5.1   Selection Bias

As elaborated at length in Sect. 6.2.1, the cases and controls in a case-control study are best viewed as resulting from outcome dependent sampling from an underlying, often idealized cohort study. The goal is to estimate the degreee of association of disease risk with exposure that would have been found had complete records been available for the entire cohort. The sampling of controls and sometimes even of cases may be stratified, for example by sex and broad categories of age, but otherwise is supposed to be random within the subpopulations of diseased and non-diseased subjects. Selection bias arises when the sampling is in fact not random. It poses a major threat to the validity of case-control studies.

The effect of sampling bias is easy to demonstrate quantitatively for an exposure variable with two levels. For simplicity, we consider the effect on the odds ratio associating exposure with the cumulative risk of disease during a defined study period. The first 2×2 subtable displayed in Table 6.4 contains the population frequencies of subjects who are exposed and become diseased during the study period (P_{11}), who are not exposed and become diseased (P_{01}) and likewise the frequences of being exposed or non-exposed and remaining disease-free (P_{10} and P_{00}, respectively). The target parameter of interest is the odds ratio ψ based on these population frequencies. As shown in the next two subtables, the odds ratio ψ^*

Table 6.4. Effect of selection bias on odds ratio measures of association

	Population frequencies		Sampling fractions		Expected sample frequencies	
	Case	Cont	Case	Cont	Case	Control
Exposed	P_{11}	P_{10}	f_{11}	f_{10}	$f_{11} \times P_{11}$	$f_{10} \times P_{10}$
Non-exposed	P_{01}	P_{00}	f_{01}	f_{00}	$f_{01} \times P_{01}$	$f_{00} \times P_{00}$
Odds ratios	$\psi = \frac{P_{11} \times P_{00}}{P_{10} \times P_{01}}$		$\psi_f = \frac{f_{11} \times f_{00}}{f_{10} \times f_{01}}$		$\psi^* = \psi_f \times \psi$	

expected from the case-control sample equals the product of the true odds ratio, ψ, times the cross products ratio of the sampling frequencies, denoted ψ_f. Hence $\psi = \psi^*$, i.e., there is no bias, provided that $\psi_f = 1$. This will occur when the sampling fractions for cases and controls are all the same, depend *only* on the disease outcome, i.e., $f_{10} = f_{00}$ and $f_{11} = f_{01}$, or depend only on exposure, i.e., $f_{01} = f_{00}$ and $f_{11} = f_{10}$. Often the sampling fractions for cases are both near 1 whereas those for the controls are much smaller. The fact that this does not matter, provided that the sampling fractions for exposed cases and non-exposed cases are the same and similarly for controls, is another way of understanding why case-control studies provide estimates of the relative risk (disease odds ratio). Bias does occur when the sampling fractions depend *jointly* on exposure and disease, usually because exposed controls are more or less likely to be sampled than non-exposed controls. In a study that ascertained all the cases, but sampled exposed persons as controls with twice the frequency as non-exposed persons, the estimated relative risk (odds ratio) would be twice the correct value. This is known as Berkson bias (Berkson 1946).

Some of the factors that contribute to selection bias are as follows.

Patient Dies Before Interview. When cases are ascertained through a population based disease registry, a significant interval of time may elapse between initial diagnosis and notification to the registry. Some patients whose disease course is rapidly fatal may therefore not be interviewed in person, but are either excluded from the study or represented by a proxy interview subject to increased measurement error. This selection factor may affect both cases *and* controls in hospital based studies. It constitutes a major problem in reproductive epidemiology (see Chap. III.5 of this handbook).

Physician Refuses Consent. Committees charged with protection of human research subjects may require that permission for participation be given by the patient's physician. This could affect control participation in hospital based studies or case participation in general.

Subject Refuses Participation. The most common reason for selection bias in case-control studies is refusal of the subject to participate, either actively by refusing to sign a consent form or passively by failure to return a questionnaire or turn up at the appointed hour for a laboratory examination. Cases with disease are often highly motivated to participate, whereas controls selected from the population are not. Unfortunately, control participation rates often depend on some correlate of exposure. Refusal rates for telephone surveys, for example, are higher for people who are older, have fewer social relationships, are less well educated and have lower income (O'Neil 1979).

Subjects Ascertained Through Their Household.   Selection bias can occur when controls are ascertained by first contacting households to determine whether a control lives there who is suitable for matching to the case, and only a single control is selected from each household. In studies of childhood disease, where controls are matched on age within two years of the case, a child with a sibling in the same age range is less likely to be selected than one who has no such siblings (Greenberg 1990).

Random Digit Dialing.   Some other problems of selection bias are associated with the use of RDD for control ascertainment besides the fact that this method identifies households rather than individuals. Households without telephones stand no chance of selection, for example, whereas those with multiple telephones will be over-represented. The absence of a telephone may particularly affect minority populations.

Adjustments for Selection Bias
6.5.2   ## in Study Design and Analysis

The most important consideration regarding selection bias is to avoid it so far as possible. At the design phase of the study, the exclusion criteria for both cases and controls may be chosen to maximize the probability of their ascertainment and participation. If RDD is used for control selection, this means taking the obvious step of excluding cases from households that lack telephones. Demographic, geographic and linguistic factors may enter into the exclusion criteria for the same reason.

If selection bias cannot be avoided, as much data as possible should be gathered on *potential* case and control subjects to allow *prediction* of which of them go on to participate and which refuse. When sampling from the general population, it may be possible to use a recent survey of the same population for this purpose, provided of course that the survey itself had nearly complete response. If cases and controls are drawn from an enumerated population such as an HMO, data may already exist in medical or other records that can be used for this purpose.

At the time of analysis, one may attempt to adjust for selection bias in the same way that one adjusts for missing data. This is to use sampling weights for each participating subject, i.e., those with "complete data", equal to the inverse predicted probability that the subject would have been selected given the data collected for this purpose at the design stage. This is only useful, of course, if there is substantial variability in the predicted probabilities. Alternatively, or additionally, one may statistically adjust the analysis for factors that are thought to be associated with selection but for which data are only available for participating subjects. Such adjustment would consist of stratification of the analysis on factor levels, or inclusion of the factor in a regression model for disease given exposure, just as one adjusts for confounders (Breslow and Day 1980, Sect. 3.8). However, if there is a substantial degree of nonresponse, it is quite unlikely that any adjustment will mitigate the serious biases that can result. There is simply no way to deal with it if selection fractions within factor levels used for adjustment purposes depend jointly on disease and exposure.

Measurement Error

A second major limitation of case-control studies is their susceptibility to measurement error. Cases and controls are often ascertained long after the relevant exposures have occurred. In spite of Dorn's (1959) admonition to use *objective* measures of exposure, most case-control studies of environmental risk factors continue today to measure exposure by interview or questionnaire. The potential for misclassification of exposure levels in such research is enormous. First, subjects may have only a vague memory of past exposures. Second, those who are diseased at the time of interview may recall these past events in a different way than those who are healthy controls. This may be in part because the early stages of their disease led to changes in behavior that made recollection of past practices more difficult. Interviewers may solicit and record answers differently if they have knowledge of the diagnosis or of the patient's status as case or control.

Austin et al. (1994) reviewed published reports of nine case-control studies of diet and cancer in which an attempt had been made to assess the accuracy of recall of dietary histories separately for cases and controls. According to their authors, three studies provided "weak" and four "moderate" evidence for recall bias. However, these results themselves were likely subject to measurement error and may have been understated in consequence.

Measurement error, whether or not it is differential between cases and controls, can compromise conclusions by seriously biasing the relative risk estimates from case-control studies that use dietary self reports or similarly error-prone measurements. Prentice (1996) developed a mathematical model for measurement error that allowed for correlation of the error with the true exposure level and for systematic underreporting of exposure for persons with high exposure levels. He fitted the model to replicate measures of dietary fat intake, some taken using a four day food record and others using a food-frequency questionnaire, for control subjects enrolled in the Women's Health Trial (Henderson et al. 1990). Employing results from international geographic correlation studies to generate the "true model", in which subjects at the 90th percentile of the distribution of dietary fat intake had 3 or 4 times the risk of disease as those at the 10th percentile, he showed that measurement error could plausibly reduce the relative risks to 1.1. The obvious conclusion from these calculations was that "dietary self-report instruments may be inadequate for analytic epidemiologic studies of dietary fat and disease risk because of measurement error biases" (Prentice 1996).

A substantial and concerted effort has been made by statisticians to develop methods of data analysis that correct for the bias in relative risk estimates caused by measurement error (see Chap. II.5 of this handbook and the text by Carroll et al. 1995). Some require the availability of "gold standard", i.e., error-free, measurements on a fairly large number of subjects in the validation subsample. Others assume that statistically independent true replicate measurements are available. Unfortunately, data collected in case-control studies rarely meet these stringent requirements, at least not in their entirety. It therefore behooves us to recall Bradford Hill's (1953, p. 995) sage advice:

> One must go and seek more facts, paying less attention to techniques of handling the data and far more to the development and perfection of the methods of obtaining them.

6.6   Conclusions

The case-control study played a major, successful role during the second half of the twentieth century in identifying risk factors for chronic disease. It has also proven helpful for evaluation of the efficacy of vaccination (Comstock 1994) and screening (Weiss 1994) programs. The twenty-first century will witness its continued use as a cost-effective study design, with increasing application in genetic epidemiology (Khoury and Beaty 1994) and particularly in the study of gene-environment interactions (Andrieu and Goldstein 1998). Statisticians and epidemiologists will continue to develop more efficient study designs and methods of data analysis that take full advantage of all available data. When a case-control study is conducted in an HMO, for example, some data will likely be available on either the exposure or the control variables for all subjects in the underlying cohort. *Two-phase* sampling designs, whereby *biased* samples of cases and controls are selected using the data available for all subjects, then offer the potential for much greater efficiency than the standard case-control design (White 1982; Breslow and Cain 1988; Langholz and Borgan 1995; Breslow and Chatterjee 1999). Chapter I.7 of this handbook discusses these and other evolving study designs and analyses.

The advantages of case-control methodology in terms of speed and cost may have also contributed, ironically, to a diminished stature for epidemiology and biostatistics in the eyes both of the scientific community and of the general public (Breslow 2003). Part of the problem is an inherent aversion to the "black box" approach of risk factor epidemiology that associates cause and effect without the need for any understanding of pathogenetic mechanisms. Epidemiologic findings are most convincing when supported by relevant laboratory research. Another part of the problem is the saturation of the news media with conflicting reports based on case-control and other studies that are too small, poorly designed, improperly analyzed or overly interpreted. Taubes (1995) began his controversial and influential article on the limitations of epidemiology with the observation: "The news about health risks comes thick and fast these days, and it seems almost constitutionally contradictory." The epidemiologists he interviewed for this article cited the ability of confounding, selection bias and measurement error to overwhelm smaller exposure effects. One even suggested that no single study, no matter how well conducted, should be viewed as "persuasive" unless the lower limit of the 95% confidence interval for the rate ratio exceeded 3 or 4. Very few published studies, even when reported by the press as "suggestive" of an association, meet this stringent criterion.

Medical science and public health would be well served by fewer, larger case-control studies designed to test specific hypotheses that are carefully articulated in advance. Studies that can barely "detect" a relative risk of 2 may not provide convincing evidence of a dose-response gradient and are unlikely to enable one to determine whether an elevated relative risk in a particular disease subgroup, even one specified in advance, is evidence for the *specificity* of association that can be useful in causal interpretation (Weiss 2002). (There are of course exceptions, as when a unique exposure contributes to an outbreak of an extremely rare disease. Recall the DES-adenocarcinoma of the vagina story mentioned in the Introduction.) Investigators are also well advised to develop a strict protocol for selection of cases and controls and for collection and *analysis* of the data. Doll and Hill (1952) utilized such a protocol. They also had the advantage of working during the punch card era that discouraged "data dredging" and the inclusion of all but the most important variables in the analysis. A reasonable strategy might be to perform a maximum of three carefully planned analyses of the association between the primary exposure and disease: one without adjustment; one adjusted for a short list of confounders known a priori to be associated with disease; and the third adjusted for a specified list of known and suspected confounders. In case of conflict, the major interpretation would be based on the second analysis though the results of all three would be reported. Flexibility would be needed in application, of course, especially to accommodate changes in the study protocol after the study had commenced. Finally, investigators would be well advised to exercise greater caution in advertising their findings to the press before confirmation was forthcoming from other sources. By following basic principles of good statistical and scientific practice, the case-control study can gain credibility within the research community and enhance its standing as a basis for public health action.

Acknowledgements. I am indebted to Sander Greenland, Noel Weiss, the Editors and an anonymous referee for helpful comments on an earlier draft. This work was supported in part by grant R01-CA40644 from the US Public Health Service.

References

Aird L, Bentall HH, Roberts JAF (1953) A relationship between cancer of stomach and the ABO blood groups. British Medical Journal 1:799–801

Andrieu N, Goldstein AM (1998) Epidemiologic and genetic approaches in the study of gene-environment interaction: An overview of available methods. Epidemiologic Reviews 20:137–147

Armenian HK, Lilienfeld DE (1994) Overview and historical perspective. Epidemiologic Reviews 16:1–5

Armstrong RW, Armstrong MJ, Yu MC, Henderson BE (1983) Salted fish and inhalants as risk-factors for nasopharyngeal carcinoma in Malaysian Chinese. Cancer Research 43:2967–2970

Austin H, Hill HA, Flanders WD, Greenberg RS (1994) Limitations in the application of case-control methodology. Epidemiologic Reviews 16:65–76

Barlow WE (1994) Robust variance estimation for the case-cohort design. Biometrics 50:1064–1072

Benichou J, Gail MH (1995) Methods of inference for estimates of absolute risk derived from population-based case-control studies. Biometrics 51:182–194

Berkson J (1946) Limitations of the application of fourfold table analysis to hospital data. Biometrics Bulletin 2:47–53

Breslow N (1982) Design and analysis of case-control studies. Annual Review of Public Health 3:29–54

Breslow NE (1996) Statistics in epidemiology: The case-control study. Journal of the American Statistical Association 91:14–28

Breslow NE (2003) Are statistical contributions to medicine undervalued? Biometrics 59:1–8

Breslow NE, Cain KC (1988) Logistic regression for two-stage case-control data. Biometrika 75:11–20

Breslow NE, Chatterjee N (1999) Design and analysis of two-phase studies with binary outcomes applied to Wilms tumor prognosis. Applied Statistics 48:457–468

Breslow NE, Day NE (1980) Statistical methods in cancer research I: The analysis of case-control studies. International Agency for Research on Cancer, Lyon

Breslow NE, Lubin JH, Marek P, Langholz B (1983) Multiplicative models and cohort analysis. Journal of the American Statistical Association 78:1–12

Broders AC (1920) Squamous-cell epithelioma of the lip. A study of five hundred and thirty-seven cases. Journal of the American Medical Association 74:656–664

Carroll RJ, Ruppert D, Stefanski LA (1995) Measurement error in nonlinear models. Chapman and Hall, London

Chase G, Klauber MR (1965) A graph of sample sizes for retrospective studies. American Journal of Public Health 55:1993–1996

Cole P (1979) The evolving case-control study. Journal of Chronic Disease 32:15–27

Comstock GW (1994) Evaluating vaccination effectiveness and vaccine efficacy by means of case-control studies. Epidemiologic Reviews 16:77–89

Cornfield J (1951) A method of estimating comparative rates from clinical data. Applications to cancer of the lung, breast, and cervix. Journal of the National Cancer Institute 11:1269–1275

Correa A, Stewart WF, Yeh HC, Santos-Burgoa C (1994) Exposure measurement in case-control studies: Reported methods and recommendations. Epidemiologic Reviews 16:18–32

Cox DR (1972) Regression models and life-tables (with discussion). Journal of the Royal Statistical Society (Series B) 34:187–220

Daling JR, Weiss NS, Metch BJ, Chow WH, Soderstrom RM, Stadel BV (1985) Primary tubal infertility in relation to the use of an intrauterine-device. New England Journal of Medicine 312:937–941

Doll R, Hill AB (1950) Smoking and carcinoma of the lung. Preliminary report. British Medical Journal 2:739–748

Doll R, Hill AB (1952) A study of the aetiology of carcinoma of the lung. British Medical Journal 2:1271–1286

Dorn HF (1959) Some problems arising in prospective and retrospective studies of the etiology of disease. New England Journal of Medicine 261:571–579

Fleming PJ, Gilbert R, Azaz Y, Berry PJ, Rudd PT, Stewart A, Hall E (1990) Interaction between bedding and sleeping position in the sudden-infant-death-syndrome – a population based case-control study. British Medical Journal 301:85–89

Gordis L (1982) Should dead cases be matched to dead controls? American Journal of Epidemiology 115:1–5

Graubard BI, Fears TR, Gail MH (1989) Effects of cluster sampling on epidemiologic analysis in population-based case-control studies (Corr: V47 p. 779–780). Biometrics 45:1053–1071

Greenberg ER (1990) Random digit dialing for control selection – A review and a caution on its use in studies of childhood-cancer. American Journal of Epidemiology 131:1–5

Greenland S (1987) Estimation of exposure-specific rates from sparse case-control data. Journal of Chronic Disease 40:1087–1094

Greenland S, Robins JM (1985) Confounding and misclassification. American Journal of Epidemiology 122:495–506

Greenland S, Thomas DC (1982) On the need for the rare disease assumption in case-control studies. American Journal of Epidemiology 116:547–553

Harlow BL, Davis S (1988) Two one-step methods for household screening and interviewing using random digit dialing. American Journal of Epidemiology 127:857–863

Henderson MM, Kushi LH, Thompson DJ, Gorbach SL, Clifford CK, Thompson RS (1990) Feasibility of a randomized trial of a low-fat diet for the prevention of breast-cancer – Dietary compliance in the womens health trial vanguard study. Preventive Medicine 19:115–133

Herbst AL, Ulfelder H, Poskanzer DC (1971) Adenocarcinoma of the vagina. New England Journal of Medicine 284:878–881

Hill AB (1953) Observation and experiment. New England Journal of Medicine 248:995–1001

Hill AB (1965) The environment and disease: association or causation? Proceedings of the Royal Statistical Society of Medicine 58:295–300

Hill AB (1971) Principles of medical statistics. Oxford University Press, New York

Horvitz DG, Thompson DJ (1952) A generalization of sampling without replacement from a finite universe. Journal of the American Statistical Association 47:663–685

Hsieh DA, Manski CF, McFadden D (1985) Estimation of response probabilities from augmented retrospective observations. Journal of the American Statistical Association 80:651–662

Ibrahim MA, Spitzer WO (1979) The case-control study: The problem and the prospect. Journal of Chronic Disease 32:139–144

Jablon S, Neel JV, Gershowitz H, Atkinson GF (1967) The NAS-NRC twin panel: Methods of construction of the panel, zygosity diagnosis, and proposed use. American Journal of Human Genetics 19:133–161

Kelsey JL, Whittemore AS, Evans AS, Thompson WD (1996) Methods in observational epidemiology, 2nd edn. Oxford University Press, New York

Khoury MJ, Beaty TH (1994) Applications of the case-control method in genetic epidemiology. Epidemiologic Reviews 16:134–150

Kupper LL, McMichael AJ, Spirtas R (1975) A hybrid epidemiologic study design useful in estimating relative risk. Journal of the American Statistical Association 70:524–528

Lane-Claypon JE (1926) A further report on cancer of the breast. Her Majesty's Stationery Office, London

Langholz B, Borgan O (1995) Counter-matching: A stratified nested case-control sampling method. Biometrika 82:69–79

Langholz B, Borgan O (1997) Estimation of absolute risk from nested case-control data. Biometrics 53:767–774

Langholz B, Goldstein L (1996) Risk set sampling in epidemiologic cohort studies. Statistical Science 11:35–53

Levin ML, Goldstein H, Gerhardt PR (1950) Cancer and tobacco smoking. A preliminary report. Journal of the American Medical Association 143:336–338

Liddell FDK, McDonald JC, Thomas DC (1977) Methods of cohort analysis: Appraisal by application to asbestos mining. Journal of the Royal Statistical Society (Series A) 140:469–491

Lilienfeld AM, Lilienfeld DE (1979) A century of case-control studies: Progress? Journal of Chronic Disease 32:5–13

Lin DY, Ying Z (1993) Cox regression with incomplete covariate measurements. Journal of the American Statistical Association 88:1341–1349

Little RJA, Rubin DB (2002) Statistical analysis with missing data, 2nd edn. Wiley, New York

Lombard HL, Doering CR (1928) Cancer studies in Massachusetts. 2. Habits, characteristics and environment of individuals with and without cancer. New England Journal of Medicine 198:481–487

MacMahon B, Cole P, Lin TM, Lowe CR, Mirra AP, Ravnihar B, Salber EJ, Valaoras VG, Yuasa S (1970) Age at first birth and breast cancer risk. Bulletin of the World Health Organization 43:209–221

Mantel N, Haenszel W (1959) Statistical aspects of the analysis of data from retrospective studies of disease. Journal of the National Cancer Institute 22:719–748

Miettinen O (1982) Design options in epidemiologic research: An update. Scandinavian Journal of Work Environment and Health 8:7–14

Miettinen OS (1970) Matching and design efficiency in retrospective studies. American Journal of Epidemiology 91:111–118

Miettinen O (1976) Estimability and estimation in case-referent studies. American Journal of Epidemiology 103:226–235

Miettinen OS (1985) Theoretical epidemiology: Principles of occurrence research in medicine. Wiley, New York

Neutra RR, Drolette ME (1978) Estimating exposure-specific disease rates from case-control studies using Bayes theorem. American Journal of Epidemiology 108:214–222

Neyman J (1955) Statistics – servant of all sciences. Science 122:401–406

O'Neil MJ (1979) Estimating the nonresponse bias due to refusals in telephone surveys. Public Opinion Quarterly 43:218–232

Poole C (1987) Critical appraisal of the exposure-potential restriction rule. American Journal of Epidemiology 125:179–183

Prentice RL (1986) A case-cohort design for epidemiologic cohort studies and disease prevention trials. Biometrika 73:1–11

Prentice RL (1996) Measurement error and results from analytic epidemiology: dietary fat and breast cancer. Journal of the National Cancer Institute 88:1738–1747

Prince AM, Szmuness W, Michon J, Demaille J, Diebolt G, Linhard J, Quenum C, Sankale M (1975) A case-control study of the association between primary liver cancer and hepatitis B infection in Senegal. International Journal of Cancer 16:376–383

Robins J, Pike M (1990) The validity of case-control studies with nonrandom selection of controls. Epidemiology 1:273–284

Robins JM, Gail MH, Lubin JH (1986) More on 'biased selection of controls for case-control analyses of cohort studies'. Biometrics 42:293–29

Robison LL, Daigle A (1984) Control selection using random digit dialing for cases of childhood cancer. American Journal of Epidemiology 120:164–165

Rodrigues L, Kirkwood BR (1990) Case-control designs in the study of common diseases: Updates on the demise of the rare disease assumption and the choice of sampling scheme for controls. International Journal of Epidemiology 19:205–213

Rosenbaum PR (1987) The role of a second control group in an observational study (with discussion). Statistical Science 2:292–316

Rothman KJ (1986) Modern epidemiology. Little, Brown, Boston

Rothman KJ, Greenland S (1998) Modern epidemiology, 2nd edn. Lippincott-Raven, Philadelphia

Schlesselman JJ (1982) Case-control studies. Oxford University Press, New York

Schlesselman JJ, Stadel BV (1987) Exposure opportunity in epidemiologic studies. American Journal of Epidemiology 125:174–178

Sheehe PR (1962) Dynamic risk analysis in retrospective matched pair studies of disease. Biometrics 18:323–341

Smith DC, Prentice R, Thompson DJ, Herrmann W (1975) Association of exogenous estrogen and endometrial carcinoma. New England Journal of Medicine 293:1164–1167

Smith PG, Day NE (1984) The design of case-control studies: The influence of confounding and interaction effects. International Journal of Epidemiology 13:356–365

Smith PG, Rodrigues LC, Fine PEM (1984) Assessment of the protective efficacy of vaccines against common diseases using case-control and cohort studies. International Journal of Epidemiology 13:87–93

Taubes G (1995) Epidemiology faces its limits. Science 269:164–169

Thomas DC, Greenland S (1983) The relative efficiencies of matched and independent sample designs for case-control studies. Journal of Chronic Disease 36:685–697

Tuyns AJ, Péquignot G, Jensen OM (1977) Le cancer de l'oesophage en Ille-et-Vilaine en fonction des niveaux de consommation d'alcool et de tabac. Bulletin du Cancer 64:45–60

Wacholder S (1995) Design issues in case-control studies. Statistical Methods in Medical Research 4:293–309

Wacholder S, McLaughlin JK, Silverman DT, Mandel JS (1992) Selection of controls in case-control studies I. Principles. American Journal of Epidemiology 135:1019–1028

Wacholder S, Silverman DT, McLaughlin JK, Mandel JS (1992) Selection of controls in case-control studies II. Types of controls. American Journal of Epidemiology 135:1029–1041

Waksberg J (1978) Sampling methods for random digit dialing. Journal of the American Statistical Association 73:40–46

Weinberg CR, Wilcox AJ (1998) Reproductive epidemiology. In: Rothman KJ, Greenland S (eds) Modern epidemiology, 2nd edn., Chap. 29, pp 585–608. Lippincott-Raven, Philadeplphia

Weiss NS (1994) Application of the case-control method in the evaluation of screening. Epidemiologic Reviews 16:102–108

Weiss NS (2002) Can the 'specificity' of an association be rehabilitated as a basis for supporting a causal hypothesis? Epidemiology 13:6–8

White JE (1982) A two stage design for the study of the relationship between a rare exposure and a rare disease. American Journal of Epidemiology 115:119–128

Wynder EL, Graham EA (1950) Tobacco smoking as a possible etiologic factor in bronchogenic carcinoma. A study of six hundred and eighty-four proved cases. Journal of the American Medical Association 143:329–336

Yu MC, Ho JHC, Lai SH, Henderson BE (1986) Cantonese-style salted fish as a cause of nasopharyngeal carcinoma - Report of a case-control study in Hong-Kong. Cancer Research 46:956–961

Ziel HK, Finkle WD (1975) Increased risk of endometrial carcinoma among users of conjugated estrogens. New England Journal of Medicine 293:1167–1170

Modern Epidemiologic Study Designs

Philip H. Kass, Ellen B. Gold

Introduction

A fundamental challenge pervasive to all experimental and nonexperimental (observational) research is valid inference of causal effects. Although actions (through undefined mechanisms, but conventionally denoted by treatment, exposure, etc.) and reactions (e.g., disease, remission, cure) must occur by definition in individuals, the realm of epidemiology principally lies in the study of individuals in the aggregate, such as patients enrolled in clinical trials, participants in cohorts, and populations. Until recently, advancements in epidemiological methods developed in the last half-century have hence largely fallen into the domain of the two major observational study designs used: cohort and case-control studies (cf. Chap. I.5 and I.6 of this handbook).

The justification for these two designs has seemingly rested on their ability to approximate – albeit observationally – the widely accepted paradigm of applied biomedical research: the randomized trial. But the potentially exquisite control that study investigators can often exercise to approach comparability of groups, and hence (in the absence of other biases) validity, cannot in general be commensurately achieved in nonexperimental research. To compensate, some epidemiologists have invoked conventions such as the "study base" concept, which have intuitive appeal and some practical value in study design, but ultimately do little to contribute to an understanding of the theoretical underpinnings of observational studies. Whether one accepts randomized trials as models for epidemiologic designs to emulate, or envisions study bases as natural referents, however, is immaterial, because these concepts neither add to the transparency of causal inference nor do they lend themselves to further advances in modern observational study design. Clearly and by necessity, a different paradigm is required.

The premise underlying such a paradigm is that individuals potentially live in a duality of exposure and nonexposure, with a corresponding duality of observable and hypothetical outcomes. That individuals living under one exposure condition should, in theory, be compared with themselves under other counterfactual (i.e., counter to fact) conditions leads in turn to the premise of "case-only" studies. This chapter is thus predominantly concerned with those studies that juxtapose a case series (i.e., individuals that have experienced a singular health event) with a hypothetical comparison group. The legitimacy of such an approach, which implicitly precludes the need for studying an observable comparison (e.g. control) group, derives from the "potential outcomes" formulation of establishing causal inferences (Little and Rubin 2000). We proceed to show its utility in recent, and most probably future, developments in modern epidemiologic study design.

Nevertheless, not all settings are conducive to comparing cases against hypothetical distributions. When these circumstances arise, such as when exposure effects are not intermittent and transient or when induction times are not transitory (enhancing the likelihood of carryover effects), traditional case-control studies and their more modern variants take on a greater relevance. This chapter will therefore also address two of these designs: case-cohort and nested case-control studies.

They share in common a conceptual understanding of case-control studies that is somewhat at odds with the more traditional view of these designs, namely a de facto comparison of cases to noncases. Such a viewpoint fails to account for the artificial nature of this dichotomy: noncases can become cases, even during the course of a study. The issue is resolved by recognizing that incidence case-control studies are in reality cost and size-efficient modifications of cohort studies, in which cases are not simply compared with noncases, but instead with a sample from a cohort of individuals at risk, some of whom might become cases. So in reality, all case-control studies are "nested" within a cohort (though the constituents of cohorts are not always obvious, as in hospital-based case-control studies). Viewed in this unifying light, the case-control studies discussed in this chapter assume a rational connection (albeit with sometimes different validity assumptions) not only to cohort studies, but in turn to case-only, experimental, and potential outcomes research as well.

Case-Cohort Studies

7.2

To illustrate the relationship between case-control studies with differing control selection strategies, consider a study period (t_0, t_1) within which cases occur and are recruited. The traditional view of case-control studies has been to sample controls from the population at risk at the termination of the study period (t_1). Although direct estimation of exposure-specific incidence proportions is not possible without ancillary information, employment of such *cumulative incidence sampling* of controls allows the use of the exposure odds ratio for estimation of the incidence proportion ratio (IPR) under the rare disease assumption (Cornfield 1951; Chap. I.6 of this handbook). An alternative control sampling approach frequently employed in nested case-control studies, *incidence density sampling*, allows odds ratio estimation of the constant incidence rate ratio without invocation of the rare disease assumption (Miettinen 1976; Greenland and Thomas 1982; Chap. I.6. Unless time is known a priori to not be a confounder, this method typically relies on riskset sampling, in which a case is matched on the basis of time of case occurrence (and potentially other confounders) to one or more members of the cohort at risk, followed by employment of an appropriate matched analysis (e.g., conditional logistic regression; cf. Chap. II.3 of this handbook). Under this design, individuals serving as controls in one riskset are eligible to become cases to be later matched with a different riskset from the remaining cohort-at-risk. Interestingly, when the parameter of interest is the incidence proportion ratio, the matched odds ratio under density sampling even generally outperforms the exposure odds ratio under cumulative incidence sampling as a better estimator (Greenland and Thomas 1982).

Several authors (Kupper et al. 1975; Miettinen 1982; Prentice 1986) envisioned yet another type of case-control study in which controls are sampled exclusively from the cohort at risk at t_0; i.e., prior to the onset of case occurrence in (t_0, t_1) and without regard to their future outcome status. This design, hereafter referred to as a case-cohort study (but also known as a case-base study), is notable not so much for its dissimilarity with other case-control design variants, but rather for what it has in common. The key feature distinguishing a nested case-control study from a case-cohort study is whether controls are matched to cases on time to outcome of the case (Wacholder and Boivin 1987). Thus, a case-cohort study can be likened to an *unmatched* nested case-control study, with controls sampled from the population at risk at t_0 (hence excluding prevalent cases) without regard to failure times. Still, a matched nested case-control study requires control sampling from the entire cohort at risk throughout (t_0, t_1), while the case-cohort study does not because controls are selected *prior* to *any* occurrence of incident cases. Exposure information, therefore, need only be obtained on those individuals sampled as controls at t_0 and any subsequent cases that may or may not be controls. This reveals another advantage of the case-cohort study: the same subset of the cohort can be employed as a control group for studies of multiple outcomes. In contrast, a nested case-control study requires different matched risksets for each outcome studied.

When an outcome is rare (i.e., most observations are censored), follow-up of a full cohort, whether closed or dynamic, can be expensive and inefficient. In contrast, by sampling only a subset of the cohort, the case-cohort study affords advantages found in both cohort and case-control studies. Table 7.1 shows how a hypothetical case-cohort study from a cohort of N individuals is implemented. In this example, an individual in the cohort has probability p of being randomly sampled (with sampling independent of exposure) and included in the subcohort when cohort membership is fixed at t_0. Thus the subcohort is comprised of pN individuals on whom exposure information is ascertained (assuming no loss to follow-up). This principle can be extended to a dynamic cohort, allowing entrance at different times. Over the study period (t_0, t_1) a total of A exposed cases + B unexposed cases occur, only some of whom $(pA + pB)$ are members of the subcohorts. The efficiency of the study is attributable to the economy of not evaluating censored individuals outside the subcohort (e.g., $(1-p)(N_1+N_0-A-B)$).

Table 7.1. Expected distribution of cases and controls in a case-cohort study with sampling fraction p, with sampling independent of exposure status

	Exposed		Nonexposed		
	Sampled subcohort	Nonsampled remainder of cohort	Sampled subcohort	Nonsampled remainder of cohort	Total
Cases	pA	$(1-p)A$	pB	$(1-p)B$	M_+
Censored individuals	$p(N_1 - A)$	$(1-p)(N_1 - A)$	$p(N_0 - B)$	$(1-p)(N_0 - B)$	$N - M_+$
Individuals at risk at t_0	pN_1	$(1-p)N_1$	pN_0	$(1-p)N_0$	N

It is noteworthy that cases occur $((1-p)(A+B))$ that are not part of the subcohort and thus are not eligible to be included in risksets for analysis prior to their failure times, but nevertheless are retained as cases in the study. Although it is advantageous to obtain a census of the cases, particularly when the outcome is rare, cases can potentially be sampled as well.

When the cohort is fixed, direct estimation of the crude IPR is possible without the rare disease assumption. Intuitively, with complete case ascertainment one would expect the case-cohort odds ratio $(A/B)/(pN_1/pN_0)$ to estimate the IPR. However, Sato (1992a) developed a maximum likelihood estimator (MLE) that is asymptotically more efficient:

$$\widehat{\text{IPR}}_{\text{MLE}} = \frac{A\left[\dfrac{BM_1}{M_+} + D\right]}{B\left[\dfrac{AM_1}{M_+} + C\right]} \tag{7.1}$$

where $A_1 = pA, A_0 = (1-p)A, B_1 = pB, B_0 = (1-p)B, C = p(N_1-A), D = p(N_0-B)$, $M_1 = A_1 + B_1$, and $M_+ = A + B$ (see Table 7.1). It is important to note that this equation does not in general algebraically simplify further because, by design, control exposure information is obtained only on the members of the subcohorts N_1' and N_0', where $N_1' = pN_1$ and $N_0' = pN_0$, and not on the entire cohort N. The key difference between the two IPR estimators lies in how the number of sampled cases is employed. For the case-cohort odds ratio, the actual exposure-specific number of sampled cases (A_1 and B_1) is used in the calculation of the size of the cohort sample (i.e., $N_1' = A_1 + C$, and $N_0' = B_1 + D$). In contrast, the MLE estimates the exposure-specific number of cases as substitutes for A_1 and B_1 by multiplying the total number of cases in the exposed or unexposed subcohorts (A or B) by the unconditional (on exposure) overall sampling fraction of cases (M_1/M_+, the proportion of cases sampled as controls in the combined exposed and unexposed subcohorts). When the exposure-specific sampling fractions are equal to the overall sampling fraction, the two IPR estimators will be equal.

To illustrate these points, consider the data from a case-cohort study by Miettinen (1982) and cited by Sato (1992a). The study included 10 individuals sampled in the exposed subcohort (N_1'), 5 of which became cases (A_1), and an additional 5 exposed cases occurred that were not in the subcohort (A_0). It also included 90 individuals sampled in the unexposed cohort (N_0'), 15 of which became cases (B_1); an additional 35 unexposed cases occurred (B_0). The intuitive estimator of the IPR for these data is 1.8, while the MLE is 2.2. However, if for example the quantity of 35 unexposed cases not in the sampled subcohort is changed to 15 unexposed cases, then the ratio of sampled to unsampled cases is constant for both exposure levels, and both IPR estimates equal 3.0.

When the outcome is not rare, random sampling of cases may be utilized. Sato (1992a) provides further details about incorporating such sampling into the analysis. When the outcome is rare, then few if any cases would be expected in the cohort sample ($M_1 \ll M_+$), and (7.1) reduces to the case-control odds ratio (AD/BC).

A large sample variance estimate of $\ln(\widehat{\mathrm{IPR}}_{\mathrm{MLE}})$ (Sato 1992a) is given by:

$$\widehat{\mathrm{Var}}[\ln(\widehat{\mathrm{IPR}}_{\mathrm{MLE}})] = \frac{1}{A} + \frac{1}{B} + \left[1 - 2\left(\frac{M_1}{M_+}\right)\left(\frac{1}{\frac{AM_1}{M_+} + C} + \frac{1}{\frac{BM_1}{M_+} + D}\right)\right]$$

$$- \frac{N'^2 A\, B(A_0 + B_0)(A_1 + B_1)}{(A+B)^3 \left(\frac{A\,M_1}{M_+} + C\right)^2 \left(\frac{BM_1}{M_+} + D\right)^2} \tag{7.2}$$

where $N' = N_1' + N_0'$.

A $(1-\alpha)\%$ confidence interval for the crude IPR can be obtained from:

$$\widehat{\mathrm{IPR}}_{\mathrm{MLE}} \exp\left\{\pm z_{1-\frac{\alpha}{2}}\left(\mathrm{var}\left[\ln\left(\widehat{\mathrm{IPR}}_{\mathrm{MLE}}\right)\right]\right)^{1/2}\right\}, \tag{7.3}$$

where $z_{1-\alpha/2}$ denotes the $(1-\alpha/2)$-quantile of the standard normal distribution.

Calculation of the IPR estimator and its large-sample distribution can be extended to stratified analyses using a Mantel-Haenszel estimator (Sato 1992b). With k strata, the estimator is given by

$$\widehat{\mathrm{IPR}}_{\mathrm{MH}} = \frac{\displaystyle\sum_k \frac{N_{0k}' A_k}{T_k}}{\displaystyle\sum_k \frac{N_{1k}' B_k}{T_k}} \tag{7.4}$$

where T_k is the total number of distinct individuals in stratum k $(A_k + B_k + C_k + D_k)$.

The variance estimator of $\ln(\widehat{\mathrm{IPR}}_{\mathrm{MH}})$, that applies to both large strata and when data are sparse, is

$$\widehat{\mathrm{Var}}\left[\ln\left(\widehat{\mathrm{IPR}}_{\mathrm{MH}}\right)\right] = \frac{\displaystyle\sum_k \frac{\left[(B_{0k} + D_k) A_k N_{1k}' + (A_{0k} + C_k) B_k N_{0k}' + A_{0k} D_k + B_{0k} C_k\right]}{(T_k)^2}}{\displaystyle\sum_k \frac{N_{1k}' B_k}{T_k} \sum_k \frac{N_{0k}' A_k}{T_k}} \tag{7.5}$$

As before, confidence limits can be obtained by applying the following formula:

$$\widehat{\mathrm{IPR}}_{\mathrm{MH}} \exp\left\{\pm z_{1-\frac{\alpha}{2}}\left(\mathrm{var}\left[\ln\left(\widehat{\mathrm{IPR}}_{\mathrm{MH}}\right)\right]\right)^{1/2}\right\}. \tag{7.6}$$

When the parameter of interest is the incidence rate ratio, the analysis becomes more complex. If all members of the cohort were followed and their exposure and outcome status, i.e. failure times measured, a Cox proportional hazards regression model could easily be employed. Instead, a modification of this model is required for case-cohort data. For further discussion about analytic issues in case-cohort studies, see Barlow et al. (1999).

The choice between which hybrid case-control study to undertake – case-cohort or nested case-control – ultimately rests less on study-specific efficiency considerations than on what primary effect measure is required, and whether the study is investigating one or multiple health outcomes. These issues are discussed in detail in Langholz and Thomas (1990) and Wacholder (1991).

Nested Case-Control Studies   7.3

Design Features   7.3.1

Nested case-control studies have received increasing attention in the last few decades, partly due to the increased number of large cohorts that have been established and followed that have permitted selection of cases and controls for such studies (Langholz and Thomas 1990). Nested case-control studies share a number of design features and advantages with case-cohort designs, most notably selection of cases and controls from the same cohort. This feature provides a number of important strengths, discussed in greater detail below, but fundamentally is designed to sample the cases and controls from the same frame, the cohort, thus minimizing the chance of lack of comparability of the cases and controls. The two designs, however, also differ in one important respect. In the case-cohort design (described in greater detail above), the controls are comprised of a random sample of the cohort at baseline, whereas in a nested case-control study, the controls are a random sample of those in the cohort at the time of diagnosis of each case, and can in addition be matched to each case on various factors at the time of diagnosis of the matched case (Szklo and Nieto 2000). Thus, as in a case-cohort design, the cases and controls in a nested case-control study are participants in a cohort, so that this design is also a form of a cohort study. The method of selection of controls in a nested case-control study is equivalent to matching controls to cases on duration of follow-up and thus on opportunity for disease occurrence, while a case-cohort study could be considered an unmatched nested case-control study. The method of control selection in a nested case-control study is thus incidence density, also known as riskset sampling (Szklo and Nieto 2000). The controls in a nested case-control study, therefore, might develop the disease of interest subsequent to the diagnosis of the cases but represent cohort members at risk of being cases when each case occurs. If controls in a nested case-control design are a random sample of the cohort at the time each case is diagnosed, then cases could have been included as controls in previous risksets, and the estimated exposure odds ratio is a statistically unbiased estimate of the constant incidence rate ratio (Greenland and Thomas 1982). However, if controls are not eligible to become subsequent cases, the analysis is that of a traditional cumulative incidence case-control study, and the effect measure is the standard exposure odds ratio, which provides an unbiased estimate of the disease risk ratio under the rare disease assumption.

7.3.2   Strengths

The nested case-control design has a number of advantages. It is more efficient than a cohort design, i.e., it can detect differences as statistically significant with a smaller sample size than that required for a cohort analysis. It shares with the case-cohort design the advantage of having measured exposures of interest at baseline entry into the cohort, so that the temporal sequence of exposure preceding disease is known and appropriate for deriving causal inferences. Exposure histories are not subject to recall bias because they are determined before the cases are diagnosed. This design also avoids the potential bias of not including fatal cases and may minimize the potential bias of non-participation, since exposure data is collected before diagnosis of disease. Both biases often occur in the traditional case-control approach. Further, since cases and controls in this design comprise a sample of the baseline cohort, and assessment of samples obtained at baseline need only be performed for this subset and not for the entire cohort, even though the cost of assembling the cohort still exists, the overall cost of the nested case-control approach is less in terms of assessing the baseline samples (e.g., serum assays for the subset in the nested case-control study) than an analysis of all the samples for the entire cohort, as would be the case for a full cohort analysis (Kelsey et al. 1996). This design also avoids the bias of the disease modifying biologic characteristics and thus not reflecting cause but rather effect of disease, as may occur when biologic samples are evaluated after diagnosis of disease in the traditional case-control approach, given that samples were obtained before disease occurrence in the nested case-control design. Finally, the nested case-control design minimizes selection biases introduced when cases and controls are not selected from the same populations, although differential losses of cases and controls from the same cohort can still introduce selection bias, just as differential loss to follow-up in a cohort study can introduce selection bias, for example, by socioeconomic status.

7.3.3   Limitations

The nested case-control design shares with the cohort design several limitations. First, data on exposure and/or specimens for exposure analysis must be collected on the entire cohort at baseline. Thus, the costs of data collection are likely to be higher than a traditional case-control study, although the costs of assaying specimens will be lower than for a cohort study analysis in which all specimens would be assayed. Further, investigators must have the foresight and resources to collect appropriate exposure data and samples to assess exposure (once disease has occurred in cases) to reap the benefits of avoiding the potential biases mentioned above. In addition, the time required for a nested case-control study, if appropriately measured from the baseline assembly of cohort information, is longer and thus less suitable for very rare diseases or those with long latent periods, than for the traditional case-control design. Just as in any observational study, exposure-disease associations may be observed due to uncontrolled confounding if inadequate data on potential covariates is collected, which may be a particular problem in nested case-control studies because the cohort study in which such a study is nested may not have been designed to collect sufficiently detailed information needed on confounding variables for the question under study in the nested case-control investigation. While additional information may be collected on confounders during the nested case-control study, it is subject to recall bias that is largely avoided by using data collected at baseline for the cohort study in which the nested case-control investigation is conducted. Finally, silent preclinical disease at baseline may affect some baseline measurements and thus result in misleading findings, although this limitation may be minimized by excluding cases diagnosed within a defined, usually short, period after baseline.

Case-Crossover Studies 7.4

Under circumstances that could be described as both ideal and impossible, it would become a trivial matter to evaluate causation within an individual, thus obviating the need for observational studies at all. This ideal, which is assumed in Table 7.2, reflects the counterfactual capacity to evaluate not only the health or disease experience of a cohort of exposed individuals (column 1), but what the experience of this cohort would have been had it been possible to evaluate these same individuals during the same time frame as when they were actually exposed, except that exposure would have been removed or its effect completely blocked (column 2).

Such a comparison between these same individuals under two identical conditions (save for the fact of exposure) could then lead not only to an individual-by-individual assessment of the causal or preventive effect of exposure, but also the average causal effect of exposure in the cohort (A/A^*). The value of the unexposed cohort (column 3) for comparison with the exposed cohort (column 1), and hence effect estimation, lies in the validity of its exchangeability property; i.e., $B/N_0 = A^*/N_1$.

Table 7.2. Hypothetical incidence data from exposed (as well as counterfactually unexposed) and not exposed cohorts. Note that $A + C$ is constrained to equal $A^* + C^*$

	Exposed	Exposed* (counterfactually unexposed)	Not exposed
Diseased	A	A^*	B
Not diseased	C	C^*	D
Total person-time at risk	N_1	N_1	N_0
Incidence proportion	A/N_1	A^*/N_1	B/N_0

Given the pragmatic limitations which epidemiologists operate under – pointedly, the inability to have study participants and investigators travel backward in time, rendering column 2 unobservable – it becomes a challenge, if not an imperative, to come as close as possible to the ideal. In experimental research, the crossover study, in which individuals crossover between periods of different exposures (possibly including nonexposure, as in a control, placebo, or sham treatment), affords the opportunity to observe different treatments within the same individual, albeit at different (and potentially confounding) time periods. The attractiveness of this experimental approach, underlying the ability to control for individual-level confounders, is offset by the assumption that neither period or carryover effects occur. Thus this design is optimally suited to exposures with both a rapid onset of action as well as a brief effect period.

The case-crossover design (Maclure 1991) is the observational study analog of the crossover study. A key distinguishing characteristic of the former is that study participants – not investigators – determine their own exposure. A very important feature of case-crossover studies, like crossover studies, is that they are best suited to episodic exposures with short induction and transient effect periods. Thus it is possible to envision, following an exposure that modifies risk in individuals, a brief induction period during which risk does not change, followed by a period subdivided into intervals characterized by varying degrees of altered risk, and ultimately a return to baseline risk. The time interval of elevated or decreased risk following exposure is known as the effect period. In practice, the effect period may not be known, but may be inferred from ancillary information (e.g., pharmacokinetic properties of a drug, duration of effect of endogenous catecholamine release following physical exertion, period of heightened immune activity following vaccination, half-life of a chemical, incubation times of a pathogen following infection, etc.). Sensitivity analyses postulating different combinations of induction time and duration of exposure effects can provide insights into periods of maximum influence. As noted by Maclure (1991), postulating effect periods that are either too brief or too long leads to nondifferential misclassification of exposure, resulting in effect measures that are biased towards the null. In the absence of other biases, the optimal choice of an effect period is that which minimizes nondifferential misclassification, and hence maximizes the effect measure.

Data from an individual i in a case-crossover study can be envisioned in Table 7.3. When the distribution of exposure is stationary over the case and control period, the Mantel–Haenszel incidence rate ratio ($\widehat{IRR}_{MH}$) is approximately unbiased (Vines and Farrington 2001). Each case occupies a unique stratum. $\widehat{IRR}_{MH}$, corresponding to the average proportionate change in the rate of the outcome resulting from exposure, can be calculated from the following formula (note: $N_{1i} + N_{0i} = T_i$):

$$\widehat{IRR}_{MH} = \frac{\sum\limits_{i} a_i N_{0i}/T_i}{\sum\limits_{i} b_i N_{1i}/T_i} \qquad (7.7)$$

Table 7.3. Representation of case-crossover data for a single individual developing an outcome event either within or outside an exposure effect period

	Time		
	within effect period	outside effect period	Total
Case occurrence	a_i	b_i	
Person-time	N_{1i}	N_{0i}	T_i

The variance of $\ln(\widehat{\text{IRR}}_{MH})$ (Greenland and Robins 1985) can be estimated by:

$$\widehat{\text{Var}}[\ln(\widehat{\text{IRR}}_{MH})] = \frac{\sum_i (a_i + b_i)N_{1i}N_{0i}/T_i^2}{\left(\sum_i a_iN_{0i}/T_i\right)\left(\sum_i b_iN_{1i}/T_i\right)}. \qquad (7.8)$$

To illustrate, consider the hypothetical data in Table 7.4 (adapted from Table 4 of Maclure 1991). The column of expected exposure odds is equivalent to Maclure's expected concurrence odds, and refers to the ratio of the expected amount of time an individual spends in the effect period, based on the usual frequency of exposure, to the expected amount of time an individual spends outside the effect period ($N_{1i}:N_{0i}$ from Table 7.3) over the duration of retrospective follow-up for cerebrovascular accidents. In this example, the period of retrospective follow-up was six months, or equivalently 4383 hours. To illustrate, for participant 1, the usual frequency of aerobic exercise was three times per week. If the effect period is assumed to be two hours beginning immediately after the cessation

Table 7.4. Data from a hypothetical case-crossover study evaluating the relationship between aerobic exercise and the onset of cerebrovascular accident. The effect period is two hours. The period of retrospective follow-up is six months or equivalently 4383 hours

Individual (i)	Usual frequency of exposure	Last exposure before cerebrovascular accident	Exposure odds	
			Observed ($a_i : b_i$)	Expected ($N_{1i} : N_{0i}$)
1	3 /week	30 min	1 : 0	156 : 4227
2	1 /week	1 day	0 : 1	52 : 4331
3	1 /month	21 days	0 : 1	12 : 4371
4	0 /month	1 year	0 : 1	0 : 4383
5	5 /week	45 min	1 : 0	260 : 4123
6	0 /month	2 years	0 : 1	0 : 4383
7	2 /month	15 hours	0 : 1	24 : 4359
8	4 /week	3 hours	0 : 1	208 : 4175
9	1 /week	6 hours	0 : 1	52 : 4331
10	0 /month	4 years	0 : 1	0 : 4383

of exercise, then the expected number of hours spent in the six-month effect (exposure) period = 2 hours/day × 3 days/week × 26 weeks = 156 hours (N_{1i} in Table 7.3), leaving 4383 − 156 = 4227 hours unexposed (N_{0i} in Table 7.3). Because participant 1's cerebrovascular accident occurred within the two hour effect period, the observed exposure odds for this individual – the ratio of the a_i and b_i cells in Table 7.3 – is 1 : 0. Using (7.7) and (7.8), the Mantel–Haenszel incidence rate ratio for cerebrovascular accidents within two hours of aerobic activity in this sample of individuals and its corresponding 95% confidence interval are 24.0 and 3.1 − 188.1, respectively.

The preceding example derived the usual frequency of exposure by utilizing a census of the information from the six months prior to the event onset. In practice, retrospective follow-up time may be briefer or longer, depending on the stability of the exposure distribution. The analysis presupposed no within-individual confounding occurred over time, and that the effect of aerobic exercise does not depend on time of day.

Mittleman et al. (1995) examined five different approaches to modeling case-crossover data from the control period, including the "usual frequency" scheme of obtaining expected exposure odds above. They also examined the relative sampling efficiencies and restrictiveness of the assumptions inherent in each approach. Four of the modeling approaches involved different methods of studying the control period in the 25 one-hour periods immediately preceding myocardial infarction, with exposure being heavy exertion. The first approach the authors evaluated was called the "Pair-Matched Interval Approach", in which the one-hour hazard period immediately prior to the onset of myocardial infarction was contrasted with the one-hour control period from the same time of day 24 hours earlier within the same subject. These data, which are analyzed using standard methods for matched-pair data (e.g., Mantel–Haenszel or conditional logistic regression estimators), control for confounding by time of day, without the need for any assumptions about baseline hazard in each of the 24 one-hour periods in the day. The analysis can be made more statistically efficient by increasing the number of control intervals sampled. However, this method is not well suited to evaluating other exposures that occur at regular and predictable intervals during a 24 hour period. For example, if an individual reliably self-administers a medication with potential cardiovascular effects to be taken at 08:00 and 20:00 hours each day, then by comparing exposure on the day of disease occurrence to the same time 24 hours earlier this approach will ensure perfect concordance between hazard and control periods, resulting in bias towards the null. A second strategy, the "Nonparametric Multiple Intervals Approach", involves explicitly modeling exposure information on each of the 24 one-hour categorical intervals in the day prior to the myo-cardial infarction. This model, besides controlling for confounding by time of day, estimates a baseline hazard for each of the 24 one-hour intervals. Although this categorical model, with indicator variables representing the one-hour intervals, makes no assumption about the functional relationship between the time of day and myocardial infarction incidence, a third model, the "Parametric Multiple Intervals Approach" does exactly that. Instead of indicator variables, the authors employed sine and cosine functions, based on consistency with prior (external) information on temporal patterns of myocardial infarction occurrence. Under the assumption that the model is correctly specified, it provides a synoptic estimate of the effect of exposure while controlling for confounding by time of day. A fourth strategy, called the "Parsimonious Multiple Intervals Approach", assumes the absence of any confounding by time of day; this is equivalent to a crude analysis that is incognizant of time of day. As noted above, the final scheme, the "Usual Frequency Approach" utilizes a census of the exposure information from an extended period of time prior to the myocardial infarction; it is, in essence, a series of distinct cohort studies of each individual, who in turn constitutes a unique stratum for analysis.

In all five of these models it was possible to estimate a single summary effect of exposure under the assumption of no effect modification of the exposure-outcome association by time of day. Each of the models could be analyzed using conditional logistic regression (with the caveats noted below). The authors showed that while the number of control periods sampled had little effect on the incidence rate ratio estimate, as the periods sampled increased, the relative efficiency (marked by a narrowing of the respective confidence intervals) concomitantly increased as well, regardless of what underlying model assumptions were invoked. The "Usual Frequency Approach" led to the smallest variance of the estimated logarithm of the incidence rate ratio, and hence narrowest confidence interval, but at the cost of assuming no within-individual confounding unless further information is available on the complex conditional relationships among all determinants of risk (Mittleman et al. 1995). Although the modeling approach by these authors may not be appropriate in all circumstances, they do underscore the point that case-crossover studies, like their case-control counterparts, can be conducted using different control period sampling schemes and employing different exposure and confounder/effect modifier assumptions.

However, it has been demonstrated by Vines and Farrington (2001) that when exposures within individuals are correlated between different time intervals (i.e., are not independent), the conditional logistic regression model can lead to biased effect estimates and is hence precarious to use. This might arise, for example, in a study of anti-inflammatory drug use in individuals allowed to self-medicate: during periods of elevated pain people would be more likely to take the medication, while during periods of relief they would be less likely. Because self-medication in one time interval is likely to provide some insight into self-medication in adjacent time intervals, the exposure information cannot be considered independent. When there is no true relationship between exposure and the outcome of interest, so long as exposure is stationary over time, the conditional logistic regression model should not erroneously suggest such a causal effect of exposure, although time of day, if explicitly modeled, could still demonstrate an effect on disease incidence. In contrast, the greater the true effect of exposure, the greater is the model's potential for bias, which can be either towards or away from the null.

It has been scarcely before the nineties of the last century since the formalization of the case-crossover study, and a deeper appreciation for its limitations – and for subsequent modifications to enhance validity – continues to evolve. One threat to validity, the lack of stationarity of exposure over time, is well-recognized and the subject of considerable recent research (e.g., Greenland 1996; Suissa 1998; Navidi 1998; Navidi and Weinhandl 2002). Likewise, information bias is particularly problematic in case-crossover studies compared to unmatched case-control studies because matched sets, by virtue of their matching on correlates of exposure, are particularly sensitive to misclassification of the study exposure (Greenland 1982, 1996). The customary sources of bias in traditional observational study designs, including confounding, selection, information, censoring, and misspecification, all have counterparts in case-crossover studies. These sources of bias are explored in more detail in Redelmeier and Tibshirani (1997) and Maclure and Mittleman (2000).

7.5   Case-Time-Control Studies

One of the assumptions – and limitations – of the case-crossover design is that of stationarity (stability) of the distribution of study exposure over time. Such an assumption takes on a reasonable legitimacy for a transient exposure assessed over a relatively short referent time interval. However, as the period of prior exposure assessment lengthens, time trends in exposure from changing external factors may become emergent and evident, precluding the measurement of "usual frequency" of exposure. Period effects lead in turn to confounding.

Suissa (1995) recognized time trends as a threat to validity in case-crossover studies, which led him to propose a modification of a case-crossover study, which he called a "case-time-control" study. The premise behind this design is that information about time trends in exposure can be obtained from individuals conventionally sampled as controls in a classical case-control study. This information can in turn be used to adjust the effect estimate from a case-crossover study, yielding less biased results by removing the confounding introduced by period effects.

To illustrate this bias practically, Suissa used as a central example in pharmacoepidemiology (cf. Chap. III.9 of this handbook) the problem of assessing drug effects in the face of confounding by indication. That is, prescription drug use is not only more likely among patients with more serious manifestations of an illness, but as disease severity progresses over time, the therapeutic indication for such drug use is also likely to commensurately change as well. Because severity is typically both an independent predictor of a health outcome and is an indication for treatment, nor is it an expected sequelae of therapeutic drug use, it fulfills the necessary criteria for confounding. Were severity an easily measurable host characteristic, it would be trivial to control for its confounding effects. However, severity within and between patients falls on a continuum that usually defies even imprecise measurement, such that even attempts to control for it would lead inevitably to meaningful residual confounding. Thus, neither conventional (i.e., case-control) nor case-only (e.g., case-crossover) studies would be capable of distinguishing drug (exposure) effects from temporal (confounding) changes in exposure.

Suissa's solution to this problem was to envision the odds of exposure (recognizing that sampling is based on outcome) in an individual as an exponential function of the following elements (retaining his notation):

$$\text{odds}(E_{ijkl} = 1) = \exp(\mu + s_{il} + \pi_j + \theta_k) \tag{7.9}$$

where E represents a binary exposure, i represents the outcome group status (case or control), j represents a current or referent time period, k represents the outcome event in a particular period, and l represents the individual in group i; $\exp(\mu)$ is the overall exposure odds, $\exp(s_{il})$ is the participant-specific odds ratio, $\exp(\pi_j)$ is the period odds, and $\exp(\theta_k)$ is the odds corresponding to the outcome event. This function can be expressed separately for cases and controls and for the current and referent time periods. As will be seen shortly, this model is notable for its lack of interactions among the different elements. It can be shown that the effect measure of interest, $\exp(\theta_k)$, is not distinguishable from the nuisance period effect, $\exp(\pi_j)$, in the cases alone, but that the addition of a control series renders the former estimable.

This model, in which each individual's current and referent period constitute a matched pair, can be envisioned within the framework of conditional logistic regression. Again, utilizing Suissa's notation, let T denote the outcome variable which is the respective time period ($1 = $ current, $0 = $ referent) for each participant's component of the matched pair, E the exposure, and G the outcome group status (case or control). The odds that the outcome T equals 1 is given by:

$$\text{odds}(T = 1) = \exp\left(\beta_0 + \beta_1 E + \beta_2 (E \times G)\right) . \tag{7.10}$$

The odds ratio corresponding to the effect of time period is $\exp(\beta_1)$, while the odds ratio corresponding to the effect of drug therapy on the outcome after removal of the period effect is $\exp(\beta_2)$.

The case-time-control study is not without its detractions, however. As Greenland (1996) pointed out, in addition to the usual assumptions of a case-crossover study (e.g., absence of carryover effects), the analysis can be confounded by the presence of unmeasured – and hence uncontrollable – confounders. Strictly speaking, for a case-time-control analysis to yield a valid point estimate of exposure, it must be assumed that there exist no interactions among any of the elements in (7.9). That is, the exposure-outcome association is unaffected by time period ($\pi_j \theta_k = 0$), the exposure-outcome association is unaffected by unmeasured confounders ($s_{il} \theta_k = 0$), and the exposure-time period association is unaffected by unmeasured confounders ($s_{il} \pi_j = 0$) (Suissa 1998). While the first assumption, that the effect measure remains stable, may be reasonable, particularly over shorter rather than longer time periods, the latter two assumptions are more problematic. The presence of unmeasured confounders is invariably a concern, though hardly unique to case-time-control studies. Those unmeasured variables may act on either the exposure effect as effect modifiers or on the time period effect as confounders.

The utility of this method, then, rests on the veracity of unverifiable assumptions of no-confounding by indicators of disease severity. Greenland (1996) points out the problem of selecting between competing study designs to cope with the problem of confounding by indication when it is unclear which design would yield a less biased result. Without a recommendation that uniformly applies to all study settings, it may ultimately be advisable when possible to employ a sensitivity analysis of two or more designs within the same cohort in order to see how their different properties and assumptions can affect conclusions.

7.6   Case-Specular Studies

It has already been shown above that when studying intermittent exposure effects with transient duration that a counterfactual paradigm is superior to a study base paradigm in motivating the choice of a comparison series for cases. More precisely, the proper conceptualization of causation as a fundamental comparison between what occurred in exposed individuals and what would have happened to the same exposed individuals had exposure been counterfactually removed or blocked can lead to a far more refined – and potentially less biased – study design. In the context of case-crossover studies, this practically meant comparing cases' recent (relative to the incident outcome event) exposure history to the same cases' customary distribution of exposure. Confounding by factors that were inherently host-related and time invariant, such as genetic predisposition or prior nutritional and environmental history, became irrelevant because each case, essentially being matched to itself, occupied a unique stratum for analysis.

By adapting counterfactual reasoning to other settings, novel study designs can emerge. An example of this is the residential case-specular method of studying the hypothesized relationship between wire codes (as a surrogate for electromagnetic fields) and childhood cancer (Zaffanella et al. 1998). Because historical information on household magnetic field exposure needed for observational studies is invariably absent, an alternative exposure metric is required. Wertheimer and Leeper (1979) proposed power line wire code categories, which are functions of wire thickness and distance from power line to residence, as a temporally stable, if imprecise, alternative measure of magnetic field exposure. However, this metric also suffers from the detraction that spatial proximity of power lines to residences is not only a proxy for exposure, but also a proxy for other unmeasured or unmeasurable characteristics of neighborhoods (e.g., socioeconomic status, traffic congestion, air pollution) that marginally or jointly may likewise be determinants of adverse health outcomes, including childhood cancer. Any residential study of the hypothesis, then, would require distinguishing two distinct, although not necessarily competing, effects: that of the household electromagnetic field, and that intrinsic yet undefined to the neighborhood. The case-specular design was proposed as one possible approach of mitigating this problem by comparing wire code exposures of case residences to counterfactual wire code exposures of purely hypothetical (specular) residences.

A specular residence is an imaginary or virtual control created by symmetrically (sagitally) reflecting a case residence across the center of its street (although other speculars, including reflecting the power lines as opposed to the residences, are possible), creating a matched case-counterfactual pair (Fig. 7.1). Specifically, the distance from the case residence to the center of the street (L_{RC}) is used for creating a specular control residence with an identical, albeit hypothetical distance ($L_{RC}{}^*$). What remains to be measured is the distance from the case residence to the electrical lines (L_{RE}) and what the distance from the specular control residence would be, had it existed, to the electrical lines ($L_{RE}{}^*$). The wire code category of the case residence can then be contrasted with the counterfactual wire code of the specular residence. The matching of this pair of residences is so spatially fine that, apart from potential discordance in wire code, it is plausible to assume that most if not all other environmental or social determinants of outcome are concordant between the pairs. If the wire code acts only as a surrogate for such neighborhood risk factors, then no residual association should exist between the higher current wire codes postulated to be related to cancer risk and case residence. The statistical analysis for this design is typical of those for matched pair data, with the polytomous exposures corresponding to wire code categories.

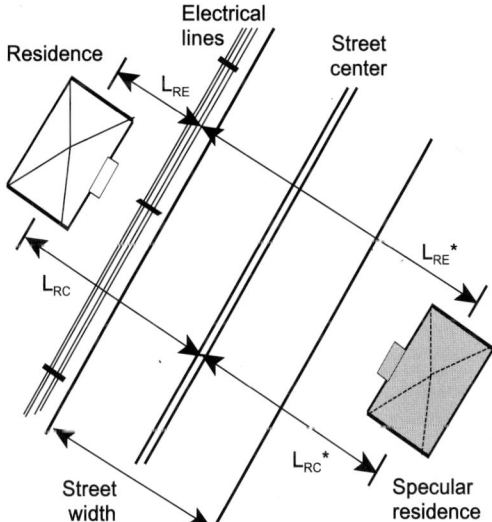

Figure 7.1. Example of construction of a specular residence on a street with case residence on the same street side as electrical lines. Note that the distance from the residence to the center of the street, L_{RC}, is equal to the distance from the center of the street to the specular residence, $L_{RC}{}^*$. Also, L_{RE} = distance from the case residence to the electrical lines, while $L_{RE}{}^*$ = distance from the specular residence to the electrical lines

Zafanella et al. (1998) note, in contrast, that if the magnetic field hypothesis is correct, a preponderance of case households should occur on the same side of a street as power lines, and that case residences should have, on average, higher wire codes than specular residences. Several assumptions are necessary for these predictions, if actually found to exist in a study, to have causal value. The first, which Zaffanella et al. called "symmetry of the residence-specular probability matrix", implies probabilistic independence between placement of power lines and placement of residences on the sides of a street. The second assumption is an implicit "randomization" of residences on both sides of a street with respect to unmeasured, unmeasurable, or unknown confounders (the usual no-confounding assumption underlying causal interpretation of all observational studies). The third assumption is no systematic misclassification of wire codes by residence type (case or specular), a problem that cannot be mitigated by blinding if only case residences are evaluated in the field. Differential misclassification may be a particular problem due to subjectivity in assigning wire codes to specular residences.

The case-specular method shares the advantage found when performing a neighbor-matched case-control study: the control of confounding attributable to intrinsic properties of the neighborhood. It also affords the economical advantage of not requiring in-situ measurements from a control group. Yet it has certain disadvantages as well, including the requirement of specifying speculars in unrealistic situations, high frequencies of concordant residence-specular pairs (particularly when power lines are located behind homes and uniform wire classes are used), and the inability to verify the assumption of symmetry of the residence-specular probability matrix without a validation control series. For further issues related to the analysis of case-specular studies, and the incorporation of controls into the study (i.e., case-control-specular analysis), see Greenland (1999).

7.7   Genetic Epidemiology Case Only Designs

7.7.1   Design Features

The discipline of genetic epidemiology has grown significantly over the past 30 years, facilitated by advances and improvements in technology and in understanding mechanisms based on molecular biology (for more details on genetic epidemiology see Chap. III.7 of this handbook). The identification of the relations of genes to clinical and subclinical disease has the potential to enable accurate and early detection of individuals at increased risk and to improve understanding of the etiology and pathophysiology of disease, which may also lead to more effective approaches to treat and prevent disease and disease transmission (Ellsworth and Manolio 1999). Traditional case-control and cohort designs have been and appropriately continue to be employed to discern genetic components of disease by detecting familial aggregation (including the special case of twin concordance) (see Table 7.5), time trends, changes in disease occurrence in migrants, linkage of genetic markers to disease and gene-environment interactions. However, some case series techniques have also proved valuable in assessing the relation of genetic characteristics to disease, as well as gene-environment interactions. For these purposes, the case series ideally consists of incident, population-based cases of the disease of interest in which mutations of interest are assessed. In recent years, methods have been published using log-linear methods to estimate relative risks for mutant alleles, to analyze case-parental control series (Yang and Khoury 1997) and case triads (mother, father and affected child) (Wilcox et al. 1998). These methods distinguish the role of genes in parent and child in disease risk, based on the asymmetric distribution of a variant allele among cases and their parents.

When investigating gene-environment interactions, if the cases are not population-based, the assumption is made that case selection for gene mutation positive or negative (negative meaning null or wild type) is not influenced by risk factors of interest. A comparison is then made of cases positive for mutation to cases with the null or wild type for the environmental risk factor of interest (see Table 7.6), and a traditional Mantel–Haenszel or logistic regression approach is used for data analyses to generate an odds ratio to test if the strength of association with the environmental risk factor differs for the two case groups (positive and negative for the mutant gene) to indicate gene-environment interaction (Begg and Zhang 1994). Gene-environment interaction can also be tested in traditional case-control studies to evaluate associations with environmental risk factors in gene mutant

Table 7.5. Estimating concordance of a discrete variable in twin studies

	Twin 1	
Twin 2	Has disease	Has no disease
Has disease	*A*	*B*
Has no disease	*C*	*D*

$$\text{Disease Concordance} = \frac{A}{A+B+C} = \frac{\text{number of concordant twin pairs}}{\text{number of twin pairs with at least one affected member}}$$

Table 7.6. Analytic design for case series

Environmental	Cases only	
exposure	Have genetic marker	Do not have genetic marker
Present	*A*	*B*
Absent	*C*	*D*

Odds Ratio = AD/BC for association of marker with exposure

Table 7.7. Expansion* of case-control study for genetic studies

Risk factor	Mutant genotype	Control	Case	Odds ratio
No	No	A	B	Reference
No	Yes	C	D	$OR_{genetic\ component} = AD/BC$
Yes	No	E	F	$OR_{environmental\ component} = AF/BE$
Yes	Yes	G	H	$OR_{gene-environment\ interaction} = AH/BG$

* When genetic marker can also be measured in the control group. Source: Khoury (1997)

Table 7.8a. Example of gene-environment interaction, with and without using controls

Environmental exposure	Cases		Controls
	Mutation positive	Mutation negative	
Present	45	50	75
Absent	15	25	60

Table 7.8b. Example of gene-environment interaction, with and without using controls

Design	Unadjusted cross products	Unadjusted odds ratios
Case series	$(45 \times 25)/(50 \times 15)$	1.5
Case-control		
Mutation positive	$(45 \times 60)/(15 \times 75)$	2.4
Mutation negative	$(50 \times 60)/(25 \times 75)$	1.6
$OR_{positive}/OR_{negative}$	2.4/1.6	1.5

positive and negative cases and controls. In this approach, polychotomous logistic regression may be used to model concurrently two separate logistic regression functions to derive separate beta coefficients for marker positive and negative and thus separate odds ratios for each relationship conditional on other risk factors. To test that the two categories possess etiologic heterogeneity with the risk factors, the equality of the two beta coefficients is tested by using the likelihood ratio tests for the difference in beta coefficients (using the natural logarithm of the ratio of the two adjusted odds ratios for the risk factors). Khoury (1997) has shown the relation of the analysis of different components of case-control studies to identify genetic and environmental components of gene-environment interactions (Table 7.7). The odds ratio from the case series described above is the same parameter as the ratio of the odds ratio from the polychotomous model in a case-control study with unmatched controls and no adjustment for other confounding factors (see Tables 7.8a and 7.8b). For example, the odds ratio in the case series in Table 7.8a for the gene-environment interaction is the same as the ratio of the two odds ratios obtained for cases and controls in Table 7.8b for mutation positive and exposure relative to mutation negative and exposure.

Strengths

The major advantages of the case series for use in genetic epidemiology and assessment of gene-environment interaction are largely ease in assembling the study population and collecting data, which reduce logistic efforts and thus cost. In addition, the case-only design is more efficient than a case-control design for detecting gene-environment interaction (assuming independence between exposure and genotype in the population) (Yang et al. 1997), since the case-only design produces more precise estimates of (due to introducing less variation since only cases, and no controls are included, thus being likely to be more homogeneous) interaction. Thus, for detecting a given odds ratio for interaction, a case-only design requires fewer cases than a case-control design. Further, since controls are often less motivated than cases to participate in studies, the case-only approach helps to minimize potential participation bias. Finally, the data analysis in a case-only design is somewhat more straightforward than in a case-control approach.

Limitations

Despite the relative ease of conducting case series studies, most are not population-based but rather convenience samples with little detail provided on methods or criteria for selection. Methods may be difficult to replicate, and misclassification of cases may occur and impede identification of true relationships. Further, if selection of cases is dependent on availability of a large enough tumor, in studies of associations of genetic markers with cancer, bias could be introduced if tumor size is related to exposure to risk factors or presence of genetic markers or both. In addition, use of prevalent cases in studies of markers can lead to biased estimates if the risk factors under study are associated with survival, just as with case-control designs. Furthermore, if sample size estimates are computed based only on main effects, but gene-environment interactions are of interest, the sample size may be underestimated and statistical power thus overestimated. Differential misclassification of environmental exposures also can modify the gene-disease association, which may result in bias either toward or away from the null of the stratum-specific odds ratios but toward the null when multiplicative interaction is present (Garcia-Closas et al. 1998). Finally, many case series studies demonstrate associations of disease with genetic markers, but, importantly, association does not necessarily connote causality and may reflect an effect of disease occurrence rather than disease causation.

Conclusions

The designs addressed in this chapter, all of relatively recent incarnation compared to their progenitor observational counterparts, should be appreciated less for their differences and more for their common lineage. These more recent designs are the evolutionary culmination of a long-held view that causal inference in populations is not fundamentally a comparison of individuals to each other, but is instead a collective comparison of single individuals to themselves. This view is rendered practical via the use of empirically-derived or hypothetical exposure distributions, such as in case-crossover and case-specular studies, respectively, thus supplanting the need for an external comparison group. It seems inevitable that future advances in both design and analysis will build upon this conceptualization. As epidemiologists employ these new designs and contrast them with older ones, the designs will undoubtedly undergo even greater scrutiny with respect to their assumptions and limitations. Such circumspection will particularly be necessary when conflicts in findings resulting from use of the different designs arise. These conflicts, however, should be regarded as the natural consequence of a progressive series of improvements in epidemiologic methods that will inevitably lead to more valid assessment of potential causal relations.

References

Barlow WE, Ichikawa L, Rosner D, Izumi S (1999) Analysis of case-cohort designs. J Clin Epidemiol 52:1165–1172

Begg CB, Zhang ZF (1994) Statistical analysis of molecular epidemiology studies employing case series. Cancer Epidemiol Biomarkers Prev 3:173–175

Cornfield J (1951) A method of estimating comparative rates from clinical data. JNCI 11:1269–1275

Ellsworth DL, Manolio TA (1999) The emerging importance of genetics in epidemiologic research. I. Basic concepts in human genetics and laboratory technology. Ann Epidemiol 9:1–16

Garcia-Closas M, Thompson WD, Robins JM (1998) Differential misclassification and the assessment of gene-environment interactions in case-control studies. Am J Epidemiol 147:426–433

Greenland S (1982) The effect of misclassification in matched-pair case-control studies. Am J Epidemiol 116:402–406

Greenland S (1996) Confounding and exposure trends in case-crossover and case-time-control designs. Epidemiol 7:231–239

Greenland S (1999) A unified approach to the analysis of case-distribution (case-only) studies. Stat Med 18:1–15

Greenland S, Thomas DC (1982) On the need for the rare disease assumption in case-control studies. Am J Epidemiol 116:547–553

Greenland S, Robins JM (1985) Estimation of a common effect parameter from sparse follow-up data. Biometrics 41:55–68

Kelsey JL, Whittemore AS, Evans AS, Thompson WD (1996) Methods in Observational Epidemiology, second edition. Oxford University Press, New York, pp 122–125

Khoury MJ (1997) Genetic epidemiology and the future of disease prevention and public health. Epidemiol Rev 19:175–180

Kupper LL, McMichael AJ, Spirtas R (1975) A hybrid epidemiologic study design useful for estimating relative risk. J Am Stat Assoc 70:524–528

Langholz B, Thomas DC (1990) Nested case-control and case-cohort methods of sampling from a cohort: a critical comparison. Am J Epidemiol 131:169–176

Little RJ, Rubin DR (2000) Causal effects in clinical and epidemiological studies via potential outcomes: concepts and analytical approaches. Annu Rev Public Health 21:121–145

Maclure M (1991) The case-crossover design: a method for studying transient effects on the risk of acute events. Am J Epidemiol 133:144–153

Maclure M, Mittleman MA (2000) Should we use a case-crossover design? Annu Rev Public Health 21:193–221

Miettinen OS (1976) Estimability and estimation in case-referent studies. Am J Epidemiol 103:226–235

Miettinen OS (1982) Design options in epidemiologic research: an update. Scand J Work Environ Health 8 (Suppl 1):7–14

Mittleman MA, Maclure M, Robins JM (1995) Control sampling strategies for case-crossover studies: an assessment of relative efficiency. Am J Epidemiol 142:91–98

Navidi W (1998) Bidirectional case-crossover designs for exposures with time trends. Biometrics 54:596–605

Navidi W, Weinhandl E (2002) Risk set sampling for case-crossover designs. Epidemiol 13:100–105

Prentice RL (1986) A case-cohort design for epidemiologic cohort studies and disease prevention trials. Biometrika 73:1–11

Redelmeier DA, Tibshirani RJ (1997) Interpretation and bias in case-crossover studies. J Clin Epidemiol 50:1281–1287

Sato T (1992a) Maximum likelihood estimation of the risk ratio in case-cohort studies. Biometrics 48:1215–1221

Sato T (1992b) Estimation of a common risk ratio in stratified case-cohort studies. Stat Med 11:1599–1605

Suissa S (1995) The case-time-control study. Epidemiol 6:248–253

Suissa S (1998) The case-time-control design: further assumptions and conditions. Epidemiol 9:441–445

Szklo M, Nieto J (2000) Epidemiology: Beyond the basics. Aspen Publishers, Gaithersburg, MD, pp 33–38

Vines SK, Farrington CP (2001) Within-subject exposure dependency in case-crossover studies. Stat Med 20:3039–3049

Wacholder S (1991) Practical considerations in choosing between case-cohort and nested case-control designs. Epidemiol 2:155–158

Wacholder S, Boivin JF (1987) External comparisons with the case-cohort design. Am J Epidemiol 126:1198–1209

Wertheimer N, Leeper E (1979) Electrical wiring configurations and childhood cancer. Am J Epidemiol 109:273–284

Wilcox AJ, Weinberg CR, Lie RT (1998) Distinguishing the effects of maternal and offspring genes through studies of "case-parent triads". Am J Epidemiol 148:893–901

Yang Q, Khoury MJ (1997) Evolving methods in genetic epidemiology. III. Gene-environment interaction in epidemiologic research. Epidemiol Rev 19:33–43

Yang Q, Khoury MJ, Flanders WD (1997) Sample size requirements in case-only designs to detect gene-environment interaction. Am J Epidemiol 146:713–720

Zaffanella LE, Savitz DA, Greenland S, Ebi KL (1998) The residential case-specular method to study wire codes, magnetic fields, and disease. Epidemiol 9:16–20

Intervention Trials

I.8

Silvia Franceschi, Martyn Plummer

Introduction

Most human diseases have avoidable causes. This is true not only of infectious diseases, but also a large proportion of cardio-vascular diseases and cancer (Doll and Peto 1981). A major goal of epidemiology is therefore to find the causes of disease in a population and then intervene to remove them.

As discussed by Doll (2002), an agent may be considered to be a cause of a disease if increased exposure to the agent is followed by an increased risk of the disease, and decreased exposure by a decreased risk. This is an empirical definition which may be tested without reference to a specific mechanism. It is particularly useful for chronic diseases, such as cancer, which may take decades to develop, and in which the disease process may involve a variety of preclinical changes before the disease manifests itself. Intervention to remove a cause of disease may then range from behavioural changes, such as tobacco control (IARC 2003), to minimizing consequences of accumulated damages by, for example, regression of precancerous lesions using anti-oxidant vitamins (Stewart et al. 1996).

Descriptive and observational epidemiological studies have provided considerable evidence for causal relationships and have, in some instances, provided the final answer (Doll 2002). However, observational studies are not always sufficient to motivate large scale public health interventions as they have some important limitations. Firstly, when relative risks of the order 2 or less are observed, it is difficult to rule out bias and confounding as possible explanations for the association. A second limitation of observational studies is that they rely on "experiments of nature" – unplanned variation in exposure within and between populations – and cannot therefore evaluate the effect of interventions that attempt to block the disease process in a way that is not found in nature. Two examples are a cholesterol lowering drug (Heart Protection Study Collaborative Group 2002b) or a prophylactic vaccine against human papillomavirus (HPV) (Koutsky et al. 2002). Both of these interventions are motivated by a large body of observational evidence as well as understanding of the mechanism of disease. However, the magnitude of the benefit from intervention cannot be evaluated from observational data. The third limitation of observational studies is that it is very difficult to balance the benefits of intervention against possible risks. Finally, observational data does not always provide evidence that exposure to an agent preceded incidence, which is an indispensable requirement for establishing causality. All of these limitations can be overcome by a properly conducted intervention trial. An intervention trial is an experiment to evaluate the efficacy of an intervention so that its more widespread use can be justified.

Intervention trials ideally take the form of a randomized controlled trial (RCT) in which the intervention is compared with a control (which may consist of no intervention at all, or a placebo) and the allocation to treatment or control is randomized. RCTs are often used for *therapeutic trials* in which different treatments for a given disease are compared in a clinical setting. This application of RCTs is beyond the scope of this chapter, which is concerned with trials on healthy, or apparently healthy individuals with the aim of preventing future morbidity or mortality. We refer to such trials as *preventive trials*. An important subclass of preventive trial is the *community intervention trial* in which the intervention is applied to groups instead of individuals.

Since RCTs offer a unique opportunity to eliminate the problems that beset observational studies, the results of such trials are generally considered to be a "gold standard", and are often taken to outweigh previous observational evidence in the case of discordant results. However, the advantages of RCTs are easily lost through poor conduct or analysis. Hence RCTs are held to much higher standards of conduct and reporting (see Sect. 8.1.1). These standards are especially important in view of the high cost of RCTs which makes them very difficult to reproduce.

Guidelines for Reporting of Clinical Trials: The CONSORT Statement 8.1.1

The CONSORT (Consolidated Standards of Reporting Trials) statement is a set of guidelines for reporting of randomized controlled trials (RCTs). These guidelines take the form of a checklist of 22 items (see Table 8.1) which should be included in a report of a randomized trial, and a model flow chart to show the flow of participants through the trial (see Fig. 8.1).

The guidelines were created by an international group of clinical trialists, statisticians, epidemiologists and biomedical journals in an effort to improve the quality of reporting of RCTs, which several reviews had shown to be inadequate. Without adequate reporting, it is not possible for a reader to judge the quality of a trial and so trust its conclusions.

Table 8.1. Checklist of items to include when reporting a randomized trial

PAPER SECTION And topic	Item	Description
TITLE AND ABSTRACT	1	*How participants were allocated to interventions* (e.g., "random allocation", "randomized", or "randomly assigned").
INTRODUCTION Background	2	*Scientific background and explanation of rationale.*
METHODS Participants	3	*Eligibility criteria for participants and the settings and locations where the data were collected.*
Interventions	4	*Precise details of the interventions intended for each group and how and when they were actually administered.*
Objectives	5	*Specific objectives and hypotheses.*

table to be continued

Table 8.1. (continued)

PAPER SECTION And topic	Item	Description
Outcomes	6	*Clearly defined primary and secondary outcome measures* and, when applicable, any *methods used to enhance the quality of measurements* (e.g., multiple observations, training of assessors).
Sample size	7	*How sample size was determined* and, when applicable, *explanation of any interim analyses and stopping rules.*
Randomization – sequence generation	8	*Method used to generate the random allocation sequence,* including *details of any restriction* (e.g., blocking, stratification).
Randomization – allocation concealment	9	*Method used to implement the random allocation sequence* (e.g., numbered containers or central telephone), clarifying whether the sequence was concealed until interventions were assigned.
Randomization – implementation	10	*Who generated the allocation sequence, who enrolled participants, and who assigned participants to their groups.*
Binding (masking)	11	*Whether or not participants, those administering the interventions, and those assessing the outcomes were blinded to group assignment.* When relevant, *how the success of blinding was evaluated.*
Statistical methods	12	*Statistical methods used to compare groups for primary outcome(s); Methods for additional analyses,* such as subgroup analyses and adjusted analyses.
Results Participant flow	13	*Flow of participants through each stage* (a diagram is strongly recommended). Specifically, for each group report the numbers of participants randomly assigned, receiving intended treatment, completing the study protocol, and analyzed for the primary outcome. *Describe protocol deviations from study as planned, together with reasons.*
Recruitment	14	*Dates defining the periods of recruitment and follow-up.*

table to be continued

Table 8.1. (continued)

PAPER SECTION And topic	Item	Description
Baseline data	15	*Baseline demographic and clinical characteristics of each group.*
Numbers analyzed	16	*Number of participants (denominator) in each group included in each analysis and whether the analysis was by "intention-to-treat".* State the results in absolute numbers when feasible (e.g., 10/20, not 50%).
Outcomes and estimation	17	*For each primary and secondary outcome, a summary of results for each group, and the estimated effect size and its precision* (e.g., 95% confidence interval).
Ancillary analyses	18	*Address multiplicity by reporting any other analyses performed,* including subgroup analyses and adjusted analyses, indicating those pre-specified and those exploratory.
Adverse events	19	*All important adverse events or side effects in each intervention group.*
DISCUSSION		
Interpretation	20	*Interpretation of the results,* taking into account study hypotheses, sources of potential bias or imprecision and the dangers associated with multiplicity of analyses and outcomes.
Generalizability	21	*Generalizability (external validity) of the trial findings.*
Overall evidence	22	*General interpretation of the results in the context of current evidence.*

(Source: http://www.consort-statement.org/)

The original CONSORT statement was published in 1996 (Begg et al. 1996). It was revised in 2001 and is available in a short form (Moher et al. 2001) and a long form with explanation and elaboration (Altman et al. 2001). The guidelines have been adopted by a growing number of biomedical journals and editorial committees.

Further details can be seen at the website: http://www.consort-statement.org/

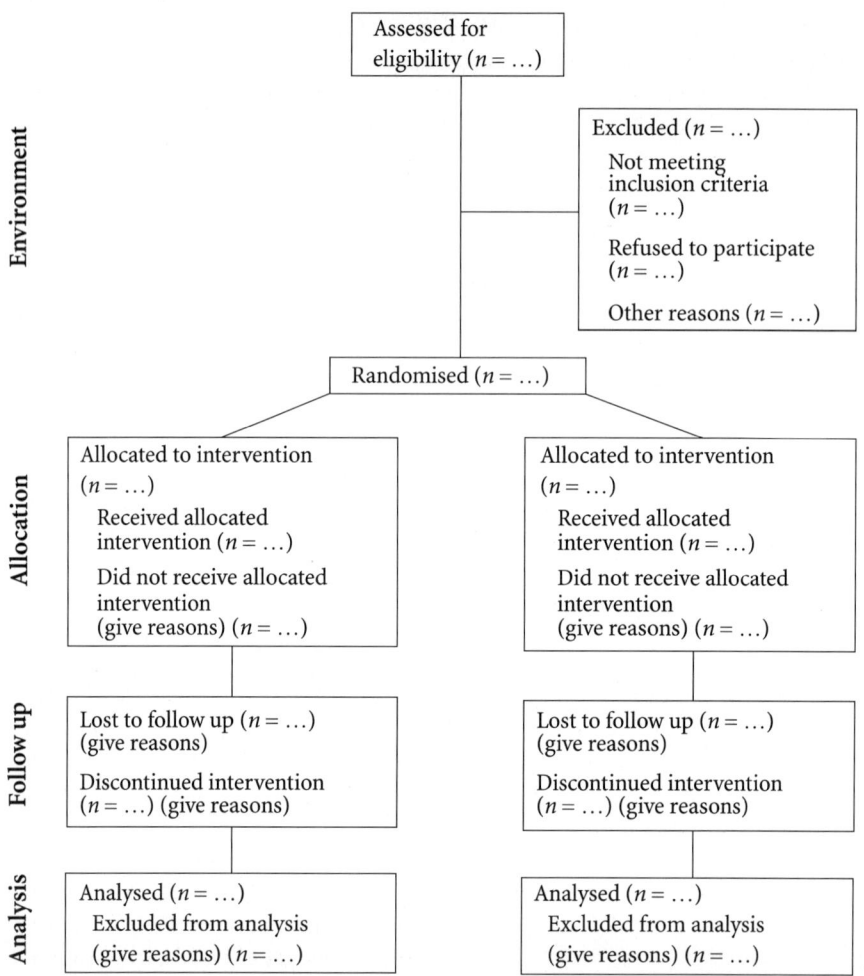

(Source: http://www.consort-statement.org/)

Figure 8.1. Revised template of the CONSORT diagram showing the flow of participants through each stage of a randomized trial

8.2   Therapeutic versus Preventive Trials

The methodological considerations for therapeutic and preventive trials are very similar. In particular, in the last two decades, therapeutic trials have grown in size. Some therapeutic trials have been able to randomize many thousands of individuals – as in breast and intestinal cancer – or even tens of thousands, as has occasionally been possible in heart disease (ISIS-2 (Second International Study of Infarct Survival) Collaborative Group 1988) and stroke (CAST (Chinese Acute Stroke Trial) Collaborative Group 1997). In this chapter, we will rely heavily upon the experience gained in the performance of therapeutic trials. (For details on prevention in general please refer to Chap. III.10 of this handbook.)

Although there is no clear dividing line between therapeutic and preventive trials, a crucial factor distinguishing the two kinds of trial is the "exposure window". In a therapeutic trial, the timing of an intervention is determined by a disease indication. In a prevention trial, the intervention may take place at any point along a disease process that may last several decades. The appropriate timing of the intervention is not always evident. Often the decision on when to intervene is determined by the practical requirement to have a sufficient number of cases of disease in the control group by the end of the trial. This limits interventions to individuals who are at an advanced stage of the preclinical disease process. Examples of such trials are the prevention of recurrence of colorectal adenomas (Bonithon-Kopp et al. 2000; Jacobs et al. 2002), and prevention of lung cancer in middle-aged heavy smokers, or workers exposed to asbestos (Omenn et al. 1996a; ATBC Cancer Prevention Study Group 1994). The paradox of such late interventions, however, is that they may miss the "exposure window" within which the intervention may possibly have a protective effect.

Surrogate Endpoints 8.2.1

Intervention may also take place at an early stage of the disease process. For example, a prophylactic vaccine against human papillomavirus given during adolescence (Koutsky et al. 2002) is intended to prevent occurrence of cervical cancer in middle age. The success of such interventions may need to be judged in terms of surrogate endpoints, since the time interval between intervention and disease outcome may be prohibitively long.

It is difficult to conduct intervention trials using disease endpoints, such as cancer, that are rare or have a long latency. Such studies may require very large numbers, or long follow-up time, or both in order to yield a sufficient number of cases to judge the efficacy of the intervention. One possible strategy to overcome this problem is to use a surrogate endpoint – a short term marker of the disease process – as a substitute for a hard endpoint such as disease incidence or death. The use of surrogate endpoints may also be necessary for ethical reasons if the hard endpoint is preventable. For example, a vaccine against human papillomavirus (HPV) may prevent cervical cancer, but this disease is already preventable by screening, in which precursors of cervical cancer are identified and treated. A trial of an HPV vaccine must therefore be based on these precursors rather than cervical cancer incidence.

The promise of surrogate endpoints is that they may make intervention trials smaller, faster or cheaper. Despite the attractiveness of this promise, the use of surrogate endpoints is fraught with difficulty. Schatzkin and colleagues have, in a series of articles, reviewed the problems of using surrogate endpoints in cancer research (Schatzkin et al. 1990, 1996; Schatzkin and Gail 2002). They suggest that there are currently only two clear candidates for surrogate endpoints in cancer research: prevention of HPV infection for subsequent cervical cancer, and prevention of colorectal adenomas for subsequent colorectal cancer. Apart from these two examples, they suggest that surrogate endpoints may have more use in phase II trials than phase III trials (for a definition of phase II and phase III trials see Table 8.2).

Table 8.2. Phases of intervention trials

Phase	Aims	Comment
I	Route of administration and dosage: maximally tolerated dose by using a dose escalation scheme	Often on volunteers
II	Evidence of "activity" of our intervention by means of "promising" outcome measures	Better randomized than not
III	Efficacy of an intervention by means of randomized comparisons and a "definite" endpoint	
IV	Effectiveness of proven interventions in wide-scale use, sometimes through post-marketing surveillance	Better randomized than not

The problem of statistical validation of surrogate endpoints is an area of active research. In a seminal paper, Prentice (1989) suggested the following definition of a valid surrogate: it must yield a valid test of the null hypothesis of no association between treatment and the true response. In operational terms, this means that the incidence rate of the true disease must be independent of the treatment history given the current value of the surrogate endpoint. Prentice's criterion is unlikely to be satisfied in practice, and some attempts have been made to broaden the definition of a surrogate endpoint by quantifying the proportion of treatment effect explained by a surrogate (Freedman et al. 1992). This extension has not been widely accepted, however. A summary of current research is given by the report of an NIH (US National Institutes of Health) workshop on surrogate endpoints (de Gruttola et al. 2001).

8.2.2 From Observation to Intervention

Another particularity of preventive trials is that, whereas the choice of intervention may be suggested by observational studies, the intervention may be a radical simplification of those observations. This is especially true in nutritional epidemiology (see Chap. III.4 of this handbook), where chemoprevention (e.g. administration of specific vitamins) has often been used as a substitute for dietary modification. This simplification involves an extra level of extrapolation – above issues of timing, dose, and duration – which makes the results of such studies particularly hard to interpret when they contradict observational studies.

Intervention studies can sometimes produce results suggesting that a treatment is harmful, increasing the risk of disease instead of decreasing it. The most notorious example is the use of beta-carotene supplements to prevent lung cancer (see Example 1).

Example 1. *Beta-Carotene and Lung Cancer: An unexpected harmful effect of treatment*

One of the most consistent findings in nutritional epidemiology is the protective effect of fresh fruit and vegetable consumption on cancer risk (World Cancer Research Fund-American Institute for Cancer Research 1997). In 1981 Peto et al. (1981) put forward the hypothesis that beta-carotene was the active agent responsible for this protective effect, and subsequently a number of cancer chemoprevention trials were conducted using supplementation with beta-carotene as an intervention. The ATBC (Alpha-Tocopherol Beta-Carotene Cancer Prevention Study Group 1994) and CARET (Omenn et al. 1996b) trials were two large chemoprevention trials using beta-carotene, in a factorial design, in subjects at high risk of lung cancer, i.e. long-term heavy smokers (ATBC/CARET) or asbestos exposed workers (CARET). The ATBC trial showed a higher incidence of lung cancer among subjects receiving beta-carotene compared with those who did not with a relative risk of 1.6 (95% CI 1.02–1.33). Subsequently, the intervention with beta-carotene in the CARET study was stopped 21 months early, after a median of 3.7 years of follow-up because of clear evidence of no benefit and substantial evidence of possible harm. The actively treated group had a relative risk of lung cancer of 1.28 (95% CI 1.04–1.57) compared with the group receiving placebo. The results of the Physicians Health Study (PHS) were published at the same time (Hennekens et al. 1996), and showed no effect of beta-carotene on lung cancer risk, with 82 cases of lung cancer in the beta-carotene group and 88 in the placebo group. However the PHS had low power to detect small changes in lung cancer risk due to the small number of cases.

The trials of beta-carotene relied on a number of extrapolations from observational data. The first extrapolation was that beta-carotene was the active agent in the protective effect observed for fresh fruits and vegetables. Although direct associations with plasma levels of beta-carotene have also been observed, it may be that beta-carotene is acting as a marker for fresh fruit and vegetable consumption and is not the active agent. The second extrapolation concerns the dose level. The dose of beta-carotene given, and the median serum beta-carotene concentration achieved in these studies exceeded by many times the level that could be achieved by normal dietary intake (IARC 1998), and it is possible that beta-carotene becomes harmful at such high doses, while remaining protective at doses associated with a healthy diet. Last, but not least, it was assumed that high-risk, middle-aged, individuals, who probably harboured pre-malignant lesions in the lung, would benefit from the same active substances that were believed to be beneficial in the prevention of early stages of carcinogenesis.

When planning an intervention study, it may be a useful exercise to consider the possible interpretations of adverse effects of treatment. This thought experiment may reveal weaknesses in the motivation for, or design of, the intervention study.

◆

8.3 The Origin of Randomized Trials

The technique of randomization was originally developed in agricultural experiments in the 1920s when individual plots of land were randomized. Trials in humans strictly controlled by random allocation date back to the mid-1940s. Many of the earliest trials were carried out in Britain by the Medical Research Council (Hill 1962). The first trial in which treatment was randomly allocated to individuals, although not the first to be reported (Doll 1998), was a prevention trial designed to test the efficacy of immunization against whooping cough (Medical Research Council Whooping-Cough Immunization Committee 1951). Parents of children aged 6–18 months were asked to volunteer to have their children entered into the trial. They were given a pamphlet describing the study, which included the information that half the inoculations would not be against whooping cough but would be "anti-catarrhal". No child was entered until a consent form had been received.

The spread of randomization, until it became an essential requirement for the licensing of new drugs, was initially slow and not without opposition. Many clinicians considered randomization to be less worthy than the use of criteria to distinguish between individuals who will and will not respond to the intervention. There is currently no competing methodology for randomized controlled trials, although there are attempts to adapt the practice of randomization to special contexts and difficulties (Lavori and Kelsey 2002).

8.4 Planning of Trials

Trials are traditionally classified into four phases (Table 8.2). In this chapter we will be dealing only with issues related to phase III and phase IV randomized trials. For design issues of phase I and phase II trials readers are referred elsewhere (Simon 2001).

The organization of a trial requires careful advance planning. This is particularly true for multi-centric trials, which have become increasingly common. The aims and methods of the trial should be described in detail in a protocol document. This will contain the scientific background of the problem under study. In topics where a substantial amount of work has already been done, a systematic review (meta-analysis, see Chap. II.7 in this handbook) of the outcomes of published randomized trials on the same type of intervention is highly preferable to a narrative review. A meta-analysis will, in fact, greatly help to evaluate the consistency of previous work, any avoidable pitfalls in study design, and the most likely effectiveness of the intervention under study. The latter information allows the trial size to be calculated (see Chap. II.1 of this handbook). The protocol should also include clear statements about: (1) preventive measures to be used (intervention); (2) types of individuals or groups to be admitted (participants); (3) assessment of response (endpoints); (4) entry criteria and treatment allocation;

(5) exclusions, withdrawals, and protocol departures; (6) size and/or duration of the trial; (7) strategy for the statistical analysis; and (8) ethical aspects.

Definition of the Intervention 8.5

The effectiveness of interventions to be compared in randomized primary prevention trials are usually known in broad terms from the outset. Many questions of primary prevention have first been evaluated in trials of treatments or secondary prevention. For example, when the Physicians' Health Study (Steering Committee of the Physicians' Health Study Research Group 1989) was begun, the hypothesis that aspirin could be effective in the primary prevention of cardiovascular disease was widely accepted, given the extensive evidence from secondary prevention or treatment trials of those who had already experienced a cardiovascular event (ISIS-2 (Second International Study of Infarct Survival) Collaborative Group 1988). Similarly, the suggestion to use tamoxifen or the new selective estrogen receptor modulators (e.g. raloxifene) in the primary prevention of breast cancer came from the observation that tamoxifen reduced the incidence of contra-lateral breast cancer when used in the adjuvant setting (Early Breast Cancer Trialists' Collaborative Group 1998). Such previous experiences in "diseased" people have generally established a "safety profile" and enabled exclusion or estimation of side effects that occur once in thousands (if not necessarily in ten thousands) of recipients of a certain type of drug. Other times, when the intervention consists in behavioral changes, clues of the benefits of certain life-style modifications (e.g., smoking cessation, dietary changes, adoption of safe sex behavior) have been brought about by consistent knowledge on risk factors accumulated in a large variety of contexts (e.g., ecological studies, studies of observational epidemiology or, as it is the case for some infectious agents, clear knowledge on the routes of transmission of the infections). Based on this background knowledge, two major questions need to be addressed in order to identify unambiguously the type of intervention study.

The first question concerns what is being compared with what. The basic design for primary prevention trials is a two-arm comparison. As discussed by Green (2002), however, this simple structure can encompass a variety of different comparisons, as shown in Table 8.3.

Table 8.3. Possible types of comparison in intervention trials

Intervention versus	No intervention
	Placebo
	Another intervention
	Same intervention at a higher dose (or longer duration)
	Same intervention, but later (only for participants who experience a certain event)

The feasibility and necessity to include a placebo arm depend on the nature of the intervention and of the outcome measure. When two drugs are being compared it is generally easy to create a placebo, provided that the route of administration is an oral one. In therapeutic trials, the use of a non-active compound has caused ethical concerns. A comparison of new treatment with old treatment is often more appropriate. As noted by Temple and Ellenberg (2000), however, placebo controls are ethical if there are no permanent adverse consequence of delaying or omitting available treatment, and if the subjects are fully informed about their alternatives. These favourable conditions typically apply to preventive trials. For intra-muscular treatments (e.g., vaccines), the use of one or more "dummy injections" is hard to justify. It has, however, been advocated in special circumstances. In a randomized trial of a prophylactic vaccine against HPV type 16, a sexually transmitted virus which is now considered a necessary cause of cervical cancer, three injections of the aluminium adjuvant used in the active vaccine were deemed justifiable in order to avoid possible imbalances in the sexual behavior of the young female participants, and to evaluate side effects attributable to the active agent (i.e. virus like particles) (Koutsky et al. 2002). Indeed, the percentage of women who discontinued the study owing to an adverse effect of treatment (0.4%), was the same in the vaccine arm and the placebo arm (Koutsky et al. 2002).

One way to avoid the use of placebo is to compare different doses or durations of a specific intervention. This is typically feasible when some type of drug or dietary supplement, whose minimal effective dose is unclear, is under evaluation. More frequently, however, in prevention trials, it is the intensity of the intervention that can be modulated. In behavioral intervention trials, it is often very useful to compare a labour-intensive and expensive package for smoking cessation or dietary changes with some simple and inexpensive message at a community or individual level (e.g., pamphlets, simple recommendations from one's practitioner, etc.).

Finally, the timing of the intervention can be randomized into an early versus delayed intervention trial. This approach is very often indicated in therapeutic trials (e.g., chemo- or radio-therapy at primary cancer diagnosis versus the same therapy at cancer recurrence), but is has some appeal in certain prevention trials as well. An example is provided by cervical cancer screening, which is currently based on use of the Papanicolaou (Pap) smear to detect abnormal cells that may indicate pre-cancerous lesions on the cervix. The majority of such lesions regress without intervention, but a few may progress to cervical cancer over the course of several years. HPV testing is now considered a more sensitive test than Pap smear in the detection of pre-cancerous lesions (Cuzick et al. 2000). Its use is already approved in the triage of cytological abnormalities. Thus, an appropriate design for testing the efficacy of HPV testing in cervical cancer screening would be to use Pap smear in both arms, and compare the concurrent use of HPV testing and Pap smear in one arm with delayed HPV testing in the other arm among women with abnormal Pap smear findings.

Factorial Design

The factorial design represents an efficient alternative to two-arm comparisons. The simplest design is the balanced 2×2 factorial but factorial designs can be generalized to more than two dimensions (Table 8.4). In a factorial design, two or more interventions are simultaneously tested in the same population. Allocation of interventions is carried out in such a way that there is no association between different interventions in the study population, and therefore no confounding, under the assumption that there is no interaction between interventions. As noted by Armitage and Berry (1987), this design contravenes a good principle of experimentation, namely that only one factor should be changed at a time. The principal advantage of the factorial design is its ability to answer two or more questions in a single trial.

Table 8.4. Illustration of the factorial design with 8000 subjects and 3 possible treatments. As the number of treatments simultaneously under test increases, the number of subjects receiving each combination of treatment diminishes, but the number receiving any given treatment (e.g. treatment A) is always 4000

Arm	Number of subjects	Treatment A	B	C
		Two arm trial of treatment A		
1	4000	yes		
2	4000	no		
		2×2 trial of treatments A and B		
1	2000	yes	yes	
2	2000	yes	no	
3	2000	no	yes	
4	2000	no	no	
		$2 \times 2 \times 2$ trial of treatments A, B and C		
1	1000	yes	yes	yes
2	1000	yes	yes	no
3	1000	yes	no	yes
4	1000	yes	no	no
5	1000	no	yes	yes
6	1000	no	yes	no
7	1000	no	no	yes
8	1000	no	no	no

In a recent trial of 20,536 UK adults with occlusive arterial disease or diabetes (Heart Protection Study Collaborative Group 2002a, b), participants were randomly allocated in a factorial design to receive 40 mg of simvastatin (a cholesterol-lowering agent) or placebo, and antioxidant vitamin supplementation or placebo.

These two interventions seemed to be, at the time the study was started, equally promising. It would have been possible to evaluate the two interventions separately in two independent trials, but this would have required twice the sample size, or over 40,000 participants. A highly significant 18% proportional reduction in the coronary death rate was found among participants who had received simvastatin. This beneficial effect was reflected also in an overall mortality reduction compared to the placebo group. Conversely, antioxidant vitamins did not produce any significant reduction in the 5-year mortality from, or incidence of, any type of vascular disease, cancer, or other major outcome. An asset of the factorial design is also the opportunity to evaluate interactions, i.e., whether two interventions in combination differ, with respect to efficacy or side effects, from either intervention alone. In the HPSCG trial, for instance, the efficacy of simvastatin was not modified by antioxidant vitamins.

The factorial design, on account of the corresponding gain in cost efficiency, is especially valuable in prevention trials that are, on average, much larger than therapeutic trials. A factorial design is often excluded out of fear of complicating trial operations. In fact, the randomization process can be easily adapted to allocate participants to different combinations of interventions. As mentioned by Buring (2002), it is, however, essential that none of the interventions under evaluation: (1) complicates eligibility criteria by, for instance, important contraindications for certain interventions; or (2) causes any side effect that could lead to poor compliance or loss to follow-up.

8.7   Definition of Participants

Eligibility criteria in intervention studies must aim at three things: (1) optimizing the potential benefit to the participants while minimizing the risk of adverse effects; (2) enrolling participants who are likely to adhere to the intervention and follow-up requirements; and most importantly (3) including a sufficiently large number of participants to produce unambiguous results even if the benefit of the intervention is small. In many types of trial, but especially in preventive trials, broad eligibility criteria are desirable because they can simplify enrolling procedures and avoid the need for complicated and expensive tests at study entry (See Box 1).

A "run-in" period can be implemented in order to allow potential participants who have difficulties adhering the protocol to withdraw prior to actual randomization. As discussed by Buring (2002), the actual format of the run-in period depends on the nature of the trial. In trials of pill-taking regimens, as in the HPSCG (Heart Protection Study Collaborative Group 2002a, 2002b) factorial trial of simvastatin and antioxidant vitamins, the run-in period involved a few-week period of placebo, to allow review of blood exams, followed by a few weeks of active treatment, to allow a pre-randomization assessment of LDL (low density lipoprotein)-lowering responsiveness of each individual and to exclude major adverse effects. In studies of behavioral interventions, the run-in period may consist of attendance at visits

Box 1. Large, Simple Randomized Trials

Many lives could be saved by moderate reductions in the common causes of death.

In a series of articles, Peto and colleagues (Collins et al. 1987; Peto et al. 1995; Peto and Baigent 1998; Yusuf et al. 1984) have promoted the idea of large, simple randomized trials to investigate the benefits of widely practicable treatments for common conditions. The essence of their argument is that only large, randomized trials can answer questions about moderate health benefits in a way that is free of bias and the play of chance. Moderate reductions in mortality may correspond to a large number of deaths prevented if the condition is common and the treatment is widely available. For example 100,000 deaths per year could be prevented or substantially delayed in developed countries by routine use of antiplatelet therapy in all patients with clinical evidence of occlusive vascular disease. This reduction corresponds to a 10% reduction in all vascular deaths in the age range 35–69 (Antiplatelet Trialists' Collaboration 1994).

Examples of the large randomized trials promoted by Peto and colleagues include the ISIS (International Study of Infarct Survival) trials ISIS-1 (First International Study of Infarct Survival) Collaborative Group 1986; ISIS-2 1988; ISIS-3 1992; ISIS-4 1995) in which tens of thousands of subjects were randomized. The need to randomize such large numbers of subjects imposes some design constraints on the trial. In particular, the entry criteria, treatment and data requirements must all be greatly simplified. In order to simplify the entry criteria into large trials, Peto et al. (1995) have proposed an "uncertainty principle", which states that the sole eligibility criterion for entry is that both patient and doctor should be substantially uncertain about the appropriateness for this particular patient of each of the trial treatments (A more complete statement is given by Peto and Baigent (1998)). Broad eligibility criteria can simplify enrolling procedures and avoid the need for complicated and expensive tests at study entry.

The principle of conducting large, simple randomized trials is not appropriate for the development of novel drugs. In this context, an extensive regulatory framework has developed, which is summarized by the guidelines of the International Conference on Harmonization of Technical Requirements for Registration of Pharmaceuticals for Human Use (http://www.ich.org). Conversely, it should be noted that the regulatory framework for drug development is not necessarily appropriate when conducting public health interventions using existing treatments.

or laboratory procedures, including completion of forms similar to those that would be used in the actual trial. Restricting a prevention trial to proven good compliers may result in a subject pool that differs from the general population with respect to outcomes. This problem may be perceived as a loss of external validity or generalizability of trial findings. As noted, however, by Hennekens and Buring (1998), the primary requirement of a generalizable study is internal validity, which may in fact be increased by the exclusion of poor compliers.

A more practical way to improve the generalizability of the results of a trial is to broaden eligibility criteria as much as possible, thus allowing the benefits of trial participation to be available more widely across populations. In the HPSCG study, for instance, substantial benefit was demonstrated not only in those already known to have had coronary disease, but also in those without diagnosed coronary disease who had cerebrovascular disease, peripheral arterial disease, or diabetes, irrespective of the blood lipid concentrations when treatment was initiated. Widespread implementation of these findings on the basis of some clinical diagnoses would therefore be relatively straightforward, without the need for extensive screening in the general population. Finally, broad eligibility criteria can also allow to enroll a larger number of participants and, in some instances, some cautious subgroup analysis.

An eligibility criterion which, however, allows substantial efficiency gain, and which must therefore be seriously considered, is high risk for the disease meant to be prevented. Age, sex, or family or personal history might be considered to identify such individuals. Since the power of the study is proportional to the number of endpoints, not simply to the number of participants enrolled, an intervention study which includes high-risk individuals will be small and of shorter duration (and, as a consequence, cheaper and likelier to be accomplished) than a study which includes lower risk participants. The demonstration of a benefit among those with high-risk characteristics will have to be applied, however, with great caution to a more heterogeneous population.

8.8   Enrollment

Enrollment of thousands participants in prevention trials is a major challenge and deserves to be monitored carefully. Since prevention studies do not require diseased people, hospitals are not frequent sources of participants. Out-patient clinics are, however, used in some secondary prevention studies.

A preliminary question in community-based enrollment is whether trial participants can be volunteers, provided they meet the eligibility criteria and can be recruited in the required number, or whether it is necessary to extend an invitation to join the study to all eligible persons in a predefined area. If the former applies, local media, pamphlet distribution, and direct contacts with special associations can be used in order to invite as many participants as required. In the previously mentioned trial of a vaccine against HPV 16, for instance, young women were recruited in the United States through advertisements on college campuses and in the surrounding communities (Koutsky et al. 2002). In order to diminish the probability of enrolling women who were infected with HPV16, only women who reported that they had no more than five male sex partners during their lifetime were eligible for participation. Obviously, in such instances, it will be impossible to evaluate accurately the fraction of the persons who eventually opted for participating in the trial, let alone any difference between participants and non-participants. This approach is, however, the only possibility when participants are defined according to life-style characteristics (e.g., current smoking habit, overweight, sleeping disorders, sexual habits, etc.) that cannot be derived from administrative records.

In other instances, however, it may be important to have access to the entire list of the population of a pre-defined area, and to make an effort to achieve, as much as possible, high participation or, at least, to estimate the participation fraction. This is necessary when the results of the trial must be generalizable to the whole of the host population, and in particular when the trial must include certain subgroups. In developed countries, complete and fairly well up-dated population lists can be found (e.g., censuses, electoral rolls, general practitioners' lists, etc.). In the latter, a direct involvement of general practitioners in the recruitment of their own patients is known to improve the yield of participants (Knatterud 2002).

In most developing countries, especially in the many areas where substantial migrations from rural to urban areas are ongoing, reliable population lists are seldom available, and a door-to-door enumeration of the target population of the trials is generally a prerequisite of the recruitment exercise. The complete enumeration of the target population is especially important in the evaluation of interventions such as immunization programs or screening programs, where a good coverage is essential for the efficacy of the intervention. The participation fraction (i.e., the acceptance of the intervention) becomes part of the evaluation of the intervention under study. A high participation rate is also especially important in cluster-randomized trials (see below).

Randomization 8.9

An eligible participant should be admitted formally to the trial, by entry of his or her name into a register and the allocation of a serial number. The random allocation of the intervention should be determined after entry or a run-in period. The fundamental reason for random allocation is to maximize the likelihood that each type of patient will be allocated in similar proportions to the different interventions being investigated. The decision to enter a participant must be made irreversibly regardless of which trial arm the participants will be allocated. This precludes systematic allocation systems and discourages easily guessable coding systems, such as one in which an active intervention is coded as A and the placebo as B, which may lead to unblinding of the study. The bias inherent in non-randomized studies may be more severe in therapeutic trials (where diseased patients can differ substantially according to prognostic factors, at least in the clinician's opinion) but is not negligible in preventive trials as well.

A common allocation technique, discussed by Knatterud (2002), is to generate a separate randomization schedule for each of the trial sites and, within each site, to have some blocking so that, after a fixed number of participants enrolled, there will be equal numbers assigned to each trial arm. It is advisable to make smaller blocks at the beginning, when the enrollment capacity of trial sites is unknown. Ideally, there should be a central office where the randomization is carried out. This ensures good record keeping and adherence to the protocol. A telephone call to the randomization office can include some verification of the patients eligibility before randomization. With current technology, it is possible to implement an automated menu-driven telephone system that is available 24 hours a day, 7 days a week (Heart Protection Study Collaborative Group 2002b). Elaborate "stratification" schemes in which a separate randomization block is made for participants with different characteristics are not encouraged in large trials (Peto et al. 1976). Proper statistical methods (see Chap. II.3 of this handbook) can make due allowance, when comparing interventions, for what was initially known about each participant.

8.10 Cluster Randomization

Interventions in communities or other groups have frequently been investigated without using randomization. Longitudinal studies of the health consequences of water fluoridation (Horowitz 1996), and initial cardiovascular disease prevention studies such as the North Karelia Project (Puska et al. 1976) provided early evidence that community-level health interventions could benefit large groups of individuals. However, non-randomized community intervention trials may be confounded by secular trends. For example, in the two studies cited above, the incidence of dental caries and cardiovascular disease may have diminished due to widespread use of fluoridated toothpaste and improvements in the treatment of hypertension, respectively.

The use of randomization is, therefore, just as important for community trials as for individual-level studies, but it is not appropriate to randomize individuals when the intervention is defined at the group level. Instead, groups of individuals or "clusters" are randomized. A cluster may be defined geographically (e.g., cities, countries, villages) or otherwise (e.g., workplaces, schools, clinical practices) (Atienza and King 2002). Cluster randomization can also avoid the potential for contamination between interventions. Furthermore, cluster randomization by village improves the chances of long duration follow-up in developing countries where personal identifiers, such as name and date of birth, are unreliable (Gambia Hepatitis Study Group 1987), but strong community links exist.

The main consequence of randomizing clusters is that the outcomes for trial participants in the same cluster are no longer independent. This lack of independence has implications for both analysis and design. The analysis of the study must take into account the presence of the clusters. Various techniques for doing so are reviewed by Donner (1998). If the clustering effect is ignored, as in 70% of cluster trials reviewed by Divine et al. (1992), p-values will be artificially small, and confidence intervals will be over-narrow. Even if a correct statistical analysis is used, the power of a cluster-randomized trial is reduced compared to an individually randomized trial. When the outcome of the trial is the mean of a continuous variable (e.g. serum cholesterol level) the increase in sample size needed to maintain the same power as an individually randomized study is given by the formula $1 + (m - 1)r$, where m is the number of subjects per cluster and r is the intra-cluster correlation coefficient (Kerry and Bland 1998), which measures the proportion of variation of the outcome in the study population that is due to differences between clusters. Typical values of r are very close to zero, but when the number of subjects per cluster (m) is large, there may be a serious loss of efficiency compared with an individually randomized study.

A large number of clusters also increases the possibility that the randomization will produce balanced intervention groups compared to trials where a small number of clusters has been allocated. "Restricted randomization" after matching or stratifying communities according to selected factors has been attempted. In the Community Intervention Trial for Smoking Cessation (COMMIT Research Group 1991), for instance, investigators examined eleven pairs of communities that were matched on socio-demographic factors. Matching is only justified for variables that are strongly related to the outcome of interest (Klar and Donner 1997). The same principle applies to case-control studies (see Chap. I.6 of this handbook).

Notwithstanding unsolved issues, cluster design can greatly contribute to the evaluation of preventive strategies and methodological advances should be pursued.

Trial Outcome(s) 8.11

Prevention trial design generally distinguishes between primary and secondary outcomes (Anderson and Prentice 1999). The primary outcome is typically the clinical disease to be prevented or controlled that provides the central justification for the trial, and determines the study size. Secondary outcomes are disease events that also motivated the trial, but that by themselves would be unlikely to justify a full-scale intervention.

The outcome measurements could be influenced by a knowledge of which intervention was used, thus producing serious bias. In a single-blinded trial, the identity of the allocated treatment is concealed from the participants. A double-blinded trial is one in which the doctor, or other technical expert, who assesses response also is unaware of the intervention identities. As discussed by Green (2002), it may not be desirable to extend blinding to the independent data and safety monitoring board (DSMB). The DSMB, as often stated in the participant's consent form, is the watcher of accumulating data and need, therefore, to be aware of the allocation.

Unlike therapeutic trials, large prevention trials cannot rely on outcomes that require frequent clinical visits for specialized tests or potential adverse reactions.

Indeed, the safety of any intervention has to be documented before the planning of any large preventive trial. Furthermore, even if participants in preventive trials are selected on the basis of elevated risk for the diseases that are targeted for the prevention, primary outcome events may constitute a small minority of the disease events experienced by study subjects during the course of the trial, and perhaps even a small minority of disease events that may in some way be affected by intervention activities. Hence, there is an obligation to define sets of outcomes to be fully ascertained, including often overall mortality, that provide an opportunity to assess the overall risks and benefits in the target population.

The International Breast Cancer Intervention Study (IBIS-I), for instance, was a double-blind placebo-controlled randomized trial of tamoxifen, 20 m/day for 5 years, in 7152 women at increased risk of breast cancer (IBIS Investigators 2002). The primary outcome measure was the frequency of the breast cancer, but outcomes other than breast cancer were found to be very important, too. A 32% reduction (95% confidence interval, CI: 8–50%) in the primary outcome was found. It was accompanied, however, by a 2.5-fold increase (95% CI: 1.5–4.4) in thromboembolic events. Eventually, there was a significant excess of deaths from all causes in the tamoxifen group (25 versus 11, $p = 0.028$). The conclusions of IBIS-I were that the overall risk to benefit ratio for the use of tamoxifen in prevention was still unclear, and continued follow-up of the trial was essential.

Although sample size determination is dealt with elsewhere in this volume (Chap. II.1 , the dangers of an inadequate statistical power on intervention studies cannot be overemphasized. More than therapeutic trials, preventive trials cannot be easily replicated, for economical and logistic reasons, and collaborative re-analyses can seldom remedy at the lack of definitive answer from a specific trial. As discussed by Buring (2002), every effort should be made during the planning phase of the trial to choose an adequate size and length of follow-up. Secular declines in disease rates within the general population, and the failure to achieve a sufficient sample size or to accrue sufficient endpoints are frequent in prevention trials. Extending the duration of the trial is often a good option to achieve a more definite result for a relatively small increase in total cost.

8.12   Follow-up, Exclusions and Withdrawal

Various aspects of the statistical analysis of follow-up data from intervention trials are dealt with elsewhere in this volume (Chaps. II.2, II.3, II.4 and II.6).

The series of articles by Peto et al. (1976, 1977) gives a clear and comprehensive overview of the analysis of long-term follow-up in randomized controlled trials. Survival analysis is the standard method of analyzing time-to-event data because it makes use of the full information and can take into account right censoring, which occurs when the study ends or when subjects are lost to follow-up. Interval censoring can also occur when the events under study are only known to have occurred in some interval in time. For example, if the event is not death but some measurement that requires a clinical examination (e.g., the appearance or the disappearance of HPV infection, which is asymptomatic and requires a specimen of exfoliated cervical cells for detection), the exact time of the event is unknown, except that it occurred between two subsequent visits. Appropriate statistical methods can take this uncertainty into account.

Censoring resulting from losses and dropouts are problematic if the censoring is "informative" (i.e., related to outcome), a situation that is difficult to rule out. As noted by Peto et al. (1977), "rigorous entry criteria are not necessary for a randomized trial, but rigorous follow-up is. Even patients who do not get the proper intervention must not be withdrawn from the analysis". Often referred to as analysis by intention to treat, this approach is the only one that provides a valid answer to a real question. It tests the "policy" (or intention) to be evaluated at the time of randomization. Every possible effort must therefore be made, at the level of trial design and implementation, to identify and, as much as possible, avoid any cause of non-adherence. This entails a run-in period and a simplified follow-up protocol.

A special problem, different from the one of losses at follow-up, is represented by participants who may be discovered to contravene the eligibility criteria after randomization. In a double-blind trial of a prophylactic vaccine against HPV 16, 2392 young women were randomized (Koutsky et al. 2002). Since the tested vaccine was not supposed to work among women who were already infected with HPV 16, 36% of the randomized trial participants were subsequently excluded, mainly because HPV tests revealed that they were already infected at enrollment. In principle, no bias should have been introduced, since the results of HPV tests became available only after the randomization. An alternative would have been to postpone the randomization, but this was considered impractical. The trial by Koutsky et al. (2002), however, was the first test of a vaccine against HPV. It was not meant to test a "policy" of vaccination in the general population, but the efficacy of a new vaccine under optimal conditions (i.e. among women unexposed to HPV). A larger, population-based trial of HPV vaccine would be necessary to evaluate the effectiveness of HPV vaccine as a tool for cervical cancer control (Plummer and Franceschi 2002). Analysis of such a trial by intention to treat would give the programmatic efficacy of the vaccine programme, which is distinct from the efficacy of the vaccine itself.

Finally, a special challenge is represented by the follow-up of community-based health interventions. As discussed by Atienza and King (2002) and Koepsell et al. (1992), it is typically not possible to assess all individuals of interest in the selected communities. Two main approaches to obtaining these longitudinal individual-level data are: (1) to follow-up groups of individuals over time and (2) to assess different cross-sections in each time period. Several large-scale community-based interventions (e.g., COMMIT) have utilized both approaches, cognizant of different strengths and weaknesses (Koepsell et al. 1992).

8.13 Conclusions

The randomized controlled trial is one of the most powerful tools available in epidemiology. It allows the evaluation of a disease risk factor that is free from the play of bias and chance and may also, with an appropriate design, give a quantitative estimate of the public health benefit that may be expected from an intervention.

Even well conducted randomized controlled trials have problems of interpretation. These problems centre on the generalizability of the findings and concern not only the selection of the study participants, but also the timing, dose and duration of the intervention and the length of time over which a beneficial effect was observed. If there are no such problems, the results of randomized controlled trials may be taken to provide a definitive answer and, in particular, overrule the results from observational studies when these disagree. In general, however, the results of intervention trials must be considered as part of the spectrum of available evidence that includes observational studies in humans and experimental data that provide mechanistic evidence.

References

Alpha-Tocopherol Beta Carotene Cancer Prevention Study Group (1994) The effect of vitamin E and beta carotene on the incidence of lung cancer and other cancers in male smokers. N Engl J Med 330:1029–1035

Altman DG, Schulz KF, Moher D, Egger M, Davidoff F, Elbourne D, Gotzsche PC, Lang T (2001) The revised CONSORT statement for reporting randomized trials: explanation and elaboration. Ann Intern Med 134:663–694

Anderson GL, Prentice RL (1999) Individually randomized intervention trials for disease prevention and control. Stat Methods Med Res 8:287–309

Antiplatelet Trialists' Collaboration (1994) Collaborative overview of randomised trials of antiplatelet therapy–I: Prevention of death, myocardial infarction, and stroke by prolonged antiplatelet therapy in various categories of patients. BMJ 308:81–106

Armitage P, Berry G (1987) Statistical methods in medical research. Blackwell, Oxford

ATBC (Alpha-Tocopherol Beta Carotene) Cancer Prevention Study Group (1994) The alpha-tocopherol, beta-carotene lung cancer prevention study: design, methods, participant characteristics, and compliance. Ann Epidemiol 4:1–10

Atienza AA, King AC (2002) Community-based health intervention trials: an overview of methodological issues. Epidemiol Rev 24:72–79

Begg C, Cho M, Eastwood S, Horton R, Moher D, Olkin I, Pitkin R, Rennie D, Schulz KF, Simel D, Stroup DF (1996) Improving the quality of reporting of randomized controlled trials. The CONSORT statement. JAMA 276:637–639

Bonithon-Kopp C, Kronborg O, Giacosa A, Rath U, Faivre J (2000) Calcium and fibre supplementation in prevention of colorectal adenoma recurrence: a randomised intervention trial. European Cancer Prevention Organisation Study Group. Lancet 356:1300–1306

Buring J E (2002) Special issues related to randomized trials of primary prevention. Epidemiol Rev 24:67–71

CAST (Chinese Acute Stroke Trial) Collaborative Group (1997) CAST: randomised placebo-controlled trial of early aspirin use in 20,000 patients with acute ischaemic stroke. Lancet 349:1641–1649

Collins R, Gray R, Godwin J, Peto R (1987) Avoidance of large biases and large random errors in the assessment of moderate treatment effects: the need for systematic overviews. Stat Med 6:245–254

COMMIT Research Group (1991) Community Intervention Trial for Smoking Cessation (COMMIT): summary of design and intervention. J Natl Cancer Inst 83:1620–1628

Cuzick J, Sasieni P, Davies P, Adams J, Normand C, Frater A, van Ballegooijen M, van den Akker-van Marle E (2000) A systematic review of the role of human papilloma virus (HPV) testing within a cervical screening programme: summary and conclusions. Br J Cancer 83:561–565

De Gruttola VG, Clax P, DeMets DL, Downing GJ, Ellenberg SS, Friedman L, Gail MH, Prentice R, Wittes J, Zeger SL (2001) Considerations in the evaluation of surrogate endpoints in clinical trials. summary of a National Institutes of Health workshop. Control Clin Trials 22:485–502

Divine GW, Brown JT, Frazier LM (1992) The unit of analysis error in studies about physicians' patient care behavior. J Gen Intern Med 7:623–629

Doll R (1998) Controlled trials: the 1948 watershed. BMJ 317:1217–1220

Doll R (2002) Proof of causality: deduction from epidemiological observation. Perspect Biol Med 45:499–515

Doll R, Peto R (1981) The causes of cancer: quantitative estimates of avoidable risks of cancer in the United States today. J Natl Cancer Inst 66:1191–1308

Donner A (1998) Some aspects of the design and analysis of cluster randomized trials. Appl Statist 47:95–113

Early Breast Cancer Trialists' Collaborative Group (1998) Tamoxifen for early breast cancer: an overview of the randomised trials. Lancet 351:1451–1467

Freedman LS, Graubard BI, Schatzkin A (1992) Statistical validation of intermediate endpoints for chronic diseases. Stat Med 11:167–178

Gambia Hepatitis Study Group (1987) The Gambia Hepatitis Intervention Study. Cancer Res 47:5782–5787

Green SB (2002) Design of randomized trials. Epidemiol Rev 24:4–11

Heart Protection Study Collaborative Group (2002a) MRC/BHF Heart Protection Study of antioxidant vitamin supplementation in 20,536 high-risk individuals: a randomised placebo-controlled trial. Lancet 360:23–33

Heart Protection Study Collaborative Group (2002b) MRC/BHF Heart Protection Study of cholesterol lowering with simvastatin in 20,536 high-risk individuals: a randomised placebo-controlled trial. Lancet 360:7–22

Hennekens CH, Buring JE (1998) Validity versus generalizability in clinical trial design and conduct. J Card Fail 4:239–241

Hennekens CH, Buring JE, Manson JE, Stampfer M, Rosner B, Cook NR, Belanger C, LaMotte F, Gaziano JM, Ridker PM, Willett W, Peto R (1996) Lack of effect of long-term supplementation with beta carotene on the incidence of malignant neoplasms and cardiovascular disease. N Engl J Med 334:1145–1149

Hill AB (1962) Statistical methods in clinical and preventive medicine. Livinstone, Edinburgh

Horowitz HS (1996) The effectiveness of community water fluoridation in the United States. J Public Health Dent 56:253–258

IARC (1998) Carotenoids. IARC handbooks of cancer prevention 2. International Agency for Research on Cancer, Lyon

IARC (2003) Tobacco smoke and involuntary smoking. IARC monographs on the evaluation of carcinogenic risks to humans 83, IARC Press, Lyon

IBIS Investigators (2002) First results from the International Breast Cancer Intervention Study (IBIS-I): a randomised prevention trial. Lancet 360:817–824

ISIS-1 (First International Study of Infarct Survival) Collaborative Group (1986) Randomised trial of intravenous atenolol among 16 027 cases of suspected acute myocardial infarction: ISIS-1. Lancet 2:57–66

ISIS-2 (Second International Study of Infarct Survival) Collaborative Group (1988) Randomised trial of intravenous streptokinase, oral aspirin, both, or neither among 17,187 cases of suspected acute myocardial infarction: ISIS-2. Lancet 2:349–360

ISIS-3 (Third International Study of Infarct Survival) Collaborative Group (1992) ISIS-3: a randomised comparison of streptokinase vs tissue plasminogen activator vs anistreplase and of aspirin plus heparin vs aspirin alone among 41,299 cases of suspected acute myocardial infarction. Lancet 339:753–770

ISIS-4 (Fourth International Study of Infarct Survival) Collaborative Group (1995) ISIS-4: a randomised factorial trial assessing early oral captopril, oral mononitrate, and intravenous magnesium sulphate in 58,050 patients with suspected acute myocardial infarction. Lancet 345:669–685

Jacobs ET, Giuliano AR, Roe DJ, Guillen-Rodriguez JM, Hess LM, Alberts DS, Martinez ME (2002) Intake of supplemental and total fiber and risk of colorectal adenoma recurrence in the wheat bran fiber trial. Cancer Epidemiol Biomarkers Prev 11:906–914

Kerry SM, Bland JM (1998) The intracluster correlation coefficient in cluster randomisation. BMJ 316:1455

Klar N, Donner A (1997) The merits of matching in community intervention trials: a cautionary tale. Stat Med 16:1753–1764

Knatterud GL (2002) Management and conduct of randomized controlled trials. Epidemiol Rev 24:12–25

Koepsell TD, Wagner EH, Cheadle AC, Patrick DL, Martin DC, Diehr PH, Perrin EB, Kristal AR, Allan-Andrilla CH, Dey LJ (1992) Selected methodological issues in evaluating community-based health promotion and disease prevention programs. Annu Rev Public Health 13:31–57

Koutsky LA, Ault KA, Wheeler CM, Brown DR, Barr E, Alvarez FB, Chiacchierini LM, Jansen KU (2002) A controlled trial of a human papillomavirus type 16 vaccine. N Engl J Med 347:1645–1651

Lavori P, Kelsey J (eds) (2002) Clinical trials. Epidemiol Rev 24:1–90

Medical Research Council Whooping-Cough Immunization Committee (1951) The prevention of whooping cough by vaccination. Br Med J 1951, i: 1463–1471

Moher D, Schulz KF, Altman DG (2001) The CONSORT statement: revised recommendations for improving the quality of reports of parallel-group randomised trials. Lancet 357:1191–1194

Omenn GS, Goodman G, Thornquist M, Barnhart S, Balmes J, Cherniack M, Cullen M, Glass A, Keogh J, Liu D, Meyskens F, Jr., Perloff M, Valanis B, Williams J, Jr. (1996a) Chemoprevention of lung cancer: the beta-Carotene and Retinol Efficacy Trial (CARET) in high-risk smokers and asbestos-exposed workers. IARC Sci Publ 67–85

Omenn GS, Goodman GE, Thornquist MD, Balmes J, Cullen MR, Glass A, Keogh JP, Meyskens FL, Valanis B, Williams J H, Barnhart S, Hammar S (1996b) Effects of a combination of beta carotene and vitamin A on lung cancer and cardiovascular disease. N Engl J Med 334:1150–1155

Peto R, Baigent C (1998) Trials: the next 50 years. Large scale randomised evidence of moderate benefits. BMJ 317:1170–1171

Peto R, Collins R, Gray R (1995) Large-scale randomized evidence: large, simple trials and overviews of trials. J Clin Epidemiol 48:23–40

Peto R, Doll R, Buckley JD, Sporn MB (1981) Can dietary beta-carotene materially reduce human cancer rates? Nature 290:201–208

Peto R, Pike MC, Armitage P, Breslow NE, Cox DR, Howard SV, Mantel N, McPherson K, Peto J, Smith PG (1976) Design and analysis of randomized clinical trials requiring prolonged observation of each patient. I. Introduction and design. Br J Cancer 34:585–612

Peto R, Pike MC, Armitage P, Breslow NE, Cox DR, Howard SV, Mantel N, McPherson K, Peto J, Smith PG (1977) Design and analysis of randomized clinical trials requiring prolonged observation of each patient. II. analysis and examples. Br J Cancer 35:1–39

Plummer M, Franceschi S (2002) Strategies for HPV prevention. Virus Res 89: 285–293

Prentice RL (1989) Surrogate endpoints in clinical trials: definition and operational criteria. Stat Med 8:431–440

Puska P, Koskela K, Pakarinen H, Puumalainen P, Soininen V, Tuomilehto J (1976) The North Karelia Project: a programme for community control of cardiovascular diseases. Scand J Soc Med 4:57–60

Schatzkin A, Freedman LS, Dorgan J, McShane LM, Schiffman MH, Dawsey SM (1996) Surrogate end points in cancer research: a critique. Cancer Epidemiol Biomarkers Prev 5:947–953

Schatzkin A, Freedman LS, Schiffman MH, Dawsey SM (1990) Validation of intermediate end points in cancer research. J Natl Cancer Inst 82:1746–1752

Schatzkin A, Gail M (2002) The promise and peril of surrogate end points in cancer research. Nat Rev Cancer 2:19–27

Simon R (2001) Clinical trials in cancer. In: DeVita VT, Hellman S, Rosenberg SA (eds) Cancer: principles and practice of oncology. Lippincott Williams & Wilkins, Philadelphia, PA, p 521

Steering Committee of the Physicians' Health Study Research Group (1989) Final report on the aspirin component of the ongoing Physicians' Health Study. N Engl J Med 321:129–135

Stewart BW, McGregor D, Kleihues P (eds) (1996) Principles of chemoprevention, IARC Scientific Publications 139. International Agency for Research on Cancer, Lyon

Temple R, Ellenberg SS (2000) Placebo-controlled trials and active-control trials in the evaluation of new treatments. Ann Int Med 133:455–463

World Cancer Research Fund – American Institute for Cancer Research (CRF-AICR) (1997) Food, nutrition and the prevention of cancer: a global perspective. American Institute for Cancer Research, Washington DC

Yusuf S, Collins R, Peto R (1984) Why do we need some large, simple randomized trials? Stat Med 3:409–422

Confounding and Interaction I.9

Neil Pearce, Sander Greenland

9.1 # Introduction

All epidemiologic studies are (or should be) based on a particular *source population* followed over a particular *risk period*. The goal is usually to estimate the effect of one or more exposures on one or more health outcomes. When we are estimating the effect of a specific exposure on a specific health outcome, *confounding* can be thought of as a mixing of the effects of the exposure being studied with the effect(s) of other factor(s) on the risk of the health outcome of interest. *Interaction* can be thought of as a modification, by other factors, of the effects of the exposure being studied on the health outcome of interest, and can be subclassified into two major concepts: *biological dependence of effects*, also known as synergism; and *effect-measure modification*, also known as heterogeneity of a measure. Both confounding and interaction can be assessed by stratification on these other factors (i.e. the potential confounders or effect modifiers). The present chapter covers the basic concepts of confounding and interaction and provides a brief overview of analytic approaches to these phenomena. Because these concepts and methods involve far more topics than we can cover in detail, we provide many references to further discussion beyond that in the present handbook, especially to relevant chapters in Modern Epidemiology by Rothman and Greenland (1998).

9.2 # Confounding

9.2.1 ## Basic Concepts

Confounding occurs when the exposed and non-exposed subpopulations of the source population have different background disease risks, which is to say: these subpopulations would have different disease risks even if exposure had been absent from both subpopulations (Greenland and Robins 1986; Rothman and Greenland 1998 Chap. 4; Greenland et al. 1999a,b). When we estimate the effect of exposure on the exposed by comparing the frequency of disease in the exposed and non-exposed groups, we assume that the disease frequency in the non-exposed group provides a valid estimate of what the disease frequency would have been in the exposed group if it had not been exposed. If this assumption is incorrect, i.e. if the exposed and non-exposed groups would have had different disease frequencies in the counterfactual situation in which the exposed group had not been exposed, then we say that the comparison of the exposed group to the non-exposed group is confounded.

More generally, confounding can arise when the exposed and non-exposed group are not completely comparable or "exchangeable" with respect to their exposure response; that is, for at least one level of exposure, the exposed and unexposed groups would exhibit different risks even if they both had experienced that exposure level (Greenland and Robins 1986). Note that the earlier definition takes this level to be that of non-exposure because it is presumed there that the effect of exposure on the exposed is the effect of interest. If instead we were interested in the effect of non-exposure on the non-exposed (as might be the case in a study of a preventive factor), we would have confounding if the exposed group failed to exhibit the risk that the non-exposed would have had if they had been exposed.

This problem of non-comparability (non-exchangeability) can also occur in randomized trials because randomization may fail, leaving the treatment groups with different characteristics (and different baseline disease risk) at the time that they enter the study, or because of differential loss and non-compliance across treatment groups. However, there is more concern about non-comparability in observational epidemiology studies because of the absence of randomization. Randomization prevents certain sources of confounding (e.g., confounding due to physician selection of treatment based on patient characteristics, also known as "confounding by indication"); also, bias due to differential loss and non-compliance can be at least partially controlled by using the randomization indicator (the "intent-to-treat" variable) as an instrumental variable (Sommer and Zeger 1991; Greenland 2000a). These benefits of randomization are not available in observational studies, and in fact confounding should be expected to occur as a by-product of ordinary life events and choices.

As an example, if we compare the risk of lung cancer in people with a low dietary beta carotene intake compared with people with a high dietary beta carotene intake, it is very likely that these two groups will differ with respect to other risk factors for lung cancer such as tobacco smoking, because people who are less health conscious are more likely to smoke as well as to neglect dietary recommendations. If this is the case (e.g. if a greater percentage of people smoke in the low beta carotene intake group than in the high beta carotene intake group), then smoking will confound the association between beta carotene intake and lung cancer: The higher smoking prevalence among those with a low beta carotene diet will lead to a higher lung-cancer risk among them compared to those with a high beta carotene diet, even if beta carotene intake itself has no effect on lung cancer risk.

Any variable that affects disease in the absence of exposure has the potential to confound the exposure-disease relationship. It will confound that relationship if, in the absence of exposure, it would have a distribution that is sufficiently different across exposure groups to produce a difference in risk across those groups even if exposure were absent. This was the case for smoking in the beta carotene example. A confounder, if not adequately controlled, will bias the estimated effect of exposure on disease. The bias will be upward if the higher-risk levels of the confounder occur more frequently among the exposed; conversely, the bias will be downward if the higher-risk levels of the confounder occur more frequently among the unexposed. Confounding may even reverse the apparent direction of an effect in extreme situations. Confounding may also occur when the main exposure under study has no effect on the risk of disease – a spurious association may be observed which is entirely due to confounding. Factors associated with confounders can also act like confounders and serve as surrogates for confounders, provided that they are not affected by exposure or disease. For example, socioeconomic status may serve as a surrogate measure of causal factors (living conditions, lifestyle, lack of preventive care, etc.) that are potential confounders.

Three conditions are traditionally given as necessary (but not sufficient) for a factor to be a confounder (Rothman and Greenland 1998, Chap. 8). First, to produce confounding, a factor has to be predictive of disease in the absence of the exposure under study. Note that a confounder need not be a genuine cause of the disease under study, but merely "predictive" within exposure levels apart from chance relations. Hence, surrogates for causal factors (e.g., ethnicity, gender, socioeconomic status) may be regarded as potential confounders, even if they are not direct causal factors. It is not always clear from the data whether an observed relation between the factor and disease represents a genuine (replicable) predictive quality, as opposed to (say) chance. In making such a determination, prior information as opposed to statistical testing should play a dominant role (Greenland and Neutra 1980; Miettinen and Cook 1981; Robins and Morgenstern 1987). This is why one almost always sees adjustment made for age and sex: these factors are known to be predictive of risk of most diseases. When prior information is not available one must of course turn to the data collected for the study as a guide as to whether the factor is predictive of disease in the source population; even in these cases, however, there are better strategies for confounder selection than those based on statistical testing. We will return to this topic below.

Second, a confounder has to be associated with the study exposure in the source population. It may occur that when participants in a case-control study are selected from the source population, then due to chance a factor may be associated with exposure in the study, even though it was not associated with exposure in the source population. In this situation, the factor is not a confounder (Miettinen and Cook 1981; Robins and Morgenstern 1987). Although in practice it is common to use the data actually collected to decide whether a factor is associated with exposure, more commonly the data are used to decide whether adjustment for the factor makes an important difference in the estimated exposure effect, a practice we will discuss below. In a case-control study, one should expect a confounder to be associated with exposure among the controls (at least if the controls are selected with no bias). If the factor is not associated with exposure among controls, an association may still occur among the cases simply because the study factor and a potential confounder are both risk factors for the disease, but this is a consequence of those effects and so does not cause confounding. A factor-exposure association will only indicate confounding by the factor if it reflects the association in the source population.

Third, a variable that is affected by the exposure or by the disease, e.g., an intermediate in the causal pathway between exposure and disease, or conditions that are caused by the health outcome of interest, should not be treated as a confounder because to do so could introduce serious bias into the results (Greenland and Neutra 1980; Robins and Morgenstern 1987; Robins and Greenland 1992; Weinberg 1993; Rothman and Greenland 1998, Chap. 8; Cole and Hernan 2002). For example, in a study of obesity and death from coronary heart disease, it would be inappropriate to control for hypertension if it was considered that hypertension was a consequence of obesity, and hence a part of the causal chain leading from obesity to death from coronary heart disease. On the other hand, if hypertension itself was of primary interest, then this would be studied directly, and obesity would be regarded as a potential confounder if it also involved exposure to other risk factors for death from coronary heart disease.

Similarly, we should avoid controlling for health outcomes that may be part of the pathogenic disease process, such as reduced pulmonary function following exposure to a respiratory hazard in a study of chronic obstructive lung disease (Checkoway et al. 2004). We would, however, be justified in controlling for baseline (i.e. pre-exposure) lung function if there were reasons to believe that baseline lung function was associated with subsequent exposure level. Evaluating whether certain factors are exposure or health outcome intermediates in causal pathways requires information external to the study. Intermediate variables can sometimes be included in the analysis, although special techniques are then required to avoid adding bias (Robins 1989; Robins and Greenland 1994; Robins et al. 1992, 2000). In no case would control of a variable affected by the disease be valid, however (Greenland et al. 1999a; Pearl 2000).

Thus, an assessment of confounding by a factor that is not an intermediate involves consideration of whether the exposed and non-exposed groups are "comparable" in the source population with respect to their disease risk in the absence of exposure. In practice, we often focus on specific potential confounders – variables that are risk predictive of disease in the absence of exposure (such as age and sex) and assess whether they are associated with exposure in the source population on which the study was based. If such an association is present, it is evidence that the two groups are not comparable or exchangeable with respect to baseline risk. If such an association is absent, however, it does not mean that the groups are comparable, because there may be other uncontrolled risk factors that confound the observed association, or the association may have been obscured by measurement error.

Because it involves judgments about causal as well as temporal ordering, the property of being a confounder cannot be determined from data alone (Miettinen and Cook 1981; Greenland and Robins 1986; Greenland et al. 1999a; Pearl 2000; Robins 2001; Hernan et al. 2002). Once that ordering is established, however, it is common to assess confounding by seeing whether the main effect estimate changes when the potential confounder is controlled in the analysis. In this approach, near-equality of the crude and adjusted effect estimates is taken as evidence that there is no confounding by the factor, and conversely, an important difference is taken as evidence of confounding by the factor. Many epidemiologists prefer to make a decision based on the basis of this "collapsibility" or "change-in-estimate" criterion (rather than the criterion of "exchangeability"), although this approach can be misleading, particularly if (as usual) there is misclassification of the adjustment factors or the exposure (Greenland 1980; Greenland and Robins 1985; Savitz and Baron 1989; Marshall and Hastrup 1996, 1999) or if the outcome is common and the measure is an odds ratio or rate ratio (Miettinen and Cook 1981; Greenland 1996;

Greenland et al. 1999b); also, this criterion does not exhibit good statistical properties, although it is no worse than significance-testing procedures (Maldonado and Greenland 1993).

The decision to control for a presumed confounder can be made with more confidence if there is supporting prior knowledge that the factor is predictive of disease, independent of its association with exposure. Such prior knowledge is usually available for well-studied factors such as age, sex, and tobacco smoking. At the very least, it is usually known if the factor is affected by exposure (in which case it is not a potential confounder and should not be controlled, at least not by conventional methods). If even this much is uncertain, the decision to control or not control a variable may be controversial, in which case analyses both with and without its control may be presented (Greenland and Neutra 1980).

As a final caution, in studies involving aggregate-level effect (such ecologic and multilevel studies), a factor at one level may, if not controlled, confound effect estimates at another level, and a factor may modify and confound effects differently at different levels of aggregation. For example, both the income of an individual and the income of his or her neighbourhood may separately predict risk of an outcome, possibly in opposite directions. Robbery rates are often higher in low-income neighbourhoods, yet within neighbourhoods it could still be that an individual's risk of robbery went up as his or her income went up. In that case both neighbourhood income and individual income could be confounders, but would confound effect estimates in opposite directions if both were positively and separately associated with the exposure under study. Thus, regardless of level of interest (e.g., country, neighbourhood, individual), it is often essential to measure and adjust for variables on other levels (Greenland 2001a).

9.2.2   Example of Confounding

Table 9.1 presents a hypothetical example of confounding in a cross-sectional study of asthma. Overall, one-half of the study participants are smokers and one-half are not. However, two-thirds of the exposed group are smokers compared with one-

Table 9.1. Hypothetical example of confounding by tobacco smoking in a study of occupational asthma

	Smokers		Non-smokers		Total	
	Exposed	Non-exposed	Exposed	Non-exposed	Exposed	Non-exposed
Asthma cases	800	400	200	400	1000	800
Non-cases	1200	600	800	1600	2000	2200
Total	2000	1000	1000	2000	3000	3000
Prevalence (%)	40	40	20	20	33.3	26.7
Prevalence ratio	1.0		1.0		1.25	

third of the non-exposed workers. Thus, although exposure is not associated with asthma either among smokers (the prevalence of asthma is 40% in the exposed and 40% in the non-exposed, PR = 1.0) or in non-smokers (the prevalence of asthma is 20% in the exposed and 20% in the non-exposed, PR = 1.0), it is associated with asthma (PR = 1.25) when the two subgroups are combined. This occurs because smoking is associated with the exposure in the source population, and is an independent risk factor for asthma. In this hypothetical example, the two stratum-specific estimates are each 1.00, thus the adjusted estimate will also be 1.00 (or very close to 1.00) whatever weights are used. Thus, the crude prevalence ratio is 1.25, whereas the adjusted prevalence ratio is 1.00, indicating that confounding has occurred (provided that there has not been biased selection of the study participants from the source population).

Control in the Study Design   9.2.3

Confounding can be controlled in the study design, in the analysis, or both. There are three common methods for control at the design stage (Rothman and Greenland 1998). The first is randomization – random allocation of participants to exposure categories. However, this is usually only an option for potentially beneficial exposures, e.g. it would be impractical and unethical to conduct a randomized trial of the health effects of smoking, and as mentioned earlier randomization may fail to prevent all confounding.

A second method of control at the design stage is to restrict the study to narrow ranges of values of the potential confounders, e.g., by restricting the study to white males aged 35–54. This approach has a number of conceptual and computational advantages, but may severely restrict the number of potential study subjects and ultimately limit the generalizability of the study.

A third method of control involves matching study subjects on potential confounders. For example, in a cohort study one could match a white male non-exposed subject aged 35–39 with an exposed white male aged 35–39. This will prevent age-gender-ethnicity confounding in a cohort study, but is seldom done because it is expensive and time-consuming. In case-control studies, matching does not prevent confounding, but does facilitate its control in the analysis in that matching on a strong confounder will usually increase the precision of effect estimates. However, matching may reduce precision in a case-control study if it is done on a factor which is associated with exposure, but is not a risk factor for the disease of interest. The matching process effectively turns such a factor into a confounder, which must then be controlled in the analysis, thus reducing precision and increasing analytical complexity. For example, in a case-control study of power-frequency electromagnetic field (EMF) exposure and childhood cancer, choosing sibling controls (i.e. for each case choosing a sibling as a control) would mean that in almost every instance, the case and control would have lived in the same house and would have similar EMF exposure, resulting in almost no exposure-discordant pairs and almost no precision in the resulting matched-pair estimates.

As already mentioned, matching may be expensive and time-consuming. Finding suitable controls becomes increasingly difficult as the number of matching factors increases beyond two or three. Moreover, when it occurs the increase in precision from matching is often modest, typically involving a 5 to 15 percent reduction in the variance of the effect estimate (Schlesselman 1982; Thomas and Greenland 1983). Therefore, although many discussions of matching stress issues of statistical efficiency, practical considerations (such as ease of finding controls) are often more important (Rothman and Greenland 1998, Chap. 10).

9.2.4   Control in the Analysis

Confounding can also be controlled in the analysis by adjusting simultaneously for all confounding factors or a sufficient subset of them. This presumes, of course, that a sufficient subset has been accurately measured, which is often not the case. Methods for controlling confounding in the analysis are discussed in more depth in the chapters on specific study designs (Chaps. I.5, I.6 and I.8 of this handbook), in Part II of this handbook and in many textbooks (e.g. Rothman and Greenland 1998, Chaps. 15–21). In the simplest situation, control of confounding in the analysis involves stratifying the data according to the levels of the confounder(s) and calculating an effect estimate that summarizes the association across strata of the confounder(s). As an example, controlling for age (grouped into 5 categories) and gender (with 2 categories) might involve grouping the data into the $10 (= 5 \times 2)$ confounder strata and calculating a summary effect estimate, which is a weighted average of the stratum-specific effect estimates. It is usually not possible to control simultaneously for more than 2 or 3 confounders in a stratified analysis, since finer stratification will often lead to many strata containing no exposed or no non-exposed persons. Such strata are uninformative; thus, too fine stratification is wasteful of information. This problem can be mitigated to some extent by the use of regression modeling (cf. Chap. II.3 of this handbook), which allows for simultaneous control of more confounders by "smoothing" the data across confounder strata.

9.2.5   Assessment of Confounding

When one lacks data on a suspected confounder, and thus cannot control confounding directly, it is still desirable to assess the likely direction and magnitude of the confounding. In particular, it may be possible to obtain information on a surrogate for the confounder of interest. For example, social class is associated with many lifestyle factors such as smoking, and may therefore be a useful surrogate for some lifestyle-related confounders. Even though confounder control will be imperfect in this situation, it is still possible to examine whether the exposure effect estimate changes when the surrogate is controlled in the analysis, and to assess the strength and direction of the change. For example, suppose the relative risk relating low dietary beta carotene intake to lung cancer actually increases (e.g. from 2.0 to 2.3) or remains stable (e.g., at 2.0) when social class is controlled. This might be taken as evidence that the observed excess risk is not entirely due to smoking, because social class is correlated with smoking (Kogevinas et al. 1997), and control for social class involves partial control for smoking. The strength of this evidence depends of course on what exposure is being studied and what sort of classification errors or other sources of bias are present.

Even if it is not possible to obtain confounder information for any study participants, it may still be possible to estimate how strong confounding is likely to be for particular risk factors. For example, this is often done in occupational studies, where tobacco smoking is a potential confounder, but smoking information is rarely available. In fact, although smoking is the strongest risk factor for lung cancer, with relative risks of 10-fold or more, it appears that smoking rarely exerts a confounding effect of greater than 1.5 times in studies of occupational disease (Axelson 1978, 1989; Siemiatycki et al. 1988; Kriebel et al. 2004) (although this degree of confounding may still be important in some contexts). There are several approaches to the assessment of potential confounding by factors such as cigarette smoking when data are lacking or incomplete. One approach is to conduct an analysis of smoking-related diseases other than the disease of primary interest (Steenland et al. 1984). If mortality from such diseases (e.g., non-malignant respiratory disease) is not elevated, this may suggest that any excess for the disease of interest is unlikely to be due to smoking. Similarly, one might be less inclined to attribute an excess of an alcohol-related cancer to unusually high drinking prevalence among the exposed if liver cirrhosis mortality is not elevated.

When detailed individual risk factor information is not available on a potential confounder, it may be possible to assess the impact of this factor on risk estimates by conducting a type of *sensitivity analysis* that estimates the potential direction and extent of confounding (Cornfield et al. 1959; Bross 1967; Axelson 1978, 1989; Schlesselman 1978; Checkoway and Waldman 1985; Axelson and Steenland 1988; Flanders and Khoury 1990; Rothman and Greenland 1998, Chap. 19). In this sensitivity analysis, the magnitude of the effect of the potential confounder on the disease should be known with some confidence, and the prevalence of the potential confounder among the exposed and comparison groups should be estimable, within reasonable bounds. Then, a range of confounding effects, including a "worst case scenario," can be calculated (Checkoway et al. 2004).

Consider the incidence rate, I, of disease in a population as consisting of two components: one being the incidence among those without the confounder, and the other the incidence among those with the confounder (assume in this simple case that the confounder is dichotomous) (Axelson 1978). Then:

$$I = I_0 \left(1 - p_c\right) + RR_c \left(I_0\right) \left(p_c\right)$$

where: I = incidence rate overall, RR_c = relative risk due to the confounder, I_0 = incidence rate among those who are confounder negative, and p_c = prevalence of the confounder in the source population from which the cases arose.

This expression can be expanded to include several levels of a confounder, for example: light, moderate, and heavy smoking. By applying the equation to two (or more) study groups (e.g., exposed and non-exposed subgroups) for which p_c is assumed to differ, one can calculate a confounding bias factor B_c comparing these two exposed groups and due to confounding alone. If there is no effect of exposure, then B_c is the magnitude of effect one would observe due to differences in p_c alone. Then, if RR_{Obs} is the observed relative risk comparing exposed to non-exposed,

$RR_{Adj} = RR_{Obs}/B_c$ is the adjusted relative risk, controlling for confounding.

To illustrate, suppose that one is concerned about smoking confounding a finding that $RR_{Obs} = 3.2$ for lung cancer and some dichotomous occupational exposure. Individual smoking data are not known. We might assume that smoking habits in the non-exposed approximate those of other typical blue-collar workers whose smoking habits have been studied. To estimate the most extreme confounding that might reasonably be expected, we might assume that the exposed were heavier smokers, with habits more like the 90th percentile of blue-collar workers. These assumptions would imply that the non-exposed might have been 50% non-smokers, 40% moderate smokers, and 10% heavy smokers, whereas the exposed were 20% non-smokers, 55% moderate smokers, and 25% heavy smokers. Assuming that moderate smoking confers a relative risk of smoking of 10 compared to non-smokers, and heavy smoking a relative risk of 20, the confounding due to smoking is $B_c = 1.65$. Thus, one would observe a relative risk of 1.65 comparing exposed to unexposed due to these smoking differences alone. One can then calculate that $RR_{Adj} = 3.2/1.65 = 1.9$ as a hypothetically "adjusted" exposure effect under a plausible, but unlikely scenario for smoking differences among exposed groups. If RR_{Adj} is elevated, one might conclude that confounding is unlikely to be the entire explanation for the elevated risk (Checkoway et al. 2004).

This method allows one to place limits on the degree of confounding that can result from failure to adjust for an unmeasured risk factor that is associated with the exposure under study. Its application is restricted however to control for factors whose risks are well established quantitatively, and for which the confounder prevalence in the population can be estimated fairly reliably. Cornfield et al. (1959) and others (Bross 1967; Flanders and Khoury 1990) showed that the relative risk that would result from differences in the prevalence of a covariate, such as smoking or alcohol consumption, may be quite limited, even in the absence of complete knowledge about the covariate. In particular, Flanders and Khoury (1990) showed that:

$$1 < B_c < \min\left\{OR, RR_c, 1/p_c, RR_c/(q_c + RR_c * p_c), OR/(q_c + RR_c * p_c)\right\}$$

where B_c, RR_c and p_c are as above, $q_c = 1-p_c$, and OR is the odds ratio measuring the association between exposure and the covariate (both measured dichotomously in this example). Using this equation, rather severe limits can be placed on the range of possible values of B_c with information about p_c and RR_c alone, making no assumption about OR at all. For example, if $p_c = 0.5$, and RR_c for esophageal cancer from 1 pack/day smoking = 5, then $B_c = 1.7$. That is, given $RR_c = 5$ an observed RR_{obs} for an exposure effect is unlikely to be confounded by more than 1.7 times. With a reasonable assumption about the likely values of OR and RR_c, the association between exposure and the confounder, the maximum value for B_c could be lower or higher. This method can be extended for the situation in which there are multiple levels of exposure and multiple levels of covariates (Schlesselman 1978; Flanders and Khoury 1990), and to other measures of association such as odds ratios (Yanagawa 1984).

A more sophisticated version of sensitivity analysis places uncertainty distributions (priors) on the unknown quantities in the sensitivity formula, repeatedly draws values from these distributions and corrects the data or estimates based on the drawn values, adds in a random-error correction, and presents the resulting distribution of corrected estimates. Such Monte-Carlo sensitivity analysis has long been a staple of risk analysis and is now finding application in epidemiology (e.g., see Greenland 2003, 2004a, 2005; Phillips 2003; Lash and Fink 2003).

Sensitivity analysis can also be useful in certain situations in which confounder information has been collected, but the validity or precision of those data are weak. Sometimes smoking data are available on only a subset of the members of a cohort. One option is to conduct an analysis that controls for smoking directly on the subset with smoking data. However, the precision of this analysis and the generalizability of findings to the entire cohort may be questionable. Instead, one might apply the data relating the confounder to exposure among this subset in a sensitivity analysis for the entire cohort (Fingerhut et al. 1991). A third option is to adjust the entire cohort based on the data from the subset, using two-stage methods or missing-data methods (Rothman and Greenland 1998, Chap. 15).

Relationship Between Confounding and Other Biases   9.2.6

In this chapter confounding has been defined as non-comparability (non-exchangeability) of the exposed and non-exposed subgroups in the source population with respect to their risk of the disease outcome in the absence of exposure. Confounding is thus a property of the source population rather than of the specific group of study participants.

Selection bias involves biases arising from the procedures by which the study participants are selected (or select themselves) from the source population. Thus, selection bias is not an issue in a cohort study (or cross-sectional study) involving complete recruitment and follow-up because in this instance the study group comprises the entire source population. However, selection bias can occur if participation in the study or follow-up is incomplete. Selection bias is usually more of an issue in case-control studies in that selection bias may occur if the case group does not include (or is not representative of) all cases in the source population, or if the control group is not representative of the population-at-risk that the cases came from.

If control selection involves only sampling at random from the entire source population with complete cooperation, *selection bias* is a minor concern. More realistically, however, selection bias is likely if response rates differ according to exposure level and disease status. When controls are selected from among persons with other diseases, considerable care must be taken in specifying the diseases that form the control group. In particular, a specific disease may not correctly reflect the exposure pattern in the source population, especially if it is caused by the study exposure. One strategy is to include only diseases that are thought to be unrelated to the exposure(s) of interest (Miettinen 1985; Rothman and Greenland 1998, Chap. 7), but this requirement may be difficult to satisfy in practice because adequate evidence for the absence of exposure effects on many diseases is frequently not available (Axelson et al. 1982). An alternative method is to select as controls a sample of all other diseases. This approach is reliable if one can be sure the factor under study does not markedly increase risk of numerous or the most common diseases. It has become common practice to exclude diseases known to be related to exposure from the pool of potential controls; however, even this restriction will not always eliminate bias (Pearce and Checkoway 1988).

Selection bias and confounding are not always clearly demarcated. In particular, selection bias in the form of non-response at baseline of a cohort can be viewed as a source of confounding, since it may produce associations of exposure with other risk factors in the study cohort and thus turn those factors into confounders (Hernan et al. 2004). A similar phenomenon occurs in case-control studies when selection is affected by a factor that itself affects exposure. An example occurs when matching on a factor that is associated with exposure in the source population; even if the factor is not a risk factor for disease in the absence of exposure, matching may turn it into a confounder which must be controlled in the data analysis, because matching will create the necessary factor-disease association if exposure affects disease (Rothman and Greenland 1998, Chap. 10). Unfortunately, as discussed earlier, if selection is affected by exposure and associated with case-control status (e.g. selection bias due to inappropriate selection of controls from persons with other diseases, or selection on factors affected by exposure), stratification on the selection-related factors will rarely produce valid estimates, and hence this type of selection bias should not be viewed as confounding.

Information bias is the result of misclassification of study participants with respect to disease or exposure status. Thus, the concept of information bias refers to those people actually included in the study, whereas selection bias refers to the selection of the study participants from the source population, and confounding generally refers to non-comparability of subgroups within the source population. There are many methods to adjust for misclassification (e.g. Copeland et al. 1977; Greenland and Kleinbaum 1983; Espeland and Hui 1987; Greenland 1988; Armstrong et al. 1992; Thomas et al. 1993; Armstrong 1998). These require estimates of sensitivity and specificity, or the reliability of the measurement, based on prior information or validation data. Estimates based on prior information are often only best guesses that may not apply to the population under study. However, it is an informative exercise to conduct sensitivity analyses that explore the range of results that might have occurred under various scenarios (Rothman and Greenland 1998, Chap. 19), and again, Monte-Carlo sensitivity analyses may be applied (Lash and Fink 2003; Phillips 2003; Greenland 2004a, 2005).

Some consider any bias that can be controlled in the analysis as confounding, but this definition is too general because any bias control requires background information for proper execution, and any bias can be controlled in the analysis given enough background information. Confounding is distinguished in that it represents a mixing or confusion of the effects of other factors with the effects of the study exposure, a concept that goes back at least as far as the writings of John Stuart Mill (Greenland et al. 1999b). Other biases are then be categorized according to whether they arise from the selection of study subjects (selection bias), or their classification (information bias). Most observational studies suffer from more than one form of bias, and the effects of multiple biases may compound error. Perhaps the best-appreciated situation is when there is misclassification of a confounder, in which case attempts to control for the confounder will not fully control that confounder and may actually increase bias (Greenland 1980; Greenland and Robins 1985; Savitz and Baron 1989; Marshall and Hastrup 1996, 1999). When (as is often the case) multiple biases are present, many complex and counterintuitive phenomena can occur, and a clear picture of the net effects of bias will require analyses that account for these bias interactions (Lash and Fink 2003; Phillips 2003; Greenland 2005).

Interaction   9.3

Basic Concepts   9.3.1

The concept of *interaction* (*effect modification*), also known as effect heterogeneity and effect variation, refers to a condition where the effect of exposure on the outcome under study varies by some other factor. In other words, in order to estimate the effect of exposure on an outcome (such as a disease time, a disease risk, or a disease rate), we must first know whether or not another factor is present (or what the level of this other factor is). This concept can be subclassified into two major concepts: *biological dependence of effects*, also known as synergism; and *effect-measure modification*, also known as heterogeneity of a measure. With regard to the latter, all secondary risk factors modify either the rate ratio or the rate difference, and uniformity over one measure implies non-uniformity over the other (Steenland and Thun 1986; Rothman and Greenland 1998, Chap. 4), e.g., an apparent additive joint effect implies a departure from a multiplicative model. A further source of ambiguity is that the term "effect modification" implies that one factor in some way biologically "modifies" the effect of the other factor but this is not necessarily the case. For this reason, the term "effect-measure modification" and "effect-measure variation" are more accurate terms, and are logically equivalent to the definition of "interaction" used in most statistics books and computer programs (Rothman and Greenland 1998, Chaps. 4 and 18).

The concepts of interaction and confounding are quite distinct. An effect-measure modifier may or may not be a confounder and a confounder may or may not be an effect-measure modifier (Miettinen 1974; Rothman and Greenland 1998, Chap. 4). For example, if we are comparing exposed and non-exposed subgroups of a population, and the percentage of people who smoke (and the intensity of smoking, and the length of time that each person has been smoking) is the same in both groups, then smoking is not a confounder. However, the rate ratio for the exposure effect may still vary by smoking status, e.g. the exposure may double the risk of disease in smokers but have no effect in non-smokers. In this situation, smoking would not be a confounder, but would be an effect-measure modifier.

9.3.2   Example of Effect-measure Modification

Table 9.2 presents a hypothetical example of effect-measure modification in a cross-sectional study of asthma. The overall findings are the same as for the study presented in Table 9.1, but the stratum-specific findings are different. Now there is no confounding by smoking because the percentage of smokers is the same in the exposed and non-exposed groups. However, there is effect modification since the prevalence ratio (for the association of exposure with disease) is 1.5 in smokers and 1.0 in non-smokers. Thus, whereas the assessment of confounding involved the comparison of the crude and adjusted effect estimates, the assessment of effect modification involves the comparison of the stratum-specific effect estimates with each other.

Table 9.2. Hypothetical example of effect modification by tobacco smoking in a study of asthma prevalence

	Smokers		Non-smokers		Total	
	Exposed	Non-exposed	Exposed	Non-exposed	Exposed	Non-exposed
Asthma cases	600	400	400	400	1000	800
Non-cases	900	1100	1100	1100	2000	2200
Total	1500	1500	1500	1500	3000	3000
Prevalence (%)	40	26.7	26.7	26.7	33.3	26.7
Prevalence ratio	1.5		1.0		1.25	

9.3.3   Concepts of Interaction

Although at first glance, the assessment of interaction is relatively straightforward, there are considerable hidden complexities. Some of the analytic issues in studying effect-measure modification will be illustrated with data (Table 9.3) from a study by Selikoff et al. (1980) of lung cancer death rates per 100,000 person-years at risk in relation to exposure to cigarette smoke and asbestos (Steenland and Thun

Table 9.3. Example of joint effects: lung cancer mortality rates per 100,000 person-years at risk in a cohort of asbestos workers compared to those in other blue collar occupations. Source: (Steenland and Thun 1986)

	Rate in smokers (RR)	Rate in non-smokers	Rate ratio
Asbestos	935.8 (RR_{11} = 32.7)	500.5 (RR_{01} = 17.5)	1.9
Non-asbestos	199.5 (RR_{10} = 7.0)	28.6 (RR_{00} = 1.0)	7.0
Rate ratio	4.7	17.5	
Rate difference	736.3	471.9	

1986). The rate difference due to asbestos exposure is 472 per 100,000 person-years in non-smokers and 736 per 100,000 person-years in smokers. Thus, the rate difference for the effect of asbestos exposure on lung cancer mortality is lower in non-smokers than in smokers. On the other hand, the rate ratio for the same effect is higher in non-smokers (asbestos rate ratio = 17.5) than in smokers (asbestos rate ratio = 4.7). Thus, both the rate difference and the rate ratio are subject to effect-measure modification in that the effect estimate depends on the presence or absence (or more generally, the level) of another factor (i.e. smoking), but the dependencies are in opposite directions: the rate difference is larger in smokers and the rate ratio is larger for non-smokers.

Several authors (Kupper and Hogan 1978; Walter and Holford 1978) have taken this dependence of interaction on the underlying effect measure to imply that the assessment of interaction is "model-dependent". Thus the authors equate all uses of the term "interaction" with effect-measure modification. In contrast to these statistically-based definitions, other authors (e.g. (Rothman and Greenland 1998, Chaps. 2 and 18)) adopt a definition of interaction in which two factors are said to exhibit interdependent effects or "biologic interaction"or "synergism" if they are component causes in the same sufficient cause (Rothman 1976; cf. Chap. I.1 of this handbook), or if individual patterns of response (the potential or counterfactual outcomes) to exposure change when the other "interacting" factor is changed (Greenland and Poole 1988; Rothman and Greenland 1998, Chap. 18). This concept of dependence of effects implies that additivity of risks will arise when no biologic interaction is present. With this concept in hand, one can show that the presence and degree of effect-measure modification depend to a large extent on the prevalence of causal cofactors of exposure, as well as the actual biologic mechanisms at work (Rothman 1976; see Chap. I.1 of this handbook for further explanation).

There was originally some confusion about the relation of biologic interaction to nonadditivity (Koopman 1977). If two factors (A and B) belong to different sufficient causes, but a third factor (C) belongs to both sufficient causes, then A and B are competing for a single pool of susceptible individuals (those who have C). Consequently the joint effect of A and B will be less than additive. Miettinen (1982) reaches a similar conclusion based on a model of individual outcomes. However, this phenomenon can be incorporated directly into the sufficient-cause model by clarifying a previous ambiguity in the description of antagonism in the model's terms. Specifically, the absence of B before A can be included in the sufficient cause involving A, and vice versa. Then, two factors would exhibit interaction, specifically antagonism, if the presence of one factor and absence of the other factor were component causes in the same sufficient cause (Greenland and Poole 1988; Rothman and Greenland 1998, Chap. 18).

Under a potential-outcomes (counterfactual) model of causation, two factors are said to exhibit interaction if the response schedule (response type) of any individual to one of the factors depended on the level of the other factor (Greenland and Poole 1988; Rothman and Greenland 1998, Chap. 18). This definition leads to the same operational (statistical) criterion for identifying the presence of interaction as that derived from the sufficient cause model, namely, departure from risk additivity.

It should be stressed that this concept of independent effects is distinct from from certain other biological concepts of no interaction. For example, Siemiatycki and Thomas (1981) give a definition in which two factors have biologically independent effects "if the qualitative nature of the mechanism of action of each is not affected by the presence of absence of the other"; this concept does not lead to an unambiguous definition of dependent effects, however (Siemiatycki and Thomas 1981), and thus does not produce clear analytic implications. In contrast, under the sufficient-cause and potential-outcome (counterfactual) models, a particular biologic model, rather than being accepted as the "baseline", is itself evaluated in terms of the co-participation of factors in a sufficient cause, or in modification of individual response. For example, two factors which act at different stages of a multistage process have dependent effects because they are joint components of at least one sufficient cause. This occurs irrespective of whether they affect each other's qualitative mechanism of action (the ambiguity in Siemiatycki and Thomas' formulation stems from the ambiguity of this concept).

9.3.4   Additive and Multiplicative Models

The sufficient-component and potential-outcome definitions of interaction (co-participation in a sufficient cause, or change in response schedule) are attractive because they are based on an explicit causal model that leads to an unambiguous definition of independence of effects, and because they lead to the additive model as the baseline for assessing interactions, just as obtained through public health (cost-benefit) considerations (Rothman et al. 1980; Rothman and Greenland 1998, Chap. 18). However, the analytic implications of these concepts are not straightforward, since assessing independence of effects is usually only one of the analytic goals of an epidemiological study. There are several other considerations which often favor the use of multiplicative models.

One is that multiplicative models have convenient statistical properties. Estimation in non-multiplicative models may have problems of convergence, and inference based on the asymptotic standard errors may be flawed unless the study size is very large (Moolgavkar and Venzon 1987). Another is that, if it is desired to keep interaction (effect-measure modification, corresponding to product terms in a regression model) to a minimum, then a multiplicative model is often most effective. It is not uncommon for joint effects to appear closer to multiplicative than to additive (Saracci 1987). In this situation there may be less masking of heterogeneity in calculating an overall rate ratio than in calculating an overall rate difference. Although there are also many instances of non-multiplicative departures from additivity (Selikoff et al. 1980; Saracci 1987), even in these cases multiplicative-model summaries are more often closer to a population-average (standardized) measure than are additive-model summaries (Greenland and Maldonado 1994). Finally, additive-risk models are not identical to additive relative-risk models when the model includes terms for confounder adjustment; unfortunately, in typical case-control studies only the latter models can be fit, thus rendering it difficult or impossible to make unconfounded assessments of risk additivity (Greenland 1993a,b). In contrast, departures from multiplicativity can be assessed in the same fashion from cohort and case-control data.

Detecting Interactions 9.4

Determining whether or not a factor is an effect-measure modifier is often done by estimating an effect measure (e.g., relative risk) for the exposure of interest separately for each level of the presumed effect modifier and testing for equality of these measures across the modifier strata (Rothman and Greenland 1998, Chap. 15). This approach lacks power, however, and so it can be quite misleading to conclude modification is absent just because the test yields a large P-value. Because of such power problems and other problems due to sample size limitations, when there are multiple possible effect-measure modifiers, such as age, ethnicity, gender, or previous employment in a hazardous industry, effect modification is usually examined for each potential modifying variable separately, or else through use of modeling methods that allow continuous modification by quantitative variables such as age. Prior selection of potential effect modifiers of greatest interest can simplify the task. Then, assessing effect-measure modification for a subset of modifying variables might be carried out, with adjustment made for other variables.

A major obstacle to interaction as well as confounding assessment is misclassification. Misclassification of any of the variables in the analysis (whether the exposure, disease, confounder, or modifier) can make a measure appear to vary across strata when in reality it does not, or make it appear nearly constant when in reality it does vary (Greenland 1980). Similarly, measurement errors can spuriously create or mask the need for product terms (interactions) in a statistical model (Greenland 1993b; cf. Chap. II.3 of this handbook). In an analogous fashion, variation in a measure across strata may be spuriously created or masked by differences in other biases (such as residual confounding or selection bias) across strata. Again, such problems can be explored using sensitivity analysis.

Conventional statistical analysis strategies often assume it is not appropriate to calculate an overall effect estimate if interaction is present. However, this principle is commonly ignored if the difference in stratum-specific effect estimates is not too great. In fact standardized rate ratios have been developed for precisely this situation, and will consistently estimate meaningful epidemiological parameters even under heterogeneity (Rothman and Greenland 1998, Chap. 15; Greenland 2004b). Furthermore, as mentioned earlier, rate ratios estimated from multiplicative models often approximate these standardized ratios (Greenland and Maldonado 1994).

As mentioned above, concluding that there is no interaction because the P-value is high can be misleading. Most studies are not designed to examine interaction, and as such, may have inadequate study sizes within strata of an effect-measure modifier to permit a useful statistical interpretation. Presentation of stratum-specific effect estimates and their confidence intervals can help to give a picture of whether the data allow any inference about effect-measure modification. Formal statistical tests may be most useful in situations where prior information suggests likely forms of effect modification (e.g., a harmful effect would only be anticipated among smokers) and the study is intentionally designed to accommodate an analysis of effect modification (e.g., sufficient numbers of smokers and non-smokers are selected).

Some authors (e.g. Kleinbaum et al. 1982) have developed modeling strategies in which the first step of an analysis involves testing for statistical interactions, where the latter are represented by product terms in the model. In the most extreme application this involves including all possible two-factor (and even three-factor) product terms in a preliminary model and retaining in subsequent analyses all products (and related lower-order terms) that meet the inclusion criterion (which might be having a p-value below a certain cut-off, such as 0.10, or having a point estimate larger than a particular magnitude). This approach often results in complex models with numerous product terms, which may lead to problems of convergence, bias in the parameter estimates, and difficulties in interpretation.

In fact, there is no logical necessity for the assessment of interaction to occur as the first step in an analysis, and there are several reasons why it can be preferable to evaluate confounding before considering interaction. One reason is that the initial aim of most analyses is to determine if there is any overall effect of exposure. It is necessary to control confounding to do this, but it is not essential to evaluate interaction when doing so (Rothman 1978). Although harmful effects in one stratum and protective effects in another stratum may yield an overall null effect, this phenomenon is presumably rare. A routine search may yield a high percentage of false positives; on the other hand, if there were a relevant a priori hypothesis then it would be appropriate to calculate stratum specific effect estimates irrespective of the value of the summary effect estimate.

Another reason to begin an analysis with confounding evaluation is that inclusion of extra stratification variables or extra product terms involving the main exposure complicates confounder assessment. With extra strata or terms, changes in either stratum-specific or in summary fitted measures must be examined; the stratum-specific measures may be numerous and unstable, and the summary of these measures can be difficult to construct from a fitted model that has product terms involving the exposure, see Rothman and Greenland (1998, pp 413–416) and Greenland (2004b) for example formulas. Measures constructed from models that omit exposure product terms are often a reasonable approximation to the formally correct and more complicated measures that allow for interactions, and so can be adequate for confounding evaluation (Greenland and Maldonado 1994).

Even if subsequent analyses concentrate on specific subgroups, it may be preferable to evaluate confounding in the whole data set, since this provides the greatest precision. If a factor is a confounder overall, then it is a risk factor, and is also associated with exposure. Thus it is necessarily a confounder in some specific subgroups, and there may be little loss of precision from control in any subgroups in which it is not a confounder (although this cannot be guaranteed). Hence, it may be preferable to evaluate confounding first, and then adjust for the same confounders in each subgroup analysis.

Some qualifications should be noted. First, confounding may be evaluated purely on a priori considerations, and as mentioned earlier has an inescapable a priori (causal) component in observational studies. Because of this causal component, purely statistical selection procedures such as stepwise regression can be even more misleading for confounder selection than they are in pure prediction problems (Greenland 1980). Second, the entire selection process and the attendant problems can be avoided by switching to hierarchical regression methods (Rothman and Greenland 1998, Chap. 21), which we discuss further below. For general principles of data analysis we refer to Chapter II.2 of this handbook and Chaps. 12 and 13 of Rothman and Greenland (1998).

Assessment of Joint Effects 9.4.1

The above considerations imply an apparent dilemma. How can an analysis be conducted that combines the advantages of ratio measures of effect with the assessment of interaction in terms of a departure from additivity? If an excess risk is found (and assumed to be causal) then attention shifts to elaborating the nature of the effect. This naturally comes toward the end of the formal presentation of the findings. Typically, the last few tables of a manuscript might examine the joint effects of the main exposure with other factors of interest, and the discussion might relate these findings to current etiologic knowledge. As noted above, it is often sufficient to evaluate only those joint effects for which there is an a priori reason for interest.

As an example, when studying asbestos and lung cancer, interaction with smoking might be expected given the powerful effects of smoking. To examine the latter interaction, relative risks might be presented for smoking (in non-asbestos workers), asbestos exposure (in non-smokers) and exposure to both factors, relative to persons exposed to neither factor. These relative risks would be adjusted for all other factors (e.g. age) that are potential confounders, but not of immediate interest as effect modifiers. The relevant table (e.g. Table 9.3) can be derived from any form of model, including the statistically convenient multiplicative models, by including product (interaction) terms as appropriate.

The estimation of separate and joint effects may be difficult when the factors of interest are closely correlated. However, when it is feasible, this approach combines the best features of multiplicative models and additive interaction assessment; it also permits readers with other concepts of independence to draw their own conclusions. It can be illustrated with the data presented above (Table 9.3) on asbestos exposure, cigarette smoking, and lung cancer. In this example, the relative risk estimates (adjusted for age and calendar period) are 7.0 for asbestos exposure alone, 17.5 for smoking alone, and 32.7 for the joint effect of both exposures. Thus, the joint effect of asbestos and smoking is more than additive (the joint effect is 32.7 times, whereas it would be $1 + (7.0 - 1) + (17.5 - 1) = 23.5$ if it were additive). This is consistent with the hypothesis that asbestos and smoking are joint components in at least one sufficient cause (it might be argued that non-additivity refutes the hypothesis that asbestos and smoking never biologically interact, assuming as usual that there is no residual confounding or bias). If their joint effect were the sum of their separate effects, the result would have favored the hypothesis that they are not joint components of a sufficient cause and do not compete for a common pool of susceptibles. However, the latter interpretation is more restricted, since additivity could arise if two factors were components of the same sufficient cause, but also had antagonistic or competitive effects that balanced their synergistic effects. Thus, even in ideal circumstances, additivity does not refute the hypothesis that asbestos and smoking interact biologically in some people (Greenland and Poole 1988; Rothman and Greenland 1998, Chap. 18).

If it is provisionally accepted that smoking and asbestos do act together in a sufficient cause of lung cancer, then attention may shift to elaborating the effect with mathematical models deduced from biologic models of the interaction. For example, Doll and Peto (1978) have suggested that smoking acts at both an early stage (probably the 2nd) and the penultimate (5th) stage of a 6-stage carcinogenic process. Asbestos appears to act at one of the later stages, probably the 4th or 5th (Pearce 1988). If asbestos acted at the same late stage as smoking, then it could be expected that its effect would add onto the late stage effect of smoking, and multiply the early stage effect of smoking. The resulting joint effect would be intermediate between additive and multiplicative. This pattern has been observed in several studies (Selikoff et al. 1980) although there are, of course, other models which predict the same result (Saracci 1987).

When interaction evaluation occurs as the last stage of an analysis, the routine evaluation (screening) of a large number of joint effects increases the number of tables, but does not necessarily complicate other aspects of the presentation (Pearce 1989). It does however raise a number of statistical problems which have been the subject of much controversy and research. The first, lesser known problem is that exposure effect estimates may be biased away from the null when too many terms (such as product terms) are entered into a risk or rate regression (Greenland et al. 2000). The second is the multiple-comparisons problem. Although many epidemiologists have denied that such problems exist (e.g. Rothman 1990), their focus concerned situations in which despite many comparisons, the investigator was interested in just one or a few exposure-disease relations. Nonetheless, screening a large number of effects (whether main effects or interactions) implies interest in many relations, and raises the issues of how one deals with the instability of the estimates and the high probability that some of the estimates are large simply because of large random errors (Greenland and Robins 1991). Classical multiple-comparisons procedures can be quite misleading, however, because they make no attempt to account for false negative error (in fact they inflate it tremendously), and are arguably inferior to making no adjustment at all if one is more concerned about false-negatives than false-positives.

An analytic solution to both problems is to employ hierarchical modeling methods (also known as multilevel methods, penalized estimation, random-coefficient regression, shrinkage estimation, Stein estimation, empirical-Bayes regression, and semi-Bayes regression) (Greenland and Robins 1991; Rothman and Greenland 1998, pp 427–432; Greenland 2000b,c; Steenland et al. 2000). Such methods are demonstrably superior to either extreme (of no adjustment versus classical adjustment) in these situations, as shown by theory, simulations, and performance in real epidemiologic examples (Efron and Morris 1977; Greenland 1993c, 2000b,c, 2001b; Steenland et al. 2000; Witte et al. 2000). Furthermore, these methods can also be applied to control of multiple confounders in place of confounder selection methods (Greenland 2000c), and can be carried out with standard software (Witte et al. 2000; Greenland 2001b).

Conclusions 9.5

Confounding occurs when the exposed and non-exposed subpopulations of the source population have different background disease risks. When we make a comparison of the frequency of disease in the exposed and non-exposed groups, we would ideally wish to be able to assume that the disease frequency in the non-exposed group provides a valid estimate of what the disease frequency would have been in the exposed group if it had not been exposed. If this assumption is incorrect, i.e. if the exposed and non-exposed groups would have had different disease frequencies in the counterfactual situation in which the exposed group had not been exposed, then we say that the comparison of the exposed and unexposed groups is confounded. A related concept is that the exposed and non-exposed group are not "exchangeable", in that the estimated effects would have been different if the exposed group had not been exposed and the non-exposed group had been exposed (i.e. if the exposure status of the subjects had been exchanged).

Interaction usually means that the exposure effect on disease risk varies by some other factor. In other words, in order to estimate the effect of exposure, we must first know whether or not another factor is present (or what the level of this other factor is). This idea turns out to subsume two separate concepts: *effect-measure modification* (statistical interaction) and *biologic interaction*. When considering an exposure that has an effect, all other causal factors will modify either the rate ratio or the rate difference, and uniformity over one measure implies non-uniformity over the other, e.g., an apparent additive joint effect implies a departure from a multiplicative model. Effect-measure modification is logically equivalent to the definition of "interaction" used in most statistics books and programs, and refers to a population measure of effect. In contrast, biologic interaction refers to effects in individuals although its absence implies absence of risk-difference modification.

In the simple case of a dichotomous main exposure (e.g. asbestos exposure), a dichotomous health outcome (e.g. lung cancer) and another categorized exposure (e.g. smoking vs. non-smoking), assessment of confounding involves stratifying on the potential confounder and assessing whether the stratum-specific effect estimates are similar to the (crude) overall effect estimate, e.g. how close are the relative risks in smokers and non-smokers (or a summary of these stratum-specific effect estimates) to the relative risk estimated when smoking is ignored? Assessment of effect-measure modification involves assessment of how the stratum specific effect estimates compare with each other, e.g. how does the relative risk in smokers compare with the relative risk in non-smokers? The two concepts are therefore often confused, because in this simple situation they are both assessed by stratification. However, confounding and interaction are completely different concepts. A factor may be a source of confounding, or effect-measure modification, or both, or neither.

Acknowledgements. The authors are grateful to Katherine J. Hoggatt and the editors for numerous helpful comments that improved this chapter. Funding for Neil Pearce's salary is from a Programme Grant from the Health Research Council of New Zealand.

References

Armstrong B, White E, Saracci R (1992) Principles of exposure measurement in epidemiology. Oxford University Press, New York

Armstrong BG (1998) Effect of measurement error on epidemiological studies of environmental and occupational exposures. Occupational & Environmental Medicine 55:651–656

Axelson O (1978) Aspects on confounding in occupational health epidemiology. Scandinavian Journal of Work, Environment & Health 4:85–89

Axelson O (1989) Confounding from smoking in occupational epidemiology. British Journal of Industrial Medicine 46:505–507

Axelson O, Steenland K (1988) Indirect methods of assessing the effects of tobacco use in occupational studies. American Journal of Industrial Medicine 13:105–118

Axelson O, Flodin U, Hardell L (1982) A comment on the reference series with regard to multiple exposure evaluations in a case-referent study. Scandinavian Journal of Work, Environment & Health 8(suppl 1):15–19

Bross IDJ (1967) Pertinency of an extraneous variable. Journal of Chronic Diseases 20:487–495

Checkoway H, Waldman GT (1985) Assessing the possible extent of confounding in occupational case-referent studies. Scandinavian Journal of Work, Environment & Health 11:131–133

Checkoway H, Pearce N, Kriebel D (2004) Research methods in occupational epidemiology. Oxford University Press, New York

Cole SR, Hernan MA (2002) Fallibility in estimating direct effects. International Journal of Epidemiology 31:163–165

Copeland KT, Checkoway H, McMichael AJ, Holbrook RH (1977) Bias due to misclassification in the estimation of relative risk. American Journal of Epidemiology 105:488–495

Cornfield J, Haenszel W, Hammond EC, Lilienfeld AM, Shimkin MB, Wynder EL (1959) Smoking and lung cancer: recent evidence and a discussion of some questions. Journal of the National Cancer Institute 22:173–203

Doll R, Peto R (1978) Cigarette smoking and bronchial carcinoma: dose and time relationships among regular smokers and lifelong non-smokers. Journal of Epidemiology & Community Health 32:303–313

Efron B, Morris C (1977) Stein's paradox in statistics. Scientific American 236:119–127

Espeland M, Hui SL (1987) A general approach to analyzing epidemiologic data that contain misclassification errors. Biometrics 43:1001–1012

Fingerhut MA, Halperin WE, Marlow DA, Piacitelli LA, Honchar PA, Sweeney MH, Greife AL, Dill PA, Steenland K, Suruda AJ (1991) Cancer mortality in workers exposed to 2,3,7,8-tetrachlorodibenzo-p-dioxin. New England Journal of Medicine 324:212–218

Flanders WD, Khoury MJ (1990) Indirect assessment of confounding: graphic description and limits on effect for adjusting for covariates. Epidemiology 1:239–246

Greenland S (1980) The effect of misclassification in the presence of covariates. American Journal of Epidemiology 112:564–569

Greenland S (1988) Variance estimation for epidemiologic effect estimates under misclassification. Statistics in Medicine 7:745–757

Greenland S (1993a) Additive-risk versus additive relative-risk models. Epidemiology 4:32–36

Greenland S (1993b) Basic problems in interaction assessment. Environmental Health Perspectives 101(suppl 4):59–66

Greenland S (1993c) Methods for epidemiologic analyses of multiple exposures: A review and a comparative study of maximum-likelihood, preliminary testing, and empirical-Bayes regression. Statistics in Medicine 12:717–736

Greenland S (1996) Absence of confounding does not correspond to collapsibility of the rate ratio or rate difference. Epidemiology 7:498–501

Greenland S (2000a) An introduction to instrumental variables for epidemiologists. International Journal of Epidemiology 29:722–729

Greenland S (2000b) Principles of multilevel modelling. International Journal of Epidemiology 29:158–167

Greenland S (2000c) When should epidemiologic regressions use random coefficients? Biometrics 56:915–921

Greenland S (2001a) Ecologic versus individual-level sources of confounding in ecologic estimates of contextual health effects. International Journal of Epidemiology 30:1343–1350

Greenland S (2001b) Putting background information about relative risks into conjugate prior distributions. Biometrics 57:663–670

Greenland S (2003) The impact of prior distributions for uncontrolled confounding and response bias: A case study of the relation of wire codes and magnetic fields to childhood leukemia. Journal of the American Statistical Association 98: 47–54

Greenland S (2004a) Interval estimation by simulation as an alternative to and extension of confidence intervals. International Journal of Epidemiology (in press)

Greenland S (2004b) Model-based estimation of relative risks and other epidemiologic measures in studies of common outcomes and in case-control studies. American Journal of Epidemiology (in press)

Greenland S (2005) Multiple-bias modeling for observational studies. Journal of the Royal Statistical Society, Series A (in press)

Greenland S, Kleinbaum D (1983) Correcting for misclassification in two-way tables and matched-pair studies. International Journal of Epidemiology 12:93–97

Greenland S, Maldonado G (1994) The interpretation of multiplicative model parameters as standardised parameters. Statistics in Medicine 13:989–999

Greenland S, Neutra RR (1980) Control of confounding in the assessment of medical technology. International Journal of Epidemiology 9:361–367

Greenland S, Poole C (1988) Invariants and noninvariants in the concept of interdependent effects. Scandinavian Journal of Work, Environment & Health. 14:125–129

Greenland S, Robins JM (1985) Confounding and misclassification. American Journal of Epidemiology 122:495–506

Greenland S, Robins JM (1986) Identifiability, exchangeability, and epidemiological confounding. International Journal of Epidemiology 15:413–419

Greenland S, Robins JM (1991) Empirical-Bayes adjustments for multiple comparisons are sometimes useful. Epidemiology 2:244–251

Greenland S, Pearl J, Robins JM (1999a) Causal diagrams for epidemiologic research. Epidemiology 10:37–48

Greenland S, Robins JM, Pearl J (1999b) Confounding and collapsibility in causal inference. Statistical Science 14:29–46

Greenland S, Schwartzbaum JA, Finkle WD (2000) Problems due to small samples and sparse data in conditional logistic regression analysis. American Journal of Epidemiology 151:531–539

Hernan MA, Hernandez-Diaz S, Werler MM, Mitchell AA (2002) Causal knowledge as a prerequisite for confounding evaluation. American Journal of Epidemiology 155:176–184

Hernan MA, Hernandez-Diaz S, Robins JM (2004) A structural approach to selection bias. Epidemiology 15:615–625

Kleinbaum DG, Kupper LL, Morgenstern H (1982) Epidemiologic research. Principles and quantitative methods. Lifetime Learning Publication, Belmont, CA

Kogevinas M, Pearce N, Susser M, Boffetta P (1997) Social inequalities and cancer. IARC Scientific Publications No. 138, Lyon

Koopman JS (1977) Causal models and sources of interaction. American Journal of Epidemiology 106:439–444

Kriebel D, Zeka A, Eisen EA, Wegman DH (2004) Quantitative evaluation of the effects of uncontrolled confounding by alcohol and tobacco in occupational cancer studies. International Journal of Epidemiology 33:1–6

Kupper LL, Hogan MD (1978) Interaction in epidemiologic studies. American Journal of Epidemiology 108:447–453

Lash TL, Fink AK (2003) Semi-automated sensitivity analysis to assess systematic errors in observational epidemiologic data. Epidemiology 14:451–458

Maldonado G, Greenland S (1993) A simulation study of confounder-selection strategies. American Journal of Epidemiology 138:923–936

Marshall JR, Hastrup JL (1996) Mismeasurement and the resonance of strong confounders: uncorrelated errors. American Journal of Epidemiology 143:1069–1078

Marshall JR, Hastrup JL (1999) Mismeasurement and the resonance of strong confounders: correlated errors. American Journal of Epidemiology 150:88–96

Miettinen OS (1974) Confounding and effect-modification. American Journal of Epidemiology 100:350–353

Miettinen OS (1982) Causal and preventive interdependence. Elementary principles. Scandinavian Journal of Work, Environment & Health 8:159–168

Miettinen OS (1985) The "case-control" study: valid selection of subjects. Journal of Chronic Diseases 38:543–548

Miettinen OS, Cook EF (1981) Confounding: essence and detection. American Journal of Epidemiology 114:593–603

Moolgavkar SH, Venzon DJ (1987) General relative risk regression models for epidemiologic studies.[comment]. American Journal of Epidemiology 126:949–961

Pearce N (1988) Multistage modelling of lung cancer mortality in asbestos textile workers. International Journal of Epidemiology 17:747–752

Pearce N (1989) Analytical implications of epidemiological concepts of interaction. International Journal of Epidemiology 18:976–980

Pearce N, Checkoway H (1988) Case-control studies using other diseases as controls: problems of excluding exposure-related diseases.[comment]. American Journal of Epidemiology 127:851–856

Pearl J (2000) Causality: models, reasoning and inference. Cambridge University Press, Cambridge

Phillips CV (2003) Quantifying and reporting uncertainty from systematic errors. Epidemiology 14:459–466

Robins JM (1989) The control of confounding by intermediate variables. Statistics in Medicine 8:679–701

Robins JM (2001) Data, design, and background knowledge in etiologic inference. Epidemiology 12:550–560

Robins JM, Greenland S (1992) Identifiability and exchangeability for direct and indirect effects. Epidemiology 3:143–155

Robins JM, Greenland S (1994) Adjusting for differential rates of prophylaxis therapy for PCP in high-dose versus low-dose AZT treatment arms in an AIDS randomized trial. Journal of the American Statistical Association 89:737–749

Robins JM, Morgenstern H (1987) The foundations of confounding in epidemiology. Computers and Mathematics with Applications 14:869–916

Robins JM, Blevins D, Ritter G, Wulfsohn M (1992) G-estimation of the effect of prophylaxis therapy for Pneumocystis carinii pneumonia on the survival of AIDS patients. Epidemiology 3:319–336

Robins JM, Hernan MA, Brumback B (2000) Marginal structural models and causal inference in epidemiology. Epidemiology 11:550–560

Rothman KJ (1976) Causes. American Journal of Epidemiology 104:587–592

Rothman KJ (1978) Occam's razor pares the choice among statistical models. American Journal of Epidemiology 108:347–349

Rothman KJ (1990) No adjustments are needed for multiple comparisons. Epidemiology 1:43–46

Rothman KJ, Greenland S (1998) Modern epidemiology, 2nd edn. Lippincott-Raven, Philadelphia

Rothman KJ, Greenland S, Walker AM (1980) Concepts of interaction. American Journal of Epidemiology 112:467–470

Saracci R (1987) The interactions of tobacco smoking and other agents in cancer etiology. Epidemiologic Reviews 9:175–193

Savitz DA, Baron EA (1989) Estimating and correcting for confounder misclassification. American Journal of Epidemiology 129:1062–1071

Schlesselman JJ (1978) Assessing effects of confounding variables. American Journal of Epidemiology 99:3–8

Schlesselman JJ (1982) Case-control studies: design, conduct, analysis. Oxford University Press, New York

Selikoff IJ, Seidman H, Hammond EC (1980) Mortality effects of cigarette smoking among amosite asbestos factory workers. Journal of the National Cancer Institute 65:507–513

Siemiatycki J, Thomas DC (1981) Biological models and statistical interactions: an example from multistage carcinogenesis. International Journal of Epidemiology 10:383–387

Siemiatycki J, Wacholder S, Dewar R, Wald L, Begin D, Richardson L, Rosenman K, Gerin M (1988) Smoking and degree of occupational exposure: are internal analyses in cohort studies likely to be confounded by smoking status? American Journal of Industrial Medicine 13:59–69

Sommer A, Zeger SL (1991) On estimating efficacy from clinical trials. Statistics in Medicine 10:45–52

Steenland K, Thun M (1986) Interaction between tobacco smoking and occupational exposures in the causation of lung cancer. Journal of Occupational Medicine 28:110–118

Steenland K, Beaumont J, Halperin W (1984) Methods of control for smoking in occupational cohort mortality studies. Scandinavian Journal of Work, Environment & Health 10:143–149

Steenland K, Bray I, Greenland S, Boffetta P (2000) Empirical Bayes adjustments for multiple results in hypothesis-generating or surveillance studies. Cancer Epidemiology Biomarkers & Prevention 9:895–903

Thomas DC, Greenland S (1983) The relative efficiencies of matched and independent sample designs for case-control studies. Journal of Chronic Diseases 36:685–697

Thomas DC, Stram D, Dwyer J (1993) Exposure-measurement error: influence on exposure-disease relationships and methods of correction. Annual Review of Public Health 14:69–93

Walter SD, Holford TR (1978) Additive, multiplicative, and other models for disease risks. American Journal of Epidemiology 108:341–346

Weinberg CR (1993) Toward a clearer definition of confounding. American Journal of Epidemiology 137:1–8

Witte JS, Greenland S, Kim L-L, Arab L (2000) Multilevel modeling in epidemiology with GLIMMIX. Epidemiology 11:684–688

Yanagawa T (1984) Case-control studies: assessing the effects of a confounding factor. Biometrika 71:191–194

Epidemiological Field Work in Population-Based Studies

Arlène Fink

Introduction

Field work in epidemiological studies consists of collecting data in natural and experimental settings to answer research questions or test hypotheses about the origins, distribution, and control of disease in populations. Field data can be collected directly and indirectly. Although direct data collection traditionally includes collecting biological samples such as blood and saliva, epidemiologists also collect data about the health of populations by contacting respondents through the telephone, mail, or online. To study a community's use of preventative health services (such as influenza vaccinations), for example, a team of epidemiologists can conduct in-person or telephone interviews or administer written, computer-assisted or online surveys. Indirect data collection includes reviewing written, oral, and visual records of respondents' thoughts and actions and observing them in their natural or experimental environment. To study the extent to which a health care system's medical providers adhere to recommended guidelines for preventative health care, for instance, a team of epidemiologists might review a sample of medical records to identify which preventative services were used and by whom. If the team were interested in understanding why preventative services were (or were not) used, it might review transcripts of audio or videotapes of selected physician and patient encounters.

This chapter focuses on providing practical tips on the spectrum of techniques epidemiologists can use in designing and administering reliable and non-biological field measures. Although the chapter focuses on direct data collection, many of the principles apply also to indirect data collection.

Asking for Information: What Are the Characteristics of Straightforward Questions and Responses?

Learning how to ask questions in written and spoken form is essential when collecting field data. A straightforward question asks for information in unambiguous way and extracts accurate and consistent data. Straightforward questions are purposeful, use correct grammar and syntax, and call for one thought at a time with mutually exclusive questions (Sudman and Bradburn 1982; Fink 2002).

Types of Questions

Purposeful Questions. Questions are purposeful when the respondent can readily identify the relationship between the intention of the question and the objectives of the study. If the objectives are to find out about the uses of health services, for instance, and some of the study's questions ask about education or place of birth, an explanation is needed of the relationship between questions and objectives. For instance, the introduction, can say something like: "We plan to compare people with differing backgrounds in their use of health services."

Concrete Questions.   A concrete question is precise and unambiguous. Adding a dimension of time can help make the question more concrete. For instance, rather than ask: "Has a physician *ever* told you that you have hypertension?" ask, "In the *past* 12 *months* has a physician told you that you have hypertension?"

Complete Sentences.   Questions should always be stated as complete sentences. Complete sentences express one entire thought, as in Example 1.

Example 1.   *Complete Sentences*
              Poor: Place of birth?
Comment: Place of birth means different things to different people. I might give the city in which I was born, but you might tell the name of the country or hospital. *Better*: Name the country in which you were born.   ◆

Make sure that experts and a sample of potential respondents review all questions even if you are using an already existing and validated instruments. Respondents' reading levels and attention spans may vary across studies.

Open and Closed Questions.   Questions can take two primary forms. When they require respondents to use their own words, they are called open or open-ended. When the answers or responses are preselected for the respondent, the question is termed closed. Both types of questions have advantages and limitations.

An open question is useful when the intricacies of an issue are still unknown, in getting unanticipated answers, and for describing the world as the respondent sees it – rather than as the questioner does. Also, some respondents prefer to state their views in their own words and may resent the questioner's preselected choices. Sometimes, when left to their own devices, respondents provide quotable material. The disadvantage is that unless the team includes a trained anthropologist or qualitative researcher, responses to open questions are often difficult to interpret and compare.

Some respondents prefer closed questions because they are either unwilling or unable to express themselves. Closed questions are more difficult to write than open ones, however, because the answers or response choices must be known in advance. But the results lend themselves more readily to statistical analysis and interpretation. This feature is particularly important in most epidemiological studies which often rely on relatively large numbers of responses and respondents. Also, because the respondent's expectations are more clearly spelled out in closed questions, the answers have a better chance of being more reliable or consistent over time. Example 2 shows a closed question.

Example 2. *A Closed Question*

How often during the past week were you irritable? Circle one.

	Please Circle One
Always or nearly always	1
Sometimes	2
Rarely or never	3

Types of Responses

The choices given to respondents for their answers may take three forms (Fink and Kosecoff 1998; McDowell and Newell 1996; Stewart and Ware 1992). The first is called nominal or categorical. (The two terms are sometimes used interchangeably.) Categorical or nominal choices have no numerical or preferential values. For example, asking respondents if they are male or female is the same as asking them to "name" themselves as belonging to one of two categories: male or female.

The second form of response choice is called ordinal. When respondents are asked to rate or order choices, say, from very positive to very negative, they are given ordinal choices. The third form of response choice results in numerical data such as when a respondent is asked to give his or her height or age at the last birthday.

A hypothetical study finding that uses nominal data results in numbers or percentages, as follows:

Five hundred respondents were interviewed in a study of preventative health. All were asked to indicate whether or not they perform four health-related activities: (1) exercise at least 30 minutes most days of the week; (2) eat 5 or 6 servings of fruits or vegetables daily; (3) smoke; (4) drink no more than 1 to 2 alcoholic drinks daily. Of the 500 respondents, 25% reported that they smoked; only 10% stated that they drank no more than 1 to 2 drinks daily. None of the respondents reported exercising at least 30 minutes per day or eating 5 or 6 servings of fruits or vegetables.

Ordinal responses are made to fit on a scale that is ordered from positive (*definitely or probably important*) to negative (*definitely or probably not important*). Ordinal data thus are often characterized by counts of the numbers and percentages of people who select each point on a graded scale.

Of 500 respondents completing the question, 250 (50.0%) rated each preventive health behavior as definitely or probably important.

Field studies often ask for numerical data as when respondents are asked for their birth date. From the date, you can calculate each respondent's age. Age is considered a numerical and continuous measure, starting with zero and ending with the age of the oldest person in the study. Numerical data lend themselves to many statistical operations. Typical findings might appear as follows: The average age of the respondents was 43 years. The oldest person was 79 years of age, and the youngest was 23.

10.3   How Are Field Study Measures and Questions Organized?

10.3.1   Length

The length of a measure depends upon what you need to know and how many questions you need to ask to get credible answers (Bourque and Fielder 2003a; Bourque and Fielder 2003b). Another consideration is the respondents. How much time do they have available, and will they pay attention? Relatively young children, for example, may only stay still for a few minutes, so shorter interviews, for example, may be better. You must also consider your resources: Longer measures may be more costly to design, validate and administer.

10.3.2   Question Order

All field measures should be preceded by an introduction, and the first set of questions should be related to the topic described in it. This is illustrated in Box 1.

Note that the interviewer starts off by saying that questions will be asked about satisfaction with the Health Clinic, and the first question calls for a rating of satisfaction.

In general, questions should proceed from easiest to answer and the most familiar to most difficult and least familiar. In a survey of needs for health services, items can first be asked about the respondent's own needs for services, then their family's, community's, and so on.

Questions of recall should also be organized according to their natural sequence. Do not ask very general questions: "When did you first start feeling dizzy?" Instead, prompt the respondent and ask: "In the past three months, how often did you felt dizzy? Think about the last time you felt dizzy. Was it in the morning, afternoon or evening?"

Sometimes the answer to one question will affect the content of another. When this happens, the value of the measure may be diminished (Example 3).

Box 1. An Introduction to a Telephone Interview and Its First Question

Hello. I am calling from the Health Clinic. We are surveying people who use the Health Clinic to find out whether it provides satisfactory services. Your name was selected at random from the Clinic's database. Our questionnaire will take no more than four minutes. You can interrupt me at any time. May I ask you the questions? [IF YES, CONTINUE. IF NO, SAY: Thank you AND HANG UP.]
CONTINUE HERE:
   The first question asks you about your overall satisfaction with the Health Clinic. Do you consider it [READ CHOICES]
a. Definitely satisfactory
b. Probably satisfactory
c. Probably not satisfactory
d. Definitely not satisfactory

[DO NOT SAY]
e. No opinion or don't know/wrong answer

Example 3. *Ordering Questions*
               Which question should come first?
   a. How efficient is the nursing staff?
Or
   b. Which improvements in nursing do you recommend?

Answer: Question b should come before Question a. If it does not, then the respondent might offer suggestions for the improvement of the nursing staff's efficiency of the nursing merely because it has been suggested.   ◆

Place relatively easy-to-answer questions at the end of the measure. When questionnaires, for instance, are long or difficult, respondents may get tired and answer the last questions carelessly or not answer them at all. You can place demographic questions (age, income, gender, and other background characteristics) at the end because these can be answered quickly.

Avoid many items that look alike. Twenty items, all of which ask the respondent to agree or disagree with statements, may lead to fatigue or boredom, and the respondent may give up. To minimize loss of interest, group the questions and provide transitions that describe the format or topic. For instance, say or print something like: "The next set of questions ask about your use of health services."

Questions that are relatively sensitive should be placed toward the end. Topics such as grooming habits, religious views, and positions on controversial subjects such as abortion and assisted suicide must be placed far enough along so there is reason to believe the respondent is willing to pay attention, but not so far that he or she is too fatigued to answer properly.

Finally, questions should appear to reasonable people to be in a logical order. Do not switch from one topic to another unless you provide a transitional statement to help the respondent make sense of the order.

Here is a checklist of points to consider in selecting the order for the questions in your field measure:

Checklist to Guide Question-Order
— For any given topic, ask relatively objective questions before the subjective ones.
— Move from the most familiar topics to the least.
— Follow the natural sequence of time.
— See to it that all questions are independent.
— Avoid many items that look alike.
— Ask sensitive questions well after the beginning.
— Place questions in a logical order.

10.3.3   Aesthetics and Other Concerns

A measure's appearance is important. A self-administered questionnaire that is hard to read can confuse or irritate respondents who may not answer accurately or at all, reducing the reliability of the responses. A poorly designed interview form with inadequate space for recording answers will reduce the efficiency of even the most skilled interviewers.

10.3.4   Branching Questions or Skip Patterns

What happens when you are concerned with getting answers to questions that you know are only appropriate for part of your group? Suppose you were interviewing older adults in a general practice to learn about their medication-use. You know that many of these patients are likely to be taking certain kinds of mediations such as antihypertensives, NSAIDs, and aspirin. However, some people will be taking all of these medications each day, while others will be taking none.

If you want to ask about a topic that you know in advance is *not* relevant to everyone in the study, you might design a form such as the one in Example 4.

Example 4.   *Skip Patterns or Branching Questions*

— Do you take any of the following medications (a list is provided)
   a. *No* (Go to question 4)
   b. *Yes*

[IF YES] How often do you take your usual dose (choices are given such as once a day; only when needed)?

OR

— Do you take any of the following medications?
   a. *Yes* (COMPLETE SECTION A)
   b. *No* (GO TO SECTION B)   ◆

Skip patterns may be confusing to people and should be avoided in self-administered printed questionnaires. Interviewers must be trained to follow the branches. Computer-assisted and online questionnaires are effective vehicles for branching because you can design the software to guide the respondent. For instance, if the questionnaire tells the respondent, "If no, go to question 6," the respondent who answers "no" will automatically be sent to question 6.

What Does It Take to Ensure Proper Administration of Field Instruments?

10.4

Self-Administered Questionnaires

10.4.1

Self-administered questionnaires take the form of written, computer-assisted, and online surveys. They require a great deal of advance preparation and subsequent monitoring to get a reasonable response rate. These questionnaires are given or sent directly to people for completion. Advance preparation, in the form of careful editing and tryouts, is necessary in helping to produce a clear, readable self-administered questionnaire (Bourque and Fielder 2003a). You should always review the returns. Are you getting the response rate you expected? Are all questions being answered? The following is a checklist for using self-administered questionnaires:

Checklist for Using Self-Administered Questionnaires
— Mail respondents a letter or email them in advance telling them the purpose of your study. The letter should inform people to expect a questionnaire, explain the importance of the study and the respondent's role, list study supporters and sources of funding, and describe procedures to ensure confidentiality.
— Prepare a short, formal letter to accompany the questionnaire form. If you have already sent an advance letter, this one should be very concise.
— Offer to send respondents a summary of the findings so they can see just how the data are used. (If you promise this, allocate resources for it.)
— If you ask questions that may be construed as personal – such as gender, age, or income – explain why the questions are necessary.

— Keep the questionnaire procedures simple. Provide stamped self-addressed envelopes for written, mailed questionnaires. Make sure no special software is needed for online surveys (e.g., to download graphics). If special software is necessary, set up a system for ensuring that all respondents who are eligible for the survey have access to the software.

— Keep questionnaires as short as you can. Ask only questions you are sure you need and do not crowd them together. Give respondents enough room to write or check boxes and be sure each question is set apart from the next.

— Consider incentives. This may encourage people to respond. Incentives may range from certificates of appreciation and money and stamps to pens, fuel and food.

— Be prepared to follow up or send reminders. These should be brief and to the point. For mailed and online surveys, it often helps to send another copy of the questionnaire to non-respondents. Do not forget to budget money and time for these additional mailings.

10.4.2   Interviews

Finding Interviewers.   Interviewers should fit in as well as possible with respondents. They should avoid flamboyant clothes, haircuts, and so on. Sometimes it is a good idea to select interviewers who are similar to respondents in gender, age or other demographic characteristics.

It is also important that the interviewers be able to speak clearly and understandably. Unusual speech patterns or accents may provoke unnecessarily favorable or unfavorable reactions. The interviewer's way of talking is of course an extremely important consideration in the telephone interview. The interviewer's attitude toward the study and the respondent will influence the results. If the interviewer does not expect much from the interview and sends this message, the response rate and reliability of responses will probably suffer. To make sure you are getting the most accurate data possible, you should systematically and frequently monitor the interviewers' progress (Bourque and Fielder 2003b).

Training Interviewers.   The key to a good telephone or face-to-face interview is training (Frey 1989). The overall goal of training should be to produce interviewers who know what is expected of them and how to answer questions and also know where to turn if problems arise unexpectedly in the field.

Whether you are training two interviewers or twenty, it is important to find a time to meet together. The advantage of meetings is that everyone can develop a standard vocabulary and share problems encountered in the field.

Once at the training site, trainees must have enough space to sit and write or perform any other activities you will require of them. If you want them to interview one another as practice for their real task, be sure the room is large enough so that two or more groups can speak without disturbing the others. You may even need several rooms.

Trainees should be taken step by step through their tasks and given an opportunity to ask questions. It is also essential to tell them some of the reasons for their tasks so they can anticipate problems and be prepared to solve them. The most efficient way to make sure the trainees have all the information they need to perform their job is to prepare a manual. Here you can explain what they are to do and when, where, why, and how they are to do it.

Conducting Interviews.   The following are suggested guidelines for conducting interviews.

— Make a brief introductory statement that will describe who is conducting the interview ("Dr. Mary Doe for Armstrong Memorial Medical Center"), tell why the interview is being conducted ("to find out how satisfied you are with our after-surgery program"), explain why the respondent is being called ("We're asking a random sample of people who were discharged from the hospital in the last two months"), and indicate whether or not answers will be kept confidential ("Your name will not be used without your written permission").
— Try to impress the person being interviewed with the importance of the interview and of the answers. People are more likely to cooperate if they appreciate the importance of the subject matter. Do not try to deal with every complaint or criticism, but suggest that all answers will receive equal attention.
— Check the hearing and "literacy" of the respondent. Although it is important to stay on schedule and ask all the questions, a few people may have trouble hearing and understanding some of the questions. If that happens, reappraise the eligibility of the respondent (perhaps an interview is not the best method of obtaining reliable data from this respondent; other methods may be more appropriate). Another option is to speak more clearly and slowly.
— Ask questions as they appear in the interview schedule. It is important to ask everyone the same questions in the same way or the results will not be comparable.

Monitoring Interview Quality.   To make sure you are getting the most accurate data possible, you should monitor the quality of the interviews. This might mean something as informal as having the interviewer call you once a week, or something as formal as having them submit to you a standardized checklist of activities they perform each day. If possible, you may actually want to go with an interviewer (if it is a face-to-face interview) or spend time with telephone interviewers to make sure that what they are doing is appropriate for the study's purposes. To prevent problems, you might want to take some or all of the following steps:

Tips for Ensuring Quality
— Establish a hot line. This means having someone available to answer any questions that might occur immediately, even at the time of an interview. Consider obtaining a toll-free number.

— Provide written scripts. If interviewers are to introduce themselves or the study, give them a script or set of topics to cover. The script may have to be approved by an Institutional Review Board.
— Make sure you give out extra copies of all supplementary materials. If data collectors are to mail completed interviews back to you, for example, make sure to give them extra forms and envelopes.
— Provide an easy-to-read handout describing the purpose of the interview and the content of the questions.
— Provide a schedule and calendar so that interviewers can keep track of their progress.
— Consider providing the interviewer with visual aids. Visual aids may be extremely important when interviewing people in-person whose ability to speak or read may be limited. The preparation of audiovisual aids for use in an interview is relatively expensive and requires that the interviewers be specially trained in using them.
— Consider the possibility that some interviewers may need to be retrained and make plans to do so.

Computer-Assisted Telephone Interviews or CATI.   Computer-assisted interviewing is becoming increasingly accepted as a useful field work tool. With CATI, the interviewer reads instructions and questions to the respondent directly from the computer monitor and enters the responses directly into the computer (Bourque and Fielder 2003b). The computer, not the interviewer, controls the progression of the interview questions. No paper copies of the interview are produced, thus eliminating the need to find secure storage place for completed questionnaires.

CATI software programs enable the researcher to enter all telephone numbers and call schedules into the computer. When the interviewer logs on, he or she will be prompted with a list of phone numbers to call, including new scheduled interviews and callbacks. For example, suppose the interviewer calls someone at 8 AM, but receives no answer. The CATI program can automatically reschedule the call for some other time. CATI programs are also available that enable specially trained interviewers to contact respondents with unique needs. For instance, suppose your study sample consists of people who speak different languages. CATI will allow multi-lingual interviewers to log on with certain keywords; the computer will then direct them to their unique set of respondents.

The major advantage of CATI is that once the data are collected they are immediately available for analysis. However, having easy access to data may not always be a blessing. Some researchers may be tempted to analyze the data before the completion of data collection, and the preliminary results may be misleading. A main value of easy access to data, certainly in the early stages of data collection, lies in having the means to check on the characteristics of the respondents and to monitor the quality of the CATI interviewers in obtaining complete data.

Intensive interviewer training is crucial when using CATI in field studies. Interviewers must first learn how to use the CATI software and handle computer problems should they arise during the course of the interview. For instance, what will the interviewer do if the computer "freezes"? Further, the interviewer needs to practice answering questions invariably posed by respondents regarding the study's objectives, methods, human subjects' protections and incentives. In fact, given the complexity of CATI, training may take up to a week. Thus, at the present time, use of CATI should probably be considered primarily when a study is well funded because it is a relatively expensive and specialized form of data collection.

CATI takes two forms. The first, which is most commonly used, consists of a lab or a facility furnished with banks of telephone calling stations that are equipped with computers linked to a central server. The costs of building the lab are extremely high and include assembling soundproof cubicles and having either a master computer that stores the data from the individual computers or linkage to a server. Additional resources are needed to cover the cost of leasing CATI software and hiring a programmer to install it. Training for this type of CATI is expensive, requiring a great deal of practice. There are also numerous incidental costs including those for headsets, seats and desks, instructional manuals and service contracts for the hardware.

A second type of computer-assisted telephone interviewing system consists of CATI software programs that are run on laptops. With this type of CATI, the researcher only needs a laptop and access to a telephone connected to the Internet. In time, we can expect that the telephone will be superseded by wireless access to the Internet, making this type of telephone interviewing a desirable method for collecting data in the field and sending them to a central server. Moreover, this second type of CATI is appropriate for studies with a variety of funding levels because it is portable and relatively inexpensive. The portability of laptops, however, raises concerns about patient privacy. Laptops are sometimes shared or stolen, providing easy access to confidential respondent data. In anticipation of these concerns, laptops that are used for CATI should be dedicated to a single study, strict privacy safeguards must be enforced, and interviewers must receive special training to ensure proper CATI implementation and respondent protection. In the U.S., patient privacy rules have become increasingly strict (e.g., through the Health Insurance Portability and Accountability Act or HIPAA), with costly penalties for violation.

How Can You Assure a Reliable and Valid Field Measure?

10.5

Pilot Testing

10.5.1

Once a field measure has been assembled, it should be tested to determine the ease with which it can be administered and to estimate the accuracy of the data. Pilot testing includes evaluating the logistics of administration as well as the ease of use of the form itself. The purpose of the pilot test is to answer these questions:

Questions Answered by Pilot Testing
— Will the measure provide the needed information? Are certain words or questions redundant or misleading?
— Are the questions appropriate for the respondents?
— Will information collectors be able to use the forms properly? Can they administer, collect, and report information using any written directions or special coding forms?
— Are the procedures standardized? Can everyone collect information in the same way?
— How consistent or reliable is the information?

10.5.2 Reliability and Validity: The Quality of the Measure

A ruler is considered to be a reliable instrument if it yields the same results every time it is used to measure the same object, assuming the object itself has not changed. A yardstick showing that you are 6 feet 1 inch tall today and 6 feet 1 inch six months from today is reliable.

People change over time. You may be more tired, angry, and tense today than you were yesterday. People also change because of their experiences or because they learned something new, but meaningful changes are not subject to random fluctuations. A reliable instrument will provide a consistent measure of important characteristics despite background fluctuations. It reflects the "true" score – one that is free from random errors.

A ruler is considered to be a valid instrument if it provides an accurate measure (free from error) of a person's height. But even if the ruler says you are 6 feet 1 inch tall today and six months from now (meaning it is reliable), it may be incorrect, that is, invalid. This would occur if the ruler were not calibrated accurately, and you are really 5 feet 6 inches tall.

If you develop an instrument that consists of nothing more than asking a hospital administrator how many beds are in a given ward, and you get the same answer on at least two occasions, you would have an instrument that is reliable. But if you claim that the same instrument reflects the quality of medical care, you have a reliable measure of questionable validity. A valid measure is always a reliable one, but a reliable one is not always valid (Bernard 2000; Dawson and Trapp 2001).

10.5.3 Ensuring Quality: Selecting Ready-to-Use Measures

One way to make sure that you have a reliable and valid measure is to use one that someone else has prepared and demonstrated to be reliable and valid through careful testing. This is particularly important to remember if you want to survey attitudes, emotions, health status, quality of life, and health beliefs (Stewart and Ware 1992; McDowell and Newell 1996). These factors, and others like them, are elusive and difficult to measure. To produce a truly satisfactory measure of health, quality of life, and human emotions and preferences thus requires a large-scale and truly scientific experimental study.

Reliability

In reviewing a published field instrument (also, in assessing the quality of a home-made form) you should ask the following questions about four types of reliability: test-retest, equivalence, internal consistency, and interobserver reliability.

Test-Retest Reliability. Does the instrument have test-retest reliability? One way to estimate reliability is to determine if someone taking the measure answers about the same on more than one occasion. Test-retest reliability is computed by administering the measure to the same group on two different occasions and then correlating the scores from one time to the next to obtain a correlation coefficient (r value). Usually, to be considered reliable, an instrument should obtain a correlation coefficient of at least 0.70 (Stewart and Ware 1992).

You can calculate test-retest reliability for single questions, subsets, or entire measures. For example, suppose you are studying the use of medications in a sample of older adults. The instrument you are using asks this question, "How many prescription medications do you usually take each day?" In order to assess the consistency of the respondents' answers, you would ask the same question twice: at baseline and then a second time, say 2–4 weeks later. Assuming medication-use rates in your sample tend to be stable over short periods of time, any differences in responses to the question can be assumed to reflect measurement error and not changes in the use of medications. To calculate test-retest reliability for an entire measure, you would administer its entire set of questions at two different points in time, score it, and then calculate the correlation coefficient for the two scores.

Equivalence. Are alternative forms equivalent? If two different forms of a questionnaire are supposed to measure the same attitude, for example, you should make sure that people are likely to obtain the same score regardless of which one they take. If you want to use Form A of the instrument as a premeasure, for example, and Form B as a postmeasure, check the equivalence of the two forms to make sure one is not different from the other.

Equivalence reliability can be computed by giving different forms of the instrument to two or more groups that have been randomly selected. The forms are created either by using differently worded questions to measure the same attributes or by reordering the questions. To test for equivalence, you can administer the different forms (reordered or reworded) at separate time points to the same population, or if the sample is large enough, you can divide it in half and administer each of the two alternate forms to half of the group. In either case, you would first compute mean scores and standard deviations on each of the forms and then correlate the two sets of scores to obtain estimates of equivalence. Equivalence reliability coefficients should be at least 0.70.

Internal Consistency.   Another measure of reliability is how internally consistent the questions are in measuring the characteristics, attitudes, or qualities that they are supposed to measure. To test for internal consistency, you calculate a statistic called coefficient alpha, or Cronbach's alpha, named for the person who first reported the statistic.(Anastasi 1982; Bernard 2000). Coefficient alpha describes how well different items complement each other in their measurement of the same quality or dimension.

Many researchers are not at all concerned with internal consistency because they are not going to be using several items to measure one attitude or characteristic. Instead, they are interested in the responses to each item. Decide if your instrument needs to consider internal consistency.

Example 5.   *Internal consistency*
        Internal consistency is important
A ten-item interview is conducted to find out patients' satisfaction with medical care in hospitals. High scores mean much satisfaction; low scores mean little satisfaction. To what extent do the ten items each measure the same dimension of satisfaction with hospital care?

   Internal consistency is not important
A ten-item interview is conducted with patients as part of a study to find out how hospitals can improve. Eight items ask about potential changes in different services such as the type of food that might be served, the availability of doctors, nurses, or other health professionals, and so on. One item asks patients for their age, and one asks about education. Since this interview is concerned with views on improving eight very different services and with providing data on age and education of respondents, each item is independent of the others.   ◆

Interobserver Reliability: Kappa.   Kappa is a statistic used to measure interrater (or intrarater) agreement for nominal measures (Cohen 1960). Suppose two researchers are asked to independently review a sample of 100 medical records to determine health services utilization among a sample of diabetic patients. Suppose also that the reviewers are required to use a standardized form containing questions about utilization. One of the questions asks the reviewer to indicate whether or not each patient has visited the emergency department (ED) within the past month. Here are the reviewers' responses to that question (Table 10.1).

   This is shown in the following formula in which O is the observed agreement and C is the chance agreement.

Measuring Agreement Between Two Coders: The *Kappa* (κ) Statistic

$$\kappa = \frac{O - C(\text{Agreement beyond chance})}{1 - C(\text{Agreement possible beyond chance})} .$$

Table 10.1. Reviewers' response

Reviewer 2	Reviewer 1		
	No, Did not Visit ED	Yes, Did Visit ED	
No	20^C	15	35^B
Yes	10	55^D	65
	30^A	70	

Reviewer 1 says that 30 (^{A}) of the 100 patients did not visit the ED, while Reviewer 2 says that 35 (^{B}) did not. The two reviewers agree that 20 (^{C}) patients did not visit the ED.
What is the best way to describe the extent of agreement between the reviewers? 20 of 100 or 20% (^{C}) is probably too low because the reviewers also agree that 55% (^{D}) of patients did visit the ED. The total agreement: 55% + 20% is an overestimate because with only two categories (yes and no), some agreement may occur by chance.

Here is how the formula works with the above example.
1. Calculate how many records the reviewers may agree by chance indicate that patents did not visit the ED. This is done by multiplying the number of no's and dividing by 100 because there are 100 interviews: $30 \times 35/100 = 10.5$
2. Calculate how many interviews they may agree by chance indicate that patients do visit the ED. This is done by multiplying the number of yes's and dividing by 100 : $70 \times 65/100 = 40.5$
3. Add the two numbers obtained in steps 1 and 2 and divide by 100 to get a proportion for *chance agreement*: $(10.5 + 45.5)/100 = 0.56$.

The *observed agreement* is 20% + 55% = 75% or 0.75. Therefore the agreement beyond chance is $0.75 - 0.56 = 0.19$: the numerator.
The *agreement possible beyond chance* is 100% minus the chance agreement of 56% or $1 - 0.56 = 0.44$: the denominator

$$\kappa = \frac{0.19}{0.44} = 0.43 .$$

What is a "high" *kappa*? Some experts have attached the following qualitative terms to *kappas*: 0.0–0.2 = slight; 0.2–0.4 = fair; 0.4–0.6 = moderate; 0.6–0.8 = substantial, and 0.8–0.10 = almost perfect.
Here are some questions to ask about a published field instrument's validity:

Questions to Ask
About a Published Instrument's Validity

1. Does the instrument have predictive validity? You can validate an instrument by proving that it predicts an individual's ability to perform a given task or behave in a certain way. For example, a medical school entrance examination has predictive validity if it accurately forecasts performance in medical school. One way of establishing predictive validity is to administer

the instrument to all students who want to enter medical school and compare these scores with their performance in school. If the two sets of scores show a high positive or negative correlation, the instrument has predictive validity.

2. Does the instrument have concurrent validity? You can validate an instrument by comparing it against a known and accepted measure. To establish the concurrent validity of a new measure of quality of care, you could administer the new instrument and an already established, validated instrument to the same group and compare the scores from both instruments. You can also administer just the new instrument to the respondents and compare their scores on it to experts' judgment of the respondents' attitudes. A high correlation between the new instrument and the criterion measure (the established instrument or expert judgment) means concurrent validity. A concurrent validity study is only valuable if the criterion measure is convincing.

3. Does the instrument have content validity? An instrument can be validated by proving that its questions accurately represent the characteristics or attitudes that they are intended to measure. An instrument that is designed to measure health beliefs has content validity, for example, if it contains a reasonable sample of facts, words, ideas, and theories commonly used when discussing or reading about the formation of beliefs about disease or health. Content validity is usually established by consulting the literature and by asking experts and prospective respondents whether the questions represent the knowledge, attitudes and behaviors you want to measure.

4. Does the instrument have construct validity? Construct validity means that the instrument measures what it purports to and not something else. Because of the difficulty of obtaining a true measure of the concepts and ideas that characterize epidemiological studies, construct validity must be established experimentally. One method of doing this is to administer the instrument to people whom selected experts say exhibit the behavior associated with the construct. Usually, the experts based their judgments on theories that have empirical support and on clinical experience. If the people chosen by the experts to be exemplars of the behavior also obtain a high score (i.e., a higher score means greater evidence of the behavior), then the instrument is considered to have construct validity. This form of validity is usually established after years of experimentation and experience with the measure.

10.5.6   Suggested Guidelines For Pilot Testing

— Try to anticipate the actual circumstances in which the instrument will be conducted and make plans to handle them. For interviews, this means reproducing the training manual and all forms; for online surveys and mailed questionnaires, you have to produce any cover letters, return envelopes, and so on. Needless to say, this requires planning and time and can be costly.

- You can start by trying out selected portions of the instrument in a very informal fashion. Just the directions on a self-administered questionnaire might be tested first, for example, or the wording of several questions in an interview might be tested. This is sometimes called a "cognitive" pretest.
- Choose respondents for the pilot who are similar to the ones who will eventually complete the measure. They should be approximately the same age, with similar education, and so on.
- Enlist as many people in the trial as seems reasonable without wasting your resources. Probably fewer people will be needed to test a five-item questionnaire than a twenty-item one.
- For reliability, focus on the clarity of the questions and the general format of the instrument. Look for:
  - failure to answer questions
  - giving several answers to the same question
  - writing comments in the margins.

Any one of these is a signal that the measure may be unreliable and needs revision. Are the choices in forced-choice questions mutually exclusive? Have you provided all possible alternatives? Is the questionnaire or interview language clear and unbiased? Do the directions and transitions make sense? Have you chosen the proper order for the questions? Is the questionnaire too long or hard to read? Does the interview take too long? For instance, you planned for a ten-minute interview, but your pilot version takes twenty.

Consider this: In a pilot of a self-administered survey of children's health behaviors, respondents were asked how often they washed their hands after eating. All six children between 8 and 10 years of age answered "always" after being given the choices "always," "never," and "I don't know." The choices were changed to "almost always," "usually," and "almost never." With the new categories, the same six children changed their answers to two "almost always" and four "usually."

Field Work Language and Culture 10.6

If you plan on translating an existing data collection instrument or measure, do not assume that you can automatically reword each question into the new language. Between the original language and the next language often lie cultural gaps. You may need to reword each question.

To avoid confusing people and even insulting them because you misunderstand their language or culture, you should follow a few simple guidelines. These involve enlisting the assistance of people who are fluent in the language (and its dialects) and pilot testing the measure with typical respondents. Suggested guidelines for translation always include the following.

10.6.1   Suggested Guidelines for Translation

- Use fluent speakers to do the first translation. If you can, use native speakers. If you can afford it, find a professional translator. The art of translation is in the subtleties – words and phrases that take years and cultural immersion to learn. If you use fluent speakers, you will minimize the time needed to revise question wording and response choices.
- Tryout the translated measure with 3 to 5 native speakers. Ask: What is this question asking you? Can you think of a better way to ask this question?
- Revise the measure with the help of the original translator.
- Translate the measure back into the original language. Use a different translator for this task. Does this "back translated" instrument match the original version? If not, the two translators should work together to make them match.
- Try the resulting measure on a small group (5–10) of target respondents. If the two translators could not agree on wording, let the group decide.
- Revise the measure.
- Pilot test the measure.
- Produce a final version.

10.7   Managing the Data

Data management consists of the methods used to store and organize information so that it can be analyzed. Data management starts with an analysis plan and ends with the final analytic operation. The analysis plan describes the hypotheses to be tested or research questions that will be answered. The plan is a guide to the data that will be collected, entered and subsequently analyzed (Example 6).

Example 6.   *A Portion of an Analysis Plan for an Interview on Health and Alcohol Use in the Elderly*
Hypothesis: More men than women will exceed drinking limits.

Variables: gender; drinking limits

Planned Analysis: Chi square to test for differences between numbers of men and women who exceed limits   ◆

Modifications to the original analysis plan can be expected, especially in large studies with a great deal of data.

A second data management activity is the creation of a code book. The contents of a code book may vary among researchers. Some researchers include in their definition only a description of study's variables (such as [DRINK]) and how they are categorized or labeled (such as 1 = 1 to 2 drinks daily; 2 = 3 or more drinks daily; 9 = no data). Increasingly, many investigators are promulgating the view that code books should include all the information needed to reproduce the study. For example (Example 7), the Field Survey, a large California polling survey group posts information like the following on its web site (http://field.com/fieldpoll/).

Example 7. *Table of Contents for A Code Book*

I. Methods
  A. *Sampling*
    1. Sampling design to include eligibility criteria (e.g., 65 years of age and older; have had at least one drink in the past month)
    2. Sampling strategies (e.g., stratified random sampling; convenience or opportunistic sampling; etc.)
    3. Sample size and justification
    4. Recruitment and enrollment
    5. Sampling statistics to include weight and sampling error calculations
  B. *Human subjects*: Informed consent
  C. *Research design* or how participants were assigned to groups (if appropriate); number and timing of instrument administration

II. Data Collection
  A. A copy of the instrument
    6. The origins of the questions (e.g., adapted from a published instrumement; created for this one)
    7. Description of how each response is coded (e.g., 1 = yes; 2 = no; 9 = no data)
  B. Training of data collectors; quality control
  C. Information on reliability and validity

III. A Data File Description
  The variable names [DRINK], Labels (quantity and frequency) and values and value labels (1 = 1 to 2 drinks daily; 2 = 3 or more drinks daily; 9 = no data) ◆

A major problem in data management is how to handle missing data. Say, you mail 100 questionnaires and get 95 back. Is this a 95% response rate? Suppose that upon close examination, you discover that half the respondents did not answer question 5, and that none of the questions was answered by all respondents. With all that missing information, you cannot claim to have a 95% response rate.

What should be done about missing responses? In some situations, you may be able to go back to the respondents and ask them to answer the questions they omitted. In small studies, where the respondents are known, the respondents may be easily re-contacted. But collecting information a second time is usually impractical, if not impossible, in most studies. Some studies are anonymous, and you do not even know who the respondents are. In institutional settings, you may have to go back to the Institutional Review Board to get permission to contact the respondents a second time. This may take too much time for your purposes.

Computerized questionnaires can be programmed so that the respondent must answer one question before proceeding to the next. Some respondents may find this approach frustrating, however, and refuse to complete the questionnaire. Although compelling respondents to answer all questions is touted as a major advantage of computer-assisted data collection, some researchers believe that forcing respondents to answer every question is coercive and unethical.

A key management activity is data entry, that is, the process of getting data into the computer. It usually takes three forms. In the first, someone enters data from a coded instrument into a database management program or spreadsheet. The data are then saved in as text or ASCII files, so that they can be exported into a statistical program like SPSS, SAS, or Stata. A second type of data entry involves entering data directly into a statistical program like SPSS, SAS, or Stata. In the third form of data entry, the respondent or interviewer enters responses directly into the computer. Data entry of this type is associated with computer-based measures including CATI and online surveys. The responses are automatically entered into database management systems or statistical programs (usually through special translation software). Programs are also available that will automatically convert one file format into another (say from SAS to Stata).

Database management programs, statistical programs and computer-assisted data collection with automatic data entry can facilitate accuracy by being programmed to allow the entry of only legal codes. For instance, if the codes should be entered as 001–010, then you can write rules so that an entry of 01 or 10 is not permitted. If you try to enter 01 or 10, you will get an error message. With minimum programming, the program can also check each entry to ensure that it is consistent with previously entered data and that skip patterns are respected. That is, the program can make sure that the fields for questions that are to be skipped by some respondents are coded as skips and not as missing data. Designing a computer-assisted protocol requires skill and time. No protocol should be regarded as error-free until it has been tested and retested in the field.

Once the data are entered, they need to be cleaned. A clean data set can be used by anyone to get the same results as you do when you run the analysis. Data become "dirty" for a number of reasons including miscoding, incorrect data entry and missing responses.

To avoid dirty data, make sure that coders or data entrers are experienced, well trained, and supervised. Check variable values against preset maximum and minimum levels, so that if someone enters 50 instead of 5, the maximum, you know there is an error. You can also minimize errors by making sure your coding scheme distinguishes among truly missing (no response or no data), from don't know and not applicable.

Run frequencies on your data as soon as you have about 10% of the responses in. Run them again and again until you are sure that the fieldwork is running smoothly. Frequencies are tabulations of the responses to each question. If your data set is relatively small, you can visually scan the frequencies for errors. For large databases with many records, variables, skip patterns, and open-ended text responses, you may need to do a systematic computerized check. All leading statistical programs provide for cleaning specifications that can be used during data entry and later as a separate cleaning process.

Several other problems may require you to clean up the data. These include having to deal with the complete absence of data because some questionnaires have not been returned, for instance, with missing data from questionnaire that have been returned, and with questionnaires that contain data that are very different form the average respondents.

What Are Reasonable Resources? 10.8

Fieldwork resources are reasonable if they adequately cover the financial costs of and time needed to conduct all activities in the time planned. This includes the costs of, and time for, hiring and training staff, preparing and validating forms, administering the instrument or measure, and analyzing, interpreting, and reporting the findings.

How much does it cost to conduct fieldwork? This question can be answered by obtaining the answers to seven other questions.

1. What are the major tasks?
2. What skills are needed to complete each task?
3. How much time do I have?
4. How much time does each task take?
5. Whom can I hire to perform each task?
6. What are the costs of each task?
7. What additional resources are needed?

Here is a checklist of typical field work tasks:

Field Work Task Checklist
— *Prepare the instrument for use in the field.*
  — Identify existing and appropriate instruments.
  — Conduct a literature review.
  — Contact other researchers.
  — Adapt some or all questions from existing instruments.
  — Prepare a new instrument.

— *Identify, enroll and recruit subjects.*
  — Determine eligibility criteria (who should be included and excluded).
  — Determine sample size.

- Identify sources for identifying respondents (e.g., existing data bases; patients in a waiting room; patients with appointments).
- Devise plans for coordinating respondents' willingness to participate and the study's field work needs. For instance, you may have to provide transportation for interviewers or participants.

- *Prepare documents for the IRB (Institutional Review Board).*
  - Develop procedures for insuring ethical principles of research. Such principles include respect for people and their autonomy; protecting people from harm and taking active steps to protect them; and balance potential risks with benefit from participation in the study.
  - Devise methods for ensuring the protection of the people who participate in field studies, including the preparation of fliers, recruitment letters, and informed consent forms.
  - Make provisions for protection against research misconduct including exaggerating findings or releasing them without permission.

- *Pretest the Instrument.*
  - Identify a relatively small sample for the pretest.
  - Conduct a "cognitive" pretest by going over the instrument question by question with each respondent.

- *Pilot test the instrument.*
  - Identify the sample for the pilot test.
  - Obtain permission for the pilot test.
  - Analyze the pilot-test data.
  - Revise the instrument to make it final.

- *Administer the instrument.*
  - Hire staff.
  - Train staff.
  - Monitor the quality of administration.
  - Retrain staff.
  - Send out mail, supervise the questionnaire, conduct interview.
  - Follow up.

- *Manage the data.*
  - Code responses.
  - Prepare code book.
  - Consult with programmer.
  - Train data enterers.
  - Enter the data.
  - Run a preliminary analysis.
  - Clean the data.
  - Prepare a final codebook.

— *Analyze the data.*
  — Prepare an analysis plan.
  — Analyze the reliability and validity of the instrument.
  — Analyze the results of the study.

— *Report the results.*
  — Write the report.
  — Have the report reviewed.
  — Modify the report based on the reviews.
  — Prepare presentation.
  — Present the report orally.

Who Will Do It, and What Resources Are Needed? Personnel, Time, And Money

Fieldwork happens because one or more persons are responsible for completing the required tasks. In a very small study, one or two persons may be in charge of developing field instruments, administering them, analyzing the data, and reporting the results. In larger studies, teams of individuals with differing skills are involved. Sometimes, a study is planned and conducted by the staff with the assistance of consultants who are called in for advice or to complete very specific activities.

First, you need to plan the activities and tasks that need to be completed. Once this is accomplished, you then decide on the skills required for each task. Next, you decide on the specific personnel or job descriptions that are likely to get you as many of the skills you need as efficiently as possible. For example, suppose your study design requires someone with experience in training interviewers and writing questions. You may just happen to know someone who needs a job and has both skills, but if you do not know the right person, knowing the skills needed will help you target your employment search.

The specific resources that are needed for each study will vary according to its size and scope and the number of skills and personnel needed to accomplish each task. Example 8 illustrates the types of skills and resources for a "typical" field study.

Example 8. *Tasks, Skills, and Resources: An Explanation*

1. *Prepare the instrument for use in the field.*
   If an instrument is to be adapted from an already existing instrument, expertise is needed in conducting literature reviews to find out if any potentially useful instruments are available. Sometimes, a reasonably good instrument is available: Why spend time and money to prepare an instrument if a valid one exists? It helps to have experience in the subject matter being addressed and to know who is working in the field and might either have instruments or questions or know where and how to get them.

Selecting items or rewording them to fit into a new measure requires special skills. You must be knowledgeable regarding the respondents' reading levels and motivation and have experience writing questions.

Preparing an entirely new instrument is daunting. A job description for an instrument writer would call for excellent writing skills and knowledge of all topics being assessed.

2. *Prepare Materials for the Institutional Review Board (IRB).*

U.S. researchers cannot perform research with funds from the U.S. government without approval from an Institutional Review Board or IRB – an independent group of people whose job is to evaluate if proposed research conforms to ethical principles (Brett and Grodin 1991). The IRB typically require a written explanation of the study plans (including rationale, purposes, and methods); the field forms and one or more informed consent forms. The following informed consent form has been approved by an IRB. As you can see, it provides potential respondents with descriptions of the study's purposes, the nature and characteristics of the tasks that will be required and describes procedures for ensuring confidentiality.

Box 2. Sample Consent Form

The Prostate Cancer Network (PROCANE)

You are asked to take part in three telephone interviews and three self-administered questionnaires on your general health, your quality of life since being diagnosed with prostate cancer, and the quality of healthcare you have received while in the PROCANE Program. XXX MD, MPH is directing the PROCANE research study. Dr. XXX works in the Department of Urology at the University of YYYY. You are being asked to take part in the interviews and questionnaires because you are enrolled in the PROCANE program. You can choose to take part in this study or not. If you volunteer to take part in this study, you may stop taking part in the study at any time. This will have no effect of any kind on the health care you receive through the PROCANE program.

Disclosure Statement

Your health care provider may be an investigator in this research protocol. As an investigator he/she is interested in both your clinical welfare and your responses to the interview questions. Before entering this study or at any time during the study, you may ask for a second opinion about your care from another doctor who is in no way associated with the PROCANE program. You are not under any agreement to take part in any research project offered by your physician.

Reason for the Telephone Interviews and Self-Administered Questionnaires

The interviews and the questionnaires are being done for the following reason: To find out if the PROCANE program is meeting the needs of the patients enrolled in the program. During the telephone interview, a trained member of the PROCANE staff will ask you a series of questions about:
— Your health
— Your quality of life since being diagnosed with prostate cancer, and
— The quality of the healthcare you have received while in the PROCANE program.

The self-administered questions will cover the same topics. But, you will be able to answer them on your own.

The PROCANE program will use your answers and the answers from other program participants to find out if the program is providing the right services to its participants and to find out if any changes need to be made to the program.

What You Will Be Asked to Do

If you agree to take part in this study, you will be asked to do the following things:

1. Answer three short (20 minutes) telephone interviews. The telephone interviews will ask you general questions about your health, your quality of life since being diagnosed with prostate cancer, and the quality of healthcare you have received while in the PROCANE program. You will be called to complete an interview when you first enroll in PROCANE, 6 months after your enrollment, and when you leave the PROCANE program. The interviews will be completed at whatever time is best for you.

    Sample questions:
    — How confident are you in your ability to know what questions to ask a doctor?

    — During the PAST 4 WEEKS, how much did pain interfere with your normal work (including both work outside the home and housework)? Would you say not at all, a little bit, moderately, quite a bit, or extremely?

    — How much of the time during the LAST 4 WEEKS have you wished that you could change your mind about the kind of treatment you chose for prostate cancer?

2. Answer three short (20 minutes) self-administered questionnaires. The self-administered questionnaires will ask you general questions about your health, your quality of life since being diagnosed with prostate cancer, and the quality of healthcare you have received while in the PROCANE program. The self-administered questionnaires will be mailed to you when you first enroll in PRO-CANE, 6 months after your enrollment, and when you leave the PROCANE program. The self-administered questionnaires can be completed at whatever time is best for you. A pre-paid envelope will be provided to you in which to return each questionnaire.

    Sample questions:
    — Over the PAST 4 WEEKS, how often have you leaked urine?

    — Overall, how big a problem have your bowel habits been for you during the LAST 4 WEEKS?

    — Overall, how would you rate your ability to function sexually during the LAST 4 WEEKS?

3. If you do not understand a question or have a problem with a self-administered questionnaire, you will be asked to call Ms. AAA at the PROCANE office at 1-800-000-000. She will be able to assist you.

Possible Risks and Discomforts

You may be sensitive about answering questions that ask about your physical and emotional health or your experiences with the PROCANE program. However, you do not have to answer any question with which you are uncomfortable.

Potential Benefits to Subjects and/or to Society

The purpose of the telephone interviews and self-administered questionnaires is to improve the services that PROCANE provides to the men enrolled in the program. Your responses might lead to changes in the program that would improve the services that PROCANE provides.

Payment for Taking Part

No payment will be given to you for completing the telephone interviews or self-administered questionnaires.

Confidentiality

Any information that is collected from you and that can be identified with you will remain confidential. Your identity will not be revealed to anyone outside the research team unless we have your permission or as required by law. You will not be identified in any reports or presentations. Confidentiality will be maintained in the following ways:
— All interviews and questionnaires will be coded with a number that identifies you. Your name will not be on any of these materials.
— A master list of names and code numbers will be kept in a completely separate, confidential, password-protected computer database.
— All copies of the self-administered questionnaires will be kept in a locked file cabinet in a locked research office.
— All telephone interviews will be recorded in a confidential computer database.
— When analysis of the data is conducted, your name will not be associated with your data in any way.
— Only research staff will have access to these files.

Taking Part and Choosing Not to Take Part in Telephone Interviews and Self-Administered Questionnaires

You can choose whether to take part in this study or not. If you decide to take part in the telephone interviews and self-administered questionnaires you may stop taking part at any time. This will have no effect of any kind on the health care you receive through the PROCANE program. The investigator may withdraw you from this research if circumstances arise which warrant doing so.

Identification of Investigators

If you have concerns or questions about this study, please contact XXX, M.D., MPH, by mailing inquires to Box 000, Los Angeles, CA 900000-9990. He can be also reached at 1-800-000-000.

Rights of Participants

You may choose to end your agreement to take part in the telephone interviews and self-administered questionnaires at any time. You may stop taking part without penalty. You are not giving up any legal claims, rights or remedies because you take part in the telephone interviews and self-administered questionnaires. If you have questions about your rights as a research subject, contact the Office for Protection of Research Subjects, 2107 QQQ Building,, Box 951694, Los Angeles, CA 90095-1694, (310) 999-9999.

I understand the events described above. My questions have been answered to my satisfaction, and I agree to take part in this study. I have been given a copy of this form.

_____
Name of Subject (Please Print)

_____
Signature of Subject   Date

Many IRB's also require detailed explanations of why each question on an instrument was chosen, how the study's participants were selected, and how you plan to ensure privacy for the respondent.

3. *Identify, recruit, and enroll patients*

Participants in field studies can be identified from existing databases (e.g., Medicare data base; physician specialty membership lists; patient appointment logs), and they can be approached in the field (e.g., a clinic's waiting room). To obtain a valid sample, the research must establish eligibility criteria that describe who will be included and excluded into the study. Effective procedures must be devised to approach potential participants, screen for eligibility, inform eligible respondents about their role in the study, and enlist their cooperation. Often, these procedures need to be tested and retested until they achieve their desired goals. In the U.S., any contact with research subjects, including letters informing potential participants about a study or "scripts" to screen or enroll participants must be approved by an IRB.

Recruitment letters are often sent in advance of a study to inform respondents of the study and its purposes. The following is an example of a recruitment letter for a study of staffing and clinical policies regarding labor and delivery in all hospitals in a single U.S. state. The letter was approved by an IRB and sent to the appropriate nurse manager at all hospitals in the state that delivered babies in a given year.

Box 3. Recruitment letter
<Letterhead and Logos>

Address

_____
_____
_____

Date _____

Dear Colleague (use name)

We are writing to invite you to participate in an exciting federally funded study of the range of clinical policies on Labor and Delivery (L&D) units in this state. Your participation includes taking part in a structured interview regarding policies and procedures on your (L&D) unit.

As you are well aware, much interest has been placed on nurse staffing policies in general, but to date most studies have centered on medical and surgical units. This will be the first study that is specifically designed to identify staffing patterns used on Labor and Delivery units, and to associate these staffing patterns with clinical policies and patient outcomes.

Likewise, there have been numerous isolated studies regarding the role of nursing support in labor, the effectiveness of doulas, nurse midwives, and various techniques of labor management (e.g. active management, "walking epidurals," hydrotherapy, etc). To date, however, there has been no systematic attempt to describe what is really happening on L&D units in the "real world." At the completion of our study, we hope to be able to answer the following types of questions:

— What does "active management" mean to you?
— How prevalent is hydrotherapy?
— What types of clinicians are trained in "teaching" hospitals?
— When do physicians need to be "in house"?
— How are L&D units staffing in the current environment of a nursing shortage?
— What strategies are being used to monitor cesarean rates?
— How are staffing and clinical policies related to maternal and neonatal outcome?

If you agree to participate, we will send you an advance copy of the L&D Clinical Policy Survey, and call to arrange a convenient interview time for you. You will be compensated $60.00 for your participation, which will take about 45 minutes to one hour. Responses will be collated and serve as the first comprehensive overview of staffing and clinical policies on L&D units in this state. This project has been reviewed and approved by the Medical Center Institutional Review Board, and an information letter has been included for your review.

This project, has been funded by the Agency for Health, and has been widely endorsed by representatives of agencies promoting a better understanding of healthcare practices, healthcare quality, and healthcare outcomes including, but not limited to the following:

— **Mary Smith**, Administrative Director of the Association of this State's Nurse Leaders
— **Tom Rodriquez**, CEO Medical Center, Current Board of the Hospital Association, and Past President of the State Hospital Association
— **Robert Johnson MD, MPH**, Center for Disease Control Director Division of Birth Defects and Developmental Disabilities
— **William Roberts, MD**, College of Obstetricians and Gynecologists, Chair District XXX

If you have any questions regarding this project, please feel free to contact us at 310 666-789. We thank you in advance for your participation in this exciting project.

Sincerely,

Yvonne Bree, RN, DrPH
Vice President & Chief Nursing Officer
YYY Medical Center

Mathilde Grun, MD, MPH Director Maternal Fetal Medicine & Women's Health Services Research
YYYY Medical Center
Department Obstetrics & Gynecology

Recruitment letters tend to be most effective if they follow these suggestions:
1. Write the letter on letterhead. If possible place one or more logos on the stationery. The logos may be of the university or agency at which the study takes place and one or more of its supporters.
2. Personalize the letter, if appropriate. In the U.S., "Dear John," is often hand-written over the "Dear Dr. Jones" to express collegiality.
3. Describe the purpose of the study. In this case, examples of study questions are included.
4. Describe the role each participant will play. This letter informs the respondent that joining the study means participation in an interview that may last up to 60 minutes.
5. Describe the incentives you are prepared to offer the respondent. In this case, the incentive is financial.
6. Inform the respondent about confidentiality. According to the letter, the Medical Center's Institutional Review Board has approved the study. An information sheet is to be included with this letter describing how confidentiality is to be ensured. If in doubt, or you do not have an information sheet, the letter should include a statement about protection of privacy.
7. Describe the source of funding for the study.
8. Give the names of any agencies or organizations that endorse or co-sponsor the study.

Sometimes, recruitment is done by telephone. As seen below, recruitment also means collecting data on refusers. Such data are used to determine if the recruitment approach is effective and to provide information on the similarity between persons who agree to participate and those who do not. If differences exist between participants and refusers, the external validity of the study may be compromised.

Box 4. Parent and Child Telephone Recruitment Script

Hello, my name is [*FIRST AND LAST NAME*] and I am calling on behalf of the LAUSD/UCLA study, *Finding Solutions Together*. May I speak to [*NAME OF PARENT*]?

1. IF SOMEONE OTHER THAN RESPONDENT ASKS WHY YOU ARE CALLING, SAY:
   I'm calling about a research study being conducted by the school district.

   (CHECK ONE ANSWER)
   a. *No one by that name is at this number* → ASK Q2
   b. *R not available* → SKIP TO Q3
   c. *I am speaking to the parent or the parent comes to the phone* → SKIP TO Q9
   d. *Refusal* → SKIP TO Q8

2. CONFIRM YOU HAVE DIALED CORRECTLY. ASK IF THE RESPONDENT WAS EVER AT THIS NUMBER AND IF THEY HAVE A NEW NUMBER FOR THE PERSON YOU ARE TRYING TO REACH. IF YOUR INFORMANT CANNOT GIVE YOU A NEW NUMBER, TRY DIRECTORY ASSISTANCE FOR A NEW LISTING. IF NO NEW NUMBER IS LISTED, NOTE AS NOT LOCATED.

3. SAY: Is there a more convenient time to reach R?
   a. *Yes* → CONTINUE
   b. *No* → GO TO Q5

4. SET CALL BACK APPOINTMENT
   Date: _____
   Time: _____
   SAY: Okay. We will try back at that time. Thank you. END CALL.

5. SAY: Is this the best number to reach R or do you have a better number for him/her?
   a. *Yes* → CONTINUE WITH Q7
   b. *No* → GO TO Q6

6. RECORD NEW NUMBER: _____ → SAY: Okay, we will try him/her at this number. Thank you for your help. END CALL.

7. SAY: Okay, thank you. We will try again another time. May I leave you my name and toll free number in case R wants to call me back?
   a. *Yes* → PROVIDE NAME AND TOLL FREE NUMBER. END CALL.
   b. *No* → THANK THE INFORMANT AND END CALL.

8. SAY: Thank you very much for your time. END CALL. FILL OUT INFORMATION BELOW:

   Refusal information

   Who did you speak to? _____

   Reason for refusal?

   _____

Hello, my name is [NAME] *(if not already introduced)* and I am calling from [NAME OF SCHOOL]. I am calling you today because your child participated in the first part of our study and [NAME OF CHILD] reported on the questionnaire that [HE/SHE] has had difficulties related to stressful experiences that may benefit from our program. I am calling to see if you and your child are interested in participating in a program that can help children learn ways of coping with stressful experiences.

9. SAY: Are you interested in hearing more about this study?
   a. *Yes* → CONTINUE
   b. *No* → END THE CALL → SKIP TO Q13

We are conducting a study of youth in middle school who have experienced a very stressful event. The goal of the study is to find out ways that young people react to stressful life events, and whether a new program might help them feel better. If you and your child volunteer to be in this study, we would ask you to do the following things:
— Your child would be given the opportunity to attend a group at school for children who have had stressful experiences and who could benefit from learning ways to improve the way that they feel and act. These groups will have 5–10 students and a group leader and will meet once a week at school for 10 weeks. The group sessions will be audio taped for research purposes

only. There will also be one meeting between your child and the counselor alone, about halfway through the program and four optional parent meetings for parents to learn more about how to help their child at home.

— Not all children who qualify for this program will be in the program right away. Children will be chosen at random, like a flip of a coin, to start right away in the program or to receive the program in about 3 months. Those children who do not get into the program right away will also be offered other services to help them while they wait to start this school program.

— In addition to the groups, we will ask that you and your child meet with an interviewer to answer questions about background about your child and family and how your child has been feeling recently. The parent interview will take about one hour and will be set up at a time and place that is convenient for you. (FILL IN DESCRIPTION OF QUESTIONS) The child interview will take about 30 minutes at school (FILL IN DESCRIP). We will ask you and your child to complete this interview before the program starts, and again at 3 months and at 6 months after starting the program, for a total of 3 times.

— We will ask your child's teacher to complete a short checklist about your child's behavior at school before the program, at 3 months, and at 6 months.

10. SAY: Are you willing to meet with me to discuss your child's participation in this study in more detail, and if interested, complete the first parent interview?
   a. *Yes* → GO TO Q11
   b. *No* → GO TO Q13

11. SAY: Would you prefer to meet at the school or at your home?
   CHECK ONE ANSWER:
   a. *School*
   b. *Home (if home, obtain address):* _____
   _____
   _____

SAY: What is a good day and time for [you and/or your child] to do the interview?

Date: _____

Time: _____

IF NECESSARY, OTHERWISE, *GO TO Q13*: SAY: Do you think you and your child are able to understand and speak English well enough to participate in this program in English?
   a. *Yes* → Go to Q13
   b. *No, cannot speak English well enough to participate* → SAY: I'm sorry to bother you. Thank you for your interest in participating in this study. Unfortunately, at this time we can only do this program in English. I would be happy to talk to you about other resources where your child can get help. Thank you for your time. END CALL.

SAY: We would like to call you the day before the interview to remind you. Is it OK to call you at this number?
   a. *Yes* → GO TO Q13
   b. *No* → RECORD DIFFERENT NUMBER → GO TO Q12

12. RECORD NEW NUMBER

　　New number: (_____) _____-_____ → GO TO Q16

　　SAY: Thank you for taking the time to speak with me today. END CALL.

13. SAY: Okay, thank you for taking the time to speak with me today. END CALL. FILL
　　OUT INFORMATION BELOW:

　　Refusal information

　　Who did you speak to? _____

　　*Reason for refusal?*_____

4. *Pretest the field instrument*
   Pretesting means identifying a relatively small sample of people who are willing
   to go through each question with you and tell you what it means to them.
   (This method is called "cognitive pretesting".) Do the participants agree with
   your interpretation of each question and response? Usually pretests are done
   using early versions of the study, and so glitches should be expected. You will
   need to find a secluded place to conduct the pretest, which is almost always an
   interview. A trained interviewer is needed. Strict rules are needed for recording
   participants' answers. Experienced personnel are needed to interpret pretest
   results and translate them into improvements.

5. *Pilot-test the instrument*
   Pilot testing means having access to a group of potential respondents that is
   willing to try out an instrument that may be difficult to understand or complete.
   Expertise is needed in analyzing the data from the pilot test, and experience
   in interpreting respondents' responses is essential. Additional knowledge is
   needed in how to feasibly incorporate the findings of the pilot test into a more
   final version of the instrument.

6. *Administer the instrument*
   Face-to-face and telephone or computer-assisted interviews require skilled and
   trained personnel. Interviewers must be able to elicit the information called
   for by the interview questionnaire and record or code the answers in the
   appropriate way. Interviewers must be able to talk to people in a courteous
   manner and listen carefully. Also, they must talk and listen efficiently. If the
   interview is to last no longer than 10 minutes, the interviewer must adhere to
   that schedule. Interviews become increasingly costly and even unreliable when
   they exceed their allotted time.
   Among the types of expertise required to put together a mail questionnaire
   is the ability to prepare a mailing that is user friendly (e.g., includes a self-
   addressed envelope) and the skill to monitor returns and conduct follow-
   ups with those not responding. Email surveys also require similar skills. The
   instrument used to collect data must be user-friendly, and you need the skills
   to keep track of responses and then follow-up non-respondents.

If you plan to conduct online studies, you should consider becoming familiar with commercial software packages that guide survey preparation and analysis. Training in their use may be necessary for projects that do not have a specialist. If the study is being done at a local site (hospital, clinic), then privacy concerns associated with the Web may be especially daunting.

Expertise is needed in defining the skills and abilities needed to administer the study's field measures and in selecting people who are likely to succeed in getting reliable and valid data. Training is the key a. For example, a poorly trained telephone interviewer is likely to get fewer responses than a well-trained interviewer. Because of the importance of training, many large studies use educational experts to assist them in designing instructional materials and programs for training.

In large and long-term studies, quality must be monitored regularly. Are interviewers continuing to follow instructions? Who is forgetting to return completed interviews at the conclusion of each 2-day session? If deficiencies in the process are noted, then retraining may be necessary.

7. *Manage the data*

    Managing data means programming, coding, and data entry. It also means setting up a database. Programming requires relatively high-level computer skills. Coding can be very complicated, too, especially if response categories are not precoded. Training and computer skills are needed to ensure that data enterers are expert in their tasks. Finally, data cleaning can be a highly skilled task involving decisions regarding what to do about missing data, for example.

8. *Analyze the data*

    Appropriate and justifiable data analysis is dependent on statistical and computer skills. Some studies are very small and require only the computation of frequencies (number and percentages) or averages. Most, however, require comparisons among groups or predictions and explanations of findings. Furthermore, measures of attitudes, values, beliefs, and social and psychological functioning also require knowledge of the statistical methods for ascertaining reliability and validity.

9. *Report the results*

    Writing the report requires communication skills, including the ability to write and present results in tables and figures. Oral presentations require ability to speak in public and to prepare presentations. It helps to have outside reviewers critique the report; time must be spent on the critique and any subsequent revisions. Expenses for reports can mount if many are to be printed and disseminated.   ♦

Use the following checklist as a guide in calculating costs and preparing field study budgets.

Costs of Field Work: A Checklist

— Learn about direct costs. These are all the expenses you will incur *because* of the fieldwork. These include all salaries and benefits, supplies, travel, equipment, and so on.

— Decide on the number of days (or hours) that constitute a working year. Commonly used numbers in the U.S. are 230 days (1840 hours) and 260 days (2080 hours). You use these numbers to show the proportion of time or "level of effort" given by each staff member. Obviously these numbers will vary from country to country.
   Example: A person who spends 20% time on the study (assuming 260 days per year) is spending 0.20 × 260, or 52 days or 416 hours.
— Formulate fieldwork tasks or activities in terms of months-to-complete each.
   Example: Prepare instrument during Months 5 and 6.
— Estimate the number of days (or hours) you need each person to complete each task.
   Example: Jones, 10 days; Smith, 8 days. If required, convert the days into hours and compute an hourly rate (e.g., Jones: 10 days, or 80 hours).
— Learn each person's daily (and hourly) rate.
   Example: Jones, US $ 320 per day, or US $ 40 per hour; Smith, US $ 200 per day, or US $ 25 per hour.
— Learn the costs of "benefits" (e.g., vacation, pension, and health) – usually a percentage of salarie.
   Example: Benefits are 25% of Jones's salary. For example, the cost of benefits for 10 days of Jones's time is 10 × 320 per day ×0.25, or US $ 800.
— Learn the costs of other expenses that are incurred specifically for *this* study.
   Example: One 2-hour focus group with 10 participants costs US $ 650. Each participant gets a US $ 25 honorarium for a total of US $ 250; refreshments cost US $ 50; a focus group expert facilitator costs US $ 300; the materials costs US $ 50 for reproduction, notebooks, nametags, and so on.
— Learn the indirect costs, or the costs that are incurred to keep the study team going. Every individual and institution has indirect costs. Indirect costs are sometimes a prescribed percentage of the total cost of the field work (e.g., 10%).
   Example: All routine costs of doing "business," such as workers' compensation and other insurance; attorney's and license fees; lights, rent, and supplies, such as paper and computer disks.
— If the fieldwork lasts more than 1 year, build in cost-of-living increases.
— Be prepared to justify all costs in writing.
   Example: The purchases include US $ 200 for 2000 labels (2 per student interviewed) at US $ 0.10 per label and US $ 486 for one copy of MIRACLE software for the data management program.

10.9   Conclusions

Fieldwork in epidemiological studies involves collecting information to describe, compare, or explain knowledge, attitudes, and behavior about the health and health care of populations. To assure reliable information, field work depends upon asking straightforward questions. Straightforward questions are purposeful, concrete and expressed as complete questions. Responses may be considered as nominal or categorical, ordinal and numerical. Open questions allow the respondent to give answers in his or her own words. Coding open responses may be difficult. Closed questions provide the respondent with choices. They are easier to interpret and analyze than open questions but may not provide in-depth information. An instrument's length is dependent upon the resources available to develop and validate a questionnaire. Keep in mind that very long instruments may tire some respondents, thereby reducing the reliability and validity of the results. Questions should be ordered logically and each such be related to the expressed purposes of the study. Relatively simple questions should go first, hardest second. Demographic information is often called for in last place.

Make certain that respondents understand the purposes of the study and each question you plan to ask. If questionnaires are to be completed by mail, include self-addressed envelopes. Try to keep questionnaires as short as possible. For online surveys, avoid the need for the respondent to follow many steps: keep the questionnaire short and easy to use. For all self-administered questionnaires, make sure they are pre tested and pilot tested; when possible look at preliminary data to check that all questions are being answered. Interviewing only succeeds with trained interviewers and a method for monitoring the quality of the process. Consider incentives to compensate respondents for their time. Pilot testing is essential to ensure the collection of reliable data. Reliability refers to the consistent with which questions are answered, while validity refers to the accuracy of the answers. Common types of reliability to consider include test-retest and internal consistency. Common types of validity are content, concurrent, predictive, and construct. To improve reliability and validity, check to see that the language and cultural assumptions of the field study are consistent with those associated with the population being studied. Consider using advance letters and incentives to encourage participation and improve response rates. Make certain all measures and the study's logistics are pre tested and pilot tested. Regardless of the methods used to collect data in the field, be ever mindful of the need to ensure confidentiality of responses. Field work tends to be costly because of its dependence upon human capital including trained field workers and data managers.

References

Anastasi A (1982) Psychological testing. Macmillan, New York

Bernard HR (2000) Social research methods: qualitative and quantitative approaches. Sage, Thousand Oaks

Bourque LB, Fielder EP (2003a) How to conduct self-administered and mail surveys. Sage, Thousand Oaks, London, New Delhi

Bourque LB, Fielder EP (2003b) How to conduct telephone surveys. Sage, Thousand Oaks, London, New Delhi

Brett A, Grodin M (1991) Ethical aspects of human experimentation in health services research. JAMA 265:1854–1857

Cohen J (1960) A coefficient of agreement for nominal scales. Educational and Psychological Measurement 20:37–48

Dawson B, Trapp RG (2001) Basic & clinical biostatistics. Lange Medical Books/McGraw-Hill, New York

Fink A (2002) How to ask survey questions. Sage, Thousand Oaks, London, New Delhi

Fink A, Kosecoff JB (1998) How to conduct surveys: a step-by-step guide. Sage, Thousand Oaks, London

Frey JH (1989) Survey research by telephone. Sage, Newbury Park

McDowell I, Newell C (1996) Measuring health: a guide to rating scales and questionnaires. Oxford University Press, New York

Stewart AL, Ware JE (1992) Measuring functioning and well-being: the medical outcomes study approach. Duke University Press, Durham

Sudman S, Bradburn NM (1982) Asking questions. Jossey-Bass, San Francisco

Exposure Assessment

I.11

Sylvaine Cordier, Patricia A. Stewart

11.1   Introduction

Accurate exposure assessment is a prerequisite for an efficient study design, more than ever before, because of the increasing challenges that epidemiology has to face to demonstrate low increases in risk, to disentangle mixed potential risk factors in disease causation, and to provide exposure-response relationships for policy makers.

Exposure assessment is the process that leads to establishing a dichotomy between exposed and non-exposed subjects, and/or introducing a level of classification between subjects. A prerequisite for any epidemiologic study is that there is variability of exposure to the agent of interest within a population and that this variability between subjects (inter-individual variability) will overcome individual variation of exposure (intra-individual variability).

This chapter will describe what choices have to be made for a proper exposure assessment depending on the pathological process under study, give an overview of the different instruments available for this assessment and highlight some specific difficulties in this process (retrospective assessment, ecological measurement or multiple exposures). Finally, measurement errors and ways for controlling them will be described.

11.2   Definition of Exposure and Exposure Assessment

Exposure can be defined as a contact of an individual with an agent through any medium or environment. An agent can also be thought of as a susceptibility characteristic. The agent is not necessarily considered to be harmful (e.g., exercise or fiber in the diet). *Exposure assessment* aims to identify whether a person is exposed or not (a dichotomous classification) to a particular agent and if the individual is exposed, to develop a ranking of subjects by exposure level.

11.2.1   Types of Exposure

An exposure may be to a chemical, a biologic, a physical, or a societal agent in the external environment (e.g., cadmium, endotoxin, ionizing radiation, and the existence of a support system, respectively). It may be a characteristic of an individual (e.g., weight or physical activity) or a perception of an individual (e.g., lack of control in the workplace). Finally, it may be a biologic agent in the body (e.g., herpes virus), a metabolite of an external agent (e.g., 1-hydroxypyrene, a metabolite of polycyclic aromatic hydrocarbons), a substance representing a pathway of action (e.g., DNA-PAH adducts), or the presence of a polymorphism (e.g., NAT wildtype). In this chapter we use the term exposure to apply to all of these, rather than separating external agents from internal agents. The concept of dose is discussed later in this chapter.

True Risk Factor or Surrogate   11.2.2

Ideally, an exposure assessment should focus on the *true risk factor*. When true risk factors have been confirmed, protective measures and monitoring of exposure can then be implemented. Medical surveillance in the work place, which usually includes some kind of biological monitoring of compounds known for their toxicity (e.g.: urinary cadmium), may be required. In many situations, however, a *surrogate* must be evaluated because the true risk factor has not yet been identified or only a surrogate can be measured. For example, the causal role of inhaled benzo[a]pyrene in the carcinogenicity of cigarette smoking for the lung may never be formally proven because the true risk factor (i.e., the total amount of inhaled benzo[a]pyrene over a period covering many decades) is impossible to measure (Rothman and Greenland 1998). The International Agency for Research on Cancer (IARC) has classified certain work environments as probably carcinogenic to humans, without identifying the specific compound(s) responsible for this health effect (e.g., the process of refining nickel). Thus, although the true risk factor(s) linked to a health effect may not yet be identified or quantified (e.g., nickel refining, tobacco smoking), measurement of a surrogate remains very useful for research and public health purpose. A surrogate is useful for identifying factors of variation for the exposure, establishing presumptive causal associations and dose-response relationships, and narrowing the search for the true risk factor(s).

Dose versus Exposure   11.2.3

The term *exposure* usually refers to contact with an agent in the external environment. (As indicated above, common nomenclature also may include agents in the body). Measuring an external agent should, but may not, take into account all the exposure sources (e.g., at home, at work, and leisure time), the time spent in each (i.e., activity patterns), and the individual susceptibility to this agent (e.g., due to physical exercise, diet, and physiological and genetic characteristics). These variables will affect the internal *dose* measured in human tissue or fluid. A biological marker of internal dose therefore comes closer to the relevant measure of exposure in some circumstances than an external exposure. This will be discussed more in Sect. 11.3.1. In the rest of the text, the term *exposure* will be used to describe agents that are being estimated for use in exposure- (or dose-) response relationships in an epidemiologic study. Dose will be used to describe the level of the true risk factor at the target organ.

Selection of Metric   11.2.4

Once the agent or a scenario to be investigated in the epidemiologic study has been selected, the relevant dimensions to quantify this exposure need to be determined. The appropriate quantification of exposure (metric) should reflect the toxic mechanism of action for the agent and disease of interest. The choice of this metric depends on the knowledge about the supposed biological mechanism inducing the health effect. Chronic diseases such as cancer, for example, are thought to be a result of lifetime exposure, so that the exposure metric often studied is *cumulative exposure*; whereas acute diseases such as asthma are thought to be due to recent high exposures, so that the metric often studied is *peak exposures.*

If there is a biological level above which detoxification processes of the organism are impaired (threshold), the *dose-rate* (*average*) of an exposure or a peak exposure may be more relevant than cumulative exposure, because exposures below such a threshold would not cause any deleterious effect.

Oftentimes, however, the biological mechanism of the disease process is not known. In such cases, it is useful to explore multiple metrics such as cumulative (life-time), highest, average (dose-rate), highest short-term (peak) exposure, and components of these (e.g., cumulative exposure level or time above a particular exposure level). For example, the induction of carcinogenesis by a mutagenic compound is, theoretically, initiated at any dose, but the mechanism necessitates a long (sometimes several decades) induction period (*latency*). In this case, recent exposure (immediately preceding diagnosis) is not pertinent, and often measurement of past exposure is "lagged", i.e. exposure occurring in years just before diagnosis of the disease is not taken into account. The exposure metric, then, may incorporate a lagged latency. When an adverse effect is expected to occur only above a certain dose (*threshold*), for instance in acute toxicity, a metric representing a quantitative level above the threshold would be more appropriate than a metric estimating the total exposure.

Often, the total exposure to a given compound received over a particular time period (cumulative exposure) is the relevant parameter in a pathological process. There are, however, several ways to receive the same cumulative exposure: a high intensity for a short period of time or a lower intensity over a longer period. For instance, the history of tobacco smoking is often summarized by a cumulative index (pack-years), i.e., the number of years of smoking times the average number of packs of cigarettes smoked every day during the smoking period. This index, or any equivalent based on the product of duration of exposure by an intensity level, does not distinguish between the roles of *duration* of exposure, irrespective of the rate of exposure, and *intensity* of exposure at every instant.

Selection of an exposure parameter that does not appropriately describe the pattern of exposure to the agent being investigated as it relates to the disease of interest will result in misclassification and loss of statistical power (see Sect. 11.5).

11.3   Exposure Data

Because exposures can have different natures, the sources of data used in exposure assessments differ. Exposure data can be thought to be of two types: measurement data (*direct*) and *indirect* information (e.g., questionnaire information, diaries, and records of surrogate information).

Measurement Data

Measurement data are generally considered the most accurate type of exposure data because they are objective measures of exposure. Measurement data include measurements of chemical hazards on the skin and chemical or radiation hazards in the food, air, or water in the general environment or in the workplace. They may be measures of quality of life, such as levels of stress. They also include measurements of human health, such as physical activity levels, physiologic measurements, such as blood pressure or weight, or measurements of agents in biologic tissues, such as drugs or nutrients. They also include measures of internal exposure or effect, such as blood lead levels and DNA adducts, respectively. For more examples of biological markers please refer to Chap. III.6 of this handbook.

Measurements may be taken for purposes of an epidemiologic study or may be available from existing records. Although individual measurement data are often thought to be the gold standard, they can be subject to substantial biases. Measurements may not represent the intensity of exposure during the relevant time window, e.g., current levels of physical activity may not reflect earlier levels of physical activity. The number of measurements on any individual is generally small, and because the variability of some exposures is large (e.g., in air and in water), one or a few measurements may not reflect the metric of interest, such as long-term exposure levels.

In addition, historical measurement data in records may not represent the true exposure level, because the purpose of the data collection was taken for reasons other than to obtain an estimate of the exposure metric of interest to the study investigator. For example, measurements of agents in the workplace often have been taken to evaluate compliance with exposure regulations, and it has been speculated that such data may reflect higher exposures than the true long-term exposure level. Moreover, the analytical method may not have measured the true risk factor (e.g., historical measurements of cholesterol did not distinguish between high and low density cholesterol, and many historical measurements of dust in the air did not distinguish respirable dust from inhalable dust).

Biological measurements of exposure (e.g., carbon monoxide in the breath) *or of effect* (e.g., cholinesterase levels in the blood) are generally thought to be the gold standard, because they most closely reflect the dose received by the target organ. (Note that biologic measurements can be both exposure data and the outcome, depending on the study design. Here, only biologic measurements used as exposure data are discussed.) There are many limitations to this type of measurement, however. The variability of the concentration of an agent in the body is often greater than that seen in the external environment, so that if the number of measurements is limited, a mean of those measurements may not accurately reflect the average exposure. Some biologic measurements may not reflect the dose at the target organ. Instead, they may reflect the amount of agent that was not received by the target organ (e.g., if the agent was measured in the urine) or the amount that was metabolized in the body (including by organs other than the target organ). In such cases it is assumed that the amount measured and the amount in the target organ are highly correlated, but this correlation is likely to vary by agent or by organ and may vary considerably by individual. There are, in addition, no long-term biomarkers for most agents, and current levels may not reflect long-term exposure levels. Moreover, biologic measurements reflect the body burden at one point in time. Even if the agent has a long half-life, the measurement may not be an accurate reflection of the total amount received due to metabolism and elimination over time (e.g., McGrail, Stewart and Schwartz 1995).

Biological measurements are often invasive and costly. For some known risk factors, only invasive techniques are available for biomonitoring, and exposure assessment, therefore, still relies on more traditional instruments. For example, asbestos is a recognized potent carcinogen. One way to evaluate asbestos exposure would be to measure the asbestos in broncho-alveolar lavage specimens. This invasive and expensive technique, however, is not routinely feasible, nor is it appropriate, because it does not reflect past exposure, which is the most relevant for cancer induction. In this example, exposure assessment must rely on indirect methods of measurement such as questionnaires or records.

If the measurement data were taken after the onset of disease (which is very difficult to determine because the onset may not be detectable), the measurements may be an effect of the disease, rather than a precursor. An example of such a measurement is serum levels of androgens and prostate cancer (Hsing 2001).

Because of their cost, biologic measurements are used more often in case-control or cross-sectional studies or in a sample of a cohort, rather than for an entire cohort. In spite of these limitations, biologic measurements can provide key insights into the toxicologic mechanisms of the agent and can be useful in estimating exposure levels if used judiciously. They can be useful in estimating recent or chronic exposure levels that have low variability over time. In addition, they represent concentrations received from all sources of exposure, so that the total amount of exposure received is better estimated. This advantage is especially important when individual work practices, such as hand washing before eating, can affect internal concentrations.

Measurements of the external environment are thought to be a lower gold standard than biologic measurements because they do not measure the internal dose received. They too represent only one point in time. This type of measurement often reflects only one source of exposure when several sources may be contributing to a study subject's overall exposure (e.g., pesticide exposures can occur from application at work, in the house and garden, from contamination of the soil from nearby farming operations and from consumption of pesticide-contaminated food and water). Thus, measurement of only one source may cause other important sources to be missed. Measuring exposures from a single source, therefore, without considering other sources, can result in lower estimates of exposure and an overestimation of disease risk. In addition, external environmental measurements do not provide an estimate of internal dose. There are several advantages of this type of measurement over biological measurements, however. External environmental measurements are non-invasive and less expensive and the number of agents for which there are analytical methods is larger. The variability of the concentration of an agent in the external environment usually is lower than the intra-individual variability in the body, meaning that when a small number of measurements is available, a small number of environmental measurements on a group of similarly exposed workers is likely to result in a better estimate of the true exposure level than a small number of biologic measurements.

Finally, when measurements are taken for the purpose of an epidemiologic study, investigators should ensure that the data are collected in a way to reflect the metric being investigated. The sampling strategy should be developed to reflect the goals of the study (e.g., randomly or randomly within strata). Strict quality control methods should be followed. When records of measurements are being used, investigators should review the collection, analytic, and quality control methods to determine the accuracy of the data and how the measurements compare to the metric being assessed in the epidemiologic study.

Indirect Exposure Data   11.3.2

The second type of exposure information, indirect data, is derived from questionnaires, diaries, or records identifying measurements of exposure surrogates. Questionnaires may describe measurement data, e.g., cigarettes consumed per week or more subjective measures, such as the perception of control at the workplace. Examples of indirect data from diaries or records of surrogates are the amount of milk products consumed or distance of a residence from a hazardous waste site, respectively. As with measurement data, information from questionnaires, diaries or records may be problematic.

Questionnaires are developed by study investigators to ensure that information is collected in a structured, standardized approach to reduce differential questioning of cases and controls and to ensure that the data are as complete as possible.

The circumstances under which the questionnaire is administered (in person, telephone, mail, at home or in a hospital) may reflect the level of response. Development and administration of the questionnaire and data entry and clean up is costly and time-consuming. Computer-assisted personal and telephone interviews (CAPI and CATI, respectively) have substantially reduced data entry and cleanup costs, but their development is more expensive than using a paper copy. They can, however, include logic checks within the questionnaire to catch errors immediately, rather than long after the interview has taken place (cf. Chap. I.10 of this handbook). Questionnaires are usually administered by professional interviewers rather than by scientists knowledgeable of the areas being investigated, so that if a respondent asks for clarification or provides a response that is unclear or inappropriate, the interviewer may not be able to respond in a way to increase the quality of the data. Interviewer training and inclusion of probing questions are means to reduce this problem. In spite of these limitations, oftentimes questionnaires are the only way to collect information on exposures.

Designing a questionnaire consists of establishing a list of questions in a pre-defined order, aimed at eliciting the presence of and often the amount of a given exposure. A questionnaire is defined by its content, the time span it covers in a subject's life, and its format and wording. Common sense principles should guide the construction of a questionnaire. Thus, each question and the flow of the questionnaire should be clear and subject to minimal misinterpretation. Administration of the question should not be a substantial burden to the subject, either in regards to the amount of time spent answering the questionnaire, the complexity of the information being collected, or the sensitivity of the questions. One hour is usually considered the maximum amount of time that respondents retain interest, but it may be much less. Aids can be used to help the respondent accurately recall information, such as lists of pesticides, logos, trademarks of products used, and pictures of medication bottles.

The list of questions in the questionnaire should include only those that the respondent can answer and that will ensure an accurate assessment of exposures. As the questions are developed, an analytical strategy also should be developed on how the responses will be used. A minimum set of questions should be asked that ensure maximum efficiency, but a small number of additional questions may be included for cross checking data. A few "red herring" questions (i.e., questions that are included to determine the accuracy of the responses, such as inserting in a list of real products, a product with a fake name) are often useful to evaluate the responses. More details on conducting interviews can be found in Chap. I.10 of this handbook.

The time span of the questionnaire is important. Respondents can more easily report on current exposures than historical ones. Past exposures, however, may be more important than current exposures in the etiology of chronic diseases, but collecting varying information over many years is problematic. Recollection of important life events at the earlier age can improve recall.

The format of the questions will determine the response rate to the question and the accuracy of the response. Open-ended questions (e.g., "What type of exercise did you do when you were in your twenties?") often gather more information than closed-ended questions because respondents can identify important exposures that are not anticipated by the investigator. Open-ended questions, however, require extensive coding, and some information collected is likely to be useless. Furthermore, important exposures may not be recalled. Close-ended questions (e.g., "Did you do any of the following in your twenties: walk? jog? play tennis? etc.") take more time, but the respondent is less likely to forget one of the identified exposures, making the information collected generally more accurate. If, however, the respondent had an important exposure to an agent not on the list, it may not be reported. Open-ended questions may be used in pilot studies to develop more standardized closed formats. Wording should be geared to the educational level of the respondents. In the US, the reading level of a 14-year old is generally considered appropriate for general population studies. When developing questionnaires, the investigator should consult one of the many references on questionnaire design (Sudman and Bradburn 1982; Armstrong et al. 1994; cf. Chap. I.10 of this handbook).

Screening questions are useful to minimize the time spent on answering inapplicable questions. Screening questions may require a simple yes or no (e.g., "Did you ever take birth control pills?"), or they may be formatted to screen out the lower exposed individuals (e.g., "Did you ever take birth control pills for at least one year?").

Diaries are another source of exposure information and have been used most frequently for diet and to a lesser extent, physical activity. In a diary, the respondent reports the amount of exposure (e.g., red meat consumption) at some identified frequency (e.g., daily). Diaries are best used when exposure occurs frequently, because if the frequency is too low, the respondent is likely to forget to complete the diary. Time spent recording the information should be minimal (e.g., less than one minute) and the time covered by the diary should be short (e.g., one to two weeks) to maximize compliance. Diaries should be formatted in a way to ease data entry as much as possible (e.g., check boxes rather than open-ended questions).

Records are often needed for retrospective exposure assessment (see Sect. 11.4.3). Records of surrogate information (including geographic information systems (GIS)) are often used in ecologic studies of the environment. Thus, amount of corn grown in various counties may be used to rank individuals with presumed exposure to herbicides. The data in such records may or may not have been accurately collected, but even if the data were accurately collected, the design of the data collection may impact the usefulness of the data in an epidemiologic study. For example, the Toxic Release Inventory of the US Environmental Protection Agency collects emissions data from private businesses. These data can be used to identify geographic areas with significant releases of agents into the air, water, and ground. However, there is a minimum amount of contaminant that must be released into the environment before reporting is required. Companies releasing smaller amounts of agents into the environment are not identified. Thus, if there are many small companies of one type in an area, the emissions reported in the database may suggest very low levels that may not, in fact, be low at all. In such cases, there may be no better data available for use in a study, but the protocol and quality control measures for the data collection should be carefully evaluated prior to use of such data, so that the investigator is aware of the strengths and limitations of the data. It may be useful to compare such data to other records systems as well. For example, a study of farmers' responses on pesticide use found reasonably good agreement with suppliers' information on pesticides bought by the farmer (Blair and Zahm 1993).

In summary, the choice of a measurement instrument is determined by knowledge of the disease (what is the true risk factor?), the feasibility of the measurement (its invasiveness and the ease of use in the exposure assessment), the cost, and its validity and reproducibility characteristics (see Sect. 11.5).

11.4 The Process of Exposure Assessment

The process of exposure assessment aims at the construction of an individual exposure estimate, from exposure data available, in order to produce a valid and efficient classification of subjects. Exposure data are usually imperfect, however, and there is a need for exposure *assessment* (rather than measurement), in order to approach the relevant dose.

The main steps for building exposure estimates and classification of subjects are described below. The specific problems resulting from the retrospective character of exposure assessment, the use of ecological estimates and the handling of multiple correlated exposures will also be presented, where ecological estimate refers to estimating an exposure level for a group of individuals, rather than for each individual separately.

The process of exposure assessment can be straightforward to relatively complicated, depending on the level of detail and the accuracy of the exposure data (e.g., surrogates of exposure may warrant less-intensive exposure assessment efforts than accurate and detailed exposure information on the true risk factor), the goal of the study (e.g., hypothesis-generating or hypothesis-testing), and the resources of the investigator.

11.4.1 Creating an Exposure Estimate

Some exposure data need little processing such as information obtained directly from answers to a questionnaire, for example smoking habits or intake of some kind of nutrients. In other investigations, some type of processing is needed. In the case of diet, for example, food composition tables allow the computation of the amount of nutrients across food groups (e.g., total vitamin A from various fruits, vegetables, meats, etc.). These tables take into account the mode of preparation and of preservation of the food. They are usually country-specific and need regular updating for an accurate translation from food groups into nutrients. For more details on assessment of micronutrients we refer to Chap. III.4 of this handbook.

Similarly, exercise can be measured using an accelerometer that measures movement, so that the total amount of energy expended can be estimated for an individual getting several types of exercise (Ainsworth et al. 1999).

In environmental studies (cf. Chap. III.3 of this handbook), the estimation process often is more complicated. These types of studies often make use of recognized pollutant dispersion models using exposure data reported by the subjects as well as exposure data from other records systems. Investigators of a study of respiratory symptoms developed exposure estimates from a model using type of vehicle, mean traffic density, emission exhaust rates, local topography, and meteorologic conditions to estimate airborne nitrogen dioxide levels (Oosterlee et al. 1996). Estimates of tricholoroethylene were developed for a municipal water system in a study of neurobehavioral effects using information on piping, flow input, water demand, and other variables, and a geographic information system (GIS) on the water distribution systems (Reif et al. 2003).

Occupational epidemiology (cf. Chap. III.2 of this handbook) also tends to estimate exposure from multiple pieces of exposure information, but to date, there are no recognized methods. In the past, experts have based their estimates on job titles and industry with little documentation as to how these estimates were derived. Recently, more attention has been paid to identifying *determinants of exposure* (e.g., factors that affect exposure) (Vermeulen et al. 2002). Examples of determinants include the presence of ventilation, the use of protective equipment, and the quantity of the contaminant in the workplace. Models to estimate an exposure score can be developed by simply assigning weights to the values of the determinants. For example, for a study of man-made mineral fibre, type of emission (active, passive), handling of fibres, presence of controls, protective equipment, and other variables were identified as affecting exposures (Cherrie et al. 1996). Variations in these variables across jobs resulted in the assignment of different scores. Use of these determinants in statistical models allows for a more rigorous and transparent estimation process, however, such as for a study of paving workers where measurement data and determinants such as the type of paving (oil, mastic) and the use of tar were used to develop a estimation model for benzo(a)pyrene exposures (Burstyn et al. 2000).

Establishing a Level of Classification 11.4.2

In deciding on a classification, a decision must be made as to whether it will be qualitative (yes/no or ever/never), semi-quantitative or ordinal (e.g., low, medium, or high, or scores of say, 1–3, with or without the quantitative levels associated with the categories identified) or quantitative (with units of measurements). This decision is usually based on the quality of the exposure data.

Continuous data (i.e., quantitative) have greater statistical power to find an association than categorical data. Continuous data, however, also provide an impression of higher quality of exposure data than categorical data do, so that if the exposure data are poor, it may be better to describe the exposures categorically.

Oftentimes, investigators believe that *categorical data* are more accurate than continuous data. In one sense, this may be true. It generally is easier to assign a study subject to one of three categories than to estimate a quantitative level. The use of categories, however, does not reduce the error of the exposure assessment because all individuals within the category are assigned the same value. To illustrate this point, when categories are used, either a score is assigned to the category or the median of the range the category represents is used. It would be rare, however, that all individuals within an exposure category actually have the same exposure level. There are likely to be some individuals exposed at the median level of the category who are therefore appropriately assigned. There are also likely to be some individuals on both the low and the high ends of the category who will be assigned the same value as those individuals at the median level. Moreover, the individuals on the edges of adjacent exposure categories (e.g., the individuals on the high end of the low exposure category and the individuals on the low end of the adjacent higher category) are assigned to different exposure categories and therefore to different median values, although they may be very similar in exposure levels. Thus, within any category of exposure, there is variability in exposure levels, and this variability will reduce the ability of the investigator to identify exposure response-relationships.

Another consideration in selecting the level of classification is the underlying assumption of the exposure-response relationship (cf. Chap. II.2 of this handbook). Using a continuous measurement of exposure in regression modelling (cf. Chap. II.3 of this handbook) assumes a linear increase of disease risk (or a transformed scale such as logit) for one unit of exposure. Use of categories of exposure, at least as a first approach, will, instead, fit observed values more closely without requiring any hypothesis about the shape of the exposure-response relationship. Categories must be developed, however, keeping in mind the limitations described above.

Grouping Strategies

Exposure groups are subsets of the population being studied that are viewed as being similarly exposed and therefore assigned the same exposure level. Exposure groups may be defined during questionnaire development, the exposure assessment process, or the analytical stage. When developing questionnaires, exposure groups are defined when responses to the questions are provided in categories. For example, if the possible responses to "At what age did you get your first menstrual period?" are < 10, $10-12$, $13-14$, ≥ 15 years of age, these categories result in four exposure groups. In some studies, exposure groups are developed during the exposure assessment process. Thus, in an environmental study a question may be asked, "How far did you live from the ABC waste site?" The exposure data that will be used in the exposure assessment may be described in three categories, e.g., concentrations of an agent within a mile, 2–5 miles, and ≥ 5 miles. The investigator, then, may develop three exposure groups: one of subjects who report living ≤ 1 mile, one of subjects living 2–5 miles, and one of subjects living ≥ 5 miles. Alternatively, the exposure data may be continuous (e.g., concentrations at various distances). In this case, the investigator may leave the question open-ended. Alternatively, he/she may prefer to use the same three response categories as indicated above because the investigator may believe that the subjects can more accurately identify the correct category than estimate a continuously measured distance. Finally, during the analytical stage, investigators may decide to group individuals into quartiles or other arbitrary or ad hoc categories. An advantage of this strategy is that categories can be developed using differing cutpoints to allow comparisons with other studies.

The definition of exposure groups is important in an epidemiologic study because the variability of exposure level within and across groups affects the power to observe an exposure-response relationship (see also Sect. 11.5). There are three types of variability in epidemiologic studies. The first is *intra-individual* or day-to-day variability. For example, a subject with a mean alcohol consumption of two glasses a day may have no drinks some days and four drinks other days. The epidemiologist has no control over this variability, but it is important to appreciate that there is variability of most exposures of individuals, which could be important when investigating threshold effects.

Intragroup variability is the variability that occurs within the exposure group. Thus, within an exposure group consuming 2–4 drinks/day, there will be some individuals who average two, some who average three and some who average four drinks/day. *Intergroup variability* is the variability across the groups (for example, with categories of 0, $\leq$ 1–2, 3–4, 5–6 and $\geq$ 6, the range is 0 $\rightarrow$ 6 drinks/day). The more intragroup variability there is compared to the intergroup variability, the more likely that an exposure-response relationship will be missed. The goal, therefore, is to have narrow ranges of exposure levels within the groups (with little to no overlap across other groups due to misreporting) and as wide a range across groups as possible. For example, in a study investigating coal dust and change in lung function (forced expiratory ventilation in one second (FEV_1)), four different exposure groups were evaluated for intragroup and intergroup variability and the effect of variability on the FEV_1. The intragroup variance ranged from 0.18–0.35 and the intergroup variance ranged from 0.20–0.23 (Heederik and Attfield 2000). The FEV_1 coefficient (in ml per mg/m^3 of coal dust) ranged from −2.0 to −5.9. The exposure group with the lowest intragroup variance (0.18) and the highest intergroup variance (0.23) was associated with the highest loss of FEV_1 per unit of dust exposure (−5.9 $ml/mg/m^3$ of dust). Intragroup and intergroup variability can be evaluated using analysis of variance techniques (e.g., Burstyn et al. 2000).

Retrospective Exposure Assessment 11.4.3

The challenges of using instruments to measure current (i.e., recent) exposures are compounded when investigating chronic disease. Because historical measurements are often lacking, investigators may collect current measurements and assume that historic levels were similar or extrapolate historic level from the current measurements. Similarly, exposure information is often asked in questionnaires in reference to a single point in time (e.g., 20 years ago or when the subject was at a certain age), which is equivalent to having only one historical measurement. For example, in the area of nutrition, questionnaires used to investigate chronic disease have traditionally collected only information on current diet. Because diets have changed over time, current diet is not necessarily highly correlated to diets of 20 to 30 years ago.

In contrast, in the occupational investigations, however, complete work histories are often collected, which is likely to result in more accurately historical exposure estimates than using only current job. There is a whole body of literature relative to retrospective exposure assessment using job exposure matrices (JEM) or expert assessment from a panel of experts (Benke et al. 2001). A JEM is a cross tabulation of jobs (or job/industry combinations) and agents by time that automatically assigns the same exposure level to all individuals having the same job. Used in association with a subject's complete work history, JEMs or expert evaluation provide an individual probability of exposure to a given agent.

11.4.4   Ecological versus Individual Exposure Assessment

Measurement data may not be available on the actual study subject, but rather on individuals thought to be similarly exposed as the individual under study. These types of measurements are called *ecologic assessments*. In contrast, assessment of individual exposures takes into account the personal characteristics of the individual. An example of an ecologic assessment is assigning the same level of trihalomethanes in a public water supply system to all individuals on that water supply, in spite of the recognition that the concentration of trihalomethanes can vary within a system. Assigning the same exposure level to individuals with different exposure levels will result in misclassification of study subjects, because in the same (macro) environment, subjects are likely, in fact, to have different exposure levels. For example, subjects living in an area with a polluted public water supply will be exposed differently to a pollutant in the water depending on whether their water resources come from a public supply or from a private well, the amount of tap water they drink, their use of tap water for cooking, etc.

An ecological evaluation is used when exposure data or resources are limited. Ecological estimates are the rule in areas such as air pollution epidemiology, where individual exposures are often defined by atmospheric measurements at the sampling location nearest to the individual's residence, or more broadly, at the city level. Ecological estimates are also popular in occupational epidemiology, where job exposure matrices have been developed. In these examples, investigators of air pollution or workplace exposures usually do not have measurement data on the individuals or individual-specific parameters such as individual work practices and protective equipment. The ecologic evaluation, therefore, assigns the same exposure value to a group of subjects sharing the same (macro) environment.

Ecologic evaluations can result in substantial misclassification of exposure levels. In the field of occupation, even among individuals thought by occupational health professionals to have similar exposure levels, the exposure level can be up to three to six times larger or smaller than estimated, as indicated by geometric standard deviations often found (van der Woord et al. 1999). It seems reasonable to assume that similar degrees of misclassification occur among other types of environmental exposures. Extrapolation of measurement data from one individual to another or from a system to an individual therefore must be done with caution.

Ecological measurements are often derived from existing records (air quality monitoring records, occupational measurement surveys) and are much cheaper to obtain and estimate than individual measurements. Using ecological measurement instead of individual measurements makes sense if the contrast of exposure between the groups (e.g., cities or jobs) is greater than variability of exposures among individuals in the same group. Studies based on ecologic measurements may also be useful for hypothesis-generation.

Individual assessment generally requires a greater assessment effort but is likely to result in less misclassification. Considerations for selecting one approach over the other include: time and financial resources, availability of exposure data and its quality and quantity, and the purpose of the study (e.g., hypothesis-generating or -testing, and investigation of an exposure-response relationship).

Dealing with Multiple Exposures 11.4.5

In many situations, exposures to various potential risk factors in human populations tend to aggregate for an individual, due to individual behaviour. An example is the correlated habits of smoking, alcohol and coffee drinking among some individuals. Similarly, in the outdoors environment, humans are exposed to mixtures of compounds originating from the same source (e.g., mercury, polychlorinated bi-phenyls (PCBs), and other organochlorines from eating fish) or from various sources (e.g., carbon monoxide from automobile and truck exhaust).

Epidemiological studies have proved to be informative about many complex mixtures such as cigarette smoke or air pollution. However, identification of the component(s) responsible for the health effects (and their joint effects) observed is still required for a better understanding of disease causation, cost-effective monitoring of the hazard, and an efficient strategy of prevention of disease.

The situation of the mixed exposures cannot be treated as a classical problem of confounding because the exposures are highly correlated. Stratified analysis or multivariate modelling is, in general, inefficient because such analytical approaches do not allow the presence of a high colinearity among different exposures. In addition, the presence of one or several agents "representative" of mixed exposures or the occurrence of interaction among exposures is not merely a statistical problem. It also requires a strategy that recognizes the different underlying biological hypotheses of the various components of the mixtures. Much of the insight about multiple exposures comes from epidemiology (for instance tobacco smoke or outdoor air pollution) because toxicological experiments often cannot replicate complex mixtures to which people are exposed across time, and such experiments are usually limited to single components or suitably chosen combinations.

To illustrate the problem of complex mixtures, we describe as an example environmental exposure to PCBs. Similar examples, however, are found in many other areas of study, including diet and occupational exposures. PCBs are a persistent type of industrial compound that includes 209 different chemical members referred to as congeners. The commercial product always is a mixture of correlated congeners, so that studying the toxicity of these compounds is not easy. For example, some PCBs act like dioxins by binding to the aryl hydrocarbon AhR receptor, and may result in cancer (Longnecker et al. 1997). Experimental work has shown the highest dioxin-like activity occurs for congeners with no chlorine in the *ortho* position. It has been speculated that neurologic effects of PCBs, on the other hand, may be caused by congeners with chlorine in the *ortho* position.

Samet (1995) has proposed five general strategies for studying such complex mixtures efficiently: (1) treating the mixture as a single agent; (2) selecting an indicator component; (3) creating a summary index; (4) identifying the separate effects of the mixture's individual components; and (5) characterizing the independent and joint effects of the components. We review these strategies with application to the problem of the toxicity of PCBs.

(1) Treating the Mixture as a Single Agent.   The early studies in Japan and Taiwan that recognized the neurotoxicity of PCBs, and the later studies in Michigan, relied on total PCBs. At that time congener-specific data were not available (Schantz et al. 2003). The exposure measurements taken in these studies were powerful enough to strongly suggest the neurotoxic potential of PCBs. There is still, however, a debate about discrepancies in health effects among studies in different countries. These discrepancies may be due to different analytical procedures, different patterns of congeners, or different co-exposures to other organochlorines, such as dioxins or furans, which have similar environmental pathways (Longnecker et al. 1997). In summary, treating the mixture of PCBs as a single agent has proved efficient for hazard identification in early work, but exposure misclassification limits the interpretation of the discrepant findings.

(2) Selecting an Indicator Component.   Several recent large studies have focussed on a small number of congeners present in relatively high concentrations (e.g.: PCB 153). The congeners present in high concentrations, however, are not necessarily the most toxic. As a rule, "a single component of a mixture may be an appropriate index of toxicity if the component mirrors the dosimetry and toxicity of other components relevant to the health effects of concern" (Samet 1995).

(3) Creating a Summary Index.   Creating a summary index implies the attribution of some type of weighting to the individual concentrations of the different components of a mixture. The weight assigned to each congener is defined according to an underlying hypothesis about the biological activity of each component. If one assumes that endocrine disruption is a relevant biological mechanism of toxicity for PCBs, a measurement of the total estrogenic xenobiotic burden in adipose tissue could provide an integrated biomarker of xeno-hormonal activity resulting from exposure to a given mixture of compounds (Soto et al. 1997). Another example of biological activity, the dioxin-like activity of a PCB congener, can be calculated using a toxic equivalency factor (TEF) (Ahlborg et al. 1994), which is assigned relative to the toxicity of the dioxin 2, 3, 7, 8 TCDD. The total toxic equivalency (TEQ) of a mixture of PCBs can then be estimated by summing across all compounds, the product of the concentration and TEF for each compound. It is likely, however, that the weighting is dependent on the state of knowledge about the relative potency of the different components at the time of calculation, and that over time it would be necessary to modify the summary index as more information becomes available.

(4) **Separating Effects of the Mixture's Components.** Creating one summary index does not reflect the heterogeneity of the mixture. There is a trade-off between measuring concentrations of the individual compounds in the mixture (which is usually time-consuming and expensive) and summarizing the mixture of highly correlated congeners. Analyzing concentrations of 38 PCBs congeners from 497 human milk samples from Canada in 1992, Gladen et al. (2003) distinguished three groups of congeners: one group of the congeners, including most of the major congeners, that were highly correlated, meaning that their individual biologic effects realistically could not be separated in an epidemiologic study; another group of congeners quantifiable in only a small fraction of the population by the assay methods used and therefore an epidemiologic analysis would be uninformative; and a third group quantifiable in a reasonable fraction of samples and not correlated with the bulk of major congeners. The authors concluded the components of this last group are worth studying separately and are good candidates for individual determination and inclusion in epidemiologic studies.

(5) **Characterizing the Independent and Joint Effects of Components.** Measurements of selected congeners allow the evaluation of health effects related to single or joint exposures. Correlations, however, exist not only between concentrations of PCBs congeners, but also with other common organochlorines, metals, and pesticides and there are strong suspicions of possible interactions among these compounds at the molecular level that affect neurobehavioral function in particular (Carpenter et al. 2002). The strategies presented earlier provide some guidelines for studying these joint effects in epidemiological studies.

Two other points regarding mixtures are appropriate. It should be recognized that while some agents within a mixture may cause a disease, it is possible that other agents in that same mixture reduce the likelihood of the disease by deactivating the active compound. For instance there is an active discussion around the beneficial impact on birthweight of seafood consumption during pregnancy, which brings high amounts of fatty acids and selenium, relative to the potential toxicity of seafood from contaminants such as mercury (Grandjean et al. 2001). This situation complicates the determination of causality in epidemiologic studies. Also, individual characteristics of the study subjects (e.g., polymorphisms) may intensify or reduce the effect of the agent. Currently, our ability to tease out these situations is limited, but investigators should at least recognize that they may be possible.

Multiple exposures can be evaluated using interaction analysis, but can also be grouped using hierarchical cluster analysis (e.g., see Hines et al. 1995 for an example). In this study fabrication workers in a semi-conductor company were exposed to multiple chemicals. Hierarchical analysis allowed the investigators to identify groups of workers exposed to the same pattern of exposures (e.g., various glycol ethers).

11.5 Measurement Errors

All types of exposure assessment in every area of investigation will have some error. Chapter II.5 of this handbook describes statistical methods to cope with measurement errors. Appreciation of the types and degree of error allows for a more appropriate interpretation of the study results. Knowing the sources of error can also provide areas for methodologic investigation within the study to allow quantification of the error. This, in turn, can allow the investigator to estimate the effect of the error on the epidemiologic findings.

11.5.1 Types of Measurement Errors

There are two types of errors that arise from measurements: random and systematic. Random error will result in the measurements being randomly distributed around the mean. Systematic error, or bias, will result in an overall mean that is erroneously high or low compared to the true mean. Both types of error are of concern in exposure assessment and they are described in terms of precision and validity. *Precision* measures random error and refers to the reproducibility or reliability of the measure. *Validity* measures systematic error and refers to the distance between the exposure measured and the target variable (ideally, the true risk factor, but practically, the surrogate).

A measurement instrument must be *reproducible*. Under ideal conditions this means that if the instrument is administered under the varying conditions, it should provide the same response within a reasonable level of variation. Generally, however, reproducibility more practically is defined as providing the same response within a reasonable level of variation under the same circumstances. Reproducibility is a necessary condition to accurately evaluate intraindividual and intragroup variability, but somewhat less necessary to accurately evaluate intergroup variability. In addition, to be useful, the measurement instrument must also be *valid* (i.e. it should measure the exposure it is supposed to measure and identify the true quantity present).

Historically, measurement error more often has been associated with categorical assessments than quantitative, probably because quantitative assessments have been limited in the past. Measurement error in either type of assessment will result in *misclassification error* when estimating the exposure levels of study subjects. For example, if a subject was assigned to a high fruit intake category, rather than a medium fruit intake category, the subject is misclassified. Misclassification of confounders can be also a serious problem since it will usually reduce the degree to which confounding can be controlled. For instance in many studies it is essential to obtain a complete smoking history including detailed periods of smoking or quitting, and quantity smoked during each period, because tobacco smoking is a risk factor, and therefore a potential confounder, for many diseases. When studying lifestyle factors associated with smoking, such as alcohol consumption, misclassification of smoking habits will result in incomplete adjustment and residual confounding. In the context of an epidemiologic study misclassification is characterized as nondifferential or differential, depending on whether it affects the comparison groups (i.e., the diseased and non-diseased subjects) similarly. *Differential misclassification,* which results from there being a different amount of error for the diseased compared to the non-diseased, can lead to underestimation or overestimation of the association between the exposure and disease. In the latter situation, misclassification can induce spurious statistically significant results. *Nondifferential misclassification* of exposure usually will bias estimates of relative risks towards the null. There are examples, however, occurring in extreme conditions, where nondifferential misclassification of exposure can produce bias away from the null (Rothman and Greenland 1998). Thus, both types of misclassification can result in incorrect conclusions.

Sources of Measurement Errors 11.5.2

Armstrong et al. (1994) classified sources of measurement error in five categories: faulty design of the instrument, errors or omissions in the protocol regarding the use of the instrument, poor execution of the protocol during data collection, limitations due to subject characteristics (e.g. poor memory of past exposures or day-to-day variability in biological characteristics), and errors during data entry and analysis. They have provided an extensive list of circumstances in which these errors may occur and these sources should be carefully evaluated before attempting to use any type of instrument.

Measurement instruments and analytical methods (such as for an air or biological measurement, blood pressure, etc.) generally are designed to be as accurate and reproducible as possible when used under similar conditions, i.e., with the same protocol. Two possible sources of systematic differences that can occur are from the measurement/analytical method itself and from the interference of other substances present in the measured environment. Reduction of these errors in the investigation of disease risks can be made by following the manufacturer's/laboratory recommendations, calibrating the instrument under the conditions being measured, using spiked and blank samples, and following other quality control procedures (cf. Chap. I.13). Random error can arise from a lack of technical precision of the instrumentation, variation introduced by the laboratory technicians, and the analytical procedures themselves. This inherent limitation of the instrument and analytical methods, however, explains only part of the variability. Other sources of variation include weather conditions, presence of other exposures, the actual concentration being out of the range of the instrument's measurement range, and the timing of the instrument's response in the relation to a change in concentration. The sources of error need to be identified in order to decrease, or at least, recognize and quantify the variability.

Questionnaires, because they also can suffer from the two types of misclassification, systematic and random, can be viewed similarly. Systematic differences can result from incorrect phrasing of questions (such that all respondents misinterpret the question similarly) or from inappropriate or misleading response categories. Random sources of misclassification can result from poor phrasing (such that different respondents interpret a question differently) and lack of interest on the part of the respondent. To collect quality data, questionnaires should be standardized, so as to ensure that all study subjects are asked the same questions. Questions must be clearly phrased, without ambiguity and use terms that are understandable to respondents. Respondents must be able to remember the events being asked about and be able to correctly respond to the questions. Thus, reporting of events that took place many years ago or that require mathematical calculations (e.g., estimating "average" amount of foods eaten on a seasonal basis) is likely to be subject to more random error than reporting of more recent events or events that do not require calculations (e.g., Bradburn et al. 1987 and Subar et al. 1995). Pilot testing of questions should be conducted on a group of individuals with the characteristics of the group who will be receiving the questions because respondents often interpret questions very differently from investigators, even if the questions were carefully developed. Questions should also be tested under the conditions that the questionnaire will be administered (e.g., in the home). Following these procedures should decrease bias and increase precision.

Diaries are prone to both systematic and random errors from the same sources as questionnaires. Records, in contrast, may have systematic and random error similar to measurement data or questionnaire data, depending on the type of record.

Both systematic and random errors may result from limited data. For example, systematic error could result in missing information from asking about sensitive issues, such as the number of sexual partners (Lindzey and Aronson 1985). Subjects may be more inclined to respond with a "don't know" if the number of partners exceeds what they consider to be acceptable. Cases with workplace-induced cancer may be so sick that proxies are used as the respondents. Proxies generally know little about workplaces of the subject. In contrast, many of the control subjects would be able to provide detailed information about the workplace.

Having limited exposure information can result in misclassification of subjects by exposure level. In the environmental area, Brunekreef et al. (1987) illustrated the effect of limited data on misclassification in a study of the relationship between environmental exposure to lead and blood lead levels in children. He found that averaging four measurements of lead on home floors increased the regression coefficient explaining blood lead levels by 69%, compared to the model using a single home floor measurement. Having only one measurement, therefore, would have increased the misclassification of subjects. Generally non-differential misclassification due to limited data will result in random error.

The problem of limited data also is evident in the use of questionnaires. For example, often investigators restrict the workplace exposure information collected to jobs, industries and dates. From these limited data, they apply job exposure matrices to assign occupational exposure estimates. When applying the matrix, individuals holding a job are considered non-exposed if the exposure occurs only in a small proportion of workers in the job. This procedure will, however, inevitably result in classifying among the "unexposed" individuals, a small proportion of workers who are, in reality, exposed. Similarly, individuals having jobs entailing a high probability of exposure will be considered exposed, even if they belong to the small proportion of nonexposed workers on this job. Detailed descriptions of tasks and work conditions of the jobs held by individual study subjects and evaluation of these data on the individual subject level are necessary for a better assessment. Thus, limited exposure data can contribute to misclassification, in that the available data (from which exposure is characterized) may not be representative of the individual's actual exposure level. This problem is more related to selection bias, is a general problem in epidemiology, and is not unique to exposure variables. The concept of bias is treated in Chap. I.12 of this handbook.

One can often recognize the circumstances in which differential misclassification may occur. Diseased subjects may have reflected more on their past exposures than the nondiseased (recall bias) or may take more care in providing correct responses. Differential bias will potentially occur when the exposure measurement instrument uses a human intermediary (e.g., the subject himself and/or an interviewer) aware of (or thinks he/she is aware of) the disease status. Thus, face-to-face interviews involve a substantial risk of producing interviewer effects. If a bias results from a different attitude of the interviewer toward the diseased compared with the non-diseased subjects, it is called interviewer bias. Self-administered questionnaires are generally believed to be less vulnerable to influences of response bias; however, the appearance of the questionnaire, the introductory letter, and the research group may all have an impact on response. The likelihood of bias from telephone interviews falls between these two data collection methods. Computer-assisted telephone interviewing has become the method of choice in many studies, and often has a high response rate and few missing data (Nybo Andersen and Olsen 2002).

Quantification of Measurement Errors – Reproducibility Studies 11.5.3

Evaluation of the reproducibility of measurement instruments can be done by comparing the same instrument under the same conditions over time or by comparing various instruments under the same conditions at the same time. An example of the first type of study evaluated the reproducibility of a self-administered lifetime physical activity questionnaire (Chasan-Taber et al. 2002). Subjects reconstructed physical activity at four ages, starting at menarche, twice in the same mail questionnaire administered one year apart. All intraclass correlation coefficients used to measure reproducibility ranged from 0.78 to 0.87, with a value of 0.83 for total lifetime estimate of exposure.

The area of nutritional epidemiology (cf. Chap. III.4 of this handbook) is one in which the design of proper questionnaire instruments has been extensively investigated. Subar et al. (2001) compared a new food frequency questionnaire and two widely used dietary questionnaires using telephone 24-hour recalls. Despite substantial differences in the length and the design of the questionnaires, correlations obtained for dietary composition (i.e., total energy intake and 26 nutrients) were very similar. This comparison provides evidence that carefully designed self-administered food frequency questionnaires can provide reasonably reproducible measures of current nutrient intakes in epidemiologic applications. There are still, however, questions about the validity of these instruments, and probably only the comparison of questionnaires with a truly uncorrelated error, such as a biochemical indicator of diet, will resolve these validity issues.

11.5.4   Quantification of Measurement Errors – Validation Studies

Ideally, an instrument should be evaluated by comparing it to a standard under the conditions the instrument is used. In evaluating the validity of any measurement instrument, the choice of the gold standard is a critical issue. Biochemical indicators of internal exposure provide an independent assessment for which measurement errors are not likely to be correlated with errors in air or water measurements or questionnaires. Biologic measurements may represent historical exposures only if the chemical of interest has a sufficiently long biological half-life and may represent recent exposures only if the chemical has a relatively short half-life. In both cases, for the biologic measure to be useful, the body burden cannot be affected by the disease or its treatment. In other situations, the biomarker may not measure the target agent of interest. Other challenges of biologic monitoring can be found in Sect. 11.3.1 of this chapter. Biochemical indicators of dietary intake have a great appeal as the gold standard to assess the validity of dietary questionnaires (Willett 1990). There are limitations, however, in that the indicators may not reflect only dietary intake, and there are many dietary factors of interest for which there is no biomarker.

Practically, however, a gold standard often does not exist, especially when exposure has to be assessed retrospectively (e.g., historical tobacco consumption of individuals). For some exposures, however, a partial validation may be possible, by comparing questionnaire results to pre-existing records. For example, reported jobs can be compared to employers' records, and smoking consumption can be compared to past medical records. Identification of gold standards that are "alloyed", and how to account for this error has been discussed (Wacholder et al. 1995). The validation of the instrument is also often measured by its ability to predict disease risk in prospective studies (Willett 1998). This approach is somewhat problematic, however, in that the epidemiologic outcome is used to test the instrument. Nonetheless, a good instrument should produce better risk estimates than a poor one (Tielemans et al. 1998).

11.5.5   Methods for Correcting Measurement Errors

The effect of a systematic difference between the actual concentration and the concentration measured can be reduced or minimized simply by applying a correction factor reflecting the difference to the exposure estimate if the difference is known. Internal validation studies have been proposed to reduce the impact of measurement error. In one approach, exposure is measured, although imperfectly, from everyone in the study, and, simultaneously, a more accurate but more expensive measurement is collected on only a small subset of cases and controls selected randomly. Sophisticated statistical methods can then be applied in order to infer the corrected odds ratio from measurement error models fitted to the parallel exposure measurements from the validation sample (Stürmer et al. 2002). These so-called two-phase designs are among others investigated by Schill et al. (1993, 1997) and have been applied by Pohlabeln et al. (2002). This method, however, has not yet been routinely implemented, and further research is needed to establish the robustness of the procedures in realistic settings and to determine optimal designs for selecting a validation sample. As quoted by Chatterjee and Wacholder (2002) in a recent commentary, "the best way to reduce bias from measurement error is to improve tools for measuring exposures including biological markers, environmental samples and questionnaires".

A second approach that is gaining popularity is to conduct an uncertainty analysis (or sensitivity analysis; Rothman and Greenland 1998). In this approach, investigators identify the uncertainty around a point estimate (e.g., 2 drinks of wine a day). For example, if a question asked "How many glasses of wine do you drink?" and the responses were < 1/day, 1–3/day, 4–5/day, > 5/day, the uncertainty ranges of these responses could be 0–0.9, 1–3, 4–5 and 6–10, respectively. Monte Carlo or other statistical simulations allow a better understanding of the uncertainty around the disease risk estimates.

Conclusions 11.6

The demand for accurate exposure assessment implies the need for development of validated and reliable tools in parallel with reduced costs and increased applicability in field studies. Sophisticated techniques are now available for direct measurement of chemicals in most mediums with excellent sensitivity and reproducibility. Similarly, questionnaires are being developed in various fields with considerable effort being put into their validation.

In some areas, such as occupational or environmental epidemiology, improvement is dependent upon additional knowledge on exposure determinants both at the personal and population levels, and on objective comparisons of the quality of various available methods for exposure assessment (Liljelind et al. 2003). Quantitative estimates of exposure using statistical modelling are currently being developed, mainly for risk assessment purposes, but their applicability to epidemiological studies has not been fully explored.

To solve the problem of mixed exposures, the trend is towards building exposure indices summarizing several exposures according to biological hypotheses about their joint mechanisms of action. In the near future, new biotechnologies (e.g., genomics, proteomics) will contribute to the development of biomarkers of gene expression, intermediate between markers of exposure and markers of early effects that will summarize the joint action of mixed exposures at the molecular level (Henry et al. 2002, cf. Chap. III.6 of this handbook). The applicability of these techniques in epidemiological studies opens a whole new area of research.

References

Ahlborg UG, Becking GC, Birnbaum LS, Brouwer A, Derks HJGM, Feeley M, Golor G, Hanberg A, Larsen JC, Liem AKD, Safe SH, Schlatter C, Waern F, Younes M, Yrjänheikki E (1994) Toxic equivalency factors for dioxin-like PCBs. Chemosphere 28:1049–1067

Ainsworth BE, Richardson MT, Jacobs DR Jr, Leon AS, Sternfeld B (1999) Accuracy of recall of occupational physical activity by questionnaire. J Clin Epidemiol 52:219–227

Armstrong BK, White E, Saracci R (1994) Principles of exposure measurement in epidemiology. Monographs in Epidemiology and Biostatistics, vol 21. Oxford University Press, Oxford

Benke G, Sim M, Fritschi L, Alfred G, Forbes A, Kauppinen T (2001) Comparison of occupational exposure using three different methods: hygiene panel, job exposure matrix (JEM) and self reports. Appl Occup Environ Hyg 16: 84–91

Blair A, Zahm SH (1993) Patterns of pesticide use among farmers: implications for epidemiologic research. Epidemiology 4:55–62

Bradburn NM, Rips LJ, Shevell SK (1987) Answering autobiographical questions: The impact of memory and inference on surveys. Science 236:157–161

Brunekreef B, Noy D, Clausing P (1987) Variability of exposure measurements in environmental epidemiology. Am J Epidemiol 125:892–898

Burstyn I, Kromhout H, Kauppinen T, Heikkila P, Boffetta P (2000) Statistical modelling of the determinants of historical exposure to bitumen and polycyclic aromatic hydrocarbons among paving workers. Ann Occup Hyg 44: 54–56

Carpenter DO, Arcaro K, Spink DC (2002) Understanding the human health effects of chemical mixtures. Environ Health Perspect 110(suppl 1):25–42

Chasan-Taber L, Erickson JB, McBride JW, Nasca PC, Chasan-Taber S, Freedson PS (2002) Reproducibility of a self-administered lifetime physical activity questionnaire among female college alumnae. Am J Epidemiol 155:282–289

Chatterjee N, Wacholder S (2002) Validation studies: bias, efficiency and exposure assessment. Epidemiology 13:503–506

Cherrie JW, Schneider T, Spankie S, Quinn M (1996) A new method for structured, subjective assessments of past concentrations. Occ Hyg 3:75–83

Gladen BC, Doucet J, Hansen LG (2003) Assessing human polychlorinated biphenyl contamination for epidemiologic studies: lessons from patterns of congener concentrations in Canadians in 1992. Environ Health Perspect 111:437–443

Grandjean P, Bjerve KS, Weihe P, Steuerwald U (2001) Birthweight in a fishing community: significance of essential fatty acids and marine food contaminants. Int J Epidemiol 30:1272–1278

Heederik D, Attfield M (2000) Characterization of dust exposure for the study of chronic occupational lung disease: A comparison of different exposure assessment strategies. Am J Epidemiol 151:982–990

Henry CJ, Phillips R, Carpanini F, Corton JC, Craig K, Igarashi K, Leboeuf R, Marchant G, Osborn K, Pennie WD, Smith LL, Teta MJ, Vu V (2002) Use of genomics in toxicology and epidemiology: findings and recommendations of a workshop. Environ Health Perspect 110:1047–1050

Hines CJ, Selvin S, Samuels SJ, Hammond SK, Woskie SR, Hallock MF, Schenker MB (1995) Hierarchical cluster analysis for exposure assessment of workers in the semiconductor health study. Am J Ind Med 28:713–722

Hsing AW (2001) Hormones and prostate cancer: what's next. Epidemiol Rev 23: 42–58

Liljelind I, Rappaport S, Eriksson K, Andersson J, Bergdahl IA, Sunesson AL, Jarvholm B (2003) Exposure assessment of monoterpenes and styrene: a comparison of air sampling and biomonitoring. Occup Environ Med 60:599–603

Lindzey G, Aronson E (1985) Handbook of social psychology, 3rd edn, vol I. Random House, New York

Longnecker MP, Rogan WJ, Lucier G (1997) The human health effects of DDT (dichlorodiphenyl-trichloroethane) and PCBs (polychlorinated biphenyls) and an overview of organochlorines in public health. Annu Rev Public Health 18:211–244

McGrail MP, Stewart W, Schwartz BS (1995) Predictors of blood lead levels in organolead manufacturing workers. J Occup Environ Med 37:1224–1229

Nybo Andersen A-M, Olsen J (2002) Do interviewer's health beliefs and habits modify responses to sensitive questions? A study using data collected from pregnant women by means of computer-assisted telephone interviews. Am J Epidemiol 155:95–100

Oosterlee A, Drijver M, Lebret E, Brunekreef B (1996) Chronic respiratory symptoms in children and adults living along streets with high traffic density. Occup Environ Med 53:241–247

Pohlabeln H, Wild P, Schill W, Ahrens W, Jahn I, Bolm-Audorff U, Jöckel K-H (2002) Asbestos fibreyears and lung cancer: a two-phase case-control study with expert exposure assessment. Occupational and Environmental Medicine 59:410–414

Reif JS, Burch JB, Nuckols JR, Metzger L, Ellington D, Anger WK (2003) Neurobehavioral effects of exposure to trichloroethylene through a municipal water supply. Environ Res 93:248–258

Rothman KJ, Greenland S (eds) (1998) Modern epidemiology, 2nd edn. Lippincott-Raven, Philadelphia, pp 115–134

Samet JM (1995) What can we expect from epidemiologic studies of chemical mixtures? Toxicology 105:307–314

Schantz SL, Widholm JJ, Rice DB (2003) Effects of PCB exposure on neuropsychological function in children. Environ Health Perspect 111:357–376

Schill W, Jöckel K-H, Drescher K, Timm J (1993) Logistic analysis in case-control studies under validation sampling. Biometrika 80:339–352

Schill W, Drescher K (1997) The analysis of case-control studies under validation subsampling: a comparison of four approaches. Statistics in Medicine 16:117–132

Soto AM, Fernandez MF, Luizzi MF, Oles-Karasko AS, Sonnenschein C (1997) Developing a marker of exposure to xenoestrogen mixtures in human serum. Environ Health Perspect 105(suppl 3):647–654

Stürmer T, Thürigen D, Spiegelman D, Blettner M, Brenner H (2002) The performance of methods for correcting measurement error in case-control studies. Epidemiology 13:507–516

Subar AF, Thompson FE, Kipnis V, Midthune D, Hurwitz P, McNutt S, McIntosh A, Rosenfeld S (2001) Comparative validation of the Block, Willett, and National Cancer Institute Food Frequency Questionnaires. The Eating at America's Table Study. Am J Epidemiol 154:1089–1099

Subar AF, Thompson FE, Smith AF, Jobe JB, Ziegler RG, Potischman N, Schatzkin A, Hartman A, Swanson C, Kruse L, Hayes RB, Lewis DR, Harlan LC (1995) Improving food frequency questionnaires: A qualitative approach using cognitive interviewing. J Am Diet Assoc 95:781–788

Sudman S, Bradburn NM (1982) Asking questions. Jossey-Bass Publishers, San Francisco

Tielemans E, Heederik D, Burdorf A, Vermeulen R, Veulemans H, Komhout H, Hartog K (1998) Assessment of occupational exposures in a general population: comparison of different methods. Occup Environ Med 56:145–151

Van der Woord MP, Kromhout H, Barregard L, Jonsson P (1999) Within-day variability of magnetic fields among electic utility workers: Consequences for measurement strategies. Am Ind Hyg Assoc J 60:713–719

Vermeulen R, Stewart P, Kromhout H (2002) Dermal exposure assessment in occupational epidemiologic research. Scand J Work Environ Health 28:371–385

Wacholder S, Hartge P, Dosemeci M, Armstrong B (1995) Validation studies using an alloyed gold standard (letter). Am J Epidemiol 141:277

Willett WC (1998) Invited commentary: comparison of food frequency questionnaires. Am J Epidemiol 148:1157–1159

Willett WC (1990) Reproducibility and validity of food-frequency questionnaires. In: Nutritional epidemiology. Oxford University Press, New York

Design and Planning of Epidemiological Studies

I.12

Pascal Wild

Introduction

This chapter deals with practical issues in designing and planning analytical epidemiological studies. Although most of the practical issues are consequences of the theoretical principles of epidemiology as presented in standard textbooks (Breslow and Day 1981, 1987; Rothman and Greenland 1998; Miettinen 1985) and in Chaps. I.1, I.5, I.6, I.9, II.1, II.5, and II.6 of this handbook, the emphasis here is on how to proceed practically when planning a study.

This chapter is based on our experience in conducting epidemiological studies and on a series of references in which many of the concerns in the practical planning of studies have been described at length. Among the key sources we used are the books by Hernberg (1992) and Armstrong et al. (1994). The series of papers by Wacholder et al. (1992a,b,c) have also inspired much of our writing. It will start with a section on early planning in which the general setting of any study is described as well as the key planning document, i.e. the study protocol. The second section is devoted to the choice and implementation of an actual design where we focus on cohort and case-control studies. The next section focuses on data collection, both, with respect to the exposure and the disease outcome. The final section is devoted to practical issues and gives a list of topics arising in all studies that may not always get the appropriate attention while planning an epidemiological study.

Early Planning

Objectives – the Concept of the Study

The first step in the planning of an epidemiological study is the definition of the problem. Researchers must ensure that they have a clear view of the problem at the abstract-general level. At this conceptual level a problem takes the form "does X cause Y?" or "how much will a certain amount of exposure to X affect Y?" (Hernberg 1992, Chap. 4). It should be stressed that in analytical studies, researchers are interested in the relationship between exposure and disease which would be valid in other circumstances. They are only interested in the particular morbidity experience of the study population as far as it can be extrapolated to other populations.

The general interest of the investigator first has to be translated into precisely formulated, written objectives. A limited number of study objectives should be defined. These objectives may be of two kinds.

A first case is when the study is focused on specific analytical questions with a predefined hypothesis. For instance "does exposure to extremely low frequency (ELF) electromagnetic fields cause childhood leukemia?". Here the hypothesis should be formulated as a series of operational questions. One can specify the ELF fields in a variety of ways both qualitative (yes/no or low/medium/high) or quantitative (e.g. present intensity, mean intensity over the last years or cumulative exposure). Other pre-defined operational hypotheses may include subgroup analyses based on the disease subtype. These operational hypotheses will have to be clarified by confirmatory tests. Additional results based on the observed data will then be clearly identified as such.

A second study type focuses on broader hypotheses generating questions that will be investigated by exploratory analyses such as "what occupations are associated with an increased risk of laryngeal cancer?". Even in this case a predefined list of questions is useful. In the present example, this would consist in a list of occupations considered. Again an unsuspected excess in an occupation not considered a priori should be identified as such.

12.2.2   Scientific Background

It is of crucial importance to undertake a thorough literature search and to know the literature in detail before planning any new project. Occasionally, the literature review may show that the answer to the study question is already available and that further data collection is not needed.

Evaluating epidemiological evidence from the literature is often challenging even for experienced researchers. Because a single positive finding may be a chance finding, a complete literature search, including negative results, should be conducted. One should consider systematic errors (biases) and confounders that may have led to a particular result in previous studies. Several independent studies using the same design and the same procedure of data collection may have similar results due to common biases or confounding. It is therefore important that the sources of spurious results are identified and controlled in subsequent investigations. It would be ineffective to simply replicate previous studies, without consideration of new research questions raised by previous studies, that could not be addressed because the information was not collected. A large literature body on how to perform a systematic literature synthesis is available, see Chap. II.7 of this handbook and references therein.

The literature search should, however, not be restricted to epidemiological studies, but may encompass a large range of topics from biological mechanisms or biomarkers related to the hypothesis under study to techniques of exposure measurement.

12.2.3   The Study Protocol

An epidemiological study is generally a complex undertaking of long duration, requiring time from study investigators and technicians, large resources in personnel and funding. The success of a study depends on a careful preparation. It is self-evident that such an undertaking cannot be done without a written study protocol.

A study protocol (study plan) should cover all aspects of the planned study. It should first state the precise objective of the study and describe the scientific rationale for undertaking a new study, based on a literature search of the relevant publications (scientific rationale: study background and objectives). It should then define the study design including the precise study base and an estimate of the corresponding statistical power to achieve the objectives. Finally it should give a detailed account of what the epidemiologists intend to do and how they intend to do it. This entails for instance procedures for identifying the outcome parameter, measuring of exposure and confounders, data management and all steps taken for quality assurance. These aspects could be contained in a separate operations manual. It should also address the strategy for statistical analysis, ethical considerations and data protection procedures, project organization, quality control, time schedule and study diary, publication, and budget.

According to Miettinen (1985) a study protocol should have five purposes:
— Crystallize the project to the researchers themselves
— Give referees the possibility to review the project (especially for funding)
— Inform and educate all those taking part in the project
— Ensure the main researchers do not forget any details of the plan in the course of the study
— Document the procedures of the project for the future.

In summary, a protocol must be so detailed that an independent researcher could carry out the study based on it. The planning of each epidemiological study needs explicit and operationalized hypotheses that have to be formulated as specific and precise as possible. The selection of the population under study has to be justified in light of the research question.

An outline of the issues to be covered in the study protocol is given in Box 1. Most of these issues will be discussed in what follows. For further details we refer to Chap. I.13 of this handbook.

Box 1. Overview of a study plan and corresponding key problems to be addressed in the planning phase

1. *Research question and working hypotheses*
   — Relevance/previous findings
   — Choice of an appropriate target population
   — Problem: Operationalizing, i.e translation of items into variables that can be quantified
   — Precise definition of endpoint
   — Precise definition of independent variables and confounders
   — Choice of statistical measures (proportions, means, risks)
   — Translation into a hypothesis that can be tested statistically
   — Confirmatory testing of hypothesis/exploratory analyses

box to be continued

2. *Study design*
   — Optimal design (theoretical)
   — Practical limitations/feasibility

3. *Study base (target population) & study population*
   — Often limited access to subjects
   — Problem: Generalization from study sample to target population

4. *Size of study & its justification*
   — Sample size determination depends on precise definition of hypothesis
   — Size of acceptable type II error to be considered (power!)
   — Often: Power calculations based on fixed sample size

5. *Selection and recruitment of study subjects*
   — Problem: Selection bias (survival bias, referral bias)
   — How to assure representativeness
   — Means to maximize response
   — Sampling procedure/
   — Data source
   — Potential problem: Finding appropriate reference groups
   — Matching, if applicable

6. *Definition of procedures for measurement & data collection of variables*
   — Problem: Information bias (recall bias, measurement bias)
   — Instruments (postal, face-to-face, telephone)
   — Structure? Comprehensible? Answerable? Length?
   — Sensitive issues?
   — "Objective" sources of data? Measurements?
   — Guidelines for measurements
   — Usefulness in the analysis
   — Coding

7. *Exposures/risk factors/potential confounders & effect modifiers*
   — Problem: Assess confounders!
   — Precise definition
   — Valid assessment
   — Quantification: What information is needed?
   — Chronological reference

box to be continued

8. *Concept for data entry and data storage*
   - Data base
   - Ergonomic layout of data entry screen
   - Validation of data entry
   - Validation of coding
   - Plausibility checks/data corrections (concurrent to data collection)
   - Documentation: Always keep raw data!
   - Merging of data

9. *Strategy for analysis including statistical models*
   - Compliance with a priori hypotheses
   - Mark and report ad hoc hypotheses accordingly
   - Problem: Adequate consideration of confounders

10. *Measures for quality assurance*
    - Guidelines for data collection, measurement, interview (interviewer and operations manual)
    - Training of staff
    - Minimal information on non-responders
    - Validation of data
    - Comparison with reference data external to the study
    - Description of changes of original study plan
    - Project diary

11. *Measures to guarantee confidentiality & ethical principles*
    - Obtain informed consent by participants
    - Anonymize data, keep names separate

12. *Time line & responsibilities*
    - Chronological sequence
    - Scientific councils
    - Agreement on publication rules

Design

12.3

The study design governs all procedures for selecting and recruiting individuals in the study sample. A design may be chosen depending on the study objectives, but may also rely on practical issues such as costs, or data availability. Most epidemiological studies, with the exception of clinical trials and intervention studies, are purely observational, in that the investigator cannot assign the exposure to the study subjects as in experimental settings. The definition of a study design includes both a definition of the study base and of the study type. The main types of observational studies are the cohort study and the case-control study (sometimes called case-referent study). Although their theoretical background is the same, as in theory every case-control study takes place within a cohort (Breslow and Day 1987, p 3), the practical implications of conducting a cohort or a case-control study are quite different. A number of other designs have been used or proposed and are mostly variations of these basic types.

12.3.1   Study Base

Once the general objective of the study has been defined (at the conceptual level), and before the study type can be described, the investigator should identify the actual setting, or study base, in which the particular scientific problem can be studied. The study base should not only be a population (a number of individuals), but the morbidity experience of this population during a certain period of time (Hernberg 1992, Chap. 4).

The definition of the study base may depend on the study aims (testing a specific hypothesis or generating hypotheses). For example, the study base may be the 10-year follow-up of workers employed for at least one year in a particular industry and exposed to a specific chemical (hypothesis testing). Another example of a study base would be the one-year incidence of a disease among individuals living in a certain geographical area and having a wide range of exposures (hypothesis generating).

The study base should be defined in terms of eligibility ("employed at least one year" – "living in a particular area"), of its size, and of distribution of exposure, confounders and modifiers (as identified from the literature review). One should also define the time period during which information on morbidity has accrued ("10-year follow-up" – "one-year incidence data").

Ideally, a study base should make possible the scientific generalization of study results (the relation between exposure and disease). This can be achieved if exposure conditions, as well as potential confounders and effect modifiers can be measured within the study base. If not, the particular morbidity experience of the study population would be mostly descriptive and would apply only to the empirical population under study.

12.3.2   Cohort Studies

The design and analysis of cohort studies is described in detail in Chap. I.5 of this handbook. In cohort studies the study sample to be included is either the whole study base or a sample of it based on some existing exposure information. Thus unlike in a case-control framework, the complete assessment of the evolution of the morbidity in the course of the follow-up time is one of the challenges of this type of studies. This can be based either on a *passive follow-up* by matching the cohort with routine records of mortality or incidence coming from registries or administrative sources (cf. Chap. I.4 of this handbook) or on an *active follow-up* by which the health status of every subject in the cohort is determined at several time points during the study period. On the contrary, at least in principle, the assessment of the exposure is less problematic than in case-control studies as it is determined before the disease arises. Conceptually, all cohort studies are prospective in the sense that one measures the exposure before disease occurrence. In practice this approach is often not realistic when the outcome of interest is a disease with a long induction period like cancer, so that a purely prospective observation of the morbidity would either imply a study duration of several decades or very large numbers of participants. One way to shorten this study time is to define the population historically, i.e. at a given time in the past and to mimic the prospective follow-up of the cohort until the present time. This design is called *a historical cohort* design in contrast to the *prospective cohort* design.

In cohort designs the main issue is the presence of study drop-outs or subjects *lost to follow-up*. When a drop-out occurs, its influence can only be controlled in the analysis assuming that the drop-out is only determined by recorded factors. In other terms, this means that we know for each missing subject, why she/he is missing and in particular that the drop-out does not depend on the unmeasured health outcome. In technically terms this is the MAR hypothesis (cf. Chap. II.6 of this handbook). This hypothesis can, however, not be tested from the data as – per definition of drop-out – we do not know the study outcome. An example of this would be a study in which the outcome of interest is smoking cessation comparing different cessation strategies. If the study participants fail to show up at later interviews aimed at investigating whether the subjects are still abstinent, this may be because they have relapsed and are ashamed of this fact or because smoking is no longer a problem as they have been abstinent for a long period. The effect of study drop-outs can then only be assessed through sensitivity studies by which one would simulate reasonable data for the missing study outcome. In the smoking cessation example one could for instance assume that all drop-outs relapsed, or a 90%, 70%, ... random proportion of the drop-outs. Preventing study drop-outs is thus the main challenge in cohort studies.

Historical Cohorts

As mentioned earlier, the historical cohort design mimics a prospective follow-up of a historically defined population. This entails that at any point in the past, it is possible to check whether a subject satisfies the cohort-inclusion criteria as defined in the protocol or not. Furthermore if a subject from this cohort developed the outcome of interest, one must be sure to detect it and to be able to determine at what time point this event of interest occurred. In historical cohorts, the operational definition of loss to follow-up is the following: if the event of interest occurs at a given time-point for a given subject one must be sure to know it. If this cannot be assured from a certain point in time onwards, the subject must be considered as lost to follow-up.

The historical cohort design has been the design of choice for industry-based epidemiology of chronic diseases especially cancer (cf. Chap. III.2 of this handbook) and we shall discuss the relevant issues in this context.

Cohort Recruitment. In a historical cohort, the first step in planning is to determine whether information exists by which one can be assured that the population satisfying the theoretical cohort definition can be collected. Completeness with respect to the cohort definition is paramount. For instance if the cohort definition is "all subjects having worked on a given industrial site since 1970", a document dated from 1970 listing all those subjects must be available as well as yearly lists of all subsequently hired subjects. Computerized files can rarely be trusted as they were usually created for administrative purposes and are often at least partially overwritten or may exclude some categories of employees. Individual files are also to be dismissed as a single source of data. Neglect, lack of place for archives or floods and fire may have led to the selective destruction of files. It cannot be assumed that these lacking data are independent from either exposure or health outcome. In order to reliably identify a historical cohort, at least two data sources which can be considered independent should be available. One example would be separate lists from the pension scheme and from the personnel department. An alternative would be an enumerated list from whatever origin and historical documents in which yearly counts of employed subjects are given.

Case Ascertainment and Loss to Follow-up. In historical cohorts the main problem is to be sure to that any case that occurred in the follow-up period was detected. As an active follow-up is impossible retrospectively, the tracing procedure of subjects must rely on the matching of the cohort data with routine records. These routine records have usually a limited recruitment area. Disease or mortality registries are regional in most countries (with the notable exception of the Scandinavian countries) and sometimes related to the place of birth or residence. When either information is incomplete or missing for some subjects or if some subjects moved out of recruitment area, these subjects are lost to follow-up i.e. from that moment on, if the event of interest had taken place, it will no longer have been recorded with certainty. In the statistical analysis henceforth the subject should no longer contribute any person-time (cf. Chap. I.5 of this handbook). Therefore it is important to set up procedures by which one can determine whether and when a subject is lost to follow-up, for instance by trying to trace the addresses of the subjects through the pension schemes. Setting up such procedures can be difficult or even impossible for selected groups. For example historical cohorts may include foreign-born subjects who may have returned to their country of origin. If a subgroup is identified, for which such loss of follow-up is likely but no individual tracing can be set up, the only solution might be to drop all members of this subgroup from the study at the time of last contact. Thus in a historical occupational cohort study without active follow-up, one may need to consider as lost to follow-up all foreign-born employees from the date of last employment.

Recording individual diseases or medical causes of death may be restricted by data protection laws in absence of an informed consent. Strategies must then be set up, often involving third parties, by which the epidemiologists will have access to anonymous but individual data (e.g. Wild et al. 1995a).

Prospective Cohorts

As mentioned, the major advantage of prospective cohorts is that the exposure information is determined before the disease occurs, which allows to precisely measure the exposure and confounders of interest. In historical cohorts the exposure is estimated retrospectively although it relies as much as possible on historical exposure data. But these data were usually not collected for this purpose with the possible consequences with respect to their validity. This leads often to missing or imprecisely measured exposure data. In the worst case, such a retrospective exposure assessment may lead to an information bias not unlike that potentially occurring in case-control studies. In prospective cohorts, the information bias is theoretically impossible.

Another advantage is that as informed consent can be obtained for each study participant, there are no legal problems with respect to access to data.

Although in some very large studies as the American Cancer Prevention Studies (Garfinkel 1985), it is possible to study long latency chronic diseases, i.e. in general diseases with long induction periods, most prospective cohorts are primarily targeted at subclinical disorders assessed by questionnaires and functional or biological measurements.

An inherent drawback of prospective studies is their practical difficulty. Such prospective follow-ups of populations require repeated contacts with each subject of the cohort and are very cost-intensive.

A first problem is that the participation proportion is often rather low, especially if that participation entails repeated contacts which might discourage taking part. For instance, participation varied between 22% and 38% in the German centres of the European Prospective Investigation into Cancer and Nutrition (EPIC) study (Boeing et al. 1999). Limited information exists (Goldberg et al. 2001) which tends to show that participants are generally in better health than non-participants. Most prospective cohorts therefore rely on voluntaries. Thus prospective cohorts are only exceptionally representative of their target populations. Fortunately, representativeness is not a key issue in analytical studies as long as the loss to follow-up is limited. In prospective cohorts, loss to follow-up occurs either due to actual loss of contact or more often due to the refusal of continued participation. An unpublished survey by Moulin (personal communication) of all large ongoing prospective cohorts in France suggested that reasonable numbers of subjects lost to follow-up can only be obtained by regular contacts, regular feedback of the results of the studies to the participants and, if possible, presence in the media. When planning prospective studies, enough resources should therefore be allocated not only to the actual contacts with the subjects (i.e. mailing of questionnaires and reminders) but also to the communication budget, both with regard to the media and the study participants.

12.3.3   Case-Control Studies

In a case-control study, incident cases of a given disease are gathered from the study base and are contrasted to a sample of controls drawn from the same base. Exposure histories are then collected from the cases and the controls. The theoretical foundations of the design of a case-control study (also called a case-referent approach as in Miettinen (1985)) are the same as for a cohort study (see also Chap. I.6 of this handbook). But instead of comparing the disease incidence between exposure groups, it compares the exposure between cases and controls.

According to the most frequent definitions, a case-control study conducted within a dynamic population may be *population-based* or *hospital-based* depending on the selection procedures of cases and controls. When the base population is an enumerated cohort, the case-control study is often called *nested within the cohort*. A case-control study designed for etiological research will belong to one of these three categories. Each of them has different practical implications which we detail below.

Population-based Case-Control Study (Primary Base)

In a population-based case-control study, the cases are all patients diagnosed with the disease during the study period among those who live within a country or a region. The controls are sampled from this population. In this design, the study base, i.e. the population living in this country or region during the study period, is precisely defined a priori before the start of the study. Another example of a primary-base case-control study would be to include all members of a given health care insurance system where all cases are also members.

Case Recruitment.   A researcher may choose a population-based case-control design if all new cases of the disease (or at least a representative sample of all cases) can be identified in the study base. As it is essential to ensure completeness of case-finding, a disease registry may be helpful for identifying the cases. The existence of a disease registry may also constitute a motivation for conducting a study in a given area. However, the value of a registry may be limited if there is a substantial time lag between diagnosis and registration, particularly if collection of data from the respondent is necessary and if the disease is rapidly fatal. Thus, a specific procedure for case identification has to be set up in most studies by the research team. For example, a case-finding network may be organized including all hospitals, clinics, and pathology departments in the study area to identify and interview the cases. This should also be extended to nearby areas as some of the diseased persons in the source population defined by residence in a given geographic area may be diagnosed and hospitalized elsewhere. It is also strongly recommended to perform an active search of the patients, by organizing periodic visits to all centres, rather than to rely on a passive notification of the cases by the medical staff of the clinics or the hospitals.

Selection of Controls. *Principles.* The controls should be selected at random from the same base population as the cases. In addition, the probability of selecting a particular control subject should be proportional to the amount of time that he contributes to the study period, or to person-time at risk (Rothman and Greenland 1998). For example, if a subject moved out of the source population at half the study period, he/she should have only half the probability of being selected as a control than a subject who stayed in the source population during the entire study period. To be eligible, a control subject should belong to the study base at the date of diagnosis of the index case. Controls who recently moved into the source population and are chosen to match cases diagnosed several years earlier should be excluded since they are outside the study base. Excluding controls who have recently moved in the base reduces the problem, but does not solve it, since people who have moved out of the base will still be missed.

A density sampling of the base population should be used. Density sampling can be achieved, for example, by selecting the controls at a steady rate throughout the study period proportional to the number of cases. In practice, the protocol may define several points in time, e.g., once a month or once a year, where controls will be selected from the population present in the study base at that time. In a design where the cases and the controls are matched individually, it is also possible to use sampling sets of possible controls, one per case, composed of all persons present in the source population at the time of case's diagnosis. The desired number of matched controls is then selected at random within each of these risk sets.

Selection of Population Controls Based on a Listing of Individuals. To be feasible, these procedures of control selection necessitate not only a fully enumerated source population, but also regular updates of this population, to take emigration and immigration during the study period into account. In Scandinavian countries, study investigators may rely on central population registers to select controls using a simple random sampling at regular intervals during the study period (see also Chap. I.4 of this handbook). More often, however, a complete population register, including the identification of individual members by name and address, as well as stratification variables such as gender and date of birth, will not be available and other methods of control selection must be used.

In the absence of a population register, the researcher may use other *lists of individuals*, such as lists of municipality residents, electoral lists, telephone books, listings of health insurance members, and so forth. Using these lists for control selection, however, may introduce bias if the probability for an individual in the source population to be listed is related to the exposure of interest. Telephone books would not be suitable for a study on cancer in relation to an occupational chemical, for example if phone numbers of highly educated and less exposed individuals are less frequently published in the directory than phone numbers of subjects of other socio-economic categories. Persons not registered in electoral rosters may also differ from those listed, and may not include immigrant workers from foreign countries. Municipal lists may not be updated regularly. The decision to use such lists for control selection must be done carefully. Beside completeness of the list, the possibility of tracing individuals based on the information provided (name, address, phone number, etc.) must also be considered. One should also check that the cases are listed on the roster. The analysis should then exclude the unlisted cases, such as those who are not citizens when using electoral lists.

Selection of Population Controls Without a Listing of Individuals.   Other sampling schemes may be used for selecting the controls when no list of individuals is available. Multistage random samplings starting with sampling of dwellings or based on random digit dialing procedures are commonly used. The controls can then be selected within each household.

Neighbourhood controls. This method implies a two-stage sampling, with a random sampling of households followed by the selection of an eligible individual within the selected residence. Households sampling may be conducted from a roster of residences, obtained for example from census data. When a roster of households is not available, controls may still be selected from residences in the case's neighbourhood. Starting from the case's residence, the interviewer may follow a predefined procedure for selecting a household, by means of a map, aerial pictures, or by a systematic walk algorithm starting at the index household (Wacholder et al. 1992b). This sampling method implies that the controls are individually matched to cases on place of residence. To avoid bias, the interviewer should not be given the flexibility to choose which house to select but a simple and unambiguous algorithm for selecting households should be developed to remove the possibility of interviewers avoiding certain areas. A potential problem of neighbourhood controls is overmatching on the exposure, due to similarities between cases and controls living in the same neighbourhood.

Random digit dialling. Random digit dialling can be used to select population controls when no roster exists and when almost every household has a telephone. Random digit dialling generates telephone numbers, and it does not rely on a telephone book where new or unpublished phone numbers are not listed. Several variants of the standard method exist (Waksberg 1978). Briefly, a phone number is created using the first numbers, including area code, of working telephone numbers provided by the telephone company, which are then completed with random numbers. The number is dialled a predetermined number of times. The first contact with a household member is used for screening and to obtain a census of the household. Based on the responses, and a predetermined sampling scheme, eligible subjects are selected to be controls. These individuals can be interviewed by telephone directly, or they can be contacted afterwards for an in-person or a telephone interview.

Random digit dialling is not appropriate if the telephone coverage is low, but this should not be a problem in most developed countries. Other problems associated with random digit dialling include residences that can be reached by more than one phone number, or if more than one person in the household is eligible to be a control, since it may lead to different selection probability of the controls. It should also be realized that random digit dialling is an expensive and time-consuming procedure, particularly when targeting subgroups of the population, since a large number of phone calls may be necessary before the desired number of eligible controls are found. Non-response and refusal is an additional problem and it may not be possible to have an exact estimate of the participation rate. It is recommended that the distribution of the final sample according to key variables such as age, sex or socio-economic status is compared to an expected distribution obtained for example from the last census. The random digit dialling has been used successfully in a large number of studies, but new technology, such as the widespread and sometimes exclusive use of mobile phones, may cause this method to be obsolete in the near future.

Hospital-based Case-Control (Secondary Base)

In hospital-based case-control studies, the cases are the patients diagnosed with the disease in a given hospital or clinic during the study period. The controls have to be selected from the population from which the cases arose, i.e. the group of individuals who would be treated in this hospital if they had developed the disease. Because the source population is not easily identified, a random sample of controls can hardly be selected directly from this population. Instead, it is usually more practical to select controls among patients with other diseases diagnosed in the same hospital, representing a non-random subset of the study base. An appropriate group of control patients should have the same referral patterns to that hospital than the cases, so that the controls would have been admitted to this hospital if they had the case disease. The possibility of selecting hospital controls rests on the assumption that they are representative of the exposure distribution in the source population. This assumption is reasonable if the control disease is not causally related to exposure, and if exposure is not related to admission to that hospital.

Case-Control Study Nested Within a Cohort

When the study base is a real enumerated cohort with available entry and exit times a case-control study may be conducted by drawing cases and controls from this cohort as the source population. It is called a "case-control study nested within a cohort". Using this design implies that the cohort has been constituted so that the controls can be selected adequately from the cohort. As this design relies on an enumerated source population, a control group can easily be identified. In a matched design for example, a set of possible controls can be constituted with all non-diseased individuals in the cohort at the time of the cases' diagnosis. One or several controls may then be selected at random from each set.

12.3.4 The Study Base Principle: Selection, Exclusion and Resulting Bias

The study base principle, the first of three principles Wacholder et al. (1992a) developed for the selection of controls in case-control studies, that also applies to the design of cohort studies, simply states that "cases and controls should be representative of the same base experience." (see also Chap. I.6 of this handbook). *Representativeness* for the general population is not needed in analytical studies of the relation between an exposure and a disease. In a representative population, an association that is limited to one group may be obscured because the effect is weaker in other groups.

Thus for the aim of scientific inference of the relation between an exposure and disease, any exclusion or inclusion criteria are valid as long as they apply equally to cases and controls.

Wacholder et al. (1992a) identified the following reasons for which exclusion criteria can be applied:

— Inconvenience: Subjects of a given subgroup might be hard to reach. Failure to exclude a priori such a group may lead to a very poor response rate and an a posteriori exclusion, with the corresponding waste of resources.

— Anticipated low or inaccurate responses, e.g. of subjects who do not speak the language of the interview sufficiently well. Failure to exclude a priori such a group may yield non-interpretable data.

— Lack of variability of the exposure: If one intends to set up a cohort investigating the dose-response effect of a potential occupational carcinogen like cobalt salts, inclusion of a large number of workers from industries which do not use these chemicals does make little sense although including a small group for stabilising the baseline category may still be justified.

— Subjects at increased risk of disease due to other causes: In a prospective study targeted on environmental effects on asthma, subjects at high asthma risk due to their occupational exposure (e.g. bakers) should be excluded because cases are likely to be attributable to the occupational exposure and therefore may not contribute to the understanding of other risk factors.

— Combination of the above: In a historical occupational cohort study based on a factory, short-time employees may be difficult to track, their exposure is likely to be determined much more by previous or subsequent work, their cumulative exposure within the company is bound to be low and they may be at increased risk for many diseases as they constitute a group of socially unstable workers who are likely to have other risk factors. It is thus standard in such settings to exclude short-time workers. This has, however, the consequence that any given subject of the study base contributes person-time only from the date on when he/she has reached the minimum employment duration.

On the other hand, if a study base is restricted the comparison with the general population is biased. The so-called Healthy Worker Effect, by which is meant that a series of extraneous factors usually lower the observed mortality among employed workers, is an example of a selection bias. A simple comparison of the mortality of a cohort with population mortality rates as expressed for instance through the standardized mortality ratio is thus of limited validity. Of course, as discussed above, internal comparisons of exposure groups are still valid but may lack the necessary power for useful scientific inference except in very large cohorts.

Another consequence of severely restricting the study base of a (cohort or case-control) study is that it can lead to reduced detection of variability of the strength of association (effect modification). If the effect of smoking were to amplify the effect of an environmental exposure, restricting the study base to non-smokers may lead to a spurious absence of effects.

In some settings representativeness is an issue. If the study is focused on attributable or absolute risks, the study must be either exhaustive or representative, or external information must be available with respect to the sampling fractions of the strata of the study population within the general population.

Choosing Between Epidemiological Designs   12.3.5

Many other etiological designs like case-cohort designs, case-only designs, two-phase sampling, counter-matched designs to cite just a few, have been proposed in the epidemiological literature (Wacholder et al. 1992c; Chap. I.7 of this handbook). These designs usually combine elements of the case-control and the cohort designs often either by making additional hypotheses (case-only design) or by making use of additional data like in two-phase designs (see e.g. Breslow and Chatterjee 1999).

Another design is the so-called ecologic design, in which the units are groups of people rather than individual subjects. The groups may be classes in a school, factories, cities or administrative areas within a country. The only requirement is that a measure of the exposure and disease distributions is available for in each group. Because the data in ecologic studies are measurements averaged over individuals, the degree of association does not reflect the association between exposure and disease among individuals (so-called ecologic bias, see Greenland and Robins (1994)). Thus, while ecologic studies can be useful for detecting associations of exposure distributions with disease occurrence, such a design should not be used for etiologic investigation.

Another possible design consists in selecting a cross-section of the study base with no time dimension (cross-sectional study). Here both exposure and disease status are collected simultaneously at one point in time. It is therefore not the incidence but rather the prevalence of the disease that is investigated, so that it is usually impossible to assess whether the exposure actually preceded its presumed effect on health. Moreover, cross-sectional studies are particularly prone to selection bias as diseased subjects may have left the study-population. A longitudinal observation of exposure and disease in a study that is the paradigm of both the cohort and the case-control design is better suited for solving etiologic problems than a cross-section of it (a prevalence study). Possible exceptions are diseases with short induction periods or exposures that cannot change such as blood type or other invariable personal characteristics (see Rothman and Greenland 1998, p 75). If, however, a prospective cohort design is not feasible for financial reasons or simply because it is impossible to follow up a large enough group of subjects, the cross-sectional design can, despite its above mentioned limitations, provide important information especially if targeted on several (non-fatal) health outcomes (see Wild et al. 1995b) or if a number of different exposures coexist.

The main study types remain the cohort and the case-control designs. Choosing one or the other design depends on a number of issues among which the incidence rate of the disease of interest and the prevalence of the exposure of interest are prominent.

If the disease is very rare (for instance a rare cancer as testicular or brain cancer), a cohort approach would necessitate huge numbers of participants and a long follow-up to identify enough cases to make useful inference. A case-control study is the more reasonable approach for rare diseases. Another situation where the case-control is the preferred approach is if the aim is to generate hypotheses concerning various exposures in relation to a given disease. Determining possible occupational origins of laryngeal cancer is such an example.

On the other hand, if the exposure is rare and restricted to easily identified subpopulations or if one is interested in all possible disease outcomes of a given exposure, a cohort study, either historical or prospective, is the most efficient choice. An example for the former reasons would be a study of the carcinogenic effects of hard metal dusts (Moulin et al. 1998b) which occurs mostly in the factories producing hard metal tools. An example of the latter would be if one were to study the health consequence of the occupational stress in call-centres.

Another aspect that can influence the choice of a design is the induction time of the disease (although it may depend on the exposure). For long induction periods, a prospective cohort study is clearly not the design of choice as this would imply waiting a long time for a sufficient number of events to occur. This problem can be circumvented by the historical cohort design. Most historical cohorts are focused on cancer, a long induction disease per se. The choice between a case-control and a historical cohort study is then dependent on whether (or not) a historical cohort can provide an answer to the research question.

Other issues which might influence the choice of a given design include the precise scientific aim of the study. Direct estimation of the population incidence would require enrolment of the target population that ideally needs a cohort design or at least a population-based case-control approach. If, on the other hand, one is interested in the precise temporal sequence, as for instance in the study of the evolution of CD4+ cell numbers in HIV infected patients (Kaslow et al. 1987), cohort studies are virtually the only available design which may, however, be supplemented by a nested case-control study.

The final choice, once a theoretically optimal design has been determined, depends on the actual feasibility of each study as well as on the practical terms of access to the data and the costs involved.

Table 12.1 summarizes strengths and weaknesses of the above study types.

Table 12.1. Strengths and limitations of different observational study designs

Investigation of ...	Study design		
	Cross-sectional	Case-control	Cohort
Rare diseases	–	+++++	–
Rare causes	–	–	+++++
Multiple endpoints	++	–	+++++
Multiple exposures including confounders	+++	++++	(+++)[a]
Temporal sequence of exposure and disease	–	(+)[b]	+++++
Direct measurement of incidence	–	(+)[c]	+++++
Long induction periods	+	++++	(+++)[d]

Suitability of study design: +++++ highly suitable; ++++ very suitable; +++ suitable; ++ moderately suitable; + limited suitability; – not suitable
[a] If prospective (multi-purpose cohorts)
[b] If nested in a cohort
[c] If population-based, combined with an incidence study
[d] If historical

Statistical Power

As mentioned in the first section any study protocol should include an evaluation of the statistical power to detect a predefined effect of the exposure with a given study base. When computing the statistical power, the need for subgrouping, based either on exposure classes or confounder classes, is important. In practice the choice of the sample size (or to be exact the size of the study base) is a compromise between what one would ideally be able to detect and the practical limits of the study. These limits are of two kinds. A first limitation occurs when there simply do not exist enough subjects in the envisaged study with either a rare disease of interest e.g. rare cancers, or with a rare exposure. An example of this would be if we were to study the interaction between a rare gene (prevalence < 0.01) and a rare environmental exposure. If the latter has a prevalence of 5%, less than 5/10,000 of controls would show both features so that the minimum sample size to investigate such an interaction would be in the tens of thousands. A second limitation is when the needed funding is not reasonable.

In general, a statistical power of 80% is considered a reasonable power to achieve objectives and any power below this arbitrary figure may be considered too low. If methods of prior assessment, either formal or intuitive, suggest that the study will be too small to be informative, there are several options:

One can lower the level of ambition. For instance instead of computing a statistical power to detect a 1.2 odds ratio, this value can be put at a 1.3 level. The drawback of this strategy is of course that if no effect of the exposure can be detected, lower risks cannot be excluded. Thus if the main interest lies in effects of low doses of exposures with expected low magnitude effects such a strategy is not recommended.

One can set-up a system with an extended follow-up time. This means that the study base is enlarged in its time dimension. This usually entails that the results will be available later.

One can try to organize a multi-centre study. This means that the study base is enlarged in its number of subject dimension. When organizing multi-centre studies, one should be reasonably sure that the gain in sample size is not offset by between-centre differences in exposure circumstances and assessment, or differences in case ascertainment. Another issue in this case is that the harmonization of centres has its costs, too.

One can abandon the project. It can be considered unethical to undertake a study which would not add to the general knowledge but costs money which could benefit other research.

Statistical power can, however, not be the only criteria by which to judge the appropriateness of a study. Other reasons like public concern or scientific background knowledge for instance based on positive animal studies are sometimes even more important.

Measures of Disease Outcome and Exposure Parameters

12.4

Measurement and Classification of Exposure

12.4.1

Introduction

Epidemiological studies are designed to assess the impact of exposure on the development of a disease. The sources of error and the ways in which exposure and disease are assessed are quite different, and thus the mechanisms by which errors arise are different as well.

The range of exposures of interest in epidemiology is broad (Savitz 2003). Exposure include exogenous agents such as drugs, diet, and chemical or physical hazards present in the environment; genetic attributes that affect ability to metabolize specific compounds; stable characteristics such as height or eye colour; physiologic attributes such as blood pressure; life habits such as physical exercise or tobacco smoking; mental states such as depression; social environment, and so forth. To this wide range of exposures of interest correspond many different methods for measuring exposure (Armstrong et al. 1994; Chap. I.11 of this handbook).

The method chosen to collect data depends on the particular exposure to study, the precision of data required, availability of existing records, sensitivity of subject to questioning about the exposure, cost of various methods, etc. The study protocol should describe the operational approach chosen for exposure ascertainment. The accuracy of an operational approach is best described in relation to the ideal measure which is always impractical or impossible to obtain.

The ultimate goal of exposure assessment is to measure the exposure that contributes to the etiologic process under investigation. Ideally, an exposure assessment should take this biologically effective exposure, and only this exposure, into consideration. Most often, however, this goal cannot be reached by an operational exposure indicator. One reason is that the biological mechanism by which exposure might cause disease is often not clearly identified. For example, in studies on the potential cancer risks associated with exposure to ELF magnetic fields, it was not clear whether the most relevant exposure indicator with respect to aetiology should be an average exposure over the entire life or over the most recent period before cancer diagnosis, or if it should be a measure of peak exposures over a certain threshold, or in a particular exposure windows. This problem could be partially overcome if a detailed exposure profile over time can be estimated, to calculate different exposure indices, each of them being related to cancer risk. Another reason is that it is often impossible to obtain the data that would reflect perfectly the biologically effective exposure. For example, the persistent organochlorine pesticide DDT and its metabolite DDE were suspected to be causally related to breast cancer risk (Wolff et al. 1993). Assume also that the biologically effective exposure is the level of DDT/DDE present in breast tissue in the time window 5–15 years before cancer diagnosis. Different exposure measures among cases and controls could be used to study the relationship between DDT/DDE exposure and breast cancer (Savitz 2003), including environmental levels measured in the area of residence at the time of diagnosis or taking into account the residential changes of the subject, present-day blood levels, or blood levels measured in the etiologically relevant period using serum specimens drawn in the past and kept in a bank. Clearly, these exposure measures are not equivalent as they correlate differently with the biologically effective exposure. Using environmental exposures as a surrogate exposure indicator is probably ineffective, since the association on breast cancer risk may fall below what can be detected. However, if blood levels are strongly correlated with breast tissue concentrations, an association with breast cancer risk can still be observed, although blood levels are not the right measure. Nevertheless, certain metabolites measured in blood may be a good indicator of past exposure if the half life of the agent is sufficiently long (Flesch-Janys et al. 1998). The choice of an operational indicator of exposure should be done in the context of a hypothesis on biological process, and a comparison of the operational and ideal exposure indicators should be provided.

All laboratory data are subject to error due to imprecise measurement. However, the conceptual error by which the measure obtained does not reflect the exposure of interest is often of much greater importance. In a study focused on effects of microbiological contamination, measurement of viable colonies may be only of marginal interest if these bacteria are not the pathogenic ones. Bacterial endotoxin has been shown to be the more relevant exposure with respect to lung diseases (Rylander 2002).

Another challenge in exposure assessment is that often different types of exposure coexist and their individual effect can only be considered in combination. The level of exposure aggregation that is chosen must, however, reflect scientific hypotheses. For instance a nutritional epidemiology study focused on the role of coffee in miscarriages could consider two relevant categorizations. The role of caffeine itself would be investigated by grouping all sources including tea, caffeine-containing medications, etc., whereas the role of constituents of the coffee other than caffeine would be investigated by grouping caffeinated and decaffeinated coffee.

Temporal Aspects

Some exposures are constant over time, such as genetic constitution, but all exogenous exposures such as diet and chemical pollutants vary substantially over time. In addition to the identification of a biologically relevant exposure, it is necessary to identify an etiologically relevant time window during which the exposure may be related to disease occurrence so that the data collection concentrates on etiologically relevant time-windows.

It has been long recognized that many diseases such as cancer appear a long time after they have been induced. The time between the beginning of the exposure and the first manifestation of the disease of interest is called the *induction* period. It serves as a surrogate for the biological induction period in epidemiological studies although the onset of exposure does not necessarily result in immediate induction. Epidemiological studies should allow for the fact that diseases with long induction periods that appear immediately after the exposure are not attributable to this exposure. In the statistical analysis of such data, the usual practice is to shift the exposure by a given *lag time* which is typically about half the usual induction period. This has the consequence to ignore the exposure of recent years. The consequences for planning is that whenever the anticipated induction period is long, the investigator must select a study base including a sufficient number of subjects for whom the exposure is ancient enough. On the other hand, if the expected effects of exposure are of a short-term nature as for instance a reversible genotoxic effect as assessed by a comet assay, it is important to precisely measure the relevant short-term exposure.

Other time-related issues may concern the temporal pattern of the exposure itself and its presupposed effects. If the exposure effect occurs through the action of peak exposure, its effects are likely to be much more important when the exposure is highly variable than in circumstances in which the exposure is virtually constant. For such presupposed effects, the exposure measurement of most interest may be an estimated number of peak exposures. On the other hand if we assume that the exposure acts through a cumulative damage, the total cumulative exposure is the adequate way to express its effects. If the disease of interest is reversible, the cumulative exposure may also be inadequate as a measure of exposure and exposure assessment in different time windows may be more relevant.

Sources of Exposure Data

The different possible sources of exposure data and their characteristics are described in Armstrong et al. (1994). The following section is mostly a summary of the issues covered in this book (see also Chap. I.11 of this handbook).

Questionnaires. A prominent and often the only way to assess an individual exposure is by an exposure questionnaire. The three main types of exposure questionnaires are self-administered questionnaires, telephone administered interviews and interviewer-administered questionnaires, also called structured personal interviews. The last two methods are the commonest methods of collecting data on exposure in epidemiological studies. Using them allows the number of errors and missing items to be reduced and more complex information to be obtained. For instance, there is a possibility of branching, i.e. specific questionnaires can be inserted after some trigger information has been recorded. This possibility has been used in occupational exposure questionnaires in which job histories are obtained and specific questionnaires are used for a limited number of jobs and/or tasks (Ahrens et al. 1993). On the other hand, the interviewer may increase error if he or she exerts a qualitative influence on the subject's responses by his or her appearance, manner, method of administration, etc. Intensive training and standardization of the interviewers is therefore very important in the planning and conduct of a study. If a series of prerequisites are fulfilled as the stressing of interview neutrality in training, the standardization of questionnaire wording and its administration, the likelihood that the interviewer's personal attitudes will affect the responses is much reduced. The main advantage of a self-administered questionnaire is its reduced cost. Armstrong et al. (1994, p 44) conclude that "there appears to be little difference between these methods (subjective recall of exposure collected through face-to-face, telephone or self-administered questionnaires) with respect to the validity of the data obtained. (…) Face-to-face interviews are the dominant approach and are clearly best for the collection of large amounts of complex data. However, where subjects are widely dispersed and the questionnaire can be kept comparatively brief, telephone interviews can be favoured. Self-administered questionnaires should be considered for low budget studies for which small amounts of reasonably simple data are required."

In setting up a questionnaire many sometimes contradictory issues arise. While obviously more details can theoretically be assessed if it is longer, long questionnaires take more time and (especially among diseased subjects) may be more difficult to apply. A questionnaire should have a clear structure and should be understandable. Questions like: "Have you been exposed to bischloromethylether?" should be avoided. Sensitive issues (religion, sexual habits, alcohol consumption, etc.) should be avoided if they are not central to the study and should be given careful consideration if necessary in order to avoid withdrawal of the interviewee. A questionnaire should always be tested before use. The use of validated instruments is of course desirable. Correspondingly, a large number of publications exists on validating existing questionnaires (see for instance Rouch et al. (2003) or Bogers et al. (2004)). It is probably a good strategy to choose, whenever possible, an already existing questionnaire that has been validated in circumstances close to its intended use. If one decides, nevertheless, to adapt a questionnaire for a given study, a pre-test should be carried out to investigate its properties, notably feasibility, clarity, and reproducibility, so that necessary adaptations can be made before applying it. If a completely new instrument has to be designed a validation study should be taken into consideration to investigate its properties as e.g. validity and responsiveness to change, i.e. its ability to reflect changes in behaviour or subjective symptoms (Bogers et al. 2004).

Diaries. Diaries refer to detailed prospective records of exposure by the subject. As such they can neither be used in case-control studies nor in historical cohort studies. This method has been used in many contexts among which their use in nutritional epidemiology for measuring dietary intake is prominent (cf. Andersen et al. 2004; Chap. III.4 of this handbook). Ongoing monitoring of symptoms of a disease is another application of diaries (cf. Goebel et al. 2002). Armstrong et al. (1994, p 219) conclude "The use of diaries may be highly accurate method of measuring present common behaviours. The limitations of diaries, in comparison with interview methods, are the greater burden on subjects, which may lead to poorer response rate and the greater cost for subject training and for coding the data. The accuracy of diary information can be enhanced by use of multiple diary days spread over a sufficient time period, and by careful training of subjects and coders."

Records of Exposures. Historical records of pre-existing data may be a valuable and sometimes the single source of early exposure data. Two types of records can be useful for exposure assessment. A first type of records contains information on the individual study subjects, for instance medical, behavioural (smoking), or physical characteristics (weight) contained in medical records but also social or occupational data contained in population registries. A second type of records contains information relevant to the exposure of groups like descriptions or measurements of environmental exposure or descriptions of histories of industrial processes in occupational epidemiology. The primary advantage of records is that they can provide prospectively recorded information, collected on information in the past. For example, use of pharmacy records in a case-control study of prescription drug use could overcome lack of recall. Exposure assessment based on historical records is immune to information or recall bias. Most important in this context is the use of data from earlier cross-sectional surveys. The main drawback is the lack of control over the availability of records for each subject and their standardized recording and the difficulty to assess the validity of the existing data.

Biological Measurements and Measurements in the Environment. In principle, measurements made directly in the human body represent the ideal approach to measuring exposure for etiological studies. In practice a number of problems exists. A first problem is to determine the measurement in terms of the correct metabolite and the appropriate point in time that is relevant for the presumed biologically effective dose. A second problem is the often large within-person variability which can be of the same size or larger than between-person variation. This has been observed repeatedly in industrial exposures (see Kromhout et al. 1994), but it is often also true for biological measurements. Liu et al. (1978) reported a ratio of within-person to between-person variances as high as 3.20 for 24-hour urinary sodium, a marker of sodium intake.

The current fast development of methods of measurement of exposures in biological materials may, however, give rise to many useful indicators. The epidemiologist should be aware of the developments in this area. Methods whose validity have been assessed should always be preferred and the operations manual should include Good Laboratory Practices. In planning laboratory work, it may be important to keep track of the internal quality control procedures and provision should be made that these informations are recorded.

Objectivity of measurements in the environment are best achieved by personal sampling over extended periods of time. Relying on samples collected over relatively short periods of time without clear sampling design may induce substantial error in the exposure assessment. While sensitivity of measurements can be very high, the measurement error is often only a small part of exposure variance which is usually dominated by the intrinsic variability in exposure. Planning exposure measurements for an epidemiological study should therefore rely on factors likely to influence the exposure (Sauleau et al. 2003). The methods for exposure measurement have to be included in the operations manual. Reliable past exposure measurements rarely exist in sufficient numbers. Moreover, their validity is in general doubtful as they were usually obtained for purposes other than an epidemiological study, typically environment control. In such cases an attempt may be made to estimate exposure by use of conversion tables such as job-exposures matrices and food tables linked to data derived from records, questionnaires or expert assessment. Moulin et al. (1998b) show an example where existing past measurements were highly variable and only scarcely related to the exposure assessed by experts. Nevertheless, using the latter, they were able to demonstrate a dose-dependent carcinogenic effect of hard-metal dusts.

Finally the use one intends to make of the exposure measurements in the analysis of the data has to be stated in the protocol. This is required in order to assess whether a certain number of measurements with a given precision and a presumed variability of exposure will be sufficient to achieve statistically valid results with respect to the association of exposure and outcome.

Measurement and Classification of Health Outcomes   12.4.2

The main distinction to be made concerning measurement and classification of health outcomes is between diseases for which a clear diagnosis can be made at a precisely defined time and health outcomes which are defined by a measurement either by questionnaire or a functional or laboratory test.

The latter case includes health outcomes like obesity or hypertension where the health outcome is better expressed on a continuous scale rather than as a classification into diseased/non diseased categories and for which no clear-cut incidence date can be obtained. This feature implies that the prospective cohort design is the only design in which it is possible to be sure that the exposure precedes the disease. In such cases determination of the point in time when to measure the health outcome is crucial. If one is interested in acute effects of an exposure, e.g. the immediate effect of the chlorine in a swimming pool on genotoxicity using the Comet assay, the health effect must be measured immediately after the exposure. If one is interested in chronic effects of an exposure, e.g. of organic solvents on chronic neurotoxicity, care must be taken to measure the health outcomes after a period of washout as for instance after the weekend in the example of a study of chronic neurotoxic effects of solvents, as the acute effects of the exposure may confuse the chronic effects. Such considerations may have serious implications on the planning, cost or even feasibility of such studies.

In the case of a well-defined disease with a defined incidence date, both historical cohorts and case-control designs can be used. Still the precise definition of the disease is one of the challenges of a clear design. The main issue is whether to group or to separate disease subtypes. Different subtypes of a same disease may have different risk factors even within a cancer site. The recent rise in adenocarcinoma of the lung has for instance been related to the increased use of "light" cigarettes. However, a too narrow definition of a disease may lead to smaller number of cases. This is even more an issue when the diagnosis is obtained from registry data or death certificates as is usually the case in historical cohorts. The precision of such data may well be fictitious and grouping of diseases thought to have similar etiologies may be the only reasonable choice.

An intermediate case would be a well-defined disease like COPD (chronic obstructive pulmonary disease) for which no systematic recording of patients is possible. For such a disease only hospital-based case-control studies with the challenge of estimating the time of onset of the disease in order to ignore all posterior irrelevant exposure, or prospective cohorts with the problem of potentially low power seem to be realistic designs.

12.4.3   Information Bias

A major bias related to data collection is the information bias that occurs if the exposure assessment is different for cases and controls or the health outcome is measured differently for exposed and non-exposed subjects. The first situation arises mainly in case-control studies when the cases know of the possible determinants of their disease (e.g. smoking or asbestos exposure among lung cancer cases) and therefore report more of their past exposure. It is possible to minimize this type of bias by standardized questionnaires and, if possible, by a data collection blinded with respect to the case-control status. The latter approach, although an option in hospital-based case-control studies, is, however, virtually impossible in population-based case-control studies. The same type of information bias is possible with historical cohorts if information is obtained a posteriori from proxies.

An information bias can also be due to the unavoidable measurement error in retrospectively measuring the exposure. The comparable accuracy principle (Wacholder et al. 1992a) states that the degree of accuracy in measuring the exposure of interest for the cases should be equivalent to the degree of accuracy for the controls unless the effect of the inaccuracy can be controlled in the analysis, as for instance by using appropriate validation data. Although adherence to this principle does not eliminate the corresponding misclassification, its rationale is to avoid that a positive finding is induced simply by differences in the accuracy of information about cases and controls (see also Chap. I.6 of this handbook).

Confounding

The *deconfounding principle*, another principle given in Wacholder et al. (1992a), states that confounding should not be allowed to distort the estimation of an effect. Confounders are per definition factors that are determinants of the disease and that are related to the exposure of interest. Setting up a list of confounders is therefore a primary task in the exploration of the scientific knowledge related to the research question of the planned study. This identification of confounders cannot only be based on statistical associations but must be thought in terms of potential causal pathways. For instance, if one were to study the effect of nutrition on coronary heart diseases (CHD), a factor that might be considered a potential confounder is obesity as it is related both to nutrition and CHD. On the other hand one might consider that obesity is on the causal pathway between nutrition and CHD in which case controlling for obesity would bias the estimation of the effect of nutrition (*overadjustment*). Careful thought should therefore be given to each factor that has to be included as a confounder. An operational result of this first step would be a list of three groups of confounders.

1. Established confounders that are known to determine disease and to be related to the exposure of interest but which are not on the causal pathways. Sex and age are virtually always included in this group.
2. Probable confounders that are established risk factors and for which there are reasons to believe that they might be related to the exposure.
3. Possible confounders including other risk factors of the disease that might be or not related to the exposure. If a given risk factor is a strong determinant of the disease (e.g. smoking for lung cancer), it might confound the association of a potential risk factor although the confounder is only weakly associated with the other risk factor in the study sample.

At the design stage, controlling for confounders can be done either by restricting the data base to certain values of the confounder (e.g. a lung cancer case-control study among non-smokers) or by matching. The latter ranges from broad frequency matching on age and sex to the individual matching on factors thought to be related to non-measurable factors (e.g. neighbourhood matching). It must be stressed at this point that controlling for confounders in the design may well be counterproductive as it is irreversible and may forbid to explore interesting post hoc hypotheses (see also Sect. 12.3 on matching in Chap. I.6 of this handbook). A last strategy is to collect the relevant data on confounders in order to be able to control them later in the analysis.

Details of how to deal with confounding using any of these methods can only be decided within the context of a given study. The main pitfall in controlling for confounders at the design stage is overmatching. Restricting the variability of the confounding variable will also reduce the variability of the exposure of interest within each matched case-control pair and will thus reduce the power of the study. This would occur if cases and controls were matched on age, sex and tight socio-economic categories. It is very likely that other variables like smoking or dietary factors would also be more similar.

12.6   Statistical Analysis

The statistical analysis of a study is an important step in the overall quality of a study and enough time and human resources should be planned from the start. Many large-scale studies we know of, are underreported because of lack of funding for the statistical analysis. It is impossible to detail all statistical analyses to be done at the planning stage. However, as already mentioned, the main research questions should be formulated in the protocol and these questions should be operationalized already at this stage, i.e. translated in a statistical hypothesis to be tested.

It is helpful at this stage to draw hypothetical causal graphs in order to formulate a priori models to be confronted with the data of the study (see Pearl 2000, Cox and Wermuth 1996). Figure 12.1 shows a very simple graph formulating a series of hypotheses on the effect of shiftwork and age on cognitive performances which may be mediated by sleep problems.

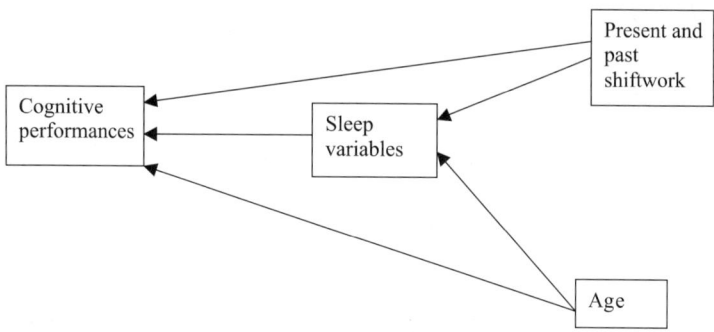

Figure 12.1. Causal hypotheses of effects of shift work and age on cognitive performances

Such a conceptual framework helps to set up a list of statistical analyses based on a priori hypotheses and additional ad hoc analyses which are more or less data driven. The minimum statistical content to be defined at the planning stage are the endpoint variable(s), the exposure variables of interest and the variables to be adjusted for (i.e. the potential confounders). The statistical measures (proportions, odds, means, standard deviations, etc.) and models (mostly regression models) to be calculated should also be enumerated including the residual and influence statistics to be applied to check the robustness of the results. Finally, all the subgroups of intrinsic interest for which separate analyses will be done should be identified.

The fact that the a priori formulated hypotheses are operationalized, means that for instance the main endpoint(s) of interest should be identified as certain values of given variables. This is relatively straightforward in case-control studies for which the endpoint is the case status whatever its definition. For cohort studies focused on the mortality or incidence of given diseases, the list of diseases possibly related to the exposure of interest should be identified. For prospective cohorts or cross-sectional studies the endpoint of interest may be less straightforward and can possibly imply a prior data transformation, e.g. a score of depression obtained from a mental health questionnaire.

The variables characterising the exposure should also be specified. These can include (possibly lagged) cumulative, peak or mean exposure. Although for power computations this exposure may have to be considered as a yes/no variable, the main message cannot be that simple. Established risk factors have to be included in the final model in any case, as long as an association of it with the exposure of interest has to be assumed. On the other hand, although all measured confounders must be tested, the list of presumed confounders to be included in the main model cannot be finalized at the planning stage as they depend to a certain extent on the data themselves. E.g. a presumed confounder may not be associated with either disease or exposure of interest, in which case its inclusion is wasteful.

Practical Issues

12.7

Fund Raising

12.7.1

Technically, the expenses must be specified as regular salaries (paid by the parent organization), salaries for temporary staff, durable equipment, travel expenses, consumables (mailing, telecommunication, office material, laboratory), fees, consultants.

It is also important to adjust the flow of payment to fit the respective stages of the project. If funding comes from a number of different sources, the tentative share of each one must be specified. Experience has shown that the situation is easier to handle if only one funding agency is involved, but very large projects may require more than one source of funding (Hernberg 1992, pp 189f).

If all real costs are considered, it can be shocking to realize how expensive the project turns out to be. At this stage, the researcher must learn how to set priorities and to lower the level of ambition.

12.7.2   Data Management

Data management is a crucial step in planning a study especially with multi-centre studies. A first task in planning the data management is to identify the different data tables which are to be set up and to plan their structure and their linkage. Added complications in this context occur if the ethical requirements imply that all names (and all direct identifiers except an anonymous study identifier) are to be kept separately from some or all data tables or even have to be completely erased.

If a protocol implies merging with an external file, be it an administrative file or a file containing causes of death or diseases as is often done in historical cohort studies, a data table must be set up containing only the minimal information for merging.

The data management of prospective cohorts and other studies where subjects have to be recruited individually is especially challenging as there are several dimensions in the data. It is nearly unavoidable in such studies to keep a separate data table for the management of all contacts. In this file for every study subject all letters sent and received, all telephone contacts, all data sets or information received should be traced. Only with such a (complex) data management structure one can quickly identify non-responders and follow them up. If a subject has moved for instance, it is easier to get the new address if this change is recent. It is also important to avoid sending repeated letters to deceased subjects. On the other hand, it is important to know at each moment if a given subject is due for another contact and whether she/he has reacted to the last mailing. This implies also that this file must be able to generate the correct letter for mailing dependent on the subject's status (questionnaire to be sent, questionnaire received, lost to follow-up, pending questionnaire, etc.). The actual data received must be kept separately from this first data base.

It is also important when planning a longitudinal study to clearly identify and label the variables containing the same information collected at different time points. If these variables have the same names, they are at risk to be overwritten. Careful a priori structuring of the data base makes life much easier when creating a data file for statistical analysis. Owing to the longer time scale of such studies, the documentation is particularly important as it is not guaranteed that the same data managers will handle the data throughout the study.

Other issues to be planned carefully are data entry and coding. Three main options exist for data entry. A first option is to input data directly when interviewing the study participants. This is mainly an option with telephone interviews; using laptops in face-to-face interview may disturb the interviewee. An important aspect with direct input is the layout of the screen; the interviewer must follow the questions she/he has to ask without being disturbed by computer problems. Issues like skip patterns, the ability to easily correct already entered data, toggling between keyboard and mouse, online detection of invalid codes or inconsistencies between different data items and so on are to be programmed carefully and to be tested in real settings. A widely used computer program is the freeware Epi-Info available from the division of public health surveillance and informatics of the

Centers of Disease Control, Atlanta (http://www.cdc.gov/epiinfo). However, it has some limitations making it unsuitable for complex large-scale studies. A large range of commercial software exists, each with its own advantages. A second option is to obtain data through paper questionnaires and input the data later. In this situation a double entry is to be recommended whenever possible, especially if the questionnaires were self-administered. The data should be entered as they are, but the data problems (errors, inconsistencies) should be documented in a log-file to be treated as soon as possible. A final option is to obtain machine-readable questionnaires and apply an automated data entry based on scanning the documents and a character recognition software. Such an approach is difficult and requires careful preparation. It has been implemented in actual large-scale studies, notably in the French part of the EPIC study (e.g. Clavel-Chapelon et al. 2002). Data coding, i.e. transforming textual information (examples are places of residence, jobs, tasks or food) in a closed list of items is also an aspect to be planned and tested. It relies often on specialized knowledge. The closed list of items and coding rules must be set up before starting the data collection. Details on the construction of instruments are given in Chap. I.10 of this handbook.

A type of data that deserves a specific discussion with respect to its management are exposure measurements since they often pertain to exposure groups rather than individuals, i.e. they characterize specific circumstances (cf. Chap. I.10 of this handbook). These circumstances include e.g. measurements of air pollution in certain areas, households or occupational tasks. The main problem with these data is to be able to link them to the subject data. It is important to include the same items (i.e. labels of the exposure group) in the exposure measurement data base as in the subjects' data base. A further complication arises when some of these exposure measurements are on individuals (e.g. exposure measurement at the workplace or in households), including subjects from the epidemiological data base. These measurements characterize both the exposure group and the specific individual. Both links must then be clearly identified from the start.

Finally a log-book of all data management tasks and files should be kept. This can be part of the overall study diary.

Quality Assurance 12.7.3

Industrial standards for quality assurance and quality management are set down in the ISO 9000 series of standards (http://www.iso.ch). Their application to epidemiological studies is not straightforward given that these standards (see Moulin et al. 1998a) are geared towards customer satisfaction and that the customers of epidemiology are not easily defined. The main ideas behind these standards are however useful.

The main principles as they apply to epidemiology are the following (although a quality assurance specialist might disagree). Write up in detail what you intend to do and document what you did. Try to be proactive in thinking of what can go wrong and plan accordingly. Set up means by which you can detect any problem as early as possible and by which you can correct your procedures accordingly. Document all changes in procedures. See also Chap. I.13 of this handbook.

We already insisted on the necessity of a detailed protocol. A protocol may furthermore be complemented by one or several standard operating procedures compiled in an mannual of operations (see below) describing the actual work to do (cook book). One main point in being proactive is to prepare the data collection in as much detail as possible. Details with respect to material conditions, e.g. hardware, software, office and storage room need to be considered in advance. Training of the data collection staff is a key to good quality data. This training should be done using the tools to be used and if possible in the setting in which the actual data collection will be conducted. It is also an important point to acknowledge that there will be non-responders and to plan how to get minimal information on those subjects from the beginning. In order to monitor errors as they arise and to be able to correct the procedures accordingly, data entry should be concurrent to the data collection and the data control and validation be done as early as possible.

Finally all changes in the protocol and in the operations manual after the start of the study must be clearly documented.

12.7.4   Study Conduct: Manual of Operations

As mentioned in the section on the study protocol, the collection of material and data as well as the methods and procedures must be described in detail. This can be done in a separate document: the manual of operations (cf. Chap. I.13 of this handbook).

The eligibility criteria must be defined in cohort studies in terms of minimum exposure, calendar time of exposure, whether or not other exposures are allowed, and so forth. If a case-control design is adopted, the eligibility criteria for both cases and controls must be well defined. For example, what histological type of cancer will be included, how will the diagnosis be confirmed? Are the controls indeed representative of the study base? Is the study a hospital-based study or a register linkage study? Who will collect the data? These questions are only examples of how detailed the description of the methods have to be. Each project has its own list of questions, so the illustration of all problems that may arise is not possible here.

The measurement methods and procedures should be described in detail. Will the indicators of disease or exposure be good measures? For example, is today's blood level of DDT a good measure of long-term exposure? Is a specially designed symptom questionnaire specific and sensitive enough to measure the neurotoxic effects of solvents? How will the interviewers be trained? Will there be a panel of radiologists for reading and interpreting the radiographs? The control and measurement of confounding should also be discussed and presented in the light of the scientific and technical background.

Time Line

The time schedule concerns the sequence and interdependency of different operational tasks and resources. It is good practice to outline the tasks and subtasks at the design stage and to plan their time flow, as well as the necessary resources required for each. Once it has been decided how many subjects will be included and what methods of examination will be used, the time needed can be estimated rather accurately. At the planning stage, one should make sure that statistical and computerizing assistance will be available when needed. The researcher must also stick to his/her original schedule, to avoid disrupting the consultants' time scheme. One should realize that the first data analysis will usually result in further analyses. Writing a manuscript takes time. Unexpected practical matters almost always disrupt the original time schedule. Enough time must be reserved for all these considerations. Hernberg (1992) recommends to make an allowance of half a year or more for unexpected complications.

The organisation of the time-line and the corresponding resources are best planned using project management tools like Gantt (after the method developed by Charles Gantt in 1917) and PERT (Program Evaluation and Review Technique) charts (see Figs. 12.2 and 12.3 for a simple fictitious example). Basically these tools decompose a project in elementary tasks with certain (possibly varying) durations and the corresponding needed human resources and the precedence of these tasks. Figure 12.2 presents the different tasks with arrows indicating which tasks must be terminated before the next task can start (e.g. the data collection can only start when the study has been approved by the ethics committee and when the staff has been trained). From this information, critical tasks (dark bars in Fig. 12.3) are identified, which if delayed will delay the whole study. Non-critical tasks such as preparation of data entry that may depend on completion of other tasks as for instance preparation of questionnaire can be delayed. However, non-critical tasks must be completed by the start of other work packages (here: data entry). This is indicated by the light bars in Fig. 12.3. For details of such tools see for instance Modell (1996). A number of sharewares easily available through the internet provides the software to draw these charts.

Project Diary

A project diary is a necessary component and should trace all aspects of the project. These aspects include the possible changes in the protocol, the data collection, and the data processing. Such a diary not only helps the investigators to keep track of the scientific realization of the operational plan of the project, but also of its administrative and economic aspects.

Changes in the original protocol may either be dictated by external circumstances but also possibly by scientific reasons, e.g. if evidence arises during the study concerning a potentially important confounder.

Documentation of data collection should not only monitor its advancement but all potentially important events. It is a particularly important issue to docu-

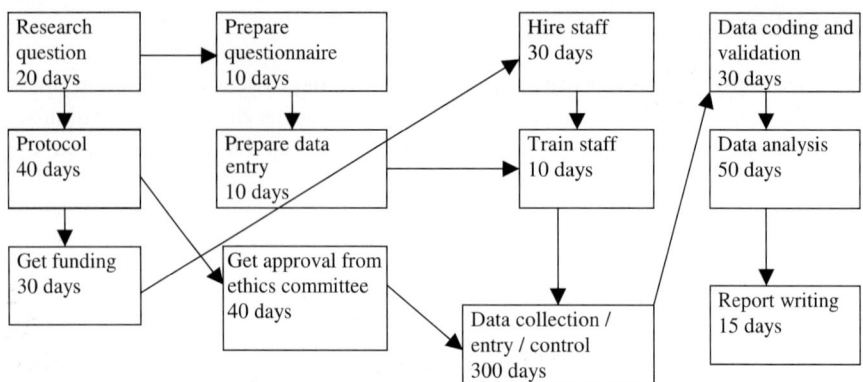

Figure 12.2. Simple fictitious example of a PERT chart for planning a study

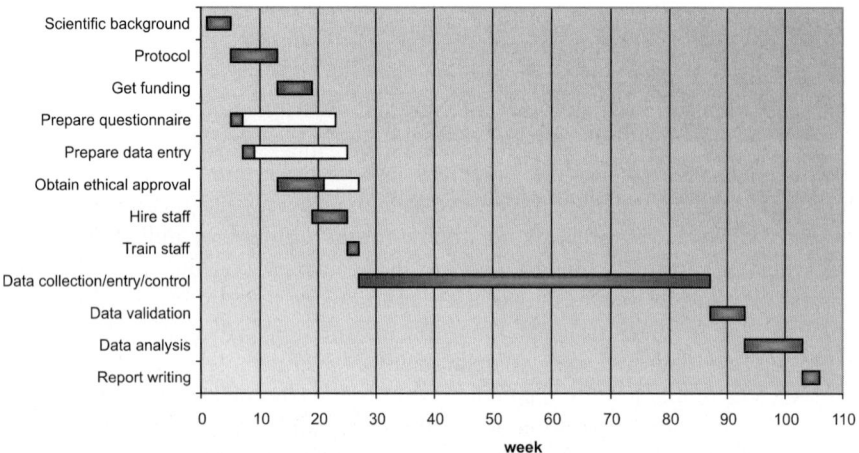

Figure 12.3. Gantt chart for planning a study

ment when and why some data could not be collected, as for instance the number of controls contacted before a control accepted to participate. It should also be documented if some technicians are on sick leave and are replaced, if some measurement instrument or computer fails and is replaced or if, at some stage, the data collection is less than optimal because of human failure. Dates and results of instrument calibration should be recorded. If some highly unlikely measurement is observed and it is redone, this information should be consigned in the diary. When some issues arise from the quality control steps (see Chap. I.13) this should also be mentioned.

Electronic data handling e.g. names of raw data files, computer transfers, merging of files, recoding, and finally all statistical data processing should all be documented including analyses which proved to be dead ends.

The project diary along with the protocol and the raw data are the central pieces of evidence with which the study can be replicated and be re-analysed, if needed.

Ethical Aspects 12.7.7

The ethical aspects are diverse and have been well covered in Chap. IV.7 of this handbook. General ethical rules for all biomedical research have been set down in the Helsinki declaration of the World Medical Organization (1996). Table 12.2 shows its central principles.

Table 12.2. General ethical principles as laid out in the declaration of Helsinki

1.	Doing good (beneficience)
2.	Not harming (nonmaleficience)
3.	Respecting persons (autonomy)
4.	Distributing goods and evils fairly (justice)

The following aspects are more specific to epidemiological research. The first ethical requirement is the respect of the data protection laws that are specific to each country. This may even require to erase part of the data, usually the personal identifiers, after a certain lapse of time. The second is the requirement that all study participants be informed of the objectives of the study, what precise medical examinations will be done and what is their purpose. The full informed consent of the participants is obligatory, at least if invasive procedures are involved. The results of each individual investigation should be made available to each study participant as well as a summary of the overall results of the study. On the contrary, confidentiality must always be adhered to and no individual results can be revealed to outsiders unless otherwise specified by law. A medical examination which might detect a hidden disease (e.g. an X-ray or a scanner might detect a lung tumor although the study was focused on pneumoconiosis) must always be medically screened before the final processing of the data in order to take the necessary medical steps. Similarly, if in the course of a prospective study it becomes evident that individual exposure levels exceed safe limits, the researcher must take the initiative to try to remove the subject from the hazardous exposure. Sensitive items in questionnaires should only be included if they are absolutely necessary. A final aspect is that the results of the study must always be made available to the community. Failing to publish the results means that the examinees have been abused and the funding has been wasted. In doing so, the interpretation of the results must be objective including a discussion of all relevant literature and all possible validity problems as well as alternative explanations of the findings.

Scientific Collaborations and Multi-centre Studies 12.7.8

An epidemiological study usually requires collaborations of the principal researcher with scientists from several fields which of course include epidemiology and usually a specialized medical field and statistics but may also include, depending on the study, genetics, molecular biology, microbiology, chemistry, industrial hygiene, psychology, sociology. Another type of collaboration occurs if a multi-centre study is set up in which several epidemiologists combine resources. Advantages and possible pitfalls have already been mentioned and the standardization of the data collection is then a major issue. The data analysis may be centralized or decentralized. For instance in multi-centre studies organized by the International Agency for Research on Cancer (IARC), the national centres may usually publish their data and/or they are in charge of a pre-defined specific analysis of a particular topic.

In any type of collaboration the respective responsibility and role of each collaborator or collaborating centre as well as the resources allocated to the project should be clear from the start so that no false expectations arise. Provisions should be made for possibly divergent interests between study partners.

12.7.9   Publication

Epidemiological research is of interest not only to epidemiologists, but also to decision makers, funding agencies, and also to the general public. The results should be published in a form and language that they are understandable to the different target groups. This often requires two or more levels of reporting, one scientific, one popular and maybe even one press release. It is worthwhile to plan responsibilities for each aspect in advance and how the information will be dispersed. Those taking part in a study have the right to know not only their personal results but also, at least in general terms, the outcome of the whole study, especially when medical examinations are involved. The correct timing of the sequence of information delivery is important. First, those examined should be informed of their own results, then summary results should be given to funding agencies, and only afterwards to the news media. Ideally, a peer-reviewed scientific article should have appeared or at least have been accepted for publication before informing the news media. However, the scientific publishing procedure is so slow that it sometimes may be unethical to withhold urgent results from the public that long.

A large project usually gives rise to several scientific publications, and it may be useful to outline their topics in advance. At the planning stage, it is advisable to agree within the team on who will be responsible, i.e., the first author, of what, and whose names should be listed as co-authors. It is usually not possible to decide the order of names at this stage, because each team member's input to the intellectual process can be judged only after the project has been successfully completed. Guidelines as to who should be considered author of a publication are included in the Vancouver guidelines (International Committee of Medical Journal Editors 2004).

Conclusions

Careful planning is a key in the successful completion of an epidemiological study. This planning should be based on up to date scientific knowledge and awareness of all possible pitfalls inherent in epidemiological studies. It should cover all aspects from study base definition, precise design used, statistical power, control of confounding, precise data collection and exposure measurement methods to quality control, statistical methods, collaborations, dissemination of study results, and ethical issues. All these issues should be written down in a study protocol which is then a "study-bible" from which the quality of the study can be assessed.

Acknowledgements. We acknowledge the important contribution of Dr. Pascal Guenel, INSERM U170, who drafted a preliminary version of this text.

References

Ahrens W, Jöckel KH, Brochard P, Bolm-Audorff U, Grossgarten K, Iwatsubo Y, Orlowski E, Pohlabeln H, Berrino F (1993) Retrospective assessment of asbestos exposure–I. Case-control analysis in a study of lung cancer: efficiency of job-specific questionnaires and job exposure matrices. Int J Epidemiol 22 Suppl 2:S83–95

Andersen LF, Bere E, Kolbjornsen N, Klepp KI (2004) Validity and reproducibility of self-reported intake of fruit and vegetable among 6th graders. Eur J Clin Nutr 58:771–777

Armstrong BK, White E, Saracci R (1994) Principles of exposure measurement in epidemiology. Oxford University Press, Lyon

Boeing H, Korfmann A, Bergmann MM (1999) Recruitment procedures of EPIC-Germany. European investigation into cancer and nutrition. Ann Nutr Metab 43:205–215

Bogers RP, Van Assema P, Kester AD, Westerterp KR, Dagnelie PC (2004) Reproducibility, validity, and responsiveness to change of a short questionnaire for measuring fruit and vegetable intake. Am J Epidemiol 159:900–909

Breslow NE, Day NE (1981) Statistical methods in cancer research, vol I-The analysis of case-control studies. IARC, Lyon

Breslow NE, Day NE (1987) Statistical methods in cancer research, vol II-The design and analysis of cohort studies. IARC, Lyon

Breslow NE, Chatterjee N (1999) Design and analysis of two-phase studies with binary outcomes applied to Wilms tumor prognosis. Appl Stat 48:457–468

Cox DR, Wermuth N (1996) Multivariate dependencies: models, analysis and interpretation. Chapman & Hall, London

Clavel-Chapelon F, E3N-EPIC Group (2002) Differential effects of reproductive factors on the risk of pre- and postmenopausal breast cancer. Results from a large cohort of French women. Br J Cancer 86:723–727

Flesch-Janys D, Steindorf K, Gurn P, Becher H (1998) Estimation of the cumulated exposure to polychlorinated dibenzo-p-dioxins/furans and standardized mortality ratio analysis of cancer mortality by dose in an occupationally exposed cohort. Environ Health Perspect 106 Suppl 2:655–662

Garfinkel L (1985) Selection, follow-up, and analysis in the American Cancer Society prospective studies. NIH Publication 85–2713, National Cancer Institute Monograph 67. Government printing office, Washington D.C., pp 49–52

Goebel A, Netal S, Schedel R, Sprotte G (2002) Human pooled immunoglobulin in the treatment of chronic pain syndromes. Pain Med 3:119–127

Goldberg M, Chastang J-F, Leclerc A, Zins M, Bonenfant S, Bugel I, Kaniewski N, Schmaus A, Niedhammer I, Piciotti M, Chevalier A, Godard C, Imbernon E (2001) Socioeconomic, demographic, occupational, and health factors associated with participation in a long-term epidemiologic survey: a prospective study of the French GAZEL cohort and its target dpopulation. Am J Epidemiol 154:373–384

Greenland S, Robins J (1994) Invited commentary: ecologic studies-biases, misconceptions, and counteraxamples. Am J Epidemiol 139:747–760

Hernberg S (1992) Introduction to occupational epidemiology. Lewis Publishers, Chelsea, Michigan

International Committee of Medical Journal Editors (ICMJE) (2004) Uniform requirements for manuscripts submitted to biomedical journals: writing and editing for biomedical publication. Haematologica 89(3):264

Kaslow RA, Ostrow DG, Detels R,Phair JP, Polk BF, Rinaldo CR Jr (1987) The Multicenter AIDS Cohort Study: rationale, organization, and selected characteristics of the participants. Am J Epidemiol 126: 310–318

Kromhout H, Symanski E, Rappaport SM (1994) A comprehensive evaluation of within- and between-worker components of occupational exposure to chemical agents. Ann Occup Hyg 37:253–270

Liu K, Stamler J, Dyer A, McKeever J, McKeever P (1978) Statistical methods to assess and minimize the role of intra-individual variability in obscuring the relationship between dietary lipids and serum cholesterol. J Chronic Dis 31:319–418

Miettinen OS (1985) Theoretical epidemiology: Principles of occurrence research in medicine. John Wiley & Sons, New-York

Modell ME (1996) A professional's guide to systems analysis, 2nd edn. McGraw Hill, New York

Moulin JJ, Clavel T, Chouaniere D, Massin N, Wild P (1998a) Implementation of ISO 9002 for research in occupational epidemiology. Accred Qual Assur 3:488–496

Moulin JJ, Wild P, Romazzini S, Lasfargues G, Perdrix A, Peltier A, Bozec C, Duguerry P, Pellet F (1998b) Lung cancer risk in hard metal workers. Am J Epidemiol 148:241–248

Pearl J (2000) Causality: models, reasoning, and inference. Cambridge University Press, Cambridge

Rothman KJ, Greenland S (1998) Modern epidemiology. Lippincott-Raven, Philadelphia

Rouch I, Wild P, Fontana JM, Chouaniere D (2003) Evaluation of the French version of EUROQUEST: a questionnaire for neurotoxic symptoms. Neurotoxicology 24:541–546

Rylander R (2002) Endotoxin in the environment-exposure and effects. J Endotox Res 8:241–252

Sauleau EA, Wild P, Hours M, Leplay A, Bergeret AR (2003) Comparison of measurement strategies for prospective occupational epidemiology. Ann Occup Hyg 47:101–110

Savitz DA (2003) Interpreting epidemiologic evidence. Strategies for study design and analysis. Oxford University Press, New York

Wacholder S, McLaughlin JK, Silverman DT, Mandel JS (1992a) Selection of controls in case-control studies I: Principles. Am J Epidemiol 135:1019–1028

Wacholder S, Silverman DT, McLaughlin JK, Mandel JS (1992b) Selection of controls in case-control studies II: Types of controls. Am J Epidemiol 135:1029–1041

Wacholder S, Silverman DT, McLaughlin JK, Mandel JS (1992c) Selection of controls in case-control studies III: Design options. Am J Epidemiol 135:1042–1050

Waksberg J (1978) Sampling methods for random digit dialing. J Am Stat Assoc 73:40–46

Wild P, Moulin JJ, Ley FX, Schaffer P (1995a) Mortality from cardiovascular diseases among potash miners exposed to heat. Epidemiology 6:243–247

Wild P, Refregier M, Auburtin G, Carton B, Moulin JJ (1995b) Survey of the respiratory health of the workers of a talc producing factory. Occup Environ Med 52:470–477

Wolff MS, Toniolo PG, Lee EW, Rivera M, Dubin N (1993) Blood levels of organochlorine residues and risk of breast cancer. J Natl Cancer Inst 85:648–652

World Medical Organization (1996) Declaration of Helsinki. Br Med J 313:1448–1449

Quality Control and Good Epidemiological Practice

I.13

Preetha Rajaraman, Jonathan M. Samet

Introduction

The use of data is fundamental in epidemiology. Epidemiologic research on causation uses data in a search for the true nature of the relationship between exposure and disease. Similarly, research on the consequences of interventions seeks an unbiased characterization of the effects of independently varying factors on the outcome measure(s). One of the most rewarding moments for a researcher is obtaining the preliminary results from his or her study. However, the question "do I believe what I see?" should immediately come to mind. The answer to this question is determined in large part by the more mundane but critical question of how good is the quality of the data, rather than by the elegance of the scientific method. Errors that occur during study population selection or in the measurement of study exposures, outcomes, or covariates can lead to a biased estimate of the effect of exposure on risk for the disease of interest. Misclassification of exposure or disease that occurs randomly between all study participants decreases the power of the study to detect an association where it exists. Data collection that is differentially biased may have more severe consequences, and can lead to an incorrect assessment of the relationship between exposure and disease.

The inherently important issue of study quality is becoming of even greater consequence as the findings of epidemiological studies gain in impact, and the field of epidemiology gains wider acceptance as an essential element of biomedical research (Samet 2000; Samet and Lee 2001). Results of epidemiological studies are routinely reported in the media, receiving widespread attention because the findings have evident relevance to the populace. Epidemiologic evidence is also used to inform regulatory and legislative policy making (Goldman 2001). The decision to set airborne standards for particulate matter in the United States, for example, was largely fueled by evidence from epidemiological studies (Greenbaum et al. 2001). Epidemiology often figures prominently in litigation, where the study methodology can become a point of debate (Bryant and Reinert 2001; Goldman 2001). Given the significance of epidemiologic evidence for decision-making, the results of epidemiological studies often face close scrutiny and questions may be raised about every aspect ranging across data quality, study methods, study conduct, data analysis and interpretation of findings.

Even if external questioning and auditing are not anticipated, the researcher nonetheless faces the responsibility of assuring the quality of the study and preventing the widespread dissemination of misleading or incorrect information. For example, findings from several cohort studies on air pollution and mortality figured prominently in a 1997 decision by the U.S. Environmental Protection Agency (EPA) to promulgate a new standard for airborne particulate matter. The great weight given to the data by the EPA led to a call for access so that others could check and analyze the data. An extensive re-analysis of the data was carried out, including validation of elements of the original data as well as replication and extension of the original analyses by an independent group (Krewski et al. 2000; Samet et al. 1997). The controversy surrounding the use of data from the air pollution cohort studies eventually led to a Congressionally-mandated requirement for sharing data with policy implications that have been collected with federal funds.

Many hypotheses of current interest in epidemiological studies call for the incorporation of data from multiple centers and involve collection of data from large populations according to centrally standardized protocols. Data sharing has also become more common, and approaches to doing so for larger grants in the United States have been mandated by the National Institutes of Health. In order to enhance statistical power, data from individual studies are often pooled, or summary results are combined using meta-analysis. These approaches to data utilization place a further demand for meticulous study documentation so that data from a study are readily usable by persons other than the original investigators.

General methods have long been available for assuring the quality of data. The idea of creating a high quality end-product using process improvement initially emerged in the context of industrial business models. Early efforts at delivering quality products to customers were based on inspecting products at the end of a factory line and eliminating those products that did not meet standards ("quality control"). The idea of improving all procedures that affect the quality of the manufactured products ("quality assurance") represented a fundamental shift in paradigm for industrial manufacture. Incorporating quality considerations into the process rather than the product has since gained widespread acceptance in the business and engineering communities (International Organization for Standardization 2003).

Although there is a vast literature on quality control in general, the issue has not received much formal attention in the epidemiological setting. Within epidemiology, much of the writing on data quality and good epidemiological practice is focused on the conduct of clinical trials (Canner et al. 1983; Cooper 1986; Dischinger and DuChene 1986; DuChene et al. 1986; Gassman et al. 1995; Hilner et al. 1992; Knatterud et al. 1998; Meinert and Tonascia 1986; Neaton et al. 1990; Vantongelen et al. 1989). While clinical and laboratory guidelines can easily be modified to make them more applicable to observational studies, few sources specifically address quality issues for the most common epidemiological study designs. In an early attempt to bridge this gap, the Epidemiology Task Group of the Chemical Manufacturers Association (CMA) compiled a set of guidelines for good epidemiology practice for occupational and environmental epidemiologic research (Cook 1991; The Chemical Manufacturers Association's Epidemiology Task Group 1991). An overview of data quality issues for epidemiological studies is also provided by Szklo and Nieto (2000) and by Whitney and colleagues (Whitney et al. 1998). Methods to improve data quality in medical registries are reviewed by Arts et al. (2002).

This chapter provides a general overview of data quality and guidelines for good practice in epidemiological research. The fundamental premise is that quality considerations should be integrated into every phase of the study from initial hypothesis formulation to the final publication of findings and archiving of data.

Obtaining data completely free from error clearly would be prohibitively expensive, and often impossible. The goal is therefore not error-free data, but rather planning and implementing cost-effective procedures that guarantee the validity of the primary results to an acceptable degree. The epidemiological researcher needs to be able to gauge the extent of any errors, and assess the consequences for interpretation of data analyses. The idea of "quality control" versus "quality assurance" is carried over from the industrial management literature into the epidemiological literature, with a distinction made between activities that take place prior to data collection (quality assurance), and activities that occur during and after data collection to correct data errors (quality control).

The ubiquitous nature of quality issues, both in terms of where these issues can arise and how they affect study results can be captured by an extended metaphor. In an article describing the causation of bias, Maclure and Schneeweiss present the idea of an "Episcope" through which an epidemiologist views a putative association between a causal agent and morbidity. Just as a user of a large telescope would be skeptical about whether and how image degradation exists, an epidemiologist should think about how and why an observed association between exposure and disease might be biased (Maclure and Schneeweiss 2001). A similar idea can be applied to data quality. As published study results are viewed through a "Datascope," a discerning epidemiologist should be wary of how the final image (the published results) may have been distorted by quality considerations during the design, conduct and dissemination of the study. Working backwards, the observer might ask a string of questions, such as "Were the observed results more likely to be published because they were positive findings? Based on the analysis, were published inferences appropriate? Were the methods of analysis suitable? Were data keyed in correctly? Has the data been collected appropriately? Was an appropriate population defined?" Each of these questions points to one or more study quality issues. Using the metaphor of the datascope, we will highlight the main issues regarding study design and conduct, and present ways in which to improve epidemiologic practice and data quality.

13.2   The Datascope

Imagine, for a moment, that published study results can be viewed only through a large telescope. As you peer into the lens, the initial picture is barely discernible. On your right is a panel with focusing controls. The first dial allows you to adjust out any distortion caused by publication bias. When you optimize this dial, the image becomes slightly clearer. The next control allows you to tune out faulty inferences. Again, you turn this knob to make the image somewhat clearer. The process continues until the results are finally sharply focused. Although we do not literally look through a telescope every time we view the results of a study, we are in fact looking at an association that may well be "out of focus" depending on how well the study was designed, conducted and interpreted. Errors in the measurement of the exposure, outcome, or other covariates can be thought of as unfocused datascope controls that contribute to degradation of the final image.

Let us consider, in some more detail, the datascope controls that manipulate sources of measurement error. The farthest dials from the observer are located in the planning phase of a study and influence purely "quality assurance" activities. For a more in-depth discussion of the planning stage see Chap. I.12 of this handbook. Errors occurring at the study planning stage are summarized below.

— *Errors in study conception*
  If the study rationale and design are not carefully formulated, the rest of the study could be rendered completely irrelevant. Errors in study conception include inadequate literature review, consideration of an inappropriate study design, and failure to plan the validation of exposure or outcome variables.

— *Errors in the selection, design, or procedures for use of instruments measuring exposure*
  The instrument selected for study exposure measurement might not cover all sources of the active agent. Conversely, the measurement instrument might include sources of exposures that are not biologically relevant, or measure exposure for a time period that is etiologically unimportant. In survey instruments, the phrasing of questions or instructions could lead to misunderstanding or bias (cf. Chap. I.10 of this handbook). Insufficient detail in the protocol for instrument use or inadequate consideration of a standardized method for dealing with unusual situations can lead to collection of poor quality data.

— *Inadequate training of study personnel*
  Even if study procedures are very well defined, inadequate training of data collection staff in the application of these procedures can introduce errors in the data (cf. Chap. I.10 of this handbook).

The next set of controls is activated during the conduct of a study and includes activities that generally fall under the categories of quality assurance as well as quality control. For instance, validation studies of instruments and equipment ensure that collected data will be accurate (quality assurance), but can also be used to correct errors in data (quality control). Sources of exposure measurement error that can occur during data collection are described in detail elsewhere (Armstrong and White 1992) and summarized below.

— *Improper execution of the study protocol*
  Errors related to study protocol execution include the misinterpretation of, or deviation from, standard operating procedures by study technicians. Mistakes in interpretation of the study protocol often arise from poor clarity of the manual of operations or inadequate training of study personnel. For example, if the standard operating procedure states that a fasting blood glucose level should be measured but does not specify the time required to have elapsed after the last meal, the interpretation of "fasting" may differ from technician to technician. Errors in data can also result from improper handling of biologic specimens, or the failure of subjects to read or understand instructions in self-administered questionnaires.

— *Errors related to study participants and intra-individual variability*
  Subjects may have poor recall of past exposures, or allow recent exposure
  to influence their memory of past exposure. Individuals also tend to over-
  report socially desirable behaviors such as exercise, and underreport socially
  undesirable habits such as smoking. Additionally, short-term variability in the
  biological characteristics of a subject can lead to unrepresentative measurement
  of exposure or outcome. For example, differences in the level of an exposure
  biomarker measured at a specified time after exposure are likely to be due
  partially to individual differences in metabolizing the agent of interest.

— *Changes in the accuracy of measurements over time*
  Failing to standardize and recalibrate laboratory equipment is likely to introduce data drift as calendar time progresses. In long-term studies, the instrument used for measurement may change over time, and the agent of interest
  in biological specimens may be subject to degradation. Also, as the study personnel get more experienced through the course of the study, changes in the
  handling of procedures and instruments may occur.

— *Mistakes in data processing*
  Data that are recorded inaccurately, illegibly, or incompletely are very difficult
  to correct after the fact. Transcription of the data to electronic files introduces
  more chances for error, both within a study site, and between field sites and the
  data coordinating center. At the coordinating center, programming or procedural errors may corrupt the database or modify data inappropriately. Errors
  can also be introduced by undocumented changes or modifications to a local
  or central database.

The final panel of controls on the datascope, closest to the observer, consists of
purely "quality control" dials, which influence study quality after the data have
been collected. Examples of these errors are presented below.

— *Inappropriate data analysis*
  If data analysis is not preceded by familiarization with the nature of the data,
  the chosen analyses may not be appropriate. Specifying the wrong model for
  analysis, for instance, can lead to completely erroneous results and inference.

— *Poor reporting of data*
  Omitting the results of important data analyses, or presenting unnecessary
  information can obfuscate the study results. Lengthy, verbose explanations
  and poorly labeled graphs and figures add to the confusion. Inappropriate
  inference given the study results can also be misleading.

In order to achieve the highest quality data possible, each of the sources of error
described in the planning, design, conduct, and conclusion of a study should
be minimized. Conceptually, this can be thought of as turning the appropriate
datascope dial to obtain the best image possible.

  A review of the different sources of error that can occur during study planning,
design and conduct informs the datascope user as to where he or she can affect
final data quality. The ultimate goal is to optimize the datascope dials in order to

minimize error and achieve the clearest possible picture of the study results. In the rest of this chapter, we present aspects of quality control and good epidemiological practice that can reduce data error. The chapter will follow the same organization as the datascope control panels, beginning with the planning phase of a study, moving onto quality considerations during study conduct, and finally describing activities that occur after data collection. Where applicable, the working of the datascope will be illustrated using the example of measuring blood pressure in a hypothetical study whose main research question is whether elevated blood pressure leads to increased risk of coronary disease.

Quality Considerations in the Planning Phase

13.3

Protocol

13.3.1

The development of a comprehensive study protocol is essential to good epidemiological practice. The *study protocol* is a narrative document that describes the general design and procedures used in the study. It can be distinguished from the study *manual of operations* (Sect. 13.3.3) by its generality and absence of specific details for day-to-day study conduct. The study protocol assists the staff in understanding the context in which their specific activities occur. A well-designed study protocol can, and should, guide all aspects of the study. In general, a protocol would include the following sections: a short descriptive title; a description of performance sites and personnel; a description of background and significance; results of preliminary studies; study design and methods; a time line for completion of major tasks; ethical considerations, and references. Quality assurance and quality control should be addressed in each relevant section of the protocol, and also summarized in a separate section. Although restrictions or recommendations provided in the guidelines for research grants applications for the U.S. National Institutes of Health may not be applicable to grants funded through other mechanisms, these guidelines nevertheless provide useful suggestions for creating study protocols (U.S. Department of Health and Human Services 2001). Recommendations for protocol write-up are also included in the Guidelines for Good Epidemiology Practices for Occupational and Environmental Epidemiologic Research (The Chemical Manufacturers Association's Epidemiology Task Force 1991). The typical sections of a study protocol are summarized in Table 13.1 (see also Chap. I.12 of this handbook).

> **Improving the Datascope Image by Choosing Appropriate Measures of Hypertension**
>
> In the planning phase of the study, investigators should make provision for collection appropriate measures of hypertension. While clinicians favor

the diagnosis and treatment of hypertension in terms of diastolic blood pressure elevation, data from the Framingham Study in Massachusetts indicate that systolic blood pressure is a better predictor of disease outcome (Kannel 2000). Additionally, ambulatory blood pressure can be measured with an automated device so that multiple measurements can be made across the course of typical activities. Studies show that such recordings provide information predictive of disease risk beyond that obtained with measurements made at a single assessment (Clement et al. 2003).

Table 13.1. Guidelines for preparation of a study protocol*

Section	Guidelines for good epidemiological practice
Title	Descriptive and to the point.
Names, titles, degrees, addresses and affiliations of the study director, principal investigator, and all co-investigators	Possible conflict of interest should be identified and resolved.
Name(s) and address(es) of the sponsor(s)	Possible conflict of interest should be identified and resolved.
Proposal abstract	Informative and succinct.
Proposed study tasks and milestones	Timetable should be realistic and identify possible sources of delay.
Statement of research objectives, rationale, and specific aims	Clearly state the purpose of the investigation, describe whether the study will be hypothesis-generating or hypothesis-testing, and whether the study will confirm previous findings or result in new findings.
Critical review of the relevant literature	Include animal, clinical, and epidemiological studies. Do not restrict search to electronic databases (e.g. PUBMED, TOXLINE), older articles might be missed. Describe the occurrence of exposure and outcome variables. Identify potential confounders and effect modifiers. Identify gaps in current knowledge.
Description of the research methods	Describe the overall research design, and why it was chosen. Consider alternative designs.
	Define exposure and outcome variables, and identify data sources for these and other variables of interest. Check whether the measure of exposure represents the biologically active agent and etiologically important time period.
	Calculate the projected study size and statistical power (if appropriate).
	Describe procedures for collecting data.

table to be continued

Table 13.1. (continued)

Section	Guidelines for good epidemiological practice
	Provide a detailed description of the methods of analysis.
	Define how exposure and outcome variables will be categorized for analysis.
	State how confounders and effect modifiers will be treated in the analysis.
	Outline the major strengths and limitations of the study design.
	Provide criteria for interpreting the study results, including ways of assessing statistical, clinical, and biological significance.
Description of plans for protecting human subjects	Describe risks and benefits of participating in the study.
	If appropriate, provide plans for obtaining informed consent.
	Describe procedures for maintaining confidentiality of subjects and data.
Description of quality assurance and control	Describe for all phases of the study.
Resources required to conduct the study	Detail the expected time, personnel, and equipment required for the study.
Bibliographic references	Include all relevant references.
Addenda, as appropriate	Examples of useful addenda include copies of collaborative agreements, institutional approvals, informed consent forms, and questionnaires.
Dated protocol review and approval sign-off sheet	Document dated amendments to the protocol.

* adapted from the Guidelines for Good Epidemiology Practices, Epidemiology Task Group (The Chemical Manufacturers Association's Epidemiology Task Force 1991).

Documentation of Operations and Procedures 13.3.2

The consistency and validity of study data are greatly enhanced by the establishment and application of *standard operating procedures* for routine data collection tasks (a *standard operating procedure* is defined here as a standardized method or process for conducting a routine research procedure). If standard procedures have been well described, variability is likely to be much lower across study sites, interviewers, or technicians. Uncorrected variability introduced by interviewers or technicians can decrease study power.

Standard procedures should be clearly described for all study procedures, including (but not limited to) raw data collection, coding of death certificates, assessment of error rates, and management of archived data. Each standard operating procedure should state the purpose of the procedure, provide a detailed description of the procedure including forms and equipment to be used, and either designate the person responsible for the procedure, or explain what training will be needed (The Chemical Manufacturers Association's Epidemiology Task Force 1991). Detailed quality control and quality assurance guidelines for the collection of laboratory samples are provided in the U.S. Toxic Substances Control Act (TSCA) standard for Good Laboratory Practices (US Environmental Protection Agency (EPA) 1989).

Once the various standard operating procedures are established, they should be integrated and summarized in the form of a study *manual of operations*. The *manual of operations* is a document or collection of documents that completely describes the procedures used in a study center. Developing a *study handbook*, which contains a series of tables, charts, figures, and specification pages that outline the main design and operating features of a study (largely without the use of a written narrative) is a useful first step in the development of the manual of operations, and can also act as a quick reference for study personnel. The study protocol, handbook, and manual of operations should be reviewed for clarity and completeness.

Since the initial version of the manual of operations is almost certain to contain some errors, pre-testing of the manual prior to finalization is essential. All aspects of the study protocol should be tested on a population similar to the one that will be studied, including the administration of surveys, sending of samples to laboratories, and the generation of and response to quality control reports. Refinements to the protocol that are identified from the pilot study can be incorporated into the final study manual of operations.

Improving the Datascope Image Using Standard Operating Procedures

Inter- and intra-technician variation in blood pressure readings viewed under the datascope can be reduced by clear and detailed descriptions of the method of measurement. Application of a standard operating procedure can also reduce variability in blood pressure measurement within a subject. Specifying details such as how the study participant should be seated, which arm the cuff should be applied to, and how long the study participant should remain quiet before the reading is taken can reduce the influence on the study measurement of factors that affect an individual's blood pressure.

13.3.3   Personnel, Training and Certification

Integral to study conduct is the availability of personnel with the necessary education, experience and training to perform assigned functions. The planning stage of the study is the appropriate time to consider personnel requirements, what kind of training will be necessary, and how often training should occur. Job descriptions should be written for each individual who will be supervising or engaging in the conduct of the study. For jobs that require training, procedures for initial and re-training of personnel should be established. Re-training may be necessary if substantial time has elapsed since the initial training, if a technician is found to be introducing a systematic error into the data, or if the study protocol changes. For each of the study personnel, a summary of relevant training and experience, including study certification and recertification, should be maintained and kept up-to-date.

Consistency in the training of personnel across sites improves comparability of data collection across different study sites. This training can be centralized, or site-specific. Often, a combination of both approaches is used (see Sect. 13.4.1 for more detail). Study personnel should be required to follow standard operating procedure. If training will be difficult or time-consuming, it is prudent to train at least two individuals for each task in case one of the trained technicians leaves the study. Certification standards should be set, and might include completion of a specified number of tests for key procedures, including some under observation.

Aside from the obvious benefit of consistency in data collection, training study personnel also increases the interviewers' or technicians' perceived value of the data that are being collected. This may influence the amount of care taken in following the protocol. Some studies use computer instruction, video cassettes, or teleconferencing to reduce the costs associated with training. While the use of computer or video training is convenient, these methods lack some of the benefits of face-to-face training, such as the opportunity for staff members to share ideas, and the opportunity for scientific presentations that remind personnel of the importance of their work (Whitney et al. 1998).

Improving the Datascope Image by Training and Certification

Some of the variation in blood pressure measurements viewed under the datascope could arise if a technician measured blood pressure in a different way each time he or she took a measurement, or if different technicians had different ways of reading the same measurement. One way to minimize these sources of error and improve the datascope image is to train and certify study technicians. In the MRFIT (Multiple Risk Factor Intervention Trial), technicians were trained in taking blood pressure measurements using training tapes and a double stethoscope (Dischinger and DuChene 1986). The training tapes consisted of two recordings of the Korotkoff sounds for twelve subjects. The first tape of Korotkoff sounds was used for training, and the second for testing. A video training film that presented twelve blood pressure readings, with sufficient time to determine and record systolic and diastolic blood pressure after each reading, was also used. Finally, supervisors and trainees took simultaneous measurements of three subjects using a double stethoscope. The differences in the readings of the trainer and technician had to fall below a certain criterion for the trainee to pass. Technicians were certified after completing the training tapes, passing a written test on procedures for taking blood pressure measurement, and passing the double stethoscope test. Recertification was required at regular intervals, or if examination of collected data indicated that a technician had a bias with respect to other technicians in a clinic.

13.3.4   Data Collection Forms and Instruments

Exposure and outcome measures for epidemiologic studies can be collected in a variety of ways. Methods of data collection include mailed self-administered questionnaires, interviewer-administered questionnaires, measures of blood or other tissues, physical measures, medical tests, use of medical or exposure records, or sampling for environmental contaminants (White et al. 1998). Most studies use more than one method of data collection.

The use of data that have been collected already ("secondary data") has the key advantage that the data already exist. Studies using secondary data are thus likely to be more cost and time-efficient than studies with primary data collection. Sources of secondary data, such as population-based registries, often allow for a much larger sample size, and can be more representative of the general population (Hearst and Hulley 1988). A substantial disadvantage of using existing data, however, is that the collected data may not adequately address the particular research question of interest. An additional drawback is that the method of collection and the quality of the secondary data are not under the researcher's control. For this reason, researchers using secondary data should carefully review data documentation and evaluate the quality and validity of these data to the extent possible (Clive et al. 1995; Gissler et al. 1995; Goldberg et al. 1980; Horbar and Leahy 1995; Maudsley and Williams 1999; Sorensen et al. 1996; Wyatt 1995). For details on the use of secondary data see Chap. I.4 of this handbook.

Most epidemiological studies collect some or all of their data using phone, mail, or self/interviewer-administered questionnaires. Data from such questionnaires, however, can be subject to various sources of bias. For instance, study participants filling out a self-administered questionnaire might report socially acceptable rather than strictly accurate results. Moreover, ways of responding to the survey may differ between participants in the study, depending on factors such as the age, gender, or racial/ethnic group of the participant. Conversely, participants may respond differently to interviewers of different age, gender or ethnic background. For further details see Chap. I.10 of this handbook. Multi-center studies encounter the additional problem of differences in data collection between study centers. In long term studies, these biases can change over time. Smoking, for example, is generally less socially acceptable today than it was 20 years ago in the United States and consequently more likely to be underreported (Ling and Glantz 2002). The acceptability of smoking also varies by ethnic groups, which may in part explain the fact that African-American high school seniors are far less likely to smoke than are white seniors (Wallace, Jr. et al. 2002). Measurement error that occurs because of the use of a survey instrument can be minimized by careful design and pre-testing of the survey, and the application of standardized interviewing techniques.

The main objective of survey design is to allow the efficient collection of data that are valid, reliable, and complete. Standardizing forms within a study is important for internal validity. Consistency of forms across studies allows more meaningful comparison with other studies, and also makes the study results more generalizable. Both internal and external form standardization can be achieved by the use of pre-existing validated study instruments. Examples of validated questionnaire instruments include the American Thoracic Society questionnaire to assess respiratory symptoms (Comstock et al. 1979), and the Willett food frequency questionnaire (Willett et al. 1985). If a validated instrument is not readily available, several sources in the literature provide guidelines for questionnaire design to maximize clarity and ease of administration. These include recommendations for physical format, as well as instructions on how to word the text of instructions and questions (Dillman 1978; Hosking et al. 1995; Knatterud et al. 1998; Meinert and Tonascia 1986; Wright and Haybittle 1979a, b, c). Studies that enroll participants of different ethnic groups may need to accommodate different languages by using interpreters, or by having translated versions of the questionnaire. However, a question might change subtly upon translation, and data generated from different languages may not be entirely comparable. For this reason, independent back-translation of questions to the original language is strongly recommended. An example of the need for back-translation is provided by data from a health survey which showed lower data reliability of data for Hispanics interviewed in Spanish than for Hispanics interviewed in English when no back-translation was done. An independent back-translation aimed at creating a linguistically equivalent version to the Spanish version indicated several instances in which the two versions were idiomatically different and appeared to have affected the seriousness with which the interview situation was perceived, in turn leading to response discrepancies (Berkanovic 1980).

Pre-testing of the survey instrument on a population similar to the study population allows the detection of flaws in the survey design and instrument before full-scale data collection begins. Separate analysis of pre-test data by language version, for example, might identify problems in translation. In the Hypertension Prevention Trial, which was designed to test the effectiveness of changes in dietary intake of calories, sodium, and potassium, a test cohort of 78 participants was enrolled, and used for the testing of forms and procedures. Data that were generated from the test cohort were used to identify problems in survey design and collection, and were not analyzed with results from the main study (Prud'homme et al. 1989).

Accuracy and consistency are also important for laboratory or clinical equipment. The study should be planned so that all study personnel and sites begin by using identical equipment. In anticipation of measurement drift over time, procedures to maintain and recalibrate equipment should be established. In the Sleep Heart Health Study (Quan et al. 1997), overnight sleep data were collected from subjects using a portable monitor. Sites were notified to have the monitor evaluated and procedures assessed when less than 85% of results scored by the monitor were of "good" or better quality (Whitney et al. 1998). Standard and random zero sphygmomanometers for blood pressure measurement in the MRFIT study (Kjelsberg et al. 1997) were maintained and calibrated according to a regular schedule, and subject to standard checks at least every other month in the case of the standard sphygmomanometer, and every week in the case of the random zero instrument (Dischinger and DuChene 1986).

As more advanced technology becomes available to measure an exposure or outcome, there may be justification to update study equipment. In such cases, data should initially be collected using both the old and new equipment to establish the comparability of the two instruments, since a change may introduce subtle differences that are only apparent as substantial data are collected using the new approach.

13.3.5   Planning Response Rate

In order to curtail the possibility of bias and increase the generalizability of study results, it is important to achieve the highest response rate possible (Gordis 2000; Wacholder et al. 1992). A recent systematic review of 292 trials found that factors which more than doubled the odds of response to surveys were: the inclusion of a monetary incentive with the questionnaire, designing surveys to be of more interest to participants, and the use of registered mail (Edwards et al. 2002). Other factors which have been reported to increase response rate are shorter questionnaire length (Dillman 1978; Eaker et al. 1998; Hoffman et al. 1998; Kalantar and Talley 1999; Kellerman and Herold 2001; Little and Davis 1984; Martinson et al. 2000; Spry et al. 1989), personalizing questionnaires (Maheux et al. 1989), using colored ink (Edwards et al. 2002), contacting participants before sending questionnaires, providing stamped return envelopes (Choi et al. 1990), and using written or telephone reminders (Asch et al. 1997). Questionnaires originating from universities are more likely to be returned than questionnaires from other sources, whereas surveys eliciting information of a sensitive nature are less likely to be returned.

While the use of a monetary incentive is probably the factor that has been shown most consistently to increase response rates (Gibson et al. 1999; Gilbart and Kreiger 1998; Hoffman et al. 1998; Kellerman and Herold 2001; Martinson et al. 2000; Parkes et al. 2000; Perneger et al. 1993), increasing the amount of the incentive results in diminishing returns of questionnaires after a certain point (Halpern et al. 2002; James and Bolstein 1992; Spry et al. 1989). In the United States, the $2.00 bill seems to be a cost-effective monetaryincentive (Asch et al. 1998; Doody et al. 2003; Shaw et al. 2001). Making a pre-payment of the incentive appears to be more cost-effective than promising payment on completion of the questionnaire (Schweitzer and Asch 1995). Including the monetary incentive in the first mailing rather than in subsequent mailings has resulted in higher response rates (John and Savitz 1994). Non-monetary incentives, while reported to increase response rates over having no incentive, do not appear as effective as monetary incentives (Kellerman and Herold 2001; Martinson et al. 2000).

Contact rates generally tend to be lower for individuals who are young, male, black, of lower socio-economic status, or employed full-time (Collins et al. 2000; Cottler et al. 1987; Moorman et al. 1999). In the context of a case-control study, response rates are often lower for controls (Moorman et al. 1999). Even within control groups, different types of controls have different response rates. For example, in the United States, controls chosen from Health Management Organizations have been shown to have a higher response rate than controls drawn from lists of licensed drivers (Slattery et al. 1995).

Long term cohort studies, in addition to having to address response rates to study questionnaires, also face the issue of loss to follow-up. The loss of cohort members to follow-up is conceptually similar to response rate, in that loss to follow-up can constitute an important source of selection bias and also limit external validity. Participants may be lost to follow up either because they drop out of the study of their own volition, or because the study investigators lose track of them. As with other types of epidemiological studies, loss to follow-up can lead to reduced study power and may result in biased estimates of risk. Strategies for minimizing loss to follow up include pre-enrollment screening of participants for willingness to participate in a long-term study, collecting names of personal contacts and proxies for participants, maintaining regular contact with study participants, using incentives for remaining participants, and maintaining tracking systems to follow participants (Hunt and White 1998). One must keep in mind, however, that populations comprised of volunteers are usually different from the population as a whole. In general, measures of relative risk are less affected by the lack of external generalizability than measures of absolute or attributable risk.

Validity and Reliability   13.3.6

The absence of bias in data measurement is called *validity*, or accuracy. The precision, or reproducibility, of collected data is known as *reliability*.

Validity Studies
The capacity of a measure to capture the true value of the exposure, outcome, confounder, or modifier of interest in the study population is known as its validity. While it is desirable to obtain the most accurate measurements possible of exposure or outcome, such measurements usually come at the price of increased cost, invasiveness, or time involvement. When faced with these constraints, epidemiologists often choose to collect less accurate measures of exposure.

The accuracy of the study's main method of exposure measurement can be assessed using validation studies which compare the study exposure measure to a more accurate measure of exposure ("gold standard"), either in a sub-sample of study participants or in a different population. For instance, evidence of validity

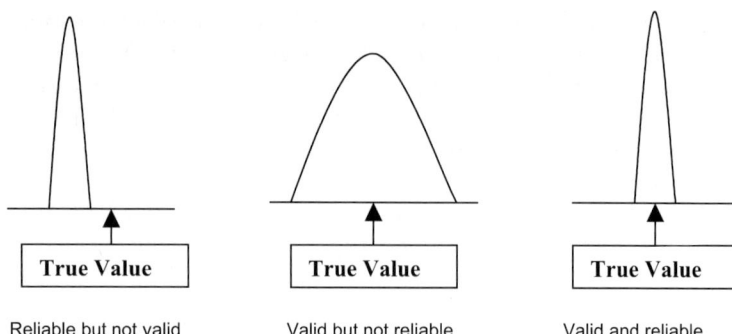

Figure 13.1. Graphs of hypothetical test results illustrating the distinction between validity and reliability

can be provided by comparing study estimates of an environmental exposure to industrial hygiene measurements or biomarkers of exposure (Cherrie and Schneider 1998; Cherrie et al. 1987; Dosemeci et al. 1997; Hawkins and Evans 1989; Kipen et al. 1989; Kromhout et al. 1987; Tielemans et al. 1999). The comparison of reported nutrient intake on a questionnaire with a biochemical indicator provides another example of this approach (Ascherio et al. 1992; Johnstone et al. 1981; Post and Kromhout 1991; Sacks et al. 1986; Willett et al. 1983).

The establishment of a serum pool can facilitate validation of biological sample processing in the study. Study measurements can be compared with results from a "gold standard" external laboratory. If study measurements deviate randomly from the gold standard, the study result would be attenuated towards the null hypothesis. However, if deviations from the gold standard are found to vary according to the presence and level of important variables such as follow-up time, or the exposure or outcome of interest, the study results may be biased.

Data from validation studies can, additionally, be used to account for uncertainty in the data analysis. Measurement error correction models can be developed that use validation study data to adjust the full data for measurement error (Holford and Stack 1995; Rosner et al. 1992; Spiegelman et al. 1997; Stram et al. 1999; Thompson 1990). In the Framingham Study (Dawber et al. 1951), for example, a small validation study was conducted to estimate the relationship between the surrogate measurement (food frequency) and the "true" measurement (diet record). Based on information from the main study relating the surrogate to disease outcome, and information from the validation study relating true and surrogate exposure, corrected point estimates of risk were calculated (Spiegelman et al. 1997). For a general discussion of statistical methods to account for measurement errors see Chap. II.5 of this handbook.

While validation studies may help form a clearer picture of the true relationship between exposure and outcome, such studies are not without their own limitations. For one, the gold standard used for comparison may itself be subject to error, thus the term "alloyed" gold standard (Wacholder et al. 1993). While calibration methods for such alloyed gold standards have been described, these complex models cannot be applied in all situations (Kaaks et al. 2002; Spiegelman et al. 1997). A second limitation of validity studies is that participants in these studies are not always representative of all participants. Subjects who volunteer to take part in a validity study are likely to be more compliant than non-volunteers would have been. Additionally, feasibility constraints often limit validity studies to small sample sizes, which can lead to statistical imprecision.

Reliability Studies

Data variation can arise within study participants (*biological variability*), or due to variation in exposure assessment or physiological measurements introduced by study technicians. Blood pressure within an individual, for example, experiences short-term changes due to factors such as activity and mood. Different blood pressure measurements taken on the same individual are thus likely to vary for physiological reasons regardless of how accurately these measurements are made. Study technicians can add an extra component of variation to the measurements, either because a given technician reads a measurement in slightly different ways each time (*intra-observer variation*), or because different technicians read a measurement in different ways (*inter-observer variation*). Variability can also be introduced as samples degrade over time.

As illustrated in the paragraph above, variability in data can arise due to true change, measurement error, or random biological variation. The component of variability in which the researcher is most interested is the true change in study exposure that might influence the outcome under consideration. The separation of desired variability in the data (true change) from undesirable variability due to measurement error or random (biological) variation can be partially assessed by incorporating into the main study a series of sub-studies that are designed to assess the reliability of the study data (cf. Chap. I.11 of this handbook).

Reliability studies can be used to assess various components of variability, such as the comparability of measurements taken by: the same technician at a given visit; different technicians at a given visit; the same/different technician at different points of time, or the same/different technician using different instruments. Inter-observer and intra-observer variability can be assessed using a set of calibration samples that are read several times by each technician, and processed by multiple technicians. Biological variability can be assessed by having a single technician perform repeat studies on a subset of participants, although some amount of variability assessed in this way would be due to technician variability (Whitney et al. 1998). For durable data, such as X-ray films or dietary recall records, variation over time can be assessed by comparing evaluation of the same samples at different times in the study. In instances where samples are limited or perishable (e.g. blood or urine), a pre-selected set of "quality control" specimens should be set aside at the beginning of the study so that small amounts of these specimens can be periodically submitted for processing. Technicians handling quality control samples should be unaware that the samples are different from other study samples being processed, in order to prevent differential handling.

Reliability studies which collect replicate measurements at the same point of time are useful in the identification of possible data errors, as well as in the calculation of more accurate measures of exposure. Averaging repeated measures has been recommended as an effective method of decreasing the measurement error associated with a single measurement (Armstrong and White 1992; Canner et al. 1991; Holford and Stack 1995; White et al. 1998).

When validity is reported, the number of samples that are deemed unacceptable for analysis should be stated, since this may indicate a bias in the remaining samples. The examination of whether reliability estimates differ according to relevant characteristics such as exposure, confounding factors, or outcome allows some assessment of whether differential misclassification is occurring in the data.

> **Improving the Datascope Image by Obtaining a More Valid Exposure Measure**
>
> Using the average of three blood pressure measurements taken on a study visit could result in a clearer picture of the individual's blood pressure than would a single blood pressure measurement.

Measures of Agreement

Quantifying the agreement between two different methods of measurement requires the use of some measure of agreement. The choice of statistic depends on the type of variables being compared, and the purpose of the comparison (Table 13.2). The calculation of different measures of agreement, and advantages and disadvantages of each measure have been reviewed by Szklo and Nieto (2000).

The basic measures of validity for binary categorical variables are sensitivity and specificity, for which the study value of the exposure or outcome is compared to the "true" value, measured by a more accurate method (Example 1). The *sensitivity* of a test is the ability to correctly identify those individuals who have the disease or exposure characteristic of interest. The test *specificity* is the ability to correctly identify those individuals who do not have the disease or exposure characteristic of interest. A limitation of the use of sensitivity and specificity is that very few diagnostic tests are inherently dichotomous. Most diagnostic tests are based on the characterization of individuals based on one or more underlying traits, such as blood pressure or serum glucose level. Values for the sensitivity and specificity would vary according to the cut-off level used to separate "diseased" (or exposed) from "undiseased" (or unexposed) individuals. In addition, if measurement error occurs, individuals with true levels of the underlying trait close to the test point are more likely to be misclassified. Since the distribution of underlying traits also determines disease prevalence, sensitivity and specificity can vary from population to population (Brenner and Gefeller 1997).

Example 1. *Calculation of Sensitivity and Specificity*

		Gold Standard Results		
		Positive	Negative	Total
Study Results	Positive	a	b	$a + b$
	Negative	c	d	$c + d$
		$a + c$	$b + d$	

Sensitivity $= a/(a + c)$
Specificity $= d/(b + d)$

Agreement for categorical variables (e.g., X-ray readings by radiologists) is generally reported using variations of the percent agreement and kappa statistics. While overall percent agreement is intuitive and easy to calculate (Example 2), it can make agreement look artificially high, since there is likely to be considerable agreement between two observers reading negative, or normal, results. An alternative approach is to disregard subjects labeled as negative by both readers, to calculate the percent positive agreement (Cicchetti and Feinstein 1990).

Example 2. *Calculation of Percent Agreement*

		Technician 2	
		Positive	Negative
Technician 1	Positive	a	b
	Negative	c	d

Percent agreement $= (a + d)/(a + b + c + d) \times 100$
Percent positive agreement $= a/(a + b + c) \times 100$

Neither overall nor percent positive agreement takes into account the fact that some amount of agreement between two observers will be due to chance alone. The extent of agreement between two readers beyond that due to chance alone can be estimated by the kappa statistic (Example 3) (Agresti 1990; Fleiss 1981; Landis and Koch 1977). In comparisons of more than two categories, a weighted kappa approach allows consideration of the fact that disagreement between some categories may be more serious than disagreement between other categories (Cohen 1968). Like the sensitivity and specificity, variations of the kappa statistic are limited by the fact that most underlying traits are not dichotomous, and different cut-off levels can affect the value of kappa (Maclure and Willett 1987). Interpretation of the kappa statistic should also take into account the fact that kappa can be affected by the prevalence of the condition: for a fixed sensitivity and specificity, kappa tends towards zero as the prevalence of the condition approaches either zero or one (Thompson and Walter 1988). Additionally, high values of kappa can be obtained if the marginal totals of the contingency table are not balanced (Feinstein and Cicchetti 1990; Maclure and Willett 1987; Thompson and Walter 1988).

Example 3. *Calculation of Kappa for a binary measurement variable*

		Technician 2		
		Positive	Negative	Totals by Technician 1
Technician 1	Positive	45	5	50 (61.0%)
	Negative	2	30	32 (39.0%)
Totals by Technician 2		47 (57.3%)	35 (42.7%)	82 (100%)

$$\text{Kappa} = \frac{(\text{Proportion Observed Agreement} - \text{Proportion Expected Agreement due to Chance})}{(1.0 - \text{Proportion Expected Agreement due to Chance})}$$

Proportion Observed Agreement, $P_o = (45 + 30)/(45 + 5 + 2 + 30) = 0.91$

Proportion Expected Agreement due to chance, $P_e = \frac{(50 \times 47)/82 + (32 \times 35)/82}{82} = 0.52$

$\text{Kappa} = \frac{P_o - P_e}{(1.0 - P_e)} = \frac{(0.91 - 0.52)}{(1.0 - 0.52)} = 0.81$

Common measures of agreement used to assess reliability for continuous measurements (such as blood pressure readings) are the *correlation coefficient*, the *intra-class coefficient*, the *average error*, and the *coefficient of variation*. *Linear regression* techniques can also be used to check for systematic differences (cf. Chap. II.3 of this handbook).

Although the *Pearson's correlation coefficient*, *r*, is one of the most frequently used measures of agreement in the medical literature, its use is often not appropriate (Altman and Bland 1983; Szklo and Nieto 2000). For one, the correlation coefficient is equally high when both observers read the exact same value, and when a systematic difference (bias) exists between observers but the readings vary simultaneously. The value of *r* is also very sensitive to extreme values and the range of values, with a broader distribution of values yielding a higher *r*. While the Spearman correlation coefficient r_s may be more appropriate to assess the comparability of the rankings of readings, and would moreover be less sensitive to outliers, it does not address the main problem of the inability to detect systemic differences between observers.

The *intra-class coefficient* (ICC), or the reliability coefficient, estimates the proportion of the total measurement variability due to the variation between individuals (Fleiss 1981). The ICC is analogous to the kappa statistic used for categorical variables, and the value can be interpreted in a similar manner. The ICC is a true measure of agreement in that it combines information on both the correlation, and the systemic differences between readings (Deyo et al. 1991). As with the correlation coefficient, however, the ICC is affected by the range of values in the study population.

Other commonly used measures of variability are the *average error*, and the *coefficient of variation* (CV). The average error is the ratio of the mean absolute difference of pairs of measurements to the overall mean value of the measurements. The coefficient of variation is the standard deviation expressed as a percentage of the mean value of sets of replicate observations. In a reliability assessment, the CV would be calculated for each pair of observations, and then averaged over all pairs of original and replicate measures. A limitation of the CV and average error is that both measures may reflect the magnitude of the mean value more than the magnitude of the measurement error (Canner et al. 1983). An alternative measure that has been suggested for assessing variability is the increase in the among-participant standard deviation, the I_{APSD} (Canner et al. 1991). This measure can directly determine the impact of measurement error on the overall among-participant variability for a variable of interest.

Linear regression techniques can estimate systematic differences between readers which are reflected in the slope and intercept of the regression model. One drawback of using regression to assess reliability, however, is that measurement error occurs in both the dependent and independent variables, violating the assumption of an error-free independent variable required for regression (Altman and Bland 1983). However, only under unusual circumstances would measurement error lead to confusing or uninformative results.

Planning Data Management 13.3.7

The management of data in a large epidemiological study can be a formidable task. The sheer volume of data for a sizeable study with extended follow-up can become quite overwhelming, as illustrated by the following example. If 100 data elements are to be collected for each participant in a cohort study with 100,000 participants, the data collected at the end of each data collection cycle are comprised of 10^6 distinct data elements. Let us say that in order to update exposure and outcome information, data are to be collected yearly for each participant for ten years. This increases the amount of data being collected by an order of magnitude, to 10^7 distinct pieces of data. Superimposing on this volume of data the errors that can occur during data recording, transcription, and transfer of data to an electronic medium, it is easy to see how data quality can be compromised without careful planning of how data are to be managed. The potential magnitude of the task of data correction is also clear.

The first step in planning a data management system is to define what data will be collected and how often data will be collected, keeping in mind that as the volume of data increases, ensuring data accuracy becomes more difficult. In order to further minimize the amount of unnecessary data collected, the chosen data variables should be prioritized, and a "tolerance" of error established for each data field. For example, it might be decided that all values of crucial

Table 13.2. Common Measures of Agreement, interpreted in the context of two separate technicians reading the same data

Statistic	Range	Type of Data	Interpretation
Sensitivity and Specificity	0 to 100%	Categorical	Sensitivity: ability to correctly identify individuals who have the disease or exposure characteristic of interest. Specificity: the ability to correctly identify individuals who do not have the disease or exposure characteristic of interest.
Overall percent agreement	0 to 100%	Paired categorical variables	The proportion of all readings that are categorized in the same way by two different observers. Higher value means better agreement.
Percent positive agreement	0 to 100%	Paired categorical variables	The proportion of all non-negative readings that are categorized in the same way by two different observers.
Kappa statistic, κ	−1 to 1 (rarely below 0)	Paired categorical variables	The extent of agreement between two readers beyond that due to chance alone. Higher value of kappa means better agreement.
Weighted Kappa	−1 to 1 (rarely below 0)	Paired categorical variables	The extent of agreement between two readers beyond that due to chance alone, allowing for consideration of partial agreement.
Pearson's correlation, r	−1 to 1	Continuous ordinal variables	The degree to which a set of paired observations in a scatter diagram approaches the situation in which every point falls exactly on a straight line. −1 is perfect negative correlation, 1 is perfect positive correlation.

Table 13.2. (continued)

Statistic	Range	Type of Data	Interpretation
Spearman's correlation, r_s	−1 to 1	Non-parametric ordinal variables	The degree to which ranking of measurements is consistent between two readers.
Intraclass Correlation Coefficient, ICC	−1 to 1 (rarely below 0)	Continuous variables	The proportion of the total measurement variability due to variation among individuals. Analogous to the kappa statistic, but for continuous variables. Higher ICC means better agreement.
Linear regression, β, c		Continuous variables	Yields a measure of the intercept c and slope β of the regression function.
Coefficient of variability, CV	0 to 100%	Continuous variables	The standard deviation expressed as a percentage of the mean value of two sets of paired observations. Lower CV means better agreement.
Average error	0 to 100%	Continuous variables	The ratio of the mean absolute difference of pairs of measurements to the overall mean value of the measurements. Lower average error means better agreement.
I_{APSD}	0 to ∞	Continuous variables	The percentage increase in among-participant standard deviation due to intra-observer measurement error.

data variables (e.g. disease outcome) should be checked against written questionnaires, but auditing a random sample of questionnaires is sufficient for other fields.

The next key step in data management planning is to define essential identifying information for the study data. *Identifiers*, generally known as *key*, *header*, or *ID* fields, are fields that allow each form to be uniquely identified and correctly related to other forms (Hosking et al. 1995; Hosking and Rochon 1982). Study identifiers are usually located in a standard header section of the form. Entry of an incorrect number into one of these fields can cause the entire data record to be processed incorrectly.

Most studies require at least four types of identifiers: study identifiers, participant identifiers, form-type identifiers, and time-point identifiers. Depending on the study, other identifiers (e.g., family identifiers) might also be necessary. *Study identifiers* designate the sponsor, study, protocol, or sub-study. *Participant identifiers* uniquely identify the study participant. In general, a study-created participant identifier is preferable to a natural identifier such as participant name or social security number, especially in a climate increasingly concerned with participant confidentiality. Encode information about participant characteristics (such as a field site code) into the participant identifier is useful, since this allows later classification of participants by their identifiers alone. *Form identifiers* identify a particular questionnaire, and often take the format of a two- or three-character abbreviation. Form identifiers in longitudinal studies should be planned so that multiple versions of each form can be accommodated. Adding a -1 at the end of the form identifier, for example, allows for future versions to end with the suffix -2 or higher. *Item identifiers* are assigned to each question on a form. While item identifiers bearing a one-to-one relationship to database fields might be useful for data analysis, this can become confusing if the study forms or database are revised. Data management systems that track the relationship between each database field and a corresponding item number in each form version provide a useful alternative.

Once data identifiers have been selected, general data management considerations that need to be addressed including identifying how data will be entered (electronically versus manually), who will do the data entry, what software will be used, what types of edits will occur during data entry, how queries will be generated, communicated and resolved, how suspicious values will be treated, and how corrections will be implemented and documented. The remainder of this section will be devoted to these considerations.

Design of a Data Management System

In a multi-center study, data are typically collected at various field centers and then sent to a coordinating center for processing, storage and analysis. Table 13.3 provides an overview of the steps involved in data management. While newer approaches to data management exist (e.g., web-based systems), these approaches rely heavily on specialized automated systems for data collection, entry and auditing. Since logistical barriers of cost, lack of expertise and low computer literacy currently render these systems impractical for many investigators, this chapter focuses on a more traditional approach to data management. Many of the underlying principles remain relevant to the newer data management approaches, which are addressed at the end of the section.

Table 13.3. Overview of the Traditional Data Management Process*

Steps in data processing	
Data collection and mailing	Complete forms at clinic/in field.
	Visually review form while participant is in clinic (visual editing).
	Mail original copy to coordinating center, keep copy at clinic.
	Create standard packing list for mailing
Receipt and conversion to electronic format	Receive forms at coordinating center.
	Acknowledge receipt of forms from clinic using postcard or electronic mail.
	Log receipt of forms into computer (including form number, ID code, date completed, date received, and unique log number).
	Key the form. Verify keying.
Forms processing, posting and backup	Process form through an edit program that checks type and range of each field, as well as internal consistency of form.
	Generate computer edit report.
	Check edit report and initiate appropriate error correction procedures.
	Back-up edited forms.
	Post forms to master file. Back up master file.
	File form.
Clearance and archiving	Run further checks on data to ensure that posted data are consistent with other data on file.
	Review edit reports that result from checks and initiate appropriate error correction procedures.
	Document master file contents and prepare file for archiving.

* adapted from DuChene et al. (1986)

Data Recording and Visual Editing

The measurement and recording of data from study participants usually occurs at the field center, and initial data checks are generally conducted by field staff personnel. Field center interviewers or technicians should check data for consistency as it is being collected, while the study participant is available to clarify any immediate discrepancies, errors, or out-of-range characteristics.

For technical measurements, an independent review of samples by two or more readers should be performed on all, or a subset of samples. This allows later assessment of validity, and enables investigators to track down sources of error. On completion of the data form, field center staff should perform a routine review of forms to establish that the questionnaire is complete, that skip patterns have been followed, and that the data values appear reasonable. If routine review of the form does not identify any unusual data, the form can be processed further. Including an indication of who reviewed the form will facilitate later examination of the editing process.

Data Entry

Almost universally, epidemiological data are entered into electronic databases for storage and analysis. The processing, storage, and analysis of study data usually occurs at the data coordinating center. Errors that can occur during the processing and storage of data include keying errors, inaccurate data transcription, and programming errors (Arts et al. 2002). In the Hypertension Prevention Trial, key error was found to be the major source of data entry error, with 5.2/1000 errors out of an overall error rate of 6.9 errors per 1000 data items being key errors (Prud'homme et al. 1989).

Most automated data entry systems allow a variety of mechanisms for checking data. As data entry is initiated, form identifiers are checked for validity and consistency. *Range checks* during data entry can be used to electronically limit the data type, or the range of possible values at entry. For example, date fields can be programmed to accept only valid dates, or table look-up systems can restrict the values of categorical data to a limited number of possible values. For continuous data, many studies use normal population ranges of a variable to flag outliers. While programmed range checks are a useful tool, retaining some flexibility to correct errors at the time of data entry is important, since too many restrictions on modifying data at entry can lead to a higher error rate (Crombie and Irving 1986).

Data accuracy can also be improved by the use of *double data-entry*. The independent keying of data twice, however, does not prevent all types of error. Examples of errors that would not be reduced by the double entry of data include errors in transcription, or misinterpretation of data in the same way by two data-entry operators.

If the data are to be manually entered, personnel should be masked regarding exposure or outcome status (depending on the study design), to prevent the possibility of observer bias. Additionally, the electronic database should have a provision to indicate who entered the data to allow for later review of data-entry performance.

The use of electronic technology for data entry as an alternative to manual data entry is gaining in popularity. Software is available for scanning forms directly into an electronic database using optical character recognition (OCR). The accuracy of scanning software is quite variable, however, and a process to check scanned data should be in place. In general, OCR is better suited to numeric or check-box responses than to hand-printed characters. Another method of electronic data entry is computer-assisted data collection (CADC), whereby interviewers directly enter participant responses into a computer file. This technology completely circumvents the need for transferring data from paper to an electronic medium, thus eliminating errors associated with this process. A CADC system can automatically enforce skip rules, require completion of required fields, and flag suspicious values for correction while the study subject is still present. Since errors in CADC data cannot be compared later with a paper form, however, these systems need to include as many ways of checking data accuracy at entry as possible. One way to allow for examination of inconsistent values is to tape record interviews while data collection is occurring.

In a pilot study of CADC, five study staff members with no prior experience using a CADC system were trained and asked to administer both CADC and paper-based interviewers to sixteen study participants. All five staff members preferred the CADC system, indicating faster and more accurate data entry and less likelihood of erroneously skipping an item. Ten of the sixteen pilot study participants had no preference between paper and CADC, and six preferred CADC. Although the median time for data collection at the reception, examination and interview stations was slightly longer for CADC than for paper interviews, the CADC data are already partially edited and in machine readable format, whereas data from the paper forms still had to be edited and keyed. The percentage of suspicious data values was similar for each method, but 21 of the 25 suspicious data values were identified and corrected at the time of collection using CADC, compared to 1 out of 23 suspicious values corrected with the paper system (Christiansen et al. 1990).

Other recent methods of data collection for epidemiological studies include the use of electronic-mail ("e-mail") (Kiesler and Sproull 1986; Paolo et al. 2000) or internet-based surveys (Baer et al. 2002; Blackmore et al. 2003; Rhodes et al. 2003; Silver et al. 2002; Turpin et al. 2003). E-mail questionnaires have been reported to have a faster rate of return and more thorough completion of returned questionnaires, but response rates have generally been lower than for mail questionnaires.

The basic process for internet-based, or web-based, data collection is the translation of the study questionnaire into an internet language (HTML, or hypertext markup language) and posting of the questionnaire onto the World Wide Web. Respondents then complete the survey using a point and click interface. The survey is generally visually and functionally similar to traditional surveys.

Web-based data collection provides several advantages over paper form data collection. For one, researchers can reach populations that previously might have been inaccesible due to geographical or cultural boundaries. Use of the web may also speed up the time of data collection, since no testing site or appointment scheduling is necessary, and the need for data entry by study personnel is eliminated. Web-based systems can also minimize the variation due to differences in survey administration, interviewer interpretation and entry of data. Since complicated branch and skip patterns can be programmed into the survey, the amount of interviewer or respondent attention necessary is reduced. Costs can drop dramatically with the use of web-based data collection, as there is no need for printing, mailing, and data collection personnel. Web-based surveys also provide a greater degree of anonymity for the collection of sensitive personal information (Baer et al. 2002).

It is important to realize, however, that depending on the situation, some advantages of web-based systems can become disadvantages. In certain populations or countries, for example, the cost of printing, mailing and administering a paper questionnaire might be considerably less than the cost of setting up a web-based system and providing training and access to study participants. Other disadvantages of web-based data collection include the possibility of selection bias when choosing a study population, and security problems during data transmission. The issue of computer users being unrepresentative of the general population can be overcome to some extent by providing internet access to a randomly sampled study population (Silver et al. 2002). Literacy or language barriers, however, may still prove to be an issue.

Incorporating strict security measures in an electronic data entry system is crucial to maintaining data confidentiality, and can require considerable time and monetary resources. In some instances, it might be possible to provide a quick solution to this problem by linking the survey security to an existing high-security system, such as a university network.

While the use of web-based systems is a promising avenue of data collection for studies, such systems require considerable expertise for adequate set-up. Often, initial versions of web-based questionnaires present frustrating technical problems to users, and may require several iterations before a working system is in place. Web-based systems may be inappropriate for populations that are not computer-literate. It may be more difficult to adress ethical concerns which arise during the course of a study in the context of web-based data collection. For example, the investigators still bear responsibility for verifying informed consent, or for providing local targeted support in case the respondent needs a referral as a result of the research. Additionally, data entry errors by users can still occur. For these reasons, the pre-testing of data instruments, post-entry error-checking, and other forms of data quality control described in this chapter are as crucial for more technologically advanced data collection as they are for more traditional forms of data collection.

Data Audits

Once data have been entered, they must be submitted to further accuracy checks. One method of assessing data accuracy is to perform a series of consistency checks, such as ensuring that the date of birth and age of a participant are in agreement. Reviewing samples that fall outside some number of standard deviations of the mean is a sensible alternative way to check data. More formal statistical methods for detecting outliers can also be used (Barnett and Lewis 1994; Vardeman and Jobe 1999). The importance of using range checks is illustrated by a simulation in which different rates of entry error were introduced into a constructed dataset, and simple range checks were used to identify and correct outliers. Even with a random entry error rate as high as 20%, population means remained very similar after the correction of unusual values, regardless of study sample size (Day et al. 1998). Error rates similar to those achieved with double data entry were achievable when extensive logic checking of fields was incorporated (Mullooly 1990; Neaton et al. 1990).

In instances where an unusual value is detected, a data quality query should be generated either manually or automatically. A system for reporting and responding to such queries needs be conceptualized during study planning, along with the designation of individuals responsible for checking and responding to questions. The automatic generation of regular quality control reports including summary statistics such as the number of queries by form and data field, or the percentage of error-free forms, can aid the systematic processing of data. Section 13.4 of this chapter addresses the processing and resolution of error queries in more detail.

Comparing the number of forms that are edited using automated checks at the data processing center to the number of forms recorded in the batch sent by the field center allows the identification of forms that are lost during keying. Additionally, a random sample of data forms should be compared to the electronic data submitted to check accuracy of data entry.

Once routine edits have been completed, the data form can be posted directly to a *master file* for smaller studies, or to a *distributor file*, for larger studies. In the Multiple Risk Factor Intervention Trial (Mr Fit), the edited form was transferred to a distributor file, which held all the forms that were edited in a day. At the end of the day, forms held in the distributor file were transferred to one or more *transaction files*, which served as temporary storage until the next scheduled update of the master file. The use of transaction files allowed investigators the flexibility to resolve discrepancies before the data were added to the master file. Transaction files were generally copied to daily backup tapes so that data could be retrieved to the time of the last back-up in case of processing errors, machine failure, or other accidents (DuChene et al. 1986).

Forms Posting

In general, it is best to keep the interval between data collection and entry as short as possible. If it is possible to process forms as they are generated, this is preferable (Meinert and Tonascia 1986). However, if batch processing is found to be more convenient, the scheduled time between subsequent postings of information from the study transaction files (raw data) to the master file should not be longer than two weeks. During forms posting, data fields from the transaction files are copied to the location in the master file(s) specified in the *data dictionary* (a database of information used to edit, document and control the processing of forms through the computer system). The data management system should be programmed to reject the form if errors are detected in the data identifiers, or if data are found to already exist in the master file (unless the form to be entered is a correction form). Personnel at the data coordinating center can then review and resolve discrepancies in rejected forms. If fields need to be modified in the master file, changes should be explained and documented in the electronic file as well as on paper.

Backup of Raw Data

Once the forms have been posted to the master file, all transaction files containing the posted forms should be copied on to a tape or other electronic medium such as compact disc (CD) or digital video display (DVD), and stored offsite. In the event of a major system failure or destruction of the master file (in a building fire, for instance), the offsite copy will allow recreation of the master file.

Clearance

After the data are posted to a master file, computer edits of the master file allow consistency checks between fields on different forms. For example, an individual's height should remain constant over forms. It is informative to flag inadmissible values, as well as unlikely values. Additional within form checks can also be performed at this time.

Archiving

When within-form verification and across-form clearance are complete, and data on the master file are finalized, the master file should be copied on to at least two tapes and stored off-site. These tapes should be read regularly to check for deterioration. If a back-up tape cannot be read, a new copy should be made.

13.3.8   Quality Assurance Committee

The most carefully designed quality assurance program cannot function efficiently without the assignation of responsibilities for various quality monitoring tasks to specific individuals, and the existence of effective communication channels between study personnel. In many large studies, a quality assurance committee is formed to oversee the quality of data collection (Knatterud et al. 1998; The Chemical Manufacturers Association's Epidemiology Task Force 1991; US Environmental Protection Agency (EPA) 1989). The quality assurance committee addresses quality issues throughout the life of the study, from protocol development to the responsible archiving of data. The quality assurance committee is also responsible for reviewing study compliance with written quality assurance/control procedures, and for evaluating interim analyses. For large studies, a data monitoring committee made up of external quality assurance auditors supportive of the protocol objectives and study design might be warranted (Fleming 1993).

13.3.9   Communications

The effective resolution of study quality issues is highly dependent on the quality of communications between study personnel. Many of the quality assurance mechanisms already described in the chapter *contribute* directly to improved communication. Examples include the training of personnel, and the definition of standard operating procedures. Other quality assurance mechanisms *depend* critically on communication for their implementation. In order for queries to be resolved effectively, study personnel need to know who to submit queries to, and how these queries should be submitted. Structures for transmitting resolved data queries back to data entry personnel are also needed. The scheduling of regular meetings between study personnel is crucial for maintaining study communications. Emphasizing the rationale for quality control and the need for wholehearted support for quality control measures is important, since quality control measures will fail if they are perceived as nit-picky and burdensome (Cooper 1986). One or more individuals should be designated responsible for preparing and disseminating the minutes of study meetings. More generally, communication structures should be in place to communicate the intent, conduct, results and interpretations of the study to study personnel, study participants, and the scientific community. In certain situations, other parties that might need to be informed of study results include health care providers, policy makers, or the media.

Cost of Quality Assurance 13.3.10

Clearly, the implementation of quality assurance and quality control measures add to the cost of a study. While some expenses, such as the cost of routine data editing, or the re-checking of statistical analyses may be impossible to estimate, cost information can be projected for other aspects of quality assurance, such as training, site visits, and external quality control programs (Knatterud et al. 1998). Considering the cost of various quality control measures early in the planning process allows for development of a realistic and feasible program that is more likely to be executed. Priorities for data quality should be set at this time. While certain aspects of data quality should not be sacrificed regardless of the expense, a compromise might be possible in other instances. For example, a costly, time-consuming measure of exposure might be collected for a sub-sample of study participants and this information can be used to validate a cheaper exposure measurement used for all study participants.

Ethical Considerations 13.3.11

Ethical considerations are perhaps the most important set of considerations in a study (for a general discussion see Chap. IV.7 of this handbook). Epidemiological research should never lose sight of the fact that data are derived from human beings. Studies such as the Tuskegee Syphilis Trial (US Department of Health Education and Welfare (DHEW) 1973) which followed the progress of untreated syphilis in black men even after effective treatment was available may now seem shocking, but it is well to keep in mind that throughout most of the trial, the investigators did not find their research particularly objectionable. The thorough consideration of ethical issues raised by a study (mandated by law in most countries) will hopefully prevent a future generation of scientists from looking back at present-day trials with regret.

The human subjects section of the protocol must describe whether the study protocol imposes any physical or psychological risk to the participants. Potential benefits of the study should also be noted, with an explanation of whether benefits will be accrued by study participants themselves, or whether the study is expected to benefit others in the future. The cost-to-benefit ratio should be weighed and discussed. Studies that involve primary data collection generally need to obtain informed consent from study participants. Consent forms should include, at a minimum: contact information for personnel available to answer questions about the research; the purpose of the study; eligibility requirements; the expected duration of participation; possible harm that the subjects could incur; expected benefits to subjects or to others; information on the voluntary nature of participation, and a statement indicating the right to withdraw from the study at any time (The Chemical Manufacturers Association's Epidemiology Task Force 1991). The study eligibility criteria are also subject to ethical considerations, both in terms of inclusions (different racial/ethnic groups and both genders should be adequately represented) and exclusions (special justification is needed for study of vulnerable groups, such as pregnant women, children, or incarcerated individuals). Adequate provisions for maintaining data confidentiality and the privacy of individuals should be described. For example, investigators might plan to store hard copies of sensitive data in locked cabinets with limited access and remove personal identifiers from datasets used for analysis. Automated data management systems should have password control, users should be logged out after a period of inactivity, and the copying of data should be discouraged (Wyatt 1995).

13.4 Quality Considerations During Study Conduct

Before data collection is initiated, all data collection procedures should be reviewed and approved by the lead investigators. Data forms and equipment should have been tested, and certified ready for use.

If rigorous quality assurance procedures have been planned prior to study initiation, quality control activities during study conduct mainly consist of the implementation of these procedures. The study protocol should be followed, personnel should be trained according to established standard procedures, and data collection should proceed with all quality assurances in place. Any deviation from standard operating procedure should be authorized by the Steering Committee.

The importance of periodic examination of data by study investigators, data coordinators, and data entry personnel while the data are being collected cannot be overstated. Examination of data trends by center, over time, or by technician (for example), can identify flaws in data collection early on. Even simple plots and graphs of data can identify sources of error. When data errors are identified, steps should be taken to correct the data in a timely manner. In some cases, statistical adjustment can be used to correct data drift. When this is not possible, data might have to be thrown out, or completely reprocessed. In order to generate a written audit trail of data, any changes made in the data should be documented.

Training and Certification

The importance of training and certifying all study personnel has already been underlined in Sect. 13.3.3. While many study investigators are aware of the need for standardized operating procedures, information regarding these procedures is often lacking in study descriptions. While 244 original research articles in three emergency medical journals (1989–1993) described data collection by means of chart review, only 18% mentioned training of abstractors, and periodic abstracter monitoring was reported in a mere 3% of these articles (Gilbert et al. 1996).

Detailed practical guidelines for training and quality control management for study interviewers, data abstractors, and biomedical technicians are available in the literature (Edwards et al. 1994; Fowler and Mangione 1986, 1990; Reisch et al. 2003). This section summarizes some of the main considerations.

Training

Training procedures should ideally involve all staff and procedures. While centralized training of all study personnel might be desirable in terms of increasing the comparability of data collection between sites and allowing study personnel from different sites to interact with each other, the expense of bringing personnel to a central training site for all their training can be considerable. Additionally, site-specific questions might arise that cannot be adequately addressed during centralized training. An optimum strategy might be to use both types of training. Table 13.4 provides an overview of the training process.

Certification

Following initial training, study personnel should be certified to perform specific procedures. Regular re-training is desirable to prevent data drift. Re-training might also be necessary if a specific study technician is found to be introducing a systematic error into the data, or if the study protocol changes. Any re-training should be accompanied by recertification.

While the interval between re-training and certification varies from study to study, the Atherosclerosis Risk in Communities study (ARIC) used a 90-day interval, since a six-month interval was found to allow too much drift to recognize and correct digit preference. More timely feedback was also needed in the Cardiovascular Health Study (CHS) (Hill 2003).

Maintenance and Calibration of Equipment

Study equipment should be inspected and calibrated at regular intervals in accordance with the study protocol. In the event of equipment breakdown, equipment

Table 13.4. Overview of Training*

Steps in data processing	
Training manual	Educational training manual is sent to all sites for review.
	The training manual consists of some or all of the following: a study overview, information on the relevant procedure, quality assessment procedures, data forms with instructions (e.g. for abstraction or interview), quick reference sheet for all variables, glossary of terms, standardized training examples, and relevant articles from the literature.
Standardized training examples	Training examples should be prepared for key study variables. For instance, study personnel might be asked to note blood pressure measurements from a training tape.
Individual orientation	Two or more individual orientation sessions should be arranged with the onsite data collection team, and with the lead study co-ordinator and/or study investigator. Additional sessions can be scheduled at the discretion of the site co-ordinators.
Double-review of initial data	The first few examples of data collected (by chart abstraction, interview, or a biomedical procedure) should be repeated by a more experienced member of the data collection team. Discrepancies can then be reviewed. Queries should be entered into an audit form and sent to the lead study co-ordinator to assist with later tracking of problematic data.
Regular double-review	Performing regular double review for a small sample of data (e.g. once a month) can prevent data drift over time. Review of data at a later time is facilitated by audio or video taping of interviews or biomedical procedures.
Regular conference calls/meetings of field staff	Regular study conference calls can include a training component if examples of data collection problems are brought up for discussion during each call. An updated decision log containing a summary of discussions held and decisions made during these conference calls can be distributed among study personnel.
Regular site visits	Review of data collection procedures during site visits by the lead study coordinator and/or lead investigator.
Retraining	Retraining of study personnel might be necessary if substantial time has passed since initial training, a systematic bias in data is detected, or the study protocol changes.

* adapted from Reisch et al. (2003)

may need to be replaced. If the new equipment is similar to the equipment already being used, then calibration before use is sufficient. When replacement of existing equipment is desirable because a new model or instrument is more accurate or efficient than the existing equipment, data should be collected using both the old and the new instrument for a defined period of time, so that comparability of measurements can be established.

Implementing Data Management 13.4.3

The data management process has already been described in detail in Sect. 13.3.7. During study conduct, the planned data management system is implemented, and refined as necessary.

Tracking and Monitoring of Data

The effective tracking and monitoring of data as data collection is in progress is essential to the timely detection and correction of errors. Monitoring should occur for subject accrual, data acquisition, and data quality. Automated tracking systems can greatly assist this process, and have been used successfully in epidemiological studies as early as 1981 (McQuade et al. 1983). Data that are collected by hand should be recorded directly, promptly, and legibly in ink. Four different types of monitoring are recommended: *pro-active efforts* to improve data, *observation of data collection, review of computer-generated checks and summary reports*, and *examination of data*.

When possible, data quality should be improved by *pro-active efforts*. Automated reminders of when patients are due for study visits for time-dependent variables (e.g. levels of an exposure biomarker) can prevent the collection of data that is later deemed of poor quality or unusable. Target dates for follow-up visits can be defined by the participant's entry date rather than the date of the last visit, in order to prevent scheduling deviations from carrying over to future visits.

Direct or indirect *observation of data collection* can also identify errors in a timely manner. An unobtrusive way to monitor interviewers for delivery and adherence to protocol is to audio-tape interviews. Measurement techniques for biomedical or laboratory technicians can either be videotaped, or directly observed by senior technicians or other qualified study personnel.

Regular *review of computer-generated queries and summary reports* of data quality can alert the investigators to a variety of data errors, including participant ineligibility, data outside the expected range, and variation in data quality by data field, site, or technician. Active examination of data during collection is crucial. Summary statistics and plots of data by technician, site or time can identify unusual trends. For example, an examination of data from the Hypertension Prevention Trial revealed that nearly 29% of the baseline systolic blood pressure readings from one clinic ended in the digit 2. This could be traced to measurements made by one technician, who recorded a number ending in the digit 2 for over 60% measurements (Canner et al. 1991). When a data collection flaw is identified, further error should be prevented by tracking down the source of the problem, and taking corrective action.

Keying errors may be identified by periodic audits of the database against source documents. Rather than check all the data, a random sample of data fields can be selected to check for keying errors. When creating the test sample, it is important to ensure that a broad cross-section of data is included (for example, both numerical and character fields should be checked). One method for sampling a variety of fields is to choose a random sub-sample of forms, and look at all fields within those forms.

Corrective Actions

Moving back to the datascope for a moment, we recall that the identification of data errors is only the first step in data quality management. In order to reach the ultimate goal of valid data, these errors need to be corrected. The process for revising data should be as systemized and well documented as the process for locating errors. While the routine correction of careless mistakes while data entry is in progress need not be reported, data errors that are identified after initial data entry should not be changed by data entry staff until the query has been checked. A paper trail should be initiated for each problem, with the initial query describing the problem, and the date it was detected (Fig. 13.2). The individual(s) responsible for query resolution should then investigate the query, and provide a response explaining why the problem occurred. Finally, the query documentation should indicate how and when the problem was resolved. If data from a form are found to be incorrect, they should be identified as incorrect rather than erased, and the correct values should be inserted (Knatterud et al. 1998). In some cases, unusual values will be confirmed to be correct, in which case they should be retained in the database with documentation.

Occasionally, errors identified during study conduct may lead to changes in the survey instrument or other study equipment. In such cases, it is crucial that the version of the form or equipment used to collect data is recorded in the database. If a new data check is added, either as a result of a query or as an additional precaution, old values in the database should be edited using the new rules in order to keep data consistent.

Tracking the time taken for corrective actions allows areas of delay to be identified and resolved for future queries. In most longitudinal studies, data are analyzed while data collection is still in progress. In such instances, one might want to exclude data that are under query from the master database until the problem is resolved. The inclusion of a "status" field for data would allow investigators to check whether values were acceptable or unacceptable (Gassman et al. 1995).

13.4.4   Site Visits

For multi-center studies, site visits to observe operations allow greater understanding of site-specific data collection issues, and provide an opportunity to recognize and correct faulty systems (Gassman et al. 1995; Knatterud et al. 1998; Prud'homme

Query

Subject ID: 111770

Form: 121   **Item Questioned:** 5, 6a
Date of Visit: 08/28/02   **Visit Number:** 2

Description: Subject claims to be a former smoker (ev_smok = 2), but reports currently smoking five cigarettes a day (cur_cig = 5).

Date: 12/6/02
Initials: PR

Response

Form to correct: 121   **Item to correct:** 6a
Old value: 5
Correct value: 0

Explanation: Checked subject's medical record and past questionnaire. Subject is a former smoker.

Date: 12/11/02
Initials: DR

Documentation

Correction: Value of cur_cig has been changed from 5 to 0.

Date: 12/20/02
Initials: TN

Figure 13.2. Example of a Data Query Form

et al. 1989). Scheduling a site visit is recommended shortly after initiation of patient recruitment, and when the data collection at the site is drawing to a close. Additional site visits should be scheduled for long-term studies.

The size of the site visit team can vary, and is dictated by the nature and purpose of the visit. A typical site visit team might include the study principal investigator (or representative), the director of another field site, the data coordinating center director, the study project officer, and selected resource personnel. During the site visit, the site visit team would meet with the director and staff of the unit, and hold private conversations with key support personnel. The site visit should include a thorough review of staffing requirements, recruiting, training and certification, and communication structures. Site visitors also have a chance to observe data collection, check data management, and review data quality monitoring. Specific activities might include observation of whether field technicians follow the study protocol, inspection of study records and documents storage, and review of the operation and maintenance of local data systems. Following the site visit, the leader of the site visit team should prepare a written report of the visit based on input from the entire team. The site visit report should describe any systematic errors that were identified in data collection, and provide recommendations on how to rectify the situation. A formal response to the report should be prepared by the staff at the study site.

13.5   Quality Considerations After Data Collection

Once data collection for the study is complete, the task of analyzing and interpreting the data begins. The study investigator should yet again consult the datascope to check for possible biases and errors that need to be resolved in order to form a clear picture of the relationship under study.

13.5.1   Reporting Response Rate

If individuals who agreed to participate in the study were different in some important way from non-respondents, the study results could well be biased. For example, non-respondents to questionnaires might be of poorer health or more likely to be smokers than respondents (Shahar et al. 1996). Studies that have followed respondents and non-respondents to questionnaires have reported that non-respondents have a significantly higher risk of myocardial infarction, cancer mortality, and all-cause mortality (Bisgard et al. 1994; Heilbrun et al. 1991).

Calculating the study *response rate* gives a first indication of whether the investigator should be concerned about possible bias in the results. Generally, the higher the study response rate, the less need to worry about selection bias affecting the results. The simplest approach to response rate calculation is to divide the number of surveys received by the number of surveys sent. However, this does not account for factors that can affect the response rate such as undelivered questionnaires, ineligibility of subjects who completed questionnaires, or substitution of the intended recipient with another subject. Typically, the numerator and denominator of the response rate are adjusted to reflect such factors. Standard definitions and methods to calculate survey response rates are provided by the American Association for Public Opinion Research (2000), or the Council of American Survey Research Organizations (CASRO).

For cohort studies, the simplest way to estimate the *follow-up rate* is to the divide the number of participants seen at the last visit by the number of participants initially enrolled. Again, different assumptions about individuals lost to follow-up yield different numbers for the follow-up rate.

Since different methods of calculating the response rate might be appropriate for different studies, the choice of the response rate formula is less critical than the identification and reporting of all the elements that enter the calculation (Table 13.5).

In general, response rates to questionnaires have been decreasing in the United States, and perhaps elsewhere (Kessler et al. 1995; Steeh 1981). Data from a nationwide survey in the United States (the Behavioral Risk Factor Surveillance System, BRFSS) indicate that response rates from random digit dialing have declined from a median of 68.4% in 1995 to a median of 55.2% in 1999 (Centers for Disease Control and Prevention (CDC) 1999). A review of 82 case-control studies published in the *American Journal of Epidemiology* (1988–1990), *Epidemiology* (1997–1999) and *Cancer Epidemiology, Biomarkers and Prevention* (1997–1999) reported a 0.2% and 0.44% decrease in reported response per year for cases and controls, respectively (Olson 2001). The same article reported an average response rate of 76.1% for cases and 71.5% for controls. A review of 321 distinct mail surveys published in a broader spectrum of United States journals in 1991 reported an average survey response rate of 62% (Asch et al. 1997).

Regardless of the exact value of the response rate, the characterization of non-respondents is crucial in order to assess whether a bias is present, and if it is, how the results of the analysis might be affected. Clearly, describing the non-respondents becomes more important when a study has a low response rate. Whenever possible, a brief survey should be administered to non-respondents to collect limited data for comparison with respondents. Otherwise, assessing available data on demographics, exposure or outcome will allow some assessment of possible bias.

Analysis 13.5.2

Before proceeding to analysis, the study data should be tested rigorously to check for *residual errors* that remain after all data processing and routine quality assurance activities are complete. Range checks provide one way to examine whether the data seem reasonable. Simple queries such as checking that the recorded age in years is consistent with the date of interview minus the recorded date of birth, can also help to detect errors.

Once the investigator feels confident that there are no obvious flaws in the data, the next step is to understand the data by conducting exploratory data analysis using univariate and bivariate summaries, as well as plots and graphs of the data. More complex exploratory analysis of the data should be guided by

Table 13.5. Reporting outcomes of recruiting respondents in case-control studies in a study of thyroid cancer in western Washington*

Units selected from sampling frame	Number
Random digit dialing screening phase	
Total	6741
Ineligible sampling unit	
Total	3589
Business, fax, government	1937
Nonworking numbers	1436
Institution, group quarters, dataline	216
Unable to determine eligibility	
Total	431
Unknown if residential	274
Residential, unknown if individual eligible	157
Answering machine on all attempts	56
Refusal to answer questions on eligibility	76
Other (language barrier)	25
Respondent not eligible	
Total	1983
Age	1749
County	216
Language	18
Respondent screened and eligible, total	738
In-Person interviews of eligible women	
Total	738
Unable to determine eligibility	0
Respondent not eligible	
Total	1
Prior thyroid cancer	1
Respondent screened and eligible	
Total	737
Not interviewed (refused)	163
Interviewed	574

* adapted from Olson et al. (2002)

the data. If assumptions implicit in the planned analysis methods are violated, alternative statistical methods must be considered. Appropriate and careful statistical analysis is integral to good epidemiological practice. A description of basic methods of analysis for epidemiological study designs can be found in Part II of this handbook "Statistical Methods in Epidemiology," and in most intermediate textbooks of epidemiology (Rothman and Greenland 1998; Szklo and Nieto 2000). Some of the key issues underlying the analysis of cohort and case-control studies are summarized in Chaps. I.5 and I.6 of this handbook and in a two-volume series published by the International Agency for Cancer Research (Breslow and Day 1980, 1987). The finer points of analysis, however, are study-specific. For this reason, it is crucial that data analysis be conducted by personnel with the necessary training and experience in statistical methods.

Once data analysis is complete, ways to check the analysis include independently reproducing the tabulations and statistical calculations from the original data, and checking different tables for consistency of the denominators. All data reduction and statistical procedures should be documented to facilitate review at a later date.

The results of any study are associated with some degree of uncertainty. To the extent possible, these uncertainties should be quantified and accounted for, or, at the minimum, characterized quantitatively. In an analysis of risk factors for coronary disease in the Framingham Heart Study, estimates of risk increased for factors measured with substantial error after correction for uncertainty (e.g. serum cholesterol), whereas risk estimates tended to remain unchanged for risk factors with little or no error, such as body mass index (Rosner et al. 1992).

The analysis of study data is followed by the task of interpreting the study results. An observed association might be due to statistical artifact, due to bias or confounding, or be truly causal. The use of statistical significance alone to guide inference is not recommended (Goodman 1999a; Goodman 1999b). If one hundred truly null associations were tested at the $\alpha = 0.05$ level, five of these associations would be significant due to chance alone. Moreover, an association might be confounded by one or more variables, or could be biased due to systematic flaws in the design or conduct of the study.

Following adequate consideration of chance, confounding and bias (cf. Chap. I.9 of this handbook), the determination of whether an association is causal will also depend on *temporality*, the *strength of the association*, the presence or absence of a *dose-response relationship*, *consistency* with prior literature, and *biological plausibility* (Gordis 2000; US Department of Health Education and Welfare (DHEW) 1964).

If an exposure is believed to cause the disease in question, this exposure must occur before the disease develops. *Temporality* is easier to establish for prospective cohort studies for which exposure information prior to disease outcome is available. For cross-sectional or case-control studies, exposure information is usually collected concurrently with disease information or has to be recreated from historical records of exposure, making the assessment of temporality more difficult.

In general, the larger the magnitude of the association, the more likely it is that the relationship between the exposure and disease is causal. In epidemiologic studies, the *strength of the association* is usually measured by the relative risk or odds ratio.

If it can be demonstrated that increasing the dose of an agent is associated with increased occurrence of disease in a well-defined relationship, this provides more evidence for causality. The absence of a *dose-response relationship*, however, does not preclude a causal relationship; since it is possible that no disease develops until a certain exposure level is reached, after which disease can occur ("threshold effect").

Consistent replication of a finding in different study populations provides further evidence for a causal relationship. However, it is possible that an association only occurs in certain population sub-groups, in which case it might be seen in some populations but not others.

Before concluding that an association is causal, it is important to consider *biological plausibility*. While it is possible that epidemiological studies can detect associations which are not yet understood on a biological level, attempting to understand how the exposure might cause the disease in question is nonetheless worthwhile.

Once the results of a study have been finalized, the investigators should consider how they plan to communicate the results, and to whom. Groups that should be informed, in general, are the study personnel, study participants, and scientific community. If the results of a study warrant immediate action, health care providers and policy makers should also be alerted. While it is important that the media is informed of the results of studies that have relevance to the general public, it is generally prudent to wait until the study is published in a peer-reviewed journal, since the process of critical review of a study allows for the identification and correction of key flaws.

A typical study report consists of the following sections: introduction, methods, results, and discussion (Table 13.6).

Regardless of the audience for the report, results should always be placed in context of the uncertainties and limitations associated with the findings. Describing results in terms of adjectives such as "definitive" or "conclusive" should be avoided. Too often, associations that receive much publicity to begin with have to be rescinded in light of further research.

Concise, simple language aids clarity of presentation. For written reports, adequately labeled tables and figures should be used to summarize information when possible. Information presented in tables should not be merely repeated in the text without additional interpretation.

It is important that results of well-designed studies are reported regardless of whether findings are negative or positive. The tendency for positive findings to be highlighted, both in terms of submission and final publication, biases the perception of the true association between exposure and outcome. This is especially problematic in the context of meta-analyses (cf. Chap. II.7 of this handbook) that attempt to quantitatively summarize published studies. A bias towards publishing positive findings results in a biased estimation of overall risk (Easterbrook et al. 1991; Egger and Smith 1998; Ioannidis 1998; Thornton and Lee 2000).

Studies with substantive findings on a research question may have implications for policies related to public health. Researchers may appropriately highlight such findings in their reports, often at the conclusion of the discussion, commenting on the extent to which new knowledge has been generated with policy implica-

Table 13.6. Guidelines for preparation of a study report*

Introduction

Review study rationale	Describe importance of problem.
	Biological plausibility.
	How does this study add to existing literature?
State hypotheses	Specify interactions of a priori interest.

Methods

Describe study population	Methods of recruitment.
	Inclusion and exclusion criteria.
Describe data collection	Include accuracy and reliability of procedures, and quality control measures.
State criteria for identification of confounders	
Describe statistical methods	Justify categorization of study variables.
	State assumptions of selected model.

Results

Describe rates of participation or response	
Provide descriptive data	Frequency distributions, means, unadjusted differences.
	Stratify by variables of interest e.g. age, sex.
	Quality control measures.
Present results of model	Use most parsimonious model.
	Additive and multiplicative interactions, if present.
Tables and figures	Should be self-explanatory.
	Use informative labels, and units.

Discussion

Review main study results	Compare and contrast with published literature.
Describe strengths and limitations of study	
Assess bias and confounding	How much would study results be affected by bias/confounding?
Address uncertainty	How precise are the study estimates, given misclassification?
Clinical, public health policy implications.	If strength and impact of study results warrants.
Future directions	How to improve on study, build on findings.

* adapted from Szklo and Nieto (2000)

tions. There has been substantial debate among epidemiologic researchers as to whether publications should also make policy recommendations (Samet 2000). In general, policy recommendations should not be made in publications providing research findings, particularly within the constraints of the policy expertise of most researchers and the space that can be devoted to such discussion in an article.

13.5.3   Storage and Retrieval of Data

Commitment to an epidemiological study does not end with the publication of the final papers. After the study is completed, sufficient material should be stored to allow future sharing of the data or auditing of the study. An index of all stored study materials should be created, along with a description of where they can be located. Materials that should be considered for archiving include source data and specimens, laboratory or research notebooks, and the study protocol. Also included should be the final study report, computer data files, copies of computer programs and statistical procedures that were used in analysis, and any printouts of analyses that formed the basis of results included in the final report (Freedland and Carney 1992; The Chemical Manufacturers Association's Epidemiology Task Force 1991; US Environmental Protection Agency (EPA) 1989). If applicable, study forms and related forms should be destroyed in accordance with local statutes and medical records. In order to ensure safety and confidentiality of study materials, storage should be in a physically secure place with limited access.

Periodic checking of stored material is recommended, to ensure that necessary updates have been made and to avoid unnecessary clutter. Original records can be transferred to microfilm for storage purposes, to conserve space. If microfilm is used, the original records should be retained until the microfilm is checked for proper identification and legibility. For very large studies, electronic storage of study data might make sense given space and cost limitations.

13.6   Conclusions

The field of epidemiology has been growing rapidly, with a vast number of epidemiologic studies published every year. A search for "Epidemiology" in the PUBMED database yielded 287 references for the year 1964. A similar search for the year 2002 yielded 46,658 references (Fig. 13.3). The results of many of these studies, however, are inconsistent. These inconsistencies are sometimes due to chance, but often can be ascribed to the variable quality of studies with respect to design, conduct, analysis or dissemination.

As a consequence of the inconsistent results reported by epidemiological studies, many consumers of epidemiological research including clinicians, policymakers, and the general public, are dismissive of new findings. The importance of

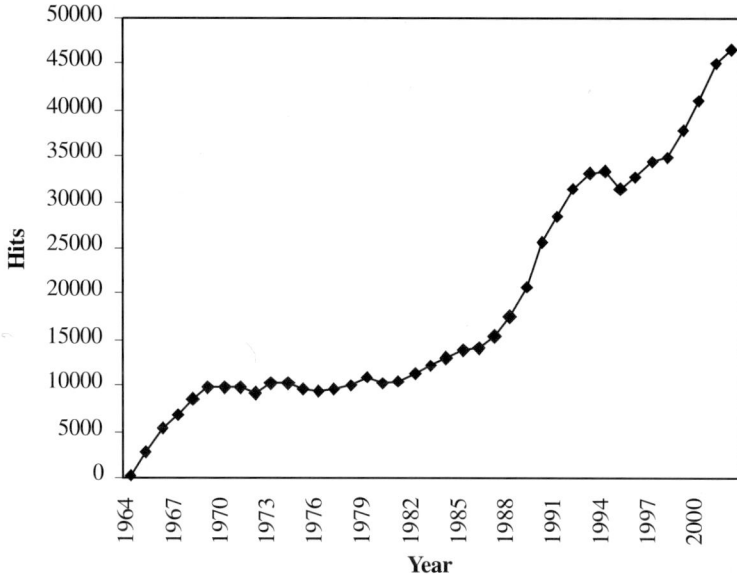

Figure 13.3. Number of references to "Epidemiology" in the PUBMED database, 1964–2002 (no delimiters)

a widespread effort to follow good epidemiologic practice and implement rigorous quality assurance and quality control procedures cannot be overstated.

Even as this chapter is being written, the methods of data collection, processing and storage are changing rapidly as technological innovations emerge. However, the basic principles of good epidemiologic practice, data quality assurance and control will not change. The increasing use of e-mail or web-based questionnaires may reduce data error due to data transfer from paper to electronic files, for example, but errors due to poor questionnaire design or data entry (to name just a few sources of error) will still exist. Similarly, electronic processing and storage of data might be helpful in identifying unusual values, but study investigators will still need to review, interpret, and correct these errors.

In this chapter, we have reviewed quality assurance and quality control activities pertinent to the planning, conduct and reporting of a study. The mental exercise of "optimizing" the dials on the datascope can be useful while conducting epidemiological studies, and when considering the results of already published studies. As high quality research becomes the norm, the field of epidemiology will gain more respect among fellow scientists, policy-makers, and the public.

References

Agresti A (1990) Categorical data analysis. John Wiley and Sons, Hoboken, NJ

Altman D, Bland J (1983) Measurements in medicine: the analysis of method comparison studies. Statistician 32:307–317

American Association for Public Opinion Research. Standard definitions (2000) Final dispositions of case codes and outcome rates for surveys. American Association for Public Opinion Research, Ann Arbor, MI

Armstrong B, White E (1992) Principles of exposure measurement in epidemiology. Oxford University Press, New York

Arts DG, De Keizer NF, Scheffer GJ (2002) Defining and improving data quality in medical registries: a literature review, case study, and generic framework. J Am Med Inform Assoc 9:600–611

Asch DA, Jedrziewski MK, Christakis NA (1997) Response rates to mail surveys published in medical journals. J Clin Epidemiol 50:1129–1136

Asch DA, Christakis NA, Ubel PA (1998) Conducting physician mail surveys on a limited budget. A randomized trial comparing $2 bill versus $5 bill incentives. Med Care 36:95–99

Ascherio A, Stampfer MJ, Colditz GA, Rimm EB, Litin L, Willet WC (1992) Correlations of vitamin A and E intakes with the plasma concentrations of carotenoids and tocopherols among American men and women. J Nutr 122: 1792–1801

Baer A, Saroiu S, Koutsky LA (2002) Obtaining sensitive data through the Web: an example of design and methods. Epidemiol 13:640–645

Barnett V, Lewis T (1994) Outliers in statistical data. John Wiley and Sons, Hoboken, N.J.

Berkanovic E (1980) The effect of inadequate language translation on Hispanics' responses to health surveys. Am J Public Health 80:1273–1276

Bisgard KM, Folsom AR, Hong CP, Sellers TA (1994) Mortality and cancer rates in nonrespondents to a prospective study of older women: 5-year follow-up. Am J Epidemiol 139:990–1000

Blackmore CC, Richardson ML, Linnau KF, Schwed AM, Lomoschitz FM, Escobedo EM, Hunter JC, Jurkovich GJ, Cummings P (2003) Web-based image review and data acquisition for multiinstitutional research. AJR Am J Roentgenol 180:1243–1246

Brenner H, Gefeller O (1997) Variation of sensitivity, specificity, likelihood ratios and predictive values with disease prevalence. Stat Med 16:981–991

Breslow N, Day N (1980) Statistical methods in cancer research. Volume I – The analysis of case-control studies. International Agency for Research on Cancer, Lyon

Breslow N, Day N (1987) Statistical methods in cancer research. Volume II – The design and analysis of cohort studies. International Agency for Research on Cancer, Lyon

Bryant AH, Reinert A (2001) Epidemiology in the legal arena and the search for truth. Am J Epidemiol 154:S27–S35

Canner PL, Krol WF, Forman SA (1983) The Coronary Drug Project. External quality control programs. Control Clin Trials 4:441–466

Canner PL, Borhani NO, Oberman A, Cutler J, Prineas RJ, Langford H, Hooper FJ (1991) The Hypertension Prevention Trial: assessment of the quality of blood pressure measurements. Am J Epidemiol 134:379–392

Centers for Disease Control and Prevention (CDC) (1999) BRFSS summary quality control report. Centers for Disease Control and Prevention, Atlanta, GA

Cherrie J, Schneider T (1998) Validation of a new method for structured subjective assessment of past concentrations. Annals Occup Hyg 43:235–245

Cherrie J, Krantz S, Schneider T, Ohberg I, Kamstrup O, Linander W (1987) An experimental simulation of an early rock wool/slag wool production process. Ann Occup Hyg 31:583–593

Choi BC, Pak AW, Purdham JT (1990) Effects of mailing strategies on response rate, response time, and cost in a questionnaire study among nurses. Epidemiol 1:72–74

Christiansen DH, Hosking JD, Dannenberg AL, Williams OD (1990) Computer-assisted data collection in multicenter epidemiologic research. The Atherosclerosis Risk in Communities Study. Control Clin Trials 11:101–115

Cicchetti DV, Feinstein AR (1990) High agreement but low kappa: II. Resolving the paradoxes. J Clin Epidemiol 43:551–558

Clement DL, De Buyzere ML, De Bacquer DA, de Leeuw PW, Duprez DA, Fagard RH, Gheeraert PJ, Missault LH, Braun JJ, Six RO, Van Der NP, O'Brien E (2003) Prognostic value of ambulatory blood-pressure recordings in patients with treated hypertension. N Engl J Med 348:2407–2415

Clive RE, Ocwieja KM, Kamell L, Hoyler SS, Seiffert JE, Young JL, Henson DE, Winchester DP, Osteen RT, Menck HR (1995) A national quality improvement effort: cancer registry data. J Surg Oncol 58:155–161

Cohen J (1968) Weighted kappa: nominal scale agreement with provision for scaled disagreement of partial credit. Psychological Bulletin 70:213–220

Collins RL, Ellickson PL, Hays RD, McCaffrey DF (2000) Effects of incentive size and timing on response rates to a follow-up wave of a longitudinal mailed survey. Eval Rev 24:347–363

Comstock GW, Tockman MS, Helsing KJ, Hennesy KM (1979) Standardized respiratory questionnaires: comparison of the old with the new. Am Rev Respir Dis 119:45–53

Cook RR (1991) Overview of good epidemiologic practices. J Occup Med 33:1216–1220

Cooper GR (1986) The importance of quality control in the Multiple Risk Factor Intervention Trial. Control Clin Trials 7:3pp

Cottler LB, Zipp JF, Robins LN, Spitznagel EL (1987) Difficult-to-recruit respondents and their effect on prevalence estimates in an epidemiologic survey. Am J Epidemiol 125:329–339

Crombie IK, Irving JM (1986) An investigation of data entry methods with a personal computer. Comput Biomed Res 19:543–550

Dawber TR, Meadors GF, Moore FE, Jr. (1951) Epidemiological approaches to heart disease: The Framingham Study. Am J Public Health 41:279–286

Day S, Fayers P, Harvey D (1998) Double data entry: what value, what price? Control Clin Trials 19:15–24

Deyo RA, Diehr P, Patrick DL (1991) Reproducibility and responsiveness of health status measures. Statistics and strategies for evaluation. Control Clin Trials 12:142S–158S

Dillman D (1978) Mail and telephone surveys: the total design method. John Wiley and Sons, New York

Dischinger P, DuChene AG (1986) Quality control aspects of blood pressure measurements in the Multiple Risk Factor Intervention Trial. Control Clin Trials 7:137S–157S

Doody MM, Sigurdson AS, Kampa D, Chimes K, Alexander BH, Ron E, Tarone RE, Linet MS (2003) Randomized trial of financial incentives and delivery methods for improving response to a mailed questionnaire. Am J Epidemiol 157:643–651

Dosemeci M, Rothman N, Yin SN, Li GL, Linet M, Wacholder S, Chow WH, Hayes RB (1997) Validation of benzene exposure assessment. Ann N Y Acad Sci 837:114–121

DuChene AG, Hultgren DH, Neaton JD, Grambsch PV, Broste SK, Aus BM, Rasmussen WL (1986) Forms control and error detection procedures used at the Coordinating Center of the Multiple Risk Factor Intervention Trial (MRFIT). Control Clin Trials 7:34S–45S

Eaker S, Bergstrom R, Bergstrom A, Adami HO, Nyren O (1998) Response rate to mailed epidemiologic questionnaires: a population-based randomized trial of variations in design and mailing routines. Am J Epidemiol 147:74–82

Easterbrook PJ, Berlin JA, Gopalan R, Matthews DR (1991) Publication bias in clinical research. Lancet 337:867–872

Edwards P, Roberts I, Clarke M, DiGuiseppi C, Pratap S, Wentz R, Kwan I (2002) Increasing response rates to postal questionnaires: systematic review. Br Med J 324:1183

Edwards S, Slattery ML, Mori M, Berry TD, Caan BJ, Palmer P, Potter JD (1994) Objective system for interviewer performance evaluation for use in epidemiologic studies. Am J Epidemiol 140:1020–1028

Egger M, Smith GD (1998) Bias in location and selection of studies. Br Med J 316:61–66

Feinstein AR, Cicchetti DV (1990) High agreement but low kappa: I. The problems of two paradoxes. J Clin Epidemiol 43:543–549

Fleiss JL (1981) Statistical methods for rates and proportions, 2nd edn. John Wiley and Sons, New York

Fleming TR (1993) Data monitoring committees and capturing relevant information of high quality. Stat Med 12:565–570

Fowler F, Mangione T (1986) Reducing interviewer effects on health survey data. Center for Survey Research, University of Massachusetts, Boston, MA

Fowler F, Mangione T (1990) Standardized survey interviewing: minimizing interviewer-related error. Sage Publications, Newberry Park, CA

Freedland KE, Carney RM (1992) Data management and accountability in behavioral and biomedical research. Am Psychol 47:640–645

Gassman JJ, Owen WW, Kuntz TE, Martin JP, Amoroso WP (1995) Data quality assurance, monitoring, and reporting. Control Clin Trials 16:104S–136S

Gibson PJ, Koepsell TD, Diehr P, Hale C (1999) Increasing response rates for mailed surveys of Medicaid clients and other low-income populations. Am J Epidemiol 149:1057–1062

Gilbart E, Kreiger N (1998) Improvement in cumulative response rates following implementation of a financial incentive. Am J Epidemiol 148:97–99

Gilbert EH, Lowenstein SR, Koziol-McLain J, Barta DC, Steiner J (1996) Chart reviews in emergency medicine research: Where are the methods? Ann Emerg Med 27:305–308

Gissler M, Teperi J, Hemminki E, Merilainen J (1995) Data quality after restructuring a national medical registry. Scand J Soc Med 23:75–80

Goldberg J, Gelfand HM, Levy PS (1980) Registry evaluation methods: a review and case study. Epidemiol Rev 2:210–220

Goldman LR (2001) Epidemiology in the regulatory arena. Am J Epidemiol 154: S18–S26

Goodman SN (1999a) Toward evidence-based medical statistics. 2: The Bayes factor. Ann Intern Med 130:1005–1013

Goodman SN (1999b) Toward evidence-based medical statistics: 1. The P value fallacy. Ann Intern Med 130:995–1004

Gordis L (2000) Epidemiology, 2nd edn. W.B. Saunders, Philadelphia

Greenbaum DS, Bachmann JD, Krewski D, Samet JM, White R, Wyzga RE (2001) Particulate air pollution standards and morbidity and mortality: case study. Am J Epidemiol 154:S78–S90

Halpern SD, Ubel PA, Berlin JA, Asch DA (2002) Randomized trial of 5 dollars versus 10 dollars monetary incentives, envelope size, and candy to increase physician response rates to mailed questionnaires. Med Care 40:834–839

Hawkins N, Evans J (1989) Subjective estimation of toluene exposures: a calibration study of industrial hygienists. Appl Ind Hygiene 4:61–68

Hearst N, Hulley SB (1988) Using secondary data. In: Hulley SB, Cummings SR (eds) Designing clinical research. Williams & Wilkins, Baltimore, MD, pp. 53–62

Heilbrun LK, Nomura A, Stemmermann GN (1991) The effects of non-response in a prospective study of cancer: 15-year follow-up. Int J Epidemiol 20:328–338

Hill J (2003) Certification in the Cardiovascular Health Study. Personal communication with Rajaraman P

Hilner JE, McDonald A, Van Horn L, Bragg C, Caan B, Slattery ML, Birch R, Smoak CG, Wittes J (1992) Quality control of dietary data collection in the CARDIA study. Control Clin Trials 13:156–169

Hoffman SC, Burke AE, Helzlsouer KJ, Comstock GW (1998) Controlled trial of the effect of length, incentives, and follow-up techniques on response to a mailed questionnaire. Am J Epidemiol 148:1007–1011

Holford TR, Stack C (1995) Study design for epidemiologic studies with measurement error. Stat Methods Med Res 4:339–358

Horbar JD, Leahy KA (1995) An assessment of data quality in the Vermont-Oxford Trials Network database. Control Clin Trials 16:51–61

Hosking JD, Rochon J (1982) A comparison of techniques for detecting and preventing key-field errors. Proceedings of the Statistical Computing Section. 82–87. American Statistical Association, Washington, D.C.

Hosking JD, Newhouse MM, Bagniewska A, Hawkins BS (1995) Data collection and transcription. Control Clin Trials 16:66S–103S

Hunt JR, White E (1998) Retaining and tracking cohort study members. Epidemiol Rev 20:57–70

International Organization for Standardization (2003) ISO 9000:2000, ISO Technical Committee ISO/TC 176

Ioannidis JP (1998) Effect of the statistical significance of results on the time to completion and publication of randomized efficacy trials. JAMA 279:281–286

James J, Bolstein R (1992) Large monetary incentives and their effect on mail survey response rates. Public Opinion Quarterly 56:442–453

John EM, Savitz DA (1994) Effect of a monetary incentive on response to a mail survey. Ann Epidemiol 4:231–235

Johnstone FD, Brown MC, Campbell D, MacGillivray I (1981) Measurement of variables: data quality control. Am J Clin Nutr 34:804–806

Kaaks R, Ferrari P, Ciampi A, Plummer M, Riboli E (2002) Uses and limitations of statistical accounting for random error correlations, in the validation of dietary questionnaire assessments. Public Health Nutr 5:969–976

Kalantar JS, Talley NJ (1999) The effects of lottery incentive and length of questionnaire on health survey response rates: a randomized study. J Clin Epidemiol 52:1117–1122

Kannel WB (2000) Risk stratification in hypertension: new insights from the Framingham Study. Am J Hypertens 13:3S–10S

Kellerman SE, Herold J (2001) Physician response to surveys. A review of the literature. Am J Prev Med 20:61–67

Kessler RC, Little RJ, Groves RM (1995) Advances in strategies for minimizing and adjusting for survey nonresponse. Epidemiol Rev 17:192–204

Kiesler S, Sproull L (1986) Response effects in the electronic survey. Public Opinion Quarterly 50:402–413

Kipen HM, Cody RP, Goldstein BD (1989) Use of longitudinal analysis of peripheral blood counts to validate historical reconstructions of benzene exposure. Environ Health Perspect 82:199–206

Kjelsberg MO, Cutler JA, Dolecek TA (1997) Brief description of the Multiple Risk Factor Intervention Trial. Am J Clin Nutr 65:191S–195S

Knatterud GL, Rockhold FW, George SL, Barton FB, Davis CE, Fairweather WR, Honohan T, Mowery R, O'Neill R (1998) Guidelines for quality assurance in multicenter trials: a position paper. Control Clin Trials 19:477–493

Krewski D, Burnett RT, Goldberg MS, Hoover K, Siemiatycki J, Abrahamowicz M, White WH (2000) Reanalysis of the Harvard Six Cities Study and the American Cancer Society Study of particulate air pollution and mortality. Investigators' reports parts I and II. Health Effects Institute, Cambridge, MA

Kromhout H, Oostendorp Y, Heederik D, Boleij JS (1987) Agreement between qualitative exposure estimates and quantitative exposure measurements. Am J Ind Med 12:551–562

Landis JR, Koch GG (1977) The measurement of observer agreement for categorical data. Biometrics 33:159–174

Ling PM, Glantz SA (2002) Using tobacco-industry marketing research to design more effective tobacco-control campaigns. JAMA 287:2983–2989

Little RE, Davis AK (1984) Effectiveness of various methods of contact and reimbursement on response rates of pregnant women to a mail questionnaire. Am J Epidemiol 120:161–163

Maclure M, Schneeweiss S (2001) Causation of bias: the episcope. Epidemiol 12: 114–122

Maclure M, Willett WC (1987) Misinterpretation and misuse of the kappa statistic. Am J Epidemiol 126:161–169

Maheux B, Legault C, Lambert J (1989) Increasing response rates in physicians' mail surveys: an experimental study. Am J Public Health 79:638–639

Martinson BC, Lazovich D, Lando HA, Perry CL, McGovern PG, Boyle RG (2000) Effectiveness of monetary incentives for recruiting adolescents to an intervention trial to reduce smoking. Prev Med 31:706–713

Maudsley G, Williams EM (1999) What lessons can be learned for cancer registration quality assurance from data users? Skin cancer as an example. Int J Epidemiol 28:809–815

McQuade CE, Kutvirt DM, Brylinski DA, Samet JM (1983) A tracking system for conducting epidemiological case-control studies. Comput Programs Biomed 16:149–153

Meinert CL, Tonascia S (1986) Controlled clinical trials: design, conduct, and analysis. Oxford University Press, New York

Moorman PG, Newman B, Millikan RC, Tse CK, Sandler DP (1999) Participation rates in a case-control study: the impact of age, race, and race of interviewer. Ann Epidemiol 9:188–195

Mullooly JP (1990) The effects of data entry error: an analysis of partial verification. Comput Biomed Res 23:259–267

Neaton JD, DuChene AG, Svendsen KH, Wentworth D (1990) An examination of the efficiency of some quality assurance methods commonly employed in clinical trials. Stat Med 9:115–123

Olson SH (2001) Reported participation in case-control studies: changes over time. Am J Epidemiol 154:574–581

Olson SH, Voigt LF, Begg CB, Weiss NS (2002) Reporting participation in case-control studies. Epidemiol 13:123–126

Paolo AM, Bonaminio GA, Gibson C, Partridge T, Kallail K (2000) Response rate comparisons of e-mail- and mail-distributed student evaluations. Teach Learn Med 12:81–84

Parkes R, Kreiger N, James B, Johnson KC (2000) Effects on subject response of information brochures and small cash incentives in a mail-based case-control study. Ann Epidemiol 10:117–124

Perneger TV, Etter JF, Rougemont A (1993) Randomized trial of use of a monetary incentive and a reminder card to increase the response rate to a mailed health survey. Am J Epidemiol 138:714–722

Post W, Kromhout H (1991) Semiquantitative estimates of exposure to methylene chloride adn styrene: the influence of quantitative exposure data. Applied Occupational and Environmental Hygiene 6:197–204

Prud'homme GJ, Canner PL, Cutler JA (1989) Quality assurance and monitoring in the Hypertension Prevention Trial. Hypertension Prevention Trial Research Group. Control Clin Trials 10:84S–94S

Quan SF, Howard BV, Iber C, Kiley JP, Nieto FJ, O'Connor GT, Rapoport DM, Redline S, Robbins J, Samet JM, Wahl PW (1997) The Sleep Heart Health Study: design, rationale, and methods. Sleep 20:1077–1085

Reisch LM, Fosse JS, Beverly K, Yu O, Barlow WE, Harris EL, Rolnick S, Barton MB, Geiger AM, Herrinton LJ, Greene SM, Fletcher SW, Elmore JG (2003) Training, quality assurance, and assessment of medical record abstraction in a multisite study. Am J Epidemiol 157:546–551

Rhodes SD, Bowie DA, Hergenrather KC (2003) Collecting behavioural data using the world wide web: considerations for researchers. J Epidemiol Community Health 57:68–73

Rosner B, Spiegelman D, Willett WC (1992) Correction of logistic regression relative risk estimates and confidence intervals for random within-person measurement error. Am J Epidemiol 136:1400–1413

Rothman KJ, Greenland S (1998) Modern epidemiology, 2nd edn. Lippincott-Raven, Philadelphia

Sacks FM, Handysides GH, Marais GE, Rosner B, Kass EH (1986) Effects of a low-fat diet on plasma lipoprotein levels. Arch Intern Med 146:1573–1577

Samet JM (2000) Epidemiology and policy: the pump handle meets the new millennium. Epidemiol Rev 22:145–154

Samet JM, Lee NL (2001) Bridging the gap: perspectives on translating epidemiologic evidence into policy. Am J Epidemiol 154:S1–S3

Samet JM, Zeger SL, Kelsall JE, Xu J, Kalkstein LS (1997) Particulate air pollution and daily mortality: analyses of the effects of weather and multiple air pollutants (The Phase IB Report of the Particle Epidemiology Evaluation Project). Health Effects Institute, Cambridge, MA

Schweitzer M, Asch DA (1995) Timing payments to subjects of mail surveys: cost-effectiveness and bias. J Clin Epidemiol 48:1325–1329

Shahar E, Folsom AR, Jackson R (1996) The effect of nonresponse on prevalence estimates for a referent population: insights from a population-based cohort study. Atherosclerosis Risk in Communities (ARIC) Study Investigators. Ann Epidemiol 6:498–506

Shaw MJ, Beebe TJ, Jensen HL, Adlis SA (2001) The use of monetary incentives in a community survey: impact on response rates, data quality, and cost. Health Serv Res 35:1339–1346

Silver RC, Holman EA, McIntosh DN, Poulin M, Gil-Rivas V (2002) Nationwide longitudinal study of psychological responses to September 11. JAMA 288: 1235–1244

Slattery ML, Edwards SL, Caan BJ, Kerber RA, Potter JD (1995) Response rates among control subjects in case-control studies. Ann Epidemiol 5:245–249

Sorensen HT, Sabroe S, Olsen J (1996) A framework for evaluation of secondary data sources for epidemiological research. Int J Epidemiol 25:435–442

Spiegelman D, Schneeweiss S, McDermott A (1997) Measurement error correction for logistic regression models with an "alloyed gold standard". Am J Epidemiol 145:184–196

Spry VM, Hovell MF, Sallis JG, Hofsteter CR, Elder JP, Molgaard CA (1989) Recruiting survey respondents to mailed surveys: controlled trials of incentives and prompts. Am J Epidemiol 130:166–172

Steeh C (1981) Trends in nonresponse rates 1952–1979. Public Opinion Quarterly 45:40–57

Stram DO, Langholz B, Huberman M, Thomas DC (1999) Correcting for exposure measurement error in a reanalysis of lung cancer mortality for the Colorado Plateau uranium miners cohort. Health Phys 77:265–275

Szklo M, Nieto FJ (2000) Epidemiology: beyond the basics. Aspen, Gaithersburg, MD

The Chemical Manufacturers Association's Epidemiology Task Force (1991) Guidelines for good epidemiological practices for occupational and environmental epidemiologic research. J Occup Med 33:1221–1229

Thompson WD (1990) Kappa and attenuation of the odds ratio. Epidemiol 1: 357–369

Thompson WD, Walter SD (1988) A reaapraisal of the kappa coefficient. J Clin Epidemiol 41:949–958

Thornton A, Lee P (2000) Publication bias in meta-analysis: its causes and consequences. J Clin Epidemiol 53:207–216

Tielemans E, Heederik D, Burdorf A, Vermeulen R, Veulemans H, Kromhout H, Hartog K (1999) Assessment of occupational exposures in a general population: comparison of different methods. Occup Environ Med 56:145–151

Turpin J, Rose R, Larsen B (2003) An adaptable, transportable web-based data acquisition platform for clinical and survey-based research. J Am Osteopath Assoc 103:182–186

US Department of Health and Human Services (2001) Application of a Public Health Service Grant. PHS 398. Public Health Service

US Department of Health Education and Welfare (DHEW) (1964) Smoking and health. Report of the Advisory Committee to the Surgeon General. DHEW Publication No. [PHS] 1103. U.S. Government Printing Office, Washington, DC

US Department of Health Education and Welfare (DHEW) (1973) Final report of the Tuskegee Syphilis STudy Ad Hoc Advisory Panel. US Public Health Service, Washington, D.C.

US Environmental Protection Agency (EPA) (1989) Toxic substances control act (TSCA): good laboratory practice standards. 40 CFR Part 792, 34034–34050

Vantongelen K, Rotmensz N, van der Schueren E (1989) Quality control of validity of data collected in clinical trials. EORTC Study Group on Data Management (SGDM). Eur J Cancer Clin Oncol 25:1241–1247

Vardeman SB, Jobe JM (1999) Statistical quality assurance methods for engineers. John Wiley and Sons, Hoboken, N.J.

Wacholder S, McLaughlin JK, Silverman DT, Mandel JS (1992) Selection of controls in case-control studies. I. Principles. Am J Epidemiol 135:1019–1028

Wacholder S, Armstrong B, Hartge P (1993) Validation studies using an alloyed gold standard. Am J Epidemiol 137:1251–1258

Wallace JM, Jr., Bachman JG, O'Malley PM, Johnston LD, Schulenberg JE, Cooper SM (2002) Tobacco, alcohol, and illicit drug use: racial and ethnic differences among U.S. high school seniors, 1976–2000. Public Health Rep 117 Suppl 1:S67–S75

White E, Hunt JR, Casso D (1998) Exposure measurement in cohort studies: the challenges of prospective data collection. Epidemiol Rev 20:43–56

Whitney CW, Lind BK, Wahl PW (1998) Quality assurance and quality control in longitudinal studies. Epidemiol Rev 20:71–80

Willett WC, Stampfer MJ, Underwood BA, Speizer FE, Rosner B, Hennekens CH (1983) Validation of a dietary questionnaire with plasma carotenoid and alpha-tocopherol levels. Am J Clin Nutr 38:631–639

Willett WC, Sampson L, Stampfer MJ, Rosner B, Bain C, Witschi J, Hennekens CH, Speizer FE (1985) Reproducibiltiy and validity of a semiquantitative food frequency questionaire. Am J Epidemiol 122:51–65

Wright P, Haybittle J (1979a) Design of forms for clinical trials (1). Br Med J 2: 529–530

Wright P, Haybittle J (1979b) Design of forms for clinical trials (2). Br Med J 2:590–592

Wright P, Haybittle J (1979c) Design of forms for clinical trials (3). Br Med J 2: 650–651

Wyatt J (1995) Acquisition and use of clinical data for audit and research. J Eval Clin Pract 1:15–27

Part II
Statistical Methods in Epidemiology

Sample Size Determination in Epidemiologic Studies

Janet D. Elashoff, Stanley Lemeshow

Introduction

When planning a research project an epidemiologist must consider how many subjects should be studied. While factors such as available budget certainly present constraints on the maximum number of subjects that might actually be included in a study, statistical considerations are extremely important. To address the statistical questions about appropriate sample size, the researcher must first specify the study design, the nature of the outcome variable, the aims of the study, the planned analysis method, and the expected results of the study. Is the goal of the study to distinguish between hypotheses about the value of a parameter or function of parameters, or is the goal to provide a confidence interval estimate of a parameter such as the odds ratio or relative risk?

This chapter is organized as follows. We introduce the issue of how to choose sample size for estimation of a parameter or for a hypothesis test regarding a parameter in the context of one-sample studies in which it is desired to estimate or test a population proportion. We continue on to two-sample studies involving comparisons between two proportions, and one and two-sample studies involving estimation or testing of population means. We conclude with a section on sample size for logistic regression.

In this chapter we will provide a brief introduction to power and sample size computation and only address sample size issues for a few of the procedures that are most commonly used in epidemiologic research. However, we do hope that the reader will gain a sense for what one can accomplish by planning a study with appropriate attention to sample size considerations.

A focus on sample size considerations when the study is first being planned is critical for the ultimate likelihood that a study proposal is accepted for funding and that the final manuscript will be accepted for publication. To ignore the issue of sample size would greatly increase the likelihood of embarking on a costly and time-consuming epidemiologic study with little likelihood of finding any definitive results.

One Group Designs, Inferences About Proportions

The simplest study design is one in which interest focuses on results for a single group. One is often interested in making inferences about the value of a population proportion. In this section we will illustrate how to choose sample size for the following examples:

Example 1. A district medical officer seeks to estimate the proportion of children in the district receiving appropriate childhood vaccinations. Assuming a simple random sample is to be selected from a community, how many children must be studied if the resulting estimate is to fall within 10 percentage points of the true proportion with 95% confidence? ◆

Example 2. Consider the information given in Example 1, only this time we will determine the sample size necessary to estimate the proportion vaccinated in the population to within 10% (not 10 percentage points) of the true value. ◆

Example 3. During a virulent outbreak of neonatal tetanus, health workers wish to determine whether the rate is decreasing after a period during which it had risen to a level of 150 cases per thousand live births. What sample size is necessary to test the null hypothesis that the population proportion is 0.15 at the 0.05 level if it is desired to have a 90% probability of detecting a decrease to a rate of 100 per thousand if that were the true proportion? ◆

The first two examples involve estimation and confidence intervals while the third involves a statistical hypothesis test.

The usual model underlying testing or estimation of a population proportion assumes that the design involves a simple independent random sample from a population in which the probability of a "success" is constant. The distribution of the number of successes in a sample of size n with a true underlying proportion of successes denoted by π is given by the binomial distribution. However, formulas are simplified when power and sample size determinations are made on the basis of using the normal approximation to the binomial.

The sampling distribution of the sample proportion "p" is approximately normal with mean of π (the expected value of p, $E(p) = \pi$) and variance of p, $\mathrm{Var}(p) = \pi(1 - \pi)/n$; the standard deviation is $\sqrt{\pi(1 - \pi)/n}$.

We begin by discussing sample size determination for estimation (the confidence interval approach) and then turn to sample size determination for hypothesis testing problems.

1.2.1   Confidence Intervals for a Single Population Proportion

Two-sided $100(1 - \alpha)\%$ confidence intervals for a parameter, θ, based on using the normal approximation can be stated in general as:

$$\widehat{\theta} \pm z_{1-\alpha/2}\widehat{SE}\left(\widehat{\theta}\right) , \tag{1.1}$$

where $z_{1-\alpha/2}$ is the $100(1-\alpha/2)$th percentile of the normal (or Gaussian) distribution. For the commonly used two-sided 95% confidence interval, $z_{1-\alpha/2} = 1.96$. The $100(1 - \alpha)\%$ confidence interval for π based on the estimated proportion, p, is given by

$$p \pm z_{1-\alpha/2}\sqrt{\frac{p(1-p)}{n}} \, . \tag{1.2}$$

Letting, ω be the half-width of the confidence interval for the expected true value π, we have

$$\omega = z_{1-\alpha/2}\sqrt{\frac{\pi(1-\pi)}{n}} \, . \tag{1.3}$$

The sample size necessary to achieve a confidence interval of width ω is given by

$$n = \left(\frac{z_{1-\alpha/2}}{\omega}\right)^2 [\pi(1-\pi)] \, . \tag{1.4}$$

Returning to Example 1, we begin by assuming that the rate of vaccinated children is expected to be about 75%. We would then set $\pi = 0.75$, $\omega = 0.10$ and $z_{1-\alpha/2} = 1.96$. From (1.4) we find that $n = 72.03$. Note that for sample size calculations we round up. We conclude that to estimate the expected population proportion to within ± 0.10, a sample of 73 children would be required.

If we don't really know what rate to expect we can make use of the fact that n will be largest for $\pi = 0.50$ and use this value to solve for n. For Example 1 we require a sample size of 97 to be sure that the confidence interval width will be no wider than plus or minus 10 percentage points no matter what the observed proportion is.

Table 1.1 presents the required sample sizes for selected values of π and ω.

Table 1.1. Sample size for 95% two-sided confidence interval for a proportion (using the normal approximation) to have expected width, ω

π	ω	
	± 0.05	$\perp 0.10$
0.50	385	97
0.25	289	73
0.10	139	35

Proceeding to Example 2, we consider the information given in Example 1, only this time we will determine the sample size necessary to estimate the proportion vaccinated in the population to within 10% (not 10 percentage points) of the true value.

Let θ be the unknown population parameter as before and let $\widehat{\theta}$ be the estimate of θ. Let ε, the desired precision, be defined as:

$$\varepsilon = \frac{|\widehat{\theta} - \theta|}{\theta} \, .$$

In the present example, based on the confidence limits using the normal approximation to the distribution of p, it follows that

$$|p - \pi| = z_{1-\alpha/2}\frac{\sqrt{\pi(1-\pi)}}{\sqrt{n}}$$

and, dividing both sides by π, an expression similar to the one presented above for ε is obtained. That is,

$$\varepsilon = \frac{|p - \pi|}{\pi} = z_{1-\alpha/2}\frac{\sqrt{1-\pi}}{\sqrt{n\pi}}$$

and squaring both sides and solving for n gives:

$$n = z^2_{1-\alpha/2}\frac{1-\pi}{\varepsilon^2\pi} \cdot \qquad (1.5)$$

Assuming $\pi = 0.75$, we would find that a sample size of 129 would be required to assure that the 95% confidence interval would be within 10% of the true value.

1.2.2 Hypothesis Testing for a Single Population Proportion

Suppose we would like to test a null hypothesis about the value of the population proportion

$$H_0 : \pi = \pi_0$$

versus the one-sided alternative hypothesis

$$H_a : \pi > \pi_0 .$$

Statistical hypothesis testing involves balancing the two types of errors that can be made. Type I error is defined as the error of rejecting the null hypothesis when it is in fact true. We denote the probability of making a Type I error as "α"; a commonly used choice for α is 0.05. The critical value of the test statistic is then chosen so that the probability of rejecting the null hypothesis when it is true will be α.

To choose the necessary sample size, we need to address Type II error as well. A Type II error is the error of failing to reject the null hypothesis when it is in fact false. To determine the probability of a Type II error (denoted by "β"), we must specify a particular value of interest for the alternative hypothesis, say, π_a. The probability of rejecting the null hypothesis when it is false is defined as the *power* of the test, $1 - \beta$. Typically, we require the power at the alternative of interest to be 80% or 90%.

Based on the normal approximation to the binomial, the test statistic for a test of the null hypothesis is given by

$$z = \frac{p - \pi_0}{\sqrt{\pi_0(1-\pi_0)/n}} \cdot$$

To set the probability of a Type I error equal to α, we plan to reject the null hypothesis if $z > z_{1-\alpha}$. To choose n, we fix the probability that $z > z_{1-\alpha}$ if the population proportion equals π_a to be $1 - \beta$. This may be represented graphically as shown in Fig. 1.1:

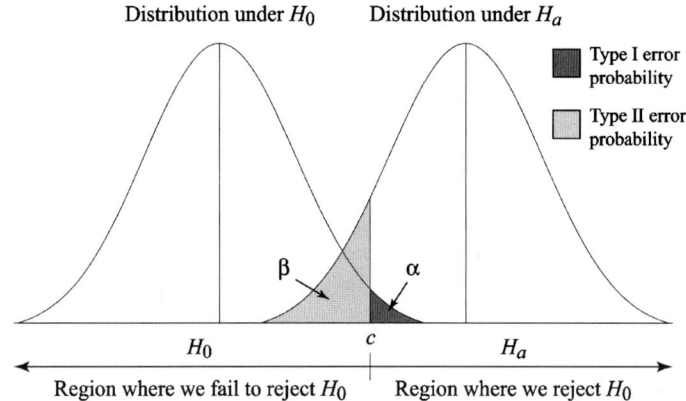

Distribution under H_0 Distribution under H_a

Type I error probability

Type II error probability

β α

H_0 c H_a

Region where we fail to reject H_0 Region where we reject H_0

Figure 1.1. Sampling distributions for one-sample hypothesis test

In this figure the point "c" represents the upper $100\,\alpha$th percent point of the distribution of p for the sampling distribution centered at π_0 (i.e., the distribution which would result if the null hypothesis were true):

$$c = \pi_0 + z_{1-\alpha}\sqrt{\pi_0\left(1 - \pi_0\right)/n}\ .$$

For the sampling distribution centered at π_a (i.e., the distribution which would result if the alternate hypothesis were true), "c" represents the lower $100\,\beta$th percent point of the distribution of p:

$$c = \pi_a + z_\beta\sqrt{\pi_a\left(1 - \pi_a\right)/n}\ .$$

In order to find n we set the two expressions equal to each other. From this, it follows that:

$$\pi_0 + z_{1-\alpha}\sqrt{\pi_0\left(1 - \pi_0\right)/n} = \pi_a + z_\beta\sqrt{\pi_a\left(1 - \pi_a\right)/n}\ .$$

Noting that $z_{1-\beta} = -z_\beta$, we find

$$\pi_a - \pi_0 = \frac{\left\{z_{1-\alpha}\sqrt{\pi_0\left(1 - \pi_0\right)} + z_{1-\beta}\sqrt{\pi_a\left(1 - \pi_a\right)}\right\}}{\sqrt{n}}$$

and, solving for n, we find that the necessary sample size, for this single sample hypothesis testing situation, is given by the formula:

$$n = \frac{\left\{ z_{1-\alpha}\sqrt{\pi_0\left(1-\pi_0\right)} + z_{1-\beta}\sqrt{\pi_a\left(1-\pi_a\right)} \right\}^2}{\left(\pi_a - \pi_0\right)^2}. \tag{1.6}$$

Notice that as π_a gets further and further away from π_0, the necessary sample size decreases.

To illustrate, we return to Example 3 in which we wish to test the null hypothesis that $\pi = 0.15$ at the one-sided 5% level and have 90% power to detect a decrease to a rate of 0.10. Using (1.6), it follows that

$$n = \frac{\left\{ 1.645\sqrt{0.15(0.85)} + 1.282\sqrt{0.10(0.90)} \right\}^2}{(0.05)^2} = 377.90 \,.$$

Hence we see that a total sample size of 378 live births would be necessary.

To plan sample size for a two-sided test, we need only substitute $z_{1-\alpha/2}$ for $z_{1-\alpha}$ in (1.6) to obtain:

$$n = \frac{\left\{ z_{1-\alpha/2}\sqrt{\pi_0\left(1-\pi_0\right)} + z_{1-\beta}\sqrt{\pi_a\left(1-\pi_a\right)} \right\}^2}{\left(\pi_a - \pi_0\right)^2}. \tag{1.7}$$

To have 90% power for a two-sided 5% level test for Example 3 would require a total of 471 subjects to detect the difference between the null hypothesis proportion, π_0, of 0.15 and the alternative proportion, π_a, of 0.10. Note that the sample size required to achieve 90% power for the specified alternative is larger when a two-sided 5% level test is planned than when a one-sided 5% level test is planned, so that the investigator needs to be clear as to whether the planned test is to be one-sided or two-sided when making sample size computations.

Table 1.2. Sample size for 0.05-level, two-sided test that the proportion equals π_0 versus the alternative π_a for specified levels of power (based on normal approximation)

		Power	
π_0	π_a	80%	90%
0.50	0.40	194	259
0.50	0.30	47	62
0.20	0.10	108	137
0.15	0.10	363	471
0.10	0.05	239	301

Table 1.2 presents the required sample sizes for selected values of π_0, π_a and power. For a two-sided test, unless the null hypothesis proportion equals 0.5, computed sample sizes for alternative proportions given by $\pi_{aL} = \pi_0 - \delta$ and

$\pi_{aU} = \pi_0 + \delta$ will differ; the larger estimate of sample size will be obtained for the alternative proportion closer to 0.5.

Additional Considerations and References

Good introductions to sample size computations for tests and confidence intervals for a single proportion can be found in Dixon and Massey (1983), Lemeshow et al. (1990), Fleiss (1981) and Lachin (1981). Books containing sample size tables are available (e.g. Machin and Campbell 1987; Machin et al. 1997; Lemeshow et al. 1990). Commercially available sample size software such as nQuery Advisor Release 5 (Elashoff 2002) can be used to compute sample size for confidence intervals or hypothesis tests (based on either the normal approximation or an exact binomial test) for a single proportion as well as for a wide variety of other sample size problems.

For values of π near 0 or 1 (or for small sample sizes), sample size methods involving a continuity correction (Fleiss et al. 1980), methods designed for rare events (e.g. Korn 1986; Louis 1981), or methods based on exact tests (Chernick and Liu 2002) may be preferable.

Note that an actual field survey is unlikely to be based on a simple random sample. As a result, the required sample size would go up by the amount of the "design effect" which is determined by the details of the actual sampling plan. The "design effect" is the ratio of the standard error of the estimated parameter under the study design to the standard error of the estimate under simple random sampling; a text on sample surveys should be consulted for details (see Levy and Lemeshow (1999)). For example, if a cluster sampling plan with a design effect of 2 were to be employed, the sample size computed using the above formulas would need to be doubled.

Comparison of Two Independent Proportions

Study Designs, Parameters, Analysis Methods

More sample size literature exists for the problem of comparing two independent proportions than for any other sample size problem. This has come about because there are several basic sampling schemes leading to problems of this type. There are different parameterizations of interest and a variety of test and estimation procedures that have been developed. Sample size formulations depend on the parameter of interest for testing or estimation as well as the specifics of the test or estimation procedure.

The basic study designs relevant to epidemiological studies are experimental trials, cohort studies, and case-control studies. We describe each study type briefly and give an example. The examples will be addressed in more detail in subsequent sections.

Experimental Trial. $2n$ subjects are recruited for a study; n are randomly assigned to group 1 and n to group 2. The intervention is applied according to the design. Subjects are followed for a fixed time and success-failure status is recorded. Experimental trials are usually randomized, often double blind, and always prospective. For example, patients with intestinal parasites are randomly assigned to receive either the standard drug or a new drug and followed to determine whether they respond favorably. The observed proportion responding favorably in group i is denoted by p_i and the true population proportion in group i by π_i.

Experimental trials are typically analyzed in terms of the difference in proportions, or the risk difference.

$$\text{Population risk difference} = \pi_1 - \pi_2 \qquad (1.8)$$

$$\text{Estimated risk difference} = p_1 - p_2 \qquad (1.9)$$

Cohort Study. n subjects are recruited from group 1 and n from group 2; subjects are followed for a fixed time and success-failure status is recorded. Cohort studies are typically prospective studies. For example, workers with asbestos exposure and workers in the same industry without asbestos exposure are followed for the development of lung disease.

Cohort studies may be analyzed in terms of the risk difference or in terms of the relative risk.

$$\text{Population relative risk} = RR = \pi_2/\pi_1 \qquad (1.10)$$

$$\text{Estimated relative risk} = rr = p_2/p_1 \qquad (1.11)$$

Referring to the example, π_1 denotes the true proportion of diseased workers in the unexposed group while π_2 denotes the true proportion of diseased workers in the exposed group, and p_1 and p_2 are the corresponding observed proportions.

Case-Control Studies. n subjects (cases) are recruited from among those who have developed a disease and n subjects (controls) are recruited from a similar group without the disease. Subjects from both groups are studied for the presence of a relevant exposure in their background. For example, tuberculosis (TB) cases and controls are assessed for whether they had been vaccinated with BCG (Bacillus Calmette-Guérin vaccine). Case-control studies are inherently retrospective studies and interest is focused on the odds ratio.

$$\text{Population odds ratio} = OR = \pi_2 \left(1 - \pi_1\right)/\left(1 - \pi_2\right)\pi_1 \qquad (1.12)$$

$$\text{Estimated odds ratio} = or = p_2 \left(1 - p_1\right)/\left(1 - p_2\right)p_1 \qquad (1.13)$$

Referring to the example, π_1 denotes the true proportion of vaccinated subjects among the controls while π_2 denotes the true proportion of vaccinated subjects among the TB cases, and p_1 and p_2 are the corresponding observed proportions.

We begin by discussing sample size determination for estimation (the confidence interval approach) and then turn to sample size determination for hypothesis testing problems.

Confidence Intervals for the Risk Difference

Example 4. A pilot study with 20 subjects randomized to receive the standard drug to control intestinal parasites and 20 to receive a new drug found that 13 subjects (65%) receiving the standard drug responded favorably while 17 (85%) of the subjects receiving the new drug responded favorably.

Question 4a: Do these data establish that the new drug is better (lower limit of confidence interval is greater than zero) and, if not, might it still be enough better to warrant a larger clinical trial? We address this question with a confidence interval below.

Question 4b: What sample size would be required for the larger clinical trial? We address this question in the context of a confidence interval later in this section, and in the context of a hypothesis test in the following section. ◆

The estimated value of the risk difference, $\pi_1 - \pi_2$, is given by $p_1 - p_2$, the observed difference in proportions. The variance of $p_1 - p_2$ for independent proportions when the sample sizes, n, in each group are equal is:

$$\text{Var}\,(p_1 - p_2) = \frac{\pi_1(1 - \pi_1) + \pi_2(1 - \pi_2)}{n}. \tag{1.14}$$

This formula is based on the assumption that the data come from independent random samples from the populations of interest. In population i, the probability of a success is a constant, π_i, and therefore the number of successes observed for each group has a binomial distribution with parameters n and π_i.

The standard error of this estimate, $p_1 - p_2$, is estimated by substituting the observed proportions for the true proportions and is given by

$$SE(p_1 - p_2) = \frac{\sqrt{p_1(1 - p_1) + p_2(1 - p_2)}}{\sqrt{n}}. \tag{1.15}$$

Referring to the basic formula for a confidence interval based on the normal approximation given in (1.1), a two-sided 95% confidence interval for the difference in the proportions responding favorably to the new drug in comparison to the old drug is given by

$$0.85 - 0.65 \pm 1.96 \frac{\sqrt{0.85(1 - 0.85) + 0.65(1 - 0.65)}}{\sqrt{20}}.$$

The limits are 0.20 ± 0.209 or -0.009 to 0.409, suggesting that although we cannot rule out a difference of zero the data indicate that the new drug might work markedly better than the standard.

The investigator wants to plan a definitive study to assess how much the success rates really do differ. What sample size would be necessary to obtain a confidence interval whose width is less than or equal to ± 0.05?

We require that the confidence interval for $\pi_1 - \pi_2$, be $p_1 - p_2 \pm \omega$, where for Example 4, $\omega \le 0.05$. To obtain a confidence interval width satisfying these conditions, we must have

$$z_{1-\alpha/2} \frac{\sqrt{\pi_1(1-\pi_1) + \pi_2(1-\pi_2)}}{\sqrt{n}} \le \omega .$$

Solving this equation for n, the sample size in each group, we obtain (1.16).

$$n = \frac{z_{1-\alpha/2}^2 \left[\pi_1(1-\pi_1) + \pi_2(1-\pi_2)\right]}{\omega^2} . \tag{1.16}$$

For Example 4, an n per group of 546 would be required to obtain an expected 95% two-sided confidence interval width of approximately ± 0.05 if we expect to see about the same proportions as we did in the pilot study.

Table 1.3 presents the sample size in each group necessary to obtain specified confidence interval widths for a few selected examples. This table should provide investigators with a quick idea of the order of magnitude of required sample sizes. Note that since the confidence interval width depends on the postulated proportions only through the terms $\pi_i(1-\pi_i)$, this table can also be used for proportions greater than 0.5.

If an investigator is a bit uncertain about what proportions to expect and wants to ensure that the confidence interval width is less than some specified amount $\pm \omega$ no matter what proportions are observed, we can use the fact that the confidence interval is widest when $\pi_1 = \pi_2 = 0.5$. In this case the sample size required for each group is

$$n \le \frac{z_{1-\alpha/2}^2}{2\omega^2} . \tag{1.17}$$

Table 1.3. Sample size per group for 95% two-sided confidence interval (using normal approximation) for risk difference to have expected width, ω

| | | ω | |
π_1	π_2	± 0.05	± 0.10
0.50	0.50	769	193
0.50	0.25	673	169
0.50	0.10	523	131
0.25	0.25	577	145
0.25	0.10	427	107
0.10	0.10	277	70

For a two-sided 95% confidence interval this becomes approximately $2/\omega^2$. For Example 4, the maximum sample size per group required for a confidence interval width of no more than ± 0.05 is 769.

Confidence Interval for Relative Risk (Ratio) 1.3.3

Example 5.   Workers with asbestos exposure and workers in the same industry without asbestos exposure are followed for the development of lung disease. Suppose that disease occurs in 20% of the unexposed group, how large a sample would be needed in each of the exposed and unexposed study groups to estimate the relative risk to within 10% of the true value with 95% confidence assuming that the relative risk is approximately 1.75?   ◆

For this purpose we define group 1 as the unexposed group and group 2 as the exposed group. The estimate of the relative risk (cf. Chap. I.2 of this handbook) is

$$\widehat{RR} = rr = p_2/p_1 \ .$$

Since we are dealing with a ratio, which can be expected to have a skewed distribution with a log-normal shape, we need to take logs to normalize the distribution so that the normal approximation can be used to construct the confidence interval.

We obtain the standard deviation for the estimate for the case where the sample sizes in the two groups are equal by using the approximation

$$\text{Var}\left(\ln(rr)\right) \approx \frac{1 - \pi_1}{n\pi_1} + \frac{1 - \pi_2}{n\pi_2} \ . \tag{1.18}$$

The estimated standard deviation is obtained by substituting the estimated proportions for the population proportions and taking the square root.

The $100(1 - \alpha)\%$ confidence limits for $\ln(RR)$ are given by $\ln(rr) \pm \omega$ where

$$\omega = z_{1-\alpha/2}\widehat{SE}\left(\ln(rr)\right) = z_{1-\alpha/2}\sqrt{\frac{1 - \pi_1}{n\pi_1} + \frac{1 - \pi_2}{n\pi_2}} \ .$$

Then the confidence limits for RR are given by $\exp\left(\ln\left(rr_L\right)\right)$ and $\exp\left(\ln\left(rr_U\right)\right)$ where $\ln\left(rr_L\right)$ and $\ln\left(rr_U\right)$ are the lower and upper confidence limits for $\ln(RR)$.

To choose the sample size necessary to obtain a confidence interval of a desired width for $\ln(RR)$, we could simply specify ω and solve for n.

$$m = \frac{z_{1-\alpha/2}^2\left[(1 - \pi_1)/\pi_1 + (1 - \pi_2)/\pi_2\right]}{\omega^2} \ . \tag{1.19}$$

Alternatively, an investigator may wish to specify the width in terms of how close the limits are to RR. For example, suppose that we are thinking in terms of values of $RR > 1$, and that we want the difference between RR and RR_L to be no greater than

εRR; that is, we set $RR - RR_L = \varepsilon RR$ which we rearrange to get $RR(1 - \varepsilon) = RR_L$. Then, taking logs, we have

$$\ln(RR) + \ln(1 - \varepsilon) = \ln\left(RR_L\right)$$

and

$$\ln(RR) - \ln\left(RR_L\right) = -\ln(1 - \varepsilon) = \omega$$

so

$$\omega = z_{1-\alpha/2}\sqrt{\frac{1 - \pi_1}{n\pi_1} + \frac{1 - \pi_2}{n\pi_2}} = -\ln(1 - \varepsilon) \, .$$

Then to find the necessary sample size for each group, we solve for n to obtain

$$n = \frac{z_{1-\alpha/2}^2\left[(1 - \pi_1)/\pi_1 + (1 - \pi_2)/\pi_2\right]}{[\ln(1 - \varepsilon)]^2} \, . \tag{1.20}$$

A version of this, which substitutes the expected RR for π_2, is

$$n = \frac{z_{1-\alpha/2}^2\left[(1 + RR)/(RR\pi_1) - 2\right]}{[\ln(1 - \varepsilon)]^2} \, . \tag{1.21}$$

Returning to Example 5, the expected $RR = 1.75$, $\pi_1 = 0.20$, and we have requested that the lower limit of the confidence interval for RR be within 10% of the true value of RR. Therefore $\varepsilon = 0.1$, $1 - \varepsilon = 0.9$ and the required sample size would be 2027 per group or 4054 total.

Table 1.4 presents the sample size in each group necessary to obtain specified confidence interval widths for a few selected examples.

Table 1.4. Sample size per group for 95% two-sided confidence interval for the relative risk to have lower limit $(1 - \varepsilon)RR$

RR	π_1	ε	
		0.10	0.20
1.25	0.20	2423	540
1.50	0.20	2192	489
1.75	0.20	2027	452
2.00	0.20	1904	424
1.25	0.40	866	193

1.3.4   Confidence Intervals for the Odds Ratio

Example 6.   The efficacy of BCG vaccine in preventing childhood tuberculosis is in doubt and a study is designed to compare the immunization coverage rates in a group of tuberculosis cases compared to a group of controls.

Available information indicated that roughly 30% of controls are not vaccinated and we wish to estimate the odds ratio to within 20% of the true value. It is believed that the odds ratio is likely to be about 2.0.   ◆

For problems involving estimation of the odds ratio (cf. Chap. I.2 of this handbook) we let group 1 denote the controls and group 2 denote the cases. Our estimate of the odds ratio is

$$or = \frac{p_2 (1 - p_1)}{(1 - p_2) p_1} .$$

Since we are dealing with a ratio we need to take logs so that the normal approximation can be used to construct the confidence interval.

We obtain the standard deviation for the estimate for the case where the sample sizes in the two groups are equal by using the approximation

$$\text{Var} \left(\ln(or) \right) \approx \frac{1}{n\pi_1(1 - \pi_1)} + \frac{1}{n\pi_2(1 - \pi_2)} . \tag{1.22}$$

The estimated standard deviation is obtained by substituting the estimated proportions for the population proportions and taking the square root.

To obtain a $100(1 - \alpha)\%$ confidence interval for $\ln(OR)$ of width ω where $\omega = z_{1-\alpha/2} SE \left(\ln(or) \right)$ when the sample sizes in the two groups are equal we require a sample size per group of

$$n = \frac{z_{1-\alpha/2}^2 \left[1/ \left(\pi_2(1 - \pi_2) \right) + 1/ \left(\pi_1(1 - \pi_1) \right) \right]}{\omega^2} . \tag{1.23}$$

In situations where we assume that the odds ratio is greater than 1.0, to specify that the lower limit of the confidence interval be no less than $(1 - \varepsilon)OR$, we would set $\omega = -\ln(1 - \varepsilon)$ as we did in the previous section for the relative risk. We then obtain

$$n = \frac{z_{1-\alpha/2}^2 \left[1/ \left(\pi_2(1 - \pi_2) \right) + 1/ \left(\pi_1(1 - \pi_1) \right) \right]}{[\ln(1 - \varepsilon)]^2} . \tag{1.24}$$

Solving for π_2 using (1.12), we have

$$\pi_2 = \frac{OR\pi_1}{OR\pi_1 + (1 - \pi_1)}$$

and we can obtain sample size expressed in terms of π_1 and OR.

$$n = z_{1-\alpha/2}^2 \left[\frac{OR + (1 - \pi_1 + OR\pi_1)^2}{\pi_1(1 - \pi_1)OR[\ln(1 - \varepsilon)]^2} \right] . \tag{1.25}$$

For Example 6, we have $OR = 2$, $\pi_1 = 0.30$, $(\pi_2 = 0.462)$ and $(1 - \varepsilon) = 0.8$, so we need 678 subjects per group.

Table 1.5 presents the sample size in each group necessary to obtain specified confidence interval widths for OR for a few selected examples.

Table 1.5. Sample size per group for 95% two-sided confidence interval for *OR* to have lower limit $(1 - \varepsilon)OR$

OR	π_1	ε 0.10	0.20
1.25	0.30	3171	708
1.50	0.30	3101	692
1.75	0.30	3061	683
2.00	0.30	3040	678
1.25	0.50	2786	621

1.3.5   Testing the Difference Between Two Proportions

The goal is to test

$$H_0 : \pi_1 = \pi_2 \quad \text{versus} \quad H_1 : \pi_1 \neq \pi_2 .$$

If it can be assumed that the samples of size n from both groups arise from independent binomial distributions, the test for H_0 can be performed using the normal approximation to the binomial.

The test statistic is

$$z = \frac{\sqrt{n}\,(p_1 - p_2)}{\sqrt{2\bar{p}\,(1 - \bar{p})}}, \tag{1.26}$$

where $z \sim N(0, 1)$, i.e. z is normally distributed with mean 0 and variance 1, and where, in the general case with unequal sample sizes in the two groups,

$$\bar{p} = \frac{n_1 p_1 + n_2 p_2}{n_1 + n_2},$$

whereas for equal sample sizes

$$\bar{p} = \frac{p_1 + p_2}{2}.$$

(Note that the two-sided z test given by (1.26) is algebraically equivalent to the standard χ^2 test.)

The sample size in each group required for a two-sided $100(1 - \alpha)\%$ test to have power $1 - \beta$ is

$$n = \frac{\left[z_{1-\alpha/2}\sqrt{2\bar{\pi}(1 - \bar{\pi})} + z_{1-\beta}\sqrt{\pi_1(1 - \pi_1) + \pi_2(1 - \pi_2)} \right]^2}{\left(\pi_1 - \pi_2\right)^2} \tag{1.27}$$

and $\bar{\pi}$ is defined by analogy with $\bar{p}$.

Example 7. Typically, the outcome measure for placebo controlled double-blind trials for acute duodenal ulcer healing is the proportion of patients whose ulcer has healed by four weeks as ascertained by endoscopy. The healing rate for the placebo group is typically about 40%. H_2-blocking active drugs usually result in 70% healed. The investigator wishes to evaluate a new drug with the expectation of seeking FDA (US Food and Drug Administration) approval; the results will be assessed by comparing observed proportions healed using the χ^2 test at the two-sided 5% significance level. Such trials are expensive to mount so that if the new drug is as effective as those currently approved, the investigator wants a 90% chance that the trial will yield a significant result.   ◆

Using (1.27) for a two-sided 5% test, a sample size of 56 patients per group or a total sample size of 112 patients would be required to achieve 90% power.

Table 1.6 presents the sample size in each group necessary for a 5% two-sided χ^2 test comparing two independent proportions to have specified power for a few selected examples.

Table 1.6. Sample size per group for 5% two-sided χ^2 test for the difference between two independent proportions to have specified power

		Power	
π_1	π_2	80%	90%
0.10	0.05	435	582
0.25	0.10	100	133
0.50	0.25	58	77
0.50	0.10	20	26

Testing the Relative Risk   1.3.6

In a cohort study, where we want to focus attention on a test of the relative risk

$$H_0 : RR = \frac{\pi_2}{\pi_1} = 1 \, ,$$

the large sample test for this null hypothesis is the same as for the null hypothesis that the difference in proportions is zero and therefore the sample size formulas are the same. If we substitute RR into (1.27) we obtain

$$n = \frac{\left[z_{1-\alpha/2}\sqrt{(1 + RR)[1 - \pi_1(1 + RR)/2]} + z_{1-\beta}\sqrt{[1 + RR - \pi_1(1 + RR^2)]} \right]^2}{\pi_1(1 - RR)^2} \, .$$

$$(1.28)$$

Example 8.   Two competing therapies for a particular cancer are to be evaluated
by the cohort study strategy in a multi-center clinical trial. Patients
are randomized to either treatment A or B and are followed for recurrence of
disease for five years following treatment. How many patients should be studied in
each of the two arms of the trial in order to have 90% power to reject $H_0 : RR = 1$
in favor of the alternative $RR = 0.5$, if the test is to be performed at the two-sided
$\alpha = 0.05$ level and it is assumed that $\pi_1 = 0.35$?   ◆

For Example 8, we substitute $\pi_1 = 0.35$ and $RR = 0.5$ into (1.28) and find that
the required sample size per group would be 131 or 262 total. Or we could have
noted that $\pi_2 = 0.175$ and used (1.27).

Table 1.7 presents the sample size in each group necessary for a 5% two-sided
normal approximation test of the null hypothesis that the relative risk is 1.0 to have
specified power for a few selected examples.

Table 1.7. Sample size per group for 5% two-sided test that the relative risk equals 1 to have specified
power

		Power	
RR	π_1	80%	90%
1.25	0.20	1094	1464
1.50	0.20	294	392
1.75	0.20	138	185
2.00	0.20	82	109
1.25	0.40	388	519

1.3.7   Testing the Odds Ratio

The null hypothesis that the odds ratio equals 1.0 can be tested using (1.26) as
for the test of difference in proportions. Sample size formulas can be modified
to be based on π_2 and OR by algebraic substitution in (1.27) if desired, however
formulas are simpler if we use (1.12) to solve for the other proportion and use (1.27)
directly.

Example 9.   The efficacy of BCG vaccine in preventing childhood tuberculosis
is in doubt and a study is designed to compare the immunization
coverage rates in a group of tuberculosis cases compared to a group of controls.
Available information indicates that roughly 30% of the controls are not vaccinated, and we wish to have an 80% chance of detecting whether the odds ratio
is significantly different from 1 at the 5% level. If an odds ratio of 2 would be
considered an important difference between the two groups, how large a sample
should be included in each study group?   ◆

For Example 9, $\pi_1 = 0.3$ and $OR = 2$ and thus $\pi_2 = 0.462$; so using (1.27) we find that to obtain 80% power for a two-sided 5% level test would require 141 subjects per group or 282 total.

Table 1.8 presents the sample size in each group necessary to obtain specified power for tests of $OR = 1$ for a few selected examples.

Table 1.8. Sample size per group for 5% two-sided test of $OR = 1$ to have specified power

		Power	
OR	π_1	80%	90%
1.25	0.30	1442	1930
1.50	0.30	425	569
1.75	0.30	219	293
2.00	0.30	141	188
1.25	0.50	1267	1695

Additional Considerations and References

1.3.8

Good introductions to sample size computations for tests and confidence intervals for comparing two independent proportions can be found in Dixon and Massey (1983), Lemeshow et al. (1990), Fleiss (1981) and Lachin (1981). Books containing sample size tables are available (e.g. Machin and Campbell 1987; Machin et al. 1997; Lemeshow et al. 1990). Commercially available sample size software such as nQuery Advisor Release 5 (Elashoff 2002) can be used to compute sample size (or width) for confidence intervals and sample size (or power) for hypothesis tests for the two proportion case (based on either the normal approximation, continuity corrected normal approximation or Fisher's exact test) as well as for a wide variety of other sample size problems.

For values of π near 0 or 1 (or for small sample sizes), sample size methods involving a continuity correction (Fleiss et al. 1980), or methods based on exact tests (Chernick and Liu 2002) may be preferable.

When plans call for the sample sizes in the two groups to be unequal, the formulas for sample size and power must incorporate the expected ratio of the sample sizes, see references above. Generally for the same total sample size, power will tend to be higher and confidence interval widths narrower when sample sizes are equal; for comparisons of proportions, total sample size will depend on whether the proportion closer to 0.5 has the larger or the smaller sample size.

Note that the sample size methods discussed above do not apply to correlation/ agreement/repeated measures (or pair-matched case-control) studies in which N subjects are recruited and each subject is measured by two different raters, or is studied under two different treatments in a cross-over design. These designs cannot be analyzed using the methods described for independent proportions; for example, sample size computations for the difference between two correlated proportions are based on the McNemar test (Lachin 1992).

One Group Designs, Inferences About a Single Mean

1.4

We turn to consideration of continuous outcomes and to inferences about the population mean. We denote the true but unknown mean in the population by μ and assume that the standard deviation for the population is given by σ. For a random sample of size n from a population with a normal (Gaussian) distribution, the distribution of the observed sample mean, $\bar{x}$, will also be normal with mean μ and standard deviation (also referred to as the standard error) given by $SE(\bar{x}) = \sigma/\sqrt{n}$. By the central limit theorem, the sampling distribution of the sample mean can usually be expected to be approximately normal for sample sizes of 30 or above even when the underlying population distribution is not normal.

1.4.1   Confidence Intervals for a Single Mean

Example 10.   Suppose an estimate is desired of the average retail price of twenty tablets of a commonly used tranquilizer. A random sample of retail pharmacies is to be selected. The estimate is required to be within 10 cents of the true average price with 95% confidence. Based on a small pilot study, the standard deviation in price, σ, can be estimated as 85 cents. How many pharmacies should be randomly selected?   ◆

Using the normal approximation, the two-sided $100(1 - \alpha)\%$ confidence interval for the true mean, μ, for the case where the standard deviation is known, is given by

$$\bar{x} \pm z_{1-\alpha/2}\sigma/\sqrt{n}. \tag{1.29}$$

So the sample size required to obtain a confidence interval of width ω is

$$n = \frac{z_{1-\alpha/2}^2 \sigma^2}{\omega^2}. \tag{1.30}$$

For Example 10, expressing costs in dollars,

$$n = \frac{(1.96)^2(0.85)^2}{(0.10)^2} = 277.6.$$

Therefore a sample size of 278 pharmacies should be selected.

We should note however that usually the standard deviation must be estimated from the sample. Then, the actual confidence interval for a sample mean would be given by

$$\bar{x} \pm t_{n-1,1-\alpha/2}s/\sqrt{n}, \tag{1.31}$$

where s is the observed standard deviation and $t_{n-1,1-\alpha/2}$ denotes the $100\left(1 - \alpha/2\right)$th percentile of the t distribution with $n-1$ degrees of freedom. The value of $t_{n-1,1-\alpha/2}$ is always greater than $z_{1-\alpha/2}$; the values are close for large n, but t may be considerably larger than z for very small samples.

The required sample size would need to be larger than given by (1.30) simply to reflect the fact that $t_{n-1,1-\alpha/2} > z_{1-\alpha/2}$. In addition, the value of the standard deviation estimated from the sample will differ from the true standard deviation. The observed value of s may be either smaller or larger than the true value of the standard deviation, σ, and it can be expected to be larger than σ in about half of samples. So, even for large n, the observed confidence interval width will be greater than the specified ω in about half of planned studies.

To ensure that the observed confidence width will be shorter than ω more than half the time, we must take the distribution of s into account in the sample size computations. To solve for the required sample size for a confidence interval whose width has a specified probability, $1-\gamma$, of being narrower than ω requires the use of sample size software since an iterative solution based on the F and χ^2 distributions must be used (Kupper and Hafner 1989).

Returning to Example 10, specifying in nQuery Advisor that the observed confidence interval width needs to be shorter than 0.1 with a probability of 50% ($1 - \gamma = 0.5$) yields a required sample size of 280, only slightly larger than that given by (1.30). However, to increase the likelihood that the observed confidence interval width will be shorter than ω from 50% to 90% would require an increase in sample size from 280 to 309 (see Table 1.9).

Table 1.10 shows the required sample sizes for two-sided 95% confidence intervals to have specified widths (expressed in terms of ω/σ).

Table 1.9. Confidence interval for mean based on t (with coverage probability)

	1	2
Confidence level, $1 - \alpha$	0.950	0.950
1 or 2 sided interval?	2	2
Coverage probability, $1 - \gamma$	0.500	0.900
Standard deviation, σ	0.850	0.850
Distance from mean to limit, ω	0.100	0.100
n	280	309

Table 1.10. Sample size for 95% two-sided confidence interval for a single mean to have width less than or equal to ω with probability

ω/σ	$100(1 - \gamma)$	
	50%	90%
0.05	1539	1609
0.10	386	421
0.20	98	116
0.30	45	56
0.50	18	24

Note that nQuery Advisor has been used to compute the sample sizes displayed in all the rest of the tables in this chapter.

Hypothesis Testing for a Single Population Mean

Suppose we would like to test the hypothesis

$$H_0 : \mu = \mu_0$$

versus the alternative hypothesis

$$H_a : \mu > \mu_0$$

and we would like to fix the level of the Type I error to equal α and the Type II error to equal β. That is, we want the power of the test to equal $1 - \beta$. We denote the actual value of the population mean under the alternative hypothesis as μ_a. Following the same development as for hypothesis testing about the population proportion (with the additional assumption that the variance of $\bar{x}$ is equal to σ^2/n under both H_0 and H_a), the necessary sample size for this hypothesis testing situation is given by:

$$n = \frac{\sigma^2 \left[z_{1-\alpha} + z_{1-\beta} \right]^2}{\left[\mu_0 - \mu_a \right]^2} . \tag{1.32}$$

Alternatively, defining the effect size as

$$\delta = \frac{\mu_0 - \mu_a}{\sigma} , \tag{1.33}$$

we have

$$n = \frac{\left[z_{1-\alpha} + z_{1-\beta} \right]^2}{\delta^2} . \tag{1.34}$$

Example 11 .   Pre and post studies with placebo in a variety of studies indicated that the standard deviation of blood pressure change was about 6 mm Hg and that the mean reduction in the placebo group was typically close to 5 mm Hg. To make a preliminary estimate of the value of a new intervention designed to lower blood pressure it was planned to enroll subjects and test the null hypothesis that mean reduction was 5 mm Hg. The new intervention would be of interest if the mean reduction was 10 or greater. How large a sample would be necessary to test, at the 5% level of significance with a power of 90%, whether the average blood pressure reduction is 5 mm Hg versus the alternative that the reduction is 10 mm Hg when it is assumed that the standard deviation is 6 mm Hg? ◆

Using (1.32) we have

$$n = \frac{6^2 (1.645 + 1.282)^2}{(10 - 5)^2} = 12.33 .$$

Therefore, a sample of 13 patients with high blood pressure would be required.

A similar approach is followed when the alternative is two-sided. That is, when we wish to test

$$H_0 : \mu = \mu_0$$

versus

$$H_a : \mu \neq \mu_0 .$$

In this situation, the null hypothesis is rejected if $\bar{x}$ is too large or too small. We assign area $\alpha/2$ to each tail of the sampling distribution under H_0. The only adjustment to (1.32) is that $z_{1-\alpha/2}$ is used in place of $z_{1-\alpha}$ resulting in

$$n = \frac{\sigma^2 \left[z_{1-\alpha/2} + z_{1-\beta} \right]^2}{\left[\mu_0 - \mu_a \right]^2} . \tag{1.35}$$

Returning to Example 11, a two-sided test could be used to test the hypothesis that the average reduction in blood pressure is 5 mm Hg versus the alternative that the average reduction in blood pressure has increased, and that a reduction of 10 mm Hg would be considered important. Using (1.35) with $z_{1-\alpha/2} = 1.960$, $z_{1-\beta} = 1.282$ and $\sigma = 6$,

$$n = \frac{6^2(1.960 + 1.282)^2}{(10 - 5)^2} = 15.1 .$$

Thus, 16 patients would be required for the sample if the alternative were two-sided.

Since usually the true standard deviation is unknown, a more accurate solution for the necessary sample size would require use of sample size software (computations are based on the central and non-central t distributions). Unlike the situation for confidence intervals, the normal approximation formula works well for computing sample size for a test; its accuracy can be improved by adding the correction factor

$$\frac{z_{1-\alpha/2}^2}{2} \tag{1.36}$$

before rounding up. For Example 11 this would lead to a sample size estimate of 18 (which agrees with the result given by nQuery Advisor).

Table 1.11 presents the sample sizes necessary for 80% or 90% power for two-sided 5% level tests for specified effect sizes, δ.

Table 1.11. Sample size for two-sided 5% level t test to detect effect size $\delta = \mu_1 - \mu_2/\sigma$

δ	80% power	90% power
0.2	199	265
0.4	52	68
0.6	24	32
0.8	15	19
1.0	10	13
1.2	8	10

Comparison of Two Independent Means

Confidence Intervals
for the Difference Between Two Means

The difference between two population means is represented by a new parameter, $\mu_1 - \mu_2$. An estimate of this parameter is given by the difference in the sample means, $\bar{x}_1 - \bar{x}_2$. The mean of the sampling distribution of $\bar{x}_1 - \bar{x}_2$ is

$$E\left(\bar{x}_1 - \bar{x}_2\right) = \mu_1 - \mu_2$$

and the variance of this distribution when the two samples are independent is

$$\text{Var}\left(\bar{x}_1 - \bar{x}_2\right) = \text{Var}\left(\bar{x}_1\right) + \text{Var}\left(\bar{x}_2\right) = \frac{\sigma_1^2}{n_1} + \frac{\sigma_2^2}{n_2},$$

where n_1 and n_2 are the sample sizes in the two groups.

In order for the distribution of the difference in sample means, $\bar{x}_1 - \bar{x}_2$ to have a t distribution, we must assume that $\sigma_1^2 = \sigma_2^2 = \sigma^2$. When the variances are equal and both sample sizes are equal to n, the formula for the variance of the difference can be simplified to

$$\text{Var}\left(\bar{x}_1 - \bar{x}_2\right) = \frac{2\sigma^2}{n}.$$

The value σ^2 is an unknown population parameter, which can be estimated from sample data by pooling the individual sample variances, s_1^2 and s_2^2 to form the *pooled variance*, s_p^2, where, in the general case,

$$s_p^2 = \frac{\left(n_1 - 1\right) s_1^2 + \left(n_2 - 1\right) s_2^2}{\left(n_1 - 1\right) + \left(n_2 - 1\right)}.$$

Example 12.   Nutritionists wish to estimate the difference in caloric intake at lunch between children in a school offering a hot school lunch program and children in a school that does not. From other nutrition studies, they estimate that the standard deviation in caloric intake among elementary school children is 75 calories, and they wish to make their estimate to within 20 calories of the true difference with 95% confidence.   ♦

Using the normal approximation, the two-sided $100\left(1 - \alpha/2\right)\%$ confidence interval for the true mean, $\mu_1 - \mu_2$, is given by

$$\bar{x}_1 - \bar{x}_2 \pm z_{1-\alpha/2} 2\sigma/\sqrt{n}. \tag{1.37}$$

So the sample size in each group required to obtain a confidence interval of width ω is

$$n = \frac{z^2_{1-\alpha/2} 2\sigma^2}{\omega^2} . \tag{1.38}$$

For Example 12,

$$n = \frac{(1.96)^2 (2)(75)^2}{(20)^2} = 108.05 .$$

Thus, a sample size of 109 children from each school should be selected.

We note, however, that the actual confidence interval for the difference in sample means would be given by

$$\bar{x}_1 - \bar{x}_2 \pm t_{2n-2,1-\alpha/2} s_p \sqrt{2}/\sqrt{n} , \tag{1.39}$$

where s_p is the observed pooled standard deviation and $t_{2n-2,1-\alpha/2}$ denotes the $100(1 - \alpha/2)$ percentile of the t distribution with $2(n - 1)$ degrees of freedom. So, as explained in the section on confidence intervals for a single mean, to solve for the required sample size for a confidence interval whose width has a specified probability, $1-\gamma$, of being narrower than ω requires the use of sample size software.

For Example 12, we show in Table 1.12 (pasted from nQuery Advisor) that a sample of 109 per group provides a 50% probability that the observed 95% confidence interval will have half-width less than 20, while to have a 90% probability that the confidence interval half-width will be less than 20 would require a sample of 123 children per school.

Table 1.12. Confidence interval for difference of two means (coverage probability) (equal *n*'s)

	1	2
Confidence level, $1 - \alpha$	0.950	0.950
1 or 2 sided interval?	2	2
Coverage probability, $1 - \gamma$	0.500	0.900
Common standard deviation, σ	75.000	75.000
Distance from difference to limit, ω	20.000	20.000
n per group	109	123

Table 1.13. Sample size per group for 95% two-sided confidence interval for the difference in means to have width less than or equal to $\pm\omega$ with probability $(1 - \gamma)$

	$100(1 - \gamma)$	
ω/σ	50%	90%
0.05	3075	3145
0.10	770	805
0.20	193	211
0.30	87	98
0.50	36	39

Table 1.13 presents the sample sizes in each group required so that the two-sided 95% confidence interval for the difference in two independent means will be no wider than $\pm\omega$ with probability $(1 - \gamma)$.

1.5.2   Testing the Difference Between Two Means (Two-Sample t Test)

The two-sample t test is used to test hypotheses about the population means in two independent groups of subjects. It is based on the assumptions that the underlying population distributions have equal standard deviations, and that the population distributions are Gaussian (normal) in shape or that the sample sizes in each group are large. (In most cases, the distribution of the sample mean will be approximately Gaussian for sample sizes greater than 30.)

We consider tests of the null hypothesis:

$$H_0 : \mu_1 = \mu_2 \quad \text{or}$$

$$H_0 : \mu_1 - \mu_2 = 0$$

versus either

$$H_a : \mu_1 \neq \mu_2 \quad \text{for a two-sided test, or}$$

$$H_a' : \mu_1 > \mu_2 \quad \text{or} \quad H_a'' : \mu_1 < \mu_2 \quad \text{for one-sided tests .}$$

To avoid repetitions of formulas with minor changes, we write formulas only in terms of a two-sided test.

The sample size required in each group, to achieve a power of $1 - \beta$ is

$$n = \frac{2\sigma^2(z_{1-\alpha/2} + z_{1-\beta})^2}{(\mu_1 - \mu_2)^2} . \tag{1.40}$$

Setting

$$\delta = \frac{\mu_1 - \mu_2}{\sigma} , \tag{1.41}$$

where δ is the effect size, we have a simpler version

$$n = \frac{2(z_{1-\alpha/2} + z_{1-\beta})^2}{\delta^2} . \tag{1.42}$$

To improve the approximation, the correction factor in (1.43) may be added to (1.42) before rounding up.

$$\frac{z_{1-\alpha/2}^2}{4} . \tag{1.43}$$

Example 13. A two-group, randomized, parallel, double-blind study is planned in elderly females after hip fracture. Patients will be studied for two weeks; each patient will be randomly assigned to receive either new drug or placebo three times per week. The sample sizes in the two groups will be equal. Plans call for a 5% level two-sided t test. The outcome variable will be change in hematocrit level during the study. Prior pilot data from several studies suggests that the standard deviation for change will be about 2.0% and it would be of interest to detect a difference of 2.2% in the changes observed in placebo and treated groups. What sample size in each group would be required to achieve a power of 90%? ◆

For Example 13, the effect size is $2.2/2 = 1.1$. Using (1.42) we find

$$n = \frac{2(1.96 + 1.28)^2}{(1.1)^2} = 17.4 \, .$$

Adding the correction factor of 0.96 and rounding up, we have a required sample size of 19 per group, which is the solution given using nQuery Advisor (computations are based on iterative methods and the central and non-central t, see Dixon and Massey 1983 or O'Brien and Muller 1983).

Table 1.14 shows the sample size needed in each group for a two-sided 5% level t test to achieve 80% or 90% power for the specified alternative, δ.

Table 1.14. Sample size in each group for two-sided 5% level t test to have specified power

δ	80% power	90% power
0.2	394	527
0.4	100	133
0.6	45	60
0.8	26	34
1.0	17	23
1.2	12	16

Additional Considerations and References

1.5.3

Good introductions to sample size computations for tests and confidence intervals for a single mean or for comparing two independent means can be found in Dixon and Massey (1983), O'Brien and Muller (1983), Lemeshow et al. (1990), Lachin (1981), and Rosner (2000). Books containing sample size tables are available (e.g. Machin and Campbell 1987; Machin et al. 1997). Commercially available sample size software such as nQuery Advisor Release 5 (Elashoff 2002) can be used to compute sample size (or width) for confidence intervals and sample size or power for hypothesis tests for means for either the single group or two group designs, as well as for a wide variety of other sample size problems.

When plans call for the sample sizes in the two groups to be unequal, the formulas for sample size and power must incorporate the expected ratio of the sample sizes, see references above. For the two-sample t test, for any given total sample size, N, power will be highest when both groups have the same sample size. For this reason we generally prefer to plan equal sample sizes for a two-group study. However, sometimes investigators wish to plan a study with unequal n's; perhaps one type of subject is easier to accrue, or perhaps the investigator wants to maximize the number of subjects receiving the presumably superior treatment, or to accumulate extra safety information for the new treatment.

When the standard deviations in the two groups are markedly unequal, the usual t test with pooled variances is no longer the appropriate test. In many situations, the standard deviations show a patterned lack of homogeneity in which groups with higher means have higher standard deviations. In such cases, it is frequently advisable that sample size predictions (and later analysis) should be done on a transformed version of the variable. If the relationship between variance and mean is linear, this suggests using the square root of the variable. Such a transformation is likely to be desirable if the data represent counts or areas (note that the variable cannot be less than zero). If the relationship between standard deviation and mean is linear, this suggests using the log of the variable. This transformation is likely to be desirable for biological measures like viral load, triglyceride level, or variables ranging over several orders of magnitude (note that the variable cannot be negative or zero). If transformation does not seem to provide a solution to the problem of inequality of variances, it is possible that comparison of means is no longer the most appropriate method of analysis to address the question of interest. Assuming that transformation is not useful and comparison of means using a two-sample t test is still deemed appropriate, a modification of the t test may be planned; see for example, Moser et al. (1989) and sample size tables for the Satterthwaite t in nQuery Advisor.

If non-normality is an issue, planning a large study or considering transformations as above may be helpful; another possibility is to plan to use a non-parametric procedure instead, such as the two-sample Mann-Whitney/Wilcoxon rank test. For a description of this test, see Rosner (2000), and for methods to determine sample size and power see Hettmansperger (1984), Noether (1987), or sample size tables in nQuery Advisor.

Note that the sample size methods for comparisons of two independent means discussed above do not apply to correlation/agreement/repeated measures (or pair-matched case-control) studies in which N subjects are recruited and each subject is measured by two different raters, or is studied under two different treatments in a cross-over design. These designs cannot be analyzed using the methods described for independent means but must be analyzed using the paired t test or a repeated measures analysis of variance; see Rosner (2000) for information on the paired t test, and Muller and Barton (1989) or sample size tables in nQuery Advisor for information about sample size and power for repeated measures tests.

Logistic Regression Models

In prior sections of this chapter, we discussed sample size problems for estimation or testing of a proportion in one or two groups. In this section, we consider study designs in which it is planned to evaluate several predictor variables for a binary outcome variable. Specifically we consider studies in which we plan to fit a logistic regression model. Readers needing an introduction to the logistic regression model and test procedures should consult Hosmer and Lemeshow (2000).

In our experience there are two sample size questions, prospective and retrospective. The prospective question is: How many subjects do I need to observe to test the significance of a specific predictor variable or set of variables? The retrospective question is: Do I have enough data to fit this model? In this section we consider methods for choosing a sample size first and then discuss the importance of having an adequate number of events per covariate.

With respect to planning sample size for logistic regression, we distinguish two situations: (1) only a single covariate is of interest, (2) the addition of one covariate to a model already containing k covariates is of interest. In addition, we must distinguish whether the covariate of interest is dichotomous or continuous.

The basic sample size question is as follows: What sample size does one need to test the null hypothesis that a particular slope coefficient, say for covariate 1, is equal to zero versus the alternative that it is equal to some specified value.

Single Dichotomous Covariate

If the logistic regression model is to contain a single dichotomous covariate, then one may use conventional sample size formulas based on testing for the equality of two proportions. Hsieh et al. (1998) recommend using the following method to obtain sample sizes for logistic regression with a dichotomous covariate. (Although Whitemore 1981 provides a sample size formula for a logistic regression model containing a single dichotomous covariate, this formula, based on the sampling distribution of the log of the odds ratio, was derived under the assumption that the logistic probabilities are small and may be less accurate than the method we outline.)

Let the covariate X define two groups; group 1 contains those subjects for which $x = 0$ and the probability that the outcome of interest $y = 1$ for the subjects in this group is π_1, while group 2 contains those subjects for which $x = 1$ and the probability that $y = 1$ for these subjects is π_2.

Example 14.   Suppose that about 1% of the population is expected to have a particular adverse reaction to a certain drug used to treat a severe illness. It is thought that those with a specific pre-existing condition (expected to be about 20% of the population) will be much more likely to have such a reaction; it will be important to detect an odds ratio of two for the likelihood of a reaction in this group using a 5% two-sided likelihood ratio test.   ◆

Table 1.15. Two group χ^2 test of equal proportions (odds ratio = 1) (unequal n's)

Test significance level, α	0.050	0.050	0.050
1 or 2 sided test?	2	2	2
No condition proportion, π_1	0.010	0.010	0.010
Pre-existing proportion, π_2	0.020	0.029	0.039
Odds ratio, $\psi = \pi_2(1-\pi_1)/[\pi_1(1-\pi_2)]$	2.000	3.000	4.000
Power (%)	90	90	90
n_1	7620	2468	1345
n_2	1905	617	337
Ratio: n_2/n_1	0.250	0.250	0.250
$N = n_1 + n_2$	9525	3085	1681

To compute the required sample size for Example 14 by hand would require using a modification of (1.27) for comparison of two proportions with unequal sample sizes, see references given in that section. Table 1.15 shows the table of results pasted from nQuery Advisor. (In this table, the symbol ψ is used to denote the odds ratio.) Defining group 1 as those without the pre-existing condition and group 2 as those with, the ratio of the sample size in group 2 to the sample size in group 1 will be $20/80 = 0.25$. Using $\pi_1 = 0.01$ for group 1 (no pre-existing condition), and $OR = 2$, we find $\pi_2 = 2(0.01)/(2(0.01) + 0.99) = 0.02$. Table 1.15 shows that to detect an odds ratio of 2 with 90% power for this example would require a sample size of 9525. Consequently, the investigator may be interested in looking at the sample sizes required to detect odds ratios of 3 or of 4 (3085 and 1681 respectively).

1.6.2   Single Continuous Covariate

If the single covariate we plan to include in the model is continuous, approximate formulas for this setting have been derived by Hsieh (1989) and implemented in sample size software packages such as nQuery Advisor. However, Hsieh et al. (1998) demonstrate that this approximate formula gives larger than required sample sizes and recommend using the following method to obtain sample sizes for logistic regression with a continuous covariate.

Let the response Y define two groups; group 1 contains cases in which $Y = 1$ with $N\pi_1$ cases expected, while group 2 contains cases in which $Y = 0$ with $N(1 - \pi_1)$ cases expected. The ratio of the expected sample size in group 2 to the expected sample size in group 1, r, is $(1 - \pi_1)/\pi_1$. The natural log of the odds ratio, the coefficient β of the covariate, x, is equal to the difference between the mean of the covariate in group 1 and the mean of the covariate in group 2 divided by the within-group standard deviation of x (denote this by δ). Therefore, a sample size formula or table for the two group t test with unequal n's can be used to estimate sample size for logistic regression with one continuous covariate.

Example 15. Patients with blocked or narrowed coronary arteries may undergo interventions designed to increase blood flow. Typically, about 30% of patients followed for a year will have renewed blockage, called "restenosis", of the artery. A study is to be planned to use logistic regression to assess factors related to the likelihood of restenosis. One such factor is serum cholesterol level. Based on the results of a large screening trial, mean serum cholesterol in middle-aged males is about 210 mg/dL; one standard deviation above the mean (which corresponds to about the 85th percentile) is approximately 250 mg/dL. In the screening study, the odds ratio for the six-year death rate for these two cholesterol levels was about 1.5. The study should be large enough to detect an effect of serum cholesterol on arterial restenosis of a size similar to that seen for death rate. We plan to conduct the test of the predictive effect of cholesterol level on the probability of restenosis using a 5% two-sided test and want to have 90% power to detect an odds ratio of 1.5 for values of cholesterol of 250 mg/dL versus 210 mg/dL. We set the effect size, $\delta = (\mu_1 - \mu_2)/\sigma = 0.405$, which is the value of the natural log of the odds ratio, 1.5. The ratio of sample sizes expected to be in the no-restenosis versus the restenosis groups, r, equals $0.7/0.3 = 2.333$. ◆

The required sample size could be computed using a version of (1.42) modified for unequal sample sizes, see references in the preceding section. In Table 1.16 we show the table of results pasted from the software nQuery Advisor.

Table 1.16. Two group t-test of equal means (unequal n's)

Test significance level, α	0.050
1 or 2 sided test?	2
Effect size, $\delta = \|\mu_1 - \mu_2\|/\sigma$	0.405
Power (%)	90
n_1	93
n_2	217
Ratio: n_2/n_1	2.333
$N = n_1 + n_2$	310

To obtain a power of 90% to detect an odds ratio of 1.5 using the covariate cholesterol to predict restenosis at one-year, we find that a total sample size of 310 is required.

Adjusting Sample Size for Inclusion of k Prior Covariates (Variance Inflation Factor)

1.6.3

It is rare in practice to have final inferences based on a univariate logistic regression model. However, the only sample size results currently available for the multivariable situation are based on very specific assumptions about the distributions of the covariates. We can however, use a "variance inflation factor" to adjust the sample size results obtained for a single covariate for the situation in which k covariates have already been added to the model before the new covariate is considered.

The sample size, N_k, required to test for the significance of a covariate after inclusion of k prior covariates in the model, is given by

$$N_k = N \left(\frac{1}{1 - \varrho^2} \right) , \tag{1.44}$$

where the factor $1/(1 - \varrho^2)$ is called the "variance inflation factor",

$$VIF = \left(\frac{1}{1 - \varrho^2} \right) , \tag{1.45}$$

and ϱ^2 is the squared multiple correlation of the covariate of interest with the covariates already included in the model. This can be estimated using any multiple regression software.

For Example 14, the total sample size was computed as $N = 1681$ for testing the significance of one dichotomous covariate. Now assume that four patient demographic variables will be entered into the logistic regression model prior to testing the covariate indicating presence or absence of the pre-existing condition (x_1 say), and that these demographic variables have a squared multiple correlation with x_1 of 0.2. Then a total sample size of at least 2100 patients would be required,

$$N_4 = 1681 \left(\frac{1}{1 - 0.2} \right) = 2101 .$$

In Example 15 if two other covariates with a squared multiple correlation with cholesterol of 0.15 are to be entered into the logistic regression first, multiply the sample size obtained for a single covariate by the variance inflation factor, (1.44), $1/(1 - \varrho^2) = 1.18$, to increase the required sample size to 365.

1.6.4   Assessing the Adequacy of Data Already Collected

So far we have discussed planning what sample size should be obtained to fit specific logistic regression models. A second consideration, and one relevant to any model being fit, is the issue of what is the maximum number of covariates it is reasonable to enter into the model and still obtain reliable estimates of the regression coefficients and avoid excessive shrinkage when the model is assessed for new cases. An ad hoc rule of thumb is to require that there be 10 "events" per variable included in the model. Here the "event" of relevance is the least frequent of the outcomes. For example, suppose the study discussed in Example 15 was planned with 365 cases. Further suppose that complete one-year follow-up was only obtained for 351 cases of which 81 had restenosis at one year. There are 81 cases with restenosis and 270 without, so the least frequent "event" is restenosis. Based on these 81 cases, only 8 variables should be fit; this means that no more than 8 covariates (or covariates plus covariate interaction terms) should be entered into the model.

This rule of thumb was evaluated and found to be reasonable by Peduzzi et al. (1996) using only discrete covariates. However, as is the case with any overly simple solution to a complex problem, the rule of 10 should only be used as a guideline and a final determination must consider the context of the total problem. This includes the actual number of events, the total sample size and, most importantly, the mix of discrete, continuous and interaction terms in the model. The "ten events per parameter" rule may work well for continuous covariates and discrete covariates with a balanced distribution. However, its applicability is less clear in settings where the distributions of discrete covariates are weighted heavily to one value.

Practical Issues in Sample Size Choice   1.7

In earlier sections, we outlined formulas for sample size computation for estimation and testing in simple designs for proportions and for means. We have shown only formulas to compute sample size from specifications of confidence interval width or desired power, but it is also possible to compute the confidence interval width or power which would be obtainable with a specified sample size. Sample size methods exist for many more complex designs and for other parameters. Software such as nQuery Advisor (Elashoff 2002) can be helpful.

For complex study designs or complex statistical methods, however, there may be no easily applied formulas or available software solutions. In such cases, sample size choices may be based on simplifications of the design or statistical methods (as we illustrated in the section on logistic regression), or in some cases a simulation study may be warranted.

For studies involving complex survey designs, sample size computations might be based on one of several approaches: (1) regarding the cluster itself as the study "subject" and using intraclass correlation values to estimate the appropriate variance to use in making computations, (2) multiplying sample sizes for a simpler design by a computed "design effect" (2 may be a sensible ad hoc choice), or (3) using simulation methods.

Although study sample sizes are usually chosen to assure desired precision or power for the primary outcome variable, investigators may also need to investigate whether that sample size choice will be adequate for evaluations of secondary outcomes, or for analyses of pre-defined subsets.

Sample size values obtained from formulas or software will generally need to be inflated to allow for expected dropout or loss to followup of study subjects or other sources of missing data (cf. Chap. II.6 of this handbook). It is important to remember however, that subjects who drop out may not be similar to those remaining in the study. This consideration may affect the parameter values which should be used for sample size computations; and even analyses using missing data techniques may not remove biases due to dropout.

Another issue of great concern to epidemiologists is that exposure or response may be misclassified. Such misclassification might have a dramatic impact on the actual power of a planned study unless sample sizes are computed based on modeling the expected type and extent of misclassification using simulation methods.

For brevity, our examples used only one set of parameter values to compute required sample sizes. In practice, investigators need to keep in mind that the estimated parameter values used in computations are only estimates and perhaps not very accurate ones. It is a good idea to compute necessary sample size for several different sets of parameter choices to evaluate sample size sensitivity to varying realistic possibilities for the true parameter values. Tables and plots can be helpful in these evaluations.

Finally, sample size justification statements in protocols, grant proposals, and manuscripts need to be complete. Details of the outcome variable, the study design, the planned analysis method, confidence level or power, one or two-sided, and all the relevant distributional parameters (proportions, means, standard deviations) need to be included in the statement. For Example 13 a minimal sample size justification might read as follows: *A sample size of 19 in each group will have 90% power to detect a difference in means of 2.2 (the difference between an active drug mean change in hematocrit of 2.2% and a placebo mean change of 0.0) assuming that the common standard deviation is 2.0 and using a two group t test with a 0.05 two-sided significance level. The planned enrollment will be 25 subjects per group (50 total) to allow for 20% dropout.* It is also desirable to provide information about sample size for other parameter choices and details about how these parameter values were selected, including references to previous studies which were consulted in selecting the values.

1.8   Conclusions

An important part of planning any research study is to assess what sample size is needed to assure that meaningful conclusions can be drawn about the primary outcome. To do this, the investigator must detail the study design, define the primary outcome variable, choose an analysis method, and specify desired or expected results of the study. Then formulas, tables, and sample size software of the sort outlined in this chapter can assist with computations. The most essential part of the process, though, is to make a thorough investigation of other information and research results concerning the outcome variable to support reasonable specification of hypothesized values for use in making computations. Beginning investigators often protest: "But this study has never been done before; how do I know what the results will be?" In most cases, however much information about rates, means, and standard deviations can be gleaned from other contexts and used to infer what kinds of outcomes would be important to detect or likely to occur. Sample size computations are not just a pro forma requirement from funding agencies but provide the basis for deciding whether a planned study is likely to be worth the expense.

References

Chernick MR, Liu CY (2002) The saw-toothed behavior of power versus sample size and software solutions: single binomial proportion using exact methods. The American Statistician 56:149–155

Dixon WJ, Massey FJ (1983) Introduction to statistical analysis. 4th edn. McGraw-Hill, New York

Elashoff JD (2002) nQuery Advisor® Release 5. Statistical Solutions, Ireland

Fleiss JL (1981) Statistical methods for rates and proportions. 2nd edn. Wiley, New York

Fleiss JL, Tytun A, Ury SH (1980) A simple approximation for calculating sample sizes for comparing independent proportions. Biometrics 36:343–346

Hettmansperger TP (1984) Statistical inference based on ranks. Wiley, New York

Hosmer DW, Lemeshow S (2000) Applied logistic regression. 2nd edn. Wiley, New York

Hsieh FY (1989) Sample size tables for logistic regression. Statistics in Medicine 8:795–802

Hsieh FY, Bloch DA, Larsen MD (1998) A simple method of sample size calculation for linear and logistic regression. Statistics in Medicine 17:1623–1634

Korn EL (1986) Sample size tables for bounding small proportions. Biometrics 42:213–216

Kupper LL, Hafner KB (1989) How appropriate are popular sample size formulas? The American Statistician 43:101–105

Lachin JM (1981) Introduction to sample size determination and power analysis for clinical trials. Controlled Clinical Trials 2:93–113

Lachin JM (1992) Power and sample size evaluation for the McNemar test with application to matched case-control studies. Statistics in Medicine 11:1239–1251

Lemeshow S, Hosmer DW, Klar J, Lwanga SK (1990) Adequacy of sample size in health studies. Wiley, Chichester

Levy PS, Lemeshow S (1999) Sampling of populations: methods and applications, 3rd edn. Wiley, New York

Louis TA (1981) Confidence intervals for a binomial parameter after observing no successes. The American Statistician 35:154

Machin D, Campbell MJ (1987) Statistical tables for design of clinical trials. Blackwell Scientific Publications, Oxford

Machin D, Campbell M, Fayers P, Pinol A (1997) Sample size tables for clinical studies. 2nd edn. Malden and Carlton: Blackwell Science, London

Moser BK, Stevens GR, Watts CL (1989) The two-sample *t* test versus Satterthwaite's approximate F test. Commun. Statist.-Theory Meth. 18:3963–3975

Muller KE, Barton CN (1989) Approximate power for repeated-measures ANOVA lacking sphericity. Journal of the American Statistical Association 84:549–555

Noether GE (1987) Sample size determination for some common nonparametric tests. Journal of the American Statistical Association 82:645–647

O'Brien RG, Muller KE (1983) Applied analysis of variance in behavioral science. Marcel Dekker, New York, pp 297–344

Peduzzi PN, Concato J, Kemper E, Holford TR, Feinstein A (1996) A simulation study of the number of events per variable in logistic regression analysis. Journal of Clinical Epidemiology 99:1373–1379

Rosner B (2000) Fundamentals of Biostatistics. 5th edn. Duxbury Press, Boston

Whitemore AS (1981) Sample size for logistic regression with small response probability. Journal of the American Statistical Association 76:27–32

General Principles of Data Analysis: Continuous Covariables in Epidemiological Studies

Heiko Becher

Introduction

When analysing data from an epidemiological study, some features are rather specific for a particular study design. Those are dealt with among others in Chaps. I.3, I.5 to I.7 and II.4. Other features are generally relevant, see Chaps. I.2 and I.9. This chapter deals with one of these, namely the analysis of continuous covariables. After a short introduction in which relevant measures used for continuous covariables are listed, we present classical methods based on categorisation and subsequent contingency table analysis. The major part of the chapter deals with the analysis of such variables in the context of regression models commonly used in epidemiology (see also Chap. II.3). These methods are then illustrated by real data examples. The chapter ends with practical recommendations and conclusions.

The sequence of action in epidemiologic research is similar to any other empirical research area and involves the following major steps:

— study planning
— data collection, data entry and data cleaning
— data analysis
— interpretation and publication

The data analysis can often be divided into
— descriptive analysis
— analytical statistical methods (modelling).

This sequence should be followed: a good, thorough and careful descriptive analysis of the data can save enormous time. The methods to be used are the same in all areas where data analysis is part of the game. This involves univariate analysis of all variables of interest, by graphical or other methods as described in textbooks on descriptive statistics (e.g. Bernstein and Bernstein 1998).

In practice, however, this sequence is often reversed, or the second part of the analysis step is started before the first is finished. This is sometimes driven by unpatient clinicians who would like to know immediately whether "the study is significant", i.e. directly after data collection is finished and before plausibility checks of the data have been performed. However, in only very rare cases the first p-value generated in the analysis step is later found in the publication. Instead, some peculiarities in the data are found such that one has to go back to the descriptive analysis. Then we have a recursive process which fortunately in most cases converges.

Many of the descriptive methods used in the analysis of epidemiological data are independent of the area of application. The mean of a continuous variable, for example, has general importance. The aim of this chapter is therefore not to give a detailed overview of measures for location of dispersion or to describe measures for dependencies between two variables. Table 2.1 summarises the most relevant of these measures. For a good introduction to descriptive methods we refer to other textbooks (Bernstein and Bernstein 1998).

Table 2.1. Some relevant measures for location and dispersion of one continuous variable, and for dependencies between two continuous variables

Measure	Definition
Arithmetic mean of n observations $x_1, x_2, \ldots, x_n$	$\bar{x} = \dfrac{1}{n}(x_1 + x_2 + x_3 + \ldots + x_n) = \dfrac{1}{n}\sum_{i=1}^{n} x_i$
Median calculated from the ordered sequence of observations $x_{(1)}, x_{(2)}, \ldots, x_{(n)}$, i.e. for all $i < j$ it holds: $x_{(i)} \leq x_{(j)}$	$x_{\text{med}} = \begin{cases} x_{\left(\frac{n+1}{2}\right)} & \text{if } n \text{ odd} \\ \dfrac{1}{2}\left(x_{\left(\frac{n}{2}\right)} + x_{\left(\frac{n}{2}+1\right)}\right) & \text{if } n \text{ even} \end{cases}$
(Sample) variance	$s^2 = \dfrac{1}{n-1}\sum (x_i - \bar{x})^2$
(Sample) standard deviation	$s = \sqrt{s^2}$
Standard error	$\text{s.e.} = s/\sqrt{n}$
Pearson correlation coefficient between variables X and Z with pairs of observations (x_1, z_1), $(x_2, z_2), \ldots, (x_n, z_n)$	$r_{XY} = \dfrac{\sum_{i=1}^{n}(x_i - \bar{x})(z_i - \bar{z})}{\sqrt{\sum_{i=1}^{n}(x_i - \bar{x})^2 \cdot \sum_{i=1}^{n}(z_i - \bar{z})^2}}$
Spearman (rank) correlation coefficient between variables X and Z with ranked pairs of observations $(R(x_1), R(z_1))$, $(R(x_2), R(z_2)), \ldots, (R(x_n), R(z_n))$	$r_{XY}(\text{Spearman}) = 1 - \dfrac{6\sum_{i=1}^{n}\left(R(x_i) - R(y_i)\right)^2}{n(n^2 - 1)}$

Instead, in this chapter we give an overview of methods to analyse continuous covariables in epidemiological studies. For a long time it has been common to categorise them into $K \geq 2$ groups and to estimate appropriate parameters (e.g. odds ratio or relative risk) that describe the effect of a certain level of the variable relative to an arbitrarily defined baseline level or to perform trend tests based on this categorisation. This procedure was exclusively used in the past because classical methods to analyse epidemiological data, for example the Mantel–Haenszel estimator were mostly based on some form of contingency table analysis and require a categorisation of continuous variables (cf. Chap. I.2 of this handbook). In the last decades they have been replaced by regression models that allow, but do not require a categorisation. With increasing computer power and availability of standard software these methods are now in common use.

We will describe and compare different methods with regard to the adequacy for the analysis of continuous covariables in classical epidemiological studies (such as case-control or cohort studies) and on the analysis of morbidity and mortality data. The aim is either (1) to analyse the relation between the outcome variable Y and the covariable X or (2) to appropriately adjust for X if one wishes to analyse the relation between Y and Z, where Z is another covariable which may be confounded by X (see also Chaps. I.1 and I.9 of this handbook). For (1), this is commonly done in epidemiology by estimating a relative risk or odds ratio function $R(\cdot)$, where $(\cdot)$ denotes dependence on an arbitrary argument. For (2), one has additionally the possibility to condition on X. Particular emphasis will also be given to the question of whether and how a trend test can be performed.

Classical Methods to Analyse Continuous Covariables Based on Contingency Tables 2.2

Before the theory of generalized linear models (Nelder and Wedderburn 1972) has been developed, which had a major influence for epidemiologic research, contingency table analysis was the common tool in our field. The famous paper by Mantel and Haenszel (1959) is still well known, mainly because the ideas developed herein facilitate the path for understanding of the modern techniques. In this section, we will therefore outline odds ratio estimation, test for trend and simple confounder adjustment based on these classical methods. Although less used today, these methods are still helpful for a general understanding of epidemiologic data analysis. It should be emphasised, however, that the methods presented here have been replaced by modern regression methods which are now the state of the art.

General Aspects 2.2.1

We assume that a continuous covariable X has been collected and that Y is a binary variable that denotes the disease or the event of interest. The classical methods first require a categorisation of X which can formally be described by the function

$$f(x) = x_k I_{x \in I_k}(x) \, ,$$

where I is the indicator function and I_k are disjoint exposure categories with $k = 1, \ldots, K$ covering the whole set M of possible values of X, i.e.

$$I_k \cap I_{k'} = \emptyset \quad \text{for} \quad k \neq k' \quad \text{and} \quad \bigcup_k I_k = M \, .$$

The most common method is to choose x_k as $k < K$, but it is also possible to assign x_k the mean exposure level in category k.

The practical questions are
1. how to choose the number of categories K and
2. how to choose the intervals I_k.

For both questions a unique or optimal answer does not exist. Since categorisation is a relevant method also in regression modelling as described later, the final result obtained from the same dataset will most likely differ, if two statisticians analyse the same dataset.

Some general rules, however, may help as a guideline for this decision:
- choose the limits and the number of categories such that a comparison with earlier studies is possible
- if a natural baseline exists (for example "0" for nonexposed), and a low exposure is a priori regarded as hazardous (e.g. smoking), choose the natural baseline (in the example: the nonsmokers) as a separate category
- K should not be larger than 10, but for small datasets fewer categories are to be preferred. Three to six categories are most frequently used in practice
- Choose the limits and number of categories a priori, i.e. do not base this choice on the resulting risk estimates.

A categorisation according to quartiles or quintiles of the distribution of the variable is often done. This is statistically correct, but then comparison with other studies is somewhat hampered since the limits follow the exact observed distribution of the covariable. It is perhaps better to report "Individuals whose diastolic blood pressure is above 90 mm Hg have a risk of ... to get disease D" than to say "Individuals in the upper quartile of the diastolic blood pressure have a risk of ... to get disease D."

2.2.2 Odds Ratio Estimation

Assume now a categorisation has been performed yielding a $2 \times K$ table. This may be denoted as follows:

Table 2.2. A $2 \times K$ table

		Cases	Controls	Total
Exposure level	x_1	a_1	c_1	m_1
	x_2	a_2	c_2	m_2
	...	...	...	...
	x_K	a_K	c_K	m_K
Total		n_1	n_0	N

Crude odds ratio estimation by exposure level is done by

$$\widehat{OR}_k = \frac{a_k c_1}{c_k a_1} , \quad k = 2, \ldots, K ,$$

and asymptotic 95% confidence intervals are given as

$$\left(\exp\left(\ln\left(\widehat{OR}_k\right) - 1.96\sqrt{\widehat{var}\left(\widehat{OR}_k\right)} \right), \exp\left(\ln\left(\widehat{OR}_k\right) + 1.96\sqrt{\widehat{var}\left(\widehat{OR}_k\right)} \right) \right)$$

with variance

$$\widehat{var}\left(\ln\left(\widehat{OR}_k\right) \right) = \frac{1}{a_k} + \frac{1}{c_1} + \frac{1}{a_1} + \frac{1}{c_k} .$$

The odds ratios can be displayed graphically such that the dose group or the average intake within each group is on the x-axis, and the odds ratio on the y-axis. This is a useful first presentation of the data.

As an example, we consider data from a laryngeal cancer case-control study (Dietz et al. 2004) where the variable X is categorised into four groups. These are of the form as depicted in Table 2.3.

Table 2.3. Alcohol consumption in males; laryngeal cancer case-control study; Germany

		Cases		Controls		
		a_k	(%)	c_k	(%)	OR
Alcohol intake	≤ 25	57	24.2	303	43.2	1.0
(g ethanol/day)	25–≤ 50	51	21.6	169	24.1	1.60
	50–≤ 75	39	16.5	113	16.1	1.83
	75+	89	37.7	117	16.7	4.04
Total		236	100.0	702	100.0	

In this study, average alcohol intake ten years before interview was assessed by asking for consumption of different alcoholic beverages (beer, wine, liqueur, spirits). Average alcohol content of these beverages yielded the estimated daily ethanol intake.

The last column gives the unadjusted (i.e. not adjusted for confounders, such as smoking) odds ratio in comparison with the baseline category (see Chap. I.2 of this handbook for an introduction of the Mantel–Haenszel estimate of the adjusted odds ratio). We observe an increasing odds ratio with increasing dose.

In the recent literature, the classical methods to analyse continuous covariables based on contingency tables have become less and less common. This is because

1. a categorisation necessarily means a loss of information
2. the classical analysis is embedded in regression models as a special case
3. the possibility to adjust for multiple confounders is limited
4. there are only limited options for a dose-response analysis.

Confounder Adjustment 2.2.3

One of the big challenges in epidemiologic data analysis is a correct adjustment for confounder. Several other chapters deal with this issue in the context of particular study designs (see especially Chaps. I.1, I.9 and I.12 of this handbook).

Suppose X is a continuous confounder and Z is the variable of main interest, i.e. one is interested in an adjusted estimate of the effect of Z with a suitable measure, for example the odds ratio. For ease of presentation we assume in the following that Z is a binary variable. In the context of classical methods, the adjustment of a continuous confounder is done through categorization of the confounder X and a stratified analysis as described below.

Suppose further that X has been categorized into K levels according to the methods described in Sect. 2.2.2 yielding K 2×2 tables of the form depicted in Table 2.4.

Table 2.4. A 2×2 table for the binary factor Z in the k-th stratum of a categorised confounder X

		Cases	Controls	Total
Z	Non-exposed	a_{1k}	c_{1k}	m_{1k}
	Exposed	a_{2k}	c_{2k}	m_{2k}
Total		n_{1k}	n_{0k}	N_k

The stratum-specific odds ratio estimate for the k-th stratum is

$$\widehat{OR}_k = \frac{a_{2k}c_{1k}}{c_{2k}a_{1k}}, \quad k = 1, \dots, K .$$

Among the several methods for adjusted odds exist for adjustment (see Breslow and Day 1980), the Mantel–Haenszel estimate is most commonly used. It is defined as:

$$\widehat{OR}_{MH} = \frac{\sum\limits_{k=1}^{K} a_{2k}c_{1k}/N_k}{\sum\limits_{k=1}^{K} c_{2k}a_{1k}/N_k}, \quad k = 1, \dots, K ,$$

this estimate is easily computed, as well as the variance for its logarithm through

$$\widehat{var}\left(\widehat{OR}_{MH}\right) = \frac{\sum\limits_{k=1}^{K} \left(a_{1k}c_{2k}/N_k\right)^2 v_k}{\sum\limits_{k=1}^{K} \left(a_{1k}c_{2k}/N_k\right)^2}, \quad k = 1, \dots, K ,$$

with

$$v_k = \frac{1}{a_{1k}} + \frac{1}{c_{1k}} + \frac{1}{a_{2k}} + \frac{1}{c_{2k}}.$$

(Dos Santos Silva 1999, p 327ff). Again, the question arises how many categories K should be used. If too few categories (e.g. $K = 2$) are used, the control of confounding is incomplete, and some "residual confounding" remains. A measure for this is described in Breslow and Day (1980, p 99ff). Five categories are usually sufficient to control for confounding. However, since in practice more than one confounder is common, a full stratified analysis would require $K_1 \times K_2 \times \dots K_\kappa$ strata, where κ denotes the number of confounders. This is usually not feasible, since this number becomes too large, and the single tables too sparse. The analysis based on classical methods has its limitation in this respect. Therefore, the Mantel–Haenszel method has been replaced by regression methods as described later in this chapter and in Chap. II.3.

Test for Trend

Instead of presenting an effect measure for separate categories, one is often interested in the general question whether the effect increases (or decreases) with increasing dose. Very often the presentation of the results goes with the presentation of a "test for trend". Although this is sometimes more specifically referred to as "test for linear trend", this is not sufficient, since there is no unique "test for (linear) trend", and it often remains unclear what the authors of a paper actually have done. Moreover, such a statistical test may yield a significant result indicating a trend even if the single risk estimates are only increased in the lower dose range but approach baseline risk at higher doses (Maclure and Greenland 1992). Also, if there is a non-monotonous relation between exposure and disease (see Example 4), does this mean "no trend"? As will become clear later in this chapter, a thorough dose-response analysis should replace the commonly used trend tests.

Based on Table 2.2, a χ^2-statistic for testing trend is

$$\chi^2 = \frac{N^2(N-1)\left[\sum\limits_{k=1}^{K} x_k(a_k - e_k)\right]^2}{n_1 n_0\left[N\sum\limits_{k=1}^{K} x_k^2 m_k - \left(\sum\limits_{k=1}^{K} x_k m_k\right)^2\right]},$$

where $e_k = E(a_k) = m_k n_1/N$ is the expected number of cases in category k.

Under the null hypothesis of no trend this test statistic has an asymptotic χ^2-distribution with one degree of freedom. This test is called *Mantel–Haenszel χ^2-test for linear trend*. As typical for χ^2-test statistics it compares the observed number in each category with the one expected under the null hypothesis where the x_k serve as weights. To achieve an asymptotic χ^2-distribution the resulting squared sum of weighted differences in the nominator has to be appropriately standardised by accounting for the weighted sample sizes for each exposure level $x_k m_k$, the numbers of cases n_1 and controls n_0 as well as the total number of subjects N. This test has been frequently used in the past. In practice, the values x_k are often chosen as k. This is appropriate when the differences of the mean levels between two adjacent categories are similar, which is for instance fulfilled if the categories are equidistant. If this is not the case, the result of a trend test can highly differ whether x_k (e.g. defined as the midpoint of the exposure category) or simply k is used in the formula above. For the last, open-ended category there is no unique best solution to assign a value x_k. Given that the rank k is not used as weight, the best solution would be to investigate the distribution of the variable and to use as x_k the expected value given the observations are larger than the lower limit of this category. Since this may be difficult, a quick and pragmatic solution is to take the lower limit of this category multiplied by 1.5. If few observations are in this category, the value used for x_k is not crucial. In any case, however, an exact description of the method used is important.

In the example presented in Table 2.3, we have $\chi^2 = 48.51$ with $x_k = k$ which is highly significant ($p < 0.001$). Thus, our observation of an increasing odds ratio with increasing dose could be confirmed by the above statistical test.

The underlying principle is identical for contingency table analysis and for regression models, but for the latter there exists a larger variety of methods to perform a trend test.

2.2.5   Concluding Remarks on Classical Methods

In summary, the above described methods, which have mainly been developed before 1980, have served in the analysis of epidemiological studies for a long time. For a more detailed treatment of classical methods of data analysis with contingency tables we refer to classical textbooks like Breslow and Day (1980). It has become apparent, however, that these methods have their limits, as best seen in the analysis of continuous covariables. The major drawbacks are:

— need to categorize continues covariables, leading to a loss of information
— limited possibilities to derive a dose-response-curve
— ambiguous interpretation
— limited options for confounder adjustment.

Nevertheless, these methods have one general advantage which should not be underestimated: They are simple and some can easily be calculated with a small pocket calculator. As a first step, following a descriptive analysis of the data, they are still useful although these results will rarely find their way into good journals today.

In the following the most relevant regression models in epidemiological research are briefly introduced (see also Chap. II.3 of this handbook) before several methods to analyse continuous covariables are presented.

2.3   Regression Models and Risk Functions

It has been mentioned at several places that regression modelling is the method of choice for the analysis of epidemiological data. The advantages of these are particularly apparent when continuous covariables are to be analysed. For the classical methods a categorisation cannot be avoided, which automatically leads to a loss of information. Regression methods, on the other hand, allow the analysis of the data as measured. In this section, we introduce relevant regression models and a notation which is useful for the subsequent presentation of the methods.

Let Y be the outcome variable, and let X and Z be two covariables (X continuous, Z unspecified). In this paper we consider (a) the logistic regression model, where the outcome variable Y is dichotomous, $Y = 1$ – (diseased), $Y = 0$ – (not diseased); (b) the Poisson regression model, where $\mu = D/PY$ is the outcome variable with D the observed number of events, e.g. deaths, and PY (person-years) the observation time for all individuals; and (c) the Cox regression model, where, $\lambda(t)$ is the hazard function and one observes the individual survival time t and a censoring indicator (for a general discussion of regression models see Chap. II.3 of this handbook; for models of the latter type we also refer to Chap. II.4).

The classical (log-linear) form of the logistic, Poisson or Cox model reads as follows for the logistic regression model:

$$P(Y = 1|x, z) = \frac{\exp\left(\beta_0 + \beta_1 x + \beta_2 z\right)}{1 + \exp\left(\beta_0 + \beta_1 x + \beta_2 z\right)} \, ,$$

the Poisson regression model:

$$\mu = \exp\left(\beta_0 + \beta_1 x + \beta_2 z\right) \, ,$$

and for the proportional hazards (Cox) regression model:

$$\lambda(t) = \lambda_0(t) \exp\left(\beta_1 x + \beta_2 z\right) \, ,$$

where β_1 and β_2 are the regression coefficients for X and Z, respectively, and β_0 is an intercept parameter. This standard form is not very flexible since a specific functional relation between the covariables and the outcome is fixed (see Sect. 2.4 for details). A more general form of these models allow transformations of X and Z with functions f and g, and the exponential function exp is replaced by R. The general form then becomes for the logistic regression model:

$$P(Y = 1|x, z) = \frac{\exp\left(\beta_0\right) R_X\left(f(x), \beta_1\right) R_Z\left(g(z), \beta_2\right)}{1 + \exp\left(\beta_0\right) R_X\left(f(x), \beta_1\right) R_Z\left(g(z), \beta_2\right)} \, ,$$

Poisson regression model:

$$\mu = \exp\left(\beta_0\right) R_X\left(f(x), \beta_1\right) R_Z\left(g(z), \beta_2\right) \, ,$$

and for the Cox regression model:

$$\lambda(t) = \lambda_0(t) R_X\left(f(x), \beta_1\right) R_Z\left(g(z), \beta_2\right) \, ,$$

where R_X and R_Z are risk functions.

For illustration, let us consider the logistic model first. In the classical form as given above, a dose-response function for the variable X, given as OR($X=x$ vs. $X = 0$) is given by

$$OR(X = x \text{ vs. } X = 0) = \frac{P(Y = 1|x, z)P(Y = 0|0, z)}{P(Y = 1|0, z)P(Y = 1|x, z)} = \exp(\beta x) \, ,$$

thus automatically yielding a specific (exponential) form of the dose-response-curve. This is not sufficient for most analyses, and the more general form is given as

$$OR(X = x \text{ vs. } X = 0) = \frac{P(Y = 1|x, z)P(Y = 0|0, z)}{P(Y = 1|0, z)P(Y = 1|x, z)} = R(\beta f(x)) \, .$$

In the history of the development, the function R has been modified first, leading to the additive relative risk model (see method (iv) in the next section). Transformations of the covariable X before entering the regression model have also been common for quite a while, but only after the development of the method of fractional polynomials this has been investigated in a more systematic way (Royston and Altman 1994). The correct functional form of the relative risk function is commonly unknown, and unless biological knowledge can be added to support a specific shape, one has to base the decision on statistical grounds. For assessing the dose-response-curve associated with X, different approaches are used in the literature which is dealt with in the next section.

It is possible in some cases to analytically derive the appropriate model if the distribution of the covariables is known. If, for instance, X is normally distributed in cases and controls with equal variance and (possibly) different mean, then the classical form $R(\cdot) = \exp(\cdot)$ and $f = \mathrm{id}$ (where id denotes identity, i.e. $f(x) = x$) is the correct one. In practice, however, it is more complex and it is necessary to find a statistical procedure for building the model and for discriminating between models.

It is noteworthy at this point that $R(\cdot) = \exp(\cdot)$ describes the odds ratio (or relative risk or rate ratio) for the value of X relative to a reference level. For example if X denotes the number of cigarettes smoked, then $R(10)$ describes the odds ratio for smoking 10 cigarettes compared to smoking zero, but likewise the odds ratio for smoking 20 cigarettes compared to 10. This is the reason why the odds ratio function often does not fit to the categorised estimates, in which the odds ratio for each exposure category in comparison to the same baseline category is estimated, a fact that is nicely described in Breslow and Day (1980, pp 220f). Here, the risk for oesophageal cancer is estimated for tobacco consumption. Compared to the baseline (non-smoker), even moderate smokers have a considerable risk (odds ratio about 4.3). The increase in risk with increasing dose, as given in four different levels of tobacco consumption, is clearly not log-linear. When estimating the risk with the classical logistic model, the odds ratio function is, however, forced to be log-linear with $\ln(\mathrm{OR}(X = x \text{ vs. } X = x_0)) = \beta(x - x_0)$ which does not fit the data well. Method (vii) below takes specific account of this problem.

The risk function R may be embedded in a similar way in the Poisson regression. However, there is one principal difference when applying this regression model. Here, a rate is modelled which results from the observed number of events in a category divided by the corresponding observed person-time (see Chap. I.5 of this handbook). Therefore, a categorisation of a continuous covariable is necessary for the allocation of person-time (see Breslow and Day 1987, pp 85–86). For example, if the effect of average daily alcohol consumption X (in g ethanol per day) on a particular disease is analysed from a cohort study with Poisson regression, then X has to be categorized first, e.g. in categories $0, > 0–10, > 10–20, > 20–40, > 40–80, 80+$ g/day. Then the observed number of cases and corresponding person-years are calculated for each exposure category, and finally the Poisson regression can be performed using one of the methods as described later. The dose-response analysis is then based on an average level within an exposure category for which the mean from all individuals falling in the respective category can be used.

Methods to Analyse Continuous Covariables in Regression Models

In this section several methods will be described to deal with continuous co-variables within regression models. For an introduction to regression models in general see Chap. II.3 of this handbook.

Categorisation of X into K Levels (Method i)

Here, we use

$$f(x) = \left(I_{x \in I_1}(x), \dots, I_{x \in I_K}(x) \right) ; \quad R(\cdot) = \exp(\cdot) ,$$

where I is the indicator function and I_K are the exposure categories $1, \dots, K$ with

$$I_k \cap I_{k'} = \emptyset \quad \text{for} \quad k \neq k' \quad \text{and} \quad \bigcup_k I_k = M ,$$

where M is the set of possible values of X.

This method is still most commonly used in epidemiology. It is the natural transformation of classical methods for the analysis of grouped data. In contrast to the classical methods, the covariable is split into K binary variables which then enter the regression model. These are also called "dummy variables". The category which shall be the baseline, usually the not or low exposed, is left out of the model. The aspects of how to choose the number of categories and the limits are the same as in the classical methods described in Sect. 2.2.

The method has the advantage that it has an easy interpretation. It is therefore popular among non-statisticians and it is "model-free" in the sense that no shape of the dose-response relationship is implicitly assumed. It is a useful step in the analysis sequence, however, it also has some serious drawbacks. Among these are an arbitrary choice of the baseline level, cutpoints and number of levels. The full information from the data is not used and the risk function is by definition a step function:

$$R(x) = \exp \left(\sum_{k=1}^{K} \beta_{1k} I_{x \in I_k}(x) \right) .$$

If X is a confounder for Z a high residual confounding may result if K is small (e.g. $K = 2$). On the other hand a high number of parameters is to be estimated if K is large which may not be feasible if the sample size is small. A frequent practice found in the literature is to choose a categorisation (dichotomisation) of X that minimizes the p-value. This procedure, however, yields incorrect p-values and must therefore not be used without p-value adjustment (Altman et al. 1994; Schulgen et al. 1994).

A "test for linear trend" which parallels the classical test introduced in Sect. 2.2.2 is given by assigning the K categories of X the values $1, 2, 3, \dots, K$ as in Sect. 2.2 and entering this variable into the regression model. The advantage here is the possibility to simultaneously adjust for other covariables which is only possible to a limited degree using the classical methods. The disadvantage, namely the restriction to a specific functional form of the dose-response function, however, is the same as before, and therefore it is not recommended for general use.

2.4.2　Leaving X Untransformed (Method ii)

Here, f is chosen as identity, i.e.

$$f(x) = x\,; \quad R(\cdot) = \exp(\cdot)\,, \quad \text{yielding} \quad R = \exp(\beta x)\,.$$

This is the standard method which uses the full information of the variable, however, it has the serious drawback that it assumes the exponential function as the dose-response-curve. This is valid only in special situations, for example if X has a normal distribution in cases and controls with equal variance. In many papers one finds statements like "odds ratio estimates are adjusted for age" which often simply means that this method has been employed to adjust for X (age). The method can easily yield false results. Example 5 in Sect. 2.5 gives data from a case-control study for which this method is not appropriate. If in this example the method is used for confounder adjustment for a second covariable Z, then residual confounding would result (Becher 1993). The simple reason is that this is an unmatched study with a special age distribution of cases and controls (see Example 5).

There are theoretical examples for which the correct form for adjustment can be derived. For example, if X is normally distributed in cases and controls with different means and variances, an additional quadratic term is required, which is a fractional polynomial of degree two (see (iv)). The risk $R(X = x$ vs. $X = x_0)$ depends on the difference $x - x_0$ only and yields $\exp(\beta(x - x_0))$ (compare with method (v)).

The p-value for $\widehat{\beta}$ as obtained from the model fit may be regarded as the result of a "test for linear trend". In that context, "linear" means that the log odds ratio increases linearly with dose.

2.4.3　Transformation of X via a Monotonous Function (Method iii)

Here, X undergoes a monotonous transformation with common functions, such as the logarithm or square root before it enters the regression model. This is a common 'ad hoc' method and directly possible with all software packages which allow the respective regression model. For choosing a particular model, one has the problem that a comparison is not easily possible through a χ^2-statistic.

Figure 2.1 shows the shape of the dose-response curve for three common transformations

$$f_1(x) = \sqrt{x}\,, \quad f_2(x) = x^2\,, \quad f_3(x) = \ln(x + 1)\,,$$

for which the regression coefficient is chosen such that $R(1) = \exp(1)$. It is seen that f_1 generates an almost linear dose-response within the given dose range, f_2

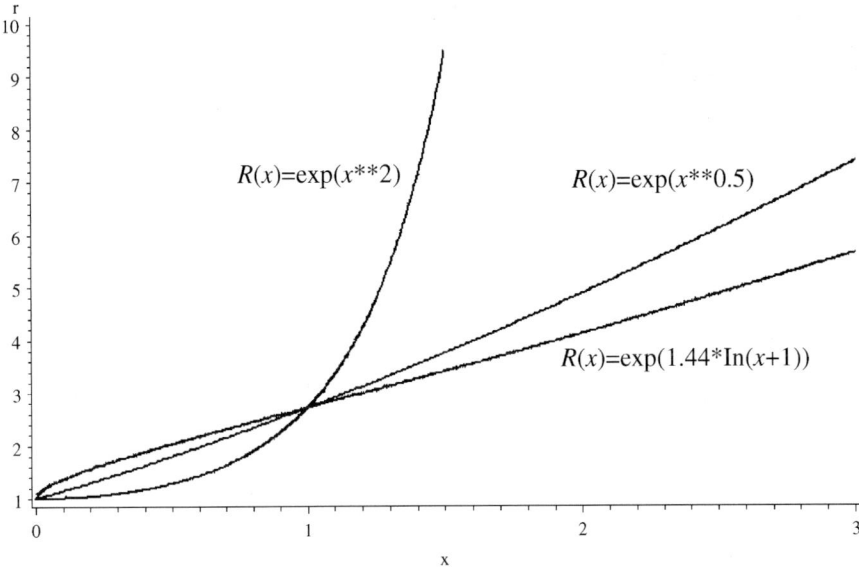

Figure 2.1. Possible shapes of dose-response curves as obtained from the transformations $f_1(x) = \sqrt{x}$, $f_2(x) = x^2$, $f_3(x) = \ln(x + 1)$

generates a strongly increasing curve, and f_3 a concave dose-response (see also method (vi) for comparison).

For f_3 a specific feature must be noted: If the covariable X can take the value 0, which is often the case (smoking, alcohol), then the simple log transformation is not possible, and instead of $\ln(x)$, $\ln(x + k)$ must be used. In order to force the dose-response to be 1 for $x = 0$ which is of course reasonable, one has to use $k = 1$ as in the function f_3 above.

Different approaches have been proposed to discriminate between such models which are called "non-nested models" (e.g. Royston and Thompson 1995; Mizon and Richard 1986) which are beyond the scope of this chapter. It is also possible to use a higher dimensional transformation, e.g. $f(x) = (x, x^2)$. Then, inclusion of X into the model is followed by adding X^2. A formal test on whether the second component significantly improves the goodness-of-fit is readily available as the difference of deviances which is asymptotically χ^2-distributed. A non-monotonous dose-response function may result from this approach. Method (vi) below is a formalized version of this method.

Use of Additive (Linear) Risk Function (Method iv)   2.4.4

Similarly to (ii), we choose f as identity, but an additive risk function instead of an exponential one

$$f(x) = x ; \quad R(x) = 1 + \beta x .$$

This method, though often described in literature and available in some software packages, is not very often used in practise. A comparison of linear and exponential relative risk function, i.e.

$$R_1(x) = \exp(\beta x) \quad \text{vs.} \quad R_2(x) = 1 + \beta x,$$

based on some goodness-of-fit statistic is desirable. However, a simple test for the hypothesis H_0: "Both models fit the data equally well" vs. H_1: "One model fits the data better than the other" is not available because the models are not nested and the difference of the deviances has an unknown distribution under the null hypothesis. The restriction $f(x) = x$ can easily be relaxed, i.e. by a transformation of X with a function as given in (iii), but this has also rarely been done in practice.

In this model, the risk when comparing two covariable values x_1 and x_2, $0 \le x_1 < x_2$, does not only depend on $x_2 - x_1$ as in method (ii):

$$R\left(X = x_2 \text{ vs. } X = x_1\right) = \frac{1 + x_2\beta}{1 + x_1\beta} < 1 + (x_2 - x_1)\beta.$$

For example, assume $\beta = 1$. Then,

$$R(X = 1 \text{ vs. } X = 0) = \frac{1 + 1}{1 + 0} = 2,$$

whereas

$$R(X = 2 \text{ vs. } X = 1) = \frac{1 + 2}{1 + 1} = 1.5,$$

although the difference of the arguments is the same in both cases.

2.4.5 Additional Dichotomous Variable (Method v)

Adding a dichotomous variable (exposed/not exposed) to the quantitative variable (level of exposure) X into the model, $f(x) = (I_{(X>0)}(x), h(x)); R(x) = \exp(\beta_0 + \beta_1 h(x))$ if compared to level zero or $R(x) = \exp(\beta_1 h(x))$ if comparing different positive levels of exposure; $h(x)$ arbitrary. For a better understanding of this method we recommend to first read Example 1.

This method was motivated by the fact that there are covariables whose distribution has a discrete and a continuous component. The most prominent example is smoking where a certain proportion of the population are non-smokers referred to as $X = 0$, i.e. $P(X = 0) > 0$, and the distribution of smoking dose within the smokers is continuous. In practice this distribution is of course also discrete since the answer options are usually integer numbers, however the underlying distribution can well be regarded as continuous. The relative risk for smoking k cigarettes daily compared to 0 may not be the same as smoking $2k$ cigarettes compared to k. To account for this fact, the above method has been applied in Jedrychowski et al. (1992) (see examples). It was more formally described in Robertson et al. (1994).

Fractional Polynomials (FP) (Method vi) 2.4.6

Here, we transform X via a fractional polynomial and use the exponential relative risk function

$$f(x) = H(x) \quad \text{(see below)} ; \quad R(\cdot) = \exp(\cdot) .$$

This method (Royston and Altman 1994) may be thought of as a formalized version of combining methods (iii) and (iv). The idea of fractional polynomials is to allow the variable to enter the model after it underwent transformations from a predefined class of eight different functions. This class is defined as $H_1(x) = x^p$ with $p \in \{-2, -1, -0.5, 0, 0.5, 1, 2, 3\}$ and x^0 is here defined as $\ln(x)$. In a FP of degree one the variable is entered successively with these eight transformations. In a FP of degree two the variable enters the model a second time with $H_2(x) = x^q$ with $q \in \{-2, -1, -0.5, 0, 0.5, 1, 2, 3\}$ and with $H_2(x) = x^p \ln(x)$ for $q = p$. Royston and Altman (1994) show that the degree two fractional polynomials cover a very rich family of dose-response curves. This means, that a huge variety of dose-response curves can be fitted. More formally, we have $R(\cdot) = \exp(\cdot)$ and as the linear predictor

$$\beta_0 + \sum_{j=1}^{J} \beta_j H_j(x) ,$$

where for a first order FP we have $J = 1$, $H_1(x) = x^p$ as defined above. For a second order FP we have $J = 2$, and the models are of the form $\beta_0 + \beta_1 x^p + \beta_2 x^q$. FPs of order larger than two rarely occur in practice.

Decision rules for a particular FP are suggested in Royston and Altman (1994) via the deviance comparison of different models. They note that often different FP's yield very similar fits with very similar dose-response curves. If X is an exposure variable which can take values smaller or equal zero, they recommend to add a constant to X in order to make the log transformation possible. A FP of degree 1 yields monotonous, a FP of degree two allows for non-monotonous dose-response functions (see Examples 3 and 4).

A Special Logarithmic Transformation (Method vii) 2.4.7

Using again the exponential relative risk function, we now perform a special logarithmic transformation of X, i.e.

$$f_k(x) = \ln(1 + \kappa x) ; \quad R(\cdot) = \exp(\cdot) ,$$

which generally yields a monotonous dose-response curve of the form

$$R(x) = \exp(\beta \ln(1 + \kappa x)) = (1 + \kappa x)^\beta .$$

It has the advantage that (a) it includes the additive and approximates the exponential relative risk function, (b) it can be applied to all regression models which are common in epidemiology, (c) monotonous concave and convex dose-response curves are possible, (d) it can be fitted with common software packages. To see (a), choose κ such that $\beta = 1$. Then we get $R(x) = 1 + kx$ as $\exp(\ln(1 + \kappa x)) = 1 + \kappa x$. Since in this case β is fixed and k is the parameter to be estimated, inference on k is made by calculating the deviance difference of the models with and without X which is under the null hypothesis asymptotically χ^2-distributed with one degree of freedom. For decreasing k, we get $R(\cdot) \approx \exp(\cdot)$. Figure 2.2 shows that this transformation allows concave, linear and convex dose-response curves.

The best fitting model within that class is obtained with an iterative search for k which results in minimal deviance (see Example 2).

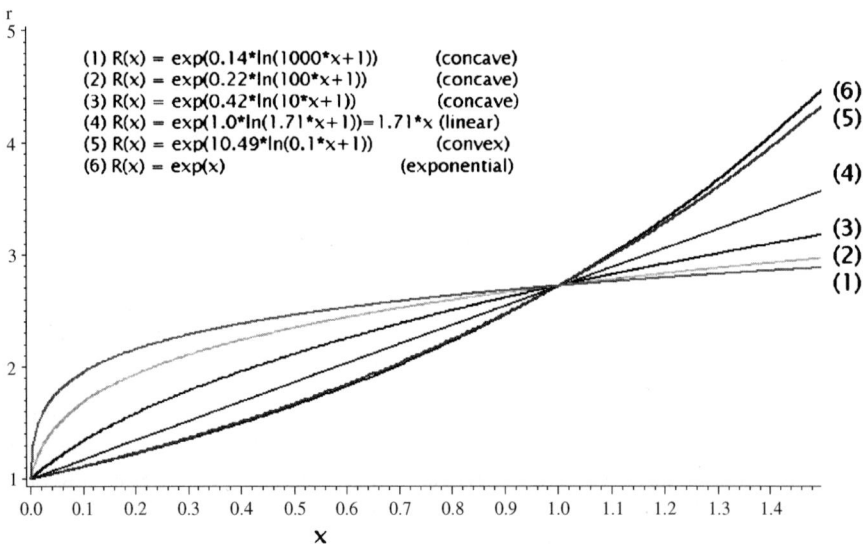

(1) R(x) = exp(0.14*ln(1000*x+1))　　(concave)
(2) R(x) = exp(0.22*ln(100*x+1))　　(concave)
(3) R(x) = exp(0.42*ln(10*x+1))　　(concave)
(4) R(x) = exp(1.0*ln(1.71*x+1))=1.71*x (linear)
(5) R(x) = exp(10.49*ln(0.1*x+1))　　(convex)
(6) R(x) = exp(x)　　(exponential)

Figure 2.2. Possible shapes of dose-response curves as obtained from the transformation (vii)

2.4.8　Conditioning (Method viii)

The method appears to be useful if X is a confounder of the variable Z. If Z is the variable of primary interest, and the main focus lies on correct and complete confounder adjustment. There is no interest in assessing the relation between X and Y. All previous methods may be applied as well, however, all these methods cannot exclude possible residual confounding. We therefore suggest to eliminate the effect of the confounder X by conditioning with fine strata. This method can readily be applied to case-control studies. It means that the regression coefficients of the logistic model are estimated by maximizing the conditional likelihood, where the conditioning is done on the observations in the matched sets which are formed post-hoc with fine strata according to X. Details may be found in Neuhäuser and Becher (1997). This method performs rather well in simulation studies with respect to bias and precision of the estimates in comparison to traditional methods to adjust for confounder through inclusion in the model as a covariable.

To further illustrate the method, consider the unconditional likelihood function of the logistic model with covariables X and Z which takes the form

$$
L_{\text{uncond}} = \prod_{i=1}^{n_0} \frac{1}{1 + \exp\left(\beta_0 + \beta'f(x) + \gamma z\right)} \prod_{i=n_0+1}^{n_0+n_1} \frac{\exp\left(\beta_0 + \beta'f(x) + \gamma z\right)}{1 + \exp\left(\beta_0 + \beta'f(x) + \gamma z\right)} ,
$$

where γ is the regression coefficient associated with z. Here we have n_0 controls and n_1 cases. To adjust for the confounding effect of X, it is common practice to include X into the model untransformed (method (ii)), or as categorical variables (method (i)), or after some other transformation (method (iii)). Instead, it is proposed to adjust for X via the conditional likelihood as

$$
L_{\text{cond}} = \prod_{h=1}^{H} \frac{\prod_{j=1}^{n_{1i}} \exp\left(\gamma z_{hj}\right)}{\sum_{l_j} \prod_{j=1}^{n_{1h}} \exp\left(\gamma z_{hl_j}\right)} .
$$

Here, we have defined H strata according to an appropriate grouping of X. Each stratum consists of n_{1i} cases and n_{0i} controls. The sum in the denominator ranges over the $l_j = \binom{n_{1h} + n_{0h}}{n_{1h}}$ choices to select n_{1h} observations from among the total observations in stratum h. It is possible to extend the method to many covariables, for example sex and age. In that case, all individuals with the same sex and the same age group form a set. Since the likelihood is conditioned on the observations of the confounder X, the variable cancels out from the likelihood (Breslow and Day 1980).

This post-hoc stratification method has a practical limitation. On one hand, one aims at defining fine strata to avoid residual confounding. On the other hand, if these strata are too fine, several of these may contain no cases or no controls. For example, if strata are defined through "year and month of birth", then in a medium sized study many will be uninformative since either cases or controls are missing. In that case they do not contribute to the estimation since they cancel out from the likelihood function above. This, in turn, yields a loss of power. See Example 5 for a practical application of the method.

For an individually matched case-control study this method can only be used to control for another confounder if the original matching is relaxed and new strata are formed according to the previous matching factors and the additional confounder. Properties of that procedure have not yet been investigated. Again, strata may become too sparse which limits the application.

2.4.9   Generalized Additive Models (GAM's) (Method ix)

The class of generalized additive models (GAM's) proposed by Hastie and Tib-shirani (1986, 1990) is a method to model an unspecified relation between a set of covariables X and a response variable Y. Using the previous notation, we have two covariables (X, Z). Here, the linear predictor $\beta_1 x + \beta_2 z$ is replaced by an ad-ditive predictor $s_1(x) + s_2(z)$, where s_i are unspecified smooth functions which are estimated by local scoring algorithms further described in Hastie and Tibshirani (1986, 1990). This method has been used in several epidemiological studies on air pollution and health effects (e.g. Stieb et al. 2000; Rossi et al. 1999). The method is intuitively appealing since it provides a flexible method for identifying non-linear covariate effects. However, this approach is more data-driven than the previous techniques described in this paper and it is not directly possible to take biologi-cal knowledge of the shape of the dose-response curve into account. In addition, since the method is rather complex, software is not commonly available and less user-friendly.

2.4.10   Spline Regression (Method x)

The last approach is also based on an exponential relative risk function, but with f chosen as a polynomial:

$$f(x) \quad \text{polynomial (see below) ;} \quad R(\cdot) = \exp(\cdot) .$$

Greenland (1995) has proposed spline regression within the logistic model (see also Chap. II.3 of this handbook). Boucher et al. (1998) use this method for analysing a case-control study on colon cancer and indicate several advantages of the method in comparison to the categorical analysis (method (i)). While in method (i) the risk is assumed to be constant within a category and jumps from category to category, with spline regression the sudden jumps of the dose-reponse function are avoided such that the fitted risk changes in a continuous manner within and across categories. The method can also be applied to the other regression models considered here. The method is formally described as follows: Let X be divided into K categories indexed by $k = 1, \ldots, K$ with $K - 1$ internal boundaries $c_1, \ldots, c_{K-1}$. In the so-called linear spline regression we have $f(x) = \alpha + \beta_1 x + \beta_2 s_2 + \ldots + \beta_K s_K$, where $s_k = 0$ if $x \le c_k$ and $s_k = x - c_k$ if $x > c_k$ and $R(\cdot) = \exp(\cdot)$. With this model one gets a continuous dose-response function with slopes changing at each cutpoint.

A more general spline regression avoids the biologically implausible fact that the first derivative of the dose-response function is not continuous. Here, a quadratic term for X is added and the s_k enter the model as squared such that $f(x) = \alpha + \beta_1 x + \gamma_1 x^2 + \beta_2 s_2^2 + \ldots + \beta_K s_K^2$. More details can be found in Greenland (1995).

Examples

In this section we demonstrate some of these methods with real data examples.

Example 1.   *Smoking and lung cancer in a case-control study*
          In a case-control study with 1432 lung cancer cases and 1343 controls
(Jedrychowski et al. 1992) we used method (v) (adding a dichotomous variable
(exposed/not exposed) in addition to the quantitative variable) for analysis. Few
individuals reported a very low dose – most individuals were either non-smokers
or smoked 10 or more cigarettes per day. This means that the effect of smoking
few cigarettes cannot be estimated with sufficient precision from the data. The
model had the form logit $P(Y = 1|x) = (\beta_0 + \beta_1 I_{X>0} + \beta_2 \ln(x + 1))$ and the
risk function is $R(x) = \exp(\beta_1 + \beta_2 \ln(x + 1))$ when compared to dose zero and
$R(x) = \exp(\beta_2[\ln(x_1 + 1) - \ln(x_0 + 1)])$ when estimating the odds ratio for dose x_1
compared to dose x_0. Since there were no individuals who reported smoking a very
low dose (say, 0.5 cigarettes per day), it is not possible to estimate the risk for
such doses. We obtained for Kreyberg type I tumors the dose-response function
$R(x) = \exp(-0.85 + 1.09 \ln(x + 1))$, x in number of cigarettes smoked per day
(Fig. 2.3). Note that this model does not allow meaningful OR estimation for low
doses compared to dose zero. This is because of the following: It can be assumed that
the "true" risk function is continuous over the full range of valid arguments, i.e. for
all positive numbers larger than or equal to zero. However, we have $R(0) = 1$, and
for small doses, say $x = 0.5$, we get $R(0.5) = \exp(-0.85 + 1.09 \ln(0.5 + 1)) = 0.665$
which is not meaningful since it would give a protective effect for a very small
dose. The advantage of the model is that the dose-response curve agreed very well

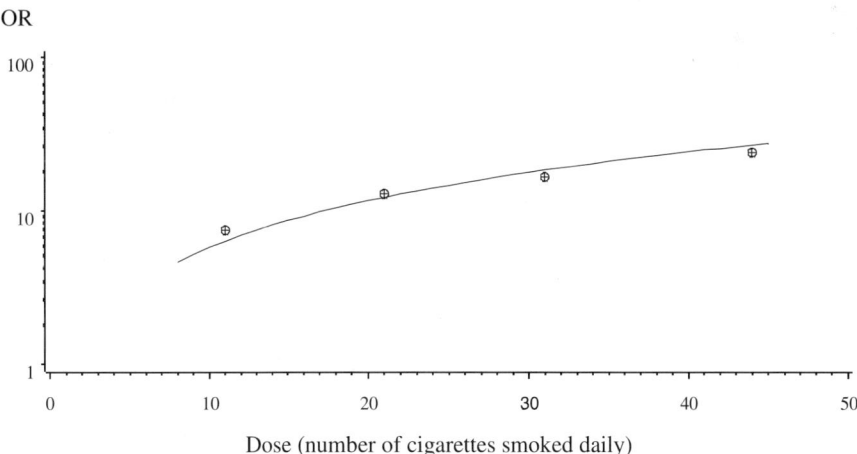

Figure 2.3. Dose-response analysis for tobacco dose and lung cancer from a Polish case-control study
(Jedrychowski et al. 1992). Point estimates indicated by dots were calculated using dummy variables;
the dose-response function was fitted as $R(x) = \exp(-0.85 + 1.09 \ln(x + 1))$

with the categorical estimates as obtained with method (i) in the observed dose range.   ◆

Example 2. *Dioxin exposure and cancer mortality in a cohort study*
             We used method (vii) $f_k(x) = \ln(kx + 1)$; $R(\cdot) = \exp(\cdot)$ within a cohort study analysis with Cox regression to investigate the relation between dioxin exposure and cancer risk. This method was chosen because monotonicity of the dose-response curve could be assumed on biological grounds. Data from 1189 workers occupationally exposed to dioxin were analysed using the Cox regression model given by $\lambda(x) = \lambda_0(x) \exp(\beta \ln(kx + 1))$. Here, X denotes the cumulative dioxin (toxic equivalencies, TEQ) exposure ranging from 0 to about 150,000 ng/kg blood fat $\times$ years which enters the model as a time-dependent covariable. Other covariables were also considered, however, they are omitted here for ease of presentation. Previous analyses showed that dioxin exposure was significantly associated with cancer risk, and the aim was to derive the most appropriate dose-response function (Becher et al. 1998). Figure 2.4 shows the resulting dose-response curves for the linear, exponential and best fitting model under the above model class. In that particular example, the best model is obtained for $\beta = 0.78$ and $k = 0.023$ yielding $RR(x) = (1 + 0.023x)^{0.78}$ with a difference of deviances to the null model of 30.49. The additive model is obtained for $k = 0.015$

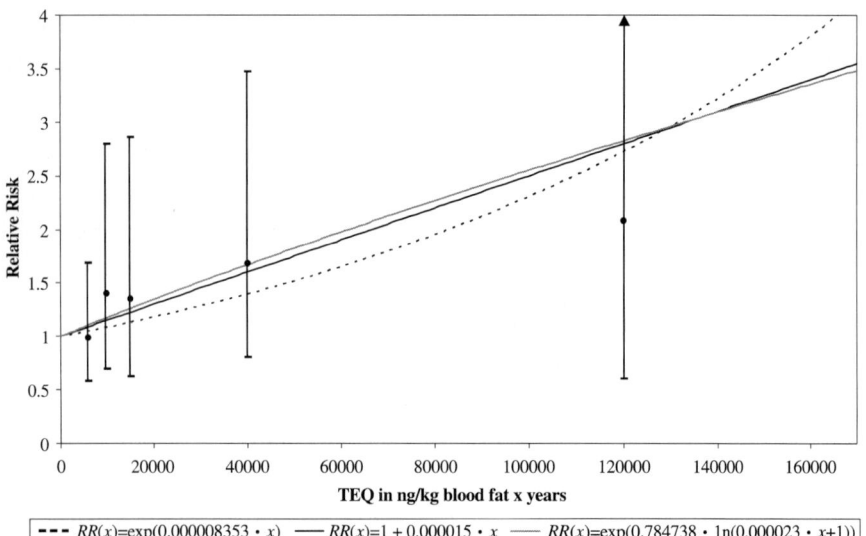

Relative Risk — TEQ in ng/kg blood fat x years

$- - -$ $RR(x)=\exp(0.000008353 \cdot x)$ ——— $RR(x)=1+0.000015 \cdot x$ ——— $RR(x)=\exp(0.784738 \cdot \ln(0.000023 \cdot x+1))$

Figure 2.4. Estimated dose-response curves and categorical risk estimates for cumulative dioxin (TEQ) – exposure and total cancer risk, cohort study on dioxin exposure and cancer mortality (from Becher et al. 1998). The point estimates give the risk estimates with corresponding 95% confidence intervals for the exposure groups categorised in quintiles of cumulative dioxin exposure in the exposed workers

which gives the risk ratio function $RR(x) = \exp(\ln(1 + 0.015x))^{1.0} = 1 + 0.015x$ with a difference of deviances to the null model of 30.47. The exponential model gives $RR(x) = \exp(0.085x)$ with a difference of deviances as 30.18. The model without the TEQ value gives a deviance of 26.935. This model includes dummy variables for age at start of employment (four categories), calendar year at start of employment (three categories) and duration of employment (four categories). Since the difference in the goodness of fit is small, it cannot be shown that one model is superior to the other. The point estimates included in the figure give the risk estimates with corresponding 95% confidence intervals for the exposure groups categorised in quintiles of cumulative dioxin exposure in the exposed workers. ◆

Example 3. *Modelling mortality by age using demographic surveillance system data*

The aim of this study was to analyse mortality data from a demographic surveillance system in Burkina Faso, West Africa (Sankoh et al. 2001). Based on a follow-up period from 1993 to 1999 in a population of about 30,000 inhabitants, vital events such as births, deaths, in and out migration were continuously monitored and age-specific mortality rates were estimated. We used Poisson regression to model the rates as a continuous function of age and employed the method of fractional polynomials. We identified the 2nd degree FP $\mu(t) = \exp(-2.66 + 0.001t + 0.646t^{0.5})$ to be the FP with the best fit according to the deviances of the respective models of degree 2. Figure 2.5 shows that the model fits the age-specific rates very well. ◆

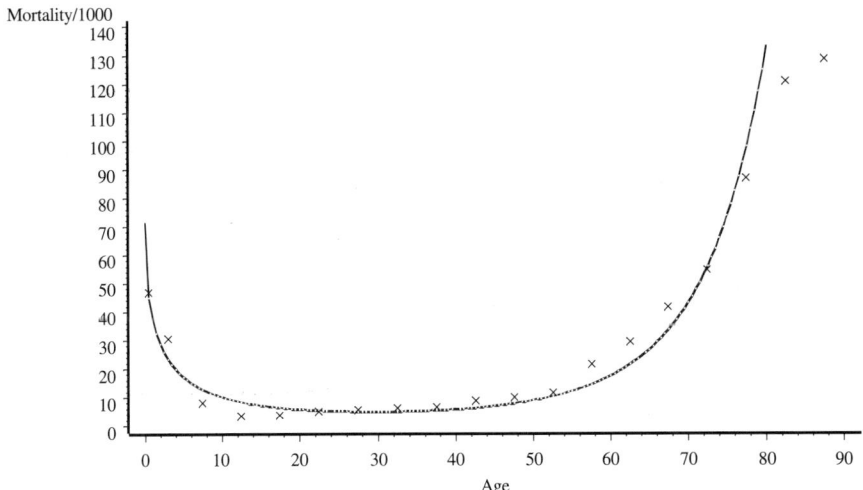

Figure 2.5. Mortality rates (all causes of death) by age, continuous and categorical, males and females, DSS population of about 30,000 inhabitants, Burkina Faso, West Africa, with a follow-up from 1993 to 1998; age-specific mortality rates fitted by $\mu(t) = \exp(-2.66 + 0.001t + 0.646t^{0.5})$

Example 4.   *Alcohol consumption and breast cancer*

In a case-control study on premenopausal breast cancer (Kropp et al. 2001) the effect of alcohol consumption was investigated. First, an analysis with the categorized variable coded as dummies was performed. Compared to abstinent women, the data indicate a decrease in risk of about 30% for consumption levels of 1–5 grams (OR 0.71, 95% CI: 0.54–0.91), 6–11 grams (OR 0.67, 95% confidence interval (95% CI): 0.50–0.91), and 12–18 grams (OR 0.73, 95% CI: 0.51–1.05) of alcohol per day. For 19–30 grams the odds ratio was 1.1 (95% CI: 0.73–1.65) and for 31 grams the OR was 1.94 (95% CI: 1.18–3.20). A dose-response-analysis was then done with fractional polynomials. This seemed particularly appropriate since a non-monotonous dose-response function was suggested by categorical analysis. The second degree polynomial $\ln(x + 1) + \sqrt{x}$ was found as the best model. The resulting function $OR(x) = \exp(-1.26 \ln(x + 1) + 0.83 \sqrt{x})$ is displayed in Fig. 2.6. The difference of deviances of this model compared to the model without alcohol was 33.1 ($p < 0.001$).   ◆

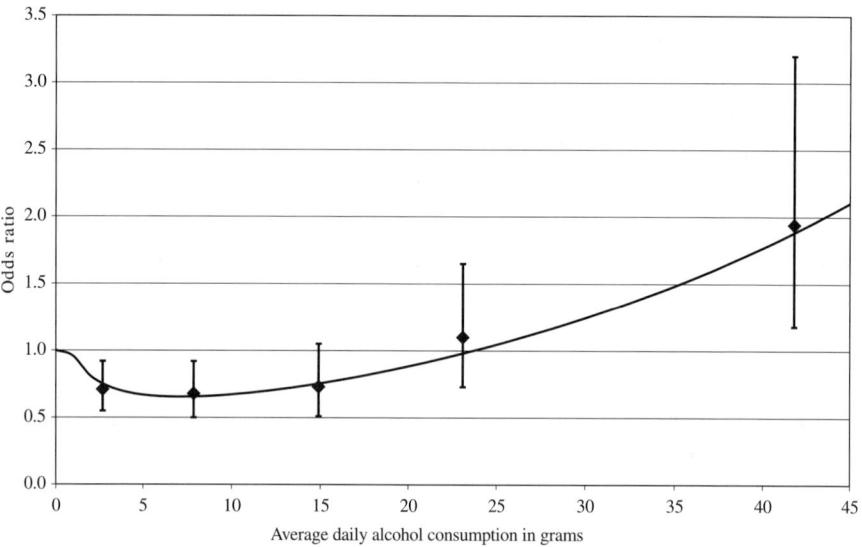

Figure 2.6. Alcohol consumption and breast cancer risk; case-control study in southwest Germany. Dose-response-analysis fitted with $OR(x) = \exp(-1.26 \ln(x + 1) + 0.83 \sqrt{x})$ and categorized estimates with 95% confidence intervals calculated for dummy variables (Kropp et al. 2001)

Example 5.   *Adjustment for the confounder "age" through conditioning*

This is an unmatched case-control study on laryngeal cancer risk factors (Zatonski et al. 1991). Here, age is the continuous covariable X and Z, smoking, is the variable of main interest. We were interested in an optimal adjustment of the confounding effect of X, not in a dose-response-analysis. The age distribution in cases and controls (Table 2.5) was extremely different. Methods (ii) and (iii) do not give satisfactory results because of a non-monotonous relation between age and

Table 2.5. Age distribution in cases and controls, Polish laryngeal cancer case-control study (Zatonski et al. 1991)

Age group (years)	Controls N	%	Cases N	%
25–34	275	28.5	7	2.8
35–39	163	16.9	7	2.8
40–44	96	10.0	19	7.6
45–49	90	9.3	27	10.9
50–54	110	11.4	71	28.5
55–59	123	12.7	62	24.9
60–65	108	11.2	56	22.5
Total	965	100.0	249	100.0

case-control status. Method (i) was used in the original paper with six age categories within an unconditional logistic regression model, however, this method may not be fully satisfactory as some residual confounding may remain with that method. Here, method (viii) „conditioning" is be advisable but the fractional polynomials also yield a good result. Table 2.6 shows the estimated regression coefficients for cigarette consumption, given as ln(no. of cigarettes smoked + 1), and standard errors, for different adjustment methods. Due to the confounding between smoking and age, the regression coefficients for smoking become smaller, the better the adjustment by age for smoking is. Method (i) with six age categories reduces the estimate for smoking from 1.732 to 1.236. The best fractional polynomials of degrees 1 and 2 yield an estimate of 1.193 and 1.185, respectively. Conditioning on age using 1-year intervals further reduces the estimate to 1.161. The difference between these latter estimates do not have practical relevance, however it confirms the simulated results by Neuhäuser and Becher (1997) that conditioning is a very appropriate method to control the confounding effect of X since (1) the confounding effect of age appears to be adjusted best and (2) the standard error of the estimate is virtually identical to that of the other models. ◆

Table 2.6. Selected regression coefficients for smoking by adjustment method, Polish laryngeal cancer case-control study (Zatonski et al. 1991)

	Method of adjustment for age	Deviance	$\widehat{\beta}_{smoking}$	s.e.
	no adjustment	960.4	1.732	0.153
(i)	categorical (2 age groups)	946.0	1.440	0.162
(i)	categorical (6 age groups)	919.7	1.236	0.163
(vi)	Fractional polynomial degree 1 (age^{-2})	931.6	1.193	0.160
(vi)	Fractional polynomial degree 2 (age^3, ln(age) × age^3)	918.7	1.185	0.159
(viii)	41 age strata (1-year intervals)	–	1.161	0.159

Conclusions

After a descriptive analysis, which may include some of the methods described in Sect. 2.2 – some of these are automatically produced by some software packages when contingency tables are generated – more elaborate methods come into play. However, it is difficult to provide recommendations in a general form of how to proceed such that each possible case is sufficiently handled.

Figure 2.7 provides a possible decision tree which is further described below.

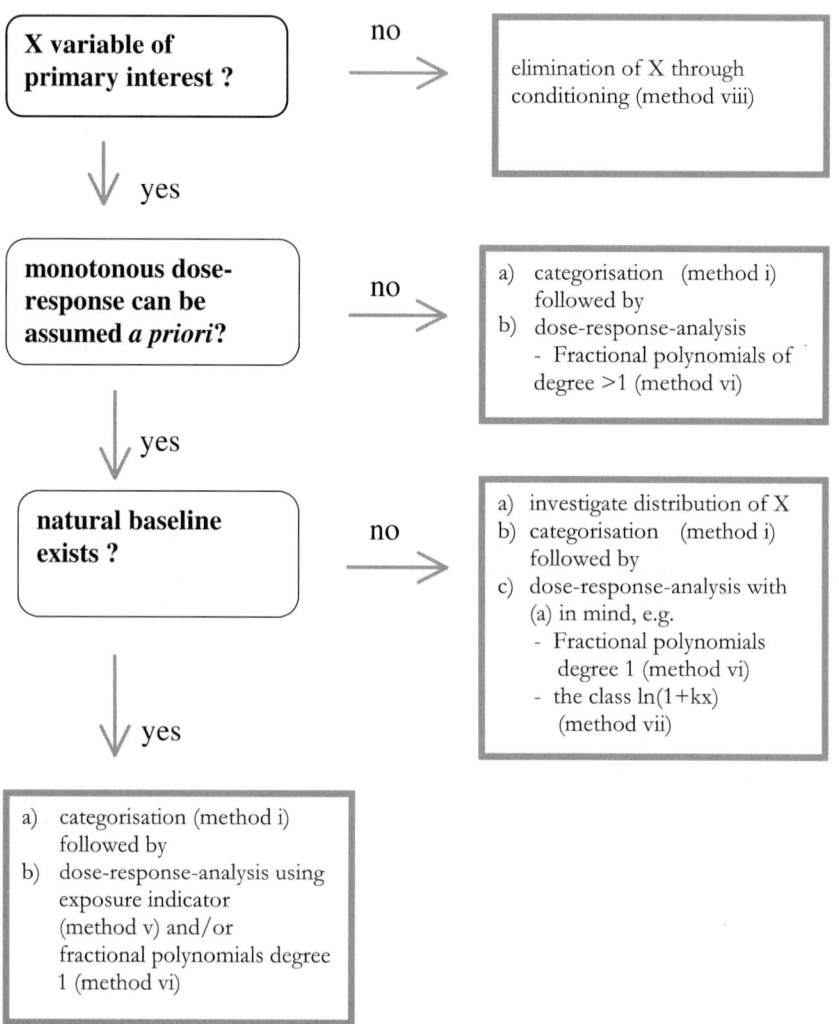

Figure 2.7. Suggested decision tree for analysing continuous covariables

The investigator is usually aware of whether X is a variable of primary interest or not. If not, conditioning is the recommended method in case-control studies to control the confounding effect of X on any other covariable since residual confounding is thus maximally reduced. Some care must be taken to define the strata appropriately. For example, if an adjustment of age is done by defining strata as "year of birth", this will result in large strata for the most frequent age groups and small strata for the extreme ages. In Neuhäuser and Becher (1997) an adaptive method which depends on the study size and distribution of X is further discussed. For other regression models, this method for control of confounding has not yet been investigated.

If X is the variable of primary interest, the situation is more complex. Biological plausibility should be taken into account. If the risk function is assumed to be non-monotonous, as in the Examples 3 and 4, fractional polynomials are a good choice. Another option would be GAM's or spline regression, however, as Royston et al. (2000) point out, the latter may exhibit artefacts which can make their interpretation difficult.

In many cases a monotonous relation can be assumed (Examples 1 and 2) and the interest is to investigate whether the dose-dependent increase in risk is linear, concave or convex (in the observed dose range). Here we have to distinguish between two cases: In Example 1 an effect is observed for which smoking is a prominent example. If the distribution of X is a mixture of a discrete and a continuous distribution, it can be shown theoretically that the correct model requires the inclusion of an exposure indicator variable. Therefore, method (v) is recommended. Of course, this method can be compared to other methods for determining the best choice of the function h.

If X is continuous and if it can be assumed on biological grounds that the relation with the disease is monotonous, method (vii) is recommended since it provides full flexibility under the constraint of monotonicity. A further feature is that the first derivative is also monotonous which does not seem to be a severe restriction. This method provides the possibility to fit a linear dose-response which is often used for regulatory risk assessment. Another option is to use fractional polynomials of degree one. Sauerbrei and Royston (1999) additionally recommend a previous transformation of the variable to guarantee a monotonous dose-response.

These recommendations give some guidance with respect to the estimation of a dose-response curve. Regarding the test of trend, these are similar. A test of linear trend within regression modelling is given by method (ii). Since this particular dose-response curve (linearity in the logarithm of the risk function) may not be the correct one, a rejection of the null hypothesis based on that test must not be interpreted as "the risk does not significantly increase (or decrease) with dose". One should rather base such a statement on the result from the most appropriate method. In the Examples 3 and 4 a trend test would not be meaningful, whereas in Example 1 a statement on increasing risk by dose should be based on the p-value for $\widehat{\beta}_2$.

Many of the methods presented above can yield very similar results although they may look very different at first sight. The models are often very closely related, and obviously the power to detect model misspecification is very small. While a categorisation into two levels (high/low exposure) is generally not recommended, a categorisation into four or more categories is, although not the optimal method, a useful first step during the analysis process because it gives a first impression on the effect of the variable for different dose levels. This is especially true if a natural baseline dose exists as for smoking where non-smokers are the natural baseline. For nutritional variables like "fat consumption" it is more difficult to define an appropriate baseline. Among the common methods are the construction of tertiles, quartiles, etc., or to use the same cutpoints as in previous studies in order to allow a comparison of the results.

The availability of software is an important aspect for practical work since statistical research is not always incorporated or intended when data are analysed for a study.

Both methods, (ix) GAM's and (x) spline regression, have drawbacks. As Royston et al. (2000) point out, "there are artefacts in the curve shapes, and possible overinterpretation of the data that may accompany them.". Royston et al. (1999) write, "we do not think that [GAM's and spline regression] are suitable as definitive models in epidemiology for the following reasons. The mathematical expressions for the curves are often very complex, so reporting of results must be by graphs or by extensive tabulation. The situation is unsatisfactory when similar studies are to be compared, and impossible if meta-analysis is intended. Data-dependence of the final model is more marked than for parametric models and the curves may be more difficult to interpret". We also think that the suggested parametric models provide sufficient flexibility on one hand, and allow inclusion of a priori assumptions on the shape of the dose-response curve (monotonous, U-shaped) on the other hand.

If a complex epidemiological study is analysed independently by different statisticians, the results will typically not be identical. This is particular true when continuous covariables are among the variables to be considered (not to mention other issues that make the analysis of epidemiological studies non-standard, such as the treatment of missing values, variable selection procedures, model building and others). Readers can be reassured, however, that if an analysis is performed with sufficient care the results and their interpretation will not differ very much.

References

Altman DG, Lausen B, Sauerbrei W, Schumacher M (1994) Dangers of using "optimal" cutpoints in the evaluation of prognostic factors. J Natl Cancer Inst 86:829–835

Becher H (1993) The concept of residual confounding in regression models and some applications. Stat Med 11:1747–1758

Becher H, Steindorf K, Flesch-Janys D (1998) Quantitative cancer risk assessment for dioxins using an occupational cohort. Env Health Persp 106 Suppl 2:663–670

Bernstein S, Bernstein R (1998) Schaum's outline of elements of statistics I: descriptive statistics and probability. McGraw–Hill, New York

Boucher KM, Slattery ML, Berry TD, Quesenberry C, Anderson K (1998) Statistical methods in epidemiology: a comparison of statistical methods to analyze dose-response and trend analysis in epidemiologic studies. J Clin Epidemiol 51:1223–1233

Breslow N, Day N (1980) Statistical methods in cancer research. Volume I – The analysis of case-control studies. IARC Scientific Publications No 32. International Agency for Research on Cancer, Lyon

Breslow N, Day N (1987) Statistical methods in cancer research. Volume II – The design and analysis of cohort studies. IARC Scientific Publications No 82. International Agency for Research on Cancer, Lyon

Dos Santos Silva I (1999) Cancer epidemiology: Principles and methods. International Agency for Research on Cancer, Lyon

Dietz A, Ramroth H, Urban T, Ahrens W, Becher H (2004) Exposure to cement dust, related occupational groups and laryngeal cancer risk: Results of a population based case-control study. International Journal of Cancer 108:907–911

Greenland S (1995) Dose-response and trend analysis in epidemiology: alternatives to categorical analysis. Epidemiology 6:356–365

Hastie T, Tibshirani R (1986) Generalized additive models. Statistical Science 1:297–318

Hastie T, Tibshirani R (1990) Generalized additive models. Chapman & Hall, London

Jedrychowski W, Becher H, Wahrendorf J, Basa-Cierpialek Z, Gomola G (1992) Effect of tobacco smoking on various histologic types of lung cancer. J Cancer Res Clin Oncol 118:276–282

Kropp S, Becher H, Nieters A, Chang-Claude J (2001) Low-to-moderate alcohol consumption and breast cancer risk by age 50 years among women in Germany. Am J Epidemiol 154:624–634

Maclure M, Greenland S (1992) Tests for trend and dose response: Misinterpretations and alternatives. Am J Epidemiol 135:96–104

Mantel N, Haenszel W (1959) Statistical aspects of the analysis of data from retrospective studies of diesease. J Natl Cancer Inst 22:719–748

Mizon GE, Richard JF (1986) The encompassing principle and its application to testing non-nested hypothesis. Econometrica 54:657–678

Nelder JA, Wedderburn RWM (1972) Generalized linear models. J Roy Statist Soc A 135:370–384

Neuhäuser M, Becher H (1997) Improved odds ratio estimation by posthoc stratification of case-control data. Stat Med 16:993–1004

Robertson C, Boyle P, Hsieh CC, Macfarlane GJ, Maisonneuve P (1994) Some statistical considerations in the analysis of case-control studies when the exposure variables are continuous measurements. Epidemiology 5:164–170

Rossi G, Vigotti MA, Zanobetti A, Repetto F, Gianelle V, Schwartz J (1999) Air pollution and cause-specific mortality in Milan, Italy, 1980–1989. Arch Environ Health 54:158–164

Royston P, Altman DG (1994) Regression using fractional polynomials of continuous covariables: Parsimonious parametric modelling. Appl Stat 43:429–467

Royston P, Thompson SG (1995) Comparing non-nested regression models. Biometrics 51:114–127

Royston P, Ambler G, Sauerbrei W (1999) The use of fractional polynomials to model continuous risk variables in epidemiology. Int J Epidemiol 28:964–974

Royston P, Sauerbrei W, Altman DG (2000) Modeling the effects of continuous risk factors [letter]. J Clin Epidemiol 53:219–221

Sankoh OA, Yé Y, Sauerborn R, Müller O, Becher H (2001) Clustering of childhood mortality in rural Burkina Faso. Int J Epidemiol 30:485–492

Sauerbrei W, Royston P (1999) Building multivariable prognostic and diagnostic models: transformation of the predictors using fractional polynomials. JRSS A 162:71–94

Schulgen G, Lausen B, Olsen JH, Schumacher M (1994) Outcome-oriented cutpoints in analysis of quantitative exposures. Am J Epidemiol 140:172–184

Stieb DM, Beveridge RC, Brook JR, Smith-Doiron M, Burnett RT, Dales RE, Beaulieu S, Judek S, Mamedov A (2000) Air pollution, aeroallergens and cardiorespiratory emergency department visits in Saint John, Canada. J Expo Anal Environ Epidemiol 10:461–477

Zatonski W, Becher H, Lissowska J, Wahrendorf J (1991) Tobacco, alcohol and diet in the etiology of laryngeal cancer – a population-based case-control study. Cancer Causes and Control 2:3–10

Regression Methods for Epidemiologic Analysis

II.3

Sander Greenland

Introduction

Basic tabular and graphical methods are an essential component of epidemiologic analysis and are often sufficient, especially when one need consider only a few variables at a time. They are, however, limited in the number of variables that they can examine simultaneously. Even sparse-strata methods (such as Mantel–Haenszel) require that some strata have two or more subjects; yet, as more and more variables or categories are added to a stratification, the number of subjects in each stratum may eventually drop to 0 or 1.

Regression analysis encompasses a vast array of techniques designed to overcome the numerical limitations of simpler methods. This advantage is purchased at a cost of stronger assumptions, which are compactly represented by a *regression model*. Such models (and hence the assumptions they represent) have the advantage of being explicit; a disadvantage is that the models may not be well understood by the intended audience or even the user. Regression models can and should be tailored by the analyst to suit the topic at hand; the latter process is sometimes called *model specification*. This process is part of the broader task of *regression modeling*.

To ensure that the assumptions underlying the regression analysis are reasonable approximations, it is essential that the modeling process be actively guided by the scientists involved in the research, rather than be left solely to mechanical algorithms. Such active guidance requires familiarity with the variety and interpretation of models. Hence, the present chapter will focus primarily on forms of models and their interpretation, rather than on the more technical issues of model fitting and testing. Because this chapter provides only outlines of key topics, it should be supplemented by readings in more detailed treatments of regression analysis, as can be found in Breslow and Day (1980, 1987), McCullagh and Nelder (1989), Clayton and Hills (1993), and Hosmer and Lemeshow (2000). For an in-depth treatment of the difficulties and limitations of regression analysis in nonexperimental studies, see Leamer (1978) or Berk (2004).

Achieving working competence in regression analysis requires comfort with basic geometry and algebra. While the ensuing discussion attempts to be self-contained, readers who feel lacking or weak in mathematical skills would do well to review a textbook in high school mathematics or college algebra (focusing especially on functions, graphs, and natural logarithms) before studying regression methods.

Regression Functions

A regression *function* is distinct from a model for that function. A regression *model* is another, simpler function used to approximate or estimate the true regression function. This distinction is often obscured and even unrecognized in elementary treatments of regression, which in turn has generated much misunderstanding of regression modeling. Therefore, this chapter provides separate discussions of *regression* functions and regression models.

There are two primary interpretations of regression functions, frequentist and Bayesian, which correspond to two different interpretations of probability (see Rothman and Greenland 1998, Chap. 12). The present chapter uses the frequentist interpretation, but briefly discusses the Bayesian interpretation at the end of this section. In both interpretations, the term *regression* is often used to refer to the regression function.

3.2.1   Frequentist Regression

In the frequentist view, the *regression* of a variable Y on another variable X is the function that describes how the average (mean) value of Y changes across population subgroups defined by levels of X. This function is often written as $E(Y|X = x)$, which should be read as "the average of Y when the variable X takes on the specific value x." The "E" part of the notation stands for "expectation", which here is just another word for "population mean".

As an example, suppose Y stands for "height" to the nearest centimeter at some time t, X stands for "weight" to the nearest kilogram at time t, and the population of interest is that of Denmark at time t. If we subclassify the Danish population at t into categories of weight X, compute the average height in each category, and tabulate or graph these average heights against the weight categories, the result displays the regression, $E(Y|X = x)$, of height Y on weight X in Denmark at time t. Several important points should be emphasized:

1. The *concept* of regression involves no modeling. Some would describe this fact by saying that the concept of regression is essentially "nonparametric". The regression of Y on X is just a graphical property of the physical world, like the orbital path of the earth around the sun.
2. There is nothing mathematically sophisticated about the regression function. Each point on a regression curve could be computed by taking the average of Y within a subpopulation defined as having a particular value of X. In the example, the value of the regression function at $X = 50$ kg, $E(Y|X = 50)$, is just average height at time t among Danes who weigh 50 kg at time t.
3. A regression function cannot be unambiguously computed until we carefully define X, Y, *and* the population over which the averages are to be taken. We will call the latter population the *target population* of the regression. This population is all too often left out of regression definitions, often resulting in confusion.

Some ambiguity is unavoidable in practice. In our example, is time t measured to the nearest year, day, minute, or millisecond? Is the Danish population all citizens, all residents, or all persons present in Denmark at t? We may decide that leaving these questions unanswered is tolerable, because varying the definitions over a modest range would not change the result to an important extent. But if we left time completely out of the definition, the regression would become hopelessly ambiguous, for now we would not have a good idea of who to include or exclude from our average: Should we include people living in Denmark in prehistoric times, or in the time of King Canute (a thousand years ago), or in the distant future (a thousand years from now)? The choice could have a strong effect on our answer, because of the large changes in height-to-weight relations that have occurred over time.

Other Concepts of Population 3.2.2

It is important to distinguish between a "target population" and a "source population". The target population of regression is defined without regard to our observations; for example, the regression of diastolic blood pressure on cigarette usage in China is defined whether or not we conduct a study in China (the target for this regression). A source population is a source of subjects for a particular study and is defined by the selection methods of the study; for example, a random-sample survey of all residents of Beijing would have Beijing as its source population. The concepts of target and source populations connect only insofar as inferences about a regression function drawn from a study are most easily justified when the source population of the study is identical to the target population of the regression. Otherwise, issues of generalization from the source to the target have to be addressed (see Rothman and Greenland 1998, Chap. 8).

In some literature, regression functions (and many other concepts) are defined in terms of averages within a "superpopulation" or "hypothetical universe". A superpopulation is an abstraction of a target population, sometimes said to represent the distribution (with respect to all variables of interest) of all possible persons that ever were or ever could be targets of inference for the analysis at hand. Because the superpopulation approach focuses on purely hypothetical distributions, it has encouraged substitution of mathematical theory for the more prosaic task of connecting study results to populations of immediate public-health concern. Thus, the present chapter defines regression functions in terms of averages within real (target) populations.

Binary Regression 3.2.3

The concept of regression applies to variables measured on any scale: The regressand and the regressor may be continuous or discrete, or even binary. For example, Y could be an indicator of diabetes ($Y = 1$ for present, $Y = 0$ for absent), and X could be an indicator for sex ($X = 1$ for female, $X = 0$ for male). Then $E(Y|X = 1)$ would represent the average of the diabetes indicator Y among females, and $E(Y|X = 0)$ would represent the average of Y among males.

When the regressand Y is a binary indicator $(0, 1)$ variable, $E(Y|X = x)$ is called a *binary regression*, and this regression simplifies in a very useful manner. Specifically, when Y can be only 0 or 1, the average $E(Y|X = x)$ equals the proportion of population members who have $Y = 1$ among those who have $X = x$. For example, if Y is the diabetes indicator, $E(Y|X = x)$ is the proportion with diabetes (i.e., with $Y = 1$) among those with $X = x$. To see this, let N_{yx} denote the number of population members who have $Y = y$ and $X = x$. Then the number of population members with $X = x$ is $N_{1x} + N_{0x} = N_{+x}$, and the average of Y among these members, $E(Y|X = x)$, is

$$\frac{N_{1x} \times 1 + N_{0x} \times 0}{N_{1x} + N_{0x}} = \frac{N_{1x}}{N_{+x}},$$

which is just the proportion with $Y = 1$ among those with $X = x$.

The epidemiologic ramifications of the preceding relation are important. Let $\Pr(Y = y|X = x)$ stand for "the proportion (of population members) with $Y = y$ among those with $X = x$" (which is often interpreted as the probability of $Y = y$ in the subpopulation with $X = x$). If Y is a binary indicator, we have just seen that

$$E(Y|X = x) = \Pr(Y = 1|X = x) ,$$

that is, the average of Y when $X = x$ equals the proportion with $Y = 1$ when $X = x$. Thus, if Y is an indicator of *disease presence* at a given time, the regression of Y on X, $E(Y|X = x)$, provides the proportion *with* the disease at that time, or prevalence proportion, given $X = x$. For example, if $Y = 1$ indicates diabetes presence on January 1, 2010 and X is weight on that day, $E(Y|X = x)$ provides diabetes prevalence as a function of weight on that day. If Y is instead an indicator of *disease incidence* over a time interval (cf. Chap. I.2 of this handbook and Chap. 3 of Rothman and Greenland, 1998), the regression of Y on X provides the proportion getting disease over that interval, or incidence proportion, given $X = x$. For example, if $Y = 1$ indicates stroke occurrence in 2010 and X is weight at the start of the year, $E(Y|X = x)$ provides the stroke incidence (proportion) in 2010 as a function of initial weight.

3.2.4 Multiple Regression

The concept of multiple regression is a simple extension of the ideas discussed above to situations in which there are multiple (two or more) regressors. To illustrate, suppose Y is a diabetes indicator, X_1 stands for "sex" (coded 1 for females, 0 for males), and X_2 stands for "weight" (in kilograms). Then the regression of Y on X_1 and X_2, written $E(Y|X_1 = x_1, X_2 = x_2)$, provides the average of Y among population members of a given sex X_1 and weight X_2. For example, $E(Y|X_1 = 1, X_2 = 70)$ is the average diabetes indicator (and, hence, the diabetes prevalence) among women who weigh 70 kg.

We can use as many regressors as we want. For example, we could include age (in years) in the last regression. Let X_3 stand for "age". Then $E(Y|X_1 = x_1, X_2 = x_2, X_3 = x_3)$ would provide the diabetes prevalence among population members of a given sex, weight, and age. Continuing to include regressors produces a very clumsy notation, however, and so we adopt a simple convention: We will let X represent the ordered list of all the regressors we want to consider. Thus, in our diabetes example, X will stand for the horizontal list (X_1, X_2, X_3) of "sex", "weight", and "age". Similarly, we will let x stand for the horizontal ordered list of values (x_1, x_2, x_3) for $X = (X_1, X_2, X_3)$. Thus, if we write $E(Y|X = x)$, it is merely a shorthand for

$$E\left(Y|X_1 = x_1, X_2 = x_2, X_3 = x_3\right),$$

when there are three regressors under consideration.

More generally, if there are n regressors $X_1, \ldots, X_n$, we will write X for the ordered list $(X_1, \ldots, X_n)$ and x for the ordered list of values $(x_1, \ldots, x_n)$. The horizontal ordered list of variables X is called a *row vector* of regressors, and the horizontal ordered list of values x is called a *row vector* of values. Above, the vector X is composed of the $n = 3$ items "sex", "weight", and "age", and the list x is composed of specific values for sex (0 or 1), weight (kilograms), and age (years). The number of items n in X is called the length or dimension of X.

The term *multivariate regression* is usually reserved for regressions in which there are multiple *regressands*. To illustrate, suppose Y_1 is an indicator of diabetes presence, Y_2 is diastolic blood pressure, and Y is the list (Y_1, Y_2) composed of these two variables. Also, let X be the list (X_1, X_2, X_3) composed of the sex indicator, weight, and age, as before. The multivariate regression of diabetes and blood pressure on sex, weight, and age provides the average diabetes indicator *and* average blood pressure for each combination of sex, weight, and age:

$$E\left(Y_1, Y_2|X_1 = x_1, X_2 = x_2, X_3 = x_3\right) = E(Y|X = x).$$

In general, there may be any number of regressands in the list Y and regressors in the list X of a multivariate regression. Multivariate regression notation allows one to express the separate regressions for each regressand in one equation.

Regression and Causation

When considering a regression function $E(Y|X = x)$, the variable Y is termed the dependent variable, outcome variable, or *regressand*, and the variable X is termed the independent variable, predictor, covariate, or *regressor*. The "dependent/independent" terminology is common but also problematic because it invites confusion of distinct probabilistic and causal concepts of dependence and independence. For example, if Y is age and X is blood pressure, $E(Y|X = x)$ represents the average age of persons given blood pressure, X. But it is blood pressure X that causally depends on age Y, not the other way around.

More generally, for any pair of variables X and Y, we can consider either the regression of Y on X, $E(Y|X = x)$, or the regression of X on Y, $E(X|Y = y)$. Thus, the concept of regression does not necessarily imply any causal or even temporal relation between the regressor and the regressand. For example, Y could be blood pressure at the start of follow-up of a cohort, and X could be blood pressure after 1 year of follow-up; then $E(Y|X = x)$ would represent the average initial blood pressure among cohort members whose blood pressure after 1 year of follow-up is x. This is an example of a noncausal regression.

Because regression functions do not involve any assumptions of time order or causal relations, regression coefficients and quantities derived from them represent measures of association, not measures of effect. To interpret the coefficients as measures of causal effects, it is important that the regression function being modeled provide a representation of the effects of interest that is approximately unconfounded (for a general discussion of the concept of confounding see Chap. I.9 of this handbook and Chap. 4 of Rothman and Greenland, 1998).

To make this no-confounding assumption more precise, suppose X contains the exposures of interest and Z contains the other regressors. Following Pearl (1995), we may then write

$$E\left[Y|\operatorname{Set}(X = x), Z = z\right]$$

for the average value Y would have *if* everyone in the target population with $Z = z$ had their X value set to x. This potentially counterfactual average can be very different from $E(Y|X = x, Z = z)$. The latter refers only to those population members with $X = x$ and $Z = z$, whereas the former refers to all population members with $Z = z$, including those who actually had X equal to values other than x.

As an example, suppose the target population is all persons born during 1901–1950 surviving to age 50, Y is an indicator of death by age 80, X contains only $X_1 =$ pack-years of cigarettes smoked by age 50, and $Z = (Z_1, Z_0)$ where $Z_1 = 1$ if female, 0 if male and $Z_2 =$ year of birth. Then

$$E\left[Y|X_1 = 20, Z = (1, 1940)\right]$$

would be the average risk of dying by age 80 (mortality proportion) among women born in 1940 and surviving to age 50 who smoked 20 pack-years by age 50. In contrast,

$$E\left[Y|\operatorname{Set}(X_1 = 20), Z = (1, 1940)\right]$$

would be the average risk of dying by age 80 among all women born in 1940 and surviving to age 50 *if* all such women had smoked 20 pack-years by age 50.

In regression analysis, we may define effect measures as contrasts of average outcomes (such as incidence) in the same population under different conditions. Consider the ratio effect measure contrasting the average of Y in the subpopulation with $Z = z$ when X is set to x^* versus that average when X is set to x:

$$\frac{E\left[Y|\operatorname{Set}(X = x^*), Z = z\right]}{E\left[Y|\operatorname{Set}(X = x), Z = z\right]}.$$

In the example,

$$\frac{E\left[Y|\operatorname{Set}(X_1 = 20), Z = (1, 1940)\right]}{E\left[Y|\operatorname{Set}(X_1 = 0), Z = (1, 1940)\right]}$$

represents the *effect* of smoking 20 pack-years by age 50 versus no smoking on the risk of dying by age 80 among women born in 1940. On the other hand, the ratio measure

$$\frac{E\left[Y|\operatorname{Set}(X_1 = 20), \boldsymbol{Z} = (1, 1940)\right]}{E\left[Y|\operatorname{Set}(X_1 = 0), \boldsymbol{Z} = (1, 1940)\right]}$$

represents only the *association* of smoking 20 pack-years by age 50 versus no smoking with the risk among women born in 1940, because it contrasts two different subpopulations (one with $X_1 = 20$, the other with $X_1 = 0$).

To infer that all associational measures estimated from our analysis equal their corresponding effect measures, we would have to make the following assumption of no confounding given $\boldsymbol{Z}$ (which is sometimes expressed by stating that there is no residual confounding):

$$E\left(Y|\boldsymbol{X} = \boldsymbol{x}, \boldsymbol{Z} = \boldsymbol{z}\right) = E\left[Y|\operatorname{Set}(\boldsymbol{X} = \boldsymbol{x}), \boldsymbol{Z} = \boldsymbol{z}\right] .$$

This assumption states that the average we observe or estimate in the subpopulation with both $\boldsymbol{X} = \boldsymbol{x}$ and $\boldsymbol{Z} = \boldsymbol{z}$ is equal to what the average in the larger subpopulation with $\boldsymbol{Z} = \boldsymbol{z}$ would have been if everyone had $\boldsymbol{X}$ set to $\boldsymbol{x}$. It is important to appreciate the strength of the assumption. In the above example, the no-confounding assumption would entail

$$E\left[Y|X_1 = 20, \boldsymbol{Z} = (1, 1940)\right] = E\left[Y|\operatorname{Set}(X_1 = 20), \boldsymbol{Z} = (1, 1940)\right] ,$$

which states that the risk we will observe among women born in 1940 who smoked 20 pack-years by age 50 equals the risk we would have observed in *all* women born in 1940 if they all had smoked 20 pack-years by age 50. The social variables associated with both smoking and death should lead us to doubt that the two quantities are even approximately equal.

If only a single summary measure of effect is desired, the covariate-specific no-confounding assumption can be replaced by a less restrictive assumption tailored to that measure. To illustrate, suppose in the above example we are only interested in what the effect of smoking 20 versus zero pack-years would be on *everyone* in the target, regardless of sex or birth year, as measured by the causal risk ratio

$$E\left[Y|\operatorname{Set}(X_1 = 20)\right] / E\left[Y|\operatorname{Set}(X_1 = 0)\right] .$$

The corresponding measure of association is the risk ratio for 20 versus 0 pack-years, standardized to the total population:

$$\frac{\sum_z E\left(Y|X_1 = 20, \boldsymbol{Z} = \boldsymbol{z}\right) \Pr(\boldsymbol{Z} = \boldsymbol{z})}{\sum_z E\left(Y|X_1 = 0, \boldsymbol{Z} = \boldsymbol{z}\right) \Pr(\boldsymbol{Z} = \boldsymbol{z})} ,$$

where $\Pr(\boldsymbol{Z} = \boldsymbol{z})$ is the proportion with $\boldsymbol{Z} = \boldsymbol{z}$ in the target. The no-confounding assumption we need here is that the standardized ratio equals the causal ratio. This summary assumption could hold even if there was confounding within levels of sex and birth year (although it would still be implausible in this example).

The dubiousness of no-confounding assumptions is often the chief limitation in using epidemiologic data for causal inference. This limitation applies to both tabular and regression methods. Randomization of persons to levels of X can largely overcome this limitation because it ensures that effect estimates follow a quantifiable probability distribution centered around the true effect. Randomization is not an option in most settings, however.

The default strategy is to ensure there are enough well-measured confounders in Z so that the no-confounding assumption is at least plausible. This strategy often leads to few subjects at each level x of X and z of Z, which in turn lead to the sparse-data problems that regression modeling attempts to address (Robins and Greenland 1986; Greenland 2000a, b; Greenland et al. 2000). A major limitation of this strategy is that, often, key confounders are poorly measured or unmeasured, and so cannot be used in ordinary modeling; prior distributions for the missing confounders must be used instead (Greenland 2003a).

3.2.6 Frequentist versus Bayesian Regression

In frequentist theory, an expectation is interpreted as an average in a specific subgroup of a specific population. The regression $E(Y|X = x)$ thus represents an objective functional relation among theoretically measurable variables (the average of Y as a function of the variables listed in X). It may be that this relation has not been observed, perhaps because it exists but we are unable to measure it, or because it does not yet exist. Examples of the former and latter are the regressions of blood pressure on weight in Spain 10 years ago and 10 years from now. In either situation, the regression is an external relation that one tries to estimate, perhaps by projecting (extrapolating) from current knowledge about presumably similar relations. For example, one might use whatever survey data one can find on blood pressure and weight to estimate what the regression of blood pressure on weight would look like in Spain 10 years ago or 10 years from now. In this approach, one tries to produce an *estimate* $\widehat{E}(Y|X = x)$ of the true regression $E(Y|X = x)$.

In subjective Bayesian theory, an expectation is what we would or should expect to see in a given target population. This notion of expectation corresponds roughly to a prediction of what we would see if we could observe the target in question. The regression $E(Y|X = x)$ does not represent an objective relation to be estimated, but instead represents a subjective (personal) expectation about how the average of Y varies across levels of X in the target population. Like the frequentist regression estimate, however, it is something one constructs from whatever data one may find that seems informative about this variation.

Both frequentist and Bayesian authors have noted that the two approaches often yield similar interval estimates (Cox and Hinkley 1974; Good 1983). It is increasingly recognized that divergences are usually due to differences in the criteria for a "good" point estimate: Frequentists traditionally prefer criteria of unbiased prediction (e.g., having an average error of zero), whereas Bayesians more often prefer criteria of closeness (e.g., having the smallest average squared error possible). When analogous criteria are adopted in both approaches, Bayesian and frequentist methods can yield similar numeric results in standard epidemiologic applications.

Nonetheless, Bayesians and frequentists interpret their results differently. The Bayesian presents a prediction, denoted by $E(Y|X = x)$, which he or she interprets as his or her "best bet" about the average of Y when $X = x$, according to some criteria for "best bet". The frequentist presents a prediction, denoted by $\widehat{E}(Y|X = x)$ (or, more commonly, $\widehat{Y}_{X=x}$), which he or she interprets as "the" best estimate of the average of Y when $X = x$, according to some criteria for "best estimate" (such as minimum variance among statistically unbiased estimators). Too often, the latter criteria are presumed to be universally shared, but are not really shared or even properly understood by epidemiologists; one could and would reach different conclusions using other defensible criteria (such as minimum mean squared error). For these reasons, when conducting regression analyses we find it valuable to consider both frequentist and Bayesian interpretations of methods and results.

Basic Regression Models

3.3

In any given instance, the true regression of Y on X, $E(Y|X = x)$, is an extremely complicated function of the regressors X. Thus, even if we observe this function without error, we may wish to formulate simplified pictures of reality that yield *models* for this regression. These models, while inevitably incorrect, can be very useful. A classic example is the representation of the distance from the earth to the sun, Y, as a function of day of the year T. To the nearest kilometer, this distance is a complex function of T because of the gravitational effects of the moon and of the other planets in the solar system. If we represent the orbit of the earth around the sun as a circle with the sun at the center, our regression model will predict the distance $E(Y|T = t)$ by a single number (about 150 million kilometers) that does not change with t. This model is adequate if we need only predict the distances to 2% accuracy. If we represent the orbit of the earth as an ellipse, our regression model will predict the earth-sun distance as smoothly and cyclically varying over the course of a year (within a range of about 147 to 153 million kilometers). Although it is not perfectly accurate, this model is adequate if we need to predict the distances to within 0.2% accuracy.

Model Specification and Model Fitting

3.3.1

Our description of the above models must be refined by distinguishing between the *form* of a model and a *fitted* model. "Circle" and "ellipse" refer to forms, that is, general classes of shapes. The circular model form corresponds to assuming a constant earth-sun distance over time; the elliptical model form allows this distance to vary over a temporal cycle. The process of deciding between these two forms is a simple example of *model specification.*

If we decide to use the circular form, we must also select a value for the radius (which is the earth-sun distance in the model). This radius specifies which circle (out of the many possible circles) to use as a representation of the earth's orbit and is an example of a model *parameter.* The process of selecting the "best" radius is an example of *model fitting,* and the circle that results is sometimes called the *fitted model* (although the latter term is sometimes used to refer to the model form instead). There are two important relations between a set of data and a model fit to those data. First, there is "distance" from the fitted model to the data; second, there is "resistance" or "stability" of the fitted model, which is the degree to which the parameter estimates change when the data themselves are changed.

Depending on our accuracy requirements, we may have on hand several simplified pictures of reality and hence several candidate models. At best, our choice might require a trade-off between simplicity and accuracy, as in the preceding example. There is an old dictum (often referred to as "Occam's razor") that one should not introduce needless complexity. According to this dictum, if we need only two percent accuracy in predicting the earth's distance from the sun, then we should not bother with the ellipse model and instead use the constant distance derived from the circle model.

There is a more subtle benefit from this advice than avoiding needless mental exertion. Suppose we are given two models, one (the more complex) containing the other (the more simple) as a special case, and some data with which to fit the two models. Then the more complex model will be able to fit the available data more closely than the simpler model, in the sense that the predictions from the more complex model will (on average) be closer to what was seen in the data than will the predictions from the simpler model. This is so in the above example because the ellipse contains the circle as a special case. Nonetheless, there is a penalty for this closeness to the data: The predictions obtained from the more complex model tend to be less stable than those obtained from the simpler model.

Consider now the use of the two different model forms to predict events outside of the data set to which the models were fit. An example would be forecasting the earth's distance from the sun; another would be predicting the incidence of AIDS five years in the future. Intuitively, we might expect that if one model is both closer to the data and more stable than the other, that model will give more accurate predictions. The problem is that the choice among models is rarely so clear-cut: Usually, one model will be closer to the data, while the other will be more stable, and it will be difficult to tell which will be more accurate. This is one dilemma we often face in a choice between a more complex and simpler model.

To summarize, model specification is the process of selecting a model form, while model fitting is the process of using data to estimate the parameters in a model form. There are many methods of model fitting, and the topic is so vast and technical that we will only superficially outline a few key elements. Nearly all commercial computer programs are based on one of just a few fitting methods, so that nearly all users (statisticians as well as epidemiologists) are forced to base their analyses on the assumptions of these methods. We will briefly discuss specification and fitting methods below.

Background Example

The following epidemiologic example will be used at various points to illustrate specific models. At the time of this writing, there is a controversy over whether women with no history of breast cancer but thought to be of high risk (due to family history and perhaps other factors) should be given the drug tamoxifen as a prophylactic regimen. Current evidence suggests that tamoxifen might prevent breast cancer but also cause or promote endometrial and liver cancer.

One measure of the net impact of tamoxifen prophylaxis up to a given age is the change in risk of death by that age. Suppose the regressand Y is an indicator of death by age 70 ($Y = 1$ for dead, 0 for alive). The regressors X include

$$X_1 = \text{years of tamoxifen therapy,}$$

$$X_2 = \text{age (in years) at start of tamoxifen therapy,}$$

$$X_3 = \text{age at menarche,}$$

$$X_4 = \text{age at menopause,}$$

$$X_5 = \text{parity.}$$

The target population is American women born during 1945–1950 who survive to age 50 and do not use tamoxifen before that age. If tamoxifen is not taken during follow-up, we set age at tamoxifen start (X_2) to 70 because women who start at 70 or later and women who never take tamoxifen have the same exposure history during the age interval under study.

In this example, the regression $E(Y|X = x)$ is just the average risk, or incidence proportion, of death by age 70 among women in the target population who have $X = x$. Therefore, we will write $R(x)$ as a shorthand for $E(Y|X = x)$. We will also write R for the crude (overall) average risk $E(Y)$, $R(x_1)$ for the average risk $E(Y|X_1 = x_1)$ in the subpopulation defined by having $X_1 = x_1$ (without regard to the other variables), and so on.

Vacuous Models

A model so general that implies nothing at all, but simply re-expresses the overall average risk R in a different notation, is

$$E(Y) = R = \alpha , \quad 0 < \alpha < 1 . \tag{3.1}$$

(this model does exclude $R = 0$ or 1, but it allows R to be arbitrarily close to 0 or 1, so this exclusion is of no practical consequence). There is only one regression parameter (or coefficient) α in this model, and it corresponds to the average risk in the target population. A model such as model (3.1) that has no implication (i.e., that imposes no restriction or constraint) is said to be *vacuous*.

Two models are said to be equivalent if they have identical implications for the regression. A model equivalent to model (3.1) is

$$E(Y) = R = \exp(\alpha) , \quad \alpha < 0 . \tag{3.2}$$

This model has no implication. In this model, α is the natural logarithm of the overall average risk:

$$\alpha = \ln(R) .$$

Another model equivalent to models (3.1) and (3.2) is

$$E(Y) = R = \text{expit}(\alpha) , \tag{3.3}$$

where $\text{expit}(\alpha)$ is the *logistic* transform of α, defined as

$$\text{expit}(\alpha) = \frac{\exp(\alpha)}{1 + \exp(\alpha)} .$$

Again, model (3.3) has no implication. Now, however, the parameter α in model (3.3) is the logit (log odds) of the overall average risk:

$$\alpha = \ln \left(\frac{R}{1 - R} \right) = \text{logit}(R) .$$

For an introduction of risk measures in general see Chap. I.2 of this handbook and Chap. 3 of Rothman and Greenland (1998).

3.3.4   Constant Models

In comparing the complexity and implications of two models A and B, we say that model A is more general, more flexible, or more complex than model B, or that A contains B, if all the implications of model A are also implications of model B, but not vice-versa (that is, if B imposes some restrictions beyond those imposed by A). Other ways of stating this relation are that B is simpler, stronger, or stricter than A, B is contained or nested within A, or B is a special case of A. The following model is superficially similar to model (3.1), but is in fact much more strict:

$$E\left(Y|X_1 = x_1\right) = R(x_1) = \alpha \tag{3.4}$$

for all x_1. This model implies that the average risks of the subpopulations defined by years of tamoxifen use are identical. The parameter α represents the common value of these risks. This model is called a *constant* regression because it allows no variation in average risks across levels of the regressor. To see that it is a special case of model (3.1), note that $E(Y)$, the overall average, is just an average of all the X_1-specific averages $E(Y|X_1 = x_1)$. Hence, if all the X_1-specific averages equal α, as in model (3.4), then the overall average must equal α as well, as in model (3.1).

The following two models are equivalent to model (3.4):

$$R(x_1) = \exp(\alpha) , \tag{3.5}$$

which can be rewritten

$$\ln[R(x_1)] = \alpha ,$$

and

$$R(x_1) = \operatorname{expit}(\alpha) = e^\alpha/(1 + e^\alpha) , \tag{3.6}$$

which can be rewritten

$$\operatorname{logit}[R(x_1)] = \alpha .$$

In model (3.5), α is the common value of the log risks $\ln[R(x_1)]$, while in model (3.6), a is the common value of the logits, $\operatorname{logit}[R(x_1)]$. Each of the equivalent models (3.4)–(3.6) is a special case of the more general models (3.1)–(3.3).

A constant regression is of course implausible in most situations. For example, age is related to most health outcomes. In the above example, we should expect the average death risk to vary across the subgroups defined by age at start (X_2). There is an infinitude of ways to model these variations. The problem of selecting a useful model from among the many choices is discussed below. For now, we only describe some of the more common choices, focusing on models for average risks (incidence proportions), incidence odds, and person-time incidence rates. The models for risks and odds can also be used to model prevalence proportions and prevalence odds.

Linear Risk Models

Consider the model

$$R(x_1) = \alpha + \beta_1 x_1 . \tag{3.7}$$

This model allows the average risk to vary across subpopulations with different values for X_1, but only in a linear fashion. The model implies that subtracting the average risk in the subpopulation with $X_1 = x_1$ from that in the subpopulation with $X_1 = x_1 + 1$ will always yield β_1, *regardless* of what x_1 is. Under model (3.7),

$$R(x_1 + 1) = a + \beta_1(x_1 + 1)$$

and

$$R(x_1) = \alpha + \beta_1 x_1 ,$$

so

$$R(x_1 + 1) - R(x_1) = \beta_1 .$$

Thus, in our example, β_1 represents the difference in risk between the subpopulation defined by having $X_1 = x_1 + 1$ and that defined by having $X_1 = x_1$. The model implies that this difference does not depend on the reference level x_1 for X_1, used for the comparison.

Model (3.7) is an example of a *linear* risk model. It is a special case of model (3.1); it also contains model (3.4) as a special case (model (3.4) is the special case of model (3.7) in which $\beta_1 = 0$ and so average risks do not vary across levels of X_1). Linear risk models (such as model (3.7)) are easy to understand, but have a severe technical problem that makes them difficult to fit in practice: There are combinations of α and β_1 that would produce impossible values (less than 0 or greater than 1) for one or more of the risks $R(x_1)$. Several models partially or wholly address this problem by transforming the linear term $\alpha + \beta_1 x_1$ before equating it to the risk. We will study two of these models below.

3.3.6   Recentering

Under model (3.7),

$$R(0) = \alpha + \beta \times 0 = \alpha ,$$

so α represents the average risk for the subpopulation with $X_1 = 0$. In the present example, 0 is a possible value for X_1 (tamoxifen) and so this interpretation of α presents no problem. Suppose, however, we modeled X_3 (age at menarche) instead of X_1:

$$R(x_3) = \alpha + \beta_3 x_3 .$$

Because age at menarche cannot equal zero, α would have no meaningful interpretation in this model. In order to avoid such interpretational problems, it is a useful practice to recenter a variable for which zero is impossible (such as X_3) by subtracting some frequently observed value from it before putting it in the model. For example, age 13 is a frequently observed value for age at menarche. We can redefine X_3 to be "age at menarche minus 13 years". With this redefinition, $R(x_3) = \alpha + \beta_3 x_3$ refers to a different model, one in which $R(0) = \alpha$ represents the average risk for women who were age 13 at menarche. We will later see that such recentering is advisable when using any model, and is especially important when product terms ("interactions") are used in a model.

3.3.7   Rescaling

A simple way of describing β_1 in model (3.7) is that it is the difference in risk per unit increase in X_1. Often the units used to measure X_1 are small relative to exposure increases of substantive interest. Suppose, for example, that X_1 was diastolic blood pressure (DBP) measured in mm Hg; β_1 would then be the risk difference per mm increase in DBP. A 1 mm Hg increase would, however, be of no clinical interest; instead, we would want to consider increases of at least 5 and possibly 10 or 20 mm Hg. Under model (3.7), the difference in risk per 10 mm Hg increase would be $10\beta_1$. If we wanted to have β_1 represent the difference in risk per 10 mm Hg, we need only redefine X_1 as DBP divided by 10; X_1 would then be DBP in cm Hg.

Division of a variable by a constant, as just described, is sometimes called *rescaling* of the variable. Such rescaling is advisable whenever it changes the measurement unit to a more meaningful value. Unfortunately, rescaling is often done in a way that makes the measurement unit *less* meaningful, by dividing the variable by its sample standard deviation (SD). The sample SD is an irregular unit unique to the study data, and depends heavily on how subjects were selected into the analysis. For example, the SD of DBP might be 12.7 mm Hg in one study and 15.3 mm Hg in another study. Suppose each study divided DBP by its SD entering it in model (3.7). In the first study β_1 would refer to the change in risk per 12.7 mm Hg increase in DBP, whereas in the second study β_1 would refer to the change in risk per 15.3 mm Hg. The rescaling would thus have rendered the coefficients interpretable only in peculiar and different units, so that they could not be compared directly to one another or to coefficients from other studies.

We will later see that rescaling is even more important when product terms are used in a model. We thus recommend that rescaling be done using simple and easily interpreted constants for the divisions. Methods that involve division by sample SDs (such as transformations of variables to Z-scores), however, should be avoided.

Exponential Risk Models

3.3.8

Consider the following model:

$$R(x_1) = \exp\left(\alpha + \beta_1 x_1\right) . \tag{3.8}$$

Since the exponential function (exp) is always positive, model (3.8) will produce positive $R(x_1)$ for any combination of $\alpha + \beta_1$. Model (3.8) is sometimes called an *exponential* risk model. It is a special case of the vacuous model (3.2); it also contains the constant model (3.5) as the special case in which $\beta_1 = 0$.

To understand the implications of the exponential risk model, we can recast it in an equivalent form by taking the natural logarithm of both sides:

$$\ln\left[R\left(x_1\right)\right] = \ln\left[\exp\left(\alpha + \beta_1 x_1\right)\right] = \alpha + \beta_1 x_1 . \tag{3.9}$$

Model (3.9) is often called a *log-linear* risk model. The exponential/log-linear model allows risk to vary across subpopulations defined by X_1, but only in an exponential fashion. To interpret the coefficients, we may compare the log risks under model (3.9) for the two subpopulations defined by $X_1 = x_1 + 1$ and $X_1 = x_1$:

$$\ln\left[R\left(x_1 + 1\right)\right] = \alpha + \beta_1\left(x_1 + 1\right)$$

and

$$\ln\left[R\left(x_1\right)\right] = \alpha + \beta_1 x_1 ,$$

so

$$\ln\left[R\left(x_1+1\right)\right]-\ln\left[R\left(x_1\right)\right]=\ln\left[R\left(x_1+1\right)/R\left(x_1\right)\right]=\beta_1 .$$

Thus, under models (3.8) and (3.9), β_1 represents the log risk ratio comparing the subpopulation defined by having $X_1 = x_1+1$ and that defined by $X_1 = x_1$, regardless of the chosen reference level x_1. Also, $\ln[R(0)] = \alpha + \beta \times 0 = \alpha$ if $X_1 = 0$; thus, α represents the log risk for the subpopulation with $X_1 = 0$ (and so is meaningful only if X_1 can be zero).

We can derive another (equivalent) interpretation of the parameters in the exponential risk model by noting that

$$R\left(x_1+1\right)=\exp\left[\alpha+\beta_1\left(x_1+1\right)\right]$$

and

$$R\left(x_1\right)=\exp\left(\alpha+\beta_1 x_1\right)$$

so

$$R\left(x_1+1\right)/R\left(x_1\right)=\exp\left[\alpha+\beta_1\left(x_1+1\right)-\left(\alpha+\beta_1 x_1\right)\right]=\exp\left(\beta_1\right) .$$

Thus, under models (3.8) and (3.9), β_1 represents the ratio of risks between the sub-populations defined by $X_1 = x_1+1$ and $X_1 = x_1$, and this ratio does not depend on the reference level x_1 (because x_1 does not appear in the final expression for the risk ratio). Also, $R(0) = \exp(\alpha + \beta \times 0) = e^\alpha$, so e^α represents the average risk for the subpopulation with $X_1 = 0$.

As with linear risk models, exponential risk models have the technical problem that some combinations of α and β_1 will yield risk values greater than 1, which are impossible. This will not be a practical concern, however, if all the fitted risks and their confidence limits fall well below 1.

3.3.9   Logistic Models

Neither linear nor exponential risk models can be used to analyze case-control data if no external information is available to allow estimation of risks in the source population, whereas the following model can be used without such information:

$$R\left(x_1\right)=\text{expit}\left(\alpha+\beta_1 x_1\right)=\frac{\exp\left(\alpha+\beta_1 x_1\right)}{1+\exp\left(\alpha+\beta_1 x_1\right)} . \tag{3.10}$$

This model is called a *logistic* risk model, after the logistic function (expit) in the core of its definition. Because the range of the logistic function is between 0 and 1, the model will only produce risks between 0 and 1, regardless of the values for α, β_1, and x_1. The logistic model is perhaps the most commonly used model in epidemiology, so we examine it in some detail. Model (3.10) is a special case of model (3.3), but unlike model (3.3) it is not vacuous because it constrains the

X_1-specific risks to follow a particular (logistic) pattern. The constant model (3.6) is the special case of the logistic model in which $\beta_1 = 0$.

To understand the implications of the logistic model, it is helpful to recast it as a model for the odds. First, note that, under the logistic model (3.10),

$$1 - R\left(x_1\right) = 1 - \frac{\exp\left(\alpha + \beta_1 x_1\right)}{1 + \exp\left(\alpha + \beta_1 x_1\right)} = \frac{1}{1 + \exp\left(\alpha + \beta_1 x_1\right)} \, .$$

Since $R(x_1)/[1 - R(x_1)]$ is the odds, we divide each side of (3.10) by the last term and find that, under the logistic model, the odds of disease $O(x_1)$ when $X_1 = x_1$ is

$$O\left(x_1\right) = \frac{R\left(x_1\right)}{1 - R\left(x_1\right)} = \frac{\dfrac{\exp\left(\alpha + \beta_1 x_1\right)}{1 + \exp\left(\alpha + \beta_1 x_1\right)}}{\dfrac{1}{1 + \exp\left(\alpha + \beta_1 x_1\right)}} = \exp\left(\alpha + \beta_1 x_1\right). \qquad (3.11)$$

This equation shows that the logistic risk model is equivalent to an exponential *odds* model.

Taking logarithms of both sides of (3.11), we see that the logistic model is also equivalent to the log-linear odds model

$$\ln\left[O\left(x_1\right)\right] = \alpha + \beta_1 x_1 \, . \qquad (3.12)$$

Recall that the logit of risk is defined as the log odds:

$$\text{logit}\left[R\left(x_1\right)\right] = \ln\left[R\left(x_1\right)/\left(1 - R(x_1)\right)\right] = \ln\left[O\left(x_1\right)\right] \, .$$

Hence, from (3.12), the logistic model can be rewritten in one more equivalent form,

$$\text{logit}\left[R\left(x_1\right)\right] = \alpha + \beta_1 x_1 \, . \qquad (3.13)$$

This equivalent of the logistic model is often called the logit-linear risk model, or *logit model*.

As a general caution regarding terms, note that "log-linear model" can refer to any of several different models, depending on the context: In addition to the log-linear risk model (3.9) and the log-linear *odds* model (3.12) given above, there are also log-linear *rate* models and log-linear *incidence-time* models, which will be described below.

We can derive two equivalent interpretations of the logistic model parameters. First,

$$\ln\left[O\left(x_1 + 1\right)\right] = \alpha + \beta\left(x_1 + 1\right) \, ,$$

$$\ln\left[O\left(x_1\right)\right] = \alpha + \beta_1 x_1 \, ,$$

so

$$\ln\left[O\left(x_1 + 1\right)\right] - \ln\left[O\left(x_1\right)\right] = \ln\left[O\left(x_1 + 1\right)/O\left(x_1\right)\right] = \beta_1 \, .$$

Thus, under the logistic model (3.10), β_1 represents the log odds ratio comparing the subpopulations with $X_1 = x_1 + 1$ and $X_1 = x_1$. Also, $\ln[O(0)] = \alpha + \beta_1 \times 0 = \alpha$; thus, α is the log odds (logit) for the subpopulation with $X_1 = 0$ (and so is meaningful only if X_1 can be zero). Equivalently, we have

$$O\left(x_1 + 1\right) / O\left(x_1\right) = \exp\left(\beta_1\right)$$

and

$$O(0) = \exp(\alpha) ,$$

so that $\exp(\beta_1)$ is the odds ratio comparing the subpopulations with $X_1 = x_1 + 1$ and $X_1 = x_1$, and $\exp(\alpha)$ is the odds for the subpopulation with $X_1 = 0$.

Logistic models may be applied to case-control studies by re-interpreting the odds $O(x)$ as the case-control ratio in the study; see Breslow and Day (1980, Chap. 6) or Rothman and Greenland (1998, pp 416–422) for details. For an introduction to case-control studies we refer to Chap. I.6 of this handbook and Chap. 7 of Rothman and Greenland (1998).

3.3.10   A Graphical Example

Suppose a particular cohort has a 1-year risk of a cardiovascular event that is 0.02 at age 50 rising to 0.32 at age 80, an absolute risk increase of 0.30, a ratio risk increase of $0.32/0.02 = 16$-fold, and a ratio odds increase of $(0.32/0.68)/(0.02/0.98) = 23.06$. The average annual absolute risk increase is $0.30/30 = 0.01$, but the way this increase is distributed over ages could be quite different under different models.

If the risk increase is linear in age and x is age, the linear model for the risk from age 51 to 80 would be $R(x) = \alpha_1 + \beta_1(x - 50)$. Solving $R(50) = 0.02$ and $R(80) = 0.32$ we get $\alpha_1 = 0.02$ and $\beta_1 = 0.30/30$ year $= 0.01/$ year, a constant absolute increase in risk of 0.01 for each of age.

Now suppose the increase is exponential rather than linear. The loglinear form of the exponential model would be $\ln[R(x)] = \alpha_1 + \beta_1(x - 50)$. Solving $R(50) = 0.02$ and $R(80) = 0.32$ we now get $\alpha_1 = \ln(0.02) = -3.912$ and $\beta_1 = \ln(16)/30$ year $= 0.09242/$ year, corresponding to a constant proportionate risk increase of $e^{0.09242} = 1.097$ or about 9.7% for each year of age. This corresponds to an absolute risk increase of only about 0.002 going from age 50 to 51, but of about 0.03 (15 times more) going from age 79 to 80.

Finally, suppose the increase is logistic. The logit version of the logistic model would be $\text{logit}[R(x)] = \alpha_1 + \beta_1(x - 50)$. Solving $R(50) = 0.02$ and $R(80) = 0.32$ we now get $\alpha_1 = \text{logit}(0.02) = -3.892$ and $\beta_1 = \ln(23.06)/30$ years $= 0.1046/$ years, corresponding to a constant proportionate odds increase of $e^{0.1046} = 1.11$ or about 11% for each year of age. This corresponds to an absolute risk increase of only about 0.002 going from age 50 to 51, but of about 0.022 (11 times more) going from age 79 to 80.

Figure 3.1a gives plots of the risks from the above three models from age 50 to 80. The linear model produces a straight line, whereas the exponential model produces

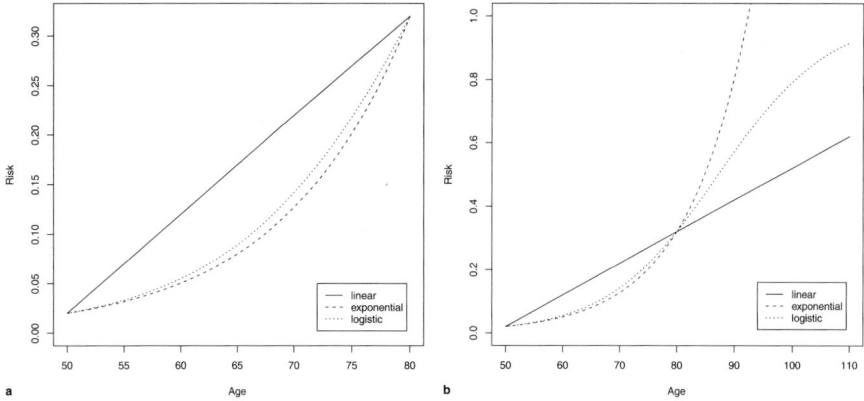

Figure 3.1. (a) Risks from linear, exponential and logistic model from age 50 to age 80 with a 1-year risk of 0.02 at age 50 and 0.32 at age 80; (b) risks from linear, exponential and logistic model extrapolated to age 110 with a 1-year risk of 0.02 at age 50 and 0.32 at age 80

an exponential curve; these shapes will always hold when x is not transformed. The logistic curve is between the two, but is much closer in shape to the exponential for risks below 0.25, and almost the same as the exponential for risks below 10%. As shown in Fig. 3.1b as a projection of the above example, the logistic curve gradually straightens out and is close to linear for risks between 40% and 60%; above that point it begins to level off, becoming nearly flat (horizontal) as it approaches 1. In contrast, the linear and exponential curves will eventually continue on above 1, and so produce impossible values for risks (which is a problem if the actual risks could get large). For negative β_1 the curves would instead go downward from left to right.

Other Risk and Odds Models   3.3.11

In addition to those given above, several other risk models are occasionally mentioned but rarely used in epidemiology. The linear odds model is obtained by replacing the average risk by the odds in the linear risk model:

$$O(x_1) = \alpha + \beta_1 x_1 . \tag{3.14}$$

Here, β_1 is the *odds* difference between subpopulations with $X_1 = x_1 + 1$ and $X_1 = x_1$, and α is the odds for the subpopulation with $X_1 = 0$. Like risk, the odds cannot be negative; unfortunately, some combinations of α and β_1 in model (3.14) will produce negative odds. As a result, this model (like the linear risk model) is difficult to fit and gives unsatisfactory results in many settings.

Another model replaces the logistic transform (expit) in the logistic model (3.10) by the inverse of the standard normal distribution, which also has a range between 0 and 1. The resulting model, called a *probit* model, has seen much use in bioassay. Its absence from epidemiologic use may stem from the fact that (unlike the logistic) its parameters have no simple epidemiologic interpretation, and the model appears to have no general advantage over the logistic in epidemiologic applications.

Finally, several attempts have been made to use models that are mixtures of different basic models, especially for multiple regressions (discussed below). These mixtures have various drawbacks, including difficulties in fitting the models and interpreting the parameters (Moolgavkar and Venzon 1987). We thus do not discuss them here.

3.3.12   Rate Models

Instead of modeling average risks, we could model person-time incidence rates. If we let Y denote the *rate* observed in a study subpopulation (so that Y is the observed number of cases per unit of observed person-time), the regression $E(Y|X = x)$ represents the average number of cases per unit of person-time in the target subpopulation defined by $X = x$. We will denote this expected rate or "average rate" by $I(x)$.

Most rate models are analogues of risk and odds models. For example, the model

$$I(x_1) = E(Y|X_1 = x_1) = \alpha + \beta_1 x_1 \tag{3.15}$$

is a linear rate model, analogous to (but different from) the linear risk and odds models (3.7), (3.14). This rate model implies that the difference in average rates between subpopulations with $X_1 = x_1 + 1$ and $X_1 = x_1$ is β_1, regardless of x_1. Also, α is the average rate for the subpopulation with $X_1 = 0$. This model can be problematic, because some combinations of α and β_1 in model (3.15) would produce negative rate values, which are impossible.

To prevent the latter problem, most rate modeling begins with an exponential *rate* model such as

$$I(x_1) = \exp(\alpha + \beta_1 x_1). \tag{3.16}$$

Because the exponential (exp) can never be negative, this model will not produce negative rates, regardless of α, β_1, or x_1. The model is equivalent to the log-linear *rate* model

$$\ln[I(x_1)] = \alpha + \beta_1 x_1. \tag{3.17}$$

The parameter β_1 in models (3.16) and (3.17) is the log of the rate ratio comparing the subpopulation with $X_1 = x_1 + 1$ to the subpopulation with $X_1 = x_1$, regardless of x_1; hence, $\exp(\beta_1)$ is the corresponding rate ratio $I(x_1 + 1)/I(x_1)$. Also, α is the log of the rate for the subpopulation with $X_1 = 0$; hence, $\exp(\alpha)$ is the average rate $I(0)$ when $X_1 = 0$. The exponential rate model (3.16) is analogous to, but different from, the exponential risk model (3.8) and the exponential odds model (3.11).

Incidence-Time and Hazard Models   3.3.13

We can also model the average time to occurrence of an event, starting from some designated zero time such as birth (in which case "time" is age), start of treatment, or some calendar date. These are called incidence-time, waiting-time, failure-time, or survival-time models (cf. Chap II.4 of this handbook). Let T stand for time of the event measured from zero. One approach to incidence time regression is to use a linear model for log incidence time, such as

$$E[\ln(T)|X_1 = x_1] = \alpha - \beta_1 x_1 . \tag{3.18}$$

Because T is always positive, $\ln(T)$ is always defined. In this model, α is the average log incidence time in the subpopulation with $X_1 = 0$, and $-\beta_1$ is the difference in average log incidence times when comparing the subpopulation with $X_1 = x_1 + 1$ to the subpopulation with $X_1 = x_1$ (regardless of the value x_1). Model (3.18) is a generalization of the basic *accelerated-life* model (Cox and Oakes 1984).

Note that the sign of β_1 in the model is reversed from its sign in earlier models. This reversal is done so that, if the outcome event at T is undesirable, then as in earlier models positive values of β_1 will correspond to harmful effects from increasing X_1, and negative values will correspond to beneficial effects. For example, under the model, if T is death time and β_1 is positive, an increase in X_1 will be associated with earlier death.

Another generalization of the basic accelerated-life model, similar but not identical to model (3.18), is the log-linear model for expected incidence time

$$\ln[E(T|X_1 = x_1)] = \alpha - \beta_1 x_1 . \tag{3.19}$$

Model (3.19) differs from model (3.18) because the log of an average is greater than the average of the logs (unless T does not vary). Model (3.19) can be rewritten

$$E(T|X_1 = x_1) = \exp(\alpha - \beta_1 x_1) = \exp(-\beta_1 x_1) e^{\alpha} ,$$

$$= \exp(-\beta_1 x_1) T_0 ,$$

where $T_0 = E(T|X_1 = 0) = e^{\alpha}$. Under model (3.19) e^{α} is the average incidence time in the subpopulation with $X_1 = 0$, and $e^{-\beta_1}$ is the ratio of average incidence times in the subpopulation with $X_1 = x_1 + 1$ and the subpopulation with $X_1 = x_1$. As with model (3.18) the sign of β_1 is negative so that positive values of β_1 will correspond to harmful effects.

More common approaches to modeling incidence times impose a model for the risk of the event up to each point in time, or for the rate of the event at each point in time. The most famous such model is the *Cox model*, also known as the *proportional hazards model*. We can give an approximate description of this model as follows: Suppose we specify a time span Δt that is small enough so that the risk of having the event in any interval t to $t + \Delta t$ among those who survive to t without the event is very small. The Cox model then implies that the rates in any such short interval will follow an exponential model like (3.16) with α but not β_1 allowed to vary with time t.

If we write $I(t; x_1)$ for the average rate in the interval t to $t + \Delta t$ among persons who survive to t and have $X_1 = x_1$, the Cox model implies that

$$I(t; x_1) \approx \exp(\alpha_t + \beta_1 x_1). \tag{3.20}$$

Under the model, the approximation ($\approx$) improves as Δt gets smaller. Note that the intercept a_t may vary with time, but in this simple Cox model the X_1-coefficient β_1 is assumed to remain constant. This means that, at any time t, the rate ratio comparing subpopulations with $X_1 = x_1 + 1$ and $X_1 = x_1$ will be

$$I(t; x_1 + 1)/I(t; x_1) \approx \exp[\alpha_t + \beta_1(x_1 + 1)]/\exp(\alpha_t + \beta_1 x_1) = \exp(\beta_1),$$

so that β_1 is the log rate ratio per unit of X_1, regardless of either the reference level x_1 or the time t at which it is computed.

Under the Cox model (3.20) the rate at time t for the subpopulation with $X_1 = 0$ is given by $I(t; 0) = \exp(\alpha_t)$. If we denote this "baseline" rate by $\lambda_0(t)$ instead of $\exp(\alpha_t)$, we have

$$I(t; x_1) \approx \exp(\alpha_t + \beta_1 x_1) = \exp(\alpha_t + \beta_1 x_1) = \lambda_0(t) \exp(\beta_1 x_1) = \exp(\beta_1 x_1)\lambda_0(t).$$

The last expression is the standard form of the model given in most textbooks. The term "Cox model" has become fairly standard, although a special case of the model was proposed by Sheehe (1962) some 10 years before Cox (1972).

The approximate form of the Cox model (3.20) may be seen as an extension of the exponential rate model (3.16) in which the rates may vary over time. In statistical theory, the assumption is made that, at each time t, the rate $I(t; x_1)$ approaches a limit $\lambda(t; x_1)$ as Δt goes to zero. This limit is usually called the *hazard* or *intensity* of the outcome at time t. The Cox model is then defined as a model for these hazards,

$$\lambda(t; x_1) = \exp(\beta_1 x_1)\lambda_0(t).$$

In epidemiologic studies, these hazards are purely theoretical quantities; thus, it is important to understand the approximate forms of the model given above and what those forms imply about observable rates.

The Cox model may be extended to allow X_1 to vary over time. Let us write $X_1(t)$ as an abbreviation for "the exposure as of time t" and $x_1(t)$ for the actual numerical value of $X_1(t)$ at time t. Then the *Cox model with time-dependent covariates* implies that the incidence rate at time t in the subpopulation that has exposure level $x_1(t)$ at time t is

$$I[t; x_1(t)] \approx \exp[\beta_1 x_1(t)]\lambda_0(t). \tag{3.21}$$

This model may be the most widely used model for time-dependent exposures. Usually, a time-dependent exposure $X_1(t)$ is not defined as the actual amount at time t, but instead is some cumulative and lagged index of exposure up to t. For example, if time is measured in months and exposure is cumulative tamoxifen lagged 3 months, $X_1(t)$ would mean "cumulative amount of tamoxifen taken up to month $t - 3$" and $x_1(t)$ would be a value for this variable.

There are biases that can arise in use of Cox models to estimate effects of time-dependent exposures. These biases and alternative models are described in Robins et al. (1992) and Robins and Greenland (1994).

Trend Models: Univariate Exposure Transforms 3.3.14

Consider again the linear risk model (3.7). If this model were correct, a plot of average risk across the subpopulations defined by X_1 (that is, a plot of risk against X_1) would yield a line. Ordinarily, however, there is no compelling reason to think the model is correct, and we might wish to entertain other possible models for the trend in risk across exposure levels. We can generate an unlimited variety of such models by *transforming* exposure, that is, by replacing X_1 in the model by some function of X_1.

To illustrate, we could replace years exposed in model (3.7) by its logarithm, to get

$$R(x_1) = \alpha + \beta_1 \ln(x_1). \tag{3.22}$$

This is still called a linear risk model, because a plot of average risk against the new regressor $\ln(X_1)$ would yield a line. But it is a very different model from model (3.7) because if model (3.22) were correct, a plot of average risk against years exposed (X_1) would yield a *logarithmic curve* rather than a line. Such a curve starts off very steep for $X_1 < 1$, but levels off rapidly beyond $X_1 > 1$. One technical problem can arise in using the logarithmic transform: It is not defined if X_1 is negative or zero. If the original exposure measurement can be negative or zero, it is common practice to add a number c to X_1 that is big enough to insure $X_1 + c$ is always positive. The resulting model is

$$R(x_1) = \alpha + \beta_1 \ln(x_1 + c). \tag{3.23}$$

The shape of the curve represented by this model (and hence results derived using the model) can be very sensitive to the value chosen for c, especially when the values of X_1 may be less than 1. Frequently, c is set equal to 1, although there is usually no compelling reason for this choice.

Among other possibilities for exposure transforms are simple power curves of the form

$$R(x_1) = \alpha + \beta_1 x_1^p, \tag{3.24}$$

where p is some number (typically $1/2$ or 2) chosen in advance according to some desired property. For example, with X_1 as years exposed, use of $p = 1/2$ yields the *square-root* model

$$R(x_1) = \alpha + \beta_1 x_1^{1/2} ,$$

which produces a trend curve that levels off as X_1 increases above zero. In contrast, use of $p = 2$ yields the simple *quadratic* model

$$R(x_1) = \alpha + \beta_1 x_1^2 ,$$

which produces a trend that rises more and more steeply as X_1 increases above zero. One technical problem can arise when using the power model (3.24). It is not defined if p is fractional and X_1 can be negative. To get around this limitation, we may add some number c to X_1 that is big enough to insure $X_1 + c$ is never negative, and then use $(X_1 + c)^p$ in the model; again, however, the result may be sensitive to choice of c.

The trend implications of linear and exponential models are vastly different, and hence the implications of exposure transforms are also different. Consider again the exponential risk model (3.8). If this model were correct, a plot of average risk against X_1 would yield an exponential curve, rather than a line. If β_1 is positive, this curve starts out slowly but rises more and more rapidly as X_1 increases; it eventually rises more rapidly than does any power curve (3.24). Such rapid increase is often implausible and we might wish to use a slower-rising curve to model risk.

One means of moderating the trend implied by an exponential model is to replace x_1 by a fixed power x_1^p with $0 < p < 1$, for example

$$R(x_1) = \exp \left(\alpha + \beta_1 x_1^{1/2} \right) .$$

Another approach is to take the logarithm of exposure. This transform produces a new model:

$$R(x_1) = \exp[\alpha + \beta_1 \ln(x_1)] = \exp(\alpha) \exp[\beta_1 \ln(x_1)]$$

$$= e^\alpha \exp[\ln(x_1)]^{\beta_1} = e^\alpha x_1^{\beta_1} . \tag{3.25}$$

A graph of risk against exposure under this model produces a power curve, but now (unlike (3.24)), the power is the unspecified (unknown) coefficient β_1 instead of a prespecified value p, and the multiplier of the exposure power is e^α (which must be positive) instead of β_1. Model (3.25) might thus appear more appropriate than model (3.24) when we want the power of X_1 to appear as an unknown coefficient β_1 in the model, rather than as a pre-specified value p. As earlier, however, X_1 must always be positive in order to use model (3.25) otherwise, one must add a constant c to it such that $X_1 + c$ is always positive.

When β_1 is negative in model (3.25) risk declines more and more gradually across increasingly exposed subpopulations. For example, if $\beta_1 = -1$, then under model (3.25) $R(x_1) = e^\alpha x_1^{-1} = e^\alpha / x_1$, which would imply risk declines 50% (from

$e^{\alpha}/1$ to $e^{\alpha}/2$) when going from $X_1 = 1$ to $X_1 = 2$, but declines less than 10% (from $e^{\alpha}/10$ to $e^{\alpha}/11$) when going from $X_1 = 10$ to $X_1 = 11$.

The exposure transforms and implications just discussed carry over to the analogous models for odds and rates. For example, we can modify the logistic model (which is an exponential odds model) by substituting the odds $O(x_1)$ for the risk $R(x_1)$ in models (3.22) to (3.25). Similarly, we can modify the rate models by substituting the rate $I(x_1)$ for $R(x_1)$. Each model will have implications for the odds or rates analogous to those described above for the risk; because the risks, odds, and rates are functions of one another (see Rothman and Greenland 1998, Chap. 3), each model will have implications for other measures as well.

Any trend in the odds will appear more gradual when transformed into a risk trend. To see this, note that

$$R(x_1) = O(x_1)/[1 + O(x_1)] < O(x_1),$$

and hence

$$O(x_1)/R(x_1) = 1 + O(x_1).$$

This ratio of odds to risk grows as the odds (and the risks) get larger. Thus, the logistic risk model, which is an exponential odds model, implies a less-than-exponential trend in the risk. Conversely, any trend in the risks will appear steeper when transformed into an odds trend. Thus, the exponential risk model implies a greater-than-exponential trend in the odds, although when risks are uniformly low (under 10% for all possible X_1 values), the risks and odds will be close and so there will be little difference between the shape of the curves produced by analogous risk and odds models.

The relation of risk and odds trends to rate trends is more complex in general, but in typical applications follows the simple rule that rate trends tend to fall between the less steep risk and more steep odds trends. For example, an exponential rate model typically implies a less than exponential risk trend but more than exponential odds trend. To see why these relations can be reasonable to expect, recall that, if incidence is measured over a span of time Δt in a closed cohort, then $R(x_1) < I(x_1)\Delta t < O(x_1)$. When the risks are uniformly low, we obtain $R(x_1) \doteq I(x_1)\Delta t \doteq O(x_1)$ (see Rothman and Greenland 1998, Chap. 3), and so there will be little difference in the curves produced by analogous risk, rate, and odds models.

Interpreting Models After Transformation   3.3.15

One drawback of models with transformed regressors is that the interpretation of the coefficients depends on the transformation. As an example, consider the model (3.25) which has $\ln(x_1)$ in place of x_1. Under this model, the risk ratio for a one-unit increase in X_1 is

$$R(x_1 + 1)/R(x_1) = e^{\alpha}(x_1 + 1)^{\beta_1}/e^{\alpha}(x_1)^{\beta_1} = [(x_1 + 1)/x_1]^{\beta_1}.$$

which will depend on the value x_1 used as the reference level: If β_1 equals 1 and x_1 is 1, the risk ratio is 2, but if β_1 equals 1 and x_1 is 2, the ratio is 1.5. Here, β_1 is the power to which x_1 is raised, and so determines the shape of the trend. The interpretation of the intercept α is also altered by the transformation. Under model (3.25), $R(1) = e^{\alpha} 1^{\beta_1} = e^{\alpha}$, thus, α is the log risk when $X_1 = 1$, rather than when $X_1 = 0$, and so is meaningful only if 1 is a possible value for X_1.

As a contrast, consider again the model $R(x_1) = \exp\left(\alpha + \beta_1 x_1^{1/2}\right)$. Use of $x_1^{1/2}$ rather than x_1 moderates the rapid increase in the slope of the exponential dose-response curve, but also leads to difficulties in coefficient interpretation. Under the model, the risk ratio for a one-unit increase in X_1 is

$$\exp\left[\alpha + \beta_1 (x_1 + 1)^{1/2}\right] \Big/ \exp\left(\alpha + \beta_1 x_1^{1/2}\right) = \exp\left\{\beta_1\left[(x_1 + 1)^{1/2} - x_1^{1/2}\right]\right\}.$$

Here, β_1 is the log risk ratio per unit increase in the *square root* of X_1, which is rather obscure in meaning. Interpretation may better proceed by considering the shape of the curve implied by the model, for example, by plotting $\exp\left(\alpha + \beta_1 x_1^{1/2}\right)$ against possible values of X_1 for several values of β_1. (The intercept α is less important in this model, because it only determines the vertical scale of the curve, rather than its shape.) Such plotting is often needed to understand and compare different transforms.

3.4   Multiple Regression Models

Suppose now we wish to model the full multiple regression $E(Y|X = x)$. Each of the previous models for the single regression $E(Y|X_1 = x_1)$ can be extended to handle this more general situation by using the following device: In any model for the single regression, replace $\beta_1 x_1$ by

$$\beta_1 x_1 + \beta_2 x_2 + \ldots + \beta_n x_n. \tag{3.26}$$

To illustrate the idea, suppose we wish to model average risk of death by age 70 across female subpopulations defined by

$$X_1 = \text{years of tamoxifen therapy,}$$

$$X_2 = \text{age at start of tamoxifen use, and}$$

$$X_3 = \text{age at menarche,}$$

with $X = (X_1, X_2, X_3)$. Then the multiple linear risk model for $R(x)$ is

$$R(x) = \alpha + \beta_1 x_1 + \beta_2 x_2 + \beta_3 x_3,$$

while the multiple logistic risk model is

$$R(x) = \text{expit}(\alpha + \beta_1 x_1 + \beta_2 x_2 + \beta_3 x_3).$$

If instead we wished to model the death rate, we could use the multiple linear rate model

$$I(x) = \alpha + \beta_1 x_1 + \beta_2 x_2 + \beta_3 x_3$$

or a multiple exponential rate model

$$I(x) = \exp(\alpha + \beta_1 x_1 + \beta_2 x_2 + \beta_3 x_3).$$

Because (3.26) can be clumsy to write out when there are three or more regressors ($n \geq 3$), several shorthand notations are in use. Let us write $\boldsymbol{\beta}$ for the vertical list (column vector) of coefficients $\beta_1, \ldots, \beta_n$. Recall that x stands for the horizontal list (row vector) of values $x_1, \ldots, x_n$. We will let $x\boldsymbol{\beta}$ stand for $\beta_1 x_1 + \ldots + \beta_n x_n$. We can then represent the multiple linear risk model by

$$R(x) = \alpha + x\boldsymbol{\beta} = \alpha + \beta_1 x_1 + \ldots + \beta_n x_n, \qquad (3.27)$$

the multiple logistic model by

$$R(x) = \text{expit}(\alpha + x\boldsymbol{\beta}), \qquad (3.28)$$

the multiple exponential rate model by

$$I(x) = \exp(\alpha + x\boldsymbol{\beta}), \qquad (3.29)$$

and so on for all the models discussed earlier.

Relations Among Multiple-Regression Models   3.4.1

The multiple-regression models (3.27)–(3.29) are not more general than the single-regression models given earlier, nor do they contain those models as special cases. This is because they refer to entirely different subclassifications of the target population: The single-regression models refer to variations in averages across subpopulations defined by levels of just one variable; in contrast, the multiple-regression models refer to variations across the much finer subdivisions defined by the levels of several variables. For example, it is possible for $R(x_1)$ to follow the single-logistic model (3.10) without $R(x)$ following the multiple-logistic model (3.28) conversely, it is possible for $R(x)$ to follow the multiple-logistic model without $R(x_1)$ following the single-logistic model.

The preceding point is often overlooked because the single-regression models are often confused with multiple-regression models in which all regressor coefficients but one are zero. The difference is, however, analogous to the differences discussed earlier between the vacuous models (3.1)–(3.3) (which are so general as to imply nothing) and the constant regression models (3.4)–(3.6) (which are so restrictive as to be unbelievable in typical situations). To see this, consider the multiple-logistic model

$$R(\boldsymbol{x}) = \text{expit}(\alpha + \beta_1 x_1). \tag{3.30}$$

The right side of this equation is the same as in the single-logistic model (3.10) but the left side is crucially different: It is the multiple-risk regression $R(\boldsymbol{x})$, instead of the single-regression $R(x_1)$. Unlike model (3.10) model (3.30) *is* a special case of the multiple-logistic model (3.28) the one in which $\beta_2 = \beta_3 = \ldots = \beta_n = 0$. Unlike model (3.10) model (3.30) asserts that risk *does not vary* across subpopulations defined by $X_1, X_2, \ldots, X_n$ *except* to the extent that X_1 varies. This is far more strict than model (3.28) which allows risk to vary with $X_2, \ldots, X_n$ as well as X_1 (albeit only in a logistic fashion). It is also far more strict than model (3.10) which says absolutely nothing about whether or how risk varies across subpopulations defined by $X_2, \ldots, X_n$ within specific levels of X_1.

More generally, we must be careful to distinguish between models that refer to different multiple regressions. For example, compare the two exponential rate models:

$$I(x_1, x_2) = \exp(\alpha + \beta_1 x_1 + \beta_2 x_2) \tag{3.31}$$

and

$$I(x_1, x_2, x_3) = \exp(\alpha + \beta_1 x_1 + \beta_2 x_2). \tag{3.32}$$

These are different models. The first is a model for the regression of rates on X_1 and X_2 only, while the second is a model for the regression of rates on X_1, X_2, and X_3. The first model in no way refers to X_3, while the second asserts that rates do not vary across levels of X_3 if one looks within levels of X_1 and X_2. Model (3.32) is the special case of

$$I(x_1, x_2, x_3) = \exp(\alpha + \beta_1 x_1 + \beta_2 x_2 + \beta_3 x_3)$$

(the case in which $\beta_3 = 0$), while model (3.31) is not, and this special case implies model (3.31).

Many textbooks and software manuals fail to distinguish between models such as models (3.31) and (3.32), and instead focus only on the appearance of the right-hand side of the models. Most software fits the model that ignores other covariates ((3.31) in the above example) rather than the more restrictive model (3.32) when requested to fit a model with only X_1 and X_2 as regressors. Note that if the less restrictive model is inadequate, then the more restrictive model must also be inadequate.

Unfortunately, if the less restrictive model appears adequate, it does *not* follow that the more restrictive model is also adequate. For example, it is possible for the model form $\exp(\alpha + \beta_1 x_1 + \beta_2 x_2)$ to describe adequately the double regression $I(x_1, x_2)$ (which means it describes adequately rate variation across X_1 and X_2 when X_3 is ignored), and yet at the same time describe poorly the triple regression

$I(x_1, x_2, x_3)$ (which means that it describes inadequately rate variation across X_1, X_2, and X_3). That is, a model may describe poorly the rate variation across X_1, X_2, and X_3 even if it describes adequately the rate variation across X_1 and X_2 when X_3 is ignored. The decision as to whether the model is acceptable should depend on whether rate variation across X_3 is relevant to the analysis objectives. For example, if the objective is to estimate the effect of changes in X_1 on the death rate, and X_2 and X_3 are both potential confounders (as in the tamoxifen example), we would want the model to describe adequately rate variation across all three variables. But if X_3 is instead affected by the study exposure X_1 (as when X_1 is past estrogen exposure and X_3 is an indicator of current uterine bleeding), we would ordinarily not want to include X_3 in the regression model (because we would not want to adjust our exposure effect estimate for X_3).

Product Terms (Statistical Interactions) 3.4.2

Each model form described above has differing implications for measures of association derived from the models. Consider again the linear risk model with three regressors X_1, X_2, and X_3, and let x_1^* and x_1 be any two values for X_1. Under the model, the risks at $X_1 = x_1^*$ and $X_1 = x_1$ and their difference RD when $X_2 = x_2$ and $X_3 = x_3$ are

$$R\left(x_1^*, x_2, x_3\right) = \alpha + \beta_1 x_1^* + \beta_2 x_2 + \beta_3 x_3 \,,$$

$$R\left(x_1, x_2, x_3\right) = \alpha + \beta_1 x_1 + \beta_2 x_2 + \beta_3 x_3 \,,$$

$$RD = \beta_1\left(x_1^* - x_1\right) \,.$$

Thus, the model implies that the risk difference between two subpopulations with the same X_2 and X_3 levels depends only on the difference in their X_1 levels. In other words, the model implies that the risk differences for X_1 within levels of X_2 and X_3 will not vary across levels of X_2 and X_3. Such an implication may be unacceptable, in which case we can either modify the linear model or switch to another model. A simple way to modify a model is to add *product terms*. For example, suppose we want to allow the risk differences for X_1 to vary across levels of X_2. We then may add the product of X_1 and X_2 to the model as a fourth variable. The risks and their differences will then be

$$R\left(x_1^*, x_2, x_3\right) = \alpha + \beta_1 x_1^* + \beta_2 x_2 + \beta_3 x_3 + \gamma_{12} x_1^* x_2 \,,$$

$$R(x_1, x_2, x_3) = \alpha + \beta_1 x_1 + \beta_2 x_2 + \beta_3 x_3 + \gamma_{12} x_1 x_2 \,, \tag{3.33}$$

$$RD = \beta_1 (x_1^* - x_1) + \gamma_{12}(x_1^* - x_1)x_2 = (\beta_1 + \gamma_{12} x_2)(x_1^* - x_1) \,. \tag{3.34}$$

Under model (3.33), the risk difference for $X_1 = x_1^*$ versus $X_1 = x_1$ is given by (3.34), which depends on X_2.

A model (e.g., (3.33)), that allows variation of the risk difference for X_1 across levels of X_2 will also allow variation in the risk difference for X_2 across levels of X_1.

As an example, let x_2^* and x_2 be any two possible values for X_2. Under model (3.33) the risks at $X_2 = x_2^*$ and $X_2 = x_2$ and their difference RD when $X_1 = x_1$, $X_3 = x_3$ are

$$R\left(x_1, x_2^*, x_3\right) = \alpha + \beta_1 x_1 + \beta_2 x_2^* + \beta_3 x_3 + \gamma_{12} x_1 x_2^*,$$

$$R(x_1, x_2, x_3) = \alpha + \beta_1 x_1 + \beta_2 x_2 + \beta_3 x_3 + \gamma_{12} x_1 x_2,$$

$$RD = \beta_2 \left(x_2^* - x_2\right) + \gamma_{12} x_1 \left(x_2^* - x_2\right) = \left(\beta_2 + \gamma_{12} x_1\right) \left(x_2^* - x_2\right). \qquad (3.35)$$

Thus, under the model, the risk difference for $X_2 = x_2^*$ versus $X_2 = x_2$ is given by (3.35), which depends on X_1. (3.34) and (3.35) illustrate how product terms modify a model in a symmetric way. The term $\gamma_{12} x_1 x_2$ allows the risk differences for X_1 to vary with X_2 and the risk differences for X_2 to vary with X_1.

If we have three regressors in a model, we have three unique two-way regressor products $(x_1 x_2, x_1 x_3, x_2 x_3)$ that we can put in the model. More generally, with n regressors, there are $\binom{n}{2}$ pairs and hence $\binom{n}{2}$ two-way products we can use. It is also possible to add triple products (e.g., $x_1 x_2 x_3$) or even more complex combinations to the model, but such additions are rare in practice; notable exceptions are body mass indices, such as kg/m^2 (Michels et al. 1998). A model without product terms is sometimes called a "main-effects only" model, and can be viewed as the special case of a model with product terms (the special case in which all the product coefficients γ_{ij} are zero).

Consider next an exponential-risk model with the above three variables. Under this model, the risks at $X_1 = x_1^*$ and $X_1 = x_1$ and their ratio RR when $X_2 = x_2$, $X_3 = x_3$ are

$$R\left(x_1^*, x_2, x_3\right) = \exp\left(\alpha + \beta_1 x_1^* + \beta_2 x_2 + \beta_3 x_3\right),$$

$$R(x_1, x_2, x_3) = \exp(\alpha + \beta_1 x_1 + \beta_2 x_2 + \beta_3 x_3),$$

$$RR = \exp\left[\beta_1 \left(x_1^* - x_1\right)\right]. \qquad (3.36)$$

Thus, the model implies that the risk ratio comparing two subpopulations with the same X_2 and X_3 levels depends only on the difference in their X_1 levels. In other words, the model implies that the risk ratios for X_1 will be constant across levels of X_2 and X_3. If this implication is unacceptable, product terms can be inserted, as with the linear model. These terms allow the risk ratios to vary in a limited fashion across levels of other variables. The preceding discussion of product terms can be applied to linear and exponential models in which the odds or rate replace the risk. For example, without product terms, the logistic model implies that the odds ratios for each regressor are constant across levels of the other regressors (because the logistic model is an exponential odds model); we can add product terms to allow the odds ratios to vary. Likewise, without product terms, the exponential rate model implies that the rate ratios for each regressor are constant across levels of the other regressors; we can add product terms to allow the rate ratios to vary.

Although product terms can greatly increase the flexibility of a model, the type of variation allowed by product terms can be very limited. For example, model (3.33) implies that raising X_2 by one unit (i.e., comparing subpopulations that have $X_2 = x_2 + 1$ instead of $X_2 = x_2$) will yield a risk difference for X_1 of

$$[\beta_1 + \gamma_{12}(x_2 + 1)](x_1^* - x_1) = (\beta_1 + \gamma_{12}x_2)(x_1^* - x_1) + \gamma_{12}(x_1^* - x_1).$$

In other words, the model implies that shifting our comparison to subpopulations that are one unit higher in X_2 will change the risk difference for X_1 in a linear fashion, by an amount $\gamma_{12}(x_1^* - x_1)$, regardless of the reference values x_1, x_2, x_3 of X_1, X_2, X_3.

Trends and Product Terms

3.4.3

Each of the above models forces or assumes a particular shape for the graph obtained when average outcome (regression) is plotted against the regressors. Consider again the tamoxifen example. Suppose we wished to plot how the risk varies across subpopulations with different number of years exposed but with the same age at start of exposure and the same age at menarche. Under the linear risk model, this would involve plotting the average risk

$$R(x_1, x_2, x_3) = \alpha + \beta x_1 + \beta_2 x_2 + \beta_3 x_3$$

against X_1, while keeping X_2 and X_3 fixed at some values x_2 and x_3. In doing so, we would obtain a line with an intercept equal to $\alpha + \beta_2 x_2 + \beta_3 x_3$ and a slope equal to β_1. Whenever we changed X_2 and X_3 and replotted $R(x)$ against X_1, the intercept would change (unless $\beta_2 = \beta_3 = 0$), but the slope would remain β_1. Because lines with the same slope are parallel, we can say that the linear risk model given above implies *parallel linear* trends in risk with increasing tamoxifen (X_1) as one moves across subpopulations of different starting age (X_2) and menarche age (X_3). This means that each change in X_2 and X_3 adds some constant (possibly negative) amount to the X_1 curve. For this reason, the linear risk model is sometimes called an *additive* risk model.

If we next plotted risks against X_2, we would get analogous results: The linear risk model given above implies parallel linear relations between average risk and X_2 as one moves across levels of X_1 and X_3. Likewise, the model implies parallel linear relations between average risk and X_3 across levels of X_1 and X_2. Thus, the linear model implies additive (parallel) relations among all the variables.

If we are unsatisfied with the linearity assumption but we wish to retain the additivity (parallel-trend) assumption, we could transform the regressors. If we are unsatisfied with the parallel-trend assumption, we can allow the trends to vary across levels of other regressors by adding product terms to the model. For example, adding the product of X_1 and X_2 to the model yields model (3.33), which can be rewritten

$$R(x_1, x_2, x_3) = \alpha + (\beta_1 + \gamma_{12}x_2)x_1 + \beta_2 x_2 + \beta_3 x_3 \,.$$

From this reformulation, we see that the slope for the line obtained by plotting average risk against X_1 while keeping X_2, X_3 fixed at x_2, x_3 would be $\beta_1 + \gamma_{12}x_2$. Thus, the slope of the trend in risk across X_1 would vary across levels of X_2 (if $\gamma_{12} \neq 0$), and so the trend lines for X_1 would not be parallel. We also see that γ_{12} is the difference in the X_1-trend slopes between subpopulations with the same X_3-value but one unit apart in their X_2-value.

An entirely different approach to producing nonparallel trends begins with an exponential model. For example, under the exponential risk model (3.36) a plot of average risk against X_1 while keeping X_2 and X_3 fixed at x_2 and x_3 would produce an *exponential* curve rather than a line. This exponential curve would have intercept $\exp(\alpha + \beta_2 x_2 + \beta_3 x_3)$. If, however, we changed the value of X_2 or X_3 and replotted risk against X_1, we would *not* obtain a parallel risk curve. Instead, the new curve would be *proportional* to the old: A change in X_2 or X_3 *multiplies* the entire X_1 curve by some amount. For this reason, the exponential model is sometimes called a *multiplicative risk* model. If we were unsatisfied with this proportionality-of-trends assumption, we could insert product terms into the model, which would allow for certain types of nonproportional trends. Proportional trends in risk appear parallel when plotted on a logarithmic vertical scale; when product terms with nonzero coefficients are present, logarithmic trends appear nonparallel.

Analogous comments and definitions apply if we substitute odds or rates for risks in the above arguments. For example, consider the multiple-logistic model in the exponential-odds form:

$$O(\mathbf{x}) = \exp(\alpha + \beta_1 x_1 + \beta_2 x_2 + \beta_3 x_3) \,.$$

A plot of the disease odds $O(\mathbf{x})$ against X_1 while keeping X_2 and X_3 fixed would produce an exponential curve; a plot of the log odds (logit) against X_1 while keeping X_2 and X_3 fixed would produce a line. If we changed the value of X_2 or X_3 and replotted the odds against X_1, we would obtain a new curve proportional to the old; that is, the new odds curve would equal the old multiplied by some constant amount. Thus, the logistic model is sometimes called a multiplicative-odds model. For analogous reasons, the exponential rate model is sometimes called a multiplicative-rate model. In both these models, inserting product terms into the model allows certain types of departures from proportional trends.

3.4.4   Interpreting Product-Term Models

Several important cautions should be highlighted when attempting to build models with product terms and interpret coefficients in models with product terms. First, the so-called "main-effect" coefficient β_j will be meaningless when considered alone if its regressor X_j appears in a product with another variable X_k that cannot be zero. In the tamoxifen example, X_1 is years of exposure, which can be zero, while X_3 is age at menarche (in years), which is always above zero. Consider the model

$$R(x_1, x_2, x_3) = \alpha + \beta_1 x_1 + \beta_2 x_2 + \beta_3 x_3 + \gamma_{13} x_1 x_3$$

$$= \alpha + \beta_1 x_1 + \beta_2 x_2 + (\beta_3 + \gamma_{13} x_1) x_3$$

$$= \alpha + (\beta_1 + \gamma_{13} x_3) x_1 + \beta_2 x_2 + \beta_3 x_3 . \qquad (3.37)$$

Under this model, $\beta_1 + \gamma_{13} x_3$ is the slope for the trend in risks across X_1 given $X_2 = x_2$ and $X_3 = x_3$. Thus, if X_3 was 0, this slope would be $\beta_1 + (\gamma_{13} \times 0) = \beta_1$, and so β_1 could be interpreted as the slope for X_1 in subpopulations of a given X_2 and with $X_3 = 0$. But X_3 is age at menarche and so cannot be zero; thus, β_1 has no simple epidemiologic interpretation. In contrast, because X_1 is years exposed and so can be zero, β_3 does have a simple interpretation: Under model (3.37) $\beta_3 + \gamma_{13} x_1$ is the slope for X_3 given $X_1 = x_1$; hence, $\beta_3 + \gamma_{13} \times 0 = \beta_3$ is the slope for X_3 in subpopulations with no tamoxifen exposure ($X_1 = 0$).

As mentioned earlier, if a regressor X_j cannot be zero, one can insure a simple interpretation of the intercept α by recentering the regressor, that is, by subtracting a reference value from the regressor before entering it in the model. Such recentering also helps provide a simple interpretation for the coefficients of variables that appear with X_j in product terms. In the example, we could recenter by redefining X_3 to be age at menarche minus 13 years. With this change, β_1 in model (3.37) would now be the slope for X_1 (years of tamoxifen) in subpopulations of a given X_2 (age at start of tamoxifen) in which this new X_3 was 0 (that is, in which the age at menarche was 13).

Rescaling can also be important for interpretation of product-term coefficients. As an example, suppose X_1 is serum cholesterol in mg/dl and X_2 is diastolic blood pressure (DBP) in mm Hg, and that the product of X_1 and X_2 is entered into the model without rescaling, say as $\gamma_{12} x_1 x_2$ in an exponential rate model. Then γ_{12} would represent the difference in the log rate ratio for a 1 mg/dl increase in cholesterol when comparing sub-populations 1 mm Hg apart in DBP. Even if this term was important, it would appear very small in magnitude because of the small units used to measure cholesterol and DBP. To avoid such deceptive appearances, we could rescale X_1 and X_2 so that their units now represented important increases in cholesterol and DBP. For example, we could redefine X_1 as cholesterol divided by 20 and X_2 as DBP divided by 10. With this rescaling, γ_{12} would represent the difference in the log rate ratio for a 20 mg/dl increase in cholesterol when comparing subpopulations 10 mm Hg apart in DBP.

Another caution is that, in most situations, a product term in a model should be accompanied by terms for all variables and products contained within that product. For example, if one enters $\gamma_{12} x_1 x_2$ in a model, $\beta_1 x_1$ and $\beta_2 x_2$ should also be included in that model; and if one enters $\delta_{123} x_1 x_2 x_3$ in a model, all of $\beta_1 x_1, \beta_2 x_2, \beta_3 x_3, \gamma_{12} x_1 x_2, \gamma_{13} x_1 x_3$, and $\gamma_{23} x_2 x_3$ should be included in that model. This rule, sometimes called the "hierarchy principle" (Bishop et al. 1975), is useful in avoiding models with bizarre implications. As an example, suppose X_1 is serum-lead concentration and X_2 is age minus 50 years. If $\gamma_{12} > 0$, the 1-year mortality-risk model

$$R(x_1, x_2) = \exp(\alpha + \beta_2 x_2 + \gamma_{12} x_1 x_2)$$

implies that serum-lead is positively related to risk among persons above age 50 ($X_2 > 0$), is unrelated to risk among persons of age 50 ($X_2 = 0$), and is negatively related to risk among persons below age 50 ($X_2 < 0$); if $\gamma_{12} < 0$, it implies a negative relation over 50 and a positive relation below 50. Rarely (if ever) would we have grounds for assuming such unusual relations hold. To prevent use of absurd models, many regression programs automatically enter all terms contained within a product when the user instructs the program to enter the product into the model.

Models violating the hierarchy principle often arise when one variable is not defined for all subjects. As an example, suppose in a study of breast cancer in women that X_1 is age at first birth (AFB) and X_2 is parity. Because X_1 is undefined for nulliparous women ($X_2 = 0$), one sometimes sees the breast-cancer rate modeled by a function in which age at first birth appears only in a product term with parity, such as $\exp(\alpha + \beta_2 x_2 + \gamma_1 x_1 x_2)$. The rationale for this model is that the rate will remain defined even when age at first birth (X_1) is undefined, because $x_1 x_2$ will be zero when parity (X_2) is zero.

One can sometimes avoid violating the hierarchy principle if there is a reasonable way to extend variable definitions to all subjects. Thus, in the tamoxifen example, age at start of tamoxifen was extended to the untreated by setting it to age 70 (end of follow-up) for those subjects, and for those subjects who started at age 70 or later. The rationale for this extension is that, within the age interval under study, untreated subjects and subjects starting tamoxifen at age 70 or later would have identical exposures.

Our final caution is that product terms are commonly labeled "interaction terms" or "statistical interactions". We avoid these labels because they may inappropriately suggest the presence of biologic (mechanical) interactions between the variables in a product term. In practice, regression models are applied in many situations in which there is no effect of the regressors on the regressand (outcome). Even in causal analyses, the connections between product terms and biologic interactions can be very indirect, and can depend on many biologic assumptions. For descriptions of these connections see Greenland (1993) and Rothman and Greenland (1998, pp 386–387).

3.4.5   Categorical Regressors

Consider a regressor whose possible values are discrete and few, and perhaps purely nominal (that is, with no natural ordering or quantitative meaning). An example is marital status (never married, currently married, formerly married). Such regressors may be entered into a multiple-regression model using *category indicator variables*. To use this approach, we first choose one level of the regressor as the *reference level*, against which we want to compare risks or rates. For each of the remaining levels (the *index* levels), we create a binary variable that indicates whether a person is at that level (1 if at the level, 0 if not). We then enter these indicators into the regression model.

The entire set of indicators is called the *coding* of the original regressor. To code marital status, we could take "currently married" as the reference level and define

$$X_1 = 1 \quad \text{if formerly married, 0 if currently or never married,}$$

$$X_2 = 1 \quad \text{if never married, 0 if ever married}$$

$$\text{(i.e., currently or formerly married)}.$$

There are $2 \times 2 = 4$ possible numerical combinations of values for X_1 and X_2, but only three of them are logically possible. The impossible combination is $X_1 = 1$ (formerly married) and $X_2 = 1$ (never married). Note, however, that we need two indicators to distinguish the three levels of marital status, because one indicator can only distinguish two levels.

In general, we need $J - 1$ indicators to code a variable with J levels. Although these indicators will have 2^{J-1} possible numerical combinations, only J of these combinations will be logically possible. For example, we will need four indicators to code a variable with five levels. These indicators will have $2^4 = 16$ numerical combinations, but only five of the 16 combinations will be logically possible.

Interpretation of the indicator coefficients depends on the model form and the chosen coding. For example, in the logistic model

$$R(x_1, x_2) = \text{expit}(\alpha + \beta_1 x_1 + \beta_2 x_2), \tag{3.38}$$

$\exp(\beta_2)$ is the odds ratio comparing $X_2 = 1$ persons (never married) to $X_2 = 0$ persons (ever married) within levels of X_1. Because one cannot have $X_2 = 1$ (never married) and $X_1 = 1$ (formerly married), the only level of X_1 within which we can compare $X_2 = 1$ to $X_2 = 0$ is the zero level (never or currently married). Thus, $\exp(\beta_2)$ is the odds ratio comparing never married ($X_2 = 1$) to currently married ($X_2 = 0$) people among those never or currently married ($X_1 = 0$). In a similar fashion, $\exp(\beta_1)$ compares those formerly married to those currently married among those ever married.

In general, the type of indicator coding described above, called *disjoint category coding*, results in coefficients that compare each index category to the reference category. With this coding, for a given person no more than one indicator in the set can equal 1; all the indicators are zero for persons in the reference category. Another kind of coding is *nested indicator coding*. In this coding, levels of the regressor are grouped, and then codes are created to facilitate comparisons both within and across groups. For example, suppose we wish to compare those not currently married (never or formerly married) to those currently married, and also compare those never married to those formerly married. We can then use the indicators

$Z_1 = 1$ if never or formerly married (i.e., not currently married),

    0 otherwise (currently married);

$Z_2 = 1$ if never married, 0 if ever married.

Z_2 is the same as the X_2 used above, but Z_1 is different from X_1. The combination $Z_1 = 0$ (currently married), $Z_2 = 1$ (never married) is impossible; $Z_1 = Z_2 = 1$ for people who never married. In the logistic model

$$R(z_1, z_2) = \text{expit}(\alpha + \beta_1 z_1 + \beta_2 z_2), \qquad (3.39)$$

$\exp(\beta_2)$ is now the odds ratio comparing those never married ($Z_2 = 1$) to those ever married ($Z_2 = 0$) within levels of Z_1. Note that the only level of Z_1 in which this comparison can be made is $Z_1 = 1$ (never or formerly married). Similarly, $\exp(\beta_1)$ is now the odds ratio comparing those formerly married ($Z_1 = 1$) among those never married ($Z_2 = 0$).

There can be quite a large number of options for coding category indicators. The choice among these options may be dictated by which comparisons are of most interest. As long as each level of the regressor can be uniquely represented by the indicator coding, the choice of coding will not alter the assumptions represented by the model. There is, however, one technical point to consider in choosing codes. The precision of the estimated coefficient for an indicator will directly depend on the numbers of subjects at each indicator level. For example, suppose in the data there were 1000 currently married subjects, 200 formerly married subjects, and only 10 never married subjects. Then any indicator that had "never married" as one of its levels (0 or 1) would have a much less precise coefficient estimate than other indicators. If "never married" were chosen as the reference level for a disjoint coding scheme, all the indicators would have that level as its zero level, and so all would have very imprecise coefficient estimates. To maximize precision, many analysts prefer to use disjoint coding in which the largest category (currently married in the above example) is taken as the reference level.

In choosing a coding scheme, one need not let precision concerns dominate if they get in the way of interesting comparisons. Coding schemes that distinguish among the same categories produce equivalent models. Therefore, one may fit a model repeatedly using different but equivalent coding schemes, in order to easily examine all comparisons of interest. For example, one could fit model (3.38) to compare those never or formerly married with those currently married, then fit model (3.39) to compare the never with formerly married.

Although indicator coding is essential for purely nominal regressors, it can also be used to study quantitative regressors as well, especially when one expects qualitative differences between persons at different levels. Consider number of marriages as a regressor. We might suspect that people of a given age who have had one marriage tend to be qualitatively distinct from people of the same age who have had no marriage or two marriages, and that people who have had several marriages are even more distinctive. We thus might want to code number of marriages in a manner that allowed qualitative distinctions among its levels. If "one marriage" was the most common level, we might take it as the reference level and use

$$X_1 = 1 \quad \text{if never married, 0 otherwise;}$$

$$X_2 = 1 \quad \text{if two marriages, 0 otherwise;}$$

$$X_3 = 1 \quad \text{if three or more marriages, 0 otherwise.}$$

We use one variable to represent "three or more" because there might be too few subjects with three or more marriages to produce acceptably precise coefficients for a finer division of levels. The coding just given would provide comparisons of those never married, twice married, and more-than-twice married to those once married. Other codings could be used to make other comparisons.

Trend Models in Multiple Regression 3.5

Multiple regression models can be extended to produce much more flexible trend models than those provided by simple transformations. The latter restrict trends to follow basic shapes, such as quadratic or logarithmic curves. The use of multiple terms for each exposure and confounder allows more detailed assessment of trends and more complete control of confounding than possible with simple transformations.

Categorical Trends 3.5.1

One way to extend trend models is to categorize the regressor and then use a category-indicator coding such as discussed above. The resulting analysis may then parallel the categorical (tabular) trend methods discussed for example in Chap 17 of Rothman and Greenland (1998). Much of the advice given there also applies here. To the extent allowed by the data numbers and background information, the categories should represent scientifically meaningful constructs within which risk is not expected to change dramatically. Purely mathematical categorization methods such as percentiles (quantiles) can do very poorly in this regard and so are best avoided when such information is available. On the other hand, the choices of categories should *not* be dictated by the results produced; for example, manipulation of category boundaries to maximize the effect estimate will produce an estimate biased away from the null, while manipulation of boundaries to minimize a *P*-value will produce a downwardly biased *P*-value. Similarly, manipulation to minimize the estimate or maximize the *P*-value will produce a null-biased estimate or an upwardly biased *P*-value.

There are two common types of category codes used in trend models. *Disjoint coding* produces estimates that compare each index category (level) to the reference level. Consider coding weekly servings of fruits and vegetables with

$$X_1 = 1 \quad \text{for} < 15, \quad 0 \text{ otherwise;}$$
$$X_2 = 1 \quad \text{for } 36\text{--}42, \quad 0 \text{ otherwise;}$$
$$X_3 = 1 \quad \text{for} > 42, \quad 0 \text{ otherwise.}$$

In the rate model

$$\ln[I(x_1, x_2, x_3)] = \alpha + \beta_1 x_1 + \beta_2 x_2 + \beta_3 x_3 , \tag{3.40}$$

$\exp(\beta_1)$ is the rate ratio comparing the "< 15" category with the "15–35" category (which is the referent), and so on, while $\exp(\alpha)$ is the rate in the "15–35" category (the category for which all the X_j are zero). When model (3.40) is fit, we can plot the fitted rates on a graph as a step function. This plot provides a crude impression of the trends across (but not within) categories.

Confounders may be added to the model in order to control confounding, and these too may be coded using multiple indicators or any of the methods described below. We may plot the model-adjusted trends by fixing each confounder at a reference level and allowing the exposure level to vary.

Incremental coding (nested coding) can be useful when one wishes to compare each category against its immediate predecessor (Maclure and Greenland 1992). For "Number of servings per week", we could use

$$Z_1 = 1 \quad \text{for} > 14, \quad 0 \text{ otherwise;}$$
$$Z_2 = 1 \quad \text{for} > 35, \quad 0 \text{ otherwise;}$$
$$Z_3 = 1 \quad \text{for} > 42, \quad 0 \text{ otherwise.}$$

Note that if $Z_2 = 1$, then $Z_1 = 1$, and if $Z_3 = 1$, then $Z_1 = Z_2 = 1$. In the model

$$\ln[I(z_1, z_2, z_3)] = \alpha + \beta_1 z_1 + \beta_2 z_2 + \beta_3 z_3 , \tag{3.41}$$

$\exp(\beta_1)$ is the rate ratio comparing the 15–35 category ($Z_1 = 1$ and $Z_2 = Z_3 = 0$) to the < 15 category ($Z_1 = Z_2 = Z_3 = 0$). Similarly, $\exp(\beta_2)$ is the rate ratio comparing the 36–42 category ($Z_1 = Z_2 = 1$ and $Z_3 = 0$) to the 15–35 category ($Z_1 = 1$ and $Z_2 = Z_3 = 0$). Finally, $\exp(\beta_3)$ compares the > 42 category ($Z_1 = Z_2 = Z_3 = 1$) to the 36–42 category ($Z_1 = Z_2 = 1$ and $Z_3 = 0$). Thus, $\exp(\beta_1)$, $\exp(\beta_2)$, and $\exp(\beta_3)$ are the incremental rate ratios across adjacent categories. Again, we may add confounders to the model and plot adjusted trends.

3.5.2   Regression with Category Scores

A common practice in epidemiology is to divide each covariate into categories, assign a score to each category, and enter scores into the model instead of the original variable values. Ordinal scores or codes (e.g., 1, 2, 3, 4, 5 for a series of five categories) should be avoided, as they can yield quantitatively meaningless dose-response curves and harm the power and precision of the results (Lagakos 1988; Greenland 1995b, c; Rothman and Greenland 1998, pp 311–312). Category midpoints can be much less distortive but are not defined for open-ended categories; category means or medians can be even less distortive and are defined for open-ended categories. Unfortunately, if there are important nonlinear effects within categories, no simple scoring method will yield an undistorted dose-response curve, nor will it achieve the power and precision obtainable by entering the uncategorized covariates into the model (Greenland 1995b, c). We thus recommend that categories be kept narrow and that scores be derived from category means or medians, rather than category scores. We further recommend that one examine models with uncategorized covariates whenever effects are clearly present.

Power Models

3.5.3

Another approach to trend analysis and confounder control is to use multiple power terms for each regressor. Such an approach does not require categorization, but does require care in selection of terms. Traditionally, the powers used are positive integers (e.g., x_1, x_1^2, x_1^3), but fractional powers may also be used (Royston and Altman 1994). As an illustration, suppose X_1 represents the actual number of servings per week (instead of an indicator). We could model trends across this regressor by using X_1 in the model along with the following powers of X_1:

$$X_2 = X_1^{1/2} = \text{square root of } X_1 \,,$$

$$X_3 = X_1^2 = \text{square of } X_1 \,.$$

The multiple-regression model

$$\ln[I(x_1, x_2, x_3)] = \alpha + \beta_1 x_1 + \beta_2 x_2 + \beta_3 x_3 \,,$$

is now just another way of writing the power model

$$\ln[I(x_1)] = \alpha + \beta_1 x_1 + \beta_2 x_1^{1/2} + \beta_3 x_1^2 \,. \tag{3.42}$$

We can plot fitted rates from this model using very fine spacings to produce a *smooth curve* as an estimate of rate trends across X_1. As always, we may also include confounders in the model and plot model-adjusted trends.

Power models have several advantages over categorical models. Most importantly, they make use of information about differences within categories, which is ignored by categorical models and categorical analyses (Greenland 1995a, b, c). Thus, they can provide a more complete picture of trends across exposure and more thorough control of confounders. They also provide a smoother picture of trends. One disadvantage of power models is a potentially greater sensitivity of estimates to *outliers*, that is, persons with unusual values or unusual *combinations* of values for the regressors. This problem can be addressed by performing delta-beta analysis, as discussed below.

3.5.4   Regression Splines

Often it is possible to combine the advantages of categorical and power models through the use of *spline models*. Such models can be defined in a number of equivalent ways, and we present only the simplest. In all approaches, one first categorizes the regressor, as in categorical analysis (although fewer, broader categories may be sufficient in a spline model). The boundaries between these categories are called the *knots* or *join points* of the spline. Next, one chooses the *power* (or order) of the spline, according to the flexibility one desires within the categories (higher powers allow more flexibility).

Use of category indicators corresponds to a zero-power spline, in which the trend is flat within categories but may jump suddenly at the knots; thus, category-indicator models are just special and unrealistic types of spline models. In a first-power or *linear* spline, the trend is modeled by a series of connected line segments. The trend within each category corresponds to a line segment; the slope of the trend may change only at the knots, and no sudden jump in risk (discontinuity in trend) can occur.

To illustrate how a linear spline may be represented, let X_1 again be "Number of servings per week" but now define

$$X_2 = X_1 - 14 \quad \text{if } X_1 > 14, \text{ 0 otherwise;}$$
$$X_3 = X_1 - 35 \quad \text{if } X_1 > 35, \text{ 0 otherwise.}$$

Then the log-linear rate model

$$\ln[I(x_1, x_2, x_3)] = \alpha + \beta_1 x_1 + \beta_2 x_2 + \beta_3 x_3 \tag{3.43}$$

will produce a log-rate trend that is a series of three line segments that are connected at the knots (category boundaries) of 14 and 35. To see this, note that when X_1 is less than 14, X_2 and X_3 are zero, so the model simplifies to a line with slope β_1:

$$\ln[I(x_1, x_2, x_3)] = \alpha + \beta_1 x_1$$

in this range. When X_1 is greater than 14 but less than 35, the model simplifies to a line with slope $\beta_1 + \beta_2$:

$$\ln[I(x_1, x_2, x_3)] = \alpha + \beta_1 x_1 + \beta_2 x_2 = \alpha + \beta_1 x_1 + \beta_2 (x_1 - 14)$$

$$= \alpha - 14\beta_2 + (\beta_1 + \beta_2) x_1 .$$

Finally, when X_1 is greater than 35, the model becomes a line with slope $\beta_1 + \beta_2 + \beta_3$:

$$\ln[I(x_1, x_2, x_3)] = \alpha + \beta_1 x_1 + \beta_2 x_2 + \beta_3 x_3$$

$$= \alpha + \beta_1 x_1 + \beta_2 (x_1 - 14) + \beta_3 (x_1 - 35)$$

$$= a - 14\beta_2 - 35\beta_3 + (\beta_1 + \beta_2 + \beta_3) x_1 .$$

Thus, β_1 is the slope of the spline in the first category, β_2 is the change in slope in going from the first to second category, and β_3 is the change in slope in going from the second to third category.

The trend produced by a linear spline is generally more realistic than a categorical trend, but can suddenly change its slope at the knots. To smooth out such sudden changes, we may increase the order of the spline. Increasing the power to 2 produces a second-power or *quadratic* spline, which comprises a series of parabolic curve segments smoothly joined together at the knots. To illustrate how such a trend may be represented, let X_1, X_2, and X_3 be as just defined. Then the model

$$\ln[I(x_1, x_2, x_3)] = \alpha + \beta_1 x_1 + \gamma_1 x_1^2 + \gamma_2 x_2^2 + \gamma_3 x_3^2 \tag{3.44}$$

will produce a log-rate trend that is a series of three parabolic segments smoothly connected at the knots of 14 and 35. The coefficient γ_1 corresponds to the curvature of the trend in the first category, while γ_2 and γ_3 correspond to the changes in curvature when going from the first to second and second to third category. A still smoother curve could be fit by using a third-power or *cubic* spline, but for epidemiologic purposes the quadratic spline is often smooth and flexible enough.

One disadvantage of quadratic and cubic splines is that the curves in the end categories (tails) may become very unstable, especially if the category is open-ended. This instability may be reduced by *restricting* one or both of the end categories to be a line segment rather than a curve. To restrict the lower category to be linear in a quadratic spline, we need only drop the *first* quadratic term $\gamma_1 x_1^2$ from the model; to restrict the upper category, we must subtract the *last* quadratic term from all the quadratic terms, and drop the last term out of the model. To illustrate an upper category restriction, suppose we wish to restrict the above quadratic spline model for log rates (3.44) so that it is linear in the upper category only. Define

$$Z_1 - X_1 = \text{number of servings per week,}$$

$$Z_2 = X_1^2 - X_3^2,$$

$$Z_3 = X_2^2 - X_3^2.$$

Then the model

$$\ln[I(z_1, z_2, z_3)] = \alpha + \beta_1 z_1 + \beta_2 z_2 + \beta_3 z_3 \tag{3.45}$$

will produce a log-rate trend that comprises smoothly connected parabolic segments in the first two categories ("< 14" and "15–35"), and a line segment in the last category ("> 35") that is smoothly connected to the parabolic segment in the second category. (If we also wanted to force the log-rate curve in the first category to follow a line, we would drop Z_2 from the model.)

To plot or tabulate a spline curve from a given spline model, we select a set of X_1 values spaced across the range of interest, compute the set of spline terms for each X_1 value, combine these terms with the coefficients in the model to get the model-predicted outcomes, and plot these predictions. To illustrate, suppose X_1 is servings per week and we wish to plot model (3.45) with $\alpha = -6.00, \beta_1 = -0.010, \beta_2 = -0.001$, and $\beta_3 = 0.001$ over the range 0–50 servings per week in 5-serving increments. We then compute Z_1, Z_2, Z_3 at $0, 5, 10, \ldots, 50$ servings per week, and compute the predicted rate

$$\exp(-6.00 - 0.010z_1 - 0.001z_2 + 0.001z_3)$$

at each set of Z_1, Z_2, Z_3 values and plot these predictions against the corresponding X_1 values $0, 5, 10, \ldots, 50$. For example, at $X_1 = 40$ we get $Z_1 = 40, Z_2 = 40^2 - (40 - 35)^2 = 1575$, and $Z_3 = (40 - 14)^2 - (40 - 35)^2 = 651$, for a predicted rate of

$$\exp[-6.00 - 0.010(40) - 0.001(1575) + 0.001(651)] = 2/1000 \text{ year}.$$

As with other trend models, we may obtain model-adjusted trends by adding confounder terms to our spline models. The confounder terms may be splines or any other form we prefer; spline plotting will be simplified, however, if the confounders are centered before they are entered into the analysis, for then the above plotting method may be used without modification. For further discussion of splines and their application, as well as more general nonparametric regression techniques, see Hastie and Tibshirani (1990), Green and Silverman (1994), and Greenland (1995a).

3.5.5   Models for Trend Variation

We may allow trends to vary across regressor levels by entering products among regressor terms. For example, suppose X_1, X_2, X_3 are power terms for fruit and vegetable intake, while W_1, W_2, W_3, W_4 are spline terms for age. To allow the fruit-vegetable trend in log rates to vary with age, we could enter into the model all $3 \times 4 = 12$ products of the X_j and W_k, along with the X_j and W_k. If in addition there was an indicator $Z_1 = 1$ for female, 0 for males, the resulting model would be

$$\ln[R(x_1, x_2, x_3, w_1, w_2, w_3, w_4, z_1)]$$

$$= \alpha + \beta_1 x_1 + \beta_2 x_2 + \beta_3 x_3 + \beta_4 w_1 + \beta_5 w_2 + \beta_6 w_3 + \beta_7 w_4 + \beta_8 z_1$$

$$+ \gamma_{11} x_1 w_1 + \gamma_{12} x_1 w_2 + \ldots + \gamma_{33} x_3 w_3 + \gamma_{34} x_3 w_4.$$

The same model form may be used if X_1, X_2, X_3 and W_1, W_2, W_3, W_4 represent category indicators or other terms for fruit-vegetable intake and age.

Models with products among multiple trend terms can be difficult to fit and may yield quite unstable results unless large numbers of cases are observed. Given enough data, however, such models can provide more realistic pictures of dose-response relations than can simpler models. Results from such models may be easily interpreted by plotting or tabulating the fitted trends for the key exposures of interest at various levels of the "modifying" regressors. In the above example, this process would involve plotting the model-fitted rates against fruit and vegetable intake for each of several ages (e.g., for ages evenly spaced within the range of case ages).

Extensions of Logistic Models 3.6

Outcomes that are polytomous or continuous are often analyzed by reducing them to just two categories and applying a logistic model. For example, CD_4 counts might be reduced to the dichotomy ≤ 200, > 200; cancer outcomes might be reduced to cancer and no cancer. Alternatively, multiple categories may be created with one designated as a referent, and the other categories compared one at a time to the referent using separate logistic models for each comparison. While not necessarily invalid, these approaches disregard the information contained in differences within categories, in differences between non-reference categories, and in ordering among the categories. As a result, models specifically designed for polytomous or continuous outcomes can yield more precision and power than simple dichotomous-outcome analyses.

This section briefly describes several extensions of the multiple logistic model (3.28) to polytomous and ordinal outcomes. Analogous extensions of other models are possible.

Polytomous Logistic Models 3.6.1

Suppose an outcome variable Y has $I + 1$ mutually exclusive outcome categories or levels $y_0, \dots, y_I$, where category y_0 is considered the reference category. For example, in a case-control study of relations of exposures to types of cancer, Y is a disease outcome variable, with y_0 = all control as the reference category, and I other categories $y_1, \dots, y_I$, which correspond to the cancer outcomes (leukemia, lymphoma, lung cancer, etc.). Let $R_i(x)$ denote the average risk of falling in outcome category $Y_i (i = 1, \dots, I)$ given that the regressors X equal x; that is, let

$$R_i(x) = \Pr(Y = y_i | X = x).$$

The *polytomous logistic* model for this risk is then

$$R_i(x) = \frac{\exp\left(\alpha_1 + x\beta_1\right)}{1 + \sum_{j=1}^{I} \exp(\alpha_j + x\beta_j)} \tag{3.46}$$

This is a model for the risk of falling in cancer category y_i. When Y has only two levels, I equals 1, and so formula (3.46) simplifies to the binary multiple logistic model (3.28).

Model (3.46) represents I separate risk equations, one for each nonreference outcome level $y_1, \dots, y_I$. Each equation has its own intercept α_i and vector of coefficients $\boldsymbol{\beta}_i = (\beta_{i1}, \ldots, \beta_{in})$, so that there is a distinct coefficient β_{ik} corresponding to every combination of a regressor X_k and nonreference outcome level y_i ($i = 1, \ldots, I$). Thus, with n regressors in $\boldsymbol{X}$, the polytomous logistic model involves I intercepts and $I \times n$ regressor coefficients. For example, with seven nonreference outcome levels and three regressors, the model would involve seven intercepts and $7 \times 3 = 21$ regressor coefficients, for a total of 28 model parameters.

The polytomous logistic model can be written more simply as a model for the odds. To see this, note that the risk of falling in the reference category must equal one minus the sum of the risks of falling in the nonreference categories:

$$R_0(\boldsymbol{x}) = \Pr(Y = y_0 | \boldsymbol{X} = \boldsymbol{x}) = 1 - \frac{\sum_{i=1}^{I} \exp\left(\alpha_i + \boldsymbol{x}\boldsymbol{\beta}_i\right)}{1 + \sum_{j=1}^{I} \exp\left(\alpha_j + \boldsymbol{x}\boldsymbol{\beta}_j\right)}$$

$$= 1 \left/ \left[1 + \sum_{j=1}^{I} \exp\left(\alpha_j + \boldsymbol{x}\boldsymbol{\beta}_j\right) \right] \right. . \tag{3.47}$$

Dividing (3.47) into (3.46), we get a model for $O_i(\boldsymbol{x}) = R_i(\boldsymbol{x})/R_0(\boldsymbol{x}) =$ the odds of falling in outcome category y_i versus category y_0:

$$O_i(\boldsymbol{x}) = \frac{\exp(\alpha_i + \boldsymbol{x}\boldsymbol{\beta}_i)/[1 + \sum_j \exp(\alpha_j + \boldsymbol{x}\boldsymbol{\beta}_j)]}{1/[1 + \sum_j \exp(\alpha_j + \boldsymbol{x}\boldsymbol{\beta}_j)]} = \exp(\alpha_i + \boldsymbol{x}\boldsymbol{\beta}_i). \tag{3.48}$$

This form of the model provides a familiar interpretation for the coefficients. Suppose $\boldsymbol{x}_1$ and $\boldsymbol{x}_0$ are two different vectors of values for the regressors $\boldsymbol{X}$. Then the ratio of the odds of falling in category y_i versus y_0 when $\boldsymbol{X} = \boldsymbol{x}_1$ and $\boldsymbol{X} = \boldsymbol{x}_0$ is

$$\frac{O_i(\boldsymbol{x}_1)}{O_i(\boldsymbol{x}_0)} = \frac{\exp(\alpha_i + \boldsymbol{x}_1\boldsymbol{\beta}_i)}{\exp(\alpha_i + \boldsymbol{x}_0\boldsymbol{\beta}_i)} = \exp\left[(\boldsymbol{x}_1 - \boldsymbol{x}_0)\boldsymbol{\beta}_i\right] .$$

From this equation, we see that the antilog $\exp(\beta_{ik})$ of a coefficient β_{ik} corresponds to the proportionate change in the odds of outcome i when the regressor X_k increases by one unit.

The polytomous logistic model is most useful when the levels of Y have no meaningful order, as with the cancer types. For further reading about the model, see McCullagh and Nelder (1989) and Hosmer and Lemeshow (2000).

3.6.2 Ordinal Logistic Models

Suppose that the levels $y_0, \ldots, y_I$ of Y follow a natural order. Order arises, for example, when Y is a clinical scale, such as $y_0 =$ normal, $y_1 =$ dysplasia, $y_2 =$ neoplasia, rather than just a cancer indicator; Y is a count, such as number of malformations found in an individual; or the Y levels represent categories of a physical quantity, such as CD_4 count (e.g., > 500, 200–500, < 200). There are at least four different ways to extend the logistic model to such outcomes.

Recall that the logistic model is equivalent to an exponential odds model. The first extension uses an exponential model to represent the odds of falling in outcome category y_i versus falling in category y_{i-1} (the next lowest category):

$$\frac{R_i(\boldsymbol{x})}{R_{i-1}(\boldsymbol{x})} = \frac{\Pr(Y = y_i | X = \boldsymbol{x})}{\Pr(Y = y_{i-1} | X = \boldsymbol{x})} = \exp(\alpha_i^* + \boldsymbol{x}\boldsymbol{\beta}^*) \tag{3.49}$$

for $i = 1, \ldots, I$. This may be called the *adjacent-category logistic model*, because taking logarithms of both sides yields the equivalent *adjacent-category logit* model (Agresti 2002). It is a special case of the polytomous logistic model: From (3.48), the polytomous logistic model implies that

$$\frac{R_i(\boldsymbol{x})}{R_{i-1}(\boldsymbol{x})} = \frac{R_i(\boldsymbol{x})/R_0(\boldsymbol{x})}{R_{i-1}(\boldsymbol{x})/R_0(\boldsymbol{x})} = \frac{\exp\left(\alpha_i + \boldsymbol{x}\boldsymbol{\beta}_i\right)}{\exp\left(\alpha_{i-1} + \boldsymbol{x}\boldsymbol{\beta}_{i-1}\right)} = \exp[(\alpha_i - \alpha_{i-1}) + \boldsymbol{x}(\boldsymbol{\beta}_i - \boldsymbol{\beta}_{i-1})].$$

The adjacent-category logistic model sets $\alpha_i^* = \alpha_i - \alpha_{i-1}$, and forces the I coefficient differences $\boldsymbol{\beta}_i - \boldsymbol{\beta}_{i-1} (i = 1, \ldots I)$ to equal a common value $\boldsymbol{\beta}^*$. If there is a natural distance d_i between adjacent outcome categories y_i and y_{i-1} (such as the difference between the category means), the model can be modified to use these distances as follows:

$$R_i(\boldsymbol{x})/R_{i-1}(\boldsymbol{x}) = \exp(\alpha_i^* + \boldsymbol{x}\boldsymbol{\beta}^* d_i) \tag{3.50}$$

for $i = 1, \ldots, I$. This model allows the coefficient differences $\boldsymbol{\beta}_i - \boldsymbol{\beta}_{i-1}$ to vary with the distances d_i between categories. Further information on adjacent-category models may be found in Greenland (1994) and Agresti (2002).

The second extension uses an exponential model to represent the odds of falling *above category y_i* versus *falling in or below* category y_i:

$$\frac{\Pr(Y > y_i | X = \boldsymbol{x})}{\Pr(Y \leq y_i | X = \boldsymbol{x})} = \exp(\alpha_i^* + \boldsymbol{x}\boldsymbol{\beta}^*), \tag{3.51}$$

where $i = 0, \ldots, I$. This is called the *cumulative-odds* or *proportional-odds* model. It can be derived by assuming that Y was obtained by categorizing a special type of continuous variable; for more details about this and other aspects of the model, see McCullagh and Nelder (1989).

The third extension uses an exponential model to represent the odds of falling *above outcome* category y_i versus *in category* y_i:

$$\frac{\Pr(Y > y_i | X = \boldsymbol{x})}{\Pr(Y = y_i | X = \boldsymbol{x})} = \exp(\alpha_i^* + \boldsymbol{x}\boldsymbol{\beta}^*), \tag{3.52}$$

where $i = 0, \ldots, I$. This is called the *continuation-ratio* model. The fourth extension uses an exponential model to represent the odds of falling *in* category y_i versus falling *below* y_i:

$$\frac{\Pr(Y = y_i | X = \boldsymbol{x})}{\Pr(Y < y_i | X = \boldsymbol{x})} = \exp(\alpha_i^* + \boldsymbol{x}\boldsymbol{\beta}^*), \tag{3.53}$$

where $i = 1, \ldots, I$. This model may be called the *reverse continuation-ratio* model. It can be derived by reversing the order of the Y levels in model (3.52) but in any given application it is not equivalent to model (3.52) (Greenland 1994).

How does one choose from the above variety of ordinal models? Certain guidelines may be of use, although none is compelling. First, the adjacent-category and cumulative-odds models are *reversible*, in that only the signs of the coefficients change if the order of the Y levels is reversed. In contrast, the two continuation-ratio models are not reversible. This observation suggests that the continuation-ratio models may be more appropriate for modeling irreversible disease stages (e.g., osteoarthritic severity), whereas the adjacent-category and cumulative-odds models may be more appropriate for potentially reversible outcomes (e.g., blood pressure, cell counts) (Greenland 1994). Second, because the coefficients of adjacent-category models contrast pairs of categories, the model appears best suited for discrete outcomes with few levels (e.g., cell types along a normal-dysplastic-neoplastic scale). Third, because the cumulative-odds model can be derived from categorizing certain special types of continuous outcomes, it is often considered most appropriate when the outcome under study is derived by categorizing a single underlying continuum (e.g., blood pressure) (McCullagh and Nelder 1989). For a more detailed comparative discussion of ordinal logistic models and guidelines for their use, see Greenland (1994).

All the above ordinal models simplify to the ordinary logistic model when there are only two outcome categories ($I = 2$). One advantage of the continuation-ratio models over their competitors is of special importance: Estimation of the coefficients β^* in those models can be carried out if the levels of Y are numerous and sparse; Y may even be continuous. Thus, one can apply the continuation-ratio models without any categorization of Y. This advantage can be important because results from all the above models (including the cumulative-odds model) may be affected by the choice of the Y categories (Greenland 1994; Strömberg 1996). The only caution is that conditional (as opposed to unconditional) maximum likelihood must be used to fit the continuation-ratio model if the observed outcomes are sparsely scattered across the levels of Y (as would be inevitable if Y were continuous). See Greenland (1994) for further details, and Cole and Ananth (2001) for futher extensions of the model.

3.7   Generalized Linear Models

Consider again the general form of the exponential risk and rate models, $R(x) = \exp(\alpha + x\beta)$ and $I(x) = \exp(\alpha + x\beta)$ and the logistic risk model $R(x) = \text{expit}(\alpha + x\beta)$. There is no reason why we cannot replace the "exp" in the exponential models or the "expit" in the logistic model by some other reasonable function. In fact, each of these models is of the general form

$$E(Y|x) = f(\alpha + x\beta), \tag{3.54}$$

where f is some function that is smooth and strictly increasing (i.e., as $\alpha + x\beta$ gets larger, $f(\alpha + x\beta)$ gets larger, but never jumps or bends suddenly).

For any such function f, there is always an inverse function g that "undoes" f, in the sense that $g[f(u)] = u$ whenever $f(u)$ is defined. Hence, a general form equivalent to (3.54) is

$$g[E(Y|x)] = \alpha + x\beta. \tag{3.55}$$

A model of the form (3.55) is called a *generalized linear* model. The function g is called the *link function* for the model; thus, the link function is ln for the log-linear model and logit for the logit-linear model. The term $\alpha + x\beta$ in it is called the *linear predictor* for the model and is often abbreviated η; that is, $\eta = \alpha + x\beta$ by definition.

All the models we have discussed are generalized linear models. Ordinary linear models (such as the linear risk model) are the simplest examples, in which f and g are both the identity function $f(u) = g(u) = u$, so that

$$E(Y|x) = \alpha + x\beta.$$

The inverse of the exponential function exp is the natural log function $\ln(u)$. Hence, the generalized-linear forms of the exponential risk and rate models are the log-linear risk and rate models

$$\ln[R(x)] = \alpha + x\beta \quad \text{and} \quad \ln[I(x)] = \alpha + x\beta;$$

that is, the exponential risk and rate models correspond to a natural-log link function, because $\ln[\exp(u)] = u$. Similarly, the inverse of expit, the logistic function, is the logit function $\text{logit}(u)$. Hence, the generalized-linear form of the logistic-risk model is the logit-linear risk model

$$\text{logit}[R(x)] = \alpha + x\beta;$$

that is, the logistic model corresponds to the logit link function, because $\text{logit}[\text{expit}(u)] = u$.

The choices for f and g are virtually unlimited. In epidemiology, however, only the logit link $g(u) = \text{logit}(u)$ is in common use for risks, and only the log link $g(u) = \ln(u)$ is in common use for rates. In practice, these link functions are almost always the default, and are sometimes the only options in commercial software for risk and rate modeling. Some packages, however, allow easy selection of linear risk, rate, and odds models, which use the identity link. Some software (e.g., GLIM) allows the user to define their own link function.

The choice of link function can have a profound impact on the shape of the trend or dose-response surface allowed by the model, especially if exposure is represented by only one or two terms. For example, if exposure is represented by a single term $\beta_1 x_1$ in a risk model, use of the identity link results in a linear risk model and a linear trend for risk; use of the log link results in an exponential (log-linear) risk model and an exponential trend for risk; and use of a logit link results in a logistic model and an exponential trend for the odds. Generalized linear models encompass a broader range than the linear, log-linear, and logistic forms, however. One example is the complementary log-log risk model,

$$R(x) = 1 - \exp[-\exp(\alpha + x\beta)],$$

which translates to the generalized-linear form

$$\ln[-\ln(1 - R(x))] = \alpha + x\beta.$$

This model corresponds to the link function $\ln[-\ln(1-u)]$ and arises naturally in certain biology experiments. For further reading on this and other generalized linear models, see McCullagh and Nelder (1989).

3.8   Model Searching

How do we find a model or set of models acceptable for our purposes? There are far too many model forms to allow us to examine most or even much of the total realm of possibilities. There are several systematic, mechanical, and traditional algorithms for finding models (such as stepwise and best-subset regression) that lack logical or statistical justification and that perform poorly in theoretical and simulation studies; see Sclove et al. (1972), Bancroft and Han (1977), Freedman (1983), Flack and Chang (1987), Hurvich and Tsai (1990), and Weiss (1995). For example, the P-values and standard-error (SE) estimates obtained when variables are selected using significance-testing criteria (such as "F-to-enter" and "F-to-remove") will be downwardly biased. In particular, the SE estimates obtained from the selected model underestimate the standard deviations (SDs) of the point estimates obtained by applying the algorithms across different random samples. As a result, the algorithms will tend to yield P-values that are too small and confidence intervals that are too narrow (and hence fail to cover the true coefficient values with the stated frequency). Unfortunately, significance-testing criteria are the basis for most variable-selection procedures in standard packaged software.

Other criteria for selecting variables, such as "change-in-point-estimate" criteria, do not necessarily perform better than significance testing (Maldonado and Greenland 1993a). Viable alternatives to significance testing in model selection have emerged only gradually with recent advances in computing and with deeper insights into the problem of model selection. We first outline the traditional approaches after reinforcing one of the most essential and neglected starting points for good modeling: laying out existing information in a manner that can help the search avoid models in conflict with established facts. A powerful alternative to model selection is provided by hierarchical regression, also known as multilevel, mixed-model, or random-coefficient regression (Rothman and Greenland 1998, pp 427–432; Greenland 2000a, b).

Role of Prior Information

The dependence of regression results on the chosen model can be either an advantage or a drawback. The advantage comes from the fact that use of a model structure capable of reasonably approximating reality can elevate the accuracy of the estimates over those from the corresponding tabular analysis. The drawback comes from the fact that use of a model incapable of even approximating reality can decrease estimation accuracy below that of tabular analysis.

This duality underscores the desirability of using flexible (and possibly complex) models. One should take care to avoid models that are entirely unsupported by background knowledge. For example, in a cohort study of lung cancer, it is reasonable to restrict rates to increase with age, because there is enormous background literature documenting that this trend is found in all human populations. In contrast, one would want to avoid restricting cardiovascular disease (CVD) rates to strictly increase with alcohol consumption, because there are considerable data to suggest the alcohol-CVD relation is not strictly increasing (Maclure 1993).

Prior knowledge about most epidemiologic relations is usually too limited to provide much guidance in model selection. A natural response might be to use models as flexible as possible (a flexible model can reproduce a wide variety of curves and surfaces). Unfortunately, flexible models have limitations. The more flexible the model, the larger the sample needed for the usual estimation methods (such as maximum likelihood) to provide approximately unbiased coefficient estimates. Also, after a certain point, increasing flexibility may increase variability of estimates so much that the accuracy of the estimates is decreased relative to estimates from simpler models, despite the greater faithfulness of the flexible model to reality. As a result, it is usual practice to employ models that are severely restrictive in arbitrary ways, such as models without product terms (Robins and Greenland 1986). Hierarchical methods can help alleviate some of these problems by allowing one to fit larger models than one can with ordinary methods (Greenland 2000b).

Fortunately, estimates obtained from the most common epidemiologic regression models, exponential (log-linear) and logistic models, retain some interpretability even when the underlying (true) regression function is not particularly close to those forms (Maldonado and Greenland 1993b, 1994). For example, under reasonably common conditions, rate-ratio or risk-ratio estimates obtained from those models can be interpreted as approximate estimates of standardized rate or risk ratios, using the total source population as the standard (Greenland and Maldonado 1994). To ensure such interpretations are reasonable, the model used should at least be able to replicate qualitative features of the underlying regression function. For example, if the underlying regression may have a reversal in the slope of the exposure-response curve, we should want to use a model capable of exhibiting such reversal (even if it cannot replicate the exact shape of the true curve).

A major problem for epidemiology is that key variables may be unmeasured or poorly measured. No conventional method can account for these problems. Unmeasured variables may be modeled using prior information on their relation to measured variables, but the results will be entirely dependent on that information (Leamer 1978; Greenland 2003a). Occasionally, measurement-error information may be in the form of data that can be used in special correction techniques (Carroll et al. 1995; Chap. II.5 of this handbook); otherwise, sensitivity analyses will be needed (Rothman and Greenland 1998, Chap. 19; Lash and Fink 2003).

3.8.2 Selection Strategies

Even with ample prior information, there will always be an overwhelming number of model choices, and so model search strategies will be needed. Many strategies have been proposed, although none has been fully justified.

Some strategies begin by specifying a minimal model form that is among the most simple credible forms. Here "credible" means "compatible with available information". Thus, we start with a model of minimal computational or conceptual complexity that does not conflict with background information. There may be many such models; in order to help insure that our analysis is credible to the intended audience, however, the starting model form should be one that most researchers would view as a reasonable possibility.

To specify a simple yet credible model form, one needs some knowledge of the background scientific literature on the relations under study. This knowledge would include information about relations of potential confounders to the study exposures and study diseases, as well as relations of study exposures to the study diseases. Thus, specification of a simple yet credible model can demand much more initial effort than is routinely used in model specification.

Once we have specified our minimal starting model, we can add complexities that seem necessary (by some criteria) in light of the data. Such a search process is sometimes called an *expanding* search (Leamer 1978). Its chief drawback is that often there are too many possible expansions to consider within a reasonable length of time. If, however, one neglects to consider any possible expansion, one risks missing an important shortcoming of the initial model. For example, if our minimal model involves only single "first-order" terms ("main effects") for 12 variables, we would have $\binom{12}{2} = 66$ possible two-way products among these variables to consider, as well as 12 quadratic terms, for a total of 78 possible expansions with just one second-order term. An analyst may not have the time, patience, or resources to examine all the possibilities in detail; this predicament usually leads to use of automatic significance-testing procedures to select additional terms, which (as referenced above) can lead to distorted statistics.

Some strategies begin by specifying an initial model form that is flexible enough to approximate any credible model form. A flexible starting point can be less demanding than a simple one in terms of need for background information. For example, rather than concern ourselves with what the literature suggests about the shape of a dose-response curve, we can employ a starting model form that can approximate a wide range of curves. Similarly, rather than concern ourselves with what the literature suggests about joint effects, we can employ a form that can approximate a wide range of joint effects. We can then search for a simpler but adequate model by removing from the flexible model any complexities that appear unnecessary in light of the data. Such a search process, based on simplifying a complex model, is sometimes called a *contracting* or simplifying search (Leamer 1978).

The chief drawback of a purely contracting search is that a sufficiently flexible prior model may be too complex to fit to the available data. This is because more complex models generally involve more parameters; with more parameters in a model, more data are needed to produce trustworthy point and interval estimates. Standard model-fitting methods may yield biased estimates or may completely fail to yield any estimates (e.g., not converge) if the fitted model is too complex. For example, if our flexible model for 12 variables contains all first and second-order terms, there will be 12 first-order plus 12 quadratic plus 66 product terms, for a total of 90 coefficients. Fitting this model may be well beyond what our data or computing resources can support.

Because of potential fitting problems, contracting searches begin with something much less than a fully flexible model. Some begin with a model as flexible as can be fit, or maximal model. As with minimal models, maximal models are not unique. In order to produce a model that can be fit, one may have to limit flexibility of dose-response, flexibility of joint effects, or both. It is also possible to start a model search anywhere in between the extremes of minimal and maximal models, and proceed by expanding as seems necessary and contracting as seems reasonable based on the data (although again, resource limitations usually lead to mechanical use of significance tests for this process). Unsurprisingly, such *stepwise* searches share some advantages and disadvantages with purely expanding and purely contracting searches. Like other searches, care should be taken to insure that the starting and ending points do not conflict with prior information.

The results obtained from a model search can be very sensitive to the choice of starting model. One may check for this problem by conducting several searches, starting at different models. However, there are always too many possible starting models to check them all. Thus, if one has many variables (and hence many possible models) to consider, model search strategies will always risk producing a misleading conclusion.

Model Fitting 3.9

Residual Distributions 3.9.1

Different fitting methods can lead to different estimates; thus, in presenting results one should specify the method used to derive the estimates. The vast majority of programs for risk and rate modeling use *maximum-likelihood* (ML) estimation, which is based on very specific assumptions about how the observed values of Y

tend to distribute (vary) when the vector of regressors X is fixed at a given value x. This distribution is called the error distribution or *residual distribution* of Y.

If Y is the person-time rate observed at a given level x of X, and T is the corresponding observed person-time, it is conventionally assumed that the number of cases observed, $A = YT$, would tend to vary according to a Poisson distribution if the person-time were fixed at its observed value. Hence, conventional ML regression analysis of person-time rates is usually called *Poisson regression*. If, on the other hand, Y is the proportion of cases observed at a given level x of X out of a person-count total N, it is conventionally assumed that the number of cases observed, $A = YN$, would tend to vary according to a *binomial distribution* if the number of persons (person count) N was fixed at its observed value. Hence, conventional ML regression analysis of prevalence or incidence proportions (average risks) is sometimes called *binomial regression*. Note that if $N = 1$, the proportion diseased Y can be only 0 or 1; in this situation, $A = YN$ can be only 0 or 14 and is said to have a Bernoulli distribution (which is just a binomial distribution with $N = 1$). The binomial distribution can be deduced from the homogeneity and independence assumptions discussed for example in Rothman and Greenland (1998, pp 232–233). As noted there, its use is inadvisable if there are important violations of either assumption, e.g., if the disease is contagious over the study period.

If Y is the number of exposed cases in a 2×2 table, the conventionally assumed distribution for Y is the *hypergeometric*; ML fitting in this situation is usually referred to as conditional maximum likelihood (CML). CML fitting is closely related to partial-likelihood methods, which are used for fitting Cox models in survival analysis.

More details on maximum-likelihood model fitting in epidemiology can be found in Breslow and Day (1980, 1987), Hosmer and Lemeshow (2000), and Clayton and Hills (1993). More general and advanced treatments of maximum likelihood can be found in many books, including Cox and Hinkley (1974) and McCullagh and Nelder (1989).

3.9.2   Overdispersion

What if the residual distribution of the observed Y does *not* follow the conventionally assumed residual distribution? Under a broad range of conditions, it can be shown that the resulting ML fitted values (ML estimates) will remain approximately unbiased if no other source of bias is present (White 1994). Nonetheless, the estimated SDs obtained from the program will be biased. In particular, if the actual variance of Y given $X = x$ (the *residual variance*) is larger than that implied by the conventional distribution, Y is said to suffer from *overdispersion* or *extravariation*, and the estimated standard deviations and P-values obtained from an ordinary maximum-likelihood regression program will be too small.

In Poisson regression, overdispersion is sometimes called "extra-Poisson variation"; in binomial regression, overdispersion is sometimes called "extra-binomial variation". Typically, such overdispersion arises when there is dependence among the recorded outcomes, as when the outcome Y is the number infected in a group, or Y is the number of times a person gets a disease. As an example, suppose Y is the number of eyes affected by glaucoma in an individual. In a natural population, $Y = 0$ for most people and $Y = 2$ for most of the remainder, with $Y = 1$ very infrequently. In other words, the Y values would be largely limited to the extremes of 0 and 2. In contrast, a binomially distributed variable with the same possible values ($0, 1$, or 2) and the same mean as Y would have a higher probability of 1 than 2, and hence a smaller variance than Y.

Two major approaches have been developed to cope with potential overdispersion, both of which are based on modeling the residual distribution. One approach is to use maximum likelihood, but with a residual distribution that allows a broader range of variation for Y, such as the negative binomial in place of the Poisson or the beta-binomial in place of the binomial (McCullagh and Nelder 1989). Such approaches can be computationally intensive, but have been implemented in some software. The second and simpler approach is to model only the residual variance of Y, rather than completely specify the residual distribution. Fitting methods that employ this approach are discussed by various authors under the topics of quasi-likelihood, pseudo-likelihood, and generalized estimating-equation (GEE) methods; see McCullagh and Nelder (1989), McCullagh (1991), and Diggle et al. (2002) for descriptions of these methods. GEE methods are often used for logitudinal data analysis (Diggle et al. 2002), but have some serious limitations in that role (Robins et al. 1999).

Sample-Size Considerations   3.9.3

One drawback of all the above fitting methods is that they depend on "large-sample" (asymptotic) approximations, which usually require that the number of parameters in the model is much less than (roughly, not more than 10% of) the number of cases observed. Methods that do not use large sample approximations (exact methods) can also be used to fit certain models. These methods require the same strong distributional assumptions as maximum-likelihood methods. An example is exact logistic regression (Cytel 2003).

Unfortunately, exact fitting methods for incidence and prevalence models are so computationally demanding that, at the time of this writing, they can be used to fit only a narrow range of models, and do not address all the problems arising from coefficient instability in small samples (Greenland et al. 2000). *Penalized likelihood estimation* and the related methods of Stein estimation and ridge regression address these problems and permit fitting of incidence and prevalence models while retaining acceptably (though still only approximately) valid small-sample results (Efron and Morris 1975; Copas 1983; Titterington 1985; Le Cessie and van Houwelingen 1992; Greenland 1997; Rothman and Greenland 1998, pp 429–430; Greenland 2001, Greenland 2003b, Greenland and Christensen 2001).

3.10   Model Checking

It is important to check a fitted model against the data. The extent of these checks may depend on what purpose we wish the model to serve. At one extreme, we may only wish the fitted model to provide approximately valid *summary* estimates or trends for a few key relationships. For example, we might wish only to estimate the average increment in risk produced by a unit increase in exposure. At the other extreme, we may want the model to provide approximately valid *regressor-specific* predictions of outcomes, such as exposure-specific risks by age, sex, and ethnicity. The latter goal is more demanding and requires more detailed scrutiny of results, sometimes on a subject-by-subject basis.

Model diagnostics can detect discrepancies between data and a model only within the range of the data, and then only where there are enough observations to provide adequate diagnostic power. For example, there is much controversy concerning the health effects of low-dose radiation exposure (exposures that are only modestly in excess of natural background levels). This controversy arises because the natural incidence of key outcomes (such as leukemia) is low, and few cases have been observed in low-dose cohorts. As a result, several proposed dose-response models "fit the data adequately" in the low-dose region, in that each model passes the standard battery of diagnostic checks. Nonetheless, the health effects predicted by these models conflict to an important extent.

More generally, one should bear in mind that a good-fitting model is not the same as a correct model. In particular, a model may appear correct in the central range of the data, but produce grossly misleading predictions for combinations of covariate values that are poorly represented or absent in the data.

3.10.1   Tabular Checks

Both tabular methods (such as Mantel–Haenszel, Mantel and Haenszel (1959)) and regression methods produce estimates by merging assumptions about population structure (such as that of a common odds ratio or of an explicit regression model) with observed data. When an estimate is derived using a regression model, especially one with many regressors, it may become difficult to judge how much the estimate reflects the data and how much it reflects the model.

To investigate the source of results, we recommend one compare model-based results to the corresponding tabular (categorical-analysis) results. As an illustration, suppose we wish to check a logistic model in which X_1 is the exposure under study, and four other regressors X_2, X_3, X_4, X_5 appear in the model, with X_1, X_2, X_3 continuous, X_4, X_5 binary, and products among X_1, X_2, and X_4 in the model. Any regressor in a model must appear in the corresponding tabular analysis. Because X_2 and X_4 appear in products with X_1 and the model is logistic, they should be treated as modifiers of the X_1 odds ratio in the corresponding tabular analysis. X_3 and X_5 do not appear in products with X_1 and so should be treated as pure confounders (adjustment variables) in the corresponding tabular analysis. Because X_1, X_2, X_3

are continuous in the model, they must have at least three levels in the tabular analysis, so that the results can at least crudely reflect trends seen with the model. If all three of these regressors were categorized into four levels, the resulting table of disease (two levels) by all regressors would have $2 \times 4^3 \times 2^2 = 512$ cells, and perhaps many zero cells.

From this table, we would attempt to compute 3 (for exposure strata 1, 2, 3, versus 0) adjusted odds ratios (e.g., Mantel–Haenszel) for each of the $4 \times 2 = 8$ combinations of X_2 and X_4, adjusting all $3 \times 8 = 24$ odds ratios for the $4 \times 2 = 8$ pure-confounder levels. Some of these 24 adjusted odds ratios might be infinite or undefined due to small numbers, which would indicate that the corresponding regression estimates are largely model projections. Similarly, the tabular estimates might not exhibit a pattern seen in the regression estimates, which would suggest that the pattern was induced by the regression model rather than the data. For example, the regression estimates might exhibit a monotone trend with increasing exposure even if the tabular estimates did not. Interpretation of such a conflict would depend on the context: If we were certain that dose-response was monotone (e.g., smoking and esophageal cancer), the monotonicity of the regression estimates would favor their use over the tabular results; in contrast, doubts about monotonicity (e.g., as with alcohol and coronary heart disease) would lead us to use the tabular results or search for a model that did not impose monotonicity.

Tests of Regression and R^2 3.10.2

Most programs supply a "test of regression" or "test of model", which is a test of the hypothesis that all the regression coefficients (except the intercept α) are zero. For instance, in the exponential rate model

$$I(x) = \exp(\alpha + x\beta),$$

the "test of regression" provides a P-value for the null hypothesis that all the components of β are zero, that is, that $\beta_1 = \ldots = \beta_n = 0$. Similarly, the "test of R^2" provided by linear regression programs is just a test that all the regressor coefficients are zero. A small P-value from these tests suggests that the variation in outcomes observed across regressor values appears improbably large under the hypothesis that the regressors are unrelated to the outcome. Such a result suggests that at least one of the regressors is related to the outcome. It does *not*, however, imply that the model fits well or is adequate in any way.

To understand the latter point, suppose that X comprises the single indicator $X_1 = 1$ for smokers, 0 for nonsmokers, and the outcome Y is average year risk of lung cancer. In most any study of reasonable size and validity, "the test of regression" (which here is just a test of $\beta_1 = 0$) would yield a small P-value. Nonetheless, the model would be inadequate to describe variation in risk, because it neglects amount smoked, age at start, and sex. More generally, a small P-value from the test of regression only tells us that at least one of the regressors in the model should be included in some form or another; it does not tell us which regressor or what form to use, nor does it tell us anything about what was left out of the model. Conversely, a large P-value from the "test of regression" does not imply that all the regressors in the model are unimportant or that the model fits well. It is always possible that transformations of those regressors would result in a small P-value, or that their importance cannot be discerned given the random error in the data.

A closely related mistake is interpreting the squared multiple-correlation co-efficient R^2 for a regression as a goodness-of-fit measure. R^2 only indicates the proportion of Y variance that is attributable to variation in the fitted mean of Y. While $R^2 = 1$ (the largest possible value) does correspond to a perfect fit, R^2 can also be close to zero under a correct model if the residual variance of Y (i.e., the variance of Y around the true regression curve) is always close to the total variance of Y.

The preceding limitations of R^2 apply in general. Correlational measures such as R^2 can become patently absurd measures of fit or association when the regressors and regressand are discrete or bounded (Rosenthal and Rubin 1979; Greenland et al. 1986; Cox and Wermuth 1992; Greenland 1996). As an example, consider Table 3.1 showing a large association of a factor with a rare disease. The logistic model $R(x) = \text{expit}(\alpha + \beta_x)$ fits these data perfectly because it uses two parameters to describe only two proportions. Furthermore, $X = 1$ is associated with a 19-fold increase in risk. Yet the correlation coefficient for X and Y (derived using standard formulas) is only 0.09, and the R^2 for the regression is only 0.008.

Correlation coefficients and R^2 can give even more distorted impressions when multiple regressors are present (Greenland et al. 1986, 1991). For this reason, we strongly recommend against their use as measures of association or effect when modeling incidence or prevalence.

3.10.3   Tests of Fit

Tests of model fit check for nonrandom incompatibilities between the fitted regression model and the data. To do so, however, these tests must assume that the fitting method used was appropriate; in particular, test validity may be sensitive to assumptions about the residual distribution that were used in fitting. Conversely, it is possible to test assumptions about the residual distribution, but these tests usually have little power to detect violations unless a parametric regression model is assumed. Thus, useful model tests cannot be performed without making some assumptions.

Many tests of regression models are *relative*, in that they test the fit of an index model by assuming the validity of a more elaborate *reference* model that contains

Table 3.1. Hypothetical cohort data illustrating inappropriateness of R^2 for binary outcomes (see text)

	$X = 1$	$X = 0$
$Y = 1$	1900	100
Total	100,000	100,000

Risk ratio = 19, $R^2 = 0.008$.

it. A test that assumes a relatively simple reference model (i.e., one that has only a few more coefficients than the index model) will tend to have better power than a test that assumes a more complex reference model, although it will be valid only under narrower conditions.

When models are fit by maximum likelihood (ML), a standard method for testing the fit of a simpler model against a more complex model is the *deviance test*, also known as the likelihood-ratio test. Suppose that X_1 represents cumulative dose of an exposure, and that the index model we wish to test is

$$R(x_1) = \text{expit}(\alpha + \beta_1 x_1),$$

a simple linear-logistic model. When we fit this model, an ML program should supply either a "residual deviance statistic" $D(\tilde{\alpha}, \tilde{\beta}_1)$, or a "model log-likelihood" $L(\tilde{\alpha}, \tilde{\beta}_1)$, where $\tilde{\alpha}, \tilde{\beta}_1$ are the ML estimates for this simple model. Suppose we wish to test the fit of the index model taking as the reference the fractional-polynomial logistic model

$$R(x_1) = \text{expit}\left(\alpha + \beta_1 x_1 + \beta_2 x_1^{1/2} + \beta_3 x_1^2\right).$$

We then fit this model and get either the residual deviance $D(\hat{\alpha}, \hat{\beta}_1, \hat{\beta}_2, \hat{\beta}_3)$ or the log-likelihood $L(\hat{\alpha}, \hat{\beta}_1, \hat{\beta}_2, \hat{\beta}_3)$ for the model, where $\hat{\alpha}, \hat{\beta}_1, \hat{\beta}_2, \hat{\beta}_3$ are the ML estimates for this power model. The deviance statistic for testing the linear-logistic model against the power-logistic model (that is, for testing $\beta_2 = \beta_3 = 0$) is then

$$\Delta D(\beta_2, \beta_3) = D\left(\tilde{\alpha}, \tilde{\beta}_1\right) - D\left(\hat{\alpha}, \hat{\beta}_1, \hat{\beta}_2, \hat{\beta}_3\right).$$

This statistic is related to the model log-likelihoods by the equation

$$\Delta D(\beta_2, \beta_3) = -2\left[L\left(\tilde{\alpha}, \tilde{\beta}_1\right) - L\left(\hat{\alpha}, \hat{\beta}_1, \hat{\beta}_2, \hat{\beta}_3\right)\right]$$

(McCullagh and Nelder 1989; Clayton and Hills 1993). If the linear-logistic model is correct (so that $\beta_2 = \beta_3 = 0$) and the sample is large enough, this statistic has an approximate χ^2 distribution with 2 degrees of freedom, which is the difference in the number of parameters in the two models.

A small *P*-value from this statistic suggests that the linear-logistic model is inadequate or fits poorly; in some way, either or both the terms $\beta_2 x_1^{1/2}$ and $\beta_3 x_1^2$ capture deviations of the true regression from the linear-logistic model. A large *P*-value does *not*, however, imply that the linear-logistic model is adequate or fits well; it means only that no need for the terms $\beta_2 x_1^{1/2}$ and $\beta_3 x_1^2$ was detected by the test. In particular, a large *P*-value from this test leaves open the possibility that $\beta_2 x_1^{1/2}$ and $\beta_3 x_1^2$ are important for describing the true regression function, but the test failed to detect this condition; it also leaves open the possibility that some other terms not present in the reference model may be important in the same sense. These unexamined terms may involve X_1 or other regressors.

Now consider a more general description. Suppose that we wish to test an index model against a reference model in which it is nested (contained) and that this reference model contains p more unknown parameters (coefficients) than the index model. We fit both models and obtain either residual deviances of D_i and D_r for the index and reference models, or log-likelihoods L_i and L_r. If the sample is large enough and the index model is correct, the deviance statistic

$$\Delta D = D_i - D_r = -2(L_i - L_r) \tag{3.56}$$

will have an approximate χ^2 distribution with p degrees of freedom. Again, a small P-value suggests that the index model does not fit well, but a large P-value does not mean the index model fits well, except in the very narrow sense that the test did not detect a need for the extra terms in the reference model.

Whatever the size of the deviance P-value, its validity depends on three assumptions (in addition to absence of the usual biases). First, it assumes that ML fitting of the models is appropriate; in particular, there must be enough subjects to justify use of ML to fit the reference model, and the assumed residual distribution must be correct. Second, it assumes that the reference regression model is approximately correct. Third, it assumes that the index model being tested is nested within the reference model. The third is the only assumption that is easy to check: In the previous example, we can see that the linear-logistic model is just the special case of the power-logistic model in which $\beta_2 = \beta_3 = 0$. In contrast, if we used the linear-logistic model as the index model (as above) but used the power-linear model

$$R(x_1) = \alpha + \beta_1 x_1 + \beta_2 x_1^{1/2} + \beta_3 x_1^2$$

as the reference model, the resulting deviance difference would be meaningless, because the latter model does *not* contain the linear-logistic model as a special case.

Comparison of non-nested models is a more difficult task unless the compared models have the same number of parameters. In the latter case, it has been suggested that (absent other considerations) one should choose the model with the highest loglikelihood (Walker and Rothman 1982).

3.10.4   Global Tests of Fit

One special type of deviance test of fit can be performed when Y is a proportion or rate. Suppose that, for every distinct regressor level x, at least four cases would be expected if the index model were correct; also, if Y is a proportion, suppose at least four noncases would be expected if the index model were correct. (This criterion, while somewhat arbitrary, originated because it ensures that the chance of a cell count being zero is less than 2% if the cell variation is Poisson and the index model is correct.) We can then test our index model against the *saturated* regression model

$$E(Y|X = x) = \alpha_x,$$

where α_x is a distinct parameter for every distinct observed level x of X; that is, α_x may represent a different number for every level of X and may vary in any fashion as X varies. This model is so general that it contains all other regression models as special cases.

The degrees of freedom for the test of the index model against the saturated model is the number of distinct X-levels (which is the number of parameters in the saturated model) minus the number of parameters in the index model, and is often called the *residual degrees of freedom* for the model. This *residual* deviance test is sometimes called a "global test of fit" because it has some power to detect any systematic incompatibility between the index model and the data. Another well-known global test of fit is the *Pearson χ^2 test*, which has the same degrees of freedom and sample-size requirements as the saturated-model deviance test.

Suppose we observe K distinct regressor values and we list them in some order, $x_1, \ldots, x_K$. The statistic used for the Pearson test has the form of a residual sum-of-squares:

$$\text{RSS}_{\text{Pearson}} = \sum_k \left(Y_k - \hat{Y}_k \right)^2 / \hat{V}_k = \sum_k \left[\left(Y_k - \hat{Y}_k \right) / \hat{S}_k \right]^2,$$

where the sum is over all observed values $1, \ldots, K$, Y_k is the rate or risk observed at level x_k, $\hat{Y}_k$ is the rate or risk predicted (fitted) at x_k by the model, $\hat{V}_k$ is the estimated variance of $\hat{Y}_k$ when $X = x_k$, and $\hat{S}_k = \hat{V}_k^{1/2}$ is the estimated standard deviation of Y_k under the model. In Poisson regression, $\hat{Y}_k = \exp(\hat{\alpha} + x_k\hat{\beta})$ and $\hat{V}_k = \hat{Y}_k/T_k$, where T_k is the person-time observed at x_k; in binomial regression, $\hat{Y}_k = \text{expit}(\hat{\alpha} + x_k\hat{\beta})$ and $\hat{V}_k = \hat{Y}_k(1 - \hat{Y}_k)/N_k$, where N_k is the number of persons observed at x_k. The quantity $(Y_k - \hat{Y}_k)/\hat{S}_k$ is sometimes called the *standardized residual* at level x_k; it is the distance between Y_k and $\hat{Y}_k$ expressed in units of the estimated standard deviation of Y_k under the model.

Other global tests have been proposed that have fewer degrees of freedom and less restrictive sample-size requirements than the deviance and Pearson tests (Hosmer and Lemeshow 2000). A major drawback of all global tests of fit, however, is their low power to detect model problems (Hosmer et al. 1997). If any of the tests yields a low *P*-value, we can be confident the tested (index) model is unsatisfactory and needs modification or replacement (albeit the tests provide no clue as to how to proceed). If, however, they all yield a high *P*-value, it does not mean the model is satisfactory. In fact, the tests are unlikely to detect any but the most gross conflicts between the fitted model and the data. Therefore, global tests should be regarded as crude preliminary screening tests only, to allow quick rejection of grossly unsatisfactory models.

The deviance and Pearson statistics are sometimes used directly as measures of distance between the data and the model. Such use is most easily seen for the

Pearson statistic. The second form of the Pearson statistic shows that it is the sum of squared standardized residuals; in other words, it is a sum of squared distances between data values and model-fitted values of Y. The deviance and Pearson global test statistics can also be transformed into measures of prediction error under the model; for example, see McCullagh and Nelder (1989) and Hosmer and Lemeshow (2000).

3.10.5   Model Diagnostics

Suppose now we have found a model that has passed preliminary checks such as tests for additional terms and global tests of fit. Before adopting this model as a source of estimates, it is wise to further check the model against the basic data, and assess the trustworthiness of any model-based inferences we wish to draw. Such activity is subsumed under the topic of *model diagnostics*, and its subsidiary topics of residual analysis, influence analysis, and model-sensitivity analysis. These topics are vast, and we can only mention a few approaches here. In particular, we neglect the classical topic of residual analysis, largely because its proper usage involves a number of technical complexities when dealing with the censored data and nonlinear models predominant in epidemiology (McCullagh and Nelder 1989). Detailed treatments of diagnostics for such models can be found in Breslow and Day (1987), Hosmer and Lemeshow (2000), and McCullagh and Nelder (1989).

3.10.6   Delta-Beta Analysis

One important and simple diagnostic tool available in some packaged software is *delta-beta* ($\Delta\beta$) *analysis*. For a data set with N subjects total, estimated model coefficients (or approximations to them) are recomputed N times over, each time deleting exactly one of the subjects from the model fitting. Alternatively, for individually-matched data comprising N matched sets, the delta-beta analysis may be done deleting one set at a time. In either approach, the output is N different sets of coefficients estimates: These sets are then examined to see if anyone subject or matched set influences the resulting estimates to an unusual extent.

To illustrate, suppose our objective is to estimate the rate-ratio per unit increase in an exposure X_1, to be measured by $\exp(\hat{\beta}_1)$, where $\hat{\beta}_1$ is the estimated exposure coefficient in an exponential-rate model. For each subject, the entire model (confounders included) is re-fit without that subject. Let $\hat{\beta}_{1(-i)}$ be the estimate of $\hat{\beta}_1$ obtained when subject i is excluded from the data. The difference $\hat{\beta}_{1(-i)} - \hat{\beta}_1 \equiv \Delta\hat{\beta}_{1(-i)}$ is called the *delta-beta* for β_1 for subject i. The influence of subject i on the results can be assessed in several ways. One way is to examine the impact on the rate-ratio estimate. The proportionate change in the estimate from dropping subject i is

$$\exp\left(\hat{\beta}_{1(-i)}\right) / \exp\left(\hat{\beta}_1\right) = \exp\left(\hat{\beta}_{1(-i)} - \hat{\beta}_1\right) = \exp\left(\Delta\hat{\beta}_{1(-i)}\right),$$

for which a value of 1.30 indicates dropping subject i increases the estimate by 30%, and a value of 0.90 indicates dropping subject i decreases the estimate by 10%. One can also assess the impact of dropping the subject on confidence limits, *P*-values, or any other quantity of interest.

Some packages compute "standardized" delta-betas, $\Delta\hat{\beta}_{1(-i)}/\hat{s}_1$ where $\hat{s}_1$ is the estimated standard deviation for $\hat{\beta}_1$. By analogy with Z-statistics, any standardized delta-beta below -1.96 or above 1.96 is sometimes interpreted as being unusual. This interpretation can be misleading, however, because the standard deviation used in the denominator is not that of the delta-beta. A standardized delta-beta is only a measure of the influence of an observation expressed in SE units.

It is possible that one or a few subjects or matched sets are so influential that deleting them alters the conclusions of the study, even when N is in the hundreds (Pregibon 1981). In such situations, comparison of the records of those subjects to others may reveal unusual combinations of regressor values among those subjects. Such unusual combinations may arise from previously undetected data errors, and should at least lead to enhanced caution in interpretation. For instance, it may be only mildly unusual to see a woman who reports having had a child at age 45 or a woman who reports natural menopause at age 45. The combination in one subject, however, may arouse suspicion of a data error in one or both regressors, a suspicion worth the labor of further data scrutiny if that woman or her matched set disproportionately influences the results.

Delta-beta analysis must be replaced by a more complex analysis if the exposure of interest appears in multiple model terms, such as indicator terms, power terms, product terms, or spline terms. In that situation, one must focus on changes in estimates of specific effects or summaries, for example, changes in estimated risk ratios.

Conclusions 3.11

This chapter has reviewed basic principles and forms of parametric regression models and model fitting. Regression analysis is a vast subject, however, and many topics and details have been omitted. For further reading on fundamentals of parametric modeling a standard text is McCullagh and Nelder (1989). A standard introduction to nonparametric regression is Hastie and Tibshirani (1990). Non-parametric methods are connected to algorithmic modeling (machine learning) methods; for a comparison of parametric and algorithmic approaches see Breiman (2001). For an integrated coverage of parametric, nonparametric, and algorithmic methods see Hastie et al. (2001).

References

Agresti A (2002) Categorical data analysis. Wiley, New York
Bancroft TA, Han C-P (1977) Inference based on conditional specification: A note and a bibliography. Int Stat Rev 45:117–127

Berk R (2004) Regression analysis: A constructive critique. Sage publications, Thousand Oaks, CA

Bishop YMM, Fienberg SE, Holland PW (1975) Discrete multivariate analysis: theory and practice. MIT Press, Cambridge, MA

Breiman L (2001) Statistical modeling: The two cultures (with discussion). Statistical Science 16:199–231

Breslow NE, Day NE (1980) Statistical methods in cancer research. Vol I: the analysis of case-control data. IARC, Lyon

Breslow NE, Day NE (1987) Statistical methods in cancer research. Vol II: the design and analysis of cohort studies. IARC, Lyon

Carroll RJ, Ruppert D, Stefanski LA (1995) Measurement error in nonlinear models. Chapman and Hall, New York

Clayton D, Hills M (1993) Statistical models in epidemiology. Oxford University Press, New York

Cole SR, Ananth CV (2001) Regression models for unconstrained, partially or fully constrained continuation odds ratios. Int J Epidemiol 30:1379–1382

Copas JB (1983) Regression, prediction, and shrinkage (with discussion). J Royal Stat Soc B 45:311–354

Cox DR (1972) Regression models and life tables (with discussions). J Royal Stat Soc B 34:187–220

Cox DR, Hinkley DV (1974) Theoretical statistics. Chapman and Hall, New York

Cox DR, Oakes D (1984) Analysis of survival data. Chapman and Hall, New York

Cox DR, Wermuth N (1992) A comment on the coefficient of determination for binary responses. Am Statist 46:1–4

Cytel Corporation. LogXact Version 5 (software) (2003) Cytel Corp., Cambridge, MA

Diggle PJ, Heagerty P, Liang KY, Zeger SL (2002) The analysis of longitudinal data, 2nd edn. Oxford University Press, New York

Efron B, Morris CN (1975) Data analysis using Stein's estimator and its generalizations. J Am Stat Assoc 70:311–319

Flack VF, Chang PC (1987) Frequency of selecting noise variables in subset regression analysis: a simulation study. Am Statist 41:84–86

Freedman DA (1983) A note on screening regression equations. Am Statist 37:152–155

Good IJ (1983) Good thinking: The foundations of probability and its applications. University of Minnesota Press, Minneapolis, MN

Green PJ, Silverman BW (1994) Nonparametric regression and generalized linear models: A roughness penalty approach. Chapman and Hall, New York

Greenland S (1993) Basic problems in interaction assessment. Environ Health Perspect 101(suppl 4):59–66

Greenland S (1994) Alternative models for ordinal logistic regression. Stat Med 13:1665–1677

Greenland S (1995a) Dose-response and trend analysis: Alternatives to categorical analysis. Epidemiology 6:356–365

Greenland S (1995b) Avoiding power loss associated with categorization and ordinal scores in dose-response and trend analysis. Epidemiology 6:450–454

Greenland S (1995c) Problems in the average-risk interpretation of categorical dose-response analyses. Epidemiology 6:563–565

Greenland S (1996) A lower bound for the correlation of exponentiated bivariate normal pairs. Am Statist 50:163–164

Greenland S (1997) Second-stage least squares versus penalized quasi-likelihood for fitting hierarchical models in epidemiologic analyses. Stat Med 16:515–526

Greenland S (2000a) Principles of multilevel modeling. Int J Epidemiol 29:158–167

Greenland S (2000b) When should epidemiologic regressions use random coefficients? Biometrics 56:915–921

Greenland S (2001) Putting background information about relative risks into conjugate prior distributions. Biometrics 57:663–70

Greenland S (2003a) The impact of prior distributions for uncontrolled confounding and response bias: A case study of the relation of wire codes and magnetic fields towards childhood leukemia. J Am Stat Assoc 98:47–54

Greenland S (2003b) Generalized conjugate priors for Bayesian analysis of risk and survival regressions. Biometrics 59:92–99

Greenland S, Christensen R (2001) Data augmentation priors for Bayesian and semi-Bayes analyses of conditional-logistic and proportional-hazards regression. Stat Med 20:2421–2428

Greenland S, Maldonado G (1994) The interpretation of multiplicative-model parameters as standardized parameters. Stat Med 13:989–999

Greenland S, Schlesselman JJ, Criqui MH (1986) The fallacy of employing standardized regression coefficients and correlations as measures of effect. Am J Epidemiol 123:203–208

Greenland S, Maclure M, Schlesselman JJ, Poole C, Morgenstern H (1991) Standardized regression coefficients: a further critique and review of some alternatives. Epidemiology 2:387–392

Greenland S, Schwarthaum JA, Finkle WD (2000) Problems from small samples and sparse data in conditional logistic regression. Am J Epidemiol 151:531–539

Hastie T, Tibshirani R (1990) Generalized additive models. Chapman and Hall, New York

Hastie T, Tibshirani R, Friedman J (2001) The elements of statistical learning. Springer, New York

Hosmer DW, Lemeshow S (2000) Applied logistic regression, 2nd edn. Wiley, New York

Hosmer DW, Hosmer T, Le Cessie S, Lemeshow S (1997) A comparison of goodness-of-fit tests for the logistic regression model. Stat Med 16:965–980

Hurvich DM, Tsai CL (1990) The impact of model selection on inference in linear regression. Am Statist 44:214–217

Lagakos SW (1988) Effects of mismodelling and mismeasuring explanatory variables on tests of their association with a response variable. Stat Med 7:257–274

Lash TL, Fink AK (2003) Semi-automated sensitivity analysis to assess systematic errors in observational data. Epidemiology 14:451–458

Le Cessie S, van Houwelingen HC (1992) Ridge estimators in logistic regression. Appl Stat 41:191–201

Leamer EE (1978) Specification searches: Ad hoc interference with nonexperimental data. Wiley, New York

Maclure M (1993) Demonstration of deductive meta-analysis: Ethanol intake and risk of myocardial infarction. Epidemiol Rev 15:328–351

Maclure M, Greenland S (1992) Tests for trend and dose response: Misinterpretations and alternatives. Am J Epidemiol 135:96–104

Maldonado G, Greenland S (1993a) Interpreting model coefficients when the true model form is unknown. Epidemiology 4:310–318

Maldonado G, Greenland S (1993b) Simulation study of confounder-selection strategies. Am J Epidemiol 138:923–936

Maldonado G, Greenland S (1994) A comparison of the performance of model-based confidence intervals when the correct model form is unknown: coverage of asymptotic means. Epidemiology 5:171–182

Mantel N, Haenszel WH (1959) Statistical aspects of the analysis of data from retrospective studies of disease. J Natl Cancer Inst 22:719–748

McCullagh P (1991) Quasi-likelihood and estimating functions. In: Hinkley DV, Reid NM, Snell EJ (eds) Statistical theory and modelling. Chapman and Hall, London, Chap. 11

McCullagh P, Nelder JA (1989) Generalized linear models, 2nd edn. Chapman and Hall, New York

Michels KB, Greenland S, Rosner BA (1998) Does body mass index adequately capture the relation of body composition and body size to health outcomes? Am J Epidemiol 147:167–172

Moolgavkar SH, Venzon DJ (1987) General relative risk regression models for epidemiologic studies. Am J Epidemiol 126:949–961

Pearl J (1995) Causal diagrams for empirical research. Biometrika 82:669–710

Pregibon D (1981) Logistic regression diagnostics. Ann Stat 9:705–724

Robins JM, Greenland S (1986) The role of model selection in causal inference from nonexperimental data. Am J Epidemiol 123:392–402

Robins JM, Greenland S (1994) Adjusting for differential rates of prophylaxis therapy for PCP in high versus low dose AZT treatment arms in an AIDS randomized trial. J Am Stat Assoc 89:737–749

Robins JM, Blevins D, Ritter G, Wulfsohn M (1992) G-estimation of the effect of prophylaxis therapy for Pneumocystis carinii pneumonia on the survival of AIDS patients. Epidemiology 3:319–336. Errata: Epidemiology (1993) 4:189

Robins JM, Greenland S, Hu FC (1999) Estimation of the causal effect of time-varying exposure on the marginal mean of a repeated binary outcome. J Am Stat Assoc 94:687–712

Rosenthal R, Rubin DB (1979) A note on percent variance explained as a measure of importance of effects. J Appl Psychol 9:395–396

Rothman KJ, Greenland S (1998) Modern epidemiology, 2nd edn. Lippincott, Philadelphia

Royston P, Altman DG (1994) Regression using fractional polynomials of continuous covariates: parsimonious parametric modelling (with discussion). Appl Stat 43:425–467

Sclove SL, Morris C, Radhakrishna R (1972) Non-optimality of preliminary-test estimators for the mean of a multivariate normal distribution. Ann Math Stat 43:1481–1490

Sheehe P (1962) Dynamic risk analysis of matched-pair studies of disease. Biometrics 18:323–341

Strömberg U (1996) Collapsing ordered outcome categories: a note of concern. Am J Epidemiol 144:421–424

Titterington DM (1985) Common structure of smoothing techniques in statistics. Int Stat Rev 53:141–170

Walker AM, Rothman KJ (1982) Models of varying parametric form in case-referent studies. Am J Epidemiol 115:129–137

Weiss RE (1995) The influence of variable selection: A Bayesian diagnostic perspective. J Am Stat Assoc 90:619–625

White H (1994) Estimation, inference, and specification analysis. Cambridge University Press, New York

Survival Analysis

II.4

Peter D. Sasieni

Introduction

The term survival analysis originally referred to statistical study of the time to death of a group of individuals. From a mathematical perspective it is irrelevant whether one is studying time until death or time to any other event and so the term has come to be applied to methods for analysing "time to event data". Although often not explicitly stated, we are always interested in the time between two events. For instance one might be studying the age of death (the time from birth until death), survival of cancer patients (the time from diagnosis until death), or the incubation time of a virus (time from infection until the development of symptomatic disease). Survival analysis is more complicated than the analysis of other measurements because one often has only partial information regarding the survival time for some individuals. The most common form of partial information arises when a study is stopped before all participants have died. At that point we might know that Mrs Patel survived for at least 3.7 years, but have no idea whether she will die a week later or 25 years later. The observation on Mrs Patel is said to be (right) censored at 3.7 years.

The goal of a survival analysis might be to describe the survival distribution for a group of individuals. One might wish to present the median age at onset of a particular disease and add that 90% of cases occur before a certain age. More often epidemiologists might be interested in factors that influence survival. In such instances, the aim of survival analysis is to estimate the effect of the factors on survival times.

Occasionally, survival times may vary little between individuals: the vast majority of humans is born at the end of 36 to 42 weeks of gestation. More frequently, survival times can vary hugely: the duration of a detectable viral infection could be anything from a few days to many years. In such circumstances, it is convenient to describe the rate at which the event (clearance of the virus) occurs. Using rates is particularly appealing when the event will never be observed in the majority of individuals being studied. It makes sense to talk about the average rate of breast cancer in a population even though the majority of the population will never get breast cancer. Studying disease rates and the factors that influence them is indeed central to much of epidemiology.

In this chapter we consider three major objectives of survival analysis:
— The description of the survival experience of a group of individuals;
— Comparison of the survival between two or more groups;
— Regression analysis of variables that influence survival.

We describe analyses appropriate for the most common study designs in epidemiology and briefly discuss methods that can be used in more complicated settings. The chapter is intended to give the reader a broad overview of the main techniques in survival analysis and to provide examples of the sorts of epidemiological problems that are amenable to survival analysis. There is now a number of texts on survival analysis written for a non-mathematical audience. Most are written either from the perspective of clinical trials or engineering. The book by Marubini and Valsecchi (1995) is written for a clinical audience and provides detailed worked examples. The book by Breslow and Day (1987) is written specifically for cancer epidemiologists, but focuses on design and analysis of cohort studies rather than specifically on survival analysis. Two recent books on survival analysis written primarily for medical statisticians are Hosmer and Lemshow (1999) and Therneau and Grambsch (2000).

Basic Concepts

4.2

Walking Backwards Through Time

4.2.1

A key feature, perhaps the key feature, of survival analysis, is that it relates to events that occur in time. In Western cultures, we tend to think in terms of looking forward into the future or backwards into the past. When thinking about survival analysis it is useful to have the opposite picture. Imagine that you are walking backwards through time so that the past is in front of you. You can look down to see things in the present and up to view things in the distant past. In order to look into the future you would need to turn your head around, which is impossible. Rather the future is revealed as you walk backwards into it. Recalling that survival analysis is the study of the time from an initiating event to a terminating event, this picture of time is useful for deciding what is an acceptable definition of an event. For instance, clinicians are fond of defining a patient as being in remission if he has been free of symptoms for a certain number of months (3 say). This is fine. What is not permissible from a probabilistic perspective is to then claim that remission started at the beginning of the three-month period. As we walk backwards through time we need to be able to see whether or not a patient is in remission without turning around to look into the future. The difficulty is that if someone has been symptom free for two months we don't know whether or not he is in remission – that depends on what happens in the future.

Another example, this time of a poorly defined initiating event is given by the duration of pregnancy. It is impossible to be just one week pregnant! Since the duration of pregnancy is measured from a woman's last period but conception cannot occur until after ovulation (which is generally about 14 days after the previous period), one day after conception a woman is said to be 15 days pregnant.

Describing and Estimating the Distribution of Survival Times

4.2.2

In her first year, a gynaeco-oncologist treated eight women with newly diagnosed cervical cancer. One died within six months, two more died over the next three years, and one died from a stroke four years later. Six years after she started, four of the patients were still alive. How should one summarise the survival times of the eight patients? Even with 800 patients and 20 years of follow-up the problem is not trivial and there is no optimal solution. In this section we assume that survival times are observed exactly and consider various ways of describing the variety of those times. More details on these topics can be found in any book on survival analysis. Although some of this material may seem to be rather abstract and of little direct relevance to epidemiologists it is necessary to have a rudimentary understanding of the different concepts in order to be able to critically assess studies analysed using survival methods.

Kaplan–Meier Estimator

There are several equivalent ways of describing a distribution. Outside of survival analysis, one might define the distribution through its density or distribution function, or choose to describe only certain features such as the mean and variance. With time to event data, it is more usual to define the distribution in terms of either the *survival function* $S(t)$ or the *hazard* or event rate function $\lambda(t)$. If T is the random survival time, then the survival function is the probability that an event did not occur before t, i.e. T is greater or equal to t, and the hazard function is the probability of an event occurring in a small unit of time just after t, given that it has not yet happened by t. In symbols,

$$S(t) = \Pr(T \geq t) \quad \text{and} \quad \lambda(t) = \Pr(T < t + \Delta | T \geq t)/\Delta \quad \text{for small } \Delta .$$

They are related through the equation $S(t) = \exp\{-\Lambda(t)\}$, where $\Lambda(t)$ is the *cumulative hazard* defined as the integral of λ from 0 to t. There is another formula that is used when estimating the survival function. Note that the probability of an event not occurring by time t is the product of the probability of it not occurring by time s (less than t) times the probability of the event not occurring between times s and t given that it has not occurred by time s. If s is close to t, we can approximate the probability of an event occurring between s and t given that it has not occurred before s by $\lambda(s)(t - s)$ or by $\{\Lambda(t) - \Lambda(s)\}$. In symbols we have $S(t)$ is approximately $S(s)\{1 - [\Lambda(t) - \Lambda(s)]\}$ for $s < t$. More generally, for a series of times $0 = s_0 < s_1 < \ldots < s_n = t$, the survival function at t is given by the product of the probability that the event does not occur in the interval s_{i-1} to s_i given that it did not occur prior to s_{i-1}:

$$S(t) = \prod_{i=1}^{n} \{1 - [\Lambda(s_i) - \Lambda(s_{i-1})]\} .$$

This formula leads naturally to the definition of the product limit or Kaplan–Meier (1958) estimator of the survival function (see also Example 9).

Let $t_1 < t_2 < \ldots < t_n$ be distinct ordered event times observed in a cohort. Let d_j be the number of events at t_j, and n_j the number in the cohort "at risk" of having an event observed at t_j. Then d_j/n_j will be a rough estimate of the probability of an event between t_{j-1} and t_j amongst those at risk at t_{j-1}. When the event of interest is death, once an individual has had an event he is no longer at risk for further events. Similarly if an individual is only followed for two-years, he is not at risk for an *observed* event beyond two-years. More formally, the cumulative hazard between t_{j-1} and t_j is estimated by d_j/n_j, and $(n_j - d_j)/n_j$ estimates the probability of an individual at risk at t_{j-1} not dying by t_j. The Kaplan–Meier estimate of $S(t)$ is then the product over all t_j less than or equal to t of $(n_j - d_j)/n_j$. So, in particular, the estimate at t_j is given by $(n_j - d_j)/n_j$ times the estimate at t_{j-1}.

Censoring and Late-Entry

One of the advantages of working in terms of the hazard function is that it can easily be estimated even in the presence of *right-censored* data (provided the censoring is independent of the event of interest). Right-censoring is the term used to describe the situation in which some individuals are known to have survived for a particular length of time, but it is unknown when beyond that time they died (or will die). Formally, we can consider a death time and a censoring time for each individual. We observe only the smaller of the two times and the knowledge of which came first. In order to be able to interpret analyses of censored data one usually needs to assume that the censoring time imparts no information regarding the timing of the event of interest other than the fact that the event of interest had not happened by the censoring time. Censoring individuals because they become too ill to attend follow-up clinic, for instance, would create problems because censored individuals will probably have greater mortality in the short-term than uncensored individuals.

An extreme example of censoring is given by the study of disease incidence from a disease registry. The annual hazard or incidence rate is estimated by the number of events during the year divided by the number of individuals (half way through the year) at risk of getting the disease. Ideally, the incidence rate should be calculated for a cohort identified at the beginning of the year, but this is rarely done by population registries. By using the number at risk, one is able to deal not only with individuals who die without getting the disease, but also those healthy individuals who immigrate into the area covered by the disease registry. The latter are termed *left-truncated* individuals because it is assumed that had they got the disease before immigrating they would never have been recorded in the registry.

In the presence of censoring, or when not everyone will experience the second event, the mean survival time may be impossible to estimate. Instead it is useful to quote either certain percentiles of the survival distribution such as the median survival time, or the value of the survival function at certain fixed times: one- and five-year survival are popular choices in some fields such as in the survival of cancer patients.

Describing Registry Data – Standardised Rates   4.2.3

Since the rates of many diseases are highly age-dependent, it may be misleading to compare the crude disease rates in two populations. For comparison purposes it is necessary to make some adjustment for the age-distribution in the two populations. The traditional approach to comparing data from two disease registries is to use *age-standardised rates* (cf. Chap. I.3 of this handbook). That is, one uses a weighted average of the age-specific rates λ_i, with weights chosen to be proportional to the numbers p_{0i} in each age group in a standard population. This estimate $(\sum \lambda_i p_{0i} / \sum p_{0i})$ is known as the *directly standardised* rate. Indirect standardisation is introduced in Sect. 4.3.1. Two frequently quoted reference populations are the "world standard population" and the "European standard population". Another approach is to use the cumulative rate up to some age such as 74 (Day 1976). This has the advantage of dispensing with the selection of a standard population and it is straightforward to convert from the cumulative rate to the cumulative risk. If the cumulative rate is 1 in x, then, to a very close approximation, the cumulative risk is 1 in $x + 0.5$. A third, less used, approach is to take a weighted sum of the age-specific rates using standard weights (corresponding to the probability of living to that age) so that the cumulative rate has the interpretation of the lifetime risk in a population with standard mortality rates (Sasieni and Adams 1999).

Example 1. *Comparing rates of cervical cancer*

Table 4.1 extracted from Sasieni and Adams (1999) compares three measures of cervical cancer rates from various cancer registries for the years 1982–1989. The lifetime risk is calculated using all cause mortality rates from England and Wales in 1992 as the standard. It is seen that the numerical difference between the various measures is not great, but the lifetime risk has perhaps the most natural interpretation.

The age-standardised rate is an average rate for the population. It will not correspond to the crude rate unless the age-distribution of the population is identical to that of the standard population. The cumulative rate to age 74 is more easily interpreted, but most people will think of it as a probability and this is not quite correct – the difference will be particularly great when the cumulative rate is large (or in the presence of competing risks – see Sect. 4.4). The lifetime risk can be directly interpreted as the probability of being diagnosed with cervix cancer. It uses the hazard of all cause mortality from a standard population and assumes that cervical cancer incidence rates are independent of mortality rates from other causes (see competing risks).   ◆

4.2.4   Exponential Distribution

In many applications in epidemiology, it is reasonable to assume that the hazard function is constant over short intervals. The number of person-years at risk in an interval is calculated by adding up the length of time that each individual was at risk within the interval. For instance, cancer incidence data are often given in five-year age-bands, or survival data might be given in terms of the number of whole

Table 4.1. Cervical cancer rates in various populations around the world

	Age-standardised rate per 1000 (World standard)	Cumulative rate (from birth) to age 74 per 1000	Lifetime risk per 1000
Cali, Columbia	49	50	71
Trujilli, Peru	55	58	77
USA (SEER)			
White	7	7	8
Black	12	12	15
Israel			
Jews	4	4	5
Non-Jews	3	3	3
Denmark	16	16	17
Finland	4	5	6
England and Wales	12	12	13
New Zealand			
Maori	30	31	34
Non-Maori	12	12	13

years from diagnosis. The family of distributions with a constant hazard rate is known as the *exponential distribution* and a distribution with a hazard function that is constant on intervals is known as a piecewise constant exponential distribution. The likelihood for such piecewise exponential models can be written quite simply and should be the basis for statistical analysis. If one has a large number of individuals all of whom are at risk in an interval with a constant hazard λ per year, then the likelihood looks like a Poisson likelihood: the number of events observed will (to a close approximation) follow a Poisson distribution with mean λn, where n is the number of person years at risk in the interval. The approximation will be good provided the number of individuals at risk in the interval is at least 10 times λn.

Cohort Studies 4.3

In cohort studies, one typically follows a group of individuals and records the incidence of various diseases and death (cf. Chap. I.5 of this handbook). These are often studied as a function of the age of the individuals. Here we consider three statistical problems related to studies with such a design. The first is to compare the cohort to the general public. The second is to compare two or more groups within the cohort. Finally, we consider how to take account of various factors in a regression model. All these approaches assume the existence of standard rates that can be used to calibrate the exposure in the study cohort. In many countries there are good population-based records on disease incidence rates and cause-specific mortality rates as a function of age.

4.3.1   Standardised Mortality Ratio

The method of expected number of deaths has a history of over 200 years (Keiding 1987) having first been described by English actuaries in the 1780s. Groups are defined by age and sex and possibly the year of risk. For each group i, let λ_{0i} and p_{0i} denote the mortality rate and the number of person-years at risk in the reference population and λ_i and p_i be the corresponding quantities in the study cohort. The standardised mortality ratio (SMR) is defined as SMR = $\sum \lambda_i p_i / \sum \lambda_{0i} p_i$ and is equal to observed number of deaths in the study cohort divided by the expected number under the assumption that the reference population rates apply (cf. Chap. I.3 of this handbook). Corresponding to the SMR, the indirectly standardised rate is the SMR times the standardised rate in the reference population: SMR $* \sum \lambda_{0i} p_{0i} / \sum p_{0i}$. Please note that the reference population does not serve as a "standard" population for the calculation of an SMR, i.e. for the indirect standardisation. Rather, the mortality rate of the reference population is standardised by the age distribution of the study cohort. This should be contrasted with the directly standardised rate: $\sum \lambda_i p_{0i} / \sum p_{0i}$. The latter is more widely used when the study cohort is very large, but requires reasonable estimates of all the individual λ_i and should be avoided unless all the p_i are reasonably large.

Example 2.   *Cohort of individual exposed to medicinal arsenic (1)*
            A cohort of 478 patients treated with Fowler's solution (potassium arsenite) between 1945 and 1965 were followed until the end of 1990 during which period 188 patients died (Cuzick et al. 1992). Completeness of follow-up was achieved through flagging the cohort with the national population register. Cause of death was determined from the death certificates. A comparison was made between the observed number of deaths from various causes (before the age of 85) and the expected number using age-, sex and calendar year-adjusted rates from England and Wales. Treating the cohort as a whole, SMRs were calculated for various causes of death (Table 4.2). There was a slight (and non-significant) deficit of death overall (suggesting that the cohort is slightly healthier than the population as a whole). The observed number of five deaths from bladder cancer was three times greater than expected and represented a significant increase compared to the general population.   ◆

4.3.2   Conditional Inference Within a Cohort

In cohort studies one often wants to compare the number of events in two groups within a cohort. This is done by considering the observed number of events and the "expected" number of events in each group. The expected number is calculated

Table 4.2. Mortality in a cohort of 478 individuals exposed to medicinal arsenic. SMR = standardised mortality ratio. CI = confidence interval

	Observed number	Expected number	SMR	95% CI
All Causes	188	209.1	0.90	0.77–1.03
All cancers	47	49.3	0.95	0.70–1.3
All circulatory diseases	97	106.5	0.91	0.74–1.1
Bladder cancer	5	1.6	3.07	1.01–7.3

as in the SMR by $\sum \lambda_{0i} p_i$. Statistical inference is usually based on the assumption of proportional hazards. That is, it is assumed that in each group $\lambda_i = k\lambda_{0i}$ for all i. Suppose the observed and expected number of events are O_1 and E_1 in group 1, and O_2 and E_2 in group 2, respectively. Then, under the null hypothesis of equal proportional hazards in the two groups, O_1 is distributed as a binomial sample from a population of size $O_1 + O_2$ with probability of $E_1/(E_1 + E_2)$. Hence in particular, under the assumption of proportional hazards within each group, the null hypothesis of no difference between the groups can be tested using an exact binomial test.

Example 3. *Cohort of individual exposed to medicinal arsenic (2)*
　　　　Of the five bladder cancer deaths, four were in individuals with a cumulative dose of over 500 mg. The expected numbers were 0.83 for those exposed to less than 500 mg and 0.80 for those exposed to over 500 mg. Thus to test whether the risk was greater at the higher dose, one calculates the binomial probability of four or more "successes" out of five with a probability of 0.49 ($= 0.80/(0.80 + 0.83)$) each. The binomial probability is 0.18. Hence although the tendency was for the individuals who died from bladder cancer to have been exposed to a greater dose of arsenic, the association was not statistically significant. ◆

Regression Models for Rare Events   4.3.3

Regression models are important when there are several factors upon which the disease rates may depend. For a general introduction of regression models see Chap. II.3 of this handbook. The popular log-linear or Poisson regression model assumes that the observed number of events follows a Poisson distribution with a particular mean given by the number of person-years at risk multiplied by the modelled disease rates. For mathematical simplicity, the usual regression model is multiplicative, i.e., it is assumed that the logarithm of the hazard follows a linear regression model: $\ln(\lambda_i) = \sum_j x_{ij}\beta_j$. Such models can be fit in many software packages. The observed numbers of events, O_i, are the values of the outcome variable, the x_{ij}'s are the covariate values, and the logarithms of person-years at risk p_i are given as offsets – their regression coefficient is forced to be one. In symbols: $E(O_i) = \exp\{\ln(p_i) + \sum_j x_{ij}\beta_j\}$.

In practice, it is often the case that the Poisson assumption is not appropriate. For whatever reasons, mortality and disease registry data often show greater variability than implied by the Poisson model. Various sophisticated solutions to the problem of "extra-Poisson variation" have been put forwarded, but simple solutions usually suffice. One approach assumes that the variance of O_i is directly proportional to (but not necessarily equal to) the expected value of O_i. Under that assumption, one can estimate the dispersion factor (the coefficient of proportionality), by dividing the Pearson chi-squared statistic for the "saturated model" (that is the model with the most terms in it, or the one including all the explanatory variables) by the number of degrees of freedom (McCullagh and Nelder 1989). Inference proceeds by multiplying the model based standard errors by the dispersion factor. Although this quasi-likelihood approach often works well, it lacks a sound theoretical justification and in practice it may be difficult to define the saturated model. Another simple approach to dealing with extra-Poisson variation is to use the sandwich estimator of the variance instead of the model-based estimator (Huber 1967). The sandwich estimator, also known as the Huber estimator or even the robust estimator, is available in many statistical packages and provides valid asymptotic inference no matter what the true variance model (hence the name robust), provided the mean model is correct.

The basic observation for Poisson regression consists of numbers of events and numbers of person years at risk together with a number of covariates. An observation could relate to a single individual (in which case the number of events would usually be 0 or 1) or it could be the sum of the observations from a number of individuals with common covariate values.

Example 4.   *Age, period cohort modelling of cervical cancer rates*
Cervical cancer mortality rates changed considerably during the second half of the 20th century. It is well known that the rates vary with age, being essentially zero until the age of 20 then increasing slowly at first and rapidly in the 30s before reaching a plateau at about age 55. One explanation for the changing rates of cervical cancer over time is the cohort effect, whereby women's exposure to the human papillomavirus during their teens and 20s largely determines their risk of cervical cancer throughout the rest of their lives. Thus cervical cancer rates may be seen to vary as a function of the year of birth. Additionally changes in calendar time may affect the mortality rate from cervical cancer regardless of a woman's underlying risk of the disease. For example, improvements in treatment might reduce the mortality from cervical cancer at all ages. Here we estimate the age and birth-cohort effects and investigate the secular trends that may be attributed to screening using data from England and Wales (Sasieni and Adams 2000). Since screening is only offered to women aged 20–64, it will have had little effect on mortality in older women except possibly in recent times in which older women may have been screened several years earlier whilst still aged under 65 (cf. Chap. III.10 of this handbook).

The model that we used was:

$$\ln(\text{rate}) = f_1(\text{age}) + f_2(\text{cohort}) + f_{3a}(\text{year if age 20–49})$$

$$+ f_{3b}(\text{year if age 50–69}) + f_{3c}(\text{age if age 70+}).$$

Here the f's are functions that we estimate using cubic splines (f_1 and f_2) or step-functions (f_{3a}, f_{3b}, and f_{3c}). Estimates of these functions are plotted in Fig. 4.1. Results summarising the goodness of fit of this model compared to various sub-models are given in Table 4.3. The scaled deviance is the deviance divided by the dispersion factor from the full model. The dispersion factor is the Pearson chi-squared statistic divided by the degrees of freedom.

The model of a constant rate at all ages and at all times gives a hopelessly bad fit with a scaled deviance of over 40,000 on 671 degrees of freedom. Over 80% of the deviance can be explained simply by allowing the rates to vary with age, but the model still does not fit the data well. Nearly 80% of the remaining deviance (all but 1194 of 5789) can be explained by allowing the age-standardised rate to

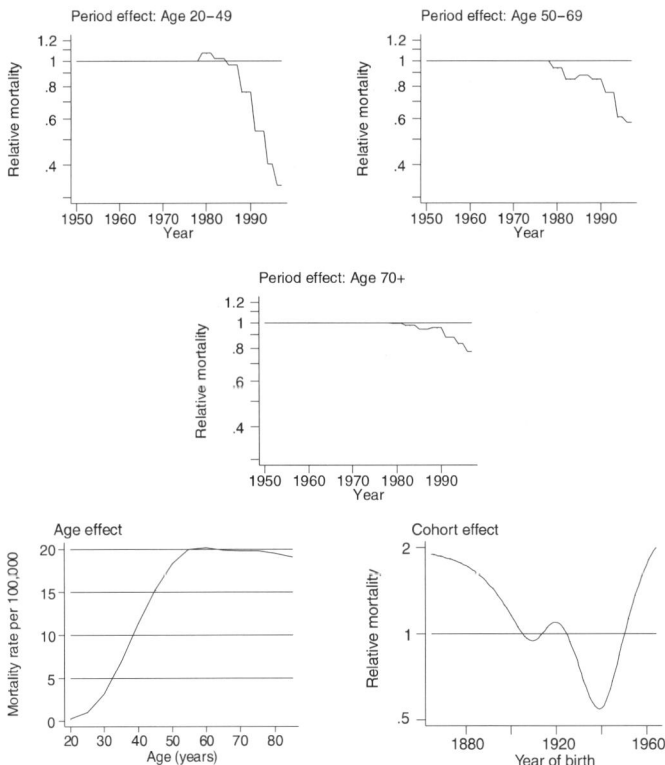

Figure 4.1. Age, cohort and age-specific period effects for cervical cancer mortality. The age effect is given as the absolute rate for a cohort born in 1905, the cohort and period effects are expressed as relative risks

Table 4.3. Age-period cohort modelling of cervical cancer mortality data from England and Wales

Model	Scaled deviance	Degrees of freedom	Chi-square/df	Change in sc. deviance	Change in df
Null	41,288	671	95.66		
f_1(age)	5789	665	14.71	35,499	6
f_1(age) + f_3(period)	2629	658	7.02	3160	7
f_1(age) + f_2(cohort)	1194	656	3.10	4595	9
f_1(age) + f_2(cohort) + f_3(period)	880	649	2.32	314	7
Full	648	635	1.74	232	14

vary with birth cohort; and adding a main effect for period (year of death) leads only to a more modest improvement in the fit. The full model, with interactions between age and period, provides further improvements in the fit suggesting that the dominant factors are age and year of birth, but that there have been significant changes over time and that these have not been the same across age groups. The usual explanation for these age-specific period effects is the widespread use of screening in women age 20–64 from the mid 1980s (see Sasieni and Adams 1999). Finally, note that even the "full" model (with 36 explanatory variables) still had considerable extra-Poisson variation – the dispersion factor was 1.74.   ◆

Example 5. *Converting survival data into Poisson regression data*
          A common problem is converting data on individuals including date of entry into the study, date of birth, date of exit and reason for exit (cause specific death or censoring) into data suitable for Poisson regression: length of time at risk and number of events in a number of risk groups. The situation can best be illustrated using a Lexis diagram (Keiding 1990; Chap. I.3 of this handbook). The horizontal axis is calendar time, the vertical axis is age and individuals in the study can be represented by diagonal lines with slope 1. For instance, an individual could enter a study at age 62.5 in May 1986 and be followed until death in August 1997. Suppose population mortality rates are available in five-year age bands (60–64, 65–69, 70–74, 75–79) for each calendar year. Then the individual's contributions to the various age-groups and calendar years are as given in Table 4.4 (see also Fig. 4.2).
          The conversion of individual data to age and calendar-year data is often referred to as person-years analysis and is fundamental to the analysis of large cohort studies. Programs exist in many software packages to facilitate the conversion of individual level data (one record per person) to a format with a separate record for each individual in each risk stratum.   ◆

Example 6. *Estimating the expected number of cancer deaths in an initially cancer free cohort*
In most applications of the person-years method, it is simply a case of multiplying the number of years at risk by the population risk (mortality rate of a particular disease) and adding these to get an expected number of events (disease-specific

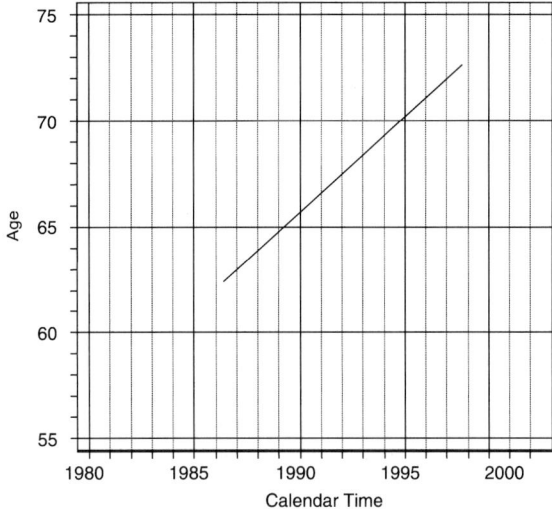

Figure 4.2. Lexis diagram illustrating the experience of one patient

Table 4.4. Example of how an individual is present in a number age-period strata

Age group	Calendar year	Months at risk	Events
60–64	1986	7.5	0
60–64	1987	12	0
60–64	1988	10.5	0
65–69	1988	1.5	0
65–69	1989	12	0
65–69	1990	12	0
65–69	1991	12	0
65–69	1992	12	0
65–69	1993	10.5	0
70–74	1993	1.5	0
70–74	1994	12	0
70–74	1995	12	0
70–74	1996	12	0
70–74	1997	7.5	1

deaths). Such estimates often overestimate the true mortality in a given study cohort because of what is known as "the healthy worker effect". Cohorts of individuals working in a particular occupation will often have low mortality rates for the first few years of follow-up simply because if they are working then they are probably healthy. A particular problem arises in cancer screening studies in which one excludes anyone who already has cancer from the study. For such a cohort it is not appropriate to simply apply the cancer specific mortality rates because individuals are all cancer-free at entry. Instead one should explicitly model the probability of first getting cancer (using population incidence rates) and then dying from cancer (using cancer survival rates). Explicit formulae are given in Sasieni et al. (2002).

♦

4.3.4   Life-Tables

We have seen that a survival function can be estimated by the product-limit or Kaplan–Meier estimate. Such an approach is standard for small and moderate cohorts. For larger cohorts, it is more usual to estimate the hazard for a year at a time and to use the hazard function to estimate survival. Sometimes people calculate the person years at risk in a given time-period exactly and then use that as the denominator for calculating the rate. Often however, the person-years at risk is approximated by multiplying the length of the interval by the mean of the number of people at risk at the beginning of the interval and the number at risk at the end of the interval. Formally one is assuming that on average anyone who "drops out" or "enters" during the interval will have been at risk for half of the interval. Dividing the number of events in an interval by this estimate of the person-years leads to the life-table estimate of survival. The probability of surviving a long period is computed by multiplying the conditional probabilities of surviving each of the intervals constituting it. Suppose the conditional probabilities have been estimated in intervals of width one and that we wish to estimate the survival at time t such that j is the largest interval that is less that or equal to t. Then the $S(t)$ is estimated by the product of $(1 - p_i)$ for $i < j$ multiplied by $(1 - p_j)^{t-j}$. This method has an extremely long history being first devised in the seventeenth century by Edmund Halley to describe the mortality of the people of Breslau (Halley 1693). The probabilities p_i are calculated by the formula $d_i/(n_i - c_i/2)$ where n_i is the number at risk at the start of the i'th interval, d_i is the number dying and c_i is the number censoring during i'th interval.

Whereas in clinical studies, it would be standard to base life tables on a group of patients followed from diagnosis to death, actuarial life tables are not constructed by observing a cohort of newborns until the last survivor dies. Rather they are based on estimates of probabilities of death, given survival to various ages, derived from the mortality experienced by the entire population over a few consecutive years. In that case there is little point in noting the numbers censored in each interval, rather one needs to keep track of the size of the risk set. The following fictitious example is provided to show the calculations involved (Table 4.5). Initially 2456 patients are followed. In the first year 543 (22%) die leaving 1913 patients at the beginning of the second year. In the second year 265 patients die and 22 are censored. In the third year 934 new patients enter the study. (This could be due to transfer from another hospital and we assume that there is no information on the numbers treated from diagnosis in that hospital, but that 934 who were diagnosed between 2 and 3 years earlier were transferred). The conditional probability

Table 4.5. Fictitious life table

Years from diagnosis	No. at start of interval	No. censored	No. new patients in interval	Deaths	Conditional probability of death	Cumulative probability of survival
j	n_j	c_j		d_j	p_j	S_j
0	2456	0	0	543	0.2211	1.0000
1	1913	22	0	265	0.1393	0.7789
2	1626	130	934	302	0.1489	0.6704
3	2128	219	0	321	0.1590	0.5706
4	1588	336	971	317	0.1664	0.4798
5	1906	447	0	278	0.1652	0.4000

of dying in the third year is calculated as $302/(1626 - 130/2 + 934/2) = 0.1489$. Thus the estimated probability of surviving until the beginning of year four is $(1 - 0.2211) * (1 - 0.1393) * (1 - 0.1489) = 0.5706$.

Estimating Survival from Population Registries 4.3.5

There is an issue as to what parts of the Lexis diagram should be used when estimating survival from population registries. In order to estimate the survival curve of colorectal cancer patients for 20 years ($S(t)$, $t \leq 20$), one might consider three approaches (see Fig. 4.3).

1. *Pooled*. Estimate the survival using the Kaplan–Meier or life-table approach using all patients who have been diagnosed with colorectal cancer over the last 20 years.
2. *Cohort*. Estimate the survival function from the cohort of patients diagnosed 20 years ago.
3. *Period*. Estimate the survival function from patients dying in a particular (recent) period. Specifically, estimate the hazard function x years from diagnosis using all patients diagnosed x years ago. Calculate the survival function from the estimated hazard function.

Approach 1 uses all available data, but if survival has improved over calendar time, the survival function will have been estimated from a mixture of patients given old and new treatments. Approach 2 has the clearest interpretation since it describes the survival experience of a particular cohort. However, using it to estimate 5-year survival will yield outdated estimates if survival has changed over the 20-years since members of the cohort were diagnosed. Approach 3 will in many circumstances provide the best prediction of the current survival experience without explicitly modelling changes in survival over time (year of diagnosis). It is possible that the estimated survival might be inappropriate, if for instance a new treatment increases the hazard of dying in the first year, but increases the proportion cured of the disease. More often the use of the most recent data to estimate the relevant hazard will mean that approach 3 will be favoured. The period

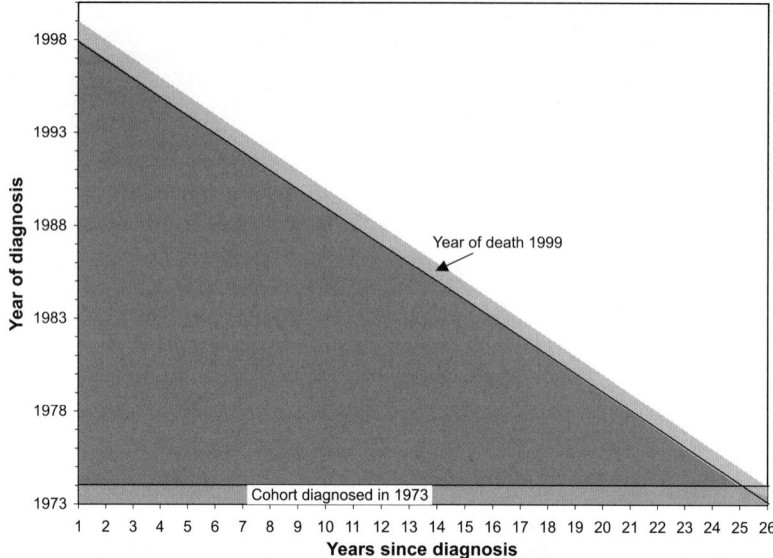

Figure 4.3. Survival experience contributing to the pooled, cohort and period estimates of survival. To estimate the survival curve up to 26 years based on follow-up until the end of 1999, one could pool all events in the *shaded part* of the diagram; or one could consider the cohort diagnosed in 1973 who have a full 26 years of follow-up (*gray strip* along the *bottom* of the diagram); or one could use the deaths from a recent period, such as all deaths in 1999 (represented by the *light-gray diagonal strip*)

method has always been favoured by demographers. It was explicitly introduced into epidemiology by Brenner and Gefeller (1996) and has been used by Brenner (2002) and by Sasieni et al. (2002) to study the long-term survival of cancer patients. Applying the period approach to data from the United States of America, Brenner (2002) estimated the 20-year relative survival for all types of cancer to be 51% compared to 40% using the cohort-based survival. The difference reflects the substantial improvement in survival over the past two decades.

4.4   # Competing Risks

In previous sections, we have assumed that there is only a single, possibly censored, event of interest. In practice study participants might die of a variety of causes or become lost to follow-up and the assumption of independent censoring may be unrealistic. When looking at cause-specific mortality one needs to think carefully about the interaction between different causes of death. The interaction may be structural as in the case when one considers the effect of coding rules on the mortality rates from pneumonia (immediate cause) and cancer (underlying cause), or on cancer of the uterus (site not otherwise specified) and cancer of the cervix uterus. In these examples an increase in one may be linked to a decrease in the other. In other examples certain causes of death will be related due to a common underlying risk factor. Smokers are at substantially increased risk of lung cancer, cardiovascular disease and respiratory disease, but at slightly reduced risk of endometrial cancer. Similarly, obesity can lead to death from a variety of causes. Despite these examples, many researchers treat different causes of death as if they are independent; they concentrate on a particular cause of death and treat all other deaths as independent censoring events. Such an approach is particularly tempting when one is interested in an event other than death: in estimating the age at natural menopause one would probably treat death as an independent source of censoring. In general however the assumption of independence may not hold and it is meaningless to ask what would happen in the absence of all other causes of death. The key is to concentrate on observable quantities and not to make unsubstantiated guesses at what might happen in the absence of a particular cause.

In many examples the issue of competing risks is at most of theoretical importance, but there are other situations in which it is impossible to ignore. The classic example is a three state model in which patients start in remission and can either relapse or die whilst in remission (Fig. 4.4). One would certainly not wish to consider death as a source of independent censoring. Kalbfleisch and Prentice (2002) identify three distinct problems in the analysis of competing risks data:

1. The estimation of the dependence of the rate of cause-specific death on a set of covariates.
2. The study of the relationship between different causes of death.
3. The estimation of mortality rates given the "removal" of competing risks.

Problem 3 is not really statistical. The solution will depend on the model, which in turn will depend on ones knowledge of the underlying biology. In general it is difficult if not impossible to conjecture about what might happen in the absence of a competing risk.

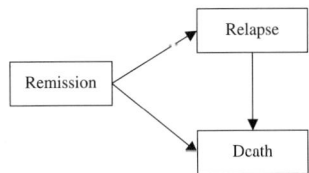

Figure 4.4. Three state model

Whenever it is not possible to ignore the competing risk problem, it is usual to estimate the cause-specific hazard and from that the *crude cause-specific cumulative incidence.* Suppose individuals can die from one of K causes and that in addition follow-up may be censored. We assume that the censoring is independent of mortality. The observed data on the i'th individual consist of a survival time T_i and a cause indicator L_i with $L_i = 0$ if T_i is a censoring time. For cause

$l \in \{0, 1, ..., K\}$, define the cause-specific hazard λ_l as one over Δ times the conditional probability of dying from cause l in the small interval between t and $t + \Delta$ conditional on surviving until time t: $\lambda_l = \Pr\{T < t + \Delta, L = l | T \geq t\}/\Delta$. The all-cause survival function S is defined in the usual way. The crude cumulative incidence function I_l for failures of type l is the probability that an individual will die from cause l (despite the possibility of dying from other causes) by time t: $I_l(t) = \Pr\{T < t, L = l\}$. Let $\widehat{S}$ denote the Kaplan–Meier estimator and d_{lj} and n_j the number of deaths of type l, and the number at risk at time T_j, respectively. Note that $\widehat{S}(T_{j-1})d_{lj}/n_j$ estimates probability of being alive at T_j times the conditional probability of dying from cause l between T_j and T_{j+1} given survival until T_j. Thus $I_l(t)$ can be estimated by $\sum_{\{j:T_j<t\}} \widehat{S}(T_{j-1})d_{lj}/n_j$.

Consider the problem of survival in patients with a particular form of cancer (breast cancer, for example). One could consider all cause-mortality, but that would dilute treatment effects by including death from causes that are not related to the cancer of interest. The temptation then is to consider deaths from breast cancer, but that could give misleading results – for instance, meta-analysis of the early trials of radiotherapy and breast cancer showed that women treated with radiotherapy had lower rates of death from breast cancer, but higher rates of death from cardiovascular disease (Cuzick et al. 1994). Later analyses showed that radiotherapy (particularly of the left breast) caused damage to the major blood vessels surrounding the heart.

A popular approach in epidemiology is to consider the excess hazard or correspondingly the relative survival function. Given a standard hazard λ_0 from a reference population, the excess hazard λ_e is the difference between the observed hazard λ and the standard hazard: $\lambda_e = \lambda - \lambda_0$. Similarly the relative survival function S_r is defined as $S_r = S/S_0$, where S_0 is the survival function from the reference population. It is useful to contrast the relative survival for patients with a particular type of cancer to the cause-specific survival. If the cause of death is well determined, one might expect the two quantities to be similar. The cause-specific survival (i.e., the survival treating death from other causes as independent censoring) might be bigger than the relative survival if patients who die *with* cancer are incorrectly recorded as having died *from* cancer. Differences will also exist if the population is heterogeneous and those who get (and survive) cancer are not representative of the whole population. For instance, breast cancer patients (particularly those that survive) tend to be of higher social class and therefore have lower rates of mortality from other causes; by contrast, lung cancer patients tend to be smokers and have higher rates of mortality form other causes.

Example 7.   *Relative survival*

Ederer et al. (1961) proposed two methods of describing the relative survival of a group of cancer patients to that of a standard population. The idea is to divide the observed survival (as estimated by the Kaplan–Meier estimate) in one group of patients by their expected survival based on the experience of a reference group. A key question is how to estimate the expected survival. The Ederer I method simply uses the mean expected survival function: $S_e(t) = \sum_{\{i=1,\ldots,n\}} S_i(t)/n$. Here the mean is calculated based on all individuals in the cohort and does not take into account the different make-up of the cohort as individuals die (or are censored). By contrast the Ederer II method takes the average hazard among those still at risk and converts that to a survival function (via the formula $S(t) = \exp[-\Lambda(t)]$). The expected or conditional cumulative hazard function is estimated by

$$\Lambda_c(t) = \int_0^t \left\{ \sum Y_i(s)\lambda_i(s) \Big/ \sum Y_i(s) \right\} \, ds$$

where $\lambda_i(s)$ is the hazard function appropriate for the i'th individual calculated from the reference population and $Y_i(s)$ is an indicator of whether the i'th individual was at risk at time s. In the Ederer II method the survival function does not correspond to the survival of an actual population, but is a measure of the excess risk in a competing-risks model. Suppose the hazard in the study population is equal to the hazard in the reference population plus some excess, then the difference between the observed cumulative hazard and the conditional expected cumulative hazard will be equal to the cumulative excess hazard.

The difference between the two methods can best be illustrated by reference to a group of cancer patients some of whom are aged 40–49 and some of whom are aged 80–89. In the Ederer I method, the 80–89 year old patients will still have an impact on the relative survival after 10 years. In the Ederer II method, the older patients will have less and less impact on the relative survival as they die. So that, if after 6 years, there are no older patients still at risk, the hazards (both observed and expected) for 7–10 years will be based exclusively on the younger patients.

A slight variation on the Ederer II method was proposed by Hakulinen (1982). Instead of using an indicator of whether the i'th individual was still at risk, he suggested using an estimate of whether the i'th individual would still be at risk if she were subject to the survival of the reference population and the censoring from the study. That is $Y_i(s)$ is replaced by $S_i(s)C_i(s)$ where $C_i(s)$ is an indicator of whether the i'th individual would still have been under follow-up at time s. A problem with this approach is that it requires knowledge of the censoring times even of those individuals who are not censored. That is not a real problem if there is no loss to follow-up and the maximal follow-up time for an individual can be calculated, for instance, from their date of entry into the study. An advantage of Hakulinen's method over Ederer II is that the expected survival function can truly be interpreted as a survival function. ◆

Example 8. *Mortality from other causes in cancer patients*

Sasieni et al. (2002) considered the probability of not dying prematurely as a measure of the proportion cured of a particular cancer. They compared (1) the probability of not dying from the excess hazard before dying from background mortality; (2) the probability of not dying from the cause-specific hazard before dying from background mortality; and (3) the probability of not dying from the excess mortality of other causes before dying from background mortality. For breast cancer these three probabilities (given as percentages) were 67%, 76% and 98%, respectively. Thus women with breast cancer are more likely to die of something other than breast cancer than are women without breast cancer, but the excess mortality due to other causes is small. By contrast, the three percentages for women with lung cancer were: 11%, 16% and 60%. So, 84% of women with lung cancer die of it, and 40% of those who don't still die prematurely.   ◆

Comparing Survival Times
4.5   # Between Groups

We have already discussed how to compare the survival experience of different groups after adjusting for their expected mortality. In this section we consider the problem of comparing survival without the use of a reference population. This approach will be most relevant when the mortality of all groups in the study is substantially greater than that of the general population so that one can almost ignore the "background mortality".

A graphical solution is achieved by plotting the estimated survival function (using the Kaplan–Meier or the life table approach) on a common set of axes. Comparison of survival at a fixed time (e.g., 3 years) can be made using Greenwood's formula for the variance of the survival estimate (Greenwood 1926). Greenwood's estimate is widely available in software packages and a formula for calculating the estimated variance can be found in any text on survival analysis. More sophisticated confidence bands, for the whole survival function, have been proposed by Hall and Wellner (1980).

Another useful summary of the survival in each group is the average event rate, which is estimated by dividing the number of events by the total person-years at risk. For instance, 12 deaths in a group of 100 patients who were followed for a total of 482 person-years would yield a rate of 12/482 or 2.5% per year. This simple approach is also amenable to hypothesis testing. Formally one is assuming a constant rate or exponential model and the problem of testing between two groups is equivalent to testing for the equally of rate parameters in an exponential regression model.

The test statistic most often used in medical statistics is a variant of the log-rank test first proposed by Mantel (1966). This is a test that is intended for use with censored survival data (including right-censoring and left-truncation) and which is most powerful when the proportional hazards model holds. The proportional hazards model is that the hazard in each group g is given by $\lambda_g(t) = \theta_g \lambda_0(t)$. In other words the ratio of the hazard functions is constant over time. Readers, who are familiar with the Mantel–Haenszel test for a series of 2×2 tables, might

Table 4.6. 2×2 table formed at time T_j

	Die at T_j	Survive T_j	At risk at T_j
Group 1	d_{1j}	$n_{1j}-d_{1j}$	n_{1j}
Group 2	d_{2j}	$n_{2j}-d_{2j}$	n_{2j}

like to know that the log-rank test for two groups is equivalent to the Mantel–Haenszel test. Consider the situation at each event time. Let d_{ij} be the number of events in group i at time T_j and n_{ij} the number at risk as illustrated in Table 4.6.

Although these 2×2 tables are not independent, they are conditionally independent (given the marginals) and the usual formula for the variance of the Mantel–Haenszel test statistic holds.

In epidemiology, it is often useful to be able to stratify the log-rank test so that a valid test can be obtained after adjusting for some other factor. Formally, the test assumes that within each stratum proportional hazards holds with the same constants of proportionality: $\lambda_{gs}(t) = \theta_g \lambda_{0s}(t)$ for each stratum s and each group g.

Example 9. *Kaplan–Meier estimates and log-rank test in a clinical trial*

This example is based on the "cancer" dataset provided by Stata. There are 48 patients who received one of three different drugs: 31 patients died during follow-up (see Fig. 4.5 and Table 4.7).

The log-rank statistic (which, under the null hypothesis of no differences in effect on survival between the three drugs, is asymptotically distributed as chi-squared with 2 degrees of freedom) was 30.2 ($p < 0.0001$). Just comparing drugs 2

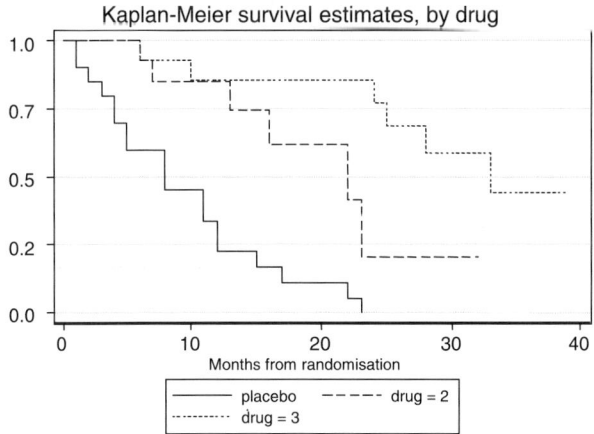

Figure 4.5. Kaplan–Meier estimates of the survival of cancer patients over 3 years. The three estimates correspond to patients on different drugs

Table 4.7. Descriptive survival in the three treatment arms

	Survival at 1 year	Survival at 2 years	Median survival (years)	Mean mortality rate
Placebo ($n = 20$)	0.23	0	0.67	1.27
Drug 2 ($n = 14$)	0.85	0.21	1.83	0.34
Drug 3 ($n = 14$)	0.86	0.77	2.75	0.21

and 3, gave a log-rank of 3.4 (1 df, $p = 0.065$). However, it was noted that older patients fared worse – the log-rank test for age under 55 versus age over 55, stratified for treatment, had $p = 0.007$ – after stratifying on age, the difference between drugs 2 and 3 became more significant ($p = 0.03$). ◆

4.6   Regression Models for Survival Data

We have already discussed the Poisson regression model, which is particularly useful when the mortality in the study population is of the same order of magnitude as that of a standard reference population. When considering a cohort of patients with a life threatening disease, the background rate of mortality is often of little interest. Additionally, when studying events other than death, there may be no reference data available. Two sorts of regression model are useful in these circumstances: ones that model the survival time itself, and ones that model the hazard or rate function.

4.6.1   Accelerated Failure Time Models

Most of the literature applying regression models to a function of the survival time assumes that the regression model is applied to the logarithm of the time. Such models are called "accelerated failure time models" because the effect of a covariate is to multiply the time-scale on which events occur. It is as if the clock is made to run either slower or faster than usual. The simplest accelerated failure time model assumes that the survival times are Exponential random variables, but other parametric models such as Weibull, Gamma, and Log-normal can also be used. For modelling all-cause adult mortality as a function of age, other distributions such as Gompertz or Makeham with hazards increasing exponentially with time are more appropriate. The book by Kalbfleisch and Prentice (2002) provides details of all these parametric distributions. All these regression models can be written as

$$\ln(T) = \beta_0 + \beta_1 Z_1 + \dots + \beta_p Z_p + \varepsilon \, , \tag{4.1}$$

where $Z_1, \ldots, Z_p$ are covariates, $\beta_0, \ldots, \beta_p$ are regression parameters to be estimated, and ε is the random component distributed according to some model. (It should be noted that in this formulation it is not ε but $\exp(\varepsilon)$ that has the named distribution). A semi-parametric variant of this model uses the same formula (4.1), but does not specify a parametric family for the distribution of ε. Parametric accelerated failure time models can be fitted using maximum likelihood estimation in a number of statistical packages. The semi-parametric model requires more advanced algorithms.

When using dummy covariates (i.e., Z_i is equal to 0 or 1), the regression parameters are easily interpreted: $\exp(\beta_i)$ is a multiplicative factor by which the "underlying" survival time is multiplied. If $\exp(\beta_i) = 3$, then on average individuals with $Z_i = 1$ take three times as long as individuals with $Z_i = 0$ to have the event of interest.

The Cox Model 4.6.2

Cox (1972) proposed modelling the conditional hazard as the product of an arbitrary baseline hazard $\lambda_0(t)$ and an exponential form that is linear in the covariates:

$$\lambda(t|Z_1, \ldots, Z_p) = \lambda_0(t) \exp\left(\beta_1 Z_1 + \ldots + \beta_p Z_p\right) . \tag{4.2}$$

The restriction $\lambda_0(t) = \lambda_0$ leads to the exponential regression model (which is also an accelerated failure time model). Such a restriction will not generally be appropriate in epidemiology where the underlying mortality rate will generally be far from constant in time. Taking $\lambda_0(t)$ to be the hazard from a reference population leads to the Poisson regression model (Breslow et al. 1983). Such modelling is particularly useful in epidemiology in which the goal may be to compare the survival of a study population to that of a reference population and to consider variables that affect the relative mortality. Alternatively, Andersen et al. (1985) proposed a Cox-type model for the relative mortality replacing $\lambda_0(t)$ by the product of the individual-specific population mortality at time t, $\lambda_i^*(t)$, and an underlying relative mortality function, $\nu_0(t)$. They applied this model to patients with diabetes mellitus. Such a model may seem reasonable when studying a cohort at increased (or decreased) mortality from a number of causes, but the proportional excess mortality model (see Sect. 4.6.3) may seem more appropriate when the cohort are at particular risk of certain causes of death and when that risk is unrelated to their underlying risk of death from other causes.

In the proportional hazards model, $\lambda_0(t)$ is the hazard for an individual with $Z_i = 0$, $i = 1, \ldots, p$ and the hazard ratio between two individuals is constant over time. If one individual has covariates Z and other has covariates Z^* then their hazard ratio is given by $\lambda_0(t|Z)/\lambda_0(t|Z^*) = \exp\{\beta(Z - Z^*)\}$. Recalling that the hazard is a measure of the instantaneous risk, one can also think of the hazard ratio as the relative risk. Such an approximation will be reasonable as long as the event of interest is rare. Consider a hazard ratio of 2.0, then when the survival in one group is S, the relative risk of death in the other group will be $1 + S$. Thus for instance, when the survival is 99% in one group it will be 98.01% in the other group yielding a relative risk of 1.99, but when the survival in one group is 20% it will be just 4% in the other group, yielding a relative risk of death of 0.96/0.80 or 1.2.

Some epidemiologists like to use other link functions such as $\lambda(t|Z_1, \ldots, Z_p) = \lambda_0(t)(1 + \beta_1 Z_1 + \ldots + \beta_p Z_p)$. This is still a proportional hazards model, but the effect of different covariates is additive rather than multiplicative. For example if in model (4.2), being male infers a hazard ratio of 2 and being black infers a hazard ratio of 3, then being a black male infers a hazard ratio of 6 (= 2 × 3) relative to white females. With the additive link, the hazard ratio for black males will be $1 + (2 - 1) + (3 - 1) = 4$.

The basic model, (4.2), has been generalized in various directions. A simple generalization is to permit different baseline hazard functions in each of a number of strata. The stratified Cox model assumes that, within each stratum, the proportional hazards assumption is justified and that the effect of the variable Z is the same in all strata:

$$\lambda(t|Z_1, \ldots, Z_p, \text{stratum } j) = \lambda_j(t) \exp\left(\beta_1 Z_1 + \ldots + \beta_p Z_p\right) . \qquad (4.3)$$

By incorporating constructed variables that are constant in some strata, the stratified model, (4.3), can be used to model interactions between explanatory variables and strata. Suppose, for example, that one is stratifying by sex and including age as an explanatory variable. Let Z_1 = (age − 50) for men, = 0 for women; and let Z_2 = (age − 50) for women, = 0 for men. Then a model stratified on sex that includes Z_1, Z_2, and a treatment indicator Z_3 permits interactions between age and sex, but assumes that the treatment acts proportionately on the hazards for any age–sex combination.

In the Cox model, there are three components to the data on each individual: the possibly censored failure time T; an indicator δ equal to 1 if T is a true failure time, 0 if it is censored; and $\mathbf{Z}$, the vector of explanatory variables. The model is flexible enough to incorporate explanatory variables that change value over the course of the study. The key censoring assumption is that the observation ($T = t, \delta = 0$) tells us nothing more than that the true failure time is greater than t. When a study ends some individuals will still be alive and will be censored. In such situations, it is necessary for survival to be independent of entry time for the above condition to be satisfied. Suppose for instance that early on after the introduction of a new type of surgery only extremely sick patients are offered the new treatment, but that once the hospital has two years experience in the technique they offer it to relatively healthy patients too. If the results of all treated patients are studied four years after the introduction of the new technique, then patients censored in under two years may have been healthier at entry, thus if follow-up were continued for a further year, their survival in the third year might be better than that of patients entered in the first two years who survived two years. Thus the censoring time tells us something about the likely survival beyond the censoring time. In such circumstances, it is necessary to include "year of treatment" as an explanatory variable in the model.

We have already discussed the effect of survival improving over calendar time when estimating survival rates, but when the duration of recruitment is short compared to the length of follow-up such administrative censoring can usually be taken to be independent of survival. Other forms of censoring are more problematic. For instance, a patient who fails to attend a follow-up clinic might be too sick to get out of bed. So the fact that she was censored at t tells us more than simply that she was alive at t.

Example 10. *Cox model fitted to clinical trial data*

Table 4.8 presents the results of fitting a Cox model to data from 216 patients with primary biliary cirrhosis in a clinical trial of azathioprine vs. placebo (Christensen et al. 1985). The six variables were selected from an initial set of 25 partly using forward stepwise selection. An additional 32 patients were excluded because they had missing values of one or more of the six variables. Recruitment was over 6 years and follow-up a further 6 years. Of the 216 patients, 113 had censored survival times. The regression coefficients may be combined with their standard errors to obtain confidence intervals that rely on the asymptotic normality of the estimates. The positive coefficient associated with treatment implies that patients on the placebo ($Z = 1$) had poorer prognosis than those on azathioprine ($Z = 0$): the hazard of those on placebo is about 1.7 times greater than that of those on active treatment. Similarly, older patients had poorer prognosis. The hazard ratio associated with two patients aged 50 and 30 is $\exp[0.007\{\exp(3) - \exp(1)\}] = 1.13$. Notice, however, that the effect on survival is not fully described by the information in Table 4.8 because, without estimating the baseline hazard, one cannot translate the regression coefficients into effects on 5-years survival nor on median survival. Most statistical software for Cox regression will also estimate the cumulative baseline hazard function $\Lambda_0(t)$ which is equal to the integral from 0 to t of $\lambda_0(u)$ and from this one can calculate the estimated survival function for a given vector of covariates using the formula

$$\widehat{S}(t|z) = \exp\{-\widehat{\Lambda}_0(t)\exp(0.007\text{Age} - 0.05\text{Albumin} + 2.51\text{Bilirubin}$$

$$+ 0.68\text{Cholestasi} + 0.88\text{Cirrhosis} + 0.52\text{Therapy})\},$$

where $\widehat{\Lambda}$ is the estimate of Λ_0. ◆

Cox Model for Excess Risk 4.6.3

When studying a cohort diagnosed with a particular disease or defined by exposure to a potential risk factor, it is often natural to model the excess mortality (or the excess cause-specific mortality). The reason is that, we may assume that members of the cohort are subject to all the usual causes of death and that their "exposure" adds an independent route of death. For instance, patients with lymphoma might die from something unrelated or they might die of their lymphoma, the former will primarily be a function of age (mortality rises steeply with age), the latter

Table 4.8. Cox model fitted to data from a clinical trial comparing the effects of azathioprine and placebo on the survival of 216 patients with primary biliary cirrhosis (se=standard error)

Variable	Coding	$\widehat{\beta}$	$se(\widehat{\beta})$	$exp(\widehat{\beta})$
Age	$exp[(\text{age in years} - 20)/10]$	0.007	0.0016	1.0
Albumin	serum value in g/l	−0.05	0.018	0.95
Bilirubin	$\log_{10}$ (serum concentration in μmol/l)	2.51	0.32	12.3
Cholestasis	0 = No central cholestasis; 1 = Yes	0.68	0.28	2.0
Cirrhosis	0 = No; 1 = Yes	0.88	0.22	2.4
Therapy	0 = azathioprine; 1 = placebo	0.52	0.20	1.7

will largely depend on the time since their diagnosis. Gore et al. (1984) considered a variety of models for the analysis of survival in breast cancer patients. Sasieni (1996) showed how the Cox model could be applied to the excess mortality. The model was applied to nearly 1000 patients with non-Hodgkins lymphoma. As one might have expected the effect of prognostic factors such as histology and stage were greater in the proportional excess model than in the usual Cox model (because these factors will not influence mortality from other causes). The model was also useful in showing that although there was still a deleterious effect of increasing age on the excess mortality, it was less than the effect estimated applying the Cox model to all cause mortality.

4.6.4 Sampling from the Risk Set

Large cohort studies with long-term follow-up are extremely expensive. Studies requiring detailed analysis of food diaries or complicated analysis of blood, urine or tissue can be prohibitively expensive. For this reason, many epidemiologists have set up cohort studies collecting questionnaires, sera or urine and storing them for later use. The idea is to nest a case-control study within the cohort study (Langholz and Goldstein 1996; cf. Chap. I.7 of this handbook). As is well known, in a matched case-control study it is rarely efficient to collect more than about 4 controls per case (Breslow and Day 1980). So in a cohort study, one might wish to select a few "controls" from the cohort each time an event (case) occurs. Another approach is to select a small sub-cohort at the beginning and to supplement it with all the cases that develop during follow-up of the main cohort. There are a number of complications related to whether one can use controls selected for one case as controls for later cases (assuming that they are still at risk) and what happens if a control later becomes a case, but such nested case-control and case-cohort designs are extremely important in very large cohort studies looking at diet, genetics, or molecular measures of exposure. The idea of the nested case-control design was first put forward by Thomas (1977) and was considered at length by Prentice (1986a) and Borgan and Langholz (1993). The case-cohort design was proposed by Prentice (1986b) and has been studied by Self and Prentice (1988) and by Chen and Lo (1999). More recent research has focused on how best to select controls (Langholz and Borgan 1995; Borgan and Olsen 1999). Chen (2002) discussed how to fit a Cox model to a study in which crude covariate information is available on the entire cohort and complete covariate information is available on a sample, but he assumed that the validation sample is chosen at random and it is not applicable to nested case-control designs.

Aalen Model

Aalen (1980, 1989, 1993) proposed an additive model for the conditional hazard function. His model is more general than the Cox model in that it has an unspecified function associated with each covariate. Although, with two or more covariates, the Cox model is *not* a special case of the Aalen model. The Aalen model is that

$$\lambda(t|Z_1, \ldots, Z_p) = \lambda_0(t) + \lambda_1(t)Z_1 + \ldots + \lambda_p(t)Z_p , \qquad (4.4)$$

where the functions $\lambda_0(t), \ldots, \lambda_p(t)$ are all unspecified and $\lambda_0(t)$ is the baseline hazard corresponding to an individual with $Z_i = 0$, $i = 1, \ldots, p$. It should be noted that if $\{Z_1, \ldots, Z_p\}$ is a set of dummy covariates for some factor, then the Aalen model is simply the non-parametric model allowing a different hazard function for each level of the factor. Biologically, the additive model may be interpreted in terms of excess risk. Such a model would be appropriate if each covariate contributed to a different route of death and these routes were independent of each other.

The fact that the Aalen model is so big (i.e., it has relative few constraints compared to a completely non-parametric model) is both to its advantage and its disadvantage. With no restriction on the relation between hazards over time, the model provides a description of the temporal influence of covariates. The Aalen model may be viewed as a one-step Taylor series approximation (i.e. a linear approximation) of an arbitrary $\lambda(t|Z_1, \ldots, Z_p)$ and will therefore provide a reasonable fit to any data provided the covariates have been centered and their effect is not too strong. For this reason, some suggest the use of the Aalen model as a diagnostic check in conjunction with the Cox model (Mau 1986; Henderson and Milner 1991). A disadvantage of the model is that the results cannot be presented in tabular form, but require graphing of the estimated functions. It should also be noted that there is no restriction to prevent $\lambda_0(t) + \lambda_1(t)Z_1 + \ldots + \lambda_p(t)Z_p$ being negative (for some combination of covariate values), but a hazard function must be non-negative, so the model should not be applied to such covariate values.

The Aalen model has been used to model the excess mortality of cancer patients compared to that in the general population by Zahl (1996). He studied the long-term survival of men with colon-cancer in Norway. A restriction of the Aalen model has been proposed by McKeague and Sasieni (1994). They suggested that some of the regression functions $\lambda_i(t)$ could be forced to be constant or a simple parametric function of time. Such a model allows parametric estimates of the constant additive effect of certain covariates. The special case $\lambda_0(t) + \beta_1 Z_1 + \ldots + \beta_p Z_p$, like the Cox model has just one (baseline) hazard function to be estimated.

4.6.6   Adjusted Survival Curves

In studying mortality in a healthy cohort it is usual to compare their survival to that of the general population. When studying a cohort of very sick individuals, or healthy individuals for an event that is not routinely registered, it may be desirable to compare their survival to a more relevant control group. For instance, suppose one wanted to see whether schizophrenic patients in a special residential environment were less likely to attempt suicide than patients cared for in the community. It might be impossible to set up a randomised study to carry out such a comparison. Instead one would like to compare the rate of attempted suicide in the two groups of patients after adjusting for known confounders – factors that would influence how likely it is that a particular patient will attempt suicide. Statistically the question is how to adjust the survival curve in patients cared for in the community so as to better reflect what one might have expected from the patients receiving residential care had they received usual care. One approach is to produce directly adjusted survival curves (Makuch 1982; Gail and Byar 1986). The idea is to estimate the survival of each individual in the residential cohort using a model fitted to the standard cohort and to take the average of these survival estimates. For instance, if a Cox model is applied to the standard data with covariates Z_1 and Z_2 and yields estimates $\widehat{\Lambda}(t)$ for the cumulate baseline hazard, $\widehat{\beta}_1$ and $\widehat{\beta}_2$, then the estimated survival curve for an individual with covariates z_{1i} and z_{2i} is

$$\widehat{S}(t) = \exp\{-\widehat{\Lambda}(t) \exp(\widehat{\beta}_1 z_{1i} + \widehat{\beta}_2 z_{2i})\} .$$

Example 11.   *Assessment of survival following liver transplantation*
              Keiding et al., (1990) compared the survival experience of 38 primary biliary cirrhosis patients treated with liver transplantation in the Nordic countries with the directly standardised survival of 82 patients receiving transplants in England. They applied a Cox model to the English data with three covariates: ln(urea), ln(bilirubin) and an indicator for diuretic-responsive ascites. About 25% of the transplanted patients died within two months of transplant, but few patients died thereafter (the median follow-up was 6 months, the maximum was 3.5 years). This was quite similar to the "expected" survival based on the English data: the expected survival at 2 months was about 75% falling to about 60% by 6 months. The authors also compared the survival of their patients to that of primary biliary cirrhosis patients without transplant from an international trial of medical treatment. Once again the expected survival was based on the results of fitting a Cox model. The expected survival based on the medically treated patients is similarly poor during the first two months, but continues to decrease at a rapid rate so that the expected survival at two years is less than 20% compared to about 60% observed in the transplanted patients.   ♦

Another method for obtaining a comparable survival curve is to use matching to identify patients from the standard cohort. With one-to-one matching, one could simply compare the two Kaplan–Meier curves. If a variable number of "controls" are selected for each patient in the "special cohort", one needs to produce a weighted Kaplan–Meier curve. Here one simply weights each control by the inverse of the number of controls in the matched set so that each matched set of controls has weight one. Estimation of the survival curve is straightforward, but estimation of its variance is more complicated (Winnett and Sasieni 2002).

Example 12.   *Assessing the benefit of bone marrow transplant in childhood leukaemia*

Galimberti et al. (2002) considered the disease-free survival of 30 children with acute lymphoblastic leukaemia (ALL) who were treated with allogenic bone marrow transplants whilst in first remission. Controls were selected from 397 ALL patients treated with chemotherapy. Matching was done on white blood cell count at diagnosis (0–10,000; 10,000–50,000; 50,000–100,000; $>100{,}000/\text{mm}^3$), age at diagnosis (<1, 1–10; >10 years), immunophenotype (T-lineage; B-lineage) as well as clinical centre and front-line chemotherapy protocol. Additionally, controls had to survive in remission at least as long as the time from remission to transplant in the patient that they matched. Each of the 30 transplant patients was matched to between one and seven controls. In all there were 130 controls and no control was matched to more than one transplanted patient. Potential controls not matching to any transplanted patients tended to have better survival, although they also included patients who died before there was time for a transplant. Similarly, when there were multiple matching controls, their survival tended to be better. Thus, compared to all 397 controls, the matched sample of 130 controls had excellent survival for the first six months, but the survival curves crossed within 12 months of remission and thereafter the smaller group had worse survival. After taking account of the variable number of controls, the weighted Kaplan–Meier showed that the expected survival of the transplanted patients was worse still (Fig. 4.6).   ♦

Censoring and Truncation   4.7

Until now we have considered only *right-censoring*. The name coming from picturing a time line that runs left to right. The actual event time lies somewhere to the right of the censoring time and information regarding what happens to the right of this time is censored. We have also discussed late-entry whereby some individuals do not join the study cohort at (their individual) time zero. Late entry is also sometimes called left-truncation. An example would arise in an epidemiological study of people living in a retirement community in which one was interested in factors influencing the age of death. In such a study, individuals only become eligible once they have moved to the retirement community. Some may move in at age 60, others

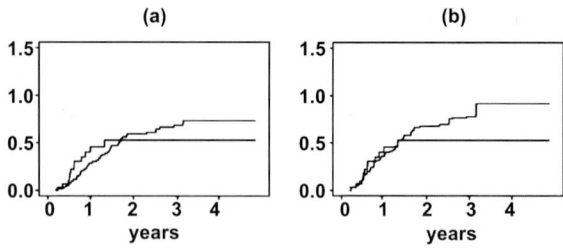

Figure 4.6. Estimates of the cumulative hazard for the bone marrow transplant (BMT) patients and the conventionally treated (CT) patients. (a) Standard estimates based on 30 BMT and a matched group of 130 CT patients. (b) Standard estimate for the 30 BMT patients and weighted estimate for the 130 matched CT patients. In both cases, the CT patients have higher cumulative hazard beyond 2 years

may not move there until they reach 80 (possibly following the death of a spouse). We observe how old individuals are when they join the community, but we do not know anything about individuals who die before they would have joined the community. If a woman joins at age 78, the fact that she lived to age 78 tells us nothing useful about events to the left of age 78 – had the individual died at age 76 she would not have been in the study. Both right-censoring and left-truncation can easily be accommodated by all the techniques that we have discussed thus far.

In epidemiology one also has data that are subject to more extreme forms of censoring. The most extreme form arises from data on prevalence rates. In a cross-sectional study one could survey whether individuals at different ages have or have not had some event in the past. For instance one might be interested in age at menarche (and survey adolescent girls as to whether or not they have had their first period), or age at infection of a particular pathogen (and test for antibodies in blood). The assumption in such studies is that the event is not reversible and that the yes/no question will reduce the recall bias associated with asking people how long ago the event occurred. Such *current status* data are also referred to as (case I) *interval-censored* data. Here the age of the individual is the censoring time and every individual is either left- or right-censored. Those who have not had the event are right-censored. But those who have are left-censored: i.e., we know that their true event time lies somewhere to the left of the censoring time. Methods exist for analysing prevalence data as reviewed by Keiding (1991). The classical problem is the non-parametric estimation of the survival function. The non-parametric maximum likelihood estimator is an extremely good estimator and it can be estimated efficiently using the "pool adjacent violators algorithm" (Barlow et al. 1972). Testing for differences in survival based on interval-censored data was first discussed by Peto and Peto (1972). More recently, several authors have considered regression models for prevalence data. Technically, fitting parametric regression models with prevalence data by maximum likelihood estimation presents no new problems (Odell et al. 1992). Semi-parametric models present more challenges

(Huang 1996). The most widely studied are the Cox (proportional hazards) model and the proportional odds model. Essentially one can alternate between estimating the baseline hazard (or odds) for fixed values of the regression parameters and estimating the regression parameters for fixed value of the baseline function. More recently, Lin et al. (1998) proposed using the additive hazards model: $\lambda_0(t|Z) = \lambda_0(t) + \beta_1 Z_1(t) + \ldots + \beta_p Z_p(t)$ for current status data. They showed that the additive hazard model for current status data was equivalent to the usual Cox model for the event "observation made and observed to have died" with the covariate equal to minus the cumulative covariate from the additive hazard model (i.e., the integral from 0 to t of $-Z(s)$). The simple approach proposed by Lin et al. is not efficient and breaks down if the observation times are not independent of the covariates. Martinussen and Scheike (2002) showed how the additive hazard model could be fit efficiently even in the presence of dependent observation times. Their method cannot simply be applied using standard Cox model software, but it is considerably simpler than efficient approaches to fitting the proportional hazards model to current status data.

In other studies, individuals are screened or questioned periodically. In such studies, event times can be left (the event happened before the first screen) or right-censored (the event happened after the last screen) or interval-censored (the event happened between two screens). This sort of data is sometimes called interval-censoring case 2 (Groeneboom and Wellner 1992) and sometimes *panel count* data. An added complication that is rarely considered is that the screening test may be less than 100% sensitive. In such circumstances, one should take into account the timing of all previous negative screens, not just the one immediately prior to the one that led to the detection of the event. For case 2 interval-censoring, the non-parametric maximum likelihood estimator of the survival function is harder to compute, but efficient algorithms exist (Groeneboom and Wellner 1992). Once again, testing has been considered (Zhang et al. 2001), and adaptation of the Cox model is possible (Kooperberg and Clarkson 1997; Goetghebeur and Ryan 2000). A simple solution is to use conditional logistic regression to fit a proportional odds model (Rabinowitz et al. 2000). More recently, rank estimation of a log-linear regression model has been proposed (Li and Pu 2003). Practical issues such as how to deal with left-truncation in addition to interval-censoring and the effect of changes in disease incidence on the analysis are considered by Williamson et al. (2001).

A further complication arises when the initiating time is also possibly censored. For instance, one might be interested in the distribution of time from an infection to the development of symptomatic disease. It is likely that the time of infection will not be observed directly, but will be interval-censored and the time of symptomatic disease may be right-censored. Such data are called *doubly-censored* (De Gruttola and Lagakos 1989).

Example 13. *Doubly censored data on AIDS*

De Gruttola and Lagakos (1989) studied a group of haemophiliacs who received blood transfusions after 1978 and before blood was screened for

HIV infection. Approximately three-quarters of patients were infected with HIV and nearly one in six developed AIDS during follow-up. The data were only available in six-month intervals. Additionally, the time of HIV infection was interval-censored. ◆

Example 14. *Doubly censored data on metastases*
Leung and Elashoff (1996) considered data on 1548 patients with melanoma. The patients were followed periodically to detect changes in disease stage. The authors were primarily interested in the time from metastasis to death, but they also wanted to investigate whether this was dependent on the time from stage II disease to metastasis. The time of metastasis was interval-censored and the time of death was right-censored. The authors used a Weibull model and looked at the effect of treatment, Breslow thickness, sex, site of the metastasis, and the time with stage II disease on survival post metastasis. ◆

4.8   Conclusions

Survival analysis is more closely associated with clinical medical research than with epidemiology, but there are a number of situations in which survival analysis is needed in epidemiological research. Some form of survival analysis will be required in any cohort study and many of the more complicated designs used in modern epidemiology require quite sophisticated analytical techniques. In this chapter, we have presented a range of survival analysis tools covering a range of study designs. Before using these techniques the reader is advised to consult an expert or to read a more complete text, but it is hoped that this chapter will help epidemiologists who come across survival analysis in the writing of others and those who think that they may need survival analysis in their own research.

The notions that events occur in time and that causes precede their effects are central to epidemiological research and the objective of understanding the causes of disease. Longitudinal studies are essential to epidemiology and the complex evolution of risk factors, disease markers and disease over time requires sophisticate statistical techniques.

References

Aalen OO (1980) A model for nonparametric regression analysis of counting processes. In: Klonecki W, Kozek A, Rosinski J (eds) Mathematical statistics and probability theory. Lecture Notes in Statistics 2. Springer, New York, pp 1–25

Aalen OO (1989) A linear regression model for the analysis of life times. Stat Med 8:907–925

Aalen OO (1993) Further results on the non-parametric linear regression model in survival analysis. Stat Med 12:1569–1588

Andersen PK, Borch-Johnsen K, Deckert T, Green A., Hougaard P, Keiding N, Kreiner S (1985) A Cox regression model for the relative mortality and its application to diabetes mellitus survival data. Biometrics 41:921–932

Barlow RE, Bartholomew DJ, Bremner JM, Brunk HD (1972) Statistical inference under order restrictions. Wiley, Chichester

Borgan O, Langholz B (1993) Nonparametric estimation of relative mortality from nested case-control studies. Biometrics 49:593–602

Borgan O, Olsen EF (1999) The efficiency of simple and counter-matched nested case-control sampling. Scand J Stat 26(4):493–509

Brenner H (2002) Long-term survival rates of cancer patients achieved by the end of the 20th century: a period analysis. Lancet 360:1131–1135

Brenner H, Gefeller O (1996) An alternative method to monitor cancer patient survival. Cancer 78:2004–2010

Breslow NE, Day NE (1980) Statistical methods in cancer research. Volume I – The analysis of case-control studies. IARC Scientific Publications No. 32. International Agency for Research on Cancer, Lyon

Breslow NE, Day NE (1987) Statistical methods in cancer research. Volume II – The design and analysis of cohort studies. IARC Scientific Publications No. 82. International Agency for Research on Cancer, Lyon

Breslow NE, Lubin JH, Marek P, Langholz B (1983) Multiplicative models and cohort analysis. J Am Stat Assoc 78:1–12

Chen K, Lo S-H (1999) Case-cohort and case-control analysis with Cox's model. Biometrika 86:755–764

Chen Y-H (2002) Cox regression in cohort studies with validation sampling. Journal of the J Roy Statist Soc, Series B 64:51–62

Christensen E, Neuberger J, Crowe J, Altman DG, Popper H, Portmann B, Doniach D, Ranek L, Tygstrup N, Williams R (1985) Beneficial effect of azathioprine and prediction of prognosis in primary biliary cirrhosis. Final results of an international trial. Gastroenterology 89:1084–1091

Cox DR (1972) Regression models and life tables (with discussion). J Roy Statist Soc, Series B 34:187–220

Cuzick J, Sasieni P, Evans S (1992) Ingested arsenic, keratoses, and bladder cancer. Am J Epidemiol 136:417–421

Cuzick J, Stewart H, Rutqvist L, Houghton J, Edwards R, Redmond C, Peto R, Baum M, Fisher B, Host H (1994) Cause-specific mortality in long-term survivors of breast cancer who participated in trials of radiotherapy. J Clin Oncol. 12(3):447–453

Day NE (1976) A new measure of age standardized incidence, the cumulative rate. In: Waterhouse JAH, Muir CS, Correa P, Powell J (eds) Cancer incidence in five continents, Volume III. IARC Scientific Publications No. 15. International Agency for Research on Cancer, Lyon, pp 443–452

De Gruttola V, Lagakos SW (1989) Analysis of doubly-censored survival data, with application to AIDS. Biometrics 45:1–11

Ederer F, Axtell LM, Cutler SJ (1961) The relative survival rate: a statistical methodology. Natl Cancer Inst Monogr 6:101–121

Gail MH, Byar DP (1986) Variance calculation for direct adjusted survival curves with application to testing for no treatment effect. Biom J 28:587–599

Galimberti S, Sasieni P, Valsecchi MG (2002) A weighted Kaplan–Meier estimator for matched data with application to the comparison of chemotherapy and bone-marrow transplant in leukaemia. Stat Med 21(24):3847–3864

Goetghebeur E, Ryan L (2000) Semiparametric regression analysis of interval-censored data. Biometrics 56:1139–1144

Gore SM, Pocock SJ, Kerr GR (1984) Regression models and non-proportional hazards in the analysis of breast cancer survival. Applied Statistics 33:176–195

Greenwood M (1926) A report on the natural duration of cancer. Reports on Public Health and Medical Subjects. 33:1–26. H. M. Stationery Office, London

Groeneboom P, Wellner J (1992) Information bounds and nonparametric Maximum Likelihood estimation. In: DMV Seminar, Band 19. Birkhauser, New York

Hakulinen T (1982) Cancer survival corrected for heterogeneity in patient withdrawal. Biometrics 38(4):933–942

Hall WJ, Wellner JA (1980) Confidence bands for a survival curve from censored data. Biometrika 67:133–143

Halley E (1693) An estimate of the degrees of the mortality of mankind, drawn from curious tables of the births and funerals at the city of Breslaw; with an attempt to ascertain the price of annuities upon lives. Philosophical Transactions of the Royal Society of London 17:596–610

Henderson R, Milner A (1991) Aalen plots under proportional hazards. Applied Statistics 40:401–409

Hosmer DW, Lemshow S (1999) Applied survival analysis: Regression modeling of time to event data. Wiley: New York

Huang J (1996) Efficient estimation for the Cox model with interval censoring. Annals of Statistics 24:540–568

Huber PJ (1967) The behavior of maximum likelihood estimates under non-standard conditions. In: Proceedings of the Fifth Berkeley Symposium on Mathematical Statistics and Probability 1:221–233. University of California Press, Berkeley CA

Kalbfleisch JD, Prentice RL (2002) The statistical analysis of failure time data, 2nd edn. Wiley, New York

Kaplan EL, Meier P (1958) Nonparametric estimation from incomplete observations. J Am Stat Assoc 58:457–481

Keiding N (1987) The method of expected number of deaths, 1786–1886-1986. Int Stat Rev 55:1–20

Keiding N (1990) Statistical inference in the Lexis diagram. Phil Trans Roy Soc London A 332:487–509

Keiding N (1991) Age-specific incidence and prevalence: A statistical perspective (with discussion). J Roy Statist Soc, Series A 154:371–412

Keiding S, Ericzon BG, Eriksson S, Flatmark A, Höckerstedt K, Isoniemi H, Karlberg I, Keiding N, Olsson R, Samela K, Schrumpf E, Söderman C (1990) Survival after liver transplantation of patients with primary biliary cirrhosis in the Nordic countries. Comparison with expected survival in another series of transplantations and in an international trial of medical treatment. Scand J Gastroenterol 25:11–18

Kooperberg C, Clarkson DB (1997) Hazard regression with interval-censored data. Biometrics 53:1485–1494

Langholz B, Borgan O (1995) Counter matching: A stratified nested case-control sampling method. Biometrika 82:69–79

Langholz B, Goldstein L (1996) Risk set sampling in epidemiologic cohort studies. Statistical Science 11:35–53

Leung KM, Elashoff RM (1996) A three-state disease model with intervalcensored data: Estimation and applications to AIDS and cancer. Lifetime Data Analysis 2:175–194

Li L, Pu Z (2003) Rank estimation of log-linear regression with interval-censored data. Lifetime Data Analysis 9:57–70

Lin DY, Oakes D, Ying Z (1998) Additive hazards regression with current status data. Biometrika 85:289–298

Makuch RW (1982) Adjusted survival curve estimation using covariates. J Chronic Dis 35:437–443

Mantel N (1966) Evaluation of survival data and two new rank order statistics arising in its consideration. Cancer Chemother Rep 50:163–170

Martinussen T, Scheike TH (2002) Efficient estimation in additive hazards regression with current status data. Biometrika 89:649–658

Marubini E, Valsecchi MG (1995) Analysing survival data from clinical trials and observational studies. Wiley, Chichester

Mau J (1986) On a graphical method for the detection of time-dependent effects of covariates in survival data. Applied Statistics 35:245–255

McCullagh P, Nelder JA (1989) Generalised linear models, 2nd edn. Chapman & Hall, London

McKeague IW, Sasieni PD (1994) A partly parametric additive risk model. Biometrika 81:501–514

Odell PM, Anderson KM, D'Agostino RB (1992) Maximum likelihood estimation for interval-censored data using a Weibull-based accelerated failure time model. Biometrics 48:951–991

Peto R, Peto J (1972) Asymptotically efficient rank invariant test procedures (with discussion). J Roy Statist Soc, Series A 135:185–206

Prentice RL (1986a) On the design of synthetic case-control studies. Biometrics 42:301–310

Prentice RL (1986b) A case-cohort design for epidemiologic cohort studies and disease prevention trials. Biometrika 73:1–11

Rabinowitz D, Betensky RA, Tsiatis AA (2000) Using conditional logistic regression to fit proportional odds models to interval censored data. Biometrics 56:511–518

Sasieni PD (1996) Proportional excess hazards. Biometrika 83:127–141

Sasieni PD, Adams J (1999) Standardized lifetime risk. Am J Epidemiol 149:869–875

Sasieni PD, Adams J (2000) Analysis of cervical cancer mortality and incidence data from England and Wales: evidence of a beneficial effect of screening. J Roy Statist Soc, Series A 163:191–209

Sasieni PD, Adams J, Cuzick J (2002) Avoidance of premature death: a new definition for the proportion cured. J Cancer Epidemiol Prev 7:165–171

Self SG, Prentice RL (1988) Asymptotic distribution theory and efficiency results for case-cohort studies. Annals of Statistics 11:804–812

Therneau TM, Grambsch PM (2000) Modeling survival data: Extending the Cox model. Springer, New York

Thomas DC (1977) Addendum to: methods of cohort analysis: Appraisal by application to asbestos mining. By FDK Liddel, JC McDonals and DC Thomas. J Roy Statist Soc, Series A 140:469–491

Williamson JM, Satten GA, Hanson JA, Weinstock H, Datta S (2001) Analysis of dynamic cohort data. Am J Epidemiol 154:366–372

Winnett A, Sasieni P (2002) Adjusted Nelson-Aalen estimates with retrospective matching. Journal of the American Statistical Association 97:245–256

Zahl P-H (1996) A linear non-parametric regression model for the excess intensity. Scandinavian Journal of Statistics 23:353–364

Zhang Y, Liu W, Zhan Y (2001) A nonparametric two-sample test of the failure function with interval censoring case 2. Biometrika 88:677–686

Measurement Error

II.5

Jeffrey S. Buzas, Leonard A. Stefanski, Tor D. Tosteson

Introduction

Factors contributing to the presence or absence of disease are not always easily determined or accurately measured. Consequently epidemiologists are often faced with the task of inferring disease patterns using noisy or indirect measurements of risk factors or covariates. Problems of measurement arise for a number of reasons, including for example: reliance on self-reported information; the use of records of suspect quality; intrinsic biological variability; sampling variability; and laboratory analysis error. Although the reasons for imprecise measurement are diverse, the inference problems they create share in common the structure that statistical models must be fit to data formulated in terms of well-defined but unobservable variables X, using information on measurements W that are less than perfectly correlated with X. Problems of this nature are called measurement error problems and the statistical models and methods for analyzing such data are called measurement error models.

This chapter focuses on statistical issues related to the problems of fitting models relating a disease response variable Y to true predictors X and error-free predictors Z, given values of measurements W, in addition to Y and Z. Although disease status may also be subject to measurement error, attention is limited to measurement error in predictor variables. We further restrict attention to measurement error in continuous predictor variables. Categorical predictors are not immune from problems of ascertainment, but misclassification is a particular form of measurement error. Consequently misclassification error is generally studied separately from measurement error, although there is clearly much overlap.

A case-control study exhibiting measurement error was described in Karagas et al. (2000, 2001, 2002) and is briefly mentioned here to exemplify the notation. The purpose of the study was to assess the risk of bladder cancer and two forms of non-melanoma skin cancer (Y's) to 'true' arsenic exposure (X), adjusting for patient age (Z). True arsenic exposure was measured imprecisely through concentrations of arsenic in toenails (W).

This chapter is organized in three main sections. Section 5.2 defines basic concepts and models of measurement error and outlines the effects of ignoring measurement error on the results of standard statistical analyses. An important aspect of most measurement error problems is the inability to estimate parameters of interest given only the information contained in a sample of (Y, Z, W) values. Some features of the joint distribution of (Y, Z, X, W) must be known or estimated in order to estimate parameters of interest. Thus additional data, depending on the type of error model, must often be collected. Consequently it is important to include measurement error considerations when planning a study, both to enable application of a measurement error analysis of the data and to ensure validity of conclusions. Planning studies in the presence of measurement error is the topic of Sect. 5.3. Methods for the analysis of data measured with error differ according to the nature of the measurement error, the additional parameter-identifying information that is available, and the strength of the modeling assumptions appropriate for a particular problem. Section 5.4 describes a number of common approaches to the analysis of data measured with error, including simple, generally applicable, bias-adjustment approaches, conditional likelihood, and full likelihood approaches.

This chapter is intended as an introduction to the topic. In depth coverage of linear measurement error models is provided by Fuller (1987). Carroll et al. (1995) provide detailed coverage of nonlinear models as well as density estimation. Other review articles addressing measurement error in epidemiology include Carroll (1998), Thomas et al. (1993), and Armstrong et al. (1992). Prior to the book by Fuller (1987) the literature on measurement error models was largely concerned with linear measurement error models and went under the name *errors-in-variables*. Chap. II.3 of this handbook presents additional topics in regression modelling.

Measurement Error and Its Effects 5.2

This section presents the basic concepts and definitions used in the literature on nonlinear measurement error models. The important distinction between differential and nondifferential error is discussed first, and is followed by a description of two important models for measurement error. The major effects of measurement error are described and illustrated in terms of multivariate normal regression models.

Differential and Nondifferential Error, and Surrogate Variables 5.2.1

The error in W as a measurement of X is *nondifferential* if the conditional distribution of Y given (Z, X, W) is the same as that of Y given (Z, X), that is, $f_{Y|ZXW} = f_{Y|ZX}$. When $f_{Y|ZXW} \neq f_{Y|ZX}$ the error is *differential*. The key feature of a nondifferential measurement is that it contains no information for predicting Y in addition to the information already contained in Z and X. When $f_{Y|ZXW} = f_{Y|ZX}$, W is said to be a *surrogate* for X.

Many statistical methods in the literature on measurement error modeling are based on the assumption that W is a surrogate. It is important to understand this concept and to recognize when it is or is not an appropriate assumption. Nondifferential error is plausible in many cases, but there are situations where it should not be assumed without careful consideration.

If measurement error is due solely to instrument or laboratory-analysis error, then it can often be argued that the error is nondifferential. However, in epidemiologic applications measurement error commonly has multiple sources and instrument and laboratory-analysis error are often minor components of the total measurement error. In these cases it is not always clear whether measurement error is nondifferential.

The potential for nondifferential error is greater in case-control studies because covariate information ascertainment and exposure measurement follow disease response determination. In such studies selective recall, or a tendency for cases to overestimate exposure, can induce dependencies between the response and the true exposure even after conditioning on true exposure.

A useful exercise for thinking about the plausibility of the assumption that W is a surrogate, is to consider whether W would have been measured (or included in a regression model) had X been available. For example, suppose that the natural predictor X is defined as the temporal or spatial average value of a time-varying risk factor or spatially-varying exposure (e.g., blood pressure, cholesterol, lead exposure, particulate matter exposure), and the observed W is a measurement at a single point in time or space. In such cases, it might be convincingly argued that the single measurement contributes little or no information in addition to that contained in the long-term average.

However, this line of reasoning is not foolproof. The surrogate status of W can depend on the particular model being fit to the data. For example, consider models where Z has two components, $Z = (Z_1, Z_2)$. It is possible to have $f_{Y|Z_1 Z_2 XW} = f_{Y|Z_1 Z_2 X}$ and $f_{Y|Z_1 XW} \neq f_{Y|Z_1 X}$. Thus W is a surrogate in the full model including Z_1 and Z_2 but not in the reduced model including only Z_1. In other words, whether a variable is a surrogate or not depends on other variables in the model. A simple example illustrates this feature. Let $X \sim N(\mu_x, \sigma_x^2)$. Assume that $\varepsilon_1, \varepsilon_2, U_1$ and U_2 are mean zero normal random variables such that $X, \varepsilon_1, \varepsilon_2, U_1, U_2$ are mutually independent. Let $Z = X + \varepsilon_1 + U_1$, $Y = \beta_1 + \beta_z Z + \beta_z X + \varepsilon_2$, and $W = X + \varepsilon_1 + U_2$. Then $E(Y|X) \neq E(Y|X, W)$ but $E(Y|Z, X, W) = E(Y|Z, X)$. The essential feature of this example is that the measurement error $W - X$ is correlated with the covariate Z. The presence or absence of Z in the model determines whether W is a surrogate or not. Such situations have the potential of arising in applications. For example, consider air pollution health effects studies. Suppose that X is the spatial-average value of an air pollutant, W is the value measured at a single location, the components of Z include meteorological variables, and Y is a spatially aggregated measure of morbidity or mortality (all variables recorded daily, with X, W and Z suitably lagged). If weather conditions influence both health and the measurement process (e.g., by influencing the spatial distribution of the pollutant), then it is possible that W would be a surrogate only for the full model containing Z.

With nondifferential measurement error, it is possible to estimate parameters in the model relating the response to the true predictor using the measured predictor only, with minimal additional information on the error distribution, i.e., it is not necessary to observe the true predictor. However, this is not generally possible with differential measurement error. In this case it is necessary to have a validation subsample in which both the measured value and the true value are recorded. Data requirements are discussed more fully in Sect. 5.3. Much of the literature on measurement error models deals with nondifferential error, and hence that is the focus of this chapter. Problems with differential error are often better analyzed via techniques for missing data.

Error Models

The number of ways a surrogate W and predictor X can be related are countless. However, in practice it is often possible to reduce most problems to one of two simple error structures. For understanding the effects of measurement error and the statistical methods for analyzing data measured with error an understanding of the two simple error structures is generally sufficient.

Classical Error Model

The standard statistical model for the case in which W is a measurement of X in the usual sense is $W = X + U$, where U has mean zero and is independent of X. As explained in the preceding section whether W is a surrogate or not depends on more than just the joint distribution of X and W. However, in the sometimes plausible case that the error U is independent of all other variables in a model, then it is nondifferential and W is a surrogate. This is often called the classical error model. More precisely, it is an independent, unbiased, additive measurement error model. Because $E(W|X) = X$, W is said to be unbiased measurement of X.

Not all measuring methods produce unbiased measurements. However, it is often possible to calibrate a biased measurement resulting in an unbiased measurement. Error calibration is discussed later in greater detail.

Berkson Error Model

For the case of Berkson error, X varies around W and the accepted statistical model is $X = W + U$ where U has mean zero and is independent of W. For this model, $E(X|W) = W$, and W is called an unbiased Berkson predictor of X, or simply an unbiased predictor of X. The terminology results from the fact that the best squared-error predictor of X given W is $E(X|W) = W$.

Berkson (1950) describes a measurement error model which is superficially similar to the classical error model, but with very different statistical properties. He describes the error model for experimental situations in which the observed variable was controlled, hence the alternative name *controlled variable model*, and the error-free variable, X, varied around W. For example, suppose that an experimental design called for curing a material in a kiln at a specified temperature W, determined by thermostat setting. Although the thermostat is set to W, the actual temperature in the kiln, X, often varies randomly from W due to less-than-perfect thermostat control. For a properly calibrated thermostat a reasonable assumption is that $E(X|W) = W$, which is the salient feature of a Berkson measurement (compare to an unbiased measurement for which $E(W|X) = X$).

Apart from experimental situations, in which W is truly a controlled variable, the unbiased Berkson error model seldom arises as a consequence of sampling design or direct measurement. However, like the classical error model, it is possible to calibrate a biased surrogate so that the calibrated measurement satisfies the assumptions of the Berkson error model.

Reduction to Unbiased Error Model

The utility of the classical and Berkson error structures is due to the fact that many error structures can be transformed to one or the other. Suppose that W^* is a surrogate for X. For the case that a linear model for the dependence of W^* on X is reasonable, that is, $W^* = \gamma_1 + \gamma_x X + U^*$, where U^* is independent of X, the transformed variable $W = (W^* - \gamma_1)/\gamma_x$ satisfies the classical error model $W = X + U$, where $U = U^*/\gamma_x$. In other words W^* can be transformed into an independent, unbiased, additive measurement.

Alternatively, for the transformation $W = E(X|W^*)$ it follows that $X = W + U$, where $U = X - E(X|W^*)$ is uncorrelated with W. Thus apart from the distinction between independence and zero correlation of the error U, any surrogate W^* can be transformed to an unbiased additive Berkson error structure.

Both types of calibration are useful. The transformation that maps an uncalibrated surrogate W^* into a classical error model is called *error calibration*. The transformation that maps W^* into a Berkson error model is called *regression calibration* (Carroll et al. 1995); see Tosteson et al. (1989) for an interesting application of regression calibration.

In theory, calibration reduces an arbitrary surrogate to a classical error measurement or a Berkson error measurement, explaining the attention given to these two unbiased error models. In practice, things are not so simple. Seldom are the parameters in the regression of W on X (error calibration) or in the regression of X on W (regression calibration) known, and these parameters have to be estimated, which is generally possible only if supplementary data are available for doing so. In these cases there is yet another source of variability introduced by the estimation of the parameters in the chosen calibration function. This is estimator variability and should be accounted for in the estimation of standard errors of the estimators calculated from the calibrated data.

5.2.3   Measurement Error in the Normal Linear Model

We now consider the effects of measurement error in a simple linear regression model with normal variation. This model has limited use in epidemiology, but it is one of the few models in which the effects of measurement error can be explicitly derived and explained. Measurement error affects relative risk coefficients in much the same way as regression coefficients, so that the insights gained from this simple model carry over to more useful epidemiologic models.

Consider the multivariate normal formulation of the simple linear regression model,

$$\begin{pmatrix} Y \\ X \end{pmatrix} \sim N \left\{ \begin{pmatrix} \beta_1 + \beta_x \mu_x \\ \mu_x \end{pmatrix}, \begin{pmatrix} \beta_x^2 \sigma_x^2 + \sigma_\varepsilon^2 & \beta_x \sigma_x^2 \\ \beta_x \sigma_x^2 & \sigma_x^2 \end{pmatrix} \right\}. \tag{5.1}$$

If, as is assumed here, the substitute variable W is jointly normally distributed with (Y, X), then in the absence of additional assumptions on the relationship between W and (Y, X) the multivariate normal model for (Y, X, W) is

$$
\begin{pmatrix} Y \\ X \\ W \end{pmatrix} \sim N \left\{ \begin{pmatrix} \beta_1 + \beta_x \mu_x \\ \mu_x \\ \mu_w \end{pmatrix}, \begin{pmatrix} \beta_x^2 \sigma_x^2 + \sigma_\varepsilon^2 & \beta_x \sigma_x^2 & \beta_x \sigma_{xw} + \sigma_{\varepsilon w} \\ \beta_x \sigma_x^2 & \sigma_x^2 & \sigma_{xw} \\ \beta_x \sigma_{xw} + \sigma_{\varepsilon w} & \sigma_{xw} & \sigma_w^2 \end{pmatrix} \right\}, \tag{5.2}
$$

where $\sigma_{xw} = \mathrm{Cov}(X, W)$ and $\sigma_{\varepsilon w} = \mathrm{Cov}(\varepsilon, W)$. In measurement error modeling the available data consist of observations (Y, W) so that the relevant sampling model is the marginal distribution of (Y, W).

We now describe biases that arise from the so-called *naive* analysis of the data, that is, the analysis of the observed data using the usual methods for error-free data. In this case the naive analysis is least squares analysis of $\{(W_i, Y_i), i = 1, \ldots, n\}$, so that the naive analysis results in unbiased estimates of the parameters in the regression model for Y on W, or what we refer to as the *naive model*. Naive-model parameters are given in Table 5.1 for some particular error models.

Differential Error

For the case of a general measurement with possibly differential error the naive estimator of slope is an unbiased estimator of $(\beta_x \sigma_{xw} + \sigma_{\varepsilon w})/\sigma_w^2$ rather than β_x. Depending on the covariances between ε and W, and X and W, and the variance of W, the naive-model slope could be less than or greater than β_x, so that no general conclusions about bias are possible. Similarly the residual variance of the naive regression could be either greater or less than the true model residual variance. It follows that for a general measurement W, the coefficient of determination for the naive analysis could be greater or less than for the true model. These results indicate the futility of trying to make generalizations about the effects of using a general measurement for X in a naive analysis.

Surrogate

For the multivariate normal model with $0 < \rho_{xw}^2 < 1$, W is a surrogate if and only if $\sigma_{\varepsilon w} = 0$. With an arbitrary surrogate measurement the naive estimator of slope unbiasedly estimates $\beta_x \sigma_{xw}/\sigma_w^2$. Depending on the covariance between X and W and the variance of W, the naive-model slope could be less or greater than β_x, so that again no general statements about bias in the regression parameters are possible. For an uncalibrated measurement, $E(W|X) = \gamma_0 + \gamma_x X$, $\sigma_{xw} = \mathrm{cov}(X, W) = \gamma_x \sigma_x^2$ and $\mathrm{Var}(X) = \gamma_x^2 \sigma_x^2 + \sigma_u^2$. In this case the relative bias, $\sigma_{xw}/\sigma_w^2 = \gamma_x \sigma_x^2/(\gamma_x^2 \sigma_x^2 + \sigma_u^2)$, is bounded in absolute value by $1/|\gamma_x|$. For an uncalibrated Berkson measurement, $E(X|W) = \alpha_1 + \alpha_w W$, $\sigma_{xw} = \alpha_w \sigma_w^2$, and the relative bias is α_w. When W is a surrogate the residual variance from the naive analysis is never less than the true-model residual variance, and is strictly greater except in the extreme case that X and W are perfectly correlated, $\rho_{xw}^2 = 1$. It follows that for an arbitrary surrogate the coefficient of determination for the naive model is always less than or equal to that for the true model. The use of a surrogate always entails a loss of predictive power.

The naive-model slope indicates that in order to recover β_x from an analysis of the observed data, only σ_{xw} would have to be known. A *validation study* in which bivariate observations (X, W) were obtained, would provide the necessary information for estimating σ_{xw}.

Classical Error

If the surrogate, W, is an unbiased measurement, $E(W|X) = X$, and the classical error model holds, then $\mu_w = \mu_x$, $\sigma_{xw} = \sigma_x^2$, and $\sigma_w^2 = \sigma_x^2 + \sigma_u^2$. In this case the naive slope estimator unbiasedly estimates $\beta_x \sigma_x^2/(\sigma_x^2 + \sigma_u^2)$. For this case the sign $(\pm)$ of $\beta_x \sigma_x^2/(\sigma_x^2 + \sigma_u^2)$ is always the same as the sign of β_x, and the inequality $\sigma_x^2/(\sigma_x^2 + \sigma_u^2)|\beta_x| \leq |\beta_x|$ shows that the naive estimator of slope is always biased toward 0. This type of bias is called *attenuation* or *attenuation toward the null*. The attenuation factor $\lambda = \sigma_x^2/(\sigma_x^2 + \sigma_u^2)$ is called the *reliability ratio* and its inverse is called the *linear correction for attenuation*. In this case the coefficient of determination is also attenuated toward zero and the term attenuation is often used to describe both attenuation in the slope coefficient and the attenuation in the coefficient of determination. *Regression dilution* has also been used in the epidemiology literature to describe attenuation (MacMahon et al. 1990; Hughes 1993). In order to recover β_x from an analysis of the observed data it would be sufficient to know σ_u^2. Either replicate measurements or validation data provide information for estimating the measurement error variance σ_u^2.

Berkson Error

With W a surrogate, the Berkson error model is embedded in the multivariate normal model by imposing the condition $E(X|W) = W$. In this case $\mu_x = \mu_w$, $\sigma_{xw} = \sigma_w^2$ and $\sigma_x^2 = \sigma_w^2 + \sigma_u^2$. When W and X satisfy the unbiased Berkson error model, $X = W + U$, the naive estimator of slope is an unbiased estimator of β_x, i.e., there is no bias. Thus there is no bias in the naive regression parameter estimators, but there is an increase in the residual variance and a corresponding decrease in the model coefficient of determination. Even though no bias is introduced there is still a penalty incurred with the use of Berkson predictors. However, with respect to valid inference on regression coefficients the linear model is robust to Berkson errors. The practical importance of this robustness property is limited because the unbiased Berkson error model seldom is appropriate without regression calibration except in certain experimental settings as described previously.

Discussion

Measurement error is generally associated with attenuation, and as Table 5.1 shows, attenuation in the coefficient of determination occurs with any surrogate measurement. However, attenuation in the regression slope is, in general, specific only to the classical error model. The fact that measurement-error-induced bias depends critically on the type of measurement error, underlies the importance of correct identification of the measurement error in applications. Incorrect specification of the measurement error component of a model can create problems as great as those caused by ignoring measurement error.

The increase in residual variance associated with surrogate measurements (including classical and Berkson) gives rise not only to a decrease in predictive power, but also contributes to reduced power for testing. The noncentrality parameter for testing $H_0 : \beta_x = 0$ with surrogate measurements is $n\beta_x^2\sigma_x^2\rho_{xw}^2 / \{\sigma_\varepsilon^2 + \beta_x^2\sigma_x^2 (1 - \rho_{xw}^2)\}$ which is less than the true-data noncentrality parameter, $n\beta_x^2\sigma_x^2/\sigma_\varepsilon^2$, whenever $\rho_{xw}^2 < 1$. These expressions give rise to the equivalent-power sample size formula

$$n_w = n_x \left[\{\sigma_\varepsilon^2 + \beta_x^2\sigma_x^2 (1 - \rho_{xw}^2)\} / \{\sigma_\varepsilon^2\rho_{xw}^2\}\right] \approx n_x/\rho_{xw}^2, \tag{5.3}$$

where n_w is the number of (W, Y) pairs required to give the same power as a sample of size n_x of (X, Y) pairs. The latter approximation is reasonable near the null value $\beta_x = 0$ (or more precisely, when $\beta_x^2\sigma_x^2 (1 - \rho_{xw}^2)$ is small).

The loss of power for testing is not always due to an increase in variability of the parameter estimates. For the classical error model the variance of the naive estimator is *less than* the variance of the true-data estimator asymptotically if and only if $\beta_x^2\sigma_x^2/(\sigma_x^2 + \sigma_u^2) < \sigma_\varepsilon^2/\sigma_x^2$, which is possible when σ_ε^2 is large, or σ_u^2 is large, or $|\beta_x|$ is small. So relative to the case of no measurement error, classical errors can result in more precise estimates of the wrong (i.e., biased) quantity. This cannot occur with Berkson errors, for which asymptotically the variance of the naive estimator is never less than the variance of the true-data estimator.

The normal linear model also illustrates the need for additional information in measurement error models. For example, for the case of an arbitrary surrogate the joint distribution of Y and W contains eight unknown parameters $(\beta_1, \beta_x, \mu_x, \mu_w, \sigma_x^2, \sigma_\varepsilon^2, \sigma_{xw}, \sigma_w^2)$, whereas a bivariate normal distribution is completely determined by only five parameters. This means that not all eight parameters can be estimated with data on (Y, W) alone. In particular, β_x is not estimable. However, from Table 5.1 it is apparent that if a consistent estimator of σ_{xw} can be constructed, say from validation data, then the method-of-moments

Table 5.1. Table entries are slopes and residual variances of the linear model relating Y to W for the cases in which W is a differential measurement, a surrogate, an unbiased classical-error measurement, an unbiased Berkson predictor, and the case of no error ($W = X$)

Error model	Slope	Residual variance
Differential	$\beta_x (\sigma_{xw}/\sigma_w^2) + (\sigma_{\varepsilon w}/\sigma_w^2)$	$\sigma_\varepsilon^2 + \beta_x^2\sigma_x^2 - \dfrac{(\sigma_{xw}\beta_x + \sigma_{\varepsilon w})^2}{\sigma_w^2}$
Surrogate	$\beta_x (\sigma_{xw}/\sigma_w^2)$	$\sigma_\varepsilon^2 + \beta_x^2\sigma_x^2(1 - \rho_{xw}^2)$
Classical	$\beta_x \dfrac{\sigma_x^2}{\sigma_x^2 + \sigma_u^2}$	$\sigma_\varepsilon^2 + \beta_x^2\sigma_x^2 \dfrac{\sigma_u^2}{\sigma_x^2 + \sigma_u^2}$
Berkson	β_x	$\sigma_\varepsilon^2 + \beta_x^2\sigma_x^2 (\sigma_u^2/\sigma_x^2)$
No error	β_x	σ_ε^2

estimator $\widehat{\beta}_x = (s_w^2/\widehat{\sigma}_{xw})\widehat{\beta}_w$, is a consistent estimator of β_x, where $\widehat{\beta}_w$ is the least squares estimator of slope in the linear regression of Y on W, s_w^2 is the sample variance of W, and $\widehat{\sigma}_{xw}$ is the validation-data estimator of σ_{xw}.

For the case of additive, unbiased, measurement error the joint distribution of Y and W contains six unknown parameters $(\beta_1, \beta_x, \mu_x, \sigma_x^2, \sigma_\varepsilon^2, \sigma_u^2)$, so that again not all of the parameters are identified. Once again β_x is not estimable. However, if a consistent estimator of σ_u^2 can be constructed, say from either replicate measurements or validation data, then the method-of-moments estimator $\widehat{\beta}_x = \{s_w^2/(s_w^2 - \widehat{\sigma}_u^2)\}\widehat{\beta}_w$, is a consistent estimator of β_x, where $\widehat{\sigma}_u^2$ is the estimator of σ_u^2.

For the Berkson error model there are also six unknown parameters in the joint distribution of Y and W, $(\beta_1, \beta_x, \mu_x, \sigma_x^2, \sigma_\varepsilon^2, \sigma_w^2)$, so that again not all of the parameters are identified. The regression parameters β_1 and β_x are estimated unbiasedly by the intercept and slope estimators from the least squares regression of Y and W. However, without additional data it is not possible to estimate σ_ε^2.

5.2.4   Multiple Linear Regression

The entries in Table 5.1 and the qualitative conclusions based on them generalize to the case of multiple linear regression with multiple predictors measured with error. For the Berkson error model it remains the case that no bias in the regression parameter estimators results from the substitution of W for X, and the major effects of measurement error are those resulting from an increase in the residual variation.

For the classical measurement error model there are important aspects of the problem that are not present in the simple linear regression model. When the model includes both covariates measured with error X and without error Z, it is possible for measurement error to bias the naive estimator of β_z as well as the naive estimator of β_x. Furthermore, attenuation in the coefficient of a variable measured with error is no longer a simple function of the variance of that variable and the measurement error variance. When there are multiple predictors measured with error, the bias in regression coefficients is a nonintuitive function of the measurement error covariance matrix and the true-predictor covariance matrix.

Suppose that the multiple linear regression model for Y given Z and X is $Y = \beta_1 + \beta_z^T Z + \beta_x^T X + \varepsilon$. For the additive error model $W = X + U$, the naive estimator of the regression coefficients is estimating

$$\begin{pmatrix} \beta_{z*} \\ \beta_{x*} \end{pmatrix} = \begin{pmatrix} \sigma_{zz} & \sigma_{zx} \\ \sigma_{xz} & \sigma_{xx} + \sigma_{uu} \end{pmatrix}^{-1} \begin{pmatrix} \sigma_{zz} & \sigma_{zx} \\ \sigma_{xz} & \sigma_{xx} \end{pmatrix} \begin{pmatrix} \beta_z \\ \beta_x \end{pmatrix} \tag{5.4}$$

and not $(\beta_z^T, \beta_x^T)^T$. For the case of multiple predictors measured with error with no restrictions on the covariance matrices of the predictors or the measurement errors, bias in individual coefficients can take almost any form. Coefficients can be attenuated toward the null, or inflated away from zero. The bias is not always multiplicative. The sign of coefficients can change, and zero coefficients can become nonzero (i.e., null predictors can appear to be significant). There is very little that can be said in general and individual cases must be analyzed separately.

However, in the case of one variable measured with error, i.e., X is a scalar, the attenuation factor in β_{x*} is $\lambda_1 = \sigma_{x|z}^2/(\sigma_{x|z}^2 + \sigma_u^2)$ where $\sigma_{x|z}^2$ is the residual variance from the regression of X on Z, that is, $\beta_{x*} = \lambda_1 \beta_x$. Because $\sigma_{x|z}^2 \leq \sigma_x^2$, attenuation is accentuated relative to the case of no covariates when the covariates in the model are correlated with X, i.e., $\lambda_1 \leq \lambda$ with strict inequality when $\sigma_{x|z}^2 < \sigma_x^2$. Also, in the case of a single variable measured with error, $\beta_{z*} = \beta_z + (1 - \lambda_1)\beta_x\Gamma_z$, where Γ_z is the coefficient vector of Z in the regression of X on Z, that is, $E(X|Z) = \Gamma_1 + \Gamma_z^T Z$. Thus measurement error in X can induce bias in the regression coefficients of Z. This has important implications for analysis of covariance models in which the continuous predictor is measured with error (Carroll 1989; Carroll et al. 1985).

The effects of measurement error on naive tests of hypotheses can be understood by exploiting the fact that in the classical error model W is a surrogate. In this case $E(Y|Z,W) = E\{E(Y|Z,X,W)|Z,W\} = E\{E(Y|Z,X)|Z,W\} = \beta_1 + \beta_z^T Z + \beta_x^T E(X|Z,W)$. With multivariate normality $E(X|Z,W)$ is linear, say $E(X|Z,W) = \alpha_0 + \alpha_z^T Z + \alpha_w W$, and thus

$$E(Y|Z,W) = \beta_0 + \beta_x^T \alpha_0 + \left(\beta_z^T + \beta_x^T \alpha_z^T\right) Z + \beta_x^T \alpha_w^T W. \tag{5.5}$$

This expression holds for any surrogate W. Our summary of hypothesis testing in the presence of measurement error is appropriate for any surrogate variable model provided α_w^T is an invertible matrix, as it is for the classical error model. Suppose that the naive model is parameterized

$$E(Y|Z,W) = \gamma_0 + \gamma_z^T Z + \gamma_w^T W. \tag{5.6}$$

A comparison of (5.5) and (5.6) reveals the main effects of measurement error on hypothesis testing.

First note that $(\beta_z^T, \beta_x^T)^T = 0$ if and only if $(\gamma_z^T, \gamma_x^T)^T = 0$. This implies that the naive-model test that none of the predictors are useful for explaining variation in Y is valid in the sense of having the desired Type I error rate. Further examination of (5.5) and (5.6) shows that $\gamma_z = 0$ is equivalent to $\beta_z = 0$, only if $\alpha_z \beta_x = 0$. It follows that the naive test of $H_0 : \beta_z = 0$ is valid only if X is unrelated to Y ($\beta_x = 0$) or if Z is unrelated to X ($\alpha_z = 0$). Finally, the fact that $\beta_x = 0$ is equivalent to $\alpha_w\beta_x = 0$ implies that the naive test of $H_0 : \beta_x = 0$ is valid. The naive tests that are valid, i.e., those that maintain the Type I error rate, will still suffer reduced power relative to the test based on the true data.

Nonlinear Regression

5.2.5

The effects of measurement error in nonlinear models are much the same qualitatively as in the normal linear model. The use of a surrogate measurement generally results in reduced power for testing associations, produces parameter bias, and results in a model with less predictive power. However, the nature of the bias depends on the model, the type of parameter, and the error model. Generally, the more nonlinear the model is, the less relevant are the results for the linear model. Parameters other than linear regression coefficients (e.g., polynomial coefficients, transformation parameters, and variance function parameters) have no counterpart in the normal linear model and the effect of measurement errors on such parameters must be studied on a case-by-case basis.

Regression coefficients in generalized linear models, including models of particular interest in epidemiology such as logistic regression and Poisson regression, are affected by measurement error in much the same manner as are linear model regression coefficients. This means that relative risks and odds ratios derived from logistic regressions models are affected by measurement error much the same as linear model regression coefficients (Rosner et al. 1989, 1990; Stefanski 1985; Stefanski and Carroll 1985). However, unlike the linear model, unbiased Berkson measurements generally produce biases in nonlinear models, although they are often much less severe than biases resulting from classical measurement errors (for comparable ρ_{xw}). This fact forms the basis for the method known as *regression calibration* in which an unbiased Berkson predictor is estimated by a preliminary calibration analysis, and then the usual (naive) analysis is performed with $E(\widehat{X|W})$ replacing X. This fact also explains why more attention is paid to the classical error model than to the Berkson error model.

The effects of classical measurement error on flexible regression models, e.g., nonparametric regression, is not easily quantified, but there are general tendencies worth noting. Measurement error generally smooths out regression functions. Nonlinear features of $E(Y|X)$ such as curvature of local extremes, points of non-differentiability, and discontinuities will generally be less pronounced or absent in $E(Y|W)$. For normal measurement error, $E(Y|W)$ is smooth whether $E(Y|X)$ is or is not, and local maxima and minima will be less extreme – measurement error tends to wear off the peaks and fill in the valleys. This can be seen in a simple parametric model. If $E(Y|X) = \beta_0 + \beta_1 X + \beta_2 X^2$ and (X, W) are jointly normal with $\mu_x = 0$, then $E(Y|W)$ is also quadratic with the quadratic coefficient attenuated by ρ_{xw}^4. The local extremes of the two regressions differ by $\beta_2 \sigma_x^2 (1 - \rho_{xw}^2)$ which is positive (negative) when $E(Y|X)$ is convex (concave). Finally we note that monotonicity of regression functions can sometimes be affected by heavy-tailed measurement error (Hwang and Stefanski 1994).

The effects of classical measurement error on density estimation is qualitatively similar to that of nonparametric regressions. Modes are attenuated and regions of low density are inflated. Measurement error can mask multimodality in the true density and will inflate the tails of the distribution. Naive estimates of tail quantiles are generally more extreme than the corresponding true-data estimates.

5.2.6   Logistic Regression Example

This section closes with an empirical example illustrating the effects of measurement error in logistic regression and the utility of the multivariate normal linear regression model results for approximating the effects of measurement error. The data used are a subset of the Framingham Heart Study data and are described in detail in Carroll et al. (1995). For these data X is long-term average systolic blood pressure after transformation via ln(SBP-50), denoted TSBP. There are replicate measurements (W_1, W_2) for each of $n = 1615$ subjects in the study. The true-data model is logistic regression of coronary heart disease $(0, 1)$ on X and covariates (Z) including age, smoking status $(0, 1)$, and cholesterol level.

Assuming the classical error model for the replicate measurements, $W_j = X + U_j$, analysis of variance produces the estimate $\widehat{\sigma}_u^2 = 0.0126$. The average $\overline{W} = (W_1 + W_2)/2$ provides the best measurement of X with an error variance of $\sigma_U^2/2$ (with estimate 0.0063).

The three measurements, W_1, W_2 and $\overline{W}$, can be used to empirically demonstrate attenuation due to measurement error. The measurement error variances of W_1 and W_2 are equal and are twice as large the measurement error variance of $\overline{W}$. Thus the attenuation in the regressions using W_1 and W_2 should be equal; whereas the regression using $\overline{W}$ should be less attenuated. Three naive logistic models,

$$\text{logit}\{\Pr(\text{CHD} = 1)\} = \beta_0 + \beta_{z_1}\text{AGE} + \beta_{z_2}\text{SMOKE} + \beta_{z_3}\text{CHOL} + \beta_x\text{TSBP}$$

were fit using each of the three measurements W_1, W_2 and $\overline{W}$. The estimates of the TSBP coefficient from the logistic regressions using W_1 and W_2 are both 1.5 (to one decimal place). The coefficient estimate from the fit using $\overline{W}$ is 1.7. The relative magnitudes of the coefficients $(1.5 < 1.7)$ are consistent with the anticipated effects of measurement error – greater attenuation associated with larger error variance. The multiple linear regression attenuation coefficient for a measurement with error variance σ^2 is $\lambda_1 = \sigma_{x|z}^2/(\sigma_{x|z}^2 + \sigma^2)$. Assuming that this applies approximately to the logistic model suggests that

$$1.7 \approx \frac{\sigma_{x|z}^2}{\sigma_{x|z}^2 + \sigma_u^2/2}\beta_x \qquad \text{and} \qquad 1.5 \approx \frac{\sigma_{x|z}^2}{\sigma_{x|z}^2 + \sigma_u^2}\beta_x.$$

Because β_x is unknown these approximations cannot be checked directly. However, a check on their consistency is obtained by taking ratios leading to $1.13 = 1.7/1.5 \approx (\sigma_{x|z}^2 + \sigma_u^2)/(\sigma_{x|z}^2 + \sigma_u^2/2)$. Using the ANOVA estimate, $\widehat{\sigma}_u^2 = 0.0126$, and the mean squared error from the linear regression of $\overline{W}$ on AGE, SMOKE and CHOL as an estimate of $\sigma_{\overline{w}|z}^2$, produces the estimate $\widehat{\sigma}_{x|z}^2 = \widehat{\sigma}_{\overline{w}|z}^2 - \widehat{\sigma}_u^2/2 = 0.0423 - 0.0063 = 0.0360$. Thus $(\sigma_{x|z}^2 + \sigma_u^2)/(\sigma_{x|z}^2 + \sigma_u^2/2)$ is estimated to be $(0.0360 + 0.0126)/(0.0360 + 0.0063) = 1.15$. In other words, the attenuation in the logistic regression coefficients is consistent $(1.13 \approx 1.15)$ with the attenuation predicted by the normal linear regression model result.

These basic statistics can also be used to calculate a simple bias-adjusted estimator as $\widehat{\beta}_x = 1.7(\widehat{\sigma}_{x|z}^2 + \widehat{\sigma}_u^2/2)/\widehat{\sigma}_{x|z}^2 = 1.7(0.0360 + 0.0063)/0.0360 = 2.0$, which is consistent with estimates reported by Carroll et al. (1995) obtained using a variety of measurement error estimation techniques. We do not recommend using linear model corrections for the logistic model because there are number of methods more suited to the task as described in Sect. 5.4. Our intent with this example is to demonstrate the general relevance of the easily-derived theoretical results for linear regression to other generalized linear models.

The odds ratio for a Δ change in transformed systolic blood pressure is $\exp(\beta_x \Delta)$. With the naive analysis this is estimated to be $\exp(1.7\Delta)$; the bias-corrected analysis produces the estimate $\exp(2.0\Delta)$. Therefore the naive odds ratio is attenuated by approximately $\exp(-0.3\Delta)$. More generally, the naive (OR_N) and true (OR_T) odd ratios are related via $OR_N/OR_T = OR_T^{\lambda_1 - 1}$, where λ_1 is the attenuation factor in the naive estimate of β_x. The naive and true relative risks have approximately the same relationship under the same conditions (small risks) that justify approximating relative risks by odds ratios.

Planning Epidemiologic Studies
5.3   **with Measurement Error**

As the previous sections have established, exposure measurement error is common in epidemiologic studies and, under certain assumptions, can be shown to have dramatic effects on the properties of relative risk estimates or other types of coefficients derived from epidemiologic regression models. It is wise therefore to include measurement error considerations in the planning of a study, both to enable the application of a measurement error analysis at the conclusion of the study and to assure scientific validity.

In developing a useful plan, one must consider a number of important questions. To begin with, what are the scientific objectives of the study? Is the goal to identify a new risk factor for disease, perhaps for the first time, or is this a study to provide improved estimates of the quantitative impact of a known risk factor? Is prediction of future risks the ultimate goal? The answers to these questions will determine the possible responses to dealing with the measurement error in the design and analysis of the study, including the choice of a criterion for statistical optimality. It is even possible that no measurement error correction is needed to achieve the purposes of the study, and in certain instances, absent other considerations such as cost, that *the most scientifically valid design would eliminate measurement error entirely.*

The nature of the measurement error should be carefully considered. For instance, is the measurement error nondifferential? What is the evidence to support this conclusion? Especially in the study of complex phenomena such as nutritional factors in disease, the nondifferential assumption deserves scrutiny. For example, much has been made of the diet "record" as the gold standard of nutritional intakes, but recent analyses have cast doubt on the nondifferential measurement error associated with substituting monthly food frequency questionnaires (Kipnis et al. 1999). On the other hand, measurement errors due to validated scientific instrument errors may be more easily justified as nondifferential.

Another thing to consider is the possible time dependency of exposure errors, and how this may affect the use of nondifferential models. This often arises in case-control studies where exposures must be assessed retrospectively (cf. Chap. I.6 of this handbook). An interesting example occurs in a recent study of arsenic exposure where both drinking water and toenail measurements are available as personal exposure measures in a cancer case-control study (Karagas et al. 1998). Toenail concentrations give a biologically time-averaged measure of exposure, but the time scale is limited and the nail concentrations are influenced by individual metabolic processes. Drinking water concentrations may be free from possible confounding due to unrelated factors affecting metabolic pathways, but could be less representative of average exposures over the time interval of interest. This kind of ambiguity is common in many epidemiologic modelling situations, and should indicate caution in the rote application of measurement error methods.

Depending on the type of nondifferential error, different study plans may be required to identify the desired relative risk parameters. For instance, replicate measurements of an exposure variable may adequately identify the necessary variance parameters in a classical measurement error model. Under certain circumstances, an "instrumental" variable may provide the information needed to correct for measurement error. This type of reliability/validity data leads to identifiable relative risk regression parameters in classical or Berkson case error.

In more complex "surrogate" variable situations with nondifferential error, an internal or external validation study may be necessary, where the "true" exposure is measured without error is available for a subset or independent sample of subjects. These designs are also useful and appropriate for classical measurement error models, but are essential in the case of surrogates which cannot be considered "unbiased". Internal validation studies have the capability of checking the nondifferential assumption, and thus are potentially more valuable. With external validation studies, there may be doubt as to whether the populations characterized by the validation and main study samples are comparable in the sense that the measurement error model is equivalent or "transportable" between the populations. The issue of whether an error model is transportable or not can arise with any type of measurement error.

The considerations described above are summarized in the following table (Table 5.2) for some of the options that should be considered when planning a study in the presence of measurement error.

Based on validity concerns alone, internal validation studies may have the greatest advantage. However, this neglects the important issue of the costs of obtaining the true exposures, which may be considerably larger than those for a more readily available surrogate. For instance, it may be the case that a classical additive error model applies and that replicate measures are easier or cheaper to get than true values. Depending on the relative impact on the optimality criterion used, the replicate design might be more cost-effective, although the internal validation study would still be valid.

A number of approaches have been suggested and used for the design of epidemiologic studies based on variables measured with error. These may be characterized broadly as sample size calculation methods, where the design decision

Table 5.2. Sampling plan options for collecting validation data in epidemiologic studies with measurement error of different types or properties

Measurement error type/property	Replicates	Validation Data		
		Instrumental variables	External study	Internal study
Classical	yes	yes	yes	yes
Berkson	no	yes	yes	yes
General surrogate	no	no	yes	yes
Differential	no	no	no	yes
Non-transportable	yes	yes	no	yes

to be made has to do mainly with the size of the main study in studies where the measurement error is known or can be ignored; and design approaches for studies using internal or external validation data where both the size of the main study and the validation sample must be chosen. In the sections that follow, we review both of these approaches.

5.3.1   Methods for Sample Size Calculations

Methods for sample size calculations are typically based on the operating characteristics of a simple hypothesis test. In the case of measurement error in a risk factor included in an epidemiologic regression model, the null hypothesis is that the regression coefficient for the risk factor equals zero, implying no association between the exposure and the health outcome. For a specific alternative one might calculate the power for a given sample size or, alternatively, the sample size required to achieve a given power.

It has been known for some time that the effect of measurement error is to reduce the power of the test for no association both in linear models (Cochran 1968) and 2×2 tables with nondifferential misclassification (Fleiss 1981). This result has been extended to survival models (Prentice 1982) and to generalized linear models with nondifferential exposure measurement error (Tosteson and Tsiatis 1988), including linear regression, logistic regression, and tests for association in 2×2 contingency tables. Using small relative risk approximations, it is possible to show that for all of these common models for epidemiologic data, the ratio of the sample size required using the data measured without error to the sample size required using the error prone exposure is approximately $n_x/n_w \approx \rho_{xw}^2$, the square of the correlation between X and W; see also (5.3), Sect. 5.2.3. This relation provides a handy method for determining sample size requirements in the presence of measurement error as

$$n_w = n_x/\rho_{xw}^2 .$$

(5.7)

If additional covariates Z are included in the calculation, a partial correlation can be used instead. The same formula has been used for sample size calculations based on regression models for prospective studies with log-linear risk functions and normal distributions for exposures and measurement error (McKeown-Eyssen and Tibshirani 1994) and case-control studies with conditionally normal exposures within the case and control groups (White et al. 1994). Recent developments have improved this approximation (Tosteson et al. 2003), but (5.7) remains a useful tool for checking sample size requirements in studies with measurement error.

For generalized linear models (Tosteson and Tsiatis 1988) and survival models (Prentice 1982), it has been shown that optimal score test can be computed by replacing the error prone exposure variable W with $E[X|W]$, a technique that was later termed regression calibration (Carroll et al. 1995). Subsequent work extended these results to a more general form of the score test incorporating a nonparametric estimate of the measurement error distribution (Stefanski and Carroll 1990a). One implication of this result is that in common measurement error models, including normally distributed exposure errors and nondifferential misclassification errors, the optimal test is computed simply by ignoring the measurement error and using the usual test based on W rather than X, the true exposure. However, the test will still suffer the loss of power implicit in (5.7).

It is interesting to consider the effects of Berkson case errors on sample size calculations. The implication for analysis are somewhat different, in as much as regression coefficients are unbiased by Berkson case errors for linear models and to the first order for all generalized linear models. However, as applied to epidemiologic research, there is no distinction with respect to the effects of this type of nondifferential sample size calculations for simple regression models without confounders, and (5.7) applies directly.

Planning for Reliability/Validation Data 5.3.2

In most epidemiologic applications, a measurement error correction will be planned, although this may be deemed unnecessary in some situations where the investigators only wish to demonstrate an association or where the measurement error is known. Information on the measurement error parameters can come from a number of possible designs, including replicate measurements, instrumental variables, external validation studies measuring the true and surrogate exposures (i.e. just X and W), or internal validation studies. A variety of statistical criteria can be used to optimize aspects of the design, most commonly the variance of the unbiased estimate of the relative risk for the exposure measured with error. Other criteria have included the power of tests of association, as in the previous section, and criteria based on the power of tests for null hypotheses other than no association (Spiegelman and Gray 1991).

To choose a design, it is usually necessary to have an estimate of the measurement error variance or other parameters. This may be difficult, since validation data are needed to derive these estimates, and will not yet have been collected at the time when the study is being planned. However, this dilemma is present in most practical design settings and can be overcome in a number of informal ways by deriving estimates from previous publications, pilot data, or theoretical considerations of the measurement error process. Certain sequential designs can be useful in this regard, and some suggestions are discussed here in the context of the design of internal validation studies.

In studies where a correction is planned for classical measurement error using replicates, the simple approach to sample size calculations may provide a guideline for choosing an appropriate number of replicates and a sample size by replacing ρ_{xw}^2 with $\rho_{x\overline{w}}^2$, where $\overline{w}$ is the mean of the n_r replicates. Depending on the relative costs of replication and obtaining a study participant, these expressions may be used to find an optimal value for the overall sample size, n, and the number of replicates, n_r. For instrumental variables, a similar calculation can be made using a variation on the regression calibration procedure as applied to the score test for no association. In this case, the inflation in sample size for (5.7) is based on $\rho_{x\widehat{x}}^2$, where $\widehat{x} = E[X|W, T]$, the predicted value of the true exposure given the unbiased surrogate W and the instrumental variable T.

External and internal validation studies both involve a main study, with a sample size of n_1 and a validation study, with sample size of n_2. The external validation study involves a independent set of measurements of the true and surrogate exposures, whereas the internal validation study is based on a subset of the subjects in the main study. Both the size of the main study and the validation study must be specified. In the internal validation study, n_2 is by necessity less than or equal to n_1, with equality implying a fully-validated design. In the external validation study, n_2 is not limited, but the impact of increasing the amount of validation data is more limited than in the internal validation study. This is because the fully validated internal validation study has no loss of power versus a study that has no measurement error, whereas the external validation study can only improve the power to the same as that of a study with measurement error where the measurement error parameters are known.

For common nonlinear epidemiologic regression analyses such as logistic regression, calculations to determine optimal values of n_1 and n_2 have typically involved specialized calculations (Spiegelman and Gray 1991; Stram et al. 1995). Less intractable expressions are available for linear discriminant models, not involving numerical integrations (Buonaccorsi 1988). The actual analysis of the data from the studies may be possible using approximations such as the regression calibration method requiring less sophisticated software (Spiegelman et al. 2001).

A variant on the internal validation study are designs which use surrogate exposures and outcomes as stratification variables to select a highly efficient validation sample. Cain and Breslow (1988) develop methods for case control studies where surrogate variables were available during the design phase for cases and controls. Tosteson and Ware (1990) develop methods for studies where surrogates were available for both exposures and a binary outcome. These designs can be analyzed with ordinary logistic regression if that model is appropriate for the population data. Methods for improving the analysis of the designs and adapting them to other regression models have been proposed (Tosteson et al. 1994; Holcroft et al. 1997; Reilly 1996).

Examples and Applications

Much of the research on methods for planning studies with measurement error has been stimulated by applications from environmental, nutritional, and occupational epidemiology. Nevertheless, it is fair to say that published examples of studies designed with measurement error in mind are relatively rare and the best source of case studies may be methods papers such as those cited in this review. This may reflect a lack of convenient statistical software other than what individual researchers have been able to make available. However, some useful calculations can be quite simple, as shown above, and a more important factor in future applications of these methods will be proper education to raise the awareness among statisticians and epidemiologists of the importance of addressing the problem of measurement error in the planning phases of health research.

Measurement Error Models and Methods

Overview

This section describes some common methods for correcting biases induced by non-differential covariate measurement error. The focus is on nonlinear regression models, and the logistic model in particular, though all the methods apply to the linear model. The intent is to familiarize the reader with the central themes and key ideas that underlie the proposals, and provide a contrast of the assumptions and types of data required to implement the procedures.

The starting point for all measurement error analyses is the disease model of interest relating the disease outcome Y to the true exposure(s) X and covariates Z, and a measurement error model relating the mismeasured exposure W to (Z, X). Measurement error methods can be grouped according to whether they employ *functional* or *structural* modeling. Functional models make no assumptions on X, beyond what are made in the absence of measurement error, e.g., $\sum_{i=1}^{n}(X_i - \overline{X})^2 > 0$ for simple linear regression. Functional modeling is compelling because often there is little information in the data on the distribution of X. For this reason, much of the initial research in measurement error methods focused on functional modeling. Methods based on functional modeling can be divided into approximately consistent (remove most bias) and fully consistent methods (remove all bias as $n \to \infty$). Fully consistent methods for nonlinear regression models typically require assumptions on the distribution of the measurement error. Regression calibration and SIMEX are examples of approximately consistent methods while corrected scores, conditional scores and some instrumental variable (IV) methods are fully consistent for large classes of models. Each of these approaches is described below.

Structural models assume X is random and require an exposure model for X, with the normal distribution as the default exposure model. Likelihood based methods are used with structural models.

Note that the terms functional and structural refer to assumptions on X, not on the measurement error model. The advantage of functional modeling is it provides valid inference regardless of the distribution of X. On the other hand, structural modeling can result in large gains in efficiency and allows construction of likelihood ratio based confidence intervals that often have coverage probabilities closer to the nominal level than large sample normal theory intervals used with functional models. The choice between functional or structural modeling depends both on the assumptions one is willing to make and, in a few cases, the form of the model relating Y to (Z, X). The type and amount of data available also plays a role. For example, validation data provides information on the distribution of X, and may make structural modeling more palatable. The remainder of the chapter describes methods for correcting for measurement error. Functional methods are described first.

5.4.2   Regression Calibration

Regression calibration is a conceptually straightforward approach to bias reduction and has been successfully applied to a broad range of regression models. It is the default approach for the linear model. The method is fully consistent in linear models and log-linear models when the conditional variance of X given (Z, W) is constant. Regression calibration is approximately consistent in non-linear models. The method was first studied in the context of proportional hazards regression (Prentice 1982). Extensions to logistic regression and a general class of regression models are studied in Rosner et al. (1989, 1990) and Carroll and Stefanski (1990), respectively. A detailed and comprehensive discussion of regression calibration can be found in Carroll et al. (1995).

When the measurement error is non-differential, the induced disease model, or regression model, relating Y to the observed exposure W and covariates Z is $E[Y|Z, W] = E[E[Y|Z, X]|Z, W]$, i.e. the induced disease model is obtained by regressing the true disease model on (Z, W). A consequence of the identity is that the form of the observed disease model depends on the conditional distribution of X given (Z, W). This distribution is typically not known, and even when known evaluating the right hand side of the identity can be difficult. For example, if the true disease model is logistic and the distribution of X conditional on (Z, W) is normal, there is no closed form expression for $E[Y|Z, W]$.

Regression calibration circumvents these problems by approximating the disease model relating Y to the observed covariates (Z, W). The approximation is obtained by replacing X with $E[X|Z, W]$ in the model relating Y to (Z, X). Because regression calibration provides a model for Y on (Z, W), the observed data can be used to assess the adequacy of the model.

To describe how to implement the method, it is useful to think of the approach as a method for imputing values for X. The idea is to estimate unobserved X

with $X^* \equiv$ predicted value of X from the regression of X on (Z, W), see the discussion of Berkson error calibration in Sect. 5.2.2. Modeling and estimating the regression of X on (Z, W) requires additional data in the form of internal/external replicate observations, instrumental variables or validation data, see the example below. The regression parameters in the true disease model are estimated by regressing Y on (Z, X^*). Note that X^* is the best estimate of X using the observed predictors (Z, W); best in the sense of minimizing mean square prediction error. To summarize, regression calibration estimation consists of two steps:

1. Model and estimate the regression of X on (Z, W) to obtain X^*;
2. Regress Y on (Z, X^*) to obtain regression parameter estimates.

A convenient feature of regression calibration is that standard software can often be used for estimation. However, standard errors for parameter estimates in Step 2 must account for the fact that X^* is estimated in Step 1, something standard software does not do. Bootstrap or asymptotic methods based on estimating equation theory are typically used, see Carroll et al. (1995) for details.

When (Z, X, W) is approximately jointly normal, or when X is strongly correlated with (Z, W), the regression of X on (Z, W) is approximately linear:

$$E[X|Z, W] \approx \mu_x + \sigma_{x|zw}\sigma_{zw}^{-1} \begin{pmatrix} Z - \mu_z \\ W - \mu_w \end{pmatrix},$$

where $\sigma_{x|zw}$ is the covariance of X with (Z, W) and σ_{zw} is the variance matrix of (Z, W). Implementing regression calibration using the linear approximation requires estimation of the calibration parameters μ_x, $\sigma_{x|zw}$, σ_{zw}, μ_w, and μ_z.

Example 1. We illustrate estimation of the calibration function when two replicate observations of X are available in the primary study (internal reliability data) and the error model is $W = X + \sigma U$. For ease of illustration, we assume there are no additional covariates Z. Let $\{W_{i1}, W_{i2}\}_{i=1}^{n}$ denote the replication data and suppose that $E[X_i|\bar{W}_i] \approx \mu_x + \sigma_{x|\bar{w}}\sigma_{\bar{w}}^{-1}(\bar{W}_i - \mu_w) = \mu_w + ((\sigma_{\bar{w}}^2 - \sigma^2/2)/\sigma_{\bar{w}}^2)(\bar{W}_i - \mu_w)$ where $\bar{W}_i = (W_{i1} + W_{i2})/2$, and the last equality follows from the form of the error model. Note that $(\sigma_{\bar{w}}^2 - \sigma^2/2)/(\sigma_{\bar{w}}^2)$ is the attenuation factor introduced in Sect. 5.2.3. The method-of-moments calibration parameter estimators are $\widehat{\mu}_w = \sum_{i=1}^{n} \bar{W}_i/n$, $\widehat{\sigma}_{\bar{w}}^2 = \sum_{i=1}^{n}(\bar{W}_i - \widehat{\mu}_w)^2/(n-1)$ and $\widehat{\sigma}^2 = \sum_{i=1}^{n}\sum_{j=1}^{2}(W_{ij} - \bar{W}_i)^2/n = \sum_{i=1}^{n}(W_{i1} - W_{i2})^2/2n$. The imputed value for X_i is $X_i^* = \widehat{\mu}_w + ((\widehat{\sigma}_{\bar{w}}^2 - \widehat{\sigma}^2/2)/\widehat{\sigma}_{\bar{w}}^2)(\bar{W}_i - \widehat{\mu}_w)$.
For the Framingham data described in Sect. 5.2.6, recall that $\{W_{i1}, W_{i2}\}_{i=1}^{1615}$ represented transformed systolic blood pressure measured for each subject at two separate exams. For these data, $\widehat{\sigma}^2 = 0.0126$, $\widehat{\sigma}_{\bar{w}}^2 = 0.0454$ and $\widehat{\mu}_w = 4.36$ so that the imputed measurement is $X_i^* = 4.36 + 0.86(\bar{W}_i - 4.36)$.
If the model relating Y to X is the simple linear regression model, $(Y = \beta_1 + \beta_x X + \varepsilon)$, regressing Y on X^* results in $\widehat{\beta}_x = (\widehat{\sigma}_{\bar{w}}^2)/(\widehat{\sigma}_{\bar{w}}^2 - \widehat{\sigma}^2/2)\widehat{\beta}_{\bar{w}}$ where $\widehat{\beta}_{\bar{w}}$ is the naive esti-

mator obtained from regressing Y on $\bar{W}$. Note for the linear model the regression calibration estimator coincides with the method-of-moments estimator given in Sect. 5.2 of this chapter.

Our illustration of calibration parameter estimation assumed exactly two replicates were available for each X_i. This estimation scheme can be easily extended to an arbitrary number of replicates for each X_i (Carroll et al. 1995).

Regression calibration is not as effective in reducing bias in nonlinear models when: (1) the effect of X on Y is large, for example large odds ratios in logistic regression; (2) the measurement error variance is large; and (3) the model relating Y to (Z, X) is not smooth. It is difficult to quantify what is meant by large in (1) and (2) because all three factors (1)–(3) can act together. In logistic regression, the method has been found to be effective in a number of applications (Rosner et al. 1989, 1990; Carroll et al. 1995). Segmented regression is an example of a model where regression calibration fails due to lack of model smoothness (Küchenhoff and Carroll 1997). Segmented models relate Y to X using separate regression models on different segments along the range of X. Extensions of regression calibration that address the potential pitfalls listed in (1)–(3) are given in Carroll and Stefanski (1990).

$\blacklozenge$

5.4.3   SIMEX

Simulation-extrapolation (SIMEX) can correct for bias in a very broad range of settings and is the only method that provides a visual display of the effects of measurement error on regression parameter estimation. SIMEX is fully consistent for linear disease models and approximate for nonlinear models. SIMEX is founded on the observation that bias in parameter estimation varies in a systematic way with the magnitude of the measurement error. Essentially, the method is to incrementally add measurement error to W using computer simulated random errors and compute the corresponding regression parameter estimate (simulation step). The extrapolation step models the relation between the parameter estimates and the magnitude of the measurement errors. The SIMEX estimate is the extrapolation of this relation to the case of zero measurement error.

The method was developed in a series of papers (Cook and Stefanski 1995; Stefanski and Cook 1995; Carroll et al. 1996) and is summarized in detail in Carroll et al. (1995). Further refinements and application of the SIMEX method appear in a number of papers (Stefanski and Bay 1996; Lin and Carroll 1999; Wang et al. 1998; Li and Lin 2003; Kim and Gleser 2000; Kim et al. 2000; Holcomb 1999; Marcus and Elais 1998).

Details of the method are best understood in the context of the classical additive measurement error model. However, the method is not limited to this model. To describe the method, suppose $W_i = X_i + \sigma U_i$ for $i = 1, \ldots, n$ and for $s = 1, \ldots, B$, define $W_{is}(\lambda) = W_i + \sqrt{\lambda}\sigma U_{is}$ where $\lambda > 0$, and $\{U_{is}\}_{s=1}^{B}$ are i.i.d. computer simulated standard normal variates. Note that the variance of the measurement error for the constructed measurement $W_{is}(\lambda)$ is $(1 + \lambda)\sigma^2$, indicating that λ regulates the magnitude of the measurement error. Let $\widehat{\beta}_s(\lambda_j)$ denote the vector of regression parameter estimators obtained by regression of Y on $\{Z, W_s(\lambda_j)\}$ for $0 = \lambda_1 < \lambda_2 < \cdots < \lambda_M$. The value $\lambda_M = 2$ is recommended (Carroll et al. 1995). The notation explicitly indicates the dependence of the estimator on λ_j. Let $\widehat{\beta}(\lambda_j) = B^{-1}\sum_{s=1}^{B}\widehat{\beta}_s(\lambda_j)$. Here we are averaging over the B simulated samples to eliminate variability due to simulation, and empirical evidence suggests $B = 100$ is sufficient. Each component of the vector $\widehat{\beta}(\lambda)$ is then modeled as a function of λ and the SIMEX estimator is the extrapolation of each model to $\lambda = -1$. Note that $\lambda = -1$ represents a measurement error variance of zero.

Consider, for example, estimation of β_x. The 'observations' produced by the simulation $\{\widehat{\beta}_x(\lambda_j), \lambda_j\}_{j=1}^{M}$ are plotted and used to develop and fit an extrapolation model relating the dependent variable $\widehat{\beta}_x(\lambda)$ to the independent variable λ. In most applications, an adequate extrapolation model is provided by either the nonlinear extrapolant function, $\widehat{\beta}_x(\lambda_j) \approx \gamma_1 + (\gamma_2/(\gamma_3 + \lambda))$, or a quadratic extrapolant function, $\widehat{\beta}_x(\lambda_j) \approx \gamma_1 + \gamma_2\lambda + \gamma_3\lambda^2$. The appropriate extrapolant function is fit to $\{\widehat{\beta}_x(\lambda_j), \lambda_j\}_{j=1}^{M}$ using ordinary least squares. It is worth noting that the nonlinear extrapolant function can be difficult to fit numerically and details for doing so are given in Carroll et al. (1995).

Analytic Example

SIMEX was developed to understand and correct for the effects of covariate measurement error in nonlinear disease models. However, it is instructive to consider the simple linear regression model to illustrate analytically the relation between $\widehat{\beta}(\lambda)$ and λ. In Sect. 5.2 the bias of the naive estimator was studied and it follows that $\widehat{\beta}_x(\lambda) = (\beta_x\sigma_x^2/(\sigma_x^2 + \sigma^2(1+\lambda))) + O_p(n^{-(1/2)})$ where the symbol $O_p(n^{-(1/2)})$ denotes terms that are negligible for n large. Therefore, the nonlinear extrapolant will result in a fully consistent estimator; $\widehat{\beta}_x(-1) = (\beta_x\sigma_x^2)/(\sigma_x^2 + \sigma^2(1 + [-1])) + O_p(n^{-(1/2)}) = \beta_x + O_p(n^{-(1/2)})$.

Graphic Example

The Framingham data described in Sect. 5.2.6 are used here to graphically illustrate the SIMEX method. In that section a logistic model was defined relating the probability of developing coronary heart disease to age, smoking status, cholesterol level and a transformation of systolic blood pressure. Figure 5.1 depicts the effect of increasing amounts of measurement error on parameter estimates (log odds ratios), and the SIMEX extrapolation to the case of no measurement error. Note that the nonlinear and quadratic extrapolants result in similar estimates.

Refinements and further details for the SIMEX method, including calculation of standard errors, have been developed, see Carroll et al. (1995).

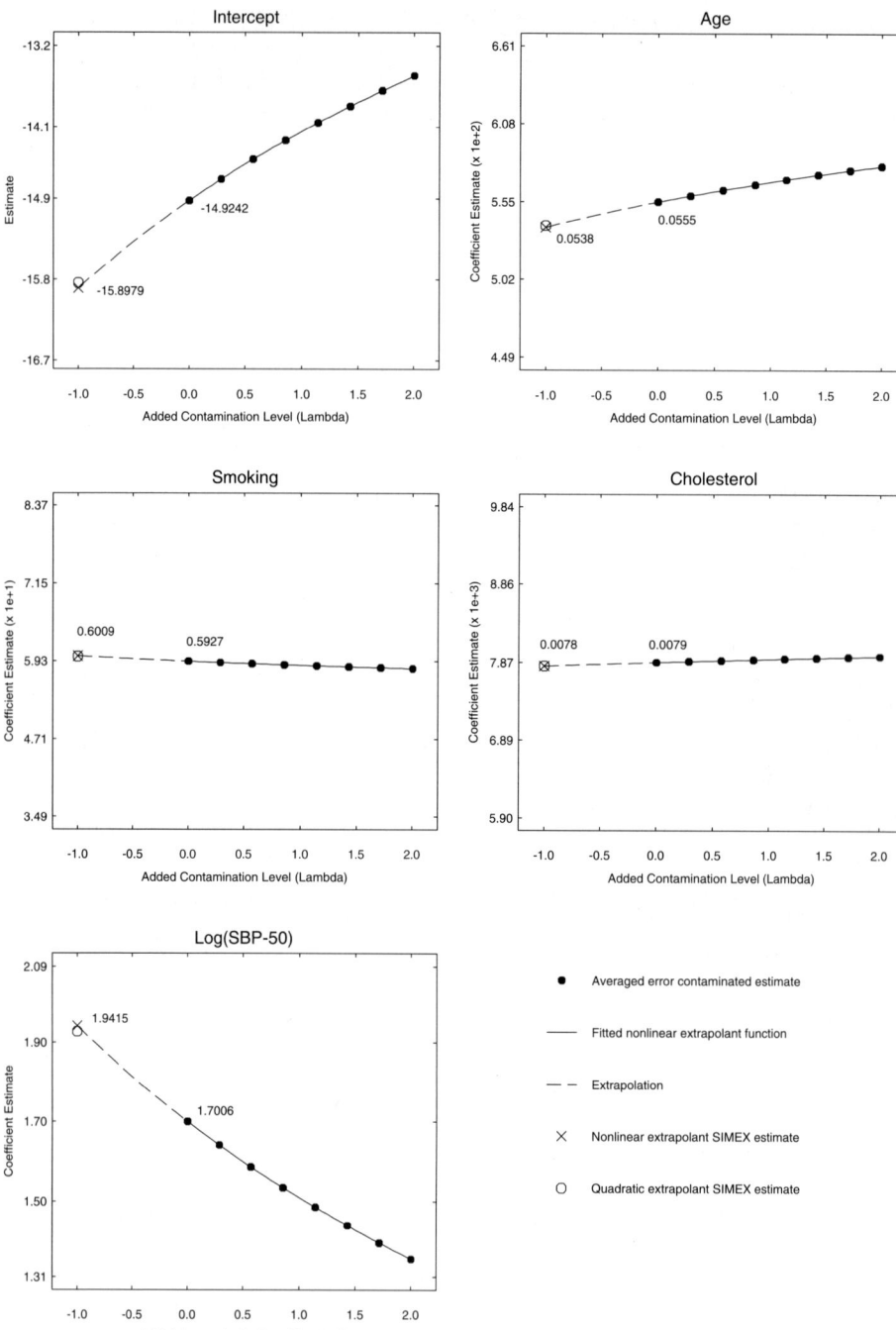

Figure 5.1. SIMEX Extrapolation Plots for the Framingham data. *Vertical axis* scaling is ± two standard errors of the naive estimates

Estimating Equations and Corrected Scores

Regression parameter estimators in nonlinear models are defined implicitly through estimating equations. Estimating equations are often based on the likelihood *score*, i.e. the derivative of the log-likelihood, or quasi-likelihood scores that only require assumptions on the first and second conditional moments of the disease model. The criterion of least squares also leads to parameter estimation based on estimating equations.

Corrected scores, conditional scores and certain instrumental variable methods have been developed starting with the estimating equations that define regression parameter estimates in the absence of measurement error. An estimating score is *unbiased* if it has expectation zero. Measurement error induces bias in estimating equations, which translates into bias in the parameter estimator. Modifying the estimating equations to remove bias produces estimators without bias. This is readily seen in the no-intercept simple linear regression model with classical measurement error; $Y = \beta_x X + \varepsilon$, $W = X + \sigma U$ and where X, ε and U have mean zero. In the absence of measurement error, the least squares estimator for β_x solves $\sum_{i=1}^{n} \psi(Y_i, X_i; \beta_x) = 0$ where $\psi(Y_i, X_i; \beta_x) = (Y_i - \beta_x X_i)X_i$ is the least squares score. The score is unbiased: $E[\psi(Y_i, X_i; \beta_x)] = \beta_x \sigma_x^2 - \beta_x \sigma_x^2 = 0$. The score is no longer unbiased when W replaces X; $E[\psi(Y_i, W_i; \beta_x)] = \beta_x \sigma_x^2 - \beta_x(\sigma_x^2 + \sigma^2) \neq 0$ whenever $\sigma^2 > 0$ and $\beta_x \neq 0$.

Corrected scores are unbiased estimators of the score that would be used in the absence of measurement error. A corrected score $\psi^*(Y_i, W_i; \beta_x)$ satisfies $E[\psi^*(Y_i, W_i; \beta_x)] = \psi(Y_i, X_i; \beta_x)$ where the expectation is with respect to the measurement error distribution. Corrected scores were first defined in Stefanski (1989a) and Nakamura (1990). Note that corrected scores are unbiased whenever the original score is unbiased. This means that estimators obtained from corrected scores are fully consistent.

The corrected score for the simple linear no-intercept regression model is easily seen to be $\psi^*(Y_i, W_i; \beta_x) = \psi(Y_i, W_i; \beta_x) + \sigma^2 \beta_x$ resulting in the estimator $\widehat{\beta}_x = \sum_{i=1}^{n} Y_i W_i / (\sum_{i=1}^{n} W_i^2 - \sigma^2)$. In applications an estimate of the measurement error variance replaces σ^2. Note that the corrected score estimator for the linear model is also the method-of-moments estimator.

For the linear model, the corrected score was identified without making an assumption on the distribution of the measurement error. For nonlinear regression models, obtaining a corrected score generally requires specification of the measurement error distribution, and typically the normal distribution is used.

Consider Poisson regression with no intercept. The likelihood score in the absence of measurement error is $\psi(Y_i, X_i; \beta_x) = (Y_i - \exp\{\beta_x X_i\})X_i$. If we assume that the measurement error satisfies $U \sim N(0, 1)$, then $\psi^*(Y_i, W_i; \beta_x) = (Y_i - \exp\{\beta_x W_i - \beta_x^2 \sigma^2/2\})W_i + \beta_x \sigma^2 \exp\{\beta_x W_i - \beta_x^2 \sigma^2/2\})$ is the corrected score. Using results for the moment generating function of a normal random variable, one can verify that $E[\psi^*(Y_i, W_i; \beta_x)] = (Y_i - \exp\{\beta_x X_i\})X_i$ where the expectation is with respect to the measurement error. The corrected score estimator solves $\sum_{i=1}^{n} \psi^*(Y_i, W_i; \beta_x) = 0$, and the solution must be obtained numerically for Poisson regression.

It is not always possible to obtain a corrected score (Stefanski 1989a). For example, the likelihood score for logistic regression does not admit a corrected score, except under certain restrictions (Buzas and Stefanski 1996c). Methods for obtaining corrected scores and approximately corrected scores via computer simulation have been recently studied (Novick and Stefanski 2002; Devanarayan and Stefanski 2002).

5.4.5   Conditional Scores

Conditional score estimation is the default method for logistic regression when the classical additive error model holds. The statistical theory of sufficient statistics and maximum likelihood underlie the derivation of conditional scores, and conditional score estimators retain certain optimality properties of likelihood estimators. Though we focus on logistic regression here, the method applies to a broader class of regression models, including Poisson and gamma regression. The method was derived in Stefanski and Carroll (1987). Construction of the conditional score estimator requires that the measurement error is normally distributed. However, the estimator remains effective in reducing bias and is surprisingly efficient for modest departures from the normality assumption (Huang and Wang 2001). Computing conditional score estimators requires an estimate of the measurement error variance.

The conditional score estimator is defined implicitly as the solution to estimating equations that are closely related to the logistic regression maximum likelihood estimating equations used in the absence of measurement error. In the absence of measurement error, the maximum likelihood estimator of $(\beta_1, \beta_z, \beta_x)$ is defined implicitly as the solution to

$$\sum_{i=1}^{n} \left\{ Y_i - F(\beta_1 + \beta_z Z_i + \beta_x X_i) \right\} \begin{pmatrix} 1 \\ Z_i \\ X_i \end{pmatrix} = 0,$$

where $F(v) = \{1 + \exp(-v)\}^{-1}$ is the logistic distribution function. The conditional score estimator is defined as the solution to the equations

$$\sum_{i=1}^{n} \left\{ Y_i - F(\beta_1 + \beta_z Z_i + \beta_x \Delta_i) \right\} \begin{pmatrix} 1 \\ Z_i \\ \Delta_i \end{pmatrix} = 0,$$

where $\Delta_i = W_i + (Y_i - (1/2))\widehat{\sigma}^2 \beta_x$ and $\widehat{\sigma}^2$ is an estimate of the measurement error variance. Conditional score estimation for logistic regression replaces the unobserved X_i with Δ_i. It can be shown that $E[Y|Z, \Delta] = F(\beta_1 + \beta_z Z + \beta_x \Delta)$ and it follows that the conditional score is unbiased. Because Δ_i depends on the parameter β_x, it is not possible to estimate $(\beta_1, \beta_z, \beta_x)$ using standard software by replacing X with Δ. Standard errors are computed using the sandwich estimator or bootstrap.

For models other than the logistic, the simple scheme of replacing X with Δ is not true generally, and conditional score estimating equations for Poisson and gamma regression are much more complicated.

The conditional score estimator for the logistic model compares favorably in terms of efficiency to the full maximum likelihood estimator that requires specification of an exposure model (Stefanski and Carroll 1990b).

Instrumental Variables

5.4.6

The methods described so far require additional data that allow estimation of the measurement error variance. Replicate observations and internal/external validation data are two sources of such additional information. Another source of additional information are instrumental variables. Instrumental variables, denoted T, are additional measurements of X that satisfy three requirements; (1) T is non-differential, i.e. $f_{Y|Z,X,T} = f_{Y|Z,X}$, (2) T is correlated with X and (3) T is independent of $W - X$. Note that a replicate observation is an instrumental variable but an instrumental variable is not necessarily a replicate. It is possible to use an instrumental variable to estimate the measurement error variance and then use one of the above methods. Doing so can be inefficient, and IV methods typically do not directly estimate the measurement error variance.

Consider the cancer case-control study of arsenic exposure mentioned in Sect. 5.3. Two measurements of arsenic exposure are available for each case/control in the form of drinking water and toenail concentrations. Neither measure is an exact measure of long-term arsenic exposure (X). Taking toenail concentration to be an unbiased measurement of X, the drinking water concentration can serve as an instrumental variable.

Instrumental variable methods have been used in linear measurement error models since the 1940s, see Fuller (1987) for a good introduction. Instrumental variable methods for nonlinear models were first studied in Amemiya (1985, 1990a,b). Extensions of regression calibration and conditional score methodology to instrumental variables are given in Carroll and Stefanski (1994), Stefanski and Buzas (1995), Buzas and Stefanski (1996a,b).

The essential idea underlying instrumental variable estimation can be understood by studying the simple linear model without intercept: $Y = \beta_x X + \varepsilon$ and $W = X + \sigma U$. Then $Y = \beta_x W + \tilde{\varepsilon}$ where $\tilde{\varepsilon} = \varepsilon - \beta_x \sigma U$ and it appears that Y and W follow a simple linear regression model. However, W and $\tilde{\varepsilon}$ are correlated, violating a standard assumption in linear regression, and the least squares estimator for β_x is biased, see Sect. 5.2. The least squares estimating equation $\sum_{i=1}^{n}\{Y_i - \beta_x W_i\}W_i = 0$ is biased because W_i and $Y_i - \beta_x W_i$ are correlated. This suggests an unbiased equation can be constructed by replacing W_i outside the brackets with a measurement uncorrelated with $Y_i - \beta_x W_i$. An IV T satisfies the requirement and the IV estimating equation $\sum_{i=1}^{n}\{Y_i - \beta_x W_i\}T_i = 0$ results in the consistent estimator $\widehat{\beta}_x = \sum_{i=1}^{n} Y_i T_i / \sum_{i=1}^{n} W_i T_i$. Non-zero correlation between X and T is required so that the denominator is not estimating zero. The key idea is that the score factors into two components where the first component $\{Y_i - \beta_x W_i\}$ has expectation zero and the second component T_i is uncorrelated with the first.

The method must be modified for nonlinear problems. Logistic regression will be used to illustrate the modification. If we ignore measurement error, the estimating equations for logistic regression are

$$\sum_{i=1}^{n} \left\{ Y_i - F(\beta_1 + \beta_z Z_i + \beta_x W_i) \right\} \begin{pmatrix} 1 \\ Z_i \\ W_i \end{pmatrix} = 0.$$

Unlike the linear case, for the logistic model and nonlinear models generally, the first term in the estimating score, $\{Y_i - F(\beta_1 + \beta_z Z_i + \beta_x W_i)\}$, does not have expectation zero, so that replacing W_i with T_i outside the brackets in the above equation does not result in an estimator that reduces bias.

Define the logistic regression instrumental variable estimating equations

$$\sum_{i=1}^{n} h(Z_i, W_i, T_i) \left\{ Y_i - F(\beta_1 + \beta_z Z_i + \beta_x W_i) \right\} \begin{pmatrix} 1 \\ Z_i \\ T_i \end{pmatrix} = 0,$$

where $h(Z_i, W_i, T_i) = \sqrt{\frac{F'(\beta_1 + \beta_z Z_i + \beta_x T_i)}{F'(\beta_1 + \beta_z Z_i + \beta_x W_i)}}$ is a scalar valued weight function and F' denotes the derivative of F. It can be shown that the estimating equation is unbiased provided the distribution of the measurement error is symmetric, implying the estimator obtained from the equations is fully consistent. See Buzas (1997) for extensions to other disease models, including the Poisson and gamma models. Huang and Wang (2001) provide an alternative approach for the logistic model.

5.4.7   Likelihood Methods

Likelihood methods for estimation and inference are appealing because of optimality properties of maximum likelihood estimates and dependability of likelihood ratio confidence intervals. In the context of measurement error problems, the advantages of likelihood methods relative to functional methods have been studied in Schafer and Purdy (1996) and Küchenhoff and Carroll (1997). However, the advantageous properties are contingent on correct specification of the likelihood. As discussed below, this is often a difficult task in measurement error problems.

The likelihood for an observed data point (Y, W) conditional on Z is

$$f_{YW|Z} = \int f_{Y|Z,X,W} f_{W|Z,X} f_{X|Z} dx = \int f_{Y|Z,X} f_{W|Z,X} f_{X|Z} dx,$$

where the second equality follows from the assumption of non-differential measurement error. The integral is replaced by a sum if X is a discrete random variable. The likelihood for the observed data is $\prod_{i=1}^{N} f_{Y_i, W_i|Z_i}$, and maximum likelihood estimates are obtained by maximizing the likelihood over all the unknown parameters in each of the three component distributions comprising the likelihood. In principle, the procedure is straightforward. However, there are several important points to be made.

1. The likelihood for the observed data requires *complete* distributional specification for the disease model ($f_{Y|Z,X}$), the error model ($f_{W|Z,X}$) and an exposure model ($f_{X|Z}$).
2. As was the case for functional models, estimation of parameters in the disease model generally requires, for all intents and purposes, observations that allow estimation of parameters in the error model, for example replicate measurements.
3. When the exposure is modeled as a continuous random variable, for example the normal distribution, the likelihood requires evaluation of an integral. For many applications the integral cannot be evaluated analytically and numerical methods must be used, typically Gaussian quadrature or Monte Carlo methods.
4. Finding the maximum of the likelihood is not always straightforward.

While the last two points must be addressed to implement the method, they are technical points and will not be discussed in detail. In principle, numerical integration followed by a maximization routine can be used, but this approach is often difficult to implement in practice, see Schafer (2002). Algorithms for computation and maximization of the likelihood in general regression models with exposure measurement error are given in Higdon and Schafer (2001) and Schafer (2002). Alternatively, a Bayesian formulation can be used to circumvent some of the computational difficulties, see Carroll et al. (1999). For the normal theory linear model and probit regression with normal distribution for the exposure model, the likelihood can be obtained analytically (Fuller 1987; Carroll et al. 1984; Schafer 1993). The analytic form of the likelihood for the probit model often provides an adequate approximation to the likelihood for the logistic model.

The first point above deserves discussion. None of the preceding methods required specification of an exposure model (functional methods). Here an exposure model is required. It is common to assume $X|Z \sim N(\alpha_1 + \alpha_x Z, \sigma_{x|z}^2)$, but, unless there are validation data, it is not possible to assess the adequacy of the exposure model using the data. Some models are robust to the normality assumption. For example, in the normal theory linear model, i.e. when (Y, Z, X, W) is jointly normal, maximum likelihood estimators are fully consistent regardless of the distribution of X. The literature is currently lacking results as to the robustness of other disease models to assumptions on X. In a Bayesian framework, Richardson and Leblond (1997) show mis-specification of the exposure model can seriously affect estimation for logistic disease models.

Semi-parametric and flexible parametric modeling are two approaches that have been explored to address potential robustness issues in specifying an exposure model. Semi-parametric methods leave the exposure model unspecified, and the exposure model is essentially considered as another parameter that needs to be estimated. These models have the advantage of model robustness but may lack efficiency relative to the full likelihood. See Roeder et al. (1996), Schafer (2001) and Taupin (2001).

Flexible parametric exposure models typically use a mixture of normal random variables to model the exposure distribution, as normal mixtures are capable of capturing moderately diversified features of distributions. Flexible parametric approaches have been studied in Küchenhoff and Carroll (1997), Carroll et al. (1999) and Schafer (2002).

The likelihood can also be obtained conditional on both W and Z. In this case the likelihood is

$$f_{Y|Z,W} = \int f_{Y|Z,X} f_{X|Z,W} dx$$

necessitating an exposure model relating X to W and Z. This form of the likelihood is natural for Berkson error models. In general, the choice of which likelihood to use is a matter of modeling convenience.

5.4.8   Survival Analysis

Analysis of survival data with exposure measurement error using proportional hazards models presents some new issues (see also Chap. II.4 of this handbook). Of the methods presented, only SIMEX can be applied without modification in the proportional hazards setting.

Many of the proposed methods for measurement error correction in proportional hazards models fall into one of two general strategies. The first strategy is to approximate the induced hazard and then use the approximated hazard in the partial likelihood equations. This strategy is analogous to the regression calibration approximation discussed earlier. The second strategy is to modify the partial likelihood estimating equations. Methods based on this strategy stem from the corrected and conditional score paradigms.

In the absence of measurement error, the proportional hazards model postulates a hazard function of the form $\lambda(t|Z, X) = \lambda_0(t) \exp(\beta_z^T Z + \beta_x X)$ where $\lambda_0(t)$ is an unspecified baseline hazard function. Estimation and inference for (β_x, β_z) are carried out through the partial likelihood function, as it does not depend on $\lambda_0(t)$.

Prentice (1982) has shown that when (Z, W) is observed, the induced hazard is $\lambda(t|Z, W) = \lambda_0(t) E[\exp(\beta_z^T Z + \beta_x X)|T \geq t, Z, W]$. The induced hazard requires a model for X conditional on $(T \geq t, Z, W)$. This is problematic because the distribution of T is left unspecified in proportional hazards models. However, when the disease is rare $\lambda(t|Z, W) \approx \lambda_0(t) E[\exp(\beta_z^T Z + \beta_x X)|Z, W]$ (Prentice 1982) and if we further assume that $X|Z, W$ is approximately normal with constant variance then the induced hazard is proportional to $\exp(\beta_z^T Z + \beta_x E[X|Z, W])$. In other words, regression calibration is appropriate in the proportional hazards setting when the disease is rare and $X|Z, W$ is approximately normal.

Modifications to the regression calibration algorithm have been developed for applications where the rare disease assumption is untenable, see Clayton (1991), Tsiatis et al. (1995), Wang et al. (1997), and Xie et al. (2001). Conditioning on $T \geq t$ cannot be ignored when the disease is not rare. The idea is to re-estimate the calibration function $E[X|Z, W]$ in each risk set, that is the set of individuals known to be at risk at time t. Clayton's proposal assumes the calibration functions across risk sets have a common slope and his method can be applied provided one has an estimate of the measurement error variance. Xie et al. (2001) extend the idea to varying slopes across the risk sets and require replication (reliability data). Tsiatis et al. (1995) consider time varying covariates and also allow for varying slopes across the risk sets.

When a validation subsample is available it is possible to estimate the induced hazard nonparametrically, that is without specifying a distribution for $X|(T \geq t, Z, W)$, see Zhou and Pepe (1995) and Zhou and Wang (2000) for cases when the exposure is discrete and continuous, respectively.

The second strategy avoids modeling the induced hazard and instead modifies the partial likelihood estimating equations. Methods based on the corrected score concept are explored in Nakamura (1992), Buzas (1998) and Huang and Wang (2000). The methods in Nakamura (1992) and Buzas (1998) assume the measurement error is normally distributed and only require an estimate of the measurement error variance. In contrast, the approach in Huang and Wang (2000) does not require assumptions on the measurement error distribution but replicate observations on the mismeasured exposure are needed to compute the estimator. Each of the methods has been shown to be effective in reducing bias in parameter estimators. Tsiatis and Davidian (2001) extend conditional score methodology to the proportional hazards setting with covariates possibly time dependent.

Conclusions 5.5

Epidemiologists have long recognized the importance of addressing problems of measurement and ascertainment in the statistical analysis of epidemiologic data. Much of the research in measurement error models has its origins in specific epidemiologic applications, and this is reflected by many of the research papers cited in this review article. The importance of measurement error modeling to epidemiologic research is on the rise, and that trend is likely to continue for the foreseeable future.

As the understanding of the etiology of disease increases, so too will the sophistication of the statistical models used to extract information from epidemiologic data. Success in these modeling endeavors will depend on the ability to accurately model ever finer sources of variability in data, and measurement error is frequently one such nonnegligible source of variation.

This chapter provides an introduction to, and a review of the literature on the problem of statistical inference in the presence of measurement error. Section 5.2 discussed the effects of measurement error in common epidemiologic models. With the inevitable increase in the sophistication of models for epidemiologic data, there will be a need to understand the effects of measurement error on parameter estimation in biologically-based and physiologically-based models of disease. The increasing ability to collect very detailed and precise information on subjects in validation samples (e.g., via continuous monitoring of biological processes, or genetic screening, etc.) means that consideration of measurement error at the design stage of a study will take on greater importance. Hence the timely relevance of the issues and methods discussed in Sect. 5.3. More elaborate modeling places greater demands on methods of estimation. Section 5.4 provided a summary and review of common approaches to estimation in the presence of measurement. Future research will necessarily have to accommodate more complex models and and possibly multiple variates measured with error.

References

Amemiya Y (1985) Instrumental variable estimator for the nonlinear errors in variables model. Journal of Econometrics 28:273–289

Amemiya Y (1990a) Instrumental variable estimation of the nonlinear measurement error model. In: Brown PJ, Fuller WA (eds) Statistical analysis of measurement error models and application. American Mathematics Society, Providence

Amemiya Y (1990b) Two-stage instrumental variable estimators for the nonlinear errors in variables model. Journal of Econometrics 44:311–332

Armstrong BK, White E, Saracci R (1992) Principles of exposure measurement error in epidemiology. Oxford University Press, Oxford

Berkson J (1950) Are there two regressions? Journal of the American Statistical Association 45:164–180

Buonaccorsi JP (1988) Errors in variables with systematic biases. Communications in Statistics – Theory and Methods 18:1001–1021

Buzas JS (1997) Instrumental variable estimation in nonlinear measurement error models. Communications in Statistics – Theory and Methods 26:2861–2877

Buzas JS (1998) Unbiased scores in proportional hazards regression with covariate measurement error. Journal of Statistical Planning and Inference 67:247–257

Buzas JS, Stefanski LA (1996a) Instrumental variable estimation in probit measurement error models. Journal of Statistical Planning and Inference 55:47–62

Buzas JS, Stefanski LA (1996b) Instrumental variable estimation in generalized linear measurement error models. Journal of the American Statistical Association 91: 999–1006

Buzas, J.S., Stefanski, L.A. (1996c) A note on corrected score estimation. Statistics and Probability Letters 28:1–8

Cain KC, Breslow, NE (1988) Logistic regression analysis and efficient design for two-stage studies. American Journal of Epidemiology 128:1198–1206

Carroll RJ (1989) Covariance analysis in generalized linear measurement error models. Statistics in Medicine 8:1075–1093

Carroll RJ (1998) Measurement error in epidemiologic studies. In: Armitage P, Colton T (eds) Encyclopedia of biostatistics. Wiley, New York, pp 2491–2519

Carroll RJ, Stefanski LA (1990) Approximate quasilikelihood estimation in models with surrogate predictors. Journal of the American Statistical Association 85:652–663

Carroll RJ, Stefanski LA (1994) Measurement error, instrumental variables and corrections for attenuation with applications to meta-analyses. Statistics in Medicine 13:1265–1282

Carroll RJ, Gallo PP, Gleser LJ (1985) Comparison of least squares and errors-in-variables regression, with special reference to randomized analysis of covariance. Journal of the American Statistical Association 80:929–932

Carroll RJ, Küchenhoff H, Lombard F, Stefanski LA (1996) Asymptotics for the SIMEX estimator in structural measurement error models. Journal of the American Statistical Association 91:242–250

Carroll RJ, Roeder K, Wasserman L (1999) Flexible parametric measurement error models. Biometrics 55:44–54

Carroll RJ, Ruppert D, Stefanski LA (1995) Measurement error in nonlinear models. Chapman & Hall, London

Carroll RJ, Spiegelman, Lan KK, Bailey KT, Abbott RD (1984) On errors-in-variables for binary regression models. Biometrika 71:19–26

Clayton DG (1991) Models for the analysis of cohort and case-control studies with inaccurately measured exposures. In: Dwyer JH, Feinleib M, Lipsert P et al. (eds.) Statistical models for longitudinal studies of health. Oxford University Press, New York , pp 301–331

Cochran WG (1968) Errors of measurement in statistics. Technometrics 10:637–666

Cook J, Stefanski LA (1995) A simulation extrapolation method for parametric measurement error models. Journal of the American Statistical Association 89:1314–1328

Devanarayan V, Stefanski LA (2002) Empirical simulation extrapolation for measurement error models with replicate measurements. Statistics and Probability Letters 59:219–225

Fleiss JL (1981) Statistical methods for rates and proportions. Wiley, New York

Fuller WA (1987) Measurement error models. Wiley, New York

Higdon R, Schafer DW (2001) Maximum likelihood computations for regression with measurement error. Computational Statistics and Data Analysis 35:283–299

Holcomb JP (1999) Regression with covariates and outcome calculated from a common set of variables measured with error: estimation using the SIMEX method. Statistics in Medicine, 18:2847–2862

Holcroft CA, Rotnitzky A, Robins JM (1997) Efficient estimation of regression parameters from multistage studies with validation of outcome and covariates. Journal of Statistical Planning and Inference 65:349–374

Huang Y, Wang CY (2000) Cox regression with accurate covariates unascertainable: a nonparametric-correction approach. Journal of the American Statistical Association 95:1209–1219

Huang Y, Wang CY (2001) Consistent functional methods for logistic regression with errors in covariates. Journal of the American Statistical Association 95:1209–1219

Hughes MD (1993) Regression dilution in the proportional hazards model. Biometrics 49:1056–1066

Hwang JT, Stefanski LA (1994) Monotonicity of regression functions in structural measurement error models. Statistics and Probability Letters 20:113–116

Karagas MR, Tosteson TD, Blum J, Morris SJ, Baron JA, Klaue B (1998) Design of an epidemiologic study of drinking water arsenic and skin and bladder cancer risk in a U.S. population. Environmental Health Perspectives 106: 1047–1050

Karagas MR, Tosteson TD, Blum J, Klaue B, Weiss JE, Stannard V, Spate V, Morris JS (2000) Measurement of low levels of arsenic exposure: a comparison of water and toenail concentrations. American Journal of Epidemiology 152:84–90

Karagas MR, Stukel TA, Morris JS, Tosteson TD, Weiss JE, Spencer SK, Greenberg ER (2001) Skin cancer risk in relation to toenail arsenic concentrations in a US population-based case-control study. American Journal of Epidemiology 153:559–565

Karagas MR, Stukel TA, Tosteson TD (2002) Assessment of cancer risk and environmental levels of arsenic in New Hampshire. International Journal of Hygiene and Environmental Health 205:85–94

Kim C, Hong C, Jeong M (2000) Simulation-extrapolation via the Bezier curve in measurement error models. Communications in Statistics – Simulation and Computation 29:1135–1147

Kim J, Gleser LJ (2000) SIMEX approaches to measurement error in ROC studies. Communications in Statistics – Theory and Methods 29:2473–2491

Kipnis V, Carroll RJ, Freedman LS, Li L (1999) Implications of a new dietary measurement error model for estimation of relative risk: application to four calibration studies. American Journal of Epidemiology 150: 642–651

Küchenhoff H, Carroll RJ (1997) Segmented regression with errors in predictors: semi-parametric and parametric methods. Statistics in Medicine 16:169–188

Li Y, Lin X (2003) Functional inference in frailty measurement error models for clustered survival data using the SIMEX approach. Journal of the American Statistical Association 98:191–203

Lin X, Carroll RJ (1999) SIMEX variance component tests in generalized linear mixed measurement error models. Biometrics 55:613–619

MacMahon S, Peto R, Cutler J, Collins R, Sorlie P, Neaton J, Abbott R, Godwin J, Dyer A, Stamler J (1990) Blood pressure, stroke and coronary heart disease: Part 1, prolonged differences in blood pressure: prospective observational studies corrected for the regression dilution bias. Lancet 335:765–774

Marcus AH, Elias RW (1998) Some useful statistical methods for model validation. Environmental Health Perspectives 106:1541–1550

McKeown-Eyssen GE, Tibshirani R (1994) Implications of measurement error in exposure for the sample sizes of case-control studies. American Journal of Epidemiology 139:415–421

Nakamura T (1990) Corrected score functions for errors-in-variables models: methodology and application to generalized linear models. Biometrika 77:127–137

Nakamura T (1992) Proportional hazards models with covariates subject to measurement error. Biometrics 48:829–838

Novick SJ, Stefanski LA (2002) Corrected score estimation via complex variable simulation extrapolation. Journal of the American Statistical Association 97:472–481

Prentice RL (1982) Covariate measurement errors and parameter estimation in a failure time regression model. Biometrika 69:331–342

Reilly M (1996) Optimal sampling strategies for two phase studies. American Journal of Epidemiology 143:92–100

Richardson S, Leblond L (1997) Some comments on misspecification of priors in Bayesian modelling of measurement error problems. Statistics in Medicine 16:203–213

Roeder K, Carroll RJ, Lindsay BG (1996) A nonparametric mixture approach to case-control studies with errors in covariables. Journal of the American Statistical Association 91:722–732

Rosner B, Willett WC, Spiegelman D (1989) Correction of logistic regression relative risk estimates and confidence intervals for systematic within-person measurement error. Statistics in Medicine 8:1051–1070

Rosner B, Spiegelman D, Willett WC (1990) Correction of logistic regression relative risk estimates and confidence intervals for measurement error: the case of multiple covariates measured with error. American Journal of Epidemiology 132:734–745

Schafer D (1993) Likelihood analysis for probit regression with measurement errors. Biometrika 80:899–904

Schafer D (2001) Semiparametric maximum likelihood for measurement error model regression. Biometrics 57:53–61

Schafer D (2002) Likelihood analysis and flexible structural modeling for measurement error model regression. Journal of Computational Statistics and Data analysis 72:33–45

Schafer D, Purdy K (1996) Likelihood analysis for errors-in-variables regression with replicate measurements. Biometrika 83:813–824

Spiegelman D, Gray R (1991) Cost-efficient study designs for binary response data with Gaussian covariate measurement error. Biometrics 47:851 869

Spiegelman D, Carroll RJ, Kipnis V (2001) Efficient regression calibration for logistic regression in mainstudy/internal validation study designs with an imperfect reference instrument. Statistics in Medicine 20:139–160

Stefanski LA (1985) The effects of measurement error on parameter estimation. Biometrika 72:583–592

Stefanski LA (1989) Unbiased estimation of a nonlinear function of a normal mean with application to measurement error models. Communications in Statistics – Theory and Methods 18:4335–4358

Stefanski LA, Bay JM (1996) Simulation extrapolation deconvolution of finite population cumulative distribution function estimators. Biometrika 83:407–417

Stefanski LA, Buzas JS (1995) Instrumental variable estimation in binary measurement error models. Journal of the American Statistical Association 90: 541–550

Stefanski LA, Carroll RJ (1985) Covariate measurement error in logistic regression. Annals of Statistics 13:1335–1351

Stefanski LA, Carroll RJ (1987) Conditional scores and optimal scores in generalized linear measurement error models. Biometrika 74:703–716

Stefanski LA, Carroll RJ (1990a) Score tests in generalized linear measurement error models. Journal of the Royal Statistical Society B 52:345–359

Stefanski LA, Carroll RJ (1990b) Structural logistic regression measurement error models. In: Brown PJ, Fuller WA (eds) Proceedings of the conference on measurement error models, Wiley, New York, pp 115–127

Stefanski LA, Cook J (1995) Simulation extrapolation: the measurement error jackknife. Journal of the American Statistical Association 90:1247–1256

Stram DO, Longnecker MP, Shames L, Kolonel LN, Wilkens LR, Pike MC, Henderson BE (1995) Cost-efficient design of a diet validation-study. American Journal of Epidemiology 142(3):353–362

Taupin M (2001) Semi-parametric estimation in the nonlinear structural errors-in-variables model. Annals of Statistics 29:66–93

Thomas D, Stram D, Dwyer J (1993) Exposure measurement error: influence on exposure-disease relationships and methods of correction. Annual Review of Public Health 14:69–93

Tosteson TD, Tsiatis AA (1988) The asymptotic relative efficiency of score tests in the generalized linear model with surrogate covariates. Biometrika 75:507–514

Tosteson TD, Ware JH (1990) Designing a logistic regression study using surrogate measures of exposure and outcome. Biometrika 77:11–20

Tosteson T, Stefanski LA, Schafer DW (1989) A measurement error model for binary and ordinal regression. Statistics in Medicine 8:1139–1147

Tosteson TD, Titus-Ernstoff L, Baron JA, Karagas MR (1994) A two-stage validation study for determining sensitivity and specificity. Environmental Health Perspectives 102:11–14

Tosteson TD, Buzas JS, Demidenko D, Karagas MR (2003) Power and sample size calculations for generalized regression models with covariate measurement error. Statistics in Medicine 22:1069–1082

Tsiatis AA, Davidian M (2001) A semiparametric estimator for the proportional hazards model with longitudinal covariates measured with error. Biometrika 88:447–458

Tsiatis AA, DeGruttola V, Wulfsohn MS (1995) Modeling the relationship of survival to longitudinal data measured with error: Applications to survival and CD4 counts in patients with AIDS. Journal of the American Statistical Association 90:27–37

Wang CY, Hsu ZD, Feng ZD, Prentice RL (1997) Regression calibration in failure time regression. Biometrics 53:131–145

Wang N, Lin X, Gutierrez R, Carroll RJ (1998) Bias analysis and the SIMEX approach in generalized linear mixed effects models. Journal of the American Statistical Association 93:249–261

White E, Kushi LH, Pepe MS (1994) The effect of exposure variance and exposure measurement error on study sample size. Implications for design of epidemiologic studies. Journal of Clinical Epidemiology 47:873–880

Xie SX, Wang CY, Prentice RL (2001) A risk set calibration method for failure time regression by using a covariate reliability sample. Journal of the Royal Statistical Society B 63:855–870

Zhou H, Pepe MS (1995) Auxiliary covariate data in failure time regression analysis. Biometrika 82:139–149

Zhou H, Wang CY (2000) Failure time regression with continuous covariates measured with error. Journal of the Royal Statistical Society, Series B 62:657–665

Missing Data

II.6

Geert Molenberghs, Caroline Beunckens, Ivy Jansen, Herbert Thijs,
Geert Verbeke, Michael G. Kenward

Introduction

The problem of dealing with missing values is common throughout statistical work and is present whenever human subjects are enrolled. Respondents may refuse participation or may be unreachable. Patients in clinical and epidemiological studies may withdraw their initial consent without further explanation. Early work on missing values was largely concerned with algorithmic and computational solutions to the induced lack of balance or deviations from the intended study design (Afifi and Elashoff 1966; Hartley and Hocking 1971). More recently general algorithms such as the Expectation-Maximisation (EM) (Dempster et al. 1977), and data imputation and augmentation procedures (Rubin 1987; Tanner and Wong 1987) combined with powerful computing resources have largely provided a solution to this aspect of the problem. There remains the very difficult and important question of assessing the impact of missing data on subsequent statistical inference. Conditions can be formulated, under which an analysis that proceeds as if the missing data are missing by design, that is, ignoring the missing value process, can provide valid answers to study questions. While such an approach is attractive from a pragmatic point of view, the difficulty is that such conditions can rarely be assumed to hold with full certainty. Indeed, assumptions will be required that cannot be assessed from the data under analysis. Hence in this setting there cannot be anything that could be termed a definitive analysis, and hence any analysis of preference is ideally to be supplemented with a so-called sensitivity analysis.

In Sect. 6.2 two key illustrative cases are introduced. Simple methods that are often used but carry quite a bit of danger in them are discussed in Sect. 6.3. Section 6.4 is devoted to a longitudinal data modeling framework for continuous outcomes, useful to further develop and illustrate practical strategies to deal with incomplete data. A general framework within which missing data ideas can be developed is presented in Sect. 6.6. Also, the concept of ignorability will be introduced within this context.

In Sects. 6.7 and 6.9 two approaches to modeling data with non-random dropout are considered: the selection model framework and the pattern-mixture modeling family.

A longitudinal data modeling framework for discrete outcomes is given in Sect. 6.11. Section 6.12 introduces weighted estimating equations, an important adaptation of generalized estimating equations to the incomplete data setting.

A perspective on the position of the various modeling strategies is provided in Sect. 6.14, summarizing important points about preceding sections, and setting the scenes for sensitivity analysis, two forms of which are described in Sects. 6.15, in the selection model context, and 6.16, using pattern mixtures.

The two case studies that were introduced in Sect. 6.2 are analysed and discussed throughout the chapter, by way of running examples.

6.2   Case Studies

In this section, two case studies are introduced, which will be analysed later in this chapter. The first one is the Vorozole study, which focuses on quality of life in breast cancer patients. The second case study is of a psychiatric type, where emphasis is on different therapies for patients with depression.

6.2.1   The Vorozole Study

This study was an open-label, multicenter, parallel group design conducted at 67 North American centers. Patients were randomized to either vorozole (2.5 mg taken once daily) or megestrol acetate (40 mg four times daily). The patient population consisted of postmenopausal patients with histologically confirmed estrogen-receptor positive metastatic breast carcinoma. All 452 randomized patients were followed until disease progression or death. The main objective was to compare the treatment groups with respect to response rate while secondary objectives included a comparison relative to duration of response, time to progression, survival, safety, pain relief, performance status and quality of life. We focus on overall quality of life, measured by the total Functional Living Index: Cancer (FLIC) (Schipper et al. 1984). Precisely, a higher FLIC score is the more desirable outcome. We analyse the change from baseline in FLIC score over time. For simplicity, we will still refer to this endpoint as 'FLIC score'. The treatment effect on this change in FLIC score will be investigated. Full details of the Vorozole study are reported in Goss et al. (1999).

Patients underwent screening and for those deemed eligible a detailed examination at baseline (occasion 0) took place. Further measurement occasions were month 1, then from month 2 at bi-monthly intervals until month 44.

Let us now graphically explore these data. The average evolution describes how the profile for a number of relevant subpopulations (or the population as a whole) evolves over time. The individual profiles are displayed in Fig. 6.1, while the mean profiles of the change in FLIC scores per treatment arm, as well as their 95% confidence intervals, are plotted in Fig. 6.2. The average profiles indicate an increase over time which is slightly stronger for the vorozole group until month 14, and afterwards, the megestrol acetate group shows a slightly higher FLIC score. As can be seen from the confidence intervals, these differences are clearly not significant.

The individual profiles augment the averaged plot with a suggestion of the variability seen within the data. The thinning of the data towards the later study times suggests that trends at later times should be treated with caution. Indeed, an extra level of complexity is added whenever not all planned measurements are observed. This results in *incompleteness* or *missingness*. Another frequently encountered term is *dropout*, which refers to the case where all observations on a subject are obtained until a certain point in time, after which all measurements are missing. Therefore, we decided to restrict attention to the first 2 years only. This leads to a maximum of 13 observations per subject (month 1, 2, 4, 6, ..., 24). While these plots also give us some indications about the variability at given times

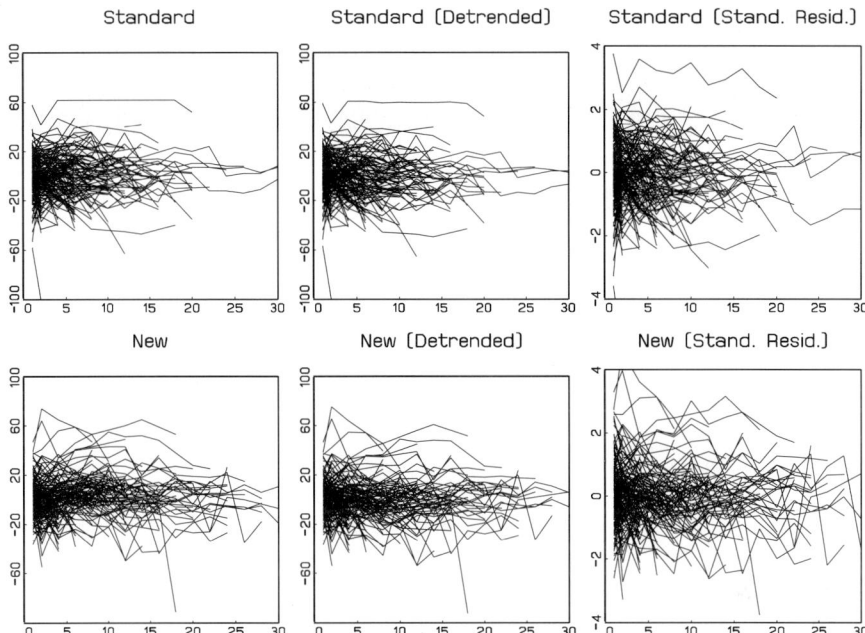

Figure 6.1. Vorozole Study. Individual profiles, raw residuals, and standardized residuals

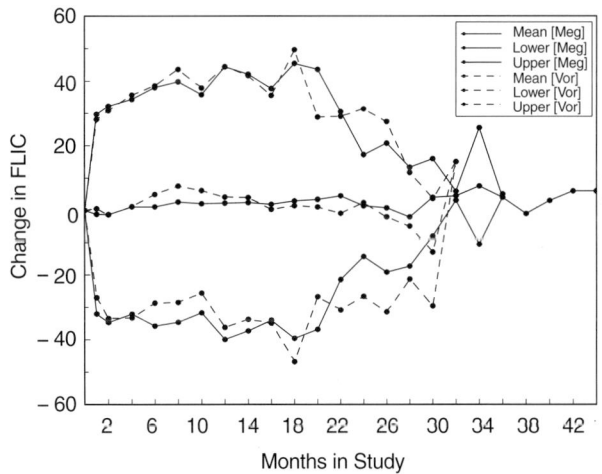

Figure 6.2. Vorozole Study. Mean profiles and 95% confidence intervals

and even about the correlation between measurements of the same individual, it is easier to base such considerations on residual profiles and standardized residual profiles.

To simplify matters, we will largely focus on dropout, but a lot of the developments made are valid also for general types of missingness.

The first issue, resulting from dropout, is evidently a depletion of the study subjects. Of course, a decreasing sample size increases variability which, in turn, decreases precision. In this respect, the Vorozole study is a dramatic example, as can be seen from Fig. 6.3 and Table 6.1, which graphically and numerically present

Table 6.1. Vorozole Study. Evolution of dropout

Month	Standard #	Standard (%)	Vorozole #	Vorozole (%)
0	226	(100)	220	(100)
1	221	(98)	216	(98)
2	203	(90)	198	(90)
4	161	(71)	146	(66)
6	123	(54)	106	(48)
8	90	(40)	90	(41)
10	73	(32)	77	(35)
12	51	(23)	64	(29)
14	39	(17)	51	(23)
16	27	(12)	44	(20)
18	19	(8)	33	(15)
20	14	(6)	27	(12)
22	6	(3)	22	(10)
24	5	(2)	17	(8)
26	4	(2)	9	(4)
28	3	(1)	7	(3)
30	3	(1)	3	(1)
32	2	(1)	1	(0)
34	2	(1)	1	(0)
36	1	(0)	1	(0)
38	1	(0)	0	(0)
40	1	(0)	0	(0)
42	1	(0)	0	(0)
44	1	(0)	0	(0)

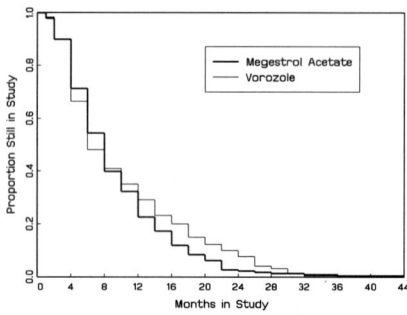

Figure 6.3. Vorozole Study. Representation of dropout

dropout in both treatment arms. Clearly, the dropout rate is high *and* there is a hint of a differential rate between the two arms. This means we have identified one potential factor that could influence a patient's probability of dropping out. Although a large part of the study scientist's interest will typically focus on the treatment effect, we should be aware that it is still a covariate and hence a design factor. Another question that will arise is whether dropout depends on observed or unobserved responses.

A different way of displaying several structural aspects is using a scatter plot matrix, such as in Fig. 6.4. The off-diagonal elements picture scatter plots of standardized residuals obtained from pairs of measurement occasions. The decay of correlation with time is studied by considering the evolution of the scatters

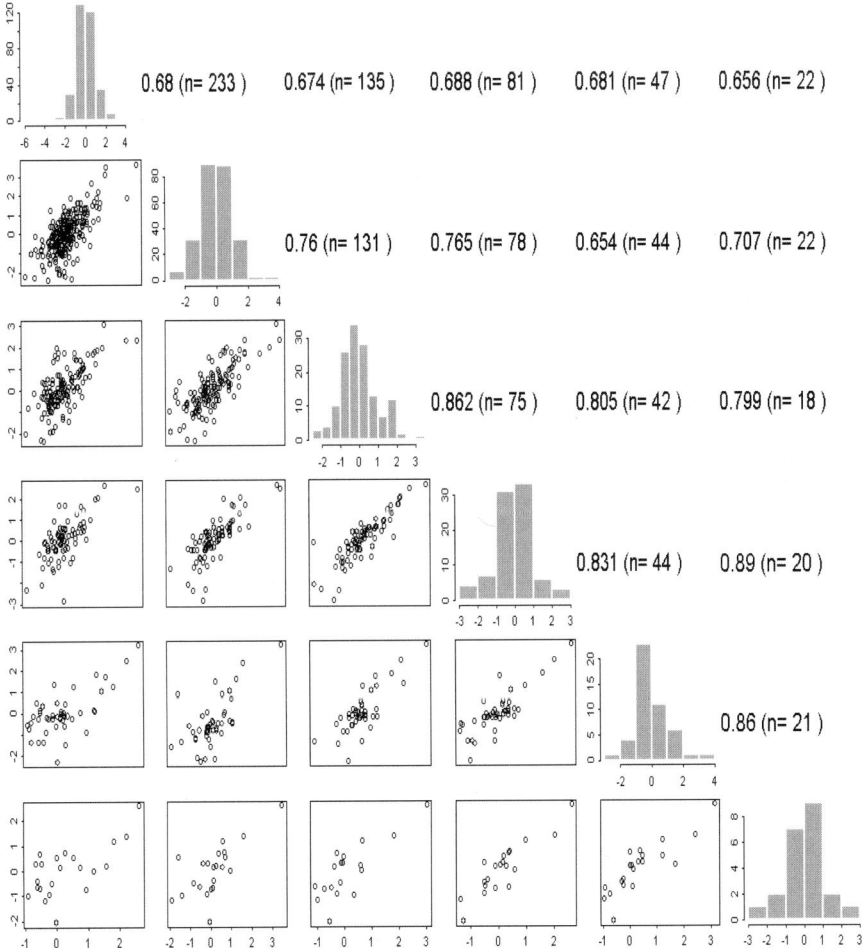

Figure 6.4. Vorozole Study. Scatter plot matrix for selected time points

with increasing distance to the main diagonal. Stationarity, on the other hand, implies that the scatter plots remain similar within diagonal bands *if measurement occasions are approximately equally spaced.* In addition to the scatter plots, we place histograms on the diagonal, capturing the variance structure. Features such as skewness, multimodality, and so forth, can then be graphically detected.

Further, the variance function is displayed in Fig. 6.5. The variance function seems to be relatively stable, except for a sharp decline near the end (at which point there are large dropout rates in both treatment groups), and hence a constant variance model is a plausible starting point.

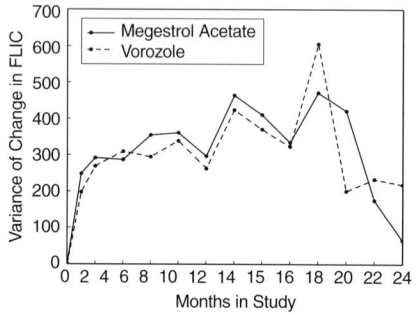

Figure 6.5. Vorozole Study. Variance function

Another aspect of the impact of dropout is also seen if we consider the average profile in each treatment arm, now with pointwise confidence limits added (Fig. 6.6). Indeed, near the end of the study, these intervals become extremely wide, as opposed to the relatively narrow intervals at the start of the experiment. Thus, it is clear that dropout leads to efficiency loss. Of course, this effect can be due in part to increasing variability over time. Modeling is needed to obtain more insight into this effect.

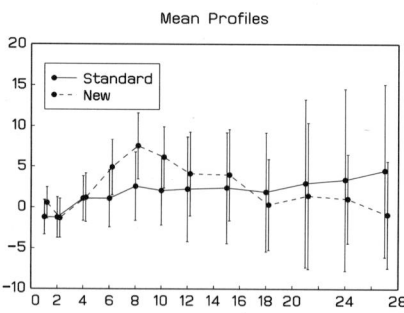

Figure 6.6. Vorozole Study. Mean profiles, with 95% pointwise confidence intervals added

To gain further insight into the impact of dropout, it is useful to construct dropout-pattern-specific plots. Figures 6.7 and 6.8 display the individual and averaged profiles per pattern.

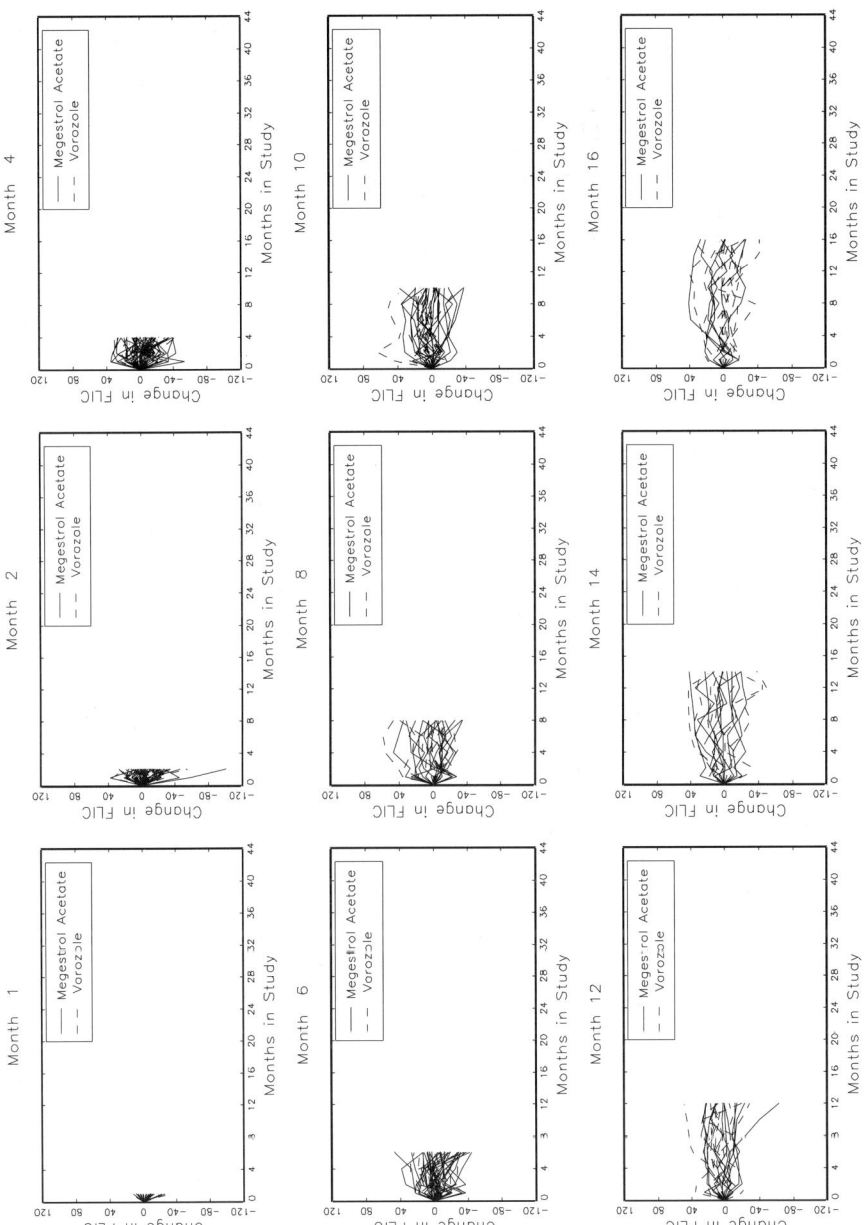

Figure 6.7. Vorozole Study. Individual profiles, per dropout pattern

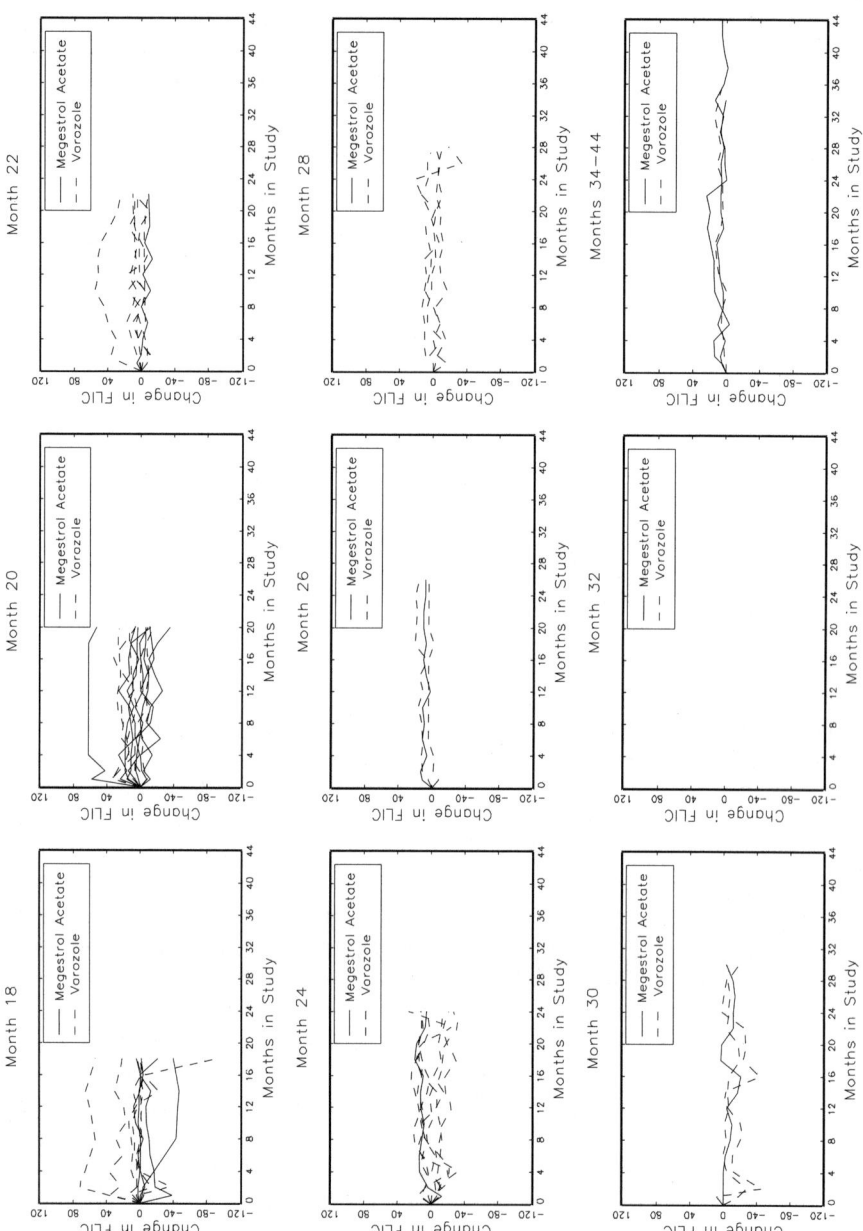

Figure 6.7. (continued)

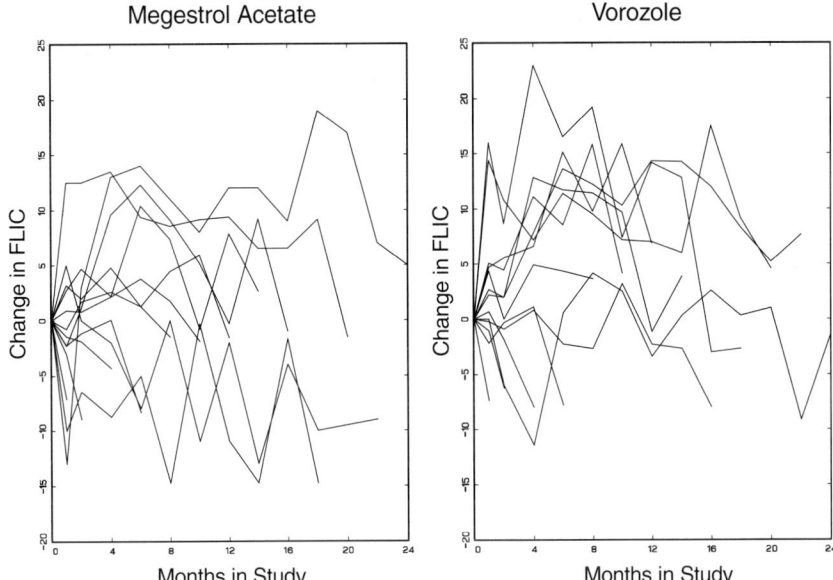

Figure 6.8. Vorozole Study. Mean profiles, per dropout pattern, grouped per treatment arm

This plot will be useful as a graphical start to a so-called pattern-mixture analysis, as described later in Sect. 6.16. The individual profiles plot, by definition displaying all available data, has some intrinsic limitations. As is the case with any individual data plot, it tends to be fairly busy. Since there is a lot of early dropout, there are many short sequences and since we decided to use the same time axis for all profiles, also for those that drop out early, very little information can be extracted. Indeed, the evolution over the first few sequences is not clear at all. In addition, the eye assigns more weight to the longer profiles, even though they are considerably less frequent.

Some of these limitations are removed in Fig. 6.8, where the pattern-specific average profiles are displayed per treatment arm. Still, care has to be taken for not overinterpreting the longer profiles and neglecting the shorter profiles. Indeed, for this study the latter represent more subjects than the longer profiles.

Several observations can be made. Most profiles clearly show a quadratic trend, which seems to be in contrast with the relatively flat nature of the average profiles in Fig. 6.6. This implies that the impression from all patterns together may differ radically from a pattern-specific look. These conclusions seem to be consistent across treatment arms.

Another important observation is that those who drop out rather early seem to decrease from the start, whereas those who remain relatively long in the study exhibit, on average and in turn, a rise, a plateau, and then a decrease. Looked upon from the standpoint of dropout, we suggest that there are at least two important characteristics that make dropout increase: (1) a low value of change versus baseline and (2) an unfavorable (downward) evolution.

Arguably, careful modeling of these data, irrespective of the approach chosen, should reflect these features. We will consider the most important routes typically taken, starting from simple ad hoc methods, and then going to more principled methods, for which we first need to develop a formal but intuitively appealing framework.

6.2.2   The Psychiatric Study

The second case study is a clinical trial, including 342 patients with post-baseline data. The Hamilton Depression Rating Scale ($HAMD_{17}$) is used to measure the

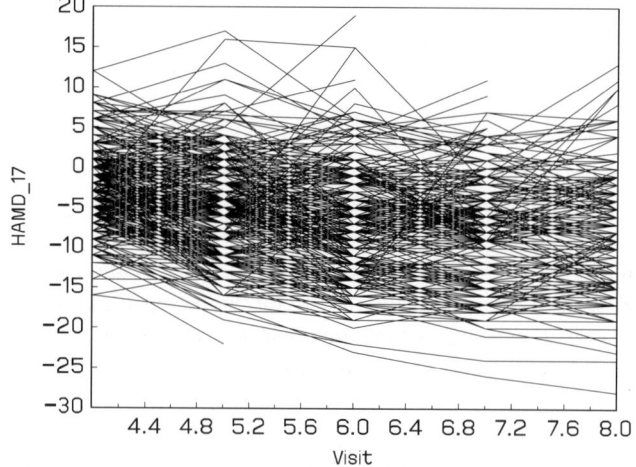

Figure 6.9. Psychiatric Study. Individual profiles

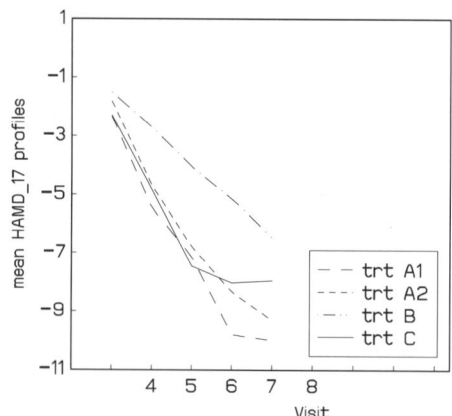

Figure 6.10. Psychiatric Study. Mean profiles per treatment arm

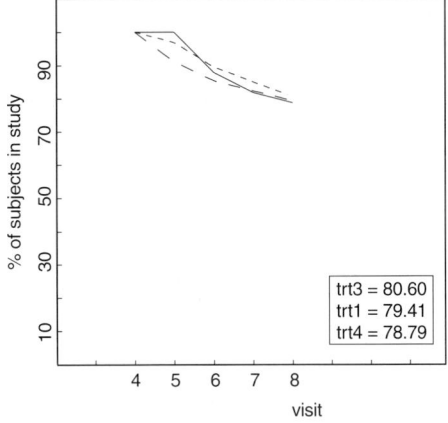

Figure 6.11. Psychiatric Study. Evolution of dropout per treatment arm. Treatment arms 1 (A1) and 4 (C), being the ones of primary interest, are shown in bolder typeface

depression status of the patients. The binary outcome of interest is 1 if the $HAMD_{17}$ score is larger than 7, and 0 otherwise. For each patient, a baseline assessment is available. Post-baseline visits are from visit 4 to 8.

For blinding purposes, therapies are recoded as A1 for primary dose of experimental drug, A2 for secondary dose of experimental drug, and B and C for non-experimental drugs. Individual profiles and mean profiles per treatment arm are shown in Figs. 6.9 and 6.10 respectively. The primary contrast is between A1 and C. Emphasis is on the difference between arms at the end of the study. A graphical representation of the dropout, per treatment arm, is given in Fig. 6.11.

Simple Ad Hoc Methods

6.3

We will briefly review a number of relatively simple methods that have been and still are in extensive use. A number of them are valid when the measurement and missing data processes are independent and their parameters are separated, which is called the missing completely at random or MCAR assumption, while for other methods this assumption is necessary but not sufficient. It is important to realize that many of these methods are used also in situations where the MCAR assumption is not tenable. This should be seen as bad practice since it will often lead to biased estimates and invalid tests and hence to erroneous conclusions. Ample detail and illustrations of several problems are provided in Verbeke and Molenberghs (1997, Chap. 5). The focus will be on the complete case method, where data are removed, on the one hand and on imputation strategies, where data are filled in on the other hand. Regarding imputation, one distinguishes between single and multiple imputation. In the first case, a single value is substituted for every "hole" in the data set and the resulting data set is analysed as if it represented the true complete data. Multiple imputation properly acknowledges the uncertainty stemming from filling in missing values rather than observing them (Rubin 1987; Schafer 1997). Last observation carried forward (LOCF) will be discussed within the context of imputation strategies, although not every author classifies the method as belonging to the imputation family. Other imputation techniques that will be described are unconditional and conditional mean imputation.

An often quoted advantage of the methods described below and related ones is that complete data software can be used. With the availability of such software like the SAS procedures GENMOD, MIXED, and NLMIXED, it is however no longer necessary to restrict oneself to complete data software, since they allow a likelihood-based ignorable analysis, using the data as they are, without deletion or imputation.

6.3.1   Complete Case Analysis

A complete case (CC) analysis includes only those cases for analysis, for which all measurements were recorded. This method has obvious advantages. It is very simple to describe and since the data structure is as would have resulted from a complete experiment, standard statistical software can be used. Further, since the entire estimation is done on the same subset of completers, there is a common basis for inference, unlike for the available case methods. Unfortunately, the method suffers from severe drawbacks. First, there is nearly always a substantial loss of information. For example, suppose there are 20 measurements, with 10% of missing data on each measurement. Suppose, further, that missingness on the different measurements is independent; then, the estimated percentage of incomplete observations is as high as 87%. The impact on precision and power is dramatic. Even though the reduction of the number of complete cases will be less dramatic in realistic settings where the missingness indicators are correlated, the effect just sketched will often undermine a complete case analysis. In addition, severe bias can result when the missingness mechanism is not MCAR. Indeed, should an estimator be consistent in the complete data problem, then the derived complete case analysis is consistent only if the missingness process is MCAR.

A simple partial check on the MCAR assumption is as follows (Little and Rubin 1987). Divide the observations on measurement j into two groups: (1) those subjects that are also observed on another measurement or set of measurements and (2) those missing on the other measurement(s). Should MCAR hold, then both groups should be random samples of the same population. Failure to reject equality of the distributional parameters of both samples increases the evidence for MCAR, but does not prove it.

6.3.2   Simple Forms of Imputation

An alternative way to obtain a data set on which complete data methods can be used is based on filling in rather then deletion. Commonly, the observed values are used to impute values for the missing observations. There are several ways to use the observed information. First, one can use information on the same subject (e.g., last observation carried forward). Second, information can be borrowed from other subjects (e.g., mean imputation). Finally, both within and between subject information can be used (e.g., conditional mean imputation, hot deck imputation). Before discussing some of these, we will point to common pitfalls. A standard reference is Little and Rubin (1987).

Indeed, great care has to be taken with these imputation strategies such as LOCF. Dempster and Rubin (1983) write: "The idea of imputation is both seductive and dangerous. It is seductive because it can lull the user into the pleasurable state of believing that the data are complete after all, and it is dangerous because it lumps together situations where the problem is sufficiently minor that it can be legitimately handled in this way and situations where standard estimators applied to the real and imputed data have substantial biases." For example, Little and Rubin (1987) show that imputation could work for a linear model with one fixed effect and one error term, but that it generally does not for hierarchical models, split-plot designs, and repeated measures (with a complicated error structure), random-effects, and mixed-effects models. For a general discussion of regression models we refer to Chap. II.3 of this handbook.

Thus, the user of imputation strategies faces several dangers. First, the imputation model could be wrong and, hence, the point estimates would be biased. Second, even for a correct imputation model, the uncertainty resulting from missingness is masked. Indeed, even when one is reasonably sure about the mean value the unknown observation *would have had*, the actual stochastic realization, depending on both the mean and error structures, is still unknown. In addition, most methods require the MCAR assumption to hold while some even require additional and often unrealistically strong assumptions.

Last Observation Carried Forward

A method that has received a lot of attention (Siddiqui and Ali 1998; Mallinckrodt et al. 2003a,b) is last observation carried forward (LOCF). In the LOCF method, whenever a value is missing, the last observed value is substituted. The technique can be applied to both monotone and nonmonotone missing data. It is typically applied to settings where incompleteness is due to attrition.

Very strong and often unrealistic assumptions have to be made to ensure validity of this method. First, one has to believe that a subjects' measurement stays at the same level from the moment of dropout onward (or during the period they are unobserved in the case of intermittent missingness). In a clinical trial setting, one might believe that the response profile *changes* as soon as a patient goes off treatment and even that it would flatten. However, the constant profile assumption is even stronger. Further, this method shares with other single imputation methods that it overestimates the precision by treating imputed and actually observed values on equal footing.

However, LOCF does not need to be seen as an imputation strategy. The situation in which the scientific question is in terms of the last observed measurement, is often considered to be the real motivation for LOCF. Though in some cases, the question defined as such, may be perceived as having an unrealistic and ad-hoc flavor. Clearly, measurements at (self-selected) dropout times are lumped together with measurements made at the (investigator defined) end of the study.

Imputing Unconditional Means

The idea behind unconditional mean imputation (Little and Rubin 1987) is to replace a missing value with the average of the observed values on the same variable over the other subjects. Thus, the term *unconditional* refers to the fact that one does not use (i.e., condition on) information on the subject for which an imputation is generated.

Buck's Method: Conditional Mean Imputation

This approach was suggested by Buck (1960) and reviewed by Little and Rubin (1987). The method is technically hardly more complex than mean imputation. Let us describe it first for a single multivariate normal sample. The first step is to estimate the mean vector μ and the covariance matrix Σ from the complete cases. This step builds on the assumption that $Y \sim N(\mu, \Sigma)$. For a subject with missing components, the regression of the missing components (Y_i^m) on the observed ones (y_i^o) is

$$Y_i^m | y_i^o \sim N\left(\mu^m + \Sigma^{mo}(\Sigma^{oo})^{-1}(y_i^o - \mu_i^o), \Sigma^{mm} - \Sigma^{mo}(\Sigma^{oo})^{-1}\Sigma^{om}\right) .$$

Superscripts o and m refer to "observed" and "missing" components, respectively. The second step calculates the conditional mean from this regression and substitutes it for the missing values. In this way, "vertical" information (estimates for μ and Σ) is combined with "horizontal" information (y_i^o).

Buck (1960) showed that under mild regularity conditions, the method is valid for MCAR mechanisms. Little and Rubin (1987) added that the method is valid under certain types of missing at random (MAR) mechanism (i.e. when conditional on the observed data, the dropout is independent of the unobserved measurements). Even though the distribution of the observed components is allowed to differ between complete and incomplete observations, it is very important that the regression of the missing components on the observed ones is constant across missingness patterns.

Again, this method shares with other single imputation strategies that, although point estimation may be consistent, the precision will be overestimated. Little and Rubin (1987, p. 46) indicated ways to correct the precision estimation for unconditional mean imputation.

6.3.3   Discussion of Imputation Techniques

The imputation methods reviewed here are clearly not the only ones. Little and Rubin (1987) and Rubin (1987) mention several others. Several methods, such as hot deck imputation, are based on filling in missing values from "matching" subjects, where an appropriate matching criterion is used.

Almost all imputation techniques suffer from the following limitations:

1. The performance of imputation techniques is unreliable. Situations where they do work are difficult to distinguish from situations were they prove misleading.
2. Imputation often requires ad hoc adjustments to yield satisfactory point estimates.
3. The methods fail to provide simple correct precision estimators.

In addition, most methods require the MCAR assumption to hold. Methods such as the last observation carried forward require additional and often unrealistically strong assumptions.

A Classic Model for Continuous Longitudinal Data

6.4

Having introduced a number of simple methods in the previous section, we would like to apply them to the Vorozole Study in the next section. To this end, we will introduce the linear mixed model (Verbeke and Molenberghs 2000) since this is undoubtedly the most commonly used model for Gaussian longitudinal data.

Assume that for subject $i = 1, \ldots, N$ in the study a sequence of responses Y_{ij} is designed to be measured at occasions $j = 1, \ldots, n$. The outcomes are grouped into a vector $Y_i = (Y_{i1}, \ldots, Y_{in})'$.

For continuous outcomes, one typically assumes a linear mixed-effects model, perhaps with serial correlation:

$$Y_i = X_i\beta + Z_i b_i + W_i + \varepsilon_i , \tag{6.1}$$

(Verbeke and Molenberghs 2000) where Y_i is the n dimensional response vector for subject i, $1 \leq i \leq N$, N is the number of subjects, X_i and Z_i are $(n \times p)$ and $(n \times q)$ known design matrices, β is the p dimensional vector containing the fixed effects, $b_i \sim N(0, D)$ is the q dimensional vector containing the random effects, $\varepsilon_i \sim N(0, \sigma^2 I_{n_i})$ is a n dimensional vector of measurement error components, and $b_1, \ldots, b_N, \varepsilon_1, \ldots, \varepsilon_N$ are assumed to be independent. Serial correlation is captured by the realization of a Gaussian stochastic process, W_i, which is assumed to follow a $N(0, \tau^2 H_i)$ law. The serial covariance matrix H_i only depends on i through the number n of observations and through the time points t_{ij} at which measurements are taken. The structure of the matrix H_i is determined through the autocorrelation function $\varrho(t_{ij} - t_{ik})$. This function decreases such that $\varrho(0) = 1$ and $\varrho(+\infty) = 0$. Finally, D is a general $(q \times q)$ covariance matrix with (i, j) element $d_{ij} = d_{ji}$. Inference is based on the marginal distribution of the response Y_i which, after integrating over random effects, can be expressed as

$$Y_i \sim N\left(X_i\beta, Z_i D Z_i' + \Sigma_i\right) . \tag{6.2}$$

Here, $\Sigma_i = \sigma^2 I_{n_i} + \tau^2 H_i$ is a $(n \times n)$ covariance matrix grouping the measurement error and serial components.

Two popular choices to capture serial correlation is by means of exponential or Gaussian decay. An exponential process is based on writing the correlation between two residuals at times t_{ij} and t_{ik} as

$$\text{Corr}\left(t_{ij}, t_{ik}\right) = \exp\left(-\frac{|t_{ij} - t_{ik}|}{\phi}\right) = \varrho^{|t_{ij} - t_{ik}|}, \tag{6.3}$$

($\phi > 0$), where $\varrho = \exp(-1/\phi)$. The Gaussian counterpart is

$$\text{Corr}\left(t_{ij}, t_{ik}\right) = \exp\left(-\frac{\left(t_{ij} - t_{ik}\right)^2}{\phi^2}\right) = \varrho^{\left(t_{ij} - t_{ik}\right)^2}, \tag{6.4}$$

($\phi > 0$), $\varrho = \exp(-1/\phi^2)$. It follows from (6.1) that, conditional on the random effect $\boldsymbol{b}_i$, $\boldsymbol{Y}_i$ is normally distributed with mean vector $X_i\boldsymbol{\beta} + Z_i\boldsymbol{b}_i$ and with covariance matrix Σ_i. Define $V_i = Z_iGZ_i' + \Sigma_i$, then the marginal distribution of $\boldsymbol{Y}_i$ is $\boldsymbol{Y}_i \sim N(X_i\boldsymbol{\beta}, V_i)$.

In a clinical-trial setting and in some epidemiological settings one often has balanced data in the sense that the measurement occasions are common to all patients. In such a case, one often considers the random effects as nuisance parameters. The focus is then, for example, on the marginal compound-symmetry model rather than on the hierarchical random-intercepts model. Or, more generally, one considers $\Sigma_i = \Sigma$ to be unstructured and then no random effects are explicitly included. Especially when the number of patients is much larger than the number of measurement occasions within a patient, such an approach is useful. In an epidemiological setting however, one is often confronted with longer measurement sequences, perhaps also unequally spaced and/or of unequal length.

6.5   Simple Methods Applied to the Vorozole Study

Let us now apply the most often used simple methods, complete case analysis and last observation carried forward, to the Vorozole study. Each method is considered twice. First, we restrict attention to the first 2 years, in line with our choice in Sect. 6.2.1, and second we only use the first year for the analyses. The linear mixed model is used to perform the analyses. As covariates we include time in months, the treatment-by-time and baseline-by-time interaction, as well as a quadratic time trend and its interaction with baseline. For the covariance structure, we consider a random intercept, together with a spatial Gaussian process and measurement error. The model selection that leads to this choice is explained in detail in Sect. 6.8.

In Tables 6.2 and 6.3, we compare the results obtained with the simple methods, CC and LOCF, with the results of a direct-likelihood analysis, which is valid under the MAR assumptions and uses all available data.

Considering the first two years, Table 6.2 shows several differences between the estimates and standard errors of the CC and LOCF analyses versus the direct-likelihood analysis. Since only few patients complete the study until the 24th month, a lot of information is excluded for the CC analysis. In the Vorozole study, many patients drop out early in the study, thus a lot of values have to be filled in. All effects become non-significant in the CC analysis, while there is not much difference between the p-values of the LOCF and direct-likelihood analyses.

Table 6.2. Vorozole Study. Estimates (Est.), standard errors (S.E.) and p-values for the fixed effect parameters, using CC, LOCF and direct-likelihood MAR analysis on data of first two years (t represents time)

	CC (2 years)			LOCF (2 years)			MAR (2 years)		
	Est.	(S.E.)	p	Est.	(S.E.)	p	Est.	(S.E.)	p
t	4.11	(3.71)	0.27	0.90	(0.22)	< 0.0001	7.29	(0.95)	< 0.0001
$t \times$ base	−0.031	(0.028)	0.27	−0.0094	(0.0018)	< 0.0001	−0.061	(0.0078)	< 0.0001
$t \times$ treat	0.20	(0.26)	0.45	−0.0064	(0.023)	0.78	0.12	(0.14)	0.39
$t \times t$	−0.073	(0.15)	0.63	−0.015	(0.0047)	0.0012	−0.28	(0.054)	< 0.0001
$t \times t \times$ base	0.00053	(0.0011)	0.64	0.00016	(0.00004)	< 0.0001	0.0023	(0.00044)	< 0.0001

Table 6.3. Vorozole Study. Estimates (Est.), standard errors (S.E.) and p-values for the fixed effect parameters, using CC, LOCF and direct-likelihood MAR analysis on data of the first year (t represents time)

	CC (1 years)			LOCF (1 years)			MAR (1 years)		
	Est.	(S.E.)	p	Est.	(S.E.)	p	Est.	(S.E.)	p
t	9.86	(2.35)	< 0.0001	3.51	(0.96)	0.0002	8.22	(1.50)	< 0.0001
$t \times$ base	−0.073	(0.019)	0.0002	−0.032	(0.0081)	< 0.0001	−0.070	(0.012)	< 0.0001
$t \times$ treat	0.41	(0.25)	0.10	0.037	(0.12)	0.75	0.17	(0.18)	0.35
$t \times t$	−0.47	(0.19)	0.012	−0.13	(0.072)	0.063	−0.37	(0.14)	0.0062
$t \times t \times$ base	0.0031	(0.0015)	0.044	0.0011	(0.00061)	0.064	0.0032	(0.0011)	0.0049

On the other hand, when performing the analyses on the data of the first year only, the results of CC analysis and direct-likelihood analysis are reasonably similar. There is no change in significance, while there still is a great difference between the LOCF and direct-likelihood analyses. Two effects become significant when switching from LOCF to a direct-likelihood analysis.

A Framework for Handling Missing Values   6.6

We assume that our aim is to make inferences about means, time evolutions, treatment differences, etc. That is, some adjustment or allowance may need to be made to recover the underlying responses that would have been observed if all the observations were available, irrespective of the occurrence of dropout. Or, in a sensitivity analysis sense, we would like to learn what range of inferences about the marginal response are plausible given the setting, observed data and pattern of missing values. An attempt is made to achieve this by jointly modeling both the response and the missing value, or dropout, mechanism.

Rubin's taxonomy (Rubin 1976; Little and Rubin 1987) of missing value processes is fundamental to modeling incomplete data. Before describing this we introduce some basic notation. Let the random vector Y correspond to the, possibly notional, complete set of measurements on a subject whether observed or not and suppose that its distribution depends on a vector of parameters θ. Let R be the associated missing value indicator, with distribution depending on parameter vector ψ. In case missingness is restricted to dropout, we define D to be the occasion of dropout. For a particular realization of this pair (y, r) the elements of r take the values 1 and 0 indicating respectively whether the corresponding values of y are observed or not. When we are dealing with dropout the information in r can be summarised in a single variable: the first time at which a value is missing. Let (y_o, y_m) denote the partition of y into the respective sets of observed and missing data. In what follows we will be attempting to fit and make inferences about models constructed for the pair (y, r) using only the observed data: (y_o, r). If $f(y, r)$ is the joint distribution of the complete data, then the marginal distribution of the observed data, which forms the basis for model fitting, is

$$f(y_o, r) = \int f(y, r)\, dy_m \; . \tag{6.5}$$

Rubin's classification essentially distinguishes settings in which important simplifications of this process are possible.

Missing Completely at Random (MCAR). Under an MCAR mechanism the probability of an observation being missing is independent of the responses: $P(R = r \mid y) = P(R = r)$. The joint distribution of the *observed* data partitions as follows: $f(y_o, r) = f(y_o; \theta)P(r; \psi)$. Under MCAR the observed data can be analysed as though the pattern of missing values were predetermined, as they are in the example just given. In whatever way the data are analysed, whether using a frequentist or likelihood procedure, the process(es) generating the missing values can be ignored. For example, in this situation simple averages of the observed data at different times provide unbiased estimates of the underlying marginal profiles.

Missing at Random (MAR). Under an MAR mechanism, the probability of an observation being missing is *conditionally* independent of the unobserved data, given the values of the observed data: $P(R = r \mid y) = P(r \mid y_o)$, and again the joint distribution of the observed data can be partitioned:

$$f(y_o, r) = f(y_o; \theta)P(r \mid y_o; \psi) \; . \tag{6.6}$$

An example of random dropout occurs in a trial in which subjects are removed when their observed response drifts outside prescribed limits, Murray and Findlay (1988) describe an instance of this. We note that the handling of the MAR assumption is much easier with dropout than with more general missing value patterns.

No mention has been made of covariates and the dependence of missing value probabilities on these. According to Little (1995), the original intention was that MCAR should refer to the case in which the probability of a value being missing does not depend on the response *or* covariates, and suggests the term "covariate-dependent" missing value mechanism for the case where it depends on the latter. This avoids the problem of having the class of mechanisms potentially changing with the addition and removal of covariates.

One can see the importance of the MAR assumption from an intuitive viewpoint. Essentially it states that once appropriate account is taken of what we have observed, there remains no dependence on unobservables, at least in terms of the probability model. We should as a consequence expect much of the missing value problem to disappear under the MAR mechanism and this is in fact the case. This can be shown more formally through consideration of the likelihood. The result (6.6) implies that the joint log-likelihood for θ and ψ partitions:

$$\ell(\theta, \psi; y_o, r) = \ell(\theta; y_o) + \ell(\psi; r) .$$

Provided that θ and ψ are not interdependent, information about the response model parameter θ is contained wholly in $\ell(\theta; y_o)$, the log-likelihood of the observed response data. This is the log-likelihood function that is used when no account is taken of the missing value mechanism, hence for a likelihood analysis under the MAR assumption, the missing value mechanism is said to be *ignorable*. It should be noted that although the correct maximum likelihood estimates and likelihood ratio statistics will be generated by the use of $\ell(\theta; y_o)$, some care needs to be taken with the choice of appropriate sampling distribution in a frequentist analysis. For this the missing value mechanism is *not* ignorable, even under MAR (Kenward and Molenberghs 1998). In practice though there is little reason for worry since this just means that estimates of precision should be based on the observed rather than the expected information matrix. More recently it has been shown how non-likelihood approaches can be developed for the MAR case (Robins et al. 1995, 1998; Fitzmaurice et al. 1995).

While the MAR assumption is particularly convenient in that it leads to considerable simplification in the issues surrounding the analysis of incomplete longitudinal data, it is rare in practice to be able to justify its adoption, and so in many situations the final class of missing value mechanisms applies.

Missing Not at Random (MNAR). In this case neither MCAR nor MAR hold. Under MNAR the probability of a measurement being missing depends on unobserved data. No simplification of the joint distribution is possible and inferences can only be made by making further assumptions, about which the observed data alone carry no information. Ideally the choice of such assumptions should be guided by external information, but the degree to which this is possible in practice varies greatly. In attempting to formulate models for the joint distribution of the response and dropout process, $f(y, r)$, two main types of model have been used and these are defined by two possible factorizations of this distribution. The first, the *selection* model, is based on

$$f(y, r) = f(y)P(r \mid y) . \tag{6.7}$$

The second, the *pattern mixture* model (PMM), uses

$$f(y, r) = f(y \mid r)P(r) . \tag{6.8}$$

The differences are important in the MNAR case, and lead to quite different, but complementary, views of the missing value problem. Little (1995) and Hogan and Laird (1997) provide detailed reviews. The term selection model originates from the econometric literature (Heckman 1976) and it can be seen that a subject's missing values are "selected" through the probability model, given their measurements, whether observed or not. Rubin's classification is defined in the selection framework, and imposition of conditions on $P(r \mid y)$ determines to which of the three classes the model belongs in the frequentist sense. On the other hand the pattern mixture model allows a different response model for each pattern of missing values, the observed data being a mixture of these weighted by the probability of each missing value or dropout pattern. At first sight such a model is less appealing in terms of probability mechanisms for generating the data, but it has other important advantages. Recently it has been shown, for dropout, how the Rubin classification can be applied in the pattern-mixture framework as well (Molenberghs et al. 1998; Kenward et al. 2003). We will consider these two approaches to modeling data with non-random dropout in Sects. 6.7 and 6.9.

6.6.1   Continuous Data and Ignorability

Let us now describe the missingness model, and then formally introduce and comment on ignorability. The measurement model will depend on whether or not a full longitudinal analysis is done. In case focus is on the last observed measurement or on the last measurement occasion only, one typically opts for classical two- or multi-group comparisons (t test, Wilcoxon, etc.). In case a longitudinal analysis is deemed necessary, the choice made depends on the nature of the outcome. For continuous outcomes, one typically assumes a linear mixed-effects model, perhaps with serial correlation as described in Sect. 6.4. Models for categorical date will be described later in this chapter.

Recall that for subject $i = 1, \ldots, N$ in the study a sequence of responses Y_{ij} is designed to be measured at occasions $j = 1, \ldots, n$ and the outcomes are grouped into a vector $Y_i = (Y_{i1}, \ldots, Y_{in})'$. In addition, define a dropout indicator D_i for the occasion at which dropout occurs and make the convention that $D_i = n + 1$ for a complete sequence.

Assume that incompleteness is due to dropout only, and that the first measurement Y_{i1} is obtained for everyone. The model for the dropout process is based on, for example, a logistic regression for the probability of dropout at occasion j, given the subject is still in the study. We denote this probability by $g(\boldsymbol{h}_{ij}, y_{ij})$ in which $\boldsymbol{h}_{ij}$ is a vector containing all responses observed up to but not including occasion j, as well as relevant covariates. We then assume that $g(\boldsymbol{h}_{ij}, y_{ij})$ satisfies

$$\text{logit}\left[g(\boldsymbol{h}_{ij}, y_{ij})\right] = \text{logit}\left[\text{pr}\left(D_i = j | D_i \geq j, \boldsymbol{y}_i\right)\right] = \boldsymbol{h}_{ij}\boldsymbol{\psi} + \omega y_{ij}. \qquad (6.9)$$

When ω equals zero, the dropout model is MAR, and all parameters can be estimated using standard software since the measurement model for which we use a linear mixed model and the dropout model, assumed to follow a logistic regression, can then be fitted separately. If $\omega \neq 0$, the posited dropout process is MNAR. Model (6.9) provides the building blocks for the dropout process $f(d_i | y_i, \boldsymbol{\psi})$. This model is often referred to as Diggle and Kenward's (1994) model.

Rubin (1976) and Little and Rubin (1987) have shown that, under MAR and mild regularity conditions (parameters $\boldsymbol{\theta}$ and $\boldsymbol{\psi}$ are functionally independent), likelihood-based inference is valid when the missing data mechanism is ignored (see also Verbeke and Molenberghs 2000). Practically speaking, the likelihood of interest is then based upon the factor $f(\boldsymbol{y}_i^o | \boldsymbol{\theta})$. This is called *ignorability*. The practical implication is that a software module with likelihood estimation facilities and with the ability to handle incompletely observed subjects manipulates the correct likelihood, providing valid parameter estimates and likelihood ratio values.

A few cautionary remarks are in place. First, when at least part of the scientific interest is directed towards the nonresponse process, obviously both processes need to be considered. Still, under MAR, both processes can be modeled and parameters estimated separately. Second, likelihood inference is often surrounded with references to the sampling distribution (e.g., to construct precision estimators and for statistical hypothesis tests; Kenward and Molenberghs 1998). However, the practical implication is that standard errors and associated tests, when based on the observed rather than the expected information matrix and given the parametric assumptions are correct, are valid. Third, it may be hard to fully rule out the operation of an MNAR mechanism. This point was brought up in the introduction and will be discussed further in Sect. 6.14. Fourth, an analysis can proceed only when a full longitudinal analysis is necessary, even when interest lies, for example, in a comparison between the two treatment groups at the last occasion. In the latter case, the fitted model can be used as the basis for inference at the last occasion.

A common criticism is that a model needs to be considered. However, it should be noted that in many clinical trial settings the repeated measures are balanced in the sense that a common (and often limited) set of measurement times is considered for all subjects, allowing the a priori specification of a saturated model (e.g., full group by time interaction model for the fixed effects and unstructured variance-covariance matrix). Such an ignorable linear mixed model specification is termed MMRM (mixed-model random missingness) by Mallinckrodt et al. (2001a,b). Thus, MMRM is a particular form of a linear mixed model, relevant for not only the clinical trials context, but also more generally for reasonably balanced studies with human subjects, and fitting within the ignorable likelihood paradigm. Such an approach is a very promising alternative for the often used simple methods described in Sect. 6.3 such as complete-case analysis or LOCF.

6.7 Selection Models

Much of the early development of, and debate about, selection models appeared in the econometrics literature in which the tobit model (Heckman 1976) played a central role. This combines a marginal Gaussian regression model for the response, as might be used in the absence of missing data, with a Gaussian based threshold model for the probability of a value being missing. For simplicity consider a single Gaussian distributed response variable $Z \sim N(\mu, \sigma^2)$. The probability of Z being missing is assumed to depend on a second Gaussian variable $Z_m \sim N(\mu_m, \sigma_m^2)$ where $P(R = 0) = P(Z_m < 0)$. Dependence of missingness on the response Z is induced by introducing a correlation between Z and Z_m. To avoid some of the complications of direct likelihood maximization, a two-stage estimation procedure was proposed by Heckman (1976) for this type of model. The use of the tobit model and associated two-stage procedure was the subject of considerable debate in the econometrics literature, much of it focusing on the issues of identifiability and sensitivity (Amemiya 1984; Little 1986). We shall see the same issues arising in developments of these ideas in the biometric and epidemiologic setting.

At first sight the tobit model does not appear to have the selection model structure specified in (6.7) in that there is no conditional partition of $f(y, r)$. However, it is simple to show from the joint Gaussian distribution of Z and Z_m, that in the tobit model $P(R = 0 \mid Z = z)$ equals $\Phi(\beta_0 + \beta_1 z)$ for suitably chosen parameters β_0 and β_1, with $\Phi(\cdot)$ the Gaussian distribution function. This can be seen as a probit regression model for the (binary) missing value process. This basic structure underlies the simplest form of selection model that has been proposed for longitudinal data in the biometric and epidemiologic setting. A suitable response model, such as the multivariate Gaussian, is combined with a binary regression model for dropout. At each time point the occurrence of dropout can be regressed on previous and current values of the response as well as covariates. We now explore such models in more detail.

Although modeling a continuous response is generally more straightforward than a categorical response, we begin by considering the latter case. By reducing the problem to a very simple setting, that of two repeated binary responses, we are able to illustrate some key points in a very explicit way. With both measurements (Y_1, Y_2) observed, a subject will generate one of four responses, with associated probabilities π_{ij}:

	Time 2		
Time 1	0	1	Total
0	π_{00}	π_{01}	$\pi_{0\cdot}$
1	π_{10}	π_{11}	$\pi_{1\cdot}$
Total	$\pi_{\cdot 0}$	$\pi_{\cdot 1}$	1

These probabilities can be parameterized in many different ways, for example using marginal or Markov representations. For the moment we are not concerned with the particular parameterization chosen and will work with the joint probabilities, noting that three of these determine the fourth. It is assumed at first that missing values are restricted to dropout and in the most general form the probability of dropout may depend on the outcome at either time, so we write for $R = 1$, the event of being observed on the second occasion:

$$P\left(R = 1 \mid Y_1 = s_1, Y_2 = s_2\right) = \phi_{s_1 s_2}, \quad s_1 = 0, 1; \quad s_2 = 0, 1.$$

There are four probabilities, making a total of seven degrees of freedom for the model that combines the response and dropout components. If we could observe the data from those who drop out, the full data could be represented as a $2 \times 2 \times 2$ contingency table, classified by the time 1 and 2 outcomes and dropout status. The model described saturates the degrees of freedom in this table. In practice, two tables of data are observed; a 2×2 table from the completers and a 2×1 table of time 1 outcomes from the dropouts, making a total of five degrees of freedom. Clearly some parameters in the full model cannot be identified, and if a model is to be estimated from the observed data some constraints must be applied. This reflects the information lost with the dropouts. The MCAR and MAR cases correspond to the simple constraints. Indeed, MCAR: $\phi_{s_1 s_2} = \phi$ and MAR: $\phi_{s_1 s_2} = \phi_{s_1}$. Allowing $\phi_{s_1 s_2}$ to depend on s_2 makes the dropout non-random. We can relate this dropout model in a simple way to the logistic regression models that have often been used in the selection model (Diggle and Kenward 1994; Baker 1995; Fitzmaurice et al. 1996a,b; Molenberghs et al. 1997) as follows:

$$\text{logit}\left(\phi_{ij}\right) = \beta_0 + \beta_1 Y_1 + \beta_2 Y_2. \tag{6.10}$$

Note that this does not saturate the dropout model; the introduction of the interaction term in $Y_1 Y_2$ would be required for this.

Selection Models Applied to the Vorozole Study 6.8

Let us consider Diggle and Kenward's (1994) selection model as introduced in Sect. 6.6.1. For the measurement model, we start by ignoring the dropout mechanism. This choice will turn out to be justified at the end of this section. Since we are modeling change versus baseline, all models are forced to pass through the origin. This is done by allowing the main covariate effects, but only through their interactions with time. The following covariates were considered for the measurement model: baseline value, treatment, dominant site, and time in months (up to a cubic time trend). Second order interactions were considered as well. Then, a backwards selection procedure was performed. For design reasons, treatment was kept in the model in spite of its non-significance. An F test for treatment effect produces a p value of 0.5822. Apart from baseline, no other time-stationary covariates were kept. A quadratic time effect provided an adequate description of the time trend. Based on the variogram, we confined the random-effects structure to random intercepts, and supplemented this with a spatial Gaussian process and measurement error. The final model is presented in Table 6.4. The total correlation between two measurements, one month apart, equals 0.696. The residual correlation, which remains after accounting for the random effects, is still equal to 0.491. The serial correlation, obtained by further ignoring the measurement error, equals $\varrho = \exp(-1/7.22^2) = 0.981$.

Table 6.4. Vorozole Study. Selection Model

Effect	Estimate (s.e.)
Fixed-Effect Parameters:	
Time	7.78 (1.05)
Time × baseline	−0.065 (0.009)
Time × treatment	0.086 (0.157)
Time × time	−0.30 (0.06)
Time × time × baseline	0.0024 (0.0005)
Variance Parameters:	
Random intercept (δ^2)	105.42
Serial variance (τ^2)	77.96
Serial association (ϕ)	7.22
Measurement error (σ^2)	77.83

Fitted profiles are displayed in Figs. 6.12 and 6.13. In Fig. 6.13, empirical Bayes estimates of the random effects are included whereas in Fig. 6.12 the purely marginal mean is used. For each treatment group, we obtain three sets of profiles. The fitted complete profile is the average curve that would be obtained, had all individuals been completely observed. If we use only those predicted values that correspond to occasions at which an observation was made, then the fitted incomplete profiles are obtained. The latter are somewhat above the former when the random effects are included, and somewhat below when they are not, suggesting that individuals with lower measurements are more likely to disappear from the study. In addition, while the fitted complete curves are very close (the treatment effect was not significant), the fitted incomplete curves are not, suggesting that there is more dropout in the standard arm than in the treatment arm. This is in agreement with the observed

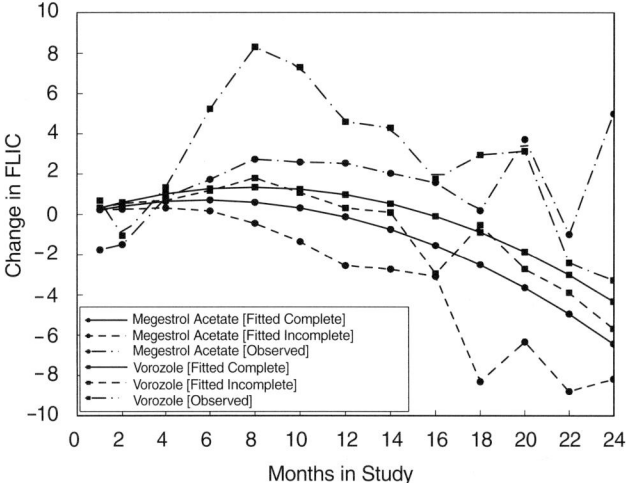

Figure 6.12. Vorozole Study. Fitted profiles (averaging the predicted means for the incomplete and complete measurement sequences, without the random effects)

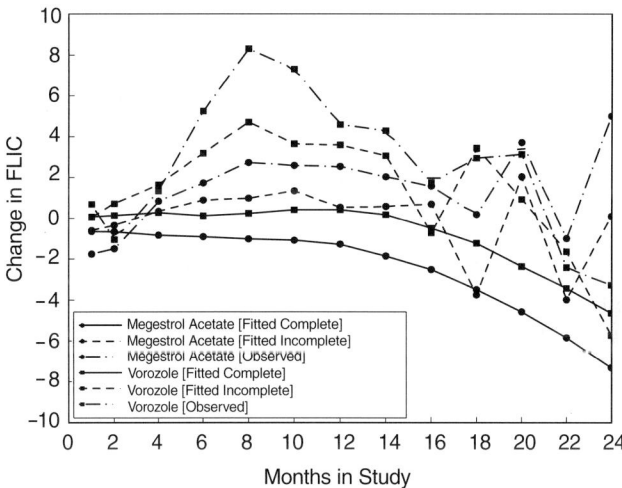

Figure 6.13. Vorozole Study. Fitted profiles (averaging the predicted means for the incomplete and complete measurement sequences, including the random effects)

dropout rate and should not be seen as evidence of a bad fit. Finally, the observed curves, based on the measurements available at each time point, are displayed. These are higher than the fitted ones, but this should be viewed with the standard errors of the observed means in mind (see Fig. 6.2).

Next, we will study factors which influence dropout. A logistic regression model, described by (6.9) and (6.29) is used. To start, we restrict attention to MAR processes, whence $\psi_d = 0$. The first model includes treatment, dominant site, baseline value, and the previous measurement but only the last two are significant, producing

$$\text{logit}\left[g(\mathbf{h}_{ij})\right] = 0.080(0.341) - 0.014(0.003)\text{base}_i - 0.033(0.004)y_{i,j-1} . \quad (6.11)$$

Diggle and Kenward (1994) and Molenberghs et al. (1997) considered non-random versions of this model by including the current, possible unobserved measurement, such as in (6.9). This requires more elaborate fitting algorithms, since the missing data process is then non-ignorable, and hence (6.5) needs to be used. Diggle and Kenward used the simplex algorithm (Nelder and Mead 1965), while Molenberghs et al. (1997) fitted their models with the EM algorithm. The algorithm of Diggle and Kenward is implemented in Oswald (Smith et al. 1996). With larger datasets such as this one, convergence can be painstakingly difficult and one has to worry about apparent convergence. Therefore, we first proceed in an alternative way. Both Diggle and Kenward, and Molenberghs et al. observed that in informative models, dropout tends to depend on the increment, i.e., the difference between the current and previous measurements $Y_{ij} - Y_{i,j-1}$. Clearly, a very similar quantity is obtained as $Y_{i,j-1} - Y_{i,j-2}$, but a major advantage of such a model is that it fits within the MAR framework. In our case, we obtain

$$\text{logit}\left[g(\mathbf{h}_{ij})\right] = 0.033(0.401) - 0.013(0.003)\text{base}_i$$

$$+ 0.012(0.006)y_{i,j-2} - 0.035(0.005)y_{i,j-1}$$

$$= 0.033(0.401) - 0.013(0.003)\text{base}_i$$

$$- 0.023(0.005)\frac{y_{i,j-2} + y_{i,j-1}}{2}$$

$$- 0.047(0.010)\frac{y_{i,j-1} - y_{i,j-2}}{2} \quad (6.12)$$

indicating that both size and increment are significant predictors for dropout. We conclude that dropout increases with a decrease in baseline, in overall level of the outcome variable, as well as with a decreasing evolution in the outcome.

Both dropout models (6.11) and (6.12) can be compared with their non-random counterparts, where y_{ij} is added to the linear predictor. The first one becomes

$$\text{logit}\left[g\left(\mathbf{h}_{ij}, y_{ij}\right)\right] = 0.53 - 0.015\text{base}_i - 0.076y_{i,j-1} + 0.057y_{ij} \quad (6.13)$$

while the second one becomes

$$\text{logit}\left[g\left(\mathbf{h}_{ij}, y_{ij}\right)\right] = 1.38 - 0.021\text{base}_i - 0.0027y_{i,j-2} - 0.064y_{i,j-1} + 0.035y_{ij} . \quad (6.14)$$

Formal testing of dropout models (6.13) versus (6.11) and for (6.14) versus (6.12) are possible in principle, but will not be carried out for two reasons. First, the likelihood function tends to be very flat for non-random dropout models and therefore the determination of the likelihood ratio is often computationally non-trivial. More fundamentally, Rubin (1994), Little (1994), Laird (1994), and Molenberghs et al. (1997) pointed out that formal testing for non-random dropout faces philosophical objections. Indeed, non-random dropout models are identified only due to strong but unverifiable assumptions. Hogan and Laird (1997) suggested pattern-mixture models as a viable alternative.

Pattern-Mixture Models   6.9

Recall that the pattern-mixture decomposition is given by (6.8). As a simple illustration consider a continuous response at three times of measurement which will be modeled using a trivariate Gaussian distribution. Assume that there may be dropout at time 2 or 3, and let the dropout indicator R take the values 1 and 2 to indicate that the last observation occurred at these times and 3 to indicate no dropout. Then, in the first instance, the model implies a different distribution for each time of dropout. We can write:

$$ y \mid r \sim N\left(\boldsymbol{\mu}^{(r)}; \boldsymbol{\Sigma}^{(r)}\right) , \tag{6.15} $$

where

$$ \boldsymbol{\mu}^{(r)} = \begin{bmatrix} \mu_1^{(r)} \\ \mu_2^{(r)} \\ \mu_3^{(r)} \end{bmatrix} \quad \text{and} \quad \boldsymbol{\Sigma}^{(r)} = \begin{bmatrix} \sigma_{11}^{(r)} & \sigma_{21}^{(r)} & \sigma_{31}^{(r)} \\ \sigma_{21}^{(r)} & \sigma_{22}^{(r)} & \sigma_{32}^{(r)} \\ \sigma_{31}^{(r)} & \sigma_{32}^{(r)} & \sigma_{33}^{(r)} \end{bmatrix} , $$

for $r = 1, 2, 3$. Let $P(r) = \pi_r$, then the marginal distribution of the response is a mixture of normals with, for example, mean

$$ \mu = \sum_{r=1}^{3} \pi_r \boldsymbol{\mu}^{(r)} . $$

However, although the π_r can be simply estimated from the observed proportions in each dropout group, only 16 of the 27 response parameters can be identified from the data without making further assumptions. These 16 comprise all the parameters from the completers plus those from the following two submodels. For $r = 2$

$$ N\left(\begin{bmatrix} \mu_1^{(2)} \\ \mu_2^{(2)} \end{bmatrix}; \begin{bmatrix} \sigma_{11}^{(2)} & \sigma_{21}^{(2)} \\ \sigma_{31}^{(3)} & \sigma_{32}^{(3)} \end{bmatrix} \right) , $$

and for $r = 1$: $N\left(\mu_1^{(2)}; \sigma_{11}^{(1)}\right)$. This is a *saturated* pattern-mixture model and the representation makes it very clear what information each dropout group provides, and consequently the assumptions that need to be made if we are to predict the behaviour of the unobserved responses, and so obtain marginal models for the response. If the three sets of parameters $\boldsymbol{\mu}^{(r)}$ are simply equated, this implies MCAR. Progress can be made with less stringent restrictions however. These identifying restrictions are considered in Sect. 6.16.1. In practice, choice of restrictions will need to be guided by the context. In addition, the form of the data will typically be more complex, requiring, for example, a more structured model for the response with the incorporation of covariates. Hence such models can be constructed in many ways.

6.10   Pattern-Mixture Models Applied to the Vorozole Study

First, we analyse the data using basic pattern-mixture models. Later in this chapter we will apply pattern-mixture models based on identifying restrictions.

Initial Pattern-Mixture Models

The dropout process simplifies to $f(d_i|\boldsymbol{\psi})$ which is a, possibly covariate-corrected, model for the probability to belong to a particular pattern. Its components describe the dropout rate at each occasion.

The measurement model has to reflect dependence on dropout. In its most general form, this implies that (6.1) is replaced by

$$
\left\{
\begin{array}{l}
Y_i = X_i\boldsymbol{\beta}(d_i) + Z_i b_i + \boldsymbol{\varepsilon}_i \, , \\[2ex]
b_i \sim N(\mathbf{0}, D(d_i)) \, , \\[2ex]
\boldsymbol{\varepsilon}_i \sim N(\mathbf{0}, \Sigma_i(d_i)) \, .
\end{array}
\right.
\tag{6.16}
$$

Thus, the fixed effects as well as the covariance parameters are allowed to change with dropout pattern and a priori no restrictions are placed on the structure of this change.

As discussed in Sect. 6.9, model family (6.16) contains underidentified members since it describes the full set of measurements in pattern d_i, even though there are not measurements after occasion $d_i - 1$. To avoid this problem, simplified (identified) models can be considered. The advantage is that the number of parameters decreases, which is generally an issue with pattern-mixture models. Hogan and Laird (1997) noted that in order to estimate the large number of parameters in general models, one has to make the awkward requirement that each dropout pattern is sufficiently "filled", in other words one has to require large numbers of dropouts.

In Sect. 6.2.1, we explored the data from a pattern-mixture point of view. Figure 6.8 displays the individual and averaged profiles per pattern and clearly shows that pattern-specific profiles are of a quadratic nature with in most cases a sharp decline prior to dropout. Note that this is in line with the fitted dropout mechanism (6.12). Therefore, this feature needs to be reflected in the pattern-mixture model. In analogy with our selection model, the profiles are forced to pass through the origin. This is done by allowing only time main effect and interactions of other covariates with time in the model.

The most complex pattern-mixture model we consider includes a different parameter vector for each of the observed patterns. This is done by including the interaction of all effects in the model with *pattern*, a factor variable calculated as 2 plus the number of observations after baseline. We then proceed by backward selection in order to simplify the model. First, we found that the covariance structure is common to all patterns, encompassing random intercept, a serial exponential process, and measurement error.

For the fixed effects we proceeded as follows. A backward selection procedure, starting from a model that includes a main effect of time and time × time, as well as interactions of time with baseline value, treatment effect, dominant site and pattern, and the interaction of pattern with time×time. This procedure revealed significant effects for nearly all included factors. The only exception was treatment effect as was the case with the selection model in Table 6.4. Indeed, a single degree of freedom F test yields a p value of 0.6868. Note that such a test is possible since treatment effect does not interact with pattern, in contrast to the model which we will describe later. The fitted profiles are displayed in Fig. 6.14. We observe that the profiles for both arms are very similar. This is due to the fact that treatment effect is not significant but perhaps also because we did not allow a more complex treatment effect. For example, we might consider an interaction of treatment with the square of time and, more importantly, a treatment effect which is pattern-specific. Some evidence for such an interaction is seen in Fig. 6.8. Our second, expanded model, allowed for up to cubic time effects, the interaction of time with dropout pattern, dominant site, baseline value and treatment, as well as their two- and three-way interactions. After a backward selection procedure, the effects included are time and time × time, the two way interaction of time and dropout pattern, as well as three factor interactions of time and dropout pattern with (1) baseline, (2) group, and (3) dominant site. Finally, time × time interacts with dropout pattern and with the interaction of baseline and dropout pattern. No cubic time effects were necessary, which is in agreement with the observed profiles in Fig. 6.8. The model is graphically represented in Fig. 6.15.

Because a pattern-specific parameter has been included, we have several options for the assessment of treatment. Since there are 13 patterns (remember we cut off the patterns at 2 years), one can test the global hypothesis, based on 13 degrees of freedom, of no treatment effect. We obtain $F = 1.25$, producing $p = 0.2403$, indicating that there is no evidence for an overall treatment effect. Each of the treatment effects separately is at a non-significant level. Alternatively, the *marginal* effect of treatment can be calculated, which is the weighted average of the pattern-specific treatment effects, with weights given by the probability of occurrence of the various patterns. Its standard error is calculated using a straightforward

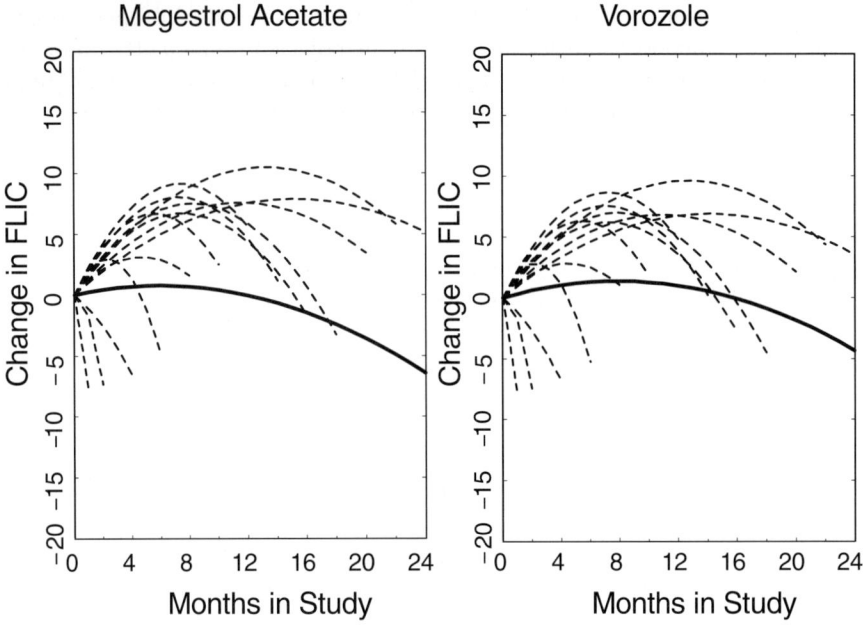

Figure 6.14. Vorozole Study. Fitted selection and first pattern-mixture model

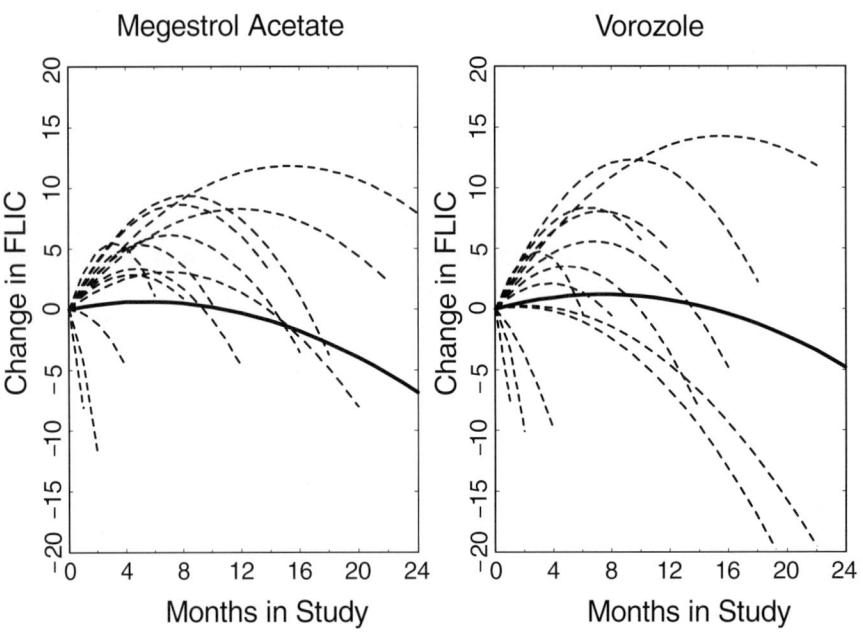

Figure 6.15. Vorozole Study. Fitted selection and second pattern-mixture models

application of the delta method. This effect is equal to $-0.286(0.288)$ producing a p value of 0.3206, which is even more non-significant.

In summary, we obtain a non-significant treatment effect from all our different models, which gives more weight to this conclusion. Further, the pattern-mixture model formulation has lead to important additional insight, which in a selection model would go unnoticed.

Non-Gaussian Repeated Measures 6.11

Marginal and random-effects models are two important sub-families of models for repeated measures. Several authors, such as Diggle et al. (2002) and Aerts et al. (2002) distinguish between three such families. Still focusing on continuous outcomes, a marginal model is characterized by the specification of a marginal mean function

$$E\left(Y_{ij}|\mathbf{x}_{ij}\right) = \mathbf{x}'_{ij}\boldsymbol{\beta} \, , \qquad (6.17)$$

whereas in a random-effects model we focus on the expectation, conditional upon the random-effects vector:

$$E\left(Y_{ij}|\mathbf{b}_i, \mathbf{x}_{ij}\right) = \mathbf{x}'_{ij}\boldsymbol{\beta} + \mathbf{z}'_{ij}\mathbf{b}_i \, . \qquad (6.18)$$

Finally, a third family of models conditions a particular outcome on the other responses or a subset thereof. In particular, a simple first-order stationary transition model focuses on expectations of the form

$$E\left(Y_{ij}|Y_{i,j-1}, \dots, Y_{i1}, \mathbf{x}_{ij}\right) = \mathbf{x}'_{ij}\boldsymbol{\beta} + \alpha Y_{i,j-1} \, . \qquad (6.19)$$

In the linear mixed model case, random-effects models imply a simple marginal model. This is due to the elegant properties of the multivariate normal distribution. In particular, the expectation (6.17) follows from (6.18) by either (1) marginalizing over the random effects or by (2) conditioning upon the random-effects vector $\mathbf{b}_i = \mathbf{0}$. Hence, the fixed-effects parameters $\boldsymbol{\beta}$ have both a marginal as well as a hierarchical model interpretation. Finally, when a conditional model is expressed in terms of residuals rather than outcomes directly, it also leads to particular forms of the general linear mixed effects model.

Such a close connection between the model families does not exist when outcomes are of a non-normal type, such as binary, categorical, or discrete. We will consider each of the model families in turn and then point to some particular issues arising within them or when comparisons are made between them.

Marginal Models 6.11.1

In marginal models, the parameters characterize the marginal probabilities of a subset of the outcomes, without conditioning on the other outcomes. Advantages and disadvantages of conditional and marginal modeling have been discussed in Diggle et al. (2002), and Fahrmeir and Tutz (2001). The specific context of clustered binary data has received treatment in Aerts et al. (2002). Apart from full likelihood approaches, non-likelihood approaches, such as generalized estimating equations (Liang and Zeger 1986) or pseudo-likelihood (le Cessie and van Houwelingen 1994; Geys et al. 1998) have been considered.

Bahadur (1961) proposed a marginal model, accounting for the association via marginal correlations. Ekholm (1991) proposed a so-called success probabilities approach. George and Bowman (1995) proposed a model for the particular case of exchangeable binary data. Ashford and Sowden (1970) considered the multivariate probit model, for repeated ordinal data, thereby extending univariate probit regression. Molenberghs and Lesaffre (1994) and Lang and Agresti (1994) have proposed models which parameterize the association in terms of marginal odds ratios. Dale (1986) defined the bivariate global odds ratio model, based on a bivariate Plackett distribution (Plackett 1965). Molenberghs and Lesaffre (1994, 1999) extended this model to multivariate ordinal outcomes. They generalize the bivariate Plackett distribution in order to establish the multivariate cell probabilities. Their 1994 method involves solving polynomials of high degree and computing the derivatives thereof, while in 1999 generalized linear models theory is exploited, together with the use of an adaption of the iterative proportional fitting algorithm. Lang and Agresti (1994) exploit the equivalence between direct modeling and imposing restrictions on the multinomial probabilities, using undetermined Lagrange multipliers. Alternatively, the cell probabilities can be fitted using a Newton iteration scheme, as suggested by Glonek and McCullagh (1995). We will now consider generalized estimating equations (GEE), while a particular extension, suitable for incomplete data where missingness is other than MCAR, is discussed in Sect. 6.12.

Generalized Estimating Equations

The main issue with full likelihood approaches is the computational complexity they entail. When we are mainly interested in first-order marginal mean parameters and pairwise interactions, a full likelihood procedure can be replaced by quasi-likelihood methods (McCullagh and Nelder 1989). In quasi-likelihood, the mean response is expressed as a parametric function of covariates; the variance is assumed to be a function of the mean up to possibly unknown scale parameters. Wedderburn (1974) first noted that likelihood and quasi-likelihood theories coincide for exponential families and that the quasi-likelihood "estimating equations" provide consistent estimates of the regression parameters β in any generalized linear model, even for choices of link and variance functions that do not correspond to exponential families.

For clustered and repeated data, Liang and Zeger (1986) proposed so-called *generalized estimating equations* (GEE or GEE1) which require only the correct specification of the univariate marginal distributions provided one is willing to adopt "working" assumptions about the association structure. They estimate the parameters associated with the expected value of an individual's vector of binary responses and phrase the working assumptions about the association between pairs of outcomes in terms of marginal correlations. The method combines estimating equations for the regression parameters β with moment-based estimating for the correlation parameters entering the working assumptions.

Prentice (1988) extended their results to allow joint estimation of probabilities and pairwise correlations. Lipsitz et al. (1991) modified the estimating equations of Prentice (1988) to allow modeling of the association through marginal odds ratios rather than marginal correlations. When adopting GEE1 one does not use information of the association structure to estimate the main effect parameters. As a result, it can be shown that GEE1 yields consistent main effect estimators, even when the association structure is misspecified. However, severe misspecification may seriously affect the efficiency of the GEE1 estimators. In addition, GEE1 should be avoided when some scientific interest is placed on the association parameters.

A second order extension of these estimating equations (GEE2) that include the marginal pairwise association as well has been studied by Liang et al. (1992). They note that GEE2 is nearly fully efficient though bias may occur in the estimation of the main effect parameters when the association structure is misspecified.

After this short overview of the GEE approach, the GEE methodology, which is based on two perceptions, will now be explained a little further. First, the score equations to be solved when computing maximum likelihood estimates under a marginal normal model $y_i \sim N(X_i\beta, V_i)$ are given by

$$\sum_{i=1}^{N} X_i' \left(A_i^{1/2} R_i A_i^{1/2} \right)^{-1} (y_i - X_i\beta) = 0 \,, \tag{6.20}$$

in which the marginal covariance matrix V_i has been decomposed in the form $A_i^{1/2} R_i A_i^{1/2}$, with A_i the matrix with the marginal variances on the main diagonal and zeros elsewhere, and with R_i equal to the marginal correlation matrix. Second, the score equations to be solved when computing maximum likelihood estimates under a marginal generalized linear model (6.17), assuming independence of the responses within units (i.e., ignoring the repeated measures structure), are given by

$$\sum_{i=1}^{N} \frac{\partial \mu_i}{\partial \beta'} \left(A_i^{1/2} I_{n_i} A_i^{1/2} \right)^{-1} (y_i - \mu_i) = 0 \,, \tag{6.21}$$

where A_i is again the diagonal matrix with the marginal variances on the main diagonal.

Note that expression (6.20) is of the form (6.21) but with the correlations between repeated measures taken into account. A straightforward extension of (6.21) that accounts for the correlation structure is

$$S(\beta) = \sum_{i=1}^{N} \frac{\partial \mu_i}{\partial \beta'} \left(A_i^{1/2} R_i A_i^{1/2} \right)^{-1} (y_i - \mu_i) = 0 \,, \tag{6.22}$$

that is obtained from replacing the identity matrix I_{n_i} by a correlation matrix $R_i = R_i(\alpha)$, often referred to as the *working* correlation matrix. Usually, the marginal covariance matrix $V_i = A_i^{1/2} R_i A_i^{1/2}$ contains a vector $\boldsymbol{\alpha}$ of unknown parameters which is replaced for practical purposes by a consistent estimate.

Assuming that the marginal mean $\boldsymbol{\mu}_i$ has been correctly specified as $h(\boldsymbol{\mu}_i) = X_i\boldsymbol{\beta}$, it can be shown that, under mild regularity conditions, the estimator $\hat{\boldsymbol{\beta}}$ obtained from solving (6.22) is asymptotically normally distributed with mean $\boldsymbol{\beta}$ and with covariance matrix

$$ I_0^{-1} I_1 I_0^{-1} , \tag{6.23} $$

where

$$ I_0 = \left(\sum_{i=1}^{N} \frac{\partial \boldsymbol{\mu}_i'}{\partial \boldsymbol{\beta}} V_i^{-1} \frac{\partial \boldsymbol{\mu}_i}{\partial \boldsymbol{\beta}'} \right) , $$

$$ I_1 = \left(\sum_{i=1}^{N} \frac{\partial \boldsymbol{\mu}_i'}{\partial \boldsymbol{\beta}} V_i^{-1} \operatorname{Var}\left(\boldsymbol{y}_i \right) V_i^{-1} \frac{\partial \boldsymbol{\mu}_i}{\partial \boldsymbol{\beta}'} \right) . $$

In practice, Var($\boldsymbol{y}_i$) in (6.23) is replaced by $(\boldsymbol{y}_i - \boldsymbol{\mu}_i)(\boldsymbol{y}_i - \boldsymbol{\mu}_i)'$, which is unbiased on the sole condition that the mean was again correctly specified.

Note that valid inferences can now be obtained for the mean structure, only assuming that the model assumptions with respect to the first-order moments are correct. Note also that, although arising from a likelihood approach, the GEE equations in (6.22) cannot be interpreted as score equations corresponding to some full likelihood for the data vector $\boldsymbol{y}_i$.

Liang and Zeger (1986) proposed moment-based estimates for the working correlation.

6.11.2   Random-Effects Models

Models with subject-specific parameters are differentiated from population-averaged models by the inclusion of parameters which are specific to the cluster. Unlike for correlated Gaussian outcomes, the parameters of the random effects and population-averaged models for correlated binary data describe different types of effects of the covariates on the response probabilities (Neuhaus 1992). The choice between population-averaged and random effects strategies should heavily depend on the scientific goals. Population-averaged models evaluate the overall risk as a function of covariates. With a subject-specific approach, the response rates are modeled as a function of covariates and parameters, specific to a subject. In such models, interpretation of fixed-effect parameters is conditional on a constant level of the random-effects parameter. Population-averaged comparisons, on the other hand, make no use of within cluster comparisons for cluster varying covariates and are therefore not useful to assess within-subject effects (Neuhaus et al. 1991).

Whereas the linear mixed model is unequivocally the most popular choice in the case of normally distributed response variables, there are more options in the case of non-normal outcomes. Stiratelli et al. (1984) assume the parameter vector to be normally distributed. This idea has been carried further in the work on so-called *generalized linear mixed models* (Breslow and Clayton 1993) which is closely related to linear and non-linear mixed models. Alternatively, Skellam (1948) introduced the beta-binomial model, in which the response probability of any response of a particular subject comes from a beta distribution. Hence, this model can also be viewed as a random-effects model. We will consider generalized linear mixed models in the following subsection.

Generalized Linear Mixed Models

Perhaps the most commonly encountered subject-specific (or random effects model) is the generalized linear mixed model. A general framework for mixed-effects models can be expressed as follows. Assume that Y_i (possibly appropriately transformed) satisfies

$$Y_i|b_i \sim F_i(\theta, b_i) , \tag{6.24}$$

i.e., conditional on b_i, Y_i follows a pre-specified distribution F_i, possibly depending on covariates, and parameterized through a vector θ of unknown parameters, common to all subjects. Further, b_i is a q-dimensional vector of subject-specific parameters, called random effects, assumed to follow a so-called mixing distribution G which may depend on a vector ψ of unknown parameters, i.e., $b_i \sim G(\psi)$. The b_i reflect the between-unit heterogeneity in the population with respect to the distribution of Y_i. In the presence of random effects, conditional independence is often assumed, under which the components Y_{ij} in Y_i are independent, conditional on b_i. The distribution function F_i in (6.24) then becomes a product over the n_i independent elements in Y_i.

In general, unless a fully Bayesian approach is followed, inference is based on the marginal model for Y_i which is obtained from integrating out the random effects, over their distribution $G(\psi)$. Let $f_i(y_i|b_i)$ and $g(b_i)$ denote the density functions corresponding to the distributions F_i and G, respectively, then the marginal density function of Y_i equals

$$f_i(y_i) = \int f_i\left(y_i|b_i\right) g(b_i) \, \mathrm{d}b_i , \tag{6.25}$$

which depends on the unknown parameters θ and ψ. Assuming independence of the units, estimates of $\widehat{\theta}$ and $\widehat{\psi}$ can be obtained from maximizing the likelihood function built from (6.25), and inferences immediately follow from classical maximum likelihood theory.

It is important to realize that the random-effects distribution G is crucial in the calculation of the marginal model (6.25). One approach is to leave G completely unspecified and to use non-parametric maximum likelihood (NPML) estimation, which maximizes the likelihood over all possible distributions G. The resulting estimate $\widehat{G}$ is then always discrete with finite support. Depending on the context, this may or may not be a realistic reflection of the true heterogeneity between units. One therefore often assumes G to be of a specific parametric form, such as a (multivariate) normal. Depending on F_i and G, the integration in (6.25) may or may not be possible analytically. Proposed solutions are based on Taylor series expansions of $f_i(y_i|b_i)$, or on numerical approximations of the integral, such as (adaptive) Gaussian quadrature.

Although in practice one is usually primarily interested in estimating the parameters in the marginal model, it is often useful to calculate estimates for the random effects b_i as well. They reflect between-subject variability, which makes them helpful for detecting special profiles (i.e., outlying individuals) or groups of individuals evolving differently in time. Also, estimates for the random effects are needed whenever interest is in prediction of subject-specific evolutions. Inference for the random effects is often based on their so-called posterior distribution $f_i(b_i|y_i)$, given by

$$f_i(b_i|y_i) = \frac{f_i(y_i|b_i)g(b_i)}{\int f_i(y_i|b_i)g(b_i)\,db_i} ,\qquad (6.26)$$

in which the unknown parameters θ and ψ are replaced by their estimates obtained earlier from maximizing the marginal likelihood. The mean or mode corresponding to (6.26) can be used as point estimates for b_i, yielding empirical Bayes (EB) estimates.

There are at least two major differences in comparison to the linear mixed model discussed in the previous section. First, the marginal distribution of Y_i can no longer be calculated analytically, such that numerical approximations to the marginal density come into play, seriously complicating the computation of the maximum likelihood estimates of the parameters in the marginal model, i.e., β, D, and the parameters in all Σ_i. A consequence is that the marginal covariance structure does not immediately follow from the model formulation, such that it is not always clear in practice what assumptions a specific model implies with respect to the underlying variance function and the underlying correlation structure in the data.

A second important difference is with respect to the interpretation of the fixed effects β. Under the linear model (6.1), $E(Y_i)$ equals $X_i\beta$, such that the fixed effects have a subject-specific as well as a population-averaged interpretation. Indeed, the elements in β reflect the effect of specific covariates, conditionally on the random effects b_i, as well as marginalized over these random effects. Under non-linear mixed models, however, this does no longer hold in general. The fixed effects now only reflect the conditional effect of covariates, and the marginal effect is not easily obtained anymore as $E(Y_i)$ which is given by

$$E(Y_i) = \int y_i \int f_i(y_i|b_i)g(b_i)\,db_i\,dy_i ,$$

which, in general, is *not* of the form $h(X_i, Z_i, \beta, 0)$, where h is the conditional mean function evaluated in the zero random effects vector.

The generalized linear mixed model (GLMM) is the most frequently used random-effects model for discrete outcomes. A general formulation is as follows. Conditionally on random effects b_i, it assumes that the elements Y_{ij} of Y_i are independent, with density function of the form

$$f\left(y|\theta_i, \phi\right) = \exp\left\{\phi^{-1}\left[y\theta_i - \psi(\theta_i)\right] + c(y, \phi)\right\},$$

with mean $E(Y_{ij}|b_i) = a'(\eta_{ij}) = \mu_{ij}(b_i)$ and variance $\text{Var}(Y_{ij}|b_i) = \phi a''(\eta_{ij})$, and where, apart from a link function h, a linear regression model with parameters β and b_i is used for the mean, i.e., $h(\mu_i(b_i)) = X_i\beta + Z_ib_i$. Note that the linear mixed model is a special case, with identity link function. The random effects b_i are again assumed to be sampled from a (multivariate) normal distribution with mean 0 and covariance matrix D. Usually, the canonical link function is used, i.e., $h = a'^{-1}$, such that $\eta_i = X_i\beta + Z_ib_i$. When the link function is chosen to be of the logit form and the random effects are assumed to be normally distributed, the familiar logistic-linear GLMM follows.

The non-linear nature of the model again implies that the marginal distribution of y_i is, in general, not easily obtained, such that model fitting requires approximation of the marginal density function. An exception to this occurs when the probit link is used. Further, as was also the case for non-linear mixed models, the parameters β have no marginal interpretation, except for some very particular models. An example where the marginal interpretation does hold is the Poisson model for count data, for which the logarithm is the canonical link function. In case the model only includes random intercepts, it follows that the only element in β which has no marginal interpretation is the intercept.

As an important example, consider the binomial model for binary data, with the logit canonical link function, and where the only random effects are intercepts b_i. It can then be shown that the marginal mean $\mu_i = E(Y_{ij})$ satisfies $h(\mu_i) \approx X_i\beta^*$ with

$$\beta^* = \left[c^2\text{Var}(b_i) + 1\right]^{-1/2}\beta, \tag{6.27}$$

in which c equals $16\sqrt{3}/15\pi$. Hence, although the parameters β in the generalized linear mixed model have no marginal interpretation, they do show a strong relation to their marginal counterparts. Note that, as a consequence of this relation, larger covariate effects are obtained under the random-effects model in comparison to the marginal model.

Weighted Generalized Estimating Equations

6.12

As Liang and Zeger (1986) pointed out, inferences under GEE are valid only under the strong assumption that the data are missing completely at random (MCAR). This is because GEE is frequentist rather than likelihood-based in nature. In such cases, it is not automatic for MCAR to imply ignorability. Hence, to allow the data to be missing at random (MAR), Robins et al. (1995) proposed a class of weighted estimating equations. They can be viewed as an extension of generalized estimating equations.

In simple terms, the idea is to weight each subject's contribution in the GEEs by the inverse probability that a subject drops out at the time he dropped out. This can be calculated as

$$\nu_{id_i} \equiv P[D_i = d_i] = \prod_{k=2}^{d_i-1} \left(1 - P\left[R_{ik} = 0|R_{i2} = \ldots = R_{i,k-1} = 1\right]\right)$$

$$\times P\left[R_{id_i} = 0|R_{i2} = \ldots = R_{i,d_i-1} = 1\right]^{I\{d_i \leq T\}} .$$

Recall that we partitioned Y_i into the unobserved components Y_i^m and the observed components Y_i^o. Similarly, we can make the same partition of μ_i into μ_i^m and μ_i^o. In the weighted GEE approach, which is proposed to reduce possible bias of $\hat{\beta}$, the score equations to be solved when taking into account the correlation structure are:

$$S(\beta) = \sum_{i=1}^{N} \frac{1}{\nu_{id}} \frac{\partial \mu_i}{\partial \beta'} \left(A_i^{1/2} R_i A_i^{1/2}\right)^{-1} (y_i - \mu_i) = 0 . \tag{6.28}$$

GLMM and WGEE
6.13   Applied to the Psychiatric Study

Let us now analyse the clinical trial, introduced in Sect. 6.2.2. The primary null hypothesis (zero difference between the treatments and placebo in mean change of the HAMD17 total score at endpoint) will be tested using both marginal models (GEE and WGEE) and random-effect models (GLMM). According to the study protocol, the models will include the fixed categorical effects of treatment, visit, and treatment-by-visit interaction, as well as the continuous, fixed covariates of baseline score and baseline score-by-visit interaction. A random intercept will be included when considering the random-effect models. Analyses are done using the SAS procedures GENMOD and NLMIXED. Apart from MAR-based analyses, complete case and LOCF analyses are considered. At the same time, three different approaches are considered, namely a full longitudinal analysis, an analysis with focus on the last planned occasion and one with focus on the last measured occasion.

We fit a generalized estimating equations model, first naively using CC and LOCF, and then using the profiles "as is" but without weighting. Finally, a weighted analysis is conducted. Results are summarized in Table 6.5.

Further, we consider generalized linear mixed effects models, again under CC, LOCF, and likelihood-based ignorable scenarios. The results are summarized in Table 6.6. Adaptive Gaussian quadrature with 50 quadrature points is used.

A few observations need to be made. First, the weighted estimating equations results, being the most general ones, are somewhat different from the others (CC, LOCF, and 'naive' MAR). This underscores that using WGEE is well in place. Further, the generalized linear mixed model parameters are quite a bit larger in absolute value than the marginal (GEE) counterparts. This is in line with theory, given 'conversion factor' (6.27) between the marginal and random-effects models, and given the estimated value for the variance of the random effects.

In terms of conclusions, we can, apart from comparing the results presented in Tables 6.5 and 6.6, also consider treatment when interest lies in the last planned occasion and when interest focuses on the last obtained measurements). The assessment of treatment effect at the last occasion is given in Table 6.7.

We reach the following conclusions. The mixed models lead to a small difference between CC and MAR, both with non-significant results. The mixed model for LOCF clearly gives a non-significant result. An endpoint analysis leads to a completely different picture, with results that are strongly different (significant) as opposed to the mixed models.

From MAR to Sensitivity Analysis   6.14

In summary, we have seen that likelihood-based inference is valid under MAR, provided a few mild regularity conditions hold. For example, a linear mixed model or a generalized linear mixed model fitted to incomplete data is valid, and it is as simple to conduct as it would be in contexts where data are complete. The situation is a little different with generalized estimating equations. However, the mild extension of GEE to weighted GEE comes to the rescue. Indeed, fitting WGEE only necessitates the construction of a model for the dropout probabilities, given covariates and previous, observed measurements. This can routinely be done using logistic regression. Thus, a number of frequently used tools for correlated data are valid in the important MAR setting. One conclusion from this is that there is little or no need for the simple methods such as complete case analysis or LOCF. On the other hand though, one can almost never rule out the possibility of missing data to be MNAR. This implies that the need may exist to consider MNAR models.

A sensible compromise between blindly shifting to MNAR models or ignoring them altogether, is to make them a component of a sensitivity analysis. In that sense, it is important to consider the effect on key parameters. One such route is to consider a selection model of the Diggle and Kenward (1994) type, and to build in devices to explore the effect of (small) changes from the posited MAR model. A further route for sensitivity analysis is to consider pattern-mixture models as a complement to selection models (Thijs et al. 2002; Michiels et al. 2002). We will consider those routes in Sects. 6.15 and 6.16.

Table 6.5. Psychiatric Study. (Weighted) Generalized Estimating Equations: parameter estimates, standard errors (model-based, empirical corrected) and p-values (model-based, empirical corrected) for each approach

	CC (GEE)		LOCF (GEE)		MAR (GEE)		MAR (WGEE)	
	Est.(S.E.)	p-value	Est.(S.E.)	p-value	Est.(S.E.)	p-value	Est.(S.E.)	p-value
intercept	2.11 (1.87; 1.09)	(0.260; 0.0528)	2.15 (1.90; 1.17)	(0.258; 0.0659)	2.04 (1.89; 1.10)	(0.281; 0.0638)	3.75 (1.33; 1.84)	(0.0048; 0.0413)
trt A1	−0.36 (1.19; 1.28)	(0.762; 0.779)	−0.39 (1.18; 1.32)	(0.743; 0.770)	−0.46 (1.19; 1.30)	(0.701; 0.727)	−0.12 (0.70; 1.31)	(0.870; 0.930)
trt B	−0.059 (1.26; 1.44)	(0.963; 0.967)	−0.16 (1.24; 1.43)	(0.899; 0.912)	−0.20 (1.25; 1.42)	(0.874; 0.889)	0.17 (0.75; 1.35)	(0.823; 0.901)
visit 5	−2.43 (1.86; 1.27)	(0.190; 0.0558)	−3.20 (1.82; 1.31)	(0.0791; 0.0145)	−3.16 (1.84; 1.30)	(0.0856; 0.0150)	−4.94 (1.29; 2.07)	(0.0001; 0.0168)
visit 6	−4.30 (1.84; 1.45)	(0.0194; 0.0031)	−4.80 (1.83; 1.48)	(0.0086; 0.0012)	−4.66 (1.85; 1.49)	(0.0119; 0.0018)	−5.98 (1.30; 2.20)	(< 0.0001; 0.0066)
visit 7	−3.84 (1.80; 1.29)	(0.0327; 0.0029)	−4.25 (1.78; 1.31)	(0.0171; 0.0012)	−4.05 (1.81; 1.31)	(0.0247; 0.0019)	−4.99 (1.28; 1.77)	(< 0.0001; 0.0049)
visit 8	−4.64 (1.80; 1.40)	(0.0100; 0.0009)	−5.15 (1.79; 1.42)	(0.0040; 0.0003)	−4.98 (1.82; 1.44)	(0.0060; 0.0005)	−5.90 (1.28; 2.13)	(< 0.0001; 0.0056)
visit 9	−4.28 (1.79; 1.44)	(0.0167; 0.0029)	−4.55 (1.78; 1.47)	(0.0103; 0.0019)	−4.33 (1.80; 1.50)	(0.0165; 0.0038)	−4.72 (1.28; 2.28)	(0.0002; 0.0389)
visit 10	−4.92 (1.79; 1.29)	(0.0059; 0.0001)	−4.71 (1.77; 1.31)	(0.0077; 0.0003)	−4.58 (1.80; 1.33)	(0.0108; 0.0006)	−4.87 (1.27; 1.99)	(0.0001; 0.0141)
visit 11	−4.74 (1.79; 1.41)	(0.0080; 0.0008)	−4.58 (1.77; 1.40)	(0.0095; 0.0011)	−4.75 (1.82; 1.46)	(0.0091; 0.0012)	−5.79 (1.28; 2.03)	(< 0.0001; 0.0043)
visit 5 * trt A1	−0.55 (1.19; 0.85)	(0.643; 0.517)	−0.11 (1.12; 0.96)	(0.921; 0.908)	−0.15 (1.14; 0.97)	(0.899; 0.881)	−0.84 (0.68; 1.00)	(0.218; 0.402)
visit 5 * trt B	−0.27 (1.26; 0.94)	(0.829; 0.773)	−0.012 (1.18; 1.04)	(0.992; 0.991)	−0.020 (1.20; 1.06)	(0.987; 0.985)	−1.37 (0.72; 1.19)	(0.0574; 0.248)
visit 6 * trt A1	0.29 (1.15; 1.31)	(0.801; 0.825)	0.51 (1.11; 1.31)	(0.644; 0.695)	0.54 (1.14; 1.36)	(0.634; 0.690)	0.27 (0.67; 1.40)	(0.691; 0.848)
visit 6 * trt B	0.15 (1.21; 1.40)	(0.902; 0.915)	0.26 (1.16; 1.36)	(0.821; 0.847)	0.38 (1.19; 1.42)	(0.751; 0.790)	−0.11 (0.72; 1.46)	(0.874; 0.938)
visit 7 * trt A1	0.47 (1.13; 1.15)	(0.680; 0.685)	0.48 (1.10; 1.17)	(0.662; 0.682)	0.52 (1.12; 1.22)	(0.646; 0.672)	−0.14 (0.67; 1.26)	(0.831; 0.910)
visit 7 * trt B	0.39 (1.19; 1.23)	(0.745; 0.753)	0.41 (1.15; 1.23)	(0.724; 0.742)	0.53 (1.18; 1.28)	(0.656; 0.681)	−0.14 (0.72; 1.29)	(0.844; 0.913)
visit 8 * trt A1	0.24 (1.13; 1.32)	(0.834; 0.857)	0.57 (1.10; 1.30)	(0.601; 0.660)	0.59 (1.13; 1.37)	(0.602; 0.670)	0.03 (0.67; 1.38)	(0.962; 0.982)
visit 8 * trt B	0.24 (1.19; 1.51)	(0.841; 0.874)	0.48 (1.15; 1.45)	(0.677; 0.741)	0.57 (1.18; 1.54)	(0.627; 0.709)	−0.28 (0.72; 1.49)	(0.692; 0.849)
visit 9 * trt A1	0.37 (1.13; 1.34)	(0.742; 0.783)	0.47 (1.09; 1.32)	(0.668; 0.722)	0.46 (1.12; 1.40)	(0.684; 0.744)	−0.12 (0.67; 1.42)	(0.859; 0.934)
visit 9 * trt B	0.21 (1.19; 1.48)	(0.861; 0.888)	0.23 (1.15; 1.42)	(0.842; 0.873)	0.26 (1.18; 1.51)	(0.825; 0.863)	−0.51 (0.72; 1.52)	(0.478; 0.737)
visit 10 * trt A1	0.11 (1.12; 1.19)	(0.922; 0.926)	0.30 (1.09; 1.21)	(0.783; 0.804)	0.31 (1.13; 1.29)	(0.783; 0.810)	−0.49 (0.67; 1.35)	(0.462; 0.715)
visit 10 * trt B	0.28 (1.18; 1.32)	(0.811; 0.830)	0.32 (1.15; 1.31)	(0.782; 0.810)	0.43 (1.18; 1.39)	(0.718; 0.759)	−0.50 (0.72; 1.42)	(0.486; 0.724)
visit 11 * trt A1	−0.70 (1.13; 1.17)	(0.535; 0.549)	−0.27 (1.09; 1.21)	(0.801; 0.820)	−0.53 (1.14; 1.27)	(0.639; 0.674)	−1.31 (0.67; 1.35)	(0.0528; 0.334)
visit 11 * trt B	−0.052 (1.18; 1.35)	(0.965; 0.969)	0.071 (1.14; 1.34)	(0.951; 0.958)	0.089 (1.19; 1.43)	(0.941; 0.950)	−0.76 (0.72; 1.43)	(0.291; 0.593)
baseline	0.054 (0.096; 0.076)	(0.575; 0.598)	0.077 (0.097; 0.11)	(0.427; 0.472)	0.085 (0.097; 0.10)	(0.380; 0.407)	0.039 (0.069; 0.15)	(0.579; 0.795)
baseline * visit 5	0.10 (0.096; 0.076)	(0.284; 0.176)	0.12 (0.095; 0.082)	(0.193; 0.133)	0.12 (0.096; 0.082)	(0.210; 0.142)	0.24 (0.068; 0.13)	(0.0006; 0.073)
baseline * visit 6	0.17 (0.096; 0.11)	(0.0830; 0.129)	0.18 (0.095; 0.11)	(0.0537; 0.104)	0.17 (0.097; 0.12)	(0.0815; 0.149)	0.24 (0.070; 0.17)	(0.0005; 0.145)
baseline * visit 7	0.10 (0.092; 0.089)	(0.268; 0.249)	0.12 (0.092; 0.093)	(0.183; 0.188)	0.10 (0.093; 0.095)	(0.281; 0.287)	0.16 (0.067; 0.13)	(0.0159; 0.221)
baseline * visit 8	0.15 (0.093; 0.11)	(0.105; 0.179)	0.16 (0.092; 0.12)	(0.0749; 0.154)	0.14 (0.094; 0.12)	(0.127; 0.234)	0.21 (0.068; 0.17)	(0.0022; 0.217)
baseline * visit 9	0.11 (0.092; 0.12)	(0.213; 0.325)	0.13 (0.091; 0.12)	(0.158; 0.275)	0.10 (0.093; 0.13)	(0.263; 0.404)	0.13 (0.067; 0.18)	(0.0575; 0.476)
baseline * visit 10	0.13 (0.091; 0.096)	(0.169; 0.189)	0.11 (0.090; 0.10)	(0.228; 0.280)	0.083 (0.093; 0.11)	(0.371; 0.434)	0.10 (0.067; 0.15)	(0.122; 0.504)
baseline * visit 11	0.13 (0.092; 0.099)	(0.163; 0.197)	0.11 (0.090; 0.10)	(0.222; 0.288)	0.11 (0.094; 0.11)	(0.253; 0.318)	0.16 (0.067; 0.15)	(0.0181; 0.293)
ℓ	−423.1		−533.0		−465.4		−2042.0	

Table 6.6. Psychiatric Study. Generalized linear mixed effects models under LOCF, CC, and MAR assumptions

	CC		LOCF		MAR	
	Est.(S.E.)	p-value	Est.(S.E.)	p-value	Est.(S.E.)	p-value
Intercept	3.56 (2.77)	0.202	3.68 (2.90)	0.207	3.39 (2.65)	0.203
Trt A1	−0.60 (1.61)	0.711	−0.71 (1.64)	0.664	−0.58 (1.51)	0.699
Trt B	−0.13 (1.68)	0.937	−0.27 (1.72)	0.876	−0.16 (1.59)	0.920
Visit 5	−3.69 (2.93)	0.211	−4.96 (2.97)	0.0975	−4.65 (2.85)	0.105
Visit 6	−6.91 (3.00)	0.0232	−7.93 (3.06)	0.0104	−7.26 (2.94)	0.0145
Visit 7	−6.30 (2.92)	0.0332	−7.26 (2.98)	0.0158	−6.52 (2.84)	0.0232
Visit 8	−8.02 (3.00)	0.0086	−9.33 (3.06)	0.0027	−8.46 (2.93)	0.0044
Visit 9	−7.42 (2.95)	0.0135	−8.19 (3.00)	0.0070	−7.29 (2.87)	0.0119
Visit 10	−9.03 (3.01)	0.0034	−9.11 (3.02)	0.0030	−8.18 (2.89)	0.0053
Visit 11	−8.61 (3.01)	0.0050	−8.84 (3.01)	0.0038	−8.47 (2.97)	0.0049
Visit 5 × trt A1	0.052 (1.77)	0.977	0.099 (1.76)	0.955	0.26 (1.70)	0.877
Visit 5 × trt B	−0.47 (1.82)	0.798	−0.19 (1.78)	0.914	−0.21 (1.71)	0.902
Visit 6 × trt A1	0.23 (1.74)	0.897	0.54 (1.74)	0.758	0.63 (1.68)	0.707
Visit 6 × trt B	0.46 (1.73)	0.791	0.35 (1.73)	0.838	0.50 (1.67)	0.763
Visit 7 × trt A1	0.45 (1.74)	0.796	0.37 (1.74)	0.832	0.50 (1.69)	0.769
Visit 7 × trt B	0.18 (1.73)	0.918	0.008 (1.73)	0.996	0.064 (1.67)	0.969
Visit 8 × trt A1	−1.16 (1.74)	0.505	−0.62 (1.68)	0.712	−0.63 (1.62)	0.698
Visit 8 × trt B	−0.24 (1.74)	0.893	−0.23 (1.73)	0.895	−0.15 (1.71)	0.928
Visit 9 × trt A1	0.38 (1.65)	0.819	0.29 (1.64)	0.861	0.30 (1.58)	0.850
Visit 9 × trt B	0.10 (1.69)	0.952	0.38 (1.67)	0.819	0.38 (1.61)	0.813
Visit 10 × trt A1	0.25 (1.66)	0.882	0.30 (1.64)	0.854	0.23 (1.59)	0.887
Visit 10 × trt B	0.006 (1.67)	0.997	0.54 (1.65)	0.742	0.48 (1.59)	0.762
Visit 11 × trt A1	−1.63 (1.68)	0.333	−1.14 (1.65)	0.491	−1.53 (1.64)	0.354
Visit 11 × trt B	−0.092 (1.67)	0.956	0.15 (1.65)	0.929	0.096 (1.61)	0.953
Baseline	0.098 (0.13)	0.469	0.17 (0.14)	0.231	0.14 (0.13)	0.295
Baseline × visit 5	0.16 (0.15)	0.269	0.20 (0.15)	0.180	0.19 (0.14)	0.194
Baseline × visit 6	0.28 (0.15)	0.0628	0.32 (0.15)	0.0386	0.28 (0.15)	0.0596
Baseline × visit 7	0.18 (0.14)	0.201	0.23 (0.15)	0.122	0.19 (0.14)	0.190
Baseline × visit 8	0.28 (0.15)	0.0559	0.32 (0.15)	0.0329	0.28 (0.15)	0.0594
Baseline × visit 9	0.22 (0.14)	0.127	0.26 (0.15)	0.0805	0.21 (0.14)	0.145
Baseline × visit 10	0.26 (0.14)	0.0781	0.24 (0.15)	0.101	0.19 (0.14)	0.192
Baseline × visit 11	0.26 (0.15)	0.0755	0.25 (0.15)	0.0912	0.23 (0.15)	0.112
σ	2.54 (0.32)	< 0.0001	3.12 (0.37)	< 0.0001	2.52 (0.30)	< 0.0001
-2ℓ	654.8		769.7		720.9	

Selection Models and Local Influence   6.15

Let us return to the Diggle and Kenward (1994) selection model, as described in Sect. 6.6.1 and consider dropout model (6.9). When ω equals zero, the dropout model is random, and all parameters can be estimated using standard software since the measurement model for which we use a linear mixed model and the

Table 6.7. Psychiatric Study. Analysis at endpoint. p-values are reported ('mixed' refers to the assessment of treatment at the last visit based on a generalized linear mixed model)

Method	Model	p-value
CC	mixed	0.0614
	Pearson's Chi-squared Test	0.0350
	Fisher's Exact Test	0.0350
LOCF	mixed	0.1067
	Pearson's Chi-squared Test	0.0384
	Fisher's Exact Test	0.0405
MAR	mixed	0.0677

dropout model, assumed to follow a logistic regression, can then be fitted separately. If $\omega \neq 0$, the dropout process is assumed to be non-random.

Model (6.9) is now used to construct the dropout process:

$$f(d_i|y_i, \boldsymbol{\psi}) = \begin{cases} \displaystyle\prod_{j=2}^{n_i} \left[1 - g\left(h_{ij}, y_{ij}\right)\right] & \text{for a complete sequence} \\[2em] \displaystyle\prod_{j=2}^{d-1} \left[1 - g\left(h_{ij}, y_{ij}\right)\right] g\left(h_{id}, y_{id}\right) & \text{for a dropout .} \end{cases} \tag{6.29}$$

Let us now shift attention to sensitivity and influence analysis issues. Whereas a global influence approach is based on case-deletion, a local influence based sensitivity assessment of the relevant quantities, such as treatment effect or time evolution parameters, with respect to assumptions about the dropout model is based on the following perturbed version of (6.9):

$$\text{logit}\left(g\left(h_{ij}, y_{ij}\right)\right) = \text{logit}\left[\text{pr}\left(D_i = j|D_i \geq j, y_i\right)\right] = h_{ij}\boldsymbol{\psi} + \omega_i y_{ij}, \tag{6.30}$$

$(i = 1, \ldots, N)$, in which different subjects give different weights to the response at time t_{ij} to predict dropout at time t_{ij}. If all ω_i equal zero, the model reduces to a MAR model. Hence (6.30) can be seen as an extension of the MAR model, which allows some individuals to drop out in a "less random" way ($|\omega_i|$ large) than others ($|\omega_i|$ small). It has to be noted that, even when ω_i is large, we still cannot conclude that the dropout model for these subjects is non-random. Rather, it is a way of pointing to subjects which, due to their strong influence, are able to distort the model parameters such that they can produce, for example, a dropout mechanism which is *seemingly* non-random. In reality, many different characteristics of such an individual's profile might be responsible for this effect. As mentioned earlier, such sensitivity has been alluded to by many authors, such as Laird (1994) and Rubin (1994).

Cook (1986) suggests that more confidence can be put in a model which is relatively stable under small modifications. The best known perturbation schemes are based on case-deletion (Cook and Weisberg 1982; Chatterjee and Hadi 1988) in which the effect is studied of completely removing cases from the analysis. They were introduced by Cook (1977, 1979) for the linear regression context. Denote the log-likelihood function, corresponding to measurement model (6.2) and dropout model (6.9) by

$$\ell(\boldsymbol{\gamma}) = \sum_{i=1}^{N} \ell_i(\boldsymbol{\gamma}) , \qquad (6.31)$$

in which $\ell_i(\boldsymbol{\gamma})$ is the contribution of the ith individual to the log-likelihood, and where $\boldsymbol{\gamma} = (\boldsymbol{\theta}, \boldsymbol{\psi}, \omega)$ is the s-dimensional vector, grouping the parameters of the measurement model and the dropout model. Further, we denote by

$$\ell_{(-i)}(\boldsymbol{\gamma}) \qquad (6.32)$$

the log-likelihood function, where the contribution of the ith subject has been removed. Cook's distances are based on measuring the discrepancy between either the maximized likelihoods (6.31) and (6.32) or (subsets of) the estimated parameter vectors $\widehat{\boldsymbol{\gamma}}$ and $\widehat{\boldsymbol{\gamma}}_{(-i)}$, with obvious notation. Precisely, we will consider both

$$CD_{1i} = 2 \left(\widehat{\ell} - \widehat{\ell}_{(-i)} \right) \qquad (6.33)$$

as well as

$$CD_{2i}(\boldsymbol{\gamma}) = 2 \left(\widehat{\boldsymbol{\gamma}} - \widehat{\boldsymbol{\gamma}}_{(-i)} \right)' \ddot{L}^{-1} \left(\widehat{\boldsymbol{\gamma}} - \widehat{\boldsymbol{\gamma}}_{(-i)} \right) , \qquad (6.34)$$

in which $\ddot{L}$ is the matrix of all second-order derivatives of $\ell(\boldsymbol{\gamma})$ with respect to $\boldsymbol{\gamma}$, evaluated at $\boldsymbol{\gamma} = \widehat{\boldsymbol{\gamma}}$. Formulation (6.34) easily allows to consider the global influence in a subvector of $\boldsymbol{\gamma}$, such as the dropout parameters $\boldsymbol{\psi}$, or the non-random parameter ω. This will be indicated using notation of the form $CD_{2i}(\boldsymbol{\psi})$, $CD_{2i}(\omega)$, etc.

In linear regression, global influence is conceptually simple, computationally straightforward and well studied. The latter two of these features do not carry over to more general settings. To overcome these limitations, *local* influence methods have been suggested. The principle is to investigate how the results of an analysis are changed under infinitesimal perturbations of the model. In the framework of the linear mixed model Beckman et al. (1987) used local influence to assess the effect of perturbing the error variances, the random-effects variances and the response vector. In the same context, Lesaffre and Verbeke (1998) have shown that the local influence approach is also useful for the detection of influential subjects in a longitudinal data analysis. Moreover, since the resulting influence diagnostics can be expressed analytically, they often can be decomposed in interpretable components, which yield additional insights in the reasons why some subjects are more influential than others.

Verbeke et al. (2001) studied the influence the non-randomness of dropout exerts on the model parameters. Let us briefly sketch the principles of local influence and then apply them to our MNAR problem.

We denote the log-likelihood function corresponding to model (6.30) by

$$\ell(\boldsymbol{\gamma}|\boldsymbol{\omega}) = \sum_{i=1}^{N} \ell_i(\boldsymbol{\gamma}|\omega_i) , \qquad (6.35)$$

in which $\ell_i(\boldsymbol{\gamma}|\omega_i)$ is the contribution of the ith individual to the log-likelihood, and where $\boldsymbol{\gamma} = (\boldsymbol{\theta}, \boldsymbol{\psi})$ is the s-dimensional vector, grouping the parameters of the measurement model and the dropout model, not including the $N \times 1$ vector $\boldsymbol{\omega} = (\omega_1, \omega_2, \dots, \omega_N)'$ of weights defining the perturbation of the MAR model. Let $\widehat{\boldsymbol{\gamma}}$ be the maximum likelihood estimator for $\boldsymbol{\gamma}$, obtained by maximizing $\ell(\boldsymbol{\gamma}|\boldsymbol{\omega}_0)$, and let $\widehat{\boldsymbol{\gamma}}_{\omega}$ denote the maximum likelihood estimator for $\boldsymbol{\gamma}$ under $\ell(\boldsymbol{\gamma}|\boldsymbol{\omega})$. Cook (1986) proposed to measure the distance between $\widehat{\boldsymbol{\gamma}}_{\omega}$ and $\widehat{\boldsymbol{\gamma}}$ by the so-called likelihood displacement, defined by $LD(\boldsymbol{\omega}) = 2\left(\ell(\widehat{\boldsymbol{\gamma}}|\boldsymbol{\omega}_0) - \ell(\widehat{\boldsymbol{\gamma}}_{\omega}|\boldsymbol{\omega})\right)$. Since this quantity can only be depicted when $N = 2$, Cook (1986) proposed to look at local influence, i.e., at the normal curvatures C_h of $\boldsymbol{\xi}(\boldsymbol{\omega})$ in $\boldsymbol{\omega}_0$, in the direction of some N dimensional vector $\boldsymbol{h}$ of unit length. It can be shown that a general form is given by

$$C_h(\boldsymbol{\theta}) = -2\boldsymbol{h}' \left[\frac{\partial^2 \ell_{i\omega}}{\partial\boldsymbol{\theta}\partial\omega_i}\bigg|_{\omega_i=0} \right]' \ddot{L}^{-1}(\boldsymbol{\theta}) \left[\frac{\partial^2 \ell_{i\omega}}{\partial\boldsymbol{\theta}\partial\omega_i}\bigg|_{\omega_i=0} \right] \boldsymbol{h}$$

$$C_h(\boldsymbol{\psi}) = -2\boldsymbol{h}' \left[\frac{\partial^2 \ell_{i\omega}}{\partial\boldsymbol{\psi}\partial\omega_i}\bigg|_{\omega_i=0} \right]' \ddot{L}^{-1}(\boldsymbol{\psi}) \left[\frac{\partial^2 \ell_{i\omega}}{\partial\boldsymbol{\psi}\partial\omega_i}\bigg|_{\omega_i=0} \right] \boldsymbol{h} ,$$

evaluated at $\boldsymbol{\gamma} = \widehat{\boldsymbol{\gamma}}$, where indeed the influence for the measurement and dropout model parameters split, since the second derivative matrix of the log-likelihood, $\ddot{L}$ is block-diagonal with blocks $\ddot{L}(\boldsymbol{\theta})$ and $\ddot{L}(\boldsymbol{\psi})$. Verbeke et al. (2001) have decomposed local influence into meaningful and interpretable components.

6.16   Pattern-Mixture Modeling Approach

Fitting pattern-mixture models (PMM) can be approached in several ways. It is important to decide whether pattern-mixture and selection modeling are to be contrasted with one another or rather the pattern-mixture modeling is the central focus. In the latter case, it is natural to conduct an analysis, and preferably a sensitivity analysis, *within* the pattern-mixture family. We will explicitly consider three strategies to deal with under-identification.

Strategy 1.   Little (1993, 1994) advocated the use of identifying restrictions and presented a number of examples. One of those, ACMV (available case missing values), is the natural counterpart of MAR in the PMM framework.

Strategy 2.   As opposed to identifying restrictions, model simplification can be done to identify the parameters. Thijs et al. (2002) discussed several sub-strategies in detail.

While the second strategy is computationally simple, it is important to note that there is a price to pay. Indeed, simplified models, qualified as "assumption rich" by Sheiner et al. (1997), are also making untestable assumptions, just as in the selection model case. In the identifying restrictions setting on the other hand, the assumptions are clear from the start.

Pattern-mixture models do not always automatically provide estimates and standard errors of marginal quantities of interest, such as overall treatment effect or overall time trend. Hogan and Laird (1997) provided a way to derive selection model quantities from the pattern-mixture model. An example of such a marginalization is given in Sect. 6.17.

Identifying Restriction Strategies   6.16.1

In line with the results obtained by Molenberghs et al. (1998), we restrict attention to monotone patterns. In general, let us assume we have $t = 1, \ldots, T$ dropout patterns where the dropout indicator, introduced earlier, is $d = t + 1$. For pattern t, the complete data density is given by

$$f_t(y_1, \ldots, y_T) = f_t(y_1, \ldots, y_t) f_t(y_{t+1}, \ldots, y_T | y_1, \ldots, y_t) . \qquad (6.36)$$

The first factor is clearly identified from the observed data, while the second factor is not. It is assumed that the first factor is known or, more realistically, modeled using the observed data. Then, identifying restrictions are applied in order to identify the second component.

While, in principle, completely arbitrary restrictions can be used by means of any valid density function over the appropriate support, strategies which relate back to the observed data deserve privileged interest. One can base identification on all patterns for which a given component, y_s say, is identified. A general expression for this is

$$f_t(y_s | y_1, \ldots, y_{s-1}) = \sum_{j=s}^{T} \omega_{sj} f_j(y_s | y_1, \ldots, y_{s-1}) , \quad s = t + 1, \ldots, T . \qquad (6.37)$$

We will use ω_s as shorthand for the set of ω_{sj}'s used. Every ω_s which sums up to one provides a valid identification scheme.

Let us incorporate (6.37) into (6.36):

$$f_t(y_1, \ldots, y_T) = f_t(y_1, \ldots, y_t) \prod_{s=0}^{T-t-1} \left[\sum_{j=T-s}^{T} \omega_{T-s,j} f_j(y_{T-s} | y_1, \ldots, y_{T-s-1}) \right] . \qquad (6.38)$$

Three special but important cases are *complete case missing values* (CCMV), *neighboring case missing values* (NCMV) and *available case missing values* (ACMV). Little (1993) introduced CCMV, in which case unavailable information is always borrowed from the completers. NCMV uses the nearest identified pattern. ACMV is the counterpart of MAR in the pattern-mixture context and uses all available patterns. More details are given in Appendix 6.A.1. It is further of interest to consider specific sub-families of the MNAR family. In the selection model context,

(6.9) restricts attention to a class of mechanisms where dropout may depend on the current, possibly unobserved, measurement, but not on future measurements. The entire class of such models will be termed non-future dependent (MNFD). While they are natural and easy to consider in a selection model context, there exist important examples of mechanisms that do not satisfy MNFD, such as shared-parameter models (Wu and Bailey 1989; Little 1995).

Kenward et al. (2003) have shown there is a counterpart to MNFD in the pattern-mixture context: non-future dependent missing value restrictions (NFMV). NFMV is not a single set of restrictions, but rather leaves one conditional distribution per incomplete pattern unidentified. Kenward et al. (2003) have shown that, for longitudinal data with dropouts, MNFD and NFMV are equivalent. See Appendix 6.A.1 for further details.

6.16.2   How to Use Restrictions?

We will briefly outline a general strategy. Several points which require further specification will be discussed in what follows. (1) Fit a model to the pattern-specific identifiable densities: $f_t(y_1, \ldots, y_t)$. This results in a parameter estimate, $\widehat{\gamma}_t$. (2) Select an identification method of choice. (3) Using this identification method, determine the conditional distributions of the unobserved outcomes, given the observed ones:

$$f_t(y_{t+1}, \ldots, y_T | y_1, \ldots, y_t) \,. \tag{6.39}$$

(4) Using standard multiple imputation methodology (Rubin 1987; Schafer 1997; Verbeke and Molenberghs 2000), draw multiple imputations for the unobserved components, given the observed outcomes and the correct pattern-specific density (6.39). (5) Analyse the multiply-imputed sets of data using the method of choice. This can be another pattern-mixture model, but also a selection model or any other desired model. (6) Inferences can be conducted in the standard multiple imputation way (Rubin 1987; Schafer 1997; Verbeke and Molenberghs 2000).

We have seen how general identifying restrictions (6.37), with CCMV, NCMV, and ACMV as special cases, lead to the conditional densities for the unobserved components, given the observed ones. This came down to deriving expressions for ω, such as in (6.42) for ACMV (see Appendix 6.A.1). In addition, we need to draw imputations from the conditional densities.

Let us proceed by studying the special case of three measurements first. To this end, we consider an identification scheme and we start off by avoiding the specification of a parametric form for these densities. The following steps are required: (1) Estimate the parameters of the identifiable densities: from pattern 3, $f_3(y_1, y_2, y_3)$; from pattern 2, $f_2(y_1, y_2)$; and from pattern 1, $f_1(y_1)$. (2) To properly account for the uncertainty with which the parameters are estimated, we need to draw from them as is customarily done in multiple imputation. It will be assumed that in all densities from which we draw, this parameter vector is used. (3) *For pattern 2.* Given an observation in this pattern, with observed values (y_1, y_2), calculate the conditional density $f_3(y_3|y_1, y_2)$ and draw from it. (4) *For pattern 1.* We now have to distinguish three substeps.

1. There is now only one ω involved: for pattern 1, in order to determine $f_1(y_2|y_1)$, as a combination of $f_2(y_2|y_1)$ and $f_3(y_2|y_1)$. Every ω in the unit interval is valid. Specific cases are: for NCMV, $\omega = 1$; for CCMV, $\omega = 0$; for ACMV, ω identifies a linear combination across patterns. Note that, given y_1, this is a constant, depending on α_2 and α_3.

    In order to pick one of the two components f_2 or f_3, we need to generate a random uniform variate, U say, except in the boundary NCMV and CCMV cases.

2. If $U \leq \omega$, calculate $f_2(y_2|y_1)$ and draw from it. Otherwise, do the same based on $f_3(y_2|y_1)$.

3. Given the observed y_1 and given y_2 which has just been drawn, calculate the conditional density $f_3(y_3|y_1, y_2)$ and draw from it.

All steps but the first one have to be repeated M times, to obtain the same number of imputed datasets. Inference then proceeds as outlined by Rubin (1987), Schafer (1997) and Verbeke and Molenberghs (2000).

In case the observed densities are assumed to be normal, the corresponding conditional densities are particularly straightforward.

In several cases, the conditional density is a mixture of normal densities. Then an additional and straightforward draw from the components of the mixture is necessary.

Pattern-Mixture Sensitivity Analysis for the Vorozole Study

6.17

Models Based on Identifying Restrictions

6.17.1

Consider those subjects with 1, 2, and 3 follow up measurements, respectively. Thus, 190 subjects are included into the analysis, with subsample sizes 35, 86, and 69, respectively. The corresponding pattern probabilities are $\hat{\pi} = (0.184, 0.453, 0.363)'$. The asymptotic variance covariance matrix can be derived without difficulty. We will now apply each of the three strategies of Sect. 6.16. We recognize a full analysis, using all patterns, is both interesting and feasible.

The patients in this study drop out mainly because they relapse or die. This in itself poses specific challenges that can be addressed within the pattern-mixture framework much easier than in the selection model framework. Indeed, if one is prepared to make the assumption that a patient who dies is representative of a slice of the population with the same characteristics, and with a certain probability to die, then identifying restrictions (i.e., extrapolation beyond the time of death) is meaningful. In case one does not want to extrapolate beyond the moment of death, one can restrict modeling to the observed data only. An intermediate approach would be to allow for extrapolation beyond relapse and not beyond death. (For the current dataset, the information needed in order to do so is unavailable.) Note that, while this may seem a disadvantage of pattern-mixture models, we believe it is an asset, because this framework not only forces one to think about such issues, it also provides a modeling solution, no matter which point of view is adopted. This contrasts with selection models where extrapolation is always done, be it explicitly by modeling the profile, averaged over all patterns.

In order to apply the identifying restriction in *Strategy 1*, one first needs to fit a model to the observed data. We will opt for a simple model, with parameters specific to each pattern. Such a model can be seen as belonging to the second modeling strategy.

We include time and time × time effects, as well as their interactions with treatment. Further, time by baseline value interaction is included as well. While we agree such a choice may seem controversial, it is consistent with the analysis plan and therefore we have opted to leave this term in. Alternatively, one could either remove this term or model raw scores rather than change scores. All effects interact with time, in order to force profiles to pass through the origin, since we are studying change versus baseline. An unstructured 3×3 covariance matrix is assumed for each pattern.

Parameter estimates are presented in Table 6.8, in the column denoted with "initial". Of course, not all parameters are estimable. This holds for the variance components, where in patterns 1 and 2 the upper 1×1 block and the upper 2×2 block are identified, respectively. In the first pattern, the effects in time × time are unidentified. The linear effects are identified by virtue of the absence of an intercept term.

Let us present this and later models graphically. Since there is one binary (treatment arm) and one continuous covariate (baseline level of FLIC score), insight can be obtained by plotting the models for selected values of baseline. Precisely, we chose the average value (Fig. 6.16). Bold line type is used for the range over which data are obtained for a particular pattern and extrapolation is indicated using thinner line type. Note that the extrapolation can have surprising and even questionable effects, even with these relatively simple models.

The initial model and its graphical representation motivate to consider identifying restriction models. Using the methodology detailed in Sect. 4, a GAUSS macro and a SAS macro, were written to conduct the multiple imputation, to fit the model to the imputed datasets, and to combine the results into a single inference. Results are presented in Table 6.8, for each of the three types of restrictions (CCMV, NCMV, ACMV). For patterns 1 and 2 there is some variability in the parameter estimates across the three strategies, although this is often consistent with random variation (see the standard errors). Since the data in pattern 3 are complete, there is of course no difference between the initial model parameters and those obtained with each of the identifying restriction techniques.

Table 6.8. Vorozole Study. Multiple imputation estimates and standard errors for CCMV, NCMV, and ACMV restrictions

Effect	initial	CCMV	NCMV	ACMV
Pattern 1:				
Time	3.40(13.94)	13.21(15.91)	7.56(16.45)	4.43(18.78)
Time×base	−0.11(0.13)	−0.16(0.16)	−0.14(0.16)	−0.11(0.17)
Time×treat	0.33(3.91)	−2.09(2.19)	−1.20(1.93)	−0.41(2.52)
Time×time		−0.84(4.21)	−2.12(4.24)	−0.70(4.22)
Time×time×treat		0.01(0.04)	0.03(0.04)	0.02(0.04)
σ_{11}	131.09(31.34)	151.91(42.34)	134.54(32.85)	137.33(34.18)
σ_{12}		59.84(40.46)	119.76(40.38)	97.86(38.65)
σ_{22}		201.54(65.38)	257.07(86.05)	201.87(80.02)
σ_{13}		55.12(58.03)	49.88(44.16)	61.87(43.22)
σ_{23}		84.99(48.54)	99.97(57.47)	110.42(87.95)
σ_{33}		245.06(75.56)	241.99(79.79)	286.16(117.90)
Pattern 2:				
Time	53.85(14.12)	29.78(10.43)	33.74(11.11)	28.69(11.37)
Time×base	−0.46(0.12)	−0.29(0.09)	−0.33(0.10)	−0.29(0.10)
Time×treat	−0.95(1.86)	−1.68(1.21)	−1.56(2.47)	−2.12(1.36)
Time×time	−18.91(6.36)	−4.45(2.87)	−7.00(3.80)	−4.22(4.20)
Time×time×treat	0.15(0.05)	0.04(0.02)	0.07(0.03)	0.05(0.04)
σ_{11}	170.77(26.14)	175.59(27.53)	176.49(27.65)	177.86(28.19)
σ_{12}	151.84(29.19)	147.14(29.39)	149.05(29.77)	146.98(29.63)
σ_{22}	292.32(44.61)	297.38(46.04)	299.40(47.22)	297.39(46.04)
σ_{13}		57.22(37.96)	89.10(34.07)	99.18(35.07)
σ_{23}		71.58(36.73)	107.62(47.59)	166.64(66.45)
σ_{33}		212.68(101.31)	264.57(76.73)	300.78(77.97)
Pattern 3:				
Time	29.91(9.08)	29.91(9.08)	29.91(9.08)	29.91(9.08)
Time×base	−0.26(0.08)	−0.26(0.08)	−0.26(0.08)	−0.26(0.08)
Time×treat	0.82(0.95)	0.82(0.95)	0.82(0.95)	0.82(0.95)
Time×time	−6.42(2.23)	−6.42(2.23)	−6.42(2.23)	−6.42(2.23)
Time×time×treat	0.05(0.02)	0.05(0.02)	0.05(0.02)	0.05(0.02)
σ_{11}	206.73(35.86)	206.73(35.86)	206.73(35.86)	206.73(35.86)
σ_{12}	96.97(26.57)	96.97(26.57)	96.97(26.57)	96.97(26.57)
σ_{22}	174.12(31.10)	174.12(31.10)	174.12(31.10)	174.12(31.10)
σ_{13}	87.38(30.66)	87.38(30.66)	87.38(30.66)	87.38(30.66)
σ_{23}	91.66(28.86)	91.66(28.86)	91.66(28.86)	91.66(28.86)
σ_{33}	262.16(44.70)	262.16(44.70)	262.16(44.70)	262.16(44.70)

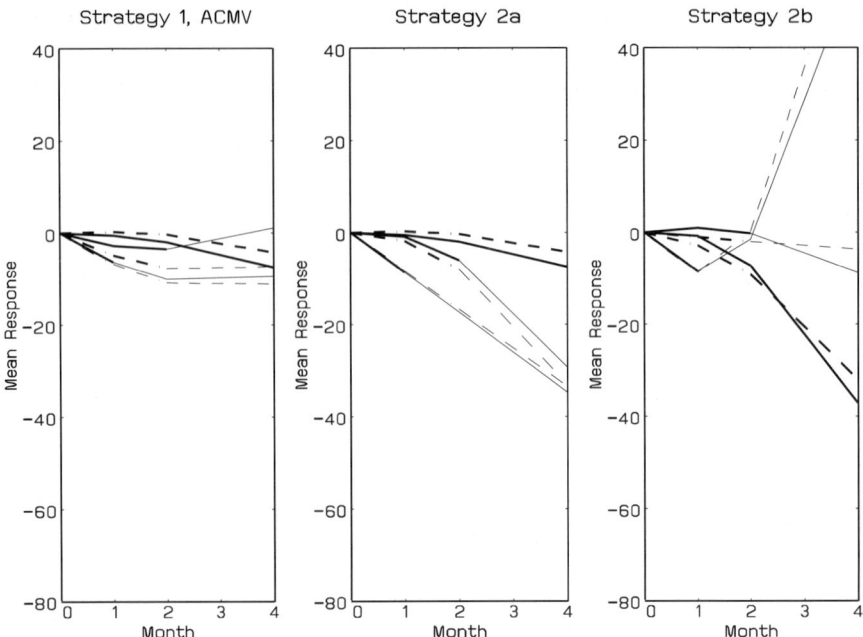

Figure 6.16. Vorozole Study. For average level of baseline value 113.57, strategies 1 (ACMV), 2a, and 2b are shown. The bold portion of the curves runs from baseline until the last obtained measurement, and the extrapolated piece is shown in thin type. The *dashed line* refers to megestrol acetate; the *solid line* is the Vorozole arm

In all of the plots, the same mean response scale was retained, illustrating that the identifying restriction strategies extrapolate much closer to the observed data mean responses. There are some differences among the identifying restriction methods, but this is not graphically represented here. This conclusion needs to be considered carefully. Since these patients drop out mainly because they relapse or die, it seems unlikely to expect a rise in quality of life. This consideration is evidence against CCMV, where missing information is always borrowed from the complete group, i.e., the one with the best prognosis. ACMV, which compromises between all strategies may be more realistic, but here NCMV is likely to be better since information is borrowed from the nearest pattern.

Nevertheless, the NCMV prediction looks more plausible since the worst baseline value shows declining profiles, whereas the best one leaves room for improvement. Should one want to explore the effect of assumptions beyond the range of (6.37), one can allow ω_s to include components outside of the unit interval. In that situation, one has to ensure that the resulting density is still non-negative over its entire support.

Strategy 2. As opposed to identifying restrictions, model simplification can be done in order to identify the parameters. The advantage is that the number of parameters decreases, which is desirable since the length of the parameter vector is a general issue with pattern-mixture models. Indeed, Hogan and Laird (1997) noted that in order to estimate the large number of parameters in general pattern-mixture models, one has to make the awkward requirement that each dropout pattern occurs sufficiently often. Broadly, we distinguish between two types of simplifications.

Strategy 2a. Trends can be restricted to functional forms supported by the information available within a pattern. For example, a linear or quadratic time trend is easily extrapolated beyond the last obtained measurement. One only needs to provide an ad hoc solution for the first or the first few patterns. In order to fit such models, one simply has to carry out a model building exercise within each of the patterns separately.

Strategy 2b. Next, one can let the parameters vary across patterns in a controlled parametric way. Thus, rather than estimating a separate time trend within each pattern, one could for example assume that the time evolution within a pattern is unstructured, but parallel across patterns. This is effectuated by treating pattern as a covariate. The available data can be used to assess whether such simplifications are supported within the time ranges for which there is information. An initial model is considered with the following effects: time, the interaction between time and treatment, baseline value, pattern, treatment × baseline, treatment × pattern, and baseline × pattern. Further time × time is included, as well as its interaction with baseline, treatment, and pattern. No interactions beyond the third order are included, and unstructured covariance matrix is common to all three patterns. This implies that the current model is *not* equivalent to a Strategy 1 model, where all parameters are pattern-specific. In order to achieve this goal, every effect would have to be made pattern-dependent. A graphical representation is given in Fig. 6.16. Early dropouts decline immediately, whereas those who stay longer in the study first show a rise and then decline thereafter. However, this is less pronounced for higher baseline values. On the other hand, the extrapolation based on the fitted model is very unrealistic, in the sense that for the early dropout sharp rises are predicted, which is totally implausible.

These findings suggest, again, that a more careful reflection on the extrapolation method is required. This is very well possible in a pattern-mixture context, but then the first strategy, rather than strategy 2a and 2b, has to be used.

In order to test for treatment effect, one can follow two strategies. In the first one, the focus is on the *marginal* treatment effect, i.e., one calculates the marginal treatment effect from the pattern-specific effects. Delta method arguments complete the procedure. We obtain p values of 0.801 (CCMV), 0.900 (NCMV), and 0.828 (ACMV). Alternatively, one can consider a 3 d.f. test, stratified for pattern. The resulting p values are 0.988 (CCMV), 0.995 (NCMV), and 0.993 (ACMV).

6.18 # Conclusions

In the Vorozole study, we have concentrated on total FLIC (i.e., change of the score versus baseline), a quality of life score measured in a multi-centric two arm study in postmenopausal women suffering from metastatic breast cancer. Since virtually all patients were followed up until disease progression or death, the amount of dropout is large. A very large group of patients drops out after just a couple of months.

It has been shown that the use of simple methods, such as complete case analysis or last observation carried forward, while historically very popular, carry major drawbacks and can and ought to be replaced with more advanced methods. One such method is a likelihood-based ignorable analysis. It has a broad basis in the sense that it is valid under MAR and compatible with general strategies such as linear or generalized linear mixed models. In the case of generalized estimating equations, a reasonably straightforward modification is needed in order to make the method suitable for the MAR setting.

While classically typical selection models are fitted, pattern-mixture models can be seen as a viable alternative. We analysed the data using both, leading to a sensitivity analysis. More confidence in the results can be gained if both models lead to similar conclusions. This is useful, since more general mechanisms than MAR are hard to exclude with certainty.

In the Vorozole study, the average profile in the selection model depends on the baseline value, as well as on time. The latter effect is mildly quadratic. There is no evidence for a treatment difference. However, it should be noted that the average profile found is the one that *would* have been observed, had no subjects dropped out, and under the additional assumption that the MAR assumption is correct. Fitting non-random dropout models, in the sense of Diggle and Kenward (1994) is possible, but computationally difficult for a fairly large trial like this one. A separate study of the dropout mechanism revealed that dropout increases with three elements: (1) an unfavourable baseline score, (2) an unfavourable value at the previous month, as well as (3) an unfavourable change in value from the penultimate to the last obtained value.

A pattern-mixture model is fitted by allowing at first a completely separate parameter vector for each observed dropout pattern, which is then simplified by using standard model selection procedures, by considering whether effects are common to all patterns. A first pattern-mixture model features a common treatment effect, of which the assessment is then straightforward. A second model includes a separate treatment effect for each dropout pattern. This leads to two distinct tests. The first one tests for the whole treatment vector to be zero. The second one first calculates the marginal treatment effect from the vector of effects, by composing a weighted sum, where the weights are the multinomially estimated probabilities of the various patterns. In all cases, there is no treatment effect. However, a graphical display of the fitted profiles per pattern is enlightening, since it clearly confirms the trend detected in the selection models, that patients tend to drop out when their quality of life score is declining. Since this feature is usually coupled to an imminent progression of the disease or to death, it should not come as a surprise. An important advantage of pattern-mixture models is that fitting them is more straightforward than non-random selection models. The additional calculations needed for the marginal treatment effect and its associated precision can be done straightforwardly using the delta method.

Further, we have illustrated three distinct strategies to fit pattern-mixture models. In this way, we have brought together several existing practices. Little (1993, 1994) has proposed identifying restrictions, which we here formalized using the connection with MAR and multiple imputation. Strategies 2a and 2b refer to fitting a model per pattern and using pattern as a covariate.

By contrasting these strategies on a single set of data, one obtains a range of conclusions rather than a single one, which provides insight into the sensitivity to the assumptions made. Especially with the identifying restrictions, one has to be very explicit about the assumptions and moreover this approach offers the possibility to consider several forms of restrictions. Special attention should go to the ACMV restrictions, since they are the MAR counterpart within the pattern-mixture context.

In addition, a comparison between the selection and pattern-mixture modeling approaches is useful to obtain additional insight into the data and/or to assess sensitivity.

The identifying restrictions strategy provides further opportunity for sensitivity analysis. Indeed, since CCMV and NCMV are extremes for the $\boldsymbol{\omega}_s$ vector in (6.37), it is very natural to consider the idea of *ranges* in the allowable space of $\boldsymbol{\omega}_s$. Clearly, any $\boldsymbol{\omega}_s$ which consists of non-negative elements that sum to one is allowable, but also the idea of extrapolation could be useful, where negative components are allowed, given they provide valid conditional densities.

We believe that our approach can play a useful role, as a member of a collection of sensitivity tools. Of course, a sensitivity analysis can be conducted within different frameworks, and there are times where the setting will determine which framework is the more appropriate one (for example Bayesian or frequentist), in conjunction with technical and computational considerations. Draper (1995) has considered ways of dealing with uncertainty in the very natural Bayesian framework and developments in the missing value setting are ongoing. A thorough comparison between the various frameworks will be interesting and worth undertaking in the future.

Acknowledgements. We gratefully acknowledge support from FWO-Vlaanderen Research Project G.0002.98: "Sensitivity Analysis for Incomplete and Coarse Data" and from Belgian IUAP/PAI network "Statistical Techniques and Modeling for Complex Substantive Questions with Complex Data". We are thankful to Janssen Research Foundation, and to Eli Lilly & Company for the kind permission to use their data.

Appendix

6.A   Pattern-Mixture Modelling

6.A.1   Identifying Restriction Strategies

Let us consider three special but important cases. Little (1993) proposes CCMV (complete case missing values) which uses the following identification:

$$f_t(y_s|y_1,\ldots,y_{s-1}) = f_T(y_s|y_1,\ldots,y_{s-1}) , \quad s = t+1,\ldots,T . \tag{6.40}$$

In other words, information which is unavailable is always borrowed from the completers. Alternatively, the nearest identified pattern can be used:

$$f_t(y_s|y_1,\ldots,y_{s-1}) = f_s(y_s|y_1,\ldots,y_{s-1}) , \quad s = t+1,\ldots,T . \tag{6.41}$$

We will refer to these restrictions as *neighboring case missing values* or NCMV.

The third special case of (6.37) will be ACMV. Thus, ACMV is reserved for the counterpart of MAR in the PMM context. The corresponding $\boldsymbol{\omega}_s$ vectors can be shown to have components:

$$\omega_{sj} = \frac{\alpha_j f_j(y_1,\ldots,y_{s-1})}{\sum_{\ell=s}^{T}\alpha_\ell f_\ell(y_1,\ldots,y_{s-1})} , \tag{6.42}$$

where α_j is the fraction of observations in pattern j (Molenberghs et al. 1998).

This MAR–ACMV link connects the selection and pattern-mixture families. It is further of interest to consider specific sub-families of the MNAR family. In the selection model context, (6.9) restricts attention to a class of mechanisms where dropout may depend on the current, possibly unobserved, measurement, but not on future measurements. The entire class of such models will be termed non-future dependent (MNFD). While they are natural and easy to consider in a selection model context, there exist important examples of mechanisms that do not satisfy MNFD, such as shared-parameter models (Wu and Bailey 1989; Little 1995).

Kenward et al. (2003) have shown there is a counterpart to MNFD in the pattern-mixture context. The MNFD selection models obviously satisfy

$$f(r = t|y_1,\ldots,y_T) = f(r = t|y_1,\ldots,y_{t+1}) . \tag{6.43}$$

Within the PMM framework, we define non-future dependent missing value restrictions (NFMV) as follows:

$$\forall t \geq 2 , \forall j < t-1 : f(y_t|y_1,\ldots,y_{t-1},r = j) = f(y_t|y_1,\ldots,y_{t-1},r \geq t-1) . \tag{6.44}$$

NFMV is not a single set of restrictions, but rather leaves one conditional distribution per incomplete pattern unidentified:

$$f(y_{t+1}|y_1,\ldots,y_t,r=t)\,. \tag{6.45}$$

In other words, the distribution of the "current" unobserved measurement, given the previous ones, is unconstrained. Note that (6.44) excludes such mechanisms as CCMV and NCMV. Kenward et al. (2003) have shown that, for longitudinal data with dropouts, MNFD and NFMV are equivalent.

For pattern t, the complete data density is given by

$$f_t(y_1,\ldots,y_T)$$
$$= f_t(y_1,\ldots,y_t)f_t(y_{t+1}|y_1,\ldots,y_t)f_t(y_{t+2},\ldots,y_T|y_1,\ldots,y_{t+1})\,. \tag{6.46}$$

It is assumed that the first factor is known or, more realistically, modelled using the observed data. Then, identifying restrictions are applied in order to identify the second and third components. First, from the data, estimate $f_t(y_1,\ldots,y_t)$. Second, the user has full freedom to choose

$$f_t(y_{t+1}|y_1,\ldots,y_t)\,. \tag{6.47}$$

Substantive considerations can be used to identify this density. Or a family of densities can be considered by way of sensitivity analysis. Third, using (6.44), the densities $f_t(y_j|y_1,\ldots,y_{j-1})$, $(j \geq t+2)$ are identified. This identification involves not only the patterns for which y_j is observed, but also the pattern for which y_j is the current, the first unobserved measurement.

Two obvious mechanisms, within the MNFD family but outside MAR, are FD1, i.e., choose (6.47) according to CCMV, and FD2, i.e., choose (6.47) according to NCMV. FD1 and FD2 are strictly different from CCMV and NCMV.

References

Aerts M, Geys H, Molenberghs G, and Ryan LM (2002) Topics in Modelling of Clustered Binary Data. Chapman & Hall, London

Afifi A, Elashoff R (1966) Missing observations in multivariate statistics I: Review of the literature. Journal of the American Statistical Association 61:595–604

Amemiya T (1984) Tobit models: a survey. Journal of Econometrics 24:3–61

Ashford JR, Sowden RR (1970) Multi-variate probit analysis. Biometrics 26:535–546

Baker SG (1995) Marginal regression for repeated binary data with outcome subject to non-ignorable non-response. Biometrics 51:1042–1052

Bahadur RR (1961) A representation of the joint distribution of responses to n dichotomous items. In: Solomon H (ed) Studies in Item Analysis and Prediction Stanford Mathematical Studies in the Social Sciences VI. Stanford University Press, Stanford CA

Beckman RJ, Nachtsheim CJ, and Cook RD (1987) Diagnostics for mixed-model analysis of variance. Technometrics 29:413–426

Breslow NE, Clayton DG (1993) Approximate inference in generalized linear mixed models. Journal of the American Statistical Association 88:9–25

Buck SF (1960) A method of estimation of missing values in multivariate data suitable for use with an electronic computer. Journal of the Royal Statistical Society Series B 22:302–306

Chatterjee S, Hadi AS (1988) Sensitivity Analysis in Linear Regression. John Wiley & Sons, New York

Cook RD (1977) Detection of influential observations in linear regression. Technometrics 19:15–18

Cook RD (1979) Influential observations in linear regression. Journal of the American Statistical Association 74:169–174

Cook RD (1986) Assessment of local influence. Journal of the Royal Statistical Society Series B 48:133–169

Cook RD, Weisberg S (1982) Residuals and Influence in Regression. Chapman & Hall, London

Dale JR (1986) Global cross-ratio models for bivariate, discrete, ordered responses. Biometrics 42:909–917

Dempster AP, Rubin DB (1983) Overview. Incomplete Data in Sample Surveys, Vol. II: Theory and Annotated Bibliography, Madow WG, Olkin I, Rubin DB (eds). Academic Press, New York, pp 3–10

Dempster AP, Laird NM, Rubin DB (1977) Maximum likelihood from incomplete data via the EM algorithm (with discussion). Journal of the Royal Statistical Society Series B 39:1–38

Diggle PJ, Kenward MG (1994) Informative drop-out in longitudinal data analysis (with discussion). Applied Statistics 43:49–93

Diggle PJ, Heagerty P, Liang K-Y, Zeger SL (2002) Analysis of Longitudinal Data. Oxford University Press, New York

Draper D (1995) Assessment and propagation of model uncertainty (with discussion). Journal of the Royal Statistical Society Series B 57:45–97

Ekholm A (1991) Algorithms versus models for analyzing data that contain misclassification errors. Biometrics 47:1171–1182

Fahrmeir L, Tutz G (2001) Multivariate Statistical Modelling Based on Generalized Linear Models. Springer-Verlag, Heidelberg

Fitzmaurice GM, Molenberghs G, Lipsitz SR (1995) Regression models for longitudinal binary responses with informative dropouts. Journal of the Royal Statistical Society Series B 57:691–704

Fitzmaurice GM, Heath G, Clifford P (1996a) Logistic regression models for binary data panel data with attrition. Journal of the Royal Statistical Society Series A 159:249–264

Fitzmaurice GM, Laird NM, Zahner GEP (1996b) Multivariate logistic models for incomplete binary response. Journal of the American Statistical Association 91:99–108

George EO, Bowman D (1995) A saturated model for analyzing exchangeable binary data: Applications to clinical and developmental toxicity studies. Journal of the American Statistical Association 90:871–879

Geys H, Molenberghs G, Lipsitz SR (1998) A note on the comparison of pseudo-likelihood and generalized estimating equations for marginal odds ratio models. Journal of Statistical Computation and Simulation 62:45–72

Glonek GFV, McCullagh P (1995) Multivariate logistic models. Journal of the Royal Statistical Society Series B 81:477–482

Goss PE, Winer EP, Tannock IF, Schwartz LH, Kremer AB (1999) Breast cancer: randomized phase III trial comparing the new potent and selective third-generation aromatase inhibitor vorozole with megestrol acetate in postmenopausal advanced breast cancer patients. Journal of Clinical Oncology 17:52–63

Hartley HO, Hocking R (1971) The analysis of incomplete data. Biometrics 27:7783–808

Heckman JJ (1976) The common structure of statistical models of truncation, sample selection and limited dependent variables and a simple estimator for such models. Annals of Economic and Social Measurement 5:475–492

Hogan JW, Laird NM (1997) Mixture models for the joint distribution of repeated measures and event times. Statistics in Medicine 16:239–258

Kenward MG, Molenberghs G (1998) Likelihood based frequentist inference when data are missing at random. Statistical Science 12:236–247

Kenward MG, Molenberghs G, Thijs H (2003) Pattern-mixture models with proper time dependence. Biometrika 90:53–71

Laird NM (1994) Discussion to Diggle PJ, Kenward MG: Informative dropout in longitudinal data analysis. Applied Statistics 43:84

Lang JB, Agresti A (1994) Simultaneously modeling joint and marginal distributions of multivariate categorical responses. Journal of the American Statistical Association 89:625–632

le Cessie S, van Houwelingen JC (1994) Logistic regression for correlated binary data. Applied Statistics 43:95–108

Lesaffre E, Verbeke G (1998) Local influence in linear mixed models. Biometrics 54:570–582

Liang K-Y, Zeger SL (1986) Longitudinal data analysis using generalized linear models. Biometrika 73:13–22

Liang K-Y, Zeger SL, Qaqish B (1992) Multivariate regression analyses for categorical data. Journal of the Royal Statistical Society Series B 54:3–40

Lipsitz SR, Laird NM, Harrington DP (1991) Generalized estimating equations for correlated binary data: using the odds ratio as a measure of association. Biometrika 78:153–160

Little RJA (1986) A note about models for selectivity bias. Econometrika 53:1469–1474

Little RJA (1993) Pattern-mixture models for multivariate incomplete data. Journal of the American Statistical Association 88:125–134

Little RJA (1994) A class of pattern-mixture models for normal incomplete data. Biometrika 81:471–483

Little RJA (1995) Modeling the drop-out mechanism in repeated measures studies. Journal of the American Statistical Association 90:1112–1121

Little RJA, Rubin DB (1987) Statistical Analysis with Missing Data. John Wiley & Sons, New York

Mallinckrodt CH, Clark WS, Stacy RD (2001a) Type I error rates from mixed-effects model repeated measures versus fixed effects analysis of variance with missing values imputed via last observation carried forward. Drug Information Journal 35:1215–1225

Mallinckrodt CH, Clark WS, Stacy RD (2001b) Accounting for dropout bias using mixed-effects models. Journal of Biopharmaceutical Statistics series 11, (1 & 2):9–21

Mallinckrodt CH, Clark WS, Carroll RJ, Molenberghs G (2003a) Assessing response profiles from incomplete longitudinal clinical trial data under regulatory considerations. Journal of Biopharmaceutical Statistics 13:179–190

Mallinckrodt CH, Sanger TM, Dube S, Debrota DJ, Molenberghs G, Carroll RJ, Zeigler Potter WM, Tollefson, GD (2003b) Assessing and interpreting treatment effects in longitudinal clinical trials with missing data. Biological Psychiatry series 53:754–760

McCullagh P, Nelder JA (1989) Generalized Linear Models. Chapman & Hall, London

Michiels B, Molenberghs G, Bijnens L, Vangeneugden T, Thijs H (2002) Selection models and pattern-mixture models to analyze longitudinal quality of life data subject to dropout. Statistics in Medicine 21:1023–1041

Molenberghs G, Lesaffre E (1994) Marginal modelling of correlated ordinal data using a multivariate Plackett distribution. Journal of the American Statistical Association 89:633–644

Molenberghs G, Lesaffre E (1999) Marginal modelling of multivariate categorical data. Statistics in Medicine 18:2237–2255

Molenberghs G, Kenward MG, Lesaffre E (1997) The analysis of longitudinal ordinal data with non-random dropout. Biometrika 84:33–44

Molenberghs G, Michiels B, Kenward MG, Diggle PJ (1998) Missing data mechanisms and pattern-mixture models. Statistica Neerlandica 52:153–161

Murray GD, Findlay JG (1988) Correcting for the bias caused by drop-outs in hypertension trials. Statististics in Medicine 7:941–946

Nelder JA, Mead R (1965) A simplex method for function minimisation. The Computer Journal 7:303–313

Neuhaus JM (1992) Statistical methods for longitudinal and clustered designs with binary responses. Statistical Methods in Medical Research 1:249–273

Neuhaus JM, Kalbfleisch JD, Hauck WW (1991) A comparison of cluster-specific and population-averaged approaches for analyzing correlated binary data. International Statistical Review 59:25–35

Plackett RL (1965) A class of bivariate distributions. Journal of the American Statistical Association 60:516–522

Prentice RL (1988) Correlated binary regression with covariates specific to each binary observation. Biometrics 44:1033–1048

Robins JM, Rotnitzky A, Zhao LP (1995) Analysis of semiparametric regression models for repeated outcomes in the presence of missing data. Journal of the American Statistical Association 90:106–121

Robins JM, Rotnitzky A, Scharfstein DO (1998) Semiparametric regression for repeated outcomes with non-ignorable non-response. Journal of the American Statistical Association 93:1321–1339

Rubin DB (1976) Inference and missing data. Biometrika 63:581–592

Rubin DB (1987) Multiple Imputation for Nonresponse in Surveys. John Wiley & Sons, New York

Rubin DB (1994) Discussion to Diggle PJ, Kenward MG: Informative dropout in longitudinal data analysis. Applied Statistics 43:80–82

Schafer JL (1997) Analysis of Incomplete Multivariate Data. Chapman & Hall, London

Schipper H, Clinch J, McMurray A (1984) Measuring the quality of life of cancer patients: the Functional-Living Index-Cancer: development and validation. Journal of Clinical Oncology 2:472–483

Sheiner LB, Beal SL, Dunne A (1997) Analysis of nonrandomly censored ordered categorical longitudinal data from analgesic trials. Journal of the American Statistical Association 92:1235–1244

Siddiqui O, Ali MW (1998) A comparison of the random-effects pattern-mixture model with last-observation-carried-forward (LOCF) analysis in longitudinal clinical trials with dropouts. Journal of Biopharmaceutical Statistics 8:545–563

Skellam JG (1948) A probability distribution derived from the binomial distribution by regarding the probability of success as variable between the sets of trials. Journal of the Royal Statistical Society Series B 10:257–261

Smith DM, Robertson B, Diggle PJ (1996) Object-oriented Software for the Analysis of Longitudinal Data in S. Technical Report MA 96/192. Department of Mathematics and Statistics, University of Lancaster, LA1 4YF, United Kingdom

Stiratelli R, Laird N, Ware J (1984) Random effects models for serial observations with dichotomous response. Biometrics 40:961–972

Tanner MA, Wong WH (1987) The calculation of posterior distributions by data augmentation. Journal of the American Statistical Association 82:528–550

Thijs H, Molenberghs G, Michiels B, Verbeke G, Curran D (2002) Strategies to fit pattern-mixture models. Biostatistics 3:245–265

Verbeke G, Molenberghs G (1997) Linear Mixed Models in Practice: A SAS-Oriented Approach. Lecture Notes in Statistics 126. Springer-Verlag, New York

Verbeke G, Molenberghs G (2000) Linear Mixed Models for Longitudinal Data. Springer-Verlag, New York

Verbeke G, Molenberghs G, Thijs H, Lesaffre E, Kenward MG (2001) Sensitivity analysis for non-random dropout: a local influence approach. Biometrics 57:7–14

Wedderburn RWM (1974) Quasi-likelihood functions, generalized linear models, and the Gauss-Newton method. Biometrika 61:439–447

Wu MC, Bailey KR (1989) Estimation and comparison of changes in the presence of informative right censoring: conditional linear model. Biometrics 45:939–955

Meta-Analysis in Epidemiology II.7

Maria Blettner, Peter Schlattmann

7.1   Introduction

The use of meta-analyses in order to synthesise the evidence from epidemiological studies has become more and more popular recently. It has been estimated by Egger et al. (1998) that from articles retrieved by MEDLINE with the medical subject heading (MeSH) term "meta-analysis" some 33% reported results of a meta-analysis from randomised clinical trials and nearly the same proportion (27%) were from observational studies, including 12% papers in which the aetiology of a disease was investigated. The remaining papers include methodological publications or review articles. Reasons for the popularity of meta-analyses are the growing information in the scientific literature and the need of timely decisions for risk assessment or in public health. While methods for meta-analyses in order to summarise or synthesise evidence from randomised controlled clinical trials have been continuously developed during the last years, and methods are now summarised in several text books for example Sutton et al. (2000), Whitehead (2002) and in a handbook by Egger et al. (2001), Dickersin (2002) argued that statistical methods for meta-analyses of epidemiological studies are still behind in comparison to the progress that has been made for randomised clinical trials. The use of meta-analyses for epidemiological research caused many controversial discussions, see for example Blettner et al. (1999), Berlin (1995), Greenland (1994), Feinstein (1995), Olkin (1994), Shapiro (1994a,b) or Weed (1997) for a detailed overview of the arguments. The most prominent arguments against meta-analyses are the fundamental issues of confounding, selection bias, as well as the large variety and heterogeneity of study designs and data collection procedures in epidemiological research. Despite these controversies, results from meta-analyses are often cited and used for decisions. They are often seen as the fundamentals for risk assessment. They are also performed to summarise the current state of knowledge often prior to designing new studies.

This chapter will first describe reasons for meta-analyses in epidemiological research and then illustrate how to perform a meta-analysis with the focus on meta-analysis of published data.

7.2   Different Types of Overviews

Approaches for summarising evidence include four different types of overviews: first, traditional narrative reviews that provide a qualitative but not a quantitative assessment of published results. Methods and guidelines for reviews have been recently published by Weed (1997).

Second, meta-analyses from literature (MAL) which are generally performed from freely available publications without the need of co-operation and without agreement of the authors from the original studies. They are comparable to a narrative review in many respects but include quantitative estimate(s) of the effect of interest. One recent example is a meta-analysis by Zeeger et al. (2003) of studies investigating some familial clustering of prostate cancer. Another meta-analysis has been recently published by Allam et al. (2003) on the association between Parkinson disease, smoking and family history.

Third, meta-analyses with individual patient data (MAP) in which individual data from published and sometimes also unpublished studies are re-analysed. Often, there is a close co-operation between the researcher performing the meta-analysis and the investigators of the individual studies. The new analysis may include specific inclusion criteria for patients and controls, new definition of the exposure and confounder variables and new statistical modeling. This re-analysis may overcome some but not all of the problems of meta-analyses of published data (Blettner et al. 1999). They have been performed in epidemiological research for many years. One of the largest investigations of this form was a recent investigation on breast cancer and oral contraceptive use, where data from 54 case-control studies were pooled and re-analysed (CGHFBC 1996). A further international collaboration led by Lubin and colleagues were set up to re-analyse data from eleven large cohort studies on lung cancer and radon among uranium miners. The re-analysis allowed a refined dose-response analysis and provided data for radiation protection issues. Pooled re-analyses are mostly performed by combining data from studies of the same type only. For example Hung et al. (2003) re-analysed data from all case-control studies in which the role of genetic polymorphisms for lung cancer in non-smokers were investigated. The role of diet for lung cancer was recently reviewed by Smith-Warner et al. (2002) in a qualitative and quantitative way by combining cohort studies. An overview of methodologic aspects for a pooled analysis of data from cohort studies was recently published by Bennett (2003).

Fourth, prospectively planned pooled meta-analyses of several studies in which pooling is already a part of the protocol. Data collection procedures, definitions of variables are as far as possible standardised for the individual studies. The statistical analysis has many similarities with the meta-analysis based on individual data. A major difference, however, is that joint planning of the data collection and analysis increase the homogeneity of the included data sets. However, in contrast to multicentre randomised clinical trials, important heterogeneity between the study centres still may exist. This heterogeneity may arise from differences in populations, in the relevant confounding variables (e.g. race may only be a confounder in some centres) and potentially differences in ascertainment of controls. For example complete listings of population controls are available in some but not all countries. In the latter siutation sometimes neighbourhood controls are used. Mainly in occupational epidemiology those studies are rather common, many of them were initiated by international bodies such as the International Agency for Research on Cancer (IARC) as the international pooled analysis by Boffetta et al. (1997) of cancer mortality among persons exposed to man-made mineral fiber. Another example for a prospectively planned pooled meta-analysis is given by a large brain tumour study initiated by the IARC including data from eight different countries (see Schlehofer et al. 1999).

Steinberg et al. (1997) compared the effort required and the results obtained of MAL and MAP with an application to ovarian cancer. Certainly, MAL are easier to perform, cheaper and faster than MAP. Their credibility may be more questionable as discussed by many authors, see for example Blettner et al. (1999) or Egger et al. (1998). Statistical issues of pooling data from case-control studies have been investigated by Stukel et al. (2001) recently. The authors proposed a two step approach and showed conditions under which the two step approach gives similar results in comparison to the pooled analysis including all data. Here the two step approach implies to estimate first the odds ratio for each study in the usual way. Then in the second step a combined estimator using either a fixed or random effects model is calculated (cf. Chap. III.8 of this handbook).

7.3   Reasons for Meta-Analysis in Epidemiology

One major issue in assessing causality in epidemiology is "consistency" as pointed out by Hill in 1965. The extent to which an observed association is similar in different studies, with different designs, using different methods of data collection and exposure assessment, by different investigators and in different regions or countries is an essential criterion for causality. If different studies with inconsistent results are known there is a need for understanding the differences. Reasons may be small sample sizes of individual studies (chance), different methods of exposure assessment (measurement errors), different statistical analyses (e.g. adjustment for confounding), or the use of different study populations (selection bias). Also, Thompson et al. (1997) showed that different baseline risks may cause heterogeneity. The goal of a meta-analysis is then to investigate, whether the available evidence is consistent and/or to which degree inconsistent results can be explained by random variation or by systematic differences between design, setting or analysis of the study as has been pointed out by Weed (2000).

Meta-analyses are often performed to obtain a combined estimator of the quantitative effect of the risk factor such as the relative risk (RR) or the odds ratio (OR). As single studies are often far too small to obtain reliable risk estimates, the combination of data of several studies may lead to more precise effect estimates and increased statistical power. This is mainly true if the exposure leads only to a small increase (or decrease) in risk or if the disease or the exposure of interest is rare. One example is the risk of developing lung cancer after the exposure to passive smoking where relative risk estimates in the order of 1.2 have been observed, see Boffetta (2002) for a summary of the epidemiological evidence. Another typical example is the association between childhood leukaemia and exposure to electromagnetic fields. Meinert and Michaelis (1996) have performed a meta-analysis of the available case-control studies as the results of the investigations were inconsistent. Although many huge case-control studies have been performed in the last decade, in each single study only a few children were categorised as "highly exposed". In most publications, a small but non-significant increase in risk was found but no single study had enough power to exclude that there is no association between EMF-exposure and childhood leukaemia.

Sometimes, meta-analyses are also used to investigate more complex dose-response functions. For example, Tweedie and Mengersen (1995) investigated the dose-response relationship of exposure to passive smoking and lung cancer. A meta-analysis was also undertaken by Longnecker et al. (1988) to study the dose-response of alcohol consumption and breast cancer risk. However, results were limited as not enough data were present in several of the included publications. Interestingly, a large group of investigators led by Hamajima et al. (2002) has recently used individual patient data from 53 studies including nearly 60,000 cases for a re-analysis. It has been shown by Sauerbrei et al. (2001) in a critique that meta-analysis from aggregated data may be too limited to perform a dose-response analysis. A major limitation is that different categories are used in different publications. Thus dose-response analyses are restricted to published values. Meta-analyses of published data have their main merits for exploring heterogeneity between studies and to provide crude quantitative estimates but probably less for investigating complex dose-response relationships.

Steps in Performing a Meta-Analysis 7.4

Each type of overview needs a clear study protocol that describes the research question and the design, including how studies are identified and selected, the statistical methods to use and how the results will be reported. This protocol should also include the exact definition of the disease of interest, the risk factors and the potential confounding variables that have to be considered. In accordance with Friedenreich (1993) and Jones (1992), the following steps are needed for a meta-analysis/pooled analysis (cf. Chap. III.8 of this handbook).

Step 1.   Define a clear and focused topic for the review: As for any other investigation, a clear protocol in which the research hypothesis, i.e. the objectives of the meta-analysis are described, is mandatory. This protocol should include the exact definition of the disease of interest, the risk factors and the potential confounding variables that have to be considered. The protocol should also include details on the steps that are described below, including specification of techniques for location of the studies, the statistical analysis and the proposed publications.

Step 2.   Establish inclusion and exclusion: It is important to define in advance which studies should be included into the meta-analysis. These criteria may include restrictions on the publication year as older studies may not be comparable to newer ones, on the design of the investigation, e.g. to exclude ecological studies. Friedenreich et al. (1994) has also proposed quality criteria to evaluate each study. Whether these criteria, however, should be used as inclusion criteria is discussed controversially. Another decision is whether studies that are only published as abstracts or internal communications should be included (Cook et al. 1993). A rule for the inclusion or exclusion of papers with repeated publication of the data is required. For example, for cohort studies, often several publications with different follow-up periods can be found. As one out of many examples, a German study among rubber workers by Straif et al. (1999, 2000) can be mentioned. In one paper, 11,633 workers were included, while the second paper is based on a subcohort of only 8933 persons. Which results are more appropriate for the meta-analysis?

Step 3.   Locate all studies (published and unpublished) that are relevant to the topic: Since the existence of electronic databases, retrieval of published studies has become much easier. Mainly systems like MEDLINE or CANCERLIT from the National Library of Medicine are valuable sources to locate publications. However, as Dickersin et al. (1994) showed for some examples as little as 50% of the publications were found by electronic searches. Therefore there is a need to extend the search by manual checks of the reference lists of retrieved papers, monographs, books and if possible by personal communications with researchers in the field. A clear goal of the search has to be to identify all relevant studies on the topic that meet the inclusion criteria. Egger et al. (2003) have pointed out that the completeness of the literature search is an important feature of the meta-analysis to avoid publication bias or selection bias. Of course, the publication should include the search strategies as well as the key-words and the databases used for electronic searches.

Step 4.   Abstract information from the publications: The data collection step in a meta-analysis needs as much care as in other studies. In the meta-analysis the unit of observation is the publication and defined variables have to be abstracted from the publication (Stock 1995). In epidemiological studies, the key parameter is often the relative risk or odds ratio. Additionally, standard error, sample size, treatment of confounders and other characteristics of the study design and data collection procedure need to be abstracted to assess the quality of the study. This is also important for subgroup analyses or for a sensitivity analysis. An abstract form has to be created before abstracting data. This form should be tested like other instruments in a pilot phase. Unfortunately, it may not always be possible to abstract the required estimates directly, e.g. standard errors are not presented and have to be calculated based on confidence intervals (Greenland 1987). It may be necessary to contact the investigators to obtain further information if results are not published in sufficient detail. Abstracting and classification of study characteristics is the most time consuming part of the meta-analysis. It has been recommended to blind the data abstractors although some authors argue that blinding may not have a major influence on the results, for further discussion see Berlin et al. (1997). Additionally, the rater may be acquainted with some of the studies and blinding can not be performed. Another requirement is that two persons should perform the abstraction in parallel. When a meta-analysis with original data is performed the major task is to obtain data from all project managers in a compatible way.

Our experience shows that this is possible in principle but time consuming as data may not be available on modern electronic devices and often adaptations between database systems are required.

Step 5. Descriptive analysis: A first step in summarising the results should be an extensive description of the single papers, including tabulation of relevant elements of each study, such as sample size, data collection procedures, confounder variables, means of statistical analysis, study design, publication year, performing year, geographical setting etc. This request is also included in the guidelines for publications of meta-analysis that were published by Stroup et al. (2000).

Step 6. Statistical analysis: This includes the analysis of the heterogeneity of the study-specific effects, the calculation of a pooled estimate and the confidence interval as well as a sensitivity analysis. Details are given in the next section on statistical methods.

Step 7. Interpretation of the results: The importance of the sources and magnitude of different biases should be taken into account when interpreting the results. Combining several studies will often give small confidence intervals and suggest a false precision (Egger et al. 1998) but estimates may be biased. For clinical studies, Thompson (1994) has pointed out that the investigation of the heterogeneity between studies will generally give more insight than inspecting the confidence intervals of the pooled estimate. This is even more true for a meta-analysis from epidemiological studies. Additionally, the possible effects of publication bias (see below) need to be considered carefully (Copas and Shi 2001).

Step 8. Publication: Guidelines for reporting meta-analyses of observational studies have been published by Stroup et al. (2000). These guidelines are quite useful for preparing the publication and are also supported by most editors of major medical journals. Especially the detailed description of methods is required so that the analysis could be replicated by others.

Statistical Analysis 7.5

The statistical analysis of aggregated data from published studies was first developed in the fields of psychology and education (Glass 1977; Smith and Glass 1977). These methods have been adopted since the mid-1980s in medicine primarily for randomized clinical trials and are also used for epidemiologic data. We will give a brief outline of some issues of the analysis using an example based on a meta-analysis performed by Sillero-Arenas et al. (1992). This study was one of the first meta-analyses which tried to summarise quantitatively the association between hormone replacement therapy (HRT) and breast cancer in women. Sillero-Arenas et al. based their meta-analysis on 23 case control and 13 cohort studies. The data extracted from their paper are given in the appendix.

The statistical analysis of MAP is more complex and not covered here.

Single Study Results.   A first step of the statistical analysis is the description of the characteristics and the results of each study. Tabulations and simple graphical methods should be employed to visualize the results of the single studies. Plotting the odds ratios and their confidence intervals (so called forest plot) is a simple way to spot obvious differences between the study results.

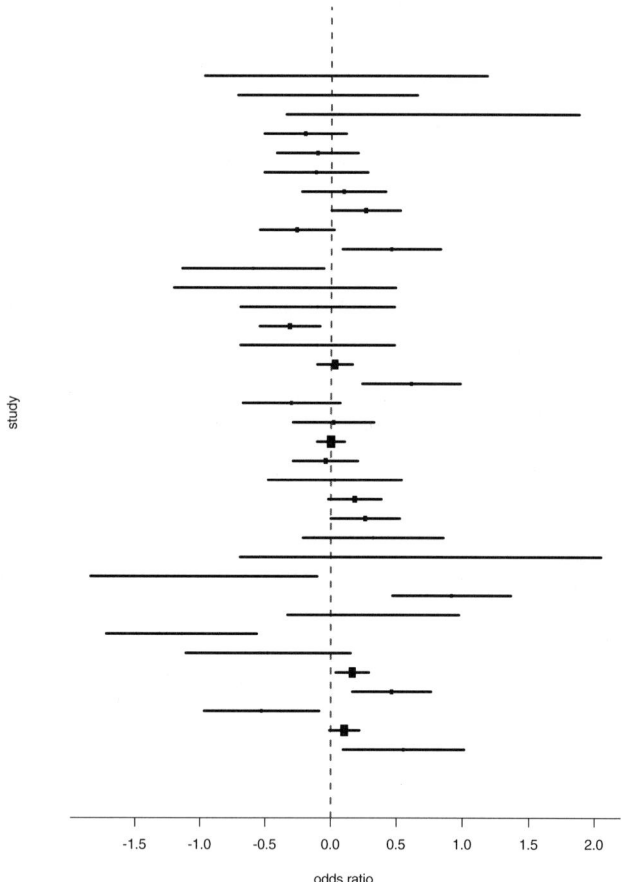

Figure 7.1. Confidence interval plot of the breast cancer data

Figure 7.1 shows a forest plot of 36 studies investigating the association of HRT and breast cancer in women. Obviously there is a high variability of effects between studies present. Later we will describe how to account for heterogeneity of studies quantitatively.

Publication Bias. An important problem of meta-analysis is publication bias. This bias has received a lot of attention particularly in the area of clinical trials. Publication bias occurs when studies that have non-significant or negative results are published less frequently than positive studies. For randomised clinical trials, it has been shown that even with a computer-aided literature search not all of the relevant studies will be identified (Dickersin et al. 1994). For epidemiologic observational studies additional problems exist, because often a large number of variables will be collected in questionnaires as potential confounders. If one or several of these potential confounders yield significant or important results, they may be published in additional papers, which have often not been planned in advance. In general, publication bias yields a non-negligible overestimation of the risk estimate. As a result prior to further statistical analyses publication bias should be investigated.

A simple graphical tool to detect publication bias is the so called funnel plot. The basic idea is that studies which do not show an effect and which are not statistically significant are less likely to published. If the sample size or alternatively the precision (i.e. the inverse of the variance) is plotted against the effect a hole in lower left quadrant is expected.

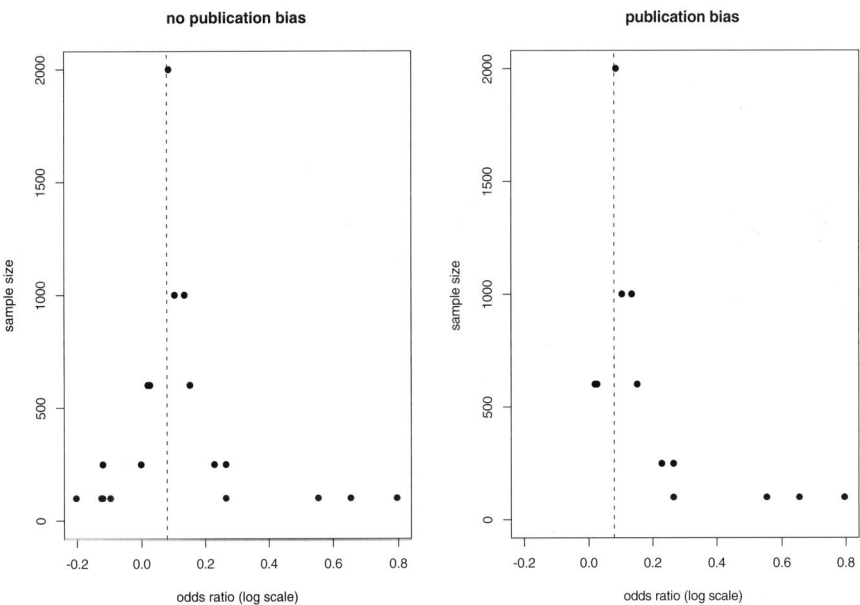

Figure 7.2. Examples of funnel plots based on simulated data with (*right figure*) and without publication bias present (*left figure*). The *dotted line* shows the true effect

Figure 7.2 shows examples of funnel plots. The left subplot of Fig. 7.2 shows a funnel plot with no indication of publication bias. The right subplot shows a so called apparent hole in the lower left corner. In the case of the right subplot of Fig. 7.2 the presence of publication bias would be assumed.

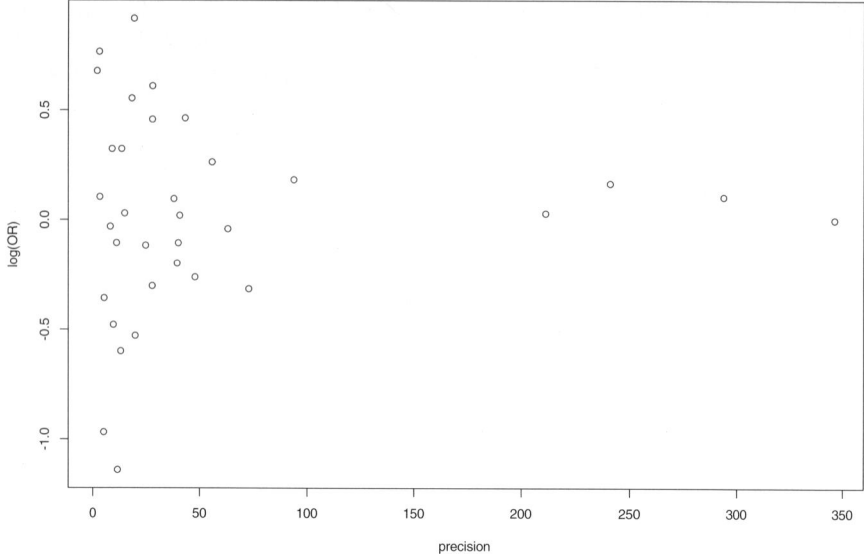

Figure 7.3. Funnel plot of the breast cancer data

Figure 7.3 shows a funnel plot for the breast cancer data. No apparent hole in the lower left corner is present. Thus based on this figure no publication bias would be assumed.

For a quantitative investigation of publication bias several methods are available. This may be based on statistical tests, see for example Begg and Mazumdar (1994) or Schwarzer et al. (2002). A recent simulation study performed by Macaskil et al. (2001) favoured the use of regression methods. The basic idea is to regress the estimated effect sizes $\hat{\theta}_i$ directly on the sample size or the inverse variance σ_i^{-2} as predictor.

$$\hat{\theta}_i = \alpha + \beta \frac{1}{\sigma_i^2} + \varepsilon_i , \quad i = 1, \ldots, k , \quad \varepsilon_i \sim N\left(0, \sigma_i^2\right) . \tag{7.1}$$

Here the number of studies to be pooled is denoted by k. In this setting it is assumed that the estimated treatment effects are independently normally distributed. With no publication bias present the regression line should be parallel to the x axis, i.e. the slope should be zero. A non zero slope would suggest an association between sample size or inverse variance, possibly due to publication bias. The estimated regression line in Fig. 7.4 shows no apparent slope. Likewise the model output (not shown) does not indicate the presence of publication bias for the data at hand.

Estimation of a Summary Effect.   Frequently, one of the aims of a meta-analysis is to provide an estimate of the overall effect of all studies combined. Methods for pooling depend on the data available. In general, a two-step procedure has to be applied. First, the risk estimates and variances from each study have to be abstracted from publications or calculated if data are available. Then, a combined

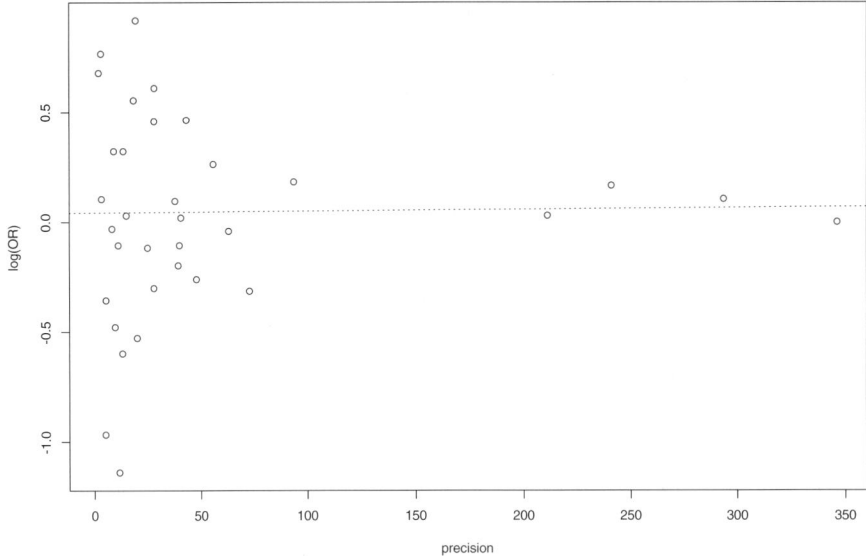

Figure 7.4. Funnel regression plot of the breast cancer data

estimate is obtained as a (variance based) weighted average of the individual estimates. The methods for pooling based on the 2×2 table include the approaches by Mantel–Haenszel and Peto (see Pettiti 1994 for details). If data are not available in a 2×2 table, but as an estimate from a more complex model (such as an adjusted relative risk estimate), the Woolf approach can be adopted using the estimates and their (published or calculated) variance resulting from the regression model. This results in a weighted average of the log-odds ratios $\hat{\theta}_i$ of the individual studies where the weights w_i are given by the inverse of the study specific variance estimates $\hat{\sigma}_i^2$. For a discussion of risk measures see Chap. I.2 of this handbook. Please note that the study specific variance is assumed to be fixed and known although they are based on estimates of the study specific variances. As a result the uncertainty associated with the estimation of σ_i^2 is ignored. Thus in the following the σ_i are treated as constants and the 'hat' notation is omitted. The estimate of the summary effect of all studies is then given by

$$\hat{\theta} = \frac{\sum_{i=1}^{k} w_i \hat{\theta}_i}{\sum_{i=1}^{k} w_i} , \tag{7.2}$$

$$w_i = \frac{1}{\sigma_i^2} . \tag{7.3}$$

The variance is given by

$$\operatorname{var}\left(\hat{\theta}\right) = \frac{1}{\sum_{i=1}^{k} 1/\sigma_i^2} . \tag{7.4}$$

Applying this approach to the HRT data leads to a pooled risk estimate of 0.05598 with an estimated variance equal to 0.00051. Transforming this back to the original scale leads to an odds ratio of 1.058 with a 95 percent confidence interval of (1.012, 1.11). Thus we would conclude combining all studies that there is a small harmful effect of hormone replacement therapy.

The major assumption here is that of a fixed model, i.e. it is assumed that the underlying true exposure effect in each study is the same. The overall variation and, therefore, the confidence intervals will reflect only the random variation within each study but not any potential heterogeneity between the studies.

Figure 7.5 displays this idea. Whether pooling of the data is appropriate should be decided after investigating the heterogeneity of the study results. If the results vary substantially, no pooled estimator should be presented or only estimators for selected subgroups should be calculated (e.g. combining results from case-control studies only).

Heterogeneity.   The investigation of heterogeneity between the different studies is a main task in each review or meta-analysis (Thompson 1994). For the quantitative assessment of heterogeneity, several statistical tests are available (Petitti 1994; Paul and Donner 1989). A simple test for heterogeneity is based on the following test statistic:

$$\chi^2_{het} = \sum_{i=1}^{k} \frac{(\hat{\theta} - \hat{\theta}_i)^2}{\sigma_i^2} \sim \chi^2_{k-1} , \tag{7.5}$$

which under the null hypothesis of heterogeneity follows a χ^2 distribution with $k-1$ degrees of freedom. Hence the null hypothesis is rejected if χ^2_{het} exceeds the $1-\alpha$ quantile of χ^2_{k-1} denoted as $\chi^2_{k-1,1-\alpha}$. For the data at hand we clearly conclude that there is heterogeneity present ($\chi^2_{het} = 116.076$, df $= 35$, p-value: 0.00000). Thus using a combined estimate is at least questionable. Pooling the individual studies and performing this test can be done with any statistical package capable of weighted least squares regression. The first part of the appendix shows a SAS-program which provides the results obtained so far. A major limitation of formal heterogeneity tests like the one presented before is, however, their low statistical power to detect any heterogeneity present.

A more powerful method is given by model based approaches. A model based approach has the advantage that it can be used to test specific alternatives and thus has a higher power to detect heterogeneity. So far we considered the following simple fixed effects model

$$\theta_i = \theta + \varepsilon_i , \quad i = 1, \ldots, k , \quad \varepsilon_i \sim N\left(0, \sigma_i^2\right) . \tag{7.6}$$

Obviously this model is not able to account for any heterogeneity, since deviations from θ_i and θ are assumed to be explained only by random error.

Thus alternatively a random effects model should be considered. This model incorporates variation between studies. It is assumed that each study has its own

Fixed effects model

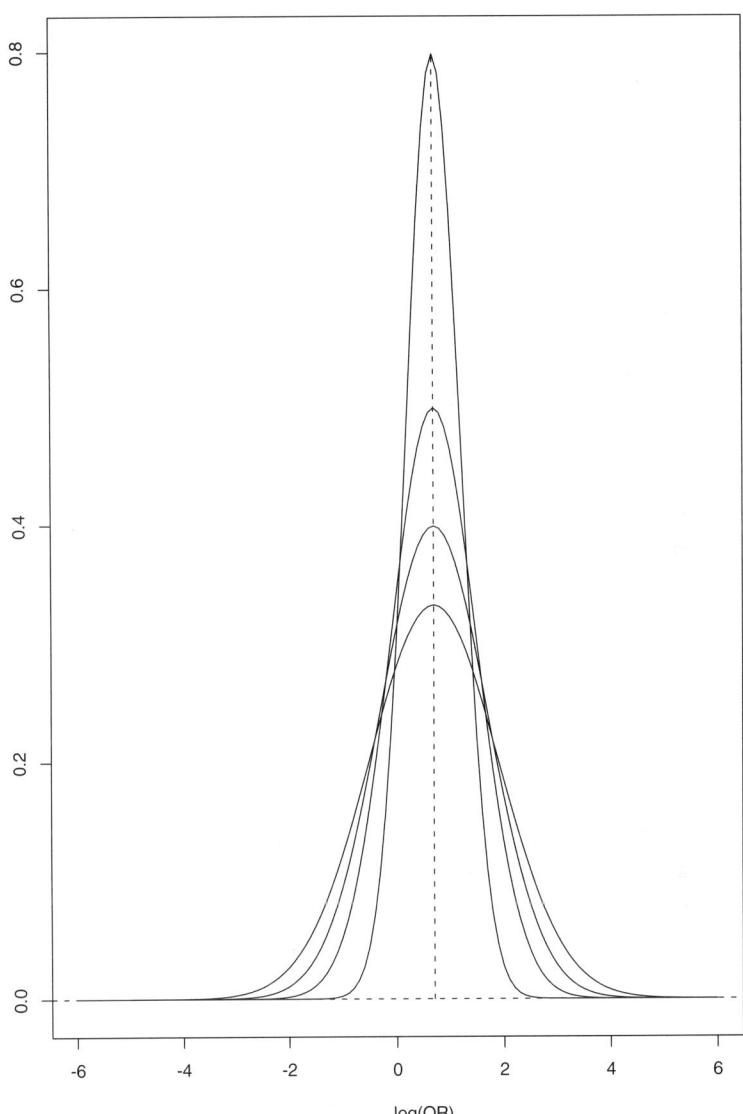

log(OR)

Figure 7.5. Fixed effects model: Common effect with different study variances

(true) exposure effect and that there is a random distribution of these true exposure effects around a central effect. This idea is presented in Fig. 7.6. Frequently it is assumed that the individual study effects follow a normal distribution with mean θ_i and variance σ_i^2 and the random distribution of the true effects is again a normal distribution with variance τ^2. In other words, the random effects model allows non-

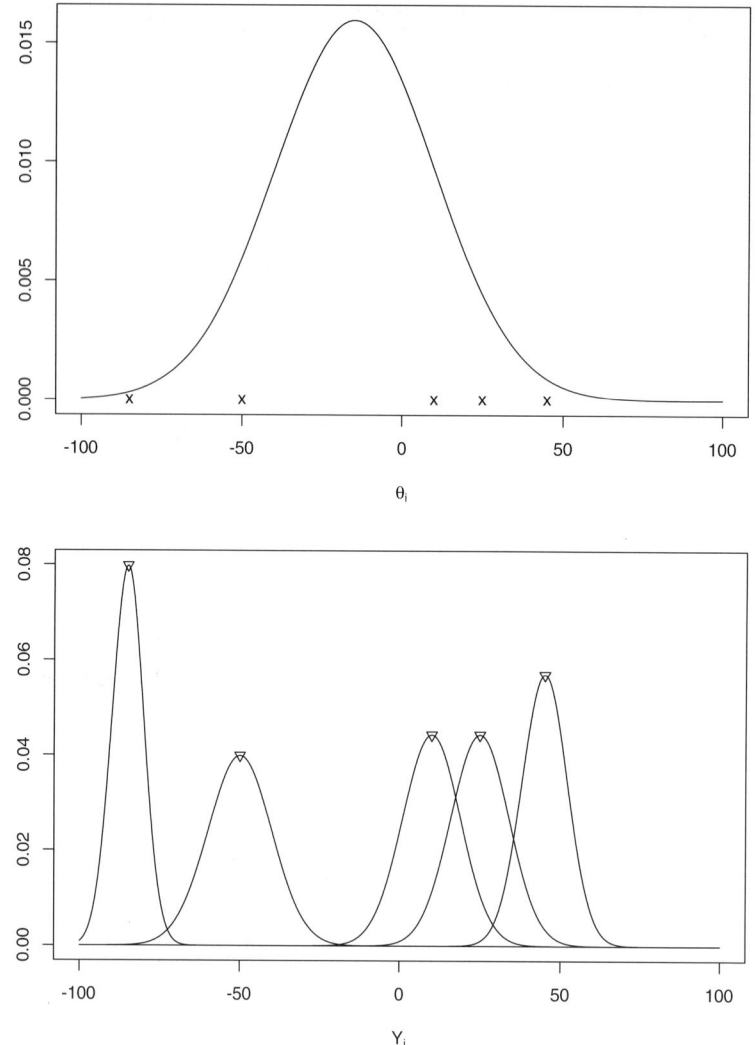

Figure 7.6. Random effects model: Variable effects drawn from a population of study effects

homogeneity between the effects of different studies. This leads to the following model:

$$\theta_i = \theta + b_i + \varepsilon_i \;, \quad i = 1, \ldots, k \;, \quad b_i \sim N\left(0, \tau^2\right) \;, \quad \varepsilon_i \sim N\left(0, \sigma_i^2\right) \;. \quad (7.7)$$

The observed effects from the different studies are used to estimate the parameters describing the fixed and random effects. This may be done using maximum-likelihood procedures. The widely used approach by DerSimonian and Laird (1986) applies a method of moments to obtain an estimate of τ^2.

Taking the expectation of (7.7) leads to $E(\theta_i) = \theta$ and calculating the variance leads to $\mathrm{var}(\theta_i) = \mathrm{var}(b_i) + \mathrm{var}(\varepsilon_i) = \tau^2 + \sigma_i^2 = \sigma_i^{*2}$ assuming that b_i and ε_i are independent. The heterogeneity variance τ^2 is unknown and has to be estimated from the data. The method by DerSimonian and Laird equates the heterogeneity test statistic (7.5) to its expected value. This expectation is calculated under the assumption of a random effects model and given by $E\left(\chi_{het}^2\right) = k - 1 + \tau^2 \left(\sum w_i - (\sum w_i^2)/(\sum w_i)\right)$. The weights w_i are those defined in (7.3). Equating χ_{het}^2 to its expectation and solving for τ^2 gives:

$$\hat{\tau}^2 = \left[\chi_{het}^2 - (k-1)\right] \Big/ \left(\sum w_i - \frac{\sum w_i^2}{\sum w_i}\right) . \tag{7.8}$$

In case $\chi_{het}^2 < k - 1$ the estimator $\hat{\tau}^2$ is truncated to zero. Thus the pooled estimator $\hat{\theta}_{DL}$ under heterogeneity can be obtained as weighted average:

$$\hat{\theta}_{DL} = \frac{\sum_{i=1}^{k} w_i^* \hat{\theta}_i}{\sum_{i=1}^{k} w_i^*} , \tag{7.9}$$

$$\text{with} \quad w_i^{*2} = \frac{1}{\sigma_i^{*2}} = \frac{1}{\hat{\tau}^2 + \sigma_i^2} \quad \text{we obtain} \tag{7.10}$$

$$\hat{\theta}_{DL} = \frac{\sum_{i=1}^{k} \hat{\theta}_i / \left(\hat{\tau}^2 + \sigma_i^2\right)}{\sum_{i=1}^{k} 1 / \left(\hat{\tau}^2 + \sigma_i^2\right)} . \tag{7.11}$$

The variance of this estimator is given by:

$$\mathrm{var}(\hat{\theta}_{DL}) = \frac{1}{\sum_{i=1}^{k} 1/\sigma_i^{*2}} , \tag{7.12}$$

$$= \frac{1}{\sum_{i=1}^{k} 1/(\hat{\tau}^2 + \sigma_i^2)} . \tag{7.13}$$

The between study variance τ^2 can also be interpreted as a measure for the heterogeneity between studies. It should be noted that in general random effects methods yield larger variance and confidence intervals than fixed effects models because a between study component τ^2 is added to the variance. If the heterogeneity between the studies is large, τ^2 will dominate the weights and all studies will be weighted more equally (in random effects model weight decreases for larger studies compared to the fixed effects model). For our example we obtain a pooled DerSimonian–Laird estimate of 0.0337 with heterogeneity variance equal to 0.0453. The variance of the pooled estimator is given by 0.0024. Transformed back to the original scale we obtain an odds ratio of OR = 1.034 with 95% CI (0.939, 1.139). Based on this analysis we would conclude that after adjusting for heterogeneity this meta-analysis does not provide evidence for an association between HRT replacement therapy and breast cancer in women.

However, two comments are in order. First, pooling in the presence of hetero-geneity may be seriously misleading. Heterogeneity between studies should yield careful investigation of the sources of the differences. If there is a sufficient number of different studies available, further analyses, such as 'meta-regression', may be used to examine the sources of heterogeneity (Greenland 1987, 1994). The second is in terms of statistical methodology. Within this approach the study specific vari-ances are assumed to be known constants. That is the reason why this approach can lead to a considerable bias when pooling estimates using the DerSimonian–Laird estimator as demonstrated by Böhning et al. (2002).

Besides the moment based method by DerSimonian and Laird estimates of τ^2 can be obtained using likelihood based methods. See for example the tuto-rials by Normand (1999) and van Houwelingen et al. (2002) for more details. The appendix gives a SAS code to estimate the fixed and random effects mod-els based on likelihood methods with the SAS program *proc mixed*. Estimates based on likelihood methods offer the advantage that they provide the option to formally test which model is appropriate for the data by applying the likeli-hood ratio test or penalized criteria such as the Bayesian Information Criterion (BIC). The BIC is obtained by the formula BIC $= -2 \times \log$ Likelihood $+ \log(k) \times q$ where q is the number of parameters in the model and k denotes the number of studies.

When using random effects models another topic of interest is the form of the random effects' distribution. Besides a parametric distribution for the random effects a discrete distribution may be assumed. Here we suppose that the study specific estimators $\hat{\theta}_1, \hat{\theta}_2, \ldots, \hat{\theta}_k$ are coming from q subpopulations $\theta_j, j = 1, \ldots, q$. Again assuming that the effect of each individual study follows a normal distribu-tion

$$f\left(\hat{\theta}_i, \theta_j, \sigma_i^2\right) = \frac{1}{\sqrt{2\pi\sigma_i^2}} e^{-(\hat{\theta}_i - \theta_j)^2/(2\sigma_i^2)} , \quad j = 1, \ldots, q . \tag{7.14}$$

we obtain a finite mixture model

$$f(\hat{\theta}_i, P) = \sum_{j=1}^{q} f\left(\hat{\theta}_i, \theta_j, \sigma_i^2\right) p_j . \tag{7.15}$$

The parameters of the distribution P

$$P \equiv \begin{bmatrix} \theta_1 & \cdots & \theta_q \\ p_1 & \cdots & p_q \end{bmatrix} \quad \text{with} \quad p_j \geq 0 \quad j = 1, \ldots, q , \tag{7.16}$$

$$p_1 + \ldots + p_q = 1 . \tag{7.17}$$

need to be estimated from the data. The mixing weights p_j denote the a priori probability of an observation of belonging to a certain subpopulation with param-eter θ_j. Please note that also the number of components q needs to be estimated as well. Estimation may be done with the program C.A.MAN (Schlattmann and

Böhning 1993; Böhning et al. 1998). For the HRT data we find a solution with three components which gives an acceptable fit to the data

```
weight:     0.2804 parameter:     -0.3365
weight:     0.5671 parameter:      0.0778
weight:     0.1524 parameter:      0.5446


Log-Likelihood at iterate:        -17.6306
```

Here the weights correspond to the mixing weights p_j and the parameter corresponds to the subpopulation mean θ_j. These results imply that about 28% of the studies show a protective effect of HRT, whereas the majority of the studies shows a harmful effect. About 57% of the studies show an increased log(risk) of 0.08 and 15% of the studies show a log(odds ratio) of 0.54. Thus using a finite mixture model (FM) we find again considerable heterogeneity where the majority of studies finds a harmful effect of hormone replacement therapy. It is noteworthy that a proportion of studies finds a beneficial effect. Of course this needs to be investigated further. One way to do this would be to classify the individual studies using the finite mixture model. Doing so we find that for example study nine from the data given in the appendix belongs to this category. This is a case-control study for which no information about confounder adjustment is available. This would be a starting point for a sensitivity analysis. Table 7.1 gives an overview about the models fitted so far. These include the fixed effects model with a BIC value of 70.0, the mixed effects model using a normal distribution for the random effects with a BIC value of 44.4. The finite mixture model (FM) has a BIC value of 53.2. Thus based on Table 7.1 it is quite obvious that a fixed effects model does not fit the data very well and that a random effects model should be used. Of course the question remains which random effects model to choose for the analysis. Based on the BIC criterion given in Table 7.1 one would choose the parametric mixture model provided the assumption of a normal distribution of the random effects is justifiable. This can be investigated for example by a normal quantile-quantile plot of the estimated individual random effects given by the parametric model. For the data at hand the assumption of normally distributed random effects appears reasonable, thus we would choose the parametric mixture model.

Table 7.1. Model comparison for the breast cancer data

Method	Residual Hetero.	Estimates (SE) Intercept	Het. ($\hat{\tau}^2$)	log Lik.	BIC
Fixed	None	0.056 (0.023)	–	−33.19	70.0
Mixed	Additive	0.027 (0.061)	0.086	−18.65	44.4
FM	Additive		0.079	−17.63	53.2

Meta-Regression.   An important method for investigating heterogeneity is sensitivity analysis, e.g. to calculate pooled estimators only for subgroups of studies (according to study type, quality of the study, period of publication, etc.) to investigate variations of the odds ratio. An extension of this approach is meta-regression as proposed by Greenland (1987), see also Thompson and Sharp (1999). The principal idea of meta-regression is once heterogeneity is detected to identify sources of heterogeneity by inclusion of known covariates.

For the breast cancer meta-analysis example a potential covariate is study type, case-control studies may show different results than cohort studies due to different exposure assessment. For our data case-control studies are coded as $x_{i1} = 0$ and cohort studies are coded as $x_{i1} = 1$.

The fixed effect model is now:

$$\theta_i = \beta_0 + \beta_1 x_{i1} + \varepsilon_i \,, \quad \varepsilon_i \sim N\left(0, \sigma_i^2\right) \,, \quad i = 1, \ldots, k \,. \tag{7.18}$$

Here we find that cohort studies identify an association between HRT and breast cancer based on the regression equation $\hat{\theta}_i = 0.0015 + 0.145$ for a cohort study. Obviously, cohort studies come to results different form case-control studies. Clearly, after adjustment for covariates the question remains if there is still residual heterogeneity present. Again we can analyse the data using a random effects model in this case with a random intercept.

$$\theta_i = \beta_0 + \beta_1 x_{i1} + b_i + \varepsilon_i \,, \quad b_i \sim N\left(0, \tau^2\right) \,, \quad \varepsilon_i \sim N\left(0, \sigma_i^2\right) \,. \tag{7.19}$$

For this model the regression equation for the fixed effects gives now for a cohort study $\hat{\theta}_i = -0.009 + 0.1080$ and the corresponding heterogeneity variance is estimated as $\hat{\tau}^2 = 0.079$.

Table 7.2. Comparison of fixed and random effects models

Method	Residual Hetero.	Estimates (SE) Intercept	Slope	Het. ($\hat{\tau}^2$)	-log Lik.	BIC
Fixed	None	0.056 (0.023)	–	–	−33.85	70.0
Fixed	None	0.0014 (0.029)	0.145 (0.046)	–	−28.36	63.9
Mixed	Additive	0.027 (0.061)	–	0.086	−18.65	44.4
Mixed	Additive	−0.009 (0.072)	0.108 (0.126)	0.079	−18.25	47.3

Table 7.2 compares fixed and random effects models for the HRT data. The table shows models with and without an estimate for the slope. Model selection can be based again on the BIC criterion. Apparently based on the BIC criterion both fixed effects models do not fit the data very well since their BIC values are considerably higher than those of the random effects models. Please note that if only the fixed effects models would be considered this meta-analysis would show that cohort studies show a harmful effect. Comparing the mixed effects models in Table 7.2 the model with the covariate does not provide an improved fit of

the data. The log-likelihood is only slighty larger and penalising the number of parameters leads to a larger BIC value for the mixed effect model with the covariate. Another interesting point is to compare the heterogeneity variance estimated by both models. Here there is no substantial portion of heterogeneity explained by the covariate, since the heterogeneity variance is reduced to 0.079 from 0.086. From a statistical point of view further covariates need to be identified and included into the model. From a public health point of view the conclusion is perhaps less straightforward. Although inclusion of the covariate study type does not explain the heterogeneity of the studies very well we find that cohort studies find a harmful effect. One might argue that although these results are far from perfect they should not be ignored as absence of evidence does not imply evidence of absence. Looking back at these data in the light of the results from the woman health initiative (WHI) study (Rossouw et al. 2002) it becomes clear that caution is required in the analysis and interpretation of meta-analyses of observational studies. The major finding of the WHI-study was that the group of subjects undergoing treatment with combined HRT in the form of Prempro (0.625 mg/day conjugated equine estrogens (CEE) +2.5 mg/day medroxyprogesterone acetate) was found to have increased risk of breast cancer (hazard ratio = 1.26, 95% CI: 1.00–1.59) and no apparent cardiac benefit. This is contradictory to the prior belief that HRT provides cardiovascular benefit. As a result, although several benefits were considered, these interim findings at 5 years were deemed sufficiently troubling to stop this arm of the trial at 5.2 years.

Interpretation of the Results of Meta-Analysis of Observational Studies 7.6

The example from above shows that the interpretation of the results of a meta-analysis should not only discuss the pooled estimator and the confidence interval but should focus on the examination of the heterogeneity between the results of the studies. Strength and weaknesses as well as potential bias should be discussed.

Bias 7.6.1

For epidemiological studies in general, the main problem is not the lack of precision and the random error but the fact that results may be distorted by different sources of bias or confounding, for an general overview of the problem of bias see Hill and Kleinbaum (2000). That means that the standard error (or the size of the study) may not be the best indicator for the weight of a study. If more or better data are collected on a smaller amount of subjects, results may be more accurate than in a large study with insufficient information on the risk factors or on confounders. The assessment of bias in individual studies is therefore crucial for the overall interpretation.

The central problem of meta-analyses of clinical trials is publication bias that has already been a topic in a paper by Berlin et al. as early as 1989 and is still a topic of recent methodological investigations (see for example Copas and Shi (2001)). This bias has received a lot of attention particularly in the area of clinical trials. Publication bias occurs when studies that have non-significant or negative results are published less frequently than positive studies. For randomized clinical trials, it has been shown that even with a computer-aided literature search only some of the relevant studies will be identified (Dickersin et al. 1994). For epidemiological observational studies additional problems exist, because often a large number of variables will be collected in questionnaires as potential confounders (Blettner et al. 1999). If one or several of these potential confounders yield significant or important results, they may be published in additional papers, which have often not been planned in advance. In general, publication bias yields a non-negligible overestimation of the risk estimate.

However, as Morris (1994) has pointed out, there exist little systematic investigations of the magnitude of the problem for epidemiological studies. A major worry is that non-significant results are neither mentioned in the title nor in the abstract and publications and may be lost in the retrieval process.

7.6.2   Confounding

Another problem arises because different studies adjust for different confounding factors. It is well known that the estimated effect of a factor of interest is (strongly) influenced by the inclusion or exclusion of other factors, in the statistical model if these factors have an influence on the outcome and if they are correlated with the risk factor of interest. Combining estimates from several studies with different ways of adjusting for confounders yields biased results. Using literature data only, crude estimates may be available for some of the studies, model-based estimates for others. However, as the adjustment for confounders is an important issue for the assessment of an effect in each single study, it is obvious that combining these different estimates in a meta-analysis may not give meaningful results. It is necessary to use 'similar' confounders in each study to adjust the estimated effect of interest in the single studies. In general that would require a re-analysis of the single studies. Obviously, that requires the original data and a MAP is needed for this purpose.

7.6.3   Heterogeneity

In epidemiological research different study designs are in use and none of them can be considered as a gold standard as the randomised clinical trial for therapy studies. Therefore it is necessary to evaluate the comparability of the single designs before summarising the results. Often, case-control studies, cohort studies and cross-sectional studies are used to investigate the same questions and results of those studies need to be combined. Egger et al. (2001) pointed out several examples in which results from case-control studies differ from those of cohort studies. E.g. in a paper by Boyd et al. (1993), it was noted that cohort studies show no association between breast cancer and saturated fat intake while the same meta-analysis using results from case-control studies only revealed an increased, statistically significant risk. Other reasons for heterogeneity may be different uses of data collection methods, different control selection (e.g. hospital vs population controls), and differences in case ascertaining. Differences could be explored in a formal sensitivity analysis but also by graphical methods (funnel plot). However, meta-analyses from published data provide only limited information if the reasons for heterogeneity shall be investigated in depth.

The problem of heterogeneity can be well demonstrated with nearly any example of published meta-analysis. For example Ursin et al. (1995) investigated the influence of the Body-Mass-Index (BMI) on the development of pre-menopausal breast cancer. They include 23 studies of which 19 are case-control studies and 4 are cohort studies. Some of these studies were designed to investigate BMI as risk factor, others measured BMI as confounders in studies investigating other risk factors. It can only be speculated that the number of unpublished studies in which BMI was mainly considered as a confounder and did not show a strong influence on pre-menopausal breast cancer is non-negligible and that this issue may result in some bias. As is usual practice in epidemiological studies relative risks were provided for several categories of BMI. To overcome this problem the authors estimated a regression coefficient for the relative risk as a function of the BMI, however, several critical assumptions are necessary for this type of approach. The authors found severe heterogeneity across all studies combined (the p-value of a corresponding test was almost zero). An influence of the type of study (cohort study or case-control study) was apparent. Therefore no overall summary is presented for case-control and cohort studies combined. One reason for the heterogeneity may be the variation in adjustment for confounders. Adjustment for confounders other than age was used only in 10 out of the 23 studies.

Conclusions 7.7

Despite the many problems, there is an immense need to summarise current knowledge, for example to assess the consequence of human exposure to environmental exposure. For this task all available data and information will be needed and meta-analysis is becoming increasingly influential. Particularly where the previously conducted epidemiological studies have provided inconsistent results a meta-analysis may give some insight. As discussed, a major impediment for meta-analysis of epidemiological data is the heterogeneity across studies in their design, data collection methods and analyses performed. The statistical combination of risk estimates should not be the central component of a meta-analysis using published data. An expert group in co-operation with the U.S. Environmental Protection Agency was recently established to discuss the use of meta-analyses in environmental health studies. One of the objectives of this group was also to develop a consensus on "when meta-analysis should or should not be used" (Blair et al. 1995). There is always a danger that meta-analysis of observational studies produces precise looking estimates which are severely biased. This should be kept in mind as more and more public health regulators and decision-makers may rely on the results of a meta-analysis.

Appendix

7.A   Data and Computer Code and Output

The listing shows the effect measure on the log-scale, the corresponding variance and the study type of each of the 36 studies analysed in the meta-analysis by Sillero-Arenas et al.

```
data sillar;
input study or est type;
cards;
  1   0.10436   0.299111   0
  2  -0.03046   0.121392   0
  3   0.76547   0.319547   0
  4  -0.19845   0.025400   0
  5  -0.10536   0.025041   0
  6  -0.11653   0.040469   0
  7   0.09531   0.026399   0
  8   0.26236   0.017918   0
  9  -0.26136   0.020901   0
 10   0.45742   0.035877   0
 11  -0.59784   0.076356   0
 12  -0.35667   0.186879   0
 13  -0.10536   0.089935   0
 14  -0.31471   0.013772   0
 15  -0.10536   0.089935   0
 16   0.02956   0.004738   0
 17   0.60977   0.035781   0
 18  -0.30111   0.036069   0
 19   0.01980   0.024611   0
 20   0.00000   0.002890   0
 21  -0.04082   0.015863   0
 22   0.02956   0.067069   0
 23   0.18232   0.010677   0
 24   0.26236   0.017918   1
 25   0.32208   0.073896   1
```

```
26  0.67803  0.489415  1
27 -0.96758  0.194768  1
28  0.91629  0.051846  1
29  0.32208  0.110179  1
30 -1.13943  0.086173  1
31 -0.47804  0.103522  1
32  0.16551  0.004152  1
33  0.46373  0.023150  1
34 -0.52763  0.050384  1
35  0.10436  0.003407  1
36  0.55389  0.054740  1
run;
```

Elementary Analysis with SAS

7.B

SAS code for the elementary analysis using weighted least squares:

```
/* calculation of weights */
data sillar;
set sillar;
weight =1./est;
run;

/* intercept only */
proc glm data=sillar;
          /* use proc GLM with data set sillar     */
model logor=/solution inverse;
          /* Show   solution                        */
          /* Show inverse of weighted design matrix */
weight weight;
          /*  weights 1./variance                   */
run;
```

This gives the following shortened output:

```
The GLM Procedure
Dependent Variable: logor
Weight: weight
                    Sum of
Source        DF    Squares        Mean Square   F Value   Pr > F
Model          1    6.1683128      6.1683128     1.86      0.1813
Error         35    116.0756869    3.3164482
Un.Total      36    122.2439997

Parameter   df   Estimate        SE            t Value   Pr > |t|
Intercept    1    0.0559813731    0.04104847    1.36      0.1813
```

Please note that for performing a meta analysis the standard error given by the program must be divided by the root mean square error in order the obtain the standard error of the pooled estimate. In order to avoid additional calculations the SAS output giving the inverse of the weighted design matrix gives the desired variance. The test of heterogeneity is given by the residual sum of squares as indicated by formula (7.5). This result can also be obtained using the SAS code for the fixed effect model based on maximum likelihood

```
proc mixed method=ml data=sillar;
   /* Use proc mixed (ML estimation)                */
class study;
   /* Specifes study as 'classificaton variable'    */
model or=/ s cl;
   /* Intercept only model, show solution and CI    */
repeated /group =study;
   /* Each trial has its own within trial variance  */
parms /parmsdata=sillar
   /* The parmsdata option reads in the variable
      EST indicating the variances from the data set
      sillar.sd2                                     */
eqcons=1 to 36;
   /* The within study variances are known and fixed */
run;
```

7.C   SAS Code for the Random Effects Model

The SAS procedure proc mixed requires the following manipulations of the data

```
data covvars; /* data set containing the variances    */
set sillar;
keep est;
run;
data start;    /* include the starting value for the   */
input est;     /* heterogeneity variance               */
cards;
0.0
run;
data start;    /* Combine both data sets                */
set start covvars;
run;
```

Obtain the model with proc mixed

```
proc mixed method=ml cl data=sillar;
      /* CL asks for confidence intervals             */
      /* of covariance parameters                     */
```

```
class study;
      /* Study is classification variable         */
model or= / s cl;
      /* Intercept only model, Fixed solution and CI  */
random int /subject=study;
      /* Study is specified as random effect        */
repeated /group =study;
      /* Each study has its own variable          */
parms /parmsdata= start
      /* start contains starting value a. trial vars. */
eqcons=2 to 37;
      /* entries 2 to 37 are the fixed study vars.    */
run;
```

References

Allam MF, Del Castillo AS, Navajas RF (2003) Parkinson's disease, smoking and family history: meta-analysis. Eur J Neurol 10:59–62

Begg CB, Mazumdar M (1994) Operating characteristics of a rank correlation test for publication bias. Biometrics 50:1088–1101

Bennett DA (2003) Review of analytical methods for prospective cohort studies using time to event data: single studies and implications for meta-analysis. Stat Methods Med Res 12:297–319

Berlin JA (1995) Invited commentary: Benefits of heterogeneity in meta-analysis of data from epidemiologic studies. Am J Epidemiol 142:383–387

Berlin JA, Begg CB, Louis TN (1989) An assessment of publication bias using a sample of published clinical trials. J Am Stat Assoc 84:381–392

Berlin JA, on behalf of University of Pennsylvania Meta-analysis Blinding Study Group (1997) Does blinding of readers affect the results of meta-analyses? Lancet 350:185–186

Blair A, Burg J, Floran J, Gibb H, Greenland S, Morris R et al. (1995) Guidelines for application of meta-analysis in environmental epidemiology. Regul Toxicol Pharmacol 22:189–197

Blettner M, Sauerbrei W, Schlehofer B, Scheuchenpflug T, Friedenreich C (1999) Traditional reviews, meta analyses and pooled analyses in epidemiology. Int J Epidemiol 28:1–9

Boffetta P (2002) Involuntary smoking and lung cancer. Scand J Work Environ Health, 28 Suppl 2:30–40

Boffetta P, Saracci R, Andersen A, Bertazzi PA, Chang-Claude J, Cherrie J, Ferro G, Frentzel-Beyme R, Hansen J, Plato N, Teppo L, Westerholm P, Winter PD, Zochetti C (1997) Cancer mortality among man-made vitreous fiber production workers. Epidemiology 8:259–268

Böhning D, Dietz E, Schlattmann P (1998) Recent developments in computer-assisted mixture analysis. Biometrics 54:283–303

Böhning D, Malzahn U, Dietz E, Schlattmann P, Viwatwongkasem C, Biggeri A (2002) Some general points in estimating heterogeneity variance with the DerSimonian–Laird estimator. Biostatistics 3:445–457

Boyd NF, Martin LJ, Noffel M, Lockwood GA, Trichler DL (1993) A meta-analysis of studies of dietary fat and breast cancer. Br J Cancer 68:627–636

CGHFBC-Collaborative Group on Hormonal Factors in Breast Cancer (1996) Breast cancer and hormonal contraceptives: collaborative reanalysis of individual data on 53,297 women with breast cancer and 100,239 women without breast cancer from 54 epidemiological studies. Lancet 347:1713–1727

Cook DJ, Guyatt GH, Ryan G, Clifton J, Buckingham L, Willan A, McLlroy W, Oxman AD (1993) Should unpublished data be included in meta-analyses? Current conflictions and controversies. JAMA 21:2749–2753

Copas JB, Shi JQ (2001) A sensitivity analysis for publication bias in systematic review. Stat Methods Med Res 10:251–265

DerSimonian R, Laird N (1986) Meta-analysis in clinical trials. Control Clin Trials 7:177–188

Dickersin K (2002) Systematic reviews in epidemiology: Why are we so far behind? Int J Epidemiol 31:6–12

Dickersin K, Scherer R, Lefebvre C (1994) Identifying relevant studies for systematic reviews. BMJ 309:1286–1291

Egger M, Davey Smith G, Altman DG (2001) Systematic reviews in health care. Meta-analysis in context, 2nd edn. BMJ Publishing Group, London

Egger M, Davey Smith G, Schneider M (2001) Systematic reviews of observational studies. In: Egger M, Davey Smith G, Altman DG Systematic reviews in health care. Meta-analysis in context, 2nd edn, BMJ Publishing Group, London, pp 211–227

Egger M, Juni P, Bartlett C, Holenstein F, Sterne J (2003) How important are comprehensive literature searches and the assessment of trial quality in systematic reviews? Empirical study. Health Technol Assess 7:1–76

Egger M, Schneider M, Davey Smith G (1998) Meta-analysis: Spurious precision? Meta-analysis of observational studies. BMJ 361:140–144

Feinstein AR (1995) Meta-analysis: statistical alchemy for the 21st century. J Clin Epidemiol 48:71–79

Friedenreich CM (1993) Methods for pooled analyses of epidemiologic studies. Epidemiology 4:295–302

Friedenreich CM, Braut RF, Riboli E (1994) Influence of methodologic factors in a pooled analysis of 13 case-control studies of colorectal cancer and dietary fiber. Epidemiology 5:66–79

Glass GV (1977) Integrating findings: The meta-analysis of research. Rev Res Educ 5:351–379

Greenland S (1987) Quantitative methods in the review of epidemiologic literature. Epidemiol Rev 9:1–302

Greenland S (1994) Invited commentary: A critical look at some popular metaanalytic methods. Am J Epidemiol 140:290–296

Hamajima N, Hirose K, Tajima K et al. (2002) Alcohol, tobacco and breast cancer-collaborative reanalysis of individual data from 53 epidemiological studies, including 58,515 women with breast cancer and 95,067 women without the disease. Br J Cancer 87:1234–1245

Hill AB (1965) The environment and disease: association or causation? Proc R Soc Med 58:295–300

Hill HA, Kleinbaum DG (2000) Bias in observational studies. In: Gail MH, Benichou J Encyclopedia of epidemiologic methods, John Wiley and Sons, Chichester, pp 94–100

Hung RJ, Boffetta P, Brockmoller J et al. (2003) CYP1A1 and GSTM1 genetic polymorphisms and lung cancer risk in Caucasian non-smokers: A pooled analysis. Carcinogenesis 24:875–882

Jones DR (1992) Meta-analysis of observational epidemiologic studies: A review. J R Soc Med 85:165–168

Longnecker MP, Berlin JA, Orza MJ, Chalmers TC (1988) A meta-analysis of alcohol consumption in relation to risk of breast cancer. JAMA 260:652–656

Lubin JH, Boice Jr JD, Edling C, Hornung RW, Howe G, Kunz E, Kusiak RA, Morrison HI, Radford EP, Samet JM, et al (1995) Radon-exposed underground miners and inverse dose-rate (protraction enhancement) effects. Health Phys 69:494–500

Macaskill P, Walter SD, Irwig L (2001) A comparison of methods to detect publication bias in meta-analysis. Stat Med 20:641–654

Meinert R, Michaelis J (1996) Meta-analyses of studies on the association between electromagnetic fields and childhood cancer. Radiat Environ Biophys 35:11–18

Morris RD (1994) Meta-analysis in cancer epidemiology. Environ Health Perspect 102 Suppl 8:61–66

Normand SL (1999) Meta-analysis: Formulating, evaluating, combining, and reporting. Stat Med 18:321–359

Olkin I (1994) Re: A critical look at some popular meta-analytic methods. Am J Epidemiol 140:297–299

Paul SR, Donner A (1989) A comparison of tests of homogeneity of odds ratios in $k2 \times 2$ tables. Stat Med 8:1455–1468

Pettiti DB (1994) Meta-analysis, decision analysis and cost-effectiveness analysis: Methods for quantitative synthesis in medicine. Oxford University Press, Oxford

Rossouw JE, Anderson GL, Prentice RL, LaCroix AZ, Kooperberg C, StefanickML, Jackson RD, Beresford SA, Howard BV, Johnson KC, Kotchen JM, Ockene J, Writing Group for the Women's Health Initiative Investigators (2002) Risks and benefits of estrogen plus progestin in healthy postmenopausal women: Principal results from the women's health initiative randomized controlled trial. JAMA 288:321–333

Sauerbrei W, Blettner M, Royston P (2001) Letter to White IR (1999): On alcohol consumption and all-cause mortality. J Clin Epidemiol 54:537–540

Schlattmann P, Böhning D (1993) Computer packages C.A.MAN (computer assisted mixture analysis) and dismap. Stat Med 12:1965

Schlehofer B, Blettner M, Preston-Martin S, Niehoff D, Wahrendorf J, Arslan A, Ahlbom A, Choi WN, Giles GG, Howe GR, Little J, Menegoz F, Ryan P (1999) Role of medical history in brain tumour development. results from the international adult brain tumour study. Int J Cancer 82:155–160

Schwarzer G, Antes G, Schumacher M (2002) Inflation of type I error rate in two statistical tests for the detection of publication bias in meta-analyses with binary outcomes. Stat Med 21:2465–2477

Shapiro S (1994a) Meta-analysis/shmeta-analysis. Am J Epidemiol 140:771–778

Shapiro S (1994b) Is there is or is there ain't no baby?: Dr Shapiro replies to Drs Petitti and Greenland. Am J Epidemiol 140:788–791

Sillero-Arenas M, Delgado-Rodriguez M, Rodigues-Canteras R, Bueno-Cavanillas A, Galvez-Vargas R (1992) Menopausal hormone replacement therapy and breast cancer: A meta-analysis. Obstet Gynecol 79:286–294

Smith ML, Glass GV (1977) Meta-analysis of psychotherapy outcome studies. Am Psychol 32(9):752–760

Smith-Warner SA, Ritz J, Hunter DJ, Albanes D et al. (2002) Dietary fat and risk of lung cancer in a pooled analysis of prospective studies. Cancer Epidemiol Biomarkers Prev 11:987–992

Steinberg KK, Smith SJ, Stroup DF, Olkin I, Lee N, Williamson GD, Thacker SB (1997) Comparison of meta-analysis to pooled analysis: an application to ovarian cancer. Am J Epidemiol 145:1917–1925

Stock WA (1995) Systematic coding for research synthesis. In: Cooper H, Hedges LV The Handbook of Research Synthesis. The Russell Sage Foundation, New York, pp 1–2

Straif K, Chambless L, Weiland SK, Wienke A, Bungers M, Taeger D, Keil U (1999) Occupational risk factors for mortality from stomach and lung cancer among rubber workers: An analysis using internal controls and refined exposure assessment. Int J Epidemiol 28:1037–1043

Straif K, Keil U, Taeger D, Holthenrich D, Sun Y, Bungers M, Weiland SK (2000) Exposure to nitrosamines, carbon black, asbestos, and talc and mortality from stomach, lung, and laryngeal cancer in a cohort of rubber workers. Am J Epidemiol 152:297–306

Stroup DF, Berlin JA, Morton SC, Olkin I, Williamson GD, Rennie D, Moher D, Becker BJ, Sipe TA, Thacker SB (2000) Meta-analysis of observational studies in epidemiology: A proposal for reporting. JAMA 283:2008–2012

Stukel TA, Demidenko E, Dykes J, Karagas MR (2001) Two-stage methods for the analysis of pooled data. Stat Med 20:2115–2130

Sutton AJ, Abram KR, Jones DR, Sheldon TA, Song F (2000) Methods for meta-analysis in medical research. John Wiley and Sons, Chichester

Thompson SG (1994) Why sources of heterogeneity in meta-analysis should be investigated. BMJ 309:1351–1355

Thompson SG, Sharp SJ (1999) Explaining heterogeneity in meta-analysis: A comparison of methods. Stat Med 18:2693–2708

Thompson SG, Smith TC, Sharp SJ (1997) Investigating underlying risk as a source of heterogeneity in meta-analysis. Stat Med 16:2741–2758

Tweedie RL, Mengersen KL (1995) Meta-analytic approaches to dose-response relationships, with application in studies of lung cancer and exposure to environmental tobacco smoke. Stat Med 14:545–569

Ursin G, Longenecker MP, Haile RW, Greenland S (1995) A meta-analysis of body mass index and risk of premenopausal breast cancer. Epidemiology 6:137–141

van Houwelingen HC, Arends LC, Stijnen T (2002) Advanced methods in meta-analyis: multivariate approach and meta-regression. Stat Med 59:589–624

Weed DL (1997) Methodologic guidelines for review papers. JNCI 89:6–7

Weed DL (2000) Interpreting epidemiological evidence: How meta-analysis and causal inference methods are related. Int J Epidemiol 29:387–390

Whitehead A (2002) Meta-analysis of controlled clinical trials. John Wiley and Sons, Chichester

Zeegers MP, Jellema A, Ostrer H (2003) Empiric risk of prostate carcinoma for relatives of patients with prostate carcinoma: A meta-analysis. Cancer 97: 1894–1903

Geographical Epidemiology

John F. Bithell

Introduction

The Nature of Geographical Epidemiology

Although, at first sight, geographical epidemiology may appear to differ substantially from other areas of epidemiology, it has many features in common. In particular, a major objective of epidemiology – to infer aetiological relationships from observed associations – applies also in geographical studies. The distinctive characteristic is of course that geographical location is an important explanatory variable, either because it reflects an environmentally determined element of risk or because people with similar risk attributes live together, so that risk varies from place to place. The two-dimensional nature of geographical location means that the standard statistical techniques for handling sets of essentially univariate variables need to be augmented by more sophisticated methods.

There are practical limitations to the scientific value of geographical studies. The data quality tends to be low – not least because population censuses are relatively infrequent – and any real effects may be attenuated by factors such as mobility, often to the point where they may not be detectable. Consideration of these difficulties may lead to the conclusion that a lot of geographical epidemiology is, in scientific terms, of very limited value. Historically, however, there have been some spectacular successes: to the famous observation of John Snow (1855) on the source of cholera infection may be added a number of more recent and equally dramatic observations, for example the identification of the cause of an outbreak of asthma in Spain (Antó and Sunyer 1992) and the implication of erionite fibres in the aetiology of mesothelioma from the very high localised rates in the Cappadocian region of Turkey (Baris et al. 1992).

Scope of the Chapter

This chapter attempts to sketch the statistical principles of the subject, with an indication of the kinds of analyses to which these principles lead quite naturally. There is a large literature on the methodology of geographical epidemiology, much of it employing a Bayesian standpoint and exploring hierarchical models analysed by Markov Chain Monte Carlo methods. It would be impossible to give a comprehensive review of this field and we adopt the less ambitious objective of outlining the fundamentals, in the hope that this will in any case provide insight into more sophisticated analyses. Nevertheless we have attempted to provide some examples of the techniques discussed and, where possible, to make recommendations for practitioners, though this latter goal is difficult in view of the large number of different analyses that have been proposed but whose properties are relatively unknown.

Our presentation will in fact be almost exclusively frequentist. To some extent, the choice between Bayesian and frequentist methods in statistics is a matter of philosophical standpoint. Frequentist arguments are undeniably limited in their scope and power and are frequently subject to misinterpretation. The limitations may, however, be argued to be intrinsic to the problem of inductive inference under uncertainty and such inference does not seem to this author to be more consistently clear-cut when derived from a Bayesian analysis. The modelling approach is admittedly more attractive than the mere detection of statistical significance, but it is not without its difficulties. For one thing the amount of data in geographical studies may often not permit the estimation of numerous parameters and, to the extent that a model makes specific assumptions about underlying phenomena, there is a risk that it may inject spurious information into the analysis, leading to the over-interpretation of the data. The limitations of the hypothesis testing approach have not prevented its widespread use in practice and an important part of the epidemiologist's role is to ensure that the tests that are carried out are chosen with due regard to maximising their power against sensible alternatives. This at least is the stand-point from which we approach this topic here; in any case the statistical framework underpins the more sophisticated analyses and forms a natural pre-requisite for their understanding.

8.1.3   Chapter Contents

We start by considering (Sect. 8.2) the models that underlie statistical methods in geographical epidemiology in order to give insight into the justification for the methods that are discussed. A key feature is the duality that exists between the two approaches to epidemiological investigations generally. To be specific, we can elect to study either the occurrence of disease conditionally on case locations or *vice versa*, i.e. to regard case location as a random variable to be compared in fixed groups of affected and unaffected individuals. This duality precisely mirrors the distinction between the cohort and case-control approaches to epidemiological surveys. The case-control approach in geographical work has only recently been recognised and is particularly relevant for the analysis of data at the individual, as opposed to the areal, level. This important approach, though not yet fully exploited, has led recently to a number of new and interesting methodological developments.

In Sect. 8.3 we develop the way in which risk may be modelled in relation to geographically referenced data, distinguishing between the analysis of areal data and data at the individual level, for which it is assumed that individual locations are known. As with any statistical modelling exercise, the objective is to explain as much of the variation as possible, up to the point where heterogeneity can be attributed to chance. There are numerous ways of approaching this subject, even within the compass of frequentist analyses, and some of the issues as to the best analysis are unresolved.

Section 8.4 is concerned with mapping. From one point of view, mapping is an end in itself and there are numerous methods available for producing maps. However, there is much scope for misinterpretation of data represented in this way and we would argue that a map should be seen as the end product of some kind of modelling process, albeit a very primitive one: no disease map can be constructed without assumptions about the underlying distribution of the disease it purports to represent.

Section 8.5 addresses the question of heterogeneity. To some extent this involves issues bound up with the problems of modelling. But the simple question of whether there is any non-uniformity of risk is a valid one that can be at least partially answered without reference to underlying models or alternatives.

In Sect. 8.6 we address the problem of clustering. This may also be seen as a violation of the twin assumptions of uniformity and independence discussed in Sect. 8.2. However, we may well be more interested in detecting small clusters of cases that are related to one another and to this extent it may be appropriate to use different methods from those in Sect. 8.5.

Finally, Sect. 8.7 considers the rather more specific problem of detecting an increase in risk near a putative point source of risk. It is argued that analyses of this kind are essentially one-dimensional and, perhaps for this reason, it is somewhat easier to determine good methods for doing so. This is in fact a problem of considerable interest and many investigations of "clustering" are really of this kind. The issue is illustrated by the incidence of childhood leukaemia around nuclear installations in the UK using data introduced in Sect. 8.3.2.

The concluding section summarises the chapter and makes suggestions for further reading.

Statistical Models 8.2

In this section we describe a statistical framework for the methods to be discussed. We start by explaining the elements that underlie the analysis of classical surveys and then show how the same starting point may be applied to geographical data.

A Statistical Framework for Epidemiological Observations 8.2.1

To describe a modelling framework for epidemiology, we start by supposing that the disease $\mathcal{D}$ in which we are interested is an essentially dichotomous entity, i.e. it is the binary outcome – affected/not affected – of some biological process applied to a finite set of individuals. Such a starting point will serve irrespective of the temporal nature of the events we are studying, be they deaths or incident cases of a disease $\mathcal{D}$ in a given time period, or the prevalence of $\mathcal{D}$ at a given epoch. We will be primarily interested in the association between $\mathcal{D}$ and various covariates $\mathcal{C}$. Some of these may represent risk factors suspected of playing a causal role: we will describe these as exposure variables and denote them by $\mathcal{E}$. Others may be of interest in their own right or because they are potential confounding variables for $\mathcal{E}$. We will treat $\mathcal{E}$ as a subset of $\mathcal{C}$ when this is convenient.

To take a specific geographical example, we cite the famous study of cardio-vascular disease $\mathcal{D}$ by Cook and Pocock (1983). The covariates $\mathcal{C}$ included water hardness $\mathcal{E}$, whose aetiological relationship to cardiovascular disease was of primary interest, and also various indicators of socio-economic status, which played the role of a confounding factor: the gradients of mortality, water hardness and socio-economic status are highly correlated with latitude in the UK. The data were analysed for males and females together, but they could equally well have been stratified by sex, which would be a covariate of interest in its own right, since one might be interested in the mortality of males and females separately.

Next we assume that occurrences of $\mathcal{D}$ are independent. This does not preclude the possibility that individuals have probabilities p of $\mathcal{D}$ that are related through their proximity, for example. Rather the condition stipulates that, *conditional on the values of $\mathcal{C}$ and $\mathcal{E}$*, the occurrence of $\mathcal{D}$ in one individual is independent of that in another, i.e. that the probability that individual A suffers from $\mathcal{D}$ is unaffected by the *fact* (as opposed to the probability) that some other individual B also suffers from it. In practice this is a reasonable mechanistic assumption for nearly all chronic disease epidemiology. It clearly breaks down for infectious diseases, for which more sophisticated models would be appropriate. In fact little theoretical foundation for modelling the epidemiology of infectious diseases at the individual level exists. This is partly because the theory is intractable, partly because it is not necessary in setting up the null hypothesis of no contagion for the purposes of testing. It is only for formulating alternative hypotheses in this situation that statistical models for a contagious mechanism are necessary. Important though this is, we will not consider the problem in this chapter.

Under this independence assumption, the individual outcomes of $\mathcal{D}$ are described by the very simple Bernoulli distribution. If all the probabilities p_i for the individuals in a group of n are the same, the number of occurrences out of the n will clearly follow the binomial distribution, while if all the p_i are different and supposed to depend on $\mathcal{C}$, we can model them through a (binary) logistic regression (Cox and Snell 1984).

Such analyses are becoming more common but they require detailed information on individuals and are not without their technical difficulties. Much of epidemiology is in practice still conducted by the more traditional approach of grouping data according to disease status and to grouped values of $\mathcal{C}$. In this approach, the assumption is that the probabilities p_i within a particular group are indeed all the same, though in practice we know that this is unlikely to be true. However, this assumption is far less troublesome than appears at first sight. For one thing, as long as the p_i are small, the difference between a binomial distribution and that of a sum of slightly different Bernoulli variables will be negligible.

A typical analysis of epidemiological data proceeds by forming a cross-tabulation into a contingency table, whose rows, columns and layers are labelled by components of $\mathcal{D}$, $\mathcal{E}$ and $\mathcal{C}$. The standard way of analysing such a table is through a log-linear model, which implicitly assumes that the counts in the table are values of Poisson distributed variables, conditioned by the requirements that certain sub-totals in the table are deemed to be fixed. For details on log-linear regressions please refer to Chap. II.3 of this handbook.

The logistic regression and log-linear modelling approaches thus described have been constructed on the assumption that $\mathcal{D}$ is a random response and the covariates $\mathcal{C}$ are fixed but we can also obtain useful analyses by conditioning on the numbers of "cases" affected by $\mathcal{D}$ and unaffected or disease-free "controls" in a suitable control group and regarding one or more of the covariates as a random response. This leads to the so-called "case-control" study (formerly termed a *retrospective* study), in distinction to a "cohort" (or *prospective*) study. Thus, for example, it might be appropriate to use a normal linear regression to model the exposure $\mathcal{E}$ of individuals to some risk factor – considered to be a continuous variable – as a function of the other variables, one of which would be an indicator for $\mathcal{D}$, the membership of the case or control group. We would then regard $\mathcal{E}$ as the factor of primary interest and the other covariates would be fitted in order to control for their possible confounding effects.

Statistical Models for Geographical Data   8.2.2

Most of the ideas outlined above carry over quite naturally to data in which geographical location plays a role. We will preserve the assumptions that $\mathcal{D}$ is a binary variable and that disease occurrences are independent conditionally on $\mathcal{C}$. We need to extend our conceptual notation to include geographical location, which we will denote by $\mathcal{G}$. There is a distinction between situations where we think of it as representing a pair of coordinates and those where it is an essentially two-dimensional location in the space representing a geographical region studied.

If $\mathcal{G}$ is thought of as representing coordinates, such as Easting and Northing, it may be meaningful to treat them like other quantitative variables, perhaps to detect a trend with latitude, for example. Alternatively, it might be meaningful to consider polar coordinates from a specified point $\mathcal{S}$ considered as a fixed origin, analysing distance and direction from it. Typically $\mathcal{S}$ would be a point of some aetiological significance, such as a putative source of pollution. We return to this topic in Sect. 8.7 below.

However, this approach implicitly reduces our analyses to consideration of essentially one-dimensional variables and it is useful to distinguish this from the *intrinsically spatial* case in which we regard two-dimensional space as a single entity. In this situation our main objective will be to depict the way in which risk varies over a region $\mathcal{R}$, usually by means of a map. It is unlikely that any kind of analytically determined trend surface, such as a polynomial, will be useful, though non-parametrically estimated surfaces might be. We return to the problems of mapping in Sect. 8.4 below.

The distinctions we made in Sect. 8.2.1 above apply for geographical data. For example, the majority of geographical analyses are effectively analyses of grouped data, in which observations have been grouped into k sub-regions $A_1, A_2, \ldots, A_k$ of $\mathcal{R}$ (which we shall refer to as "areas"). Within each area, we would hope to know the population to serve as a denominator and the number of occurrences Y_i of the disease $\mathcal{D}$ would then follow a binomial or approximately a Poisson distribution, by the arguments outlined above. The areas may be regarded as analogous to the bins of a histogram, though they will nearly always be based on administrative areas with highly irregular boundaries, so that they do not share the attractive regularity properties of the more familiar histograms formed from quantitative variables. The identities of the areas themselves typically enter the analysis through the coordinates of their population centroids and these may then be analysed by incorporating them into the model as described above, though the analysis might well take account of spatial autocorrelation.

If instead of binning or grouping the observed cases into areas we record the exact locations of the occurrences of $\mathcal{D}$, we need a rather different modelling approach. The case-independence assumption implies that the cases are located according to a non-homogenous Poisson process (Diggle 2000), which is the standard probability model for events happening at random in a continuum, though not necessarily with a uniform pattern of risk. This model supposes that the probability of an event in a small area δA at the point (x, y) is $\lambda(x, y)\delta A$, where $\lambda(x, y)$ is the "intensity function" of the process giving the rate per unit area at (x, y); it also incorporates the crucial assumption that the occurrence of such a point is independent of occurrences outside δA.

It is well known, however, that when points occur according to a Poisson process in such a way that the total number is fixed at a value n, say, the pattern of points obtained is typically exactly the same as if we had sampled from a probability distribution with density function proportional to $\lambda(x, y)$. This enables us to describe the behaviour in geographical space of a fixed sample of cases, with a view to estimating the risk at each point (x, y) or to compare the resulting risk function with that for a sample of controls. Thus we have moved to the "dual" or case-control approach, for we are effectively regarding the locations as realisations of a continuous bivariate random variable defined for our samples of cases and controls. Methods of analysing data within this framework are discussed in Sect. 8.3.4 below.

8.3   Modelling Disease Risk in Relation to Geographically Referenced Factors

8.3.1   Areal Data

One of the commonest and most straightforward analyses of geographical data consists of modelling the counts Y_i of cases in areas A_i using a Poisson regression or, equivalently, a generalised linear model (GLM) with Poisson error and log link function; see McCullagh and Nelder (1989) and Chap. II.3 of this handbook. We start by assuming that we can calculate "null expectations" e_i for the Y_i. In the simplest form these could be obtained by multiplying some global reference estimate of risk p by the population sizes in the A_i. In practice we will almost certainly wish to *standardise* for the age distribution and other known demographic factors such as socio-economic status. Part of our objective is of course to modify the assumption that the risk is the same in every area, so we will incorporate a *relative risk* (RR) θ_i, to give the model for the counts as:

$$Y_i \sim \text{Poisson}[\theta_i e_i] \ .$$

We then model the θ_i in the usual manner for a GLM through

$$\log \theta_i = \sum_{j=1}^{p} x_{ij} \beta_j \ ,$$

where the β_j are coefficients in the log-linear model and x_{ij} is the value of the jth covariate for the ith areal unit A_i.

Typical covariates in such an analysis might include intrinsically geographical features, such as altitude, geological composition or levels of background radiation, or essentially demographic features, such as the age or socio-economic composition of the population of each area. It should be emphasised that the units in the latter kind of analysis are not the individuals with a disease $\mathcal{D}$ but the areas within which they reside and the covariates are also necessarily attributes of these areas. The analysis is implicitly imputing the properties of the area to all the individuals in the area. To the extent that this is inappropriate, conclusions drawn are sometimes described as being subject to the "ecological fallacy". This is a matter of scientific interpretation rather than statistical validity and it is arguable that this kind of analysis involves no logical fallacy at all. For details on this ecological approach, please refer to Chap. I.3 of this handbook.

An Example of the Log-Linear Model for Areal Data 8.3.2

An example of this use of the log-linear model is provided by the application to childhood leukaemia data described by Bithell et al. (1995). The dataset analysed was from the UK National Registry of Childhood Tumours (NRCT) maintained by the Childhood Cancer Research Group in Oxford and related to 5359 children diagnosed with leukaemia or non-Hodgkin lymphoma under the age of 15 years between 1966 and 1987. Each of the cases was located in one of 9831 electoral wards, which are administrative areas with an average population of around 5000.

The explanatory variables fitted were "Standard Region", a classification into ten regions, and the Townsend Index, an areal index of social deprivation which is a function of unemployment, housing ownership and other socio-economic indicators. As shown in Table 8.1, there was a significant reduction in the deviance associated with each of these factors: the p-values shown in the first two lines are based on the chi-square approximation to the deviance reductions. It is interesting, incidentally, to note that the direction of the association is negative for the

Table 8.1. Analysis of deviance of childhood leukaemia data

Variation due to	d.f.	Deviance	P-value
Standard Region	9	23.1	0.0060
Townsend Index	1	23.6	10^{-6}
Residual	9820	8610.6	0.025

Townsend index, i.e. the disease is slightly commoner in less deprived families. This is a feature of childhood leukaemia that differentiates it from most other diseases.

The goodness of fit of the model can in principle be tested by the residual deviance, but because the expected numbers of cases per ward in this analysis were small (less than half on average), the chi-square approximation is unreliable. However, the theoretical mean and variance of the deviance for Poisson observations with a specified set of expectations can be calculated straightforwardly. We can therefore obtain an approximate test of the residual deviance as follows:

1. compute the values for the expectations predicted by the model for each ward;
2. compute the mean μ and variance σ^2 of the deviance statistic D as defined by

$$D = 2 \sum_i [Y_i \log(Y_i/e_i) - (Y_i - e_i)] \tag{8.1}$$

as if the contributions to D were independent;
3. refer the statistic $(D - \mu)/\sigma$ to the standard normal distribution.

The assumption of independence should be approximately true in view of the large number of degrees of freedom. Bithell et al. check the p-value by simulation of data from the fitted model and found a very good degree of approximation to the calculated value of 0.025. These results may be interpreted as meaning that the model fits much better than if the explanatory factors had not been taken into account (for which the equivalent p-value was 0.00042); though there is some evidence of residual heterogeneity, it must be remembered that this is a large data set and the level of significance observed is not indicative of a large degree of variation. We return to the issue of testing residual variation in Sect. 8.5.

8.3.3   Calculating the Expectations

The model described above involves the expectations e_i, which appear as an "offset" term in the model, i.e. $\log(e_i)$ is added to the linear function of the covariates defining $\log \theta_i$. These may be calculated from externally calculated rates, for example from national statistics. If such rates are not easily available, the data can be internally standardised by supplying the sizes of the populations at risk; any factor representing the overall risk will appear in the intercept term of the model. The expectations predicted by the model can then be used as expectations for subsequent analyses and this is a useful by-product of the modelling process. The method can be seen as an elegant and more consistent alternative to classical standardisation, permitting the flexible inclusion of covariates according to their importance, as indicated by the modelling process.

Indeed, the analysis described by Bithell et al. is part of a larger one designed to produce expected numbers of childhood leukaemias for the areal analysis of incidence near nuclear installations; this is briefly described in Sect. 8.7.3.

Continuous Data

Following the discussion in Sect. 8.2.2 above, we suppose that we have a sample of exact locations of cases of disease $\mathcal{D}$ and that we denote their density function over $\mathcal{R}$ by $\psi(x, y)$. We need an analogue of the denominators in an areal analysis to serve as a measure of how many individuals there are at risk at each point (x, y) of $\mathcal{R}$. This is provided in principle by knowledge of the population density, which we will consider to be continuous and which we will denote by $\pi(x, y)$. Then our problem becomes one of comparing the density function for the incident cases with that of the population. For a rare disease, the population density (which strictly speaking includes diseased as well as healthy individuals) will be very similar to that for all non-diseased individuals, which can in turn be estimated by a suitable *sample* of controls. The natural way to make this comparison is through the ratio and it is easily seen that this is

$$\theta(x, y) = \psi(x, y)/\pi(x, y)$$

which defines a *relative risk function* (RRF) giving the risk of being affected by $\mathcal{D}$ at each point (x, y) of $\mathcal{R}$ relative to the mean for the whole of $\mathcal{R}$ (see Bithell 1990).

A natural estimate $\widehat{\theta}(x, y)$ of $\theta(x, y)$ is provided by the ratio of estimates of $\psi(x, y)$ and $\pi(x, y)$. These may be obtained using one of the modern methods available for estimating a density function (see the books by Scott (1992) and Silverman (1986), for example). The process is not without difficulties but it can be used to provide meaningful estimates of the RRF over $\mathcal{R}$, in effect providing a map of it. We return to the problem of mapping in Sect. 8.4 below.

A more ambitious objective than merely mapping the RRF is to model it as a function of covariates x, say. These may be geographically defined at every point of $\mathcal{R}$ or they may be attributes of the cases and controls in the samples. An elegant modelling approach is due to Diggle and Rowlingson (1994) and proceeds by analogy with classical case-control studies. We condition on the coordinates of the n cases and m controls and consider the probability that, under random allocation of the cases and controls to the $m + n$ locations, an individual sampled at a given location (x, y) is a case rather than a control. This probability can then be modelled logistically as a function of x. If there appears to be unexplained variation in the RRF, it can in principle be modelled by adding a non-parametric function of (x, y) to the linear predictor. The numerical problems of the latter approach appear not to be trivial.

The inclusion of attributes of the individuals in the analysis is particularly attractive, since it provides the possibility of controlling for them within the geographical analysis. In practice it is not always straightforward to obtain suitable controls for analyses of this kind, partly because the current emphasis on data protection makes it difficult to access individual records and partly because of the number of combinations of categories with respect to which we may wish to match. Nevertheless, this methodology, though still in its infancy, would seem to have considerable potential.

8.3.5   Spatial Structure in the Residual Variation

The object of fitting a model of the kind discussed is to obtain a satisfactory explanation of the data, i.e. a residual deviance that is not statistically significant. This is not always very easy, since the risk of disease may depend on factors that we have been unable to measure. Large data sets – for example of national mortality rates – may also demonstrate a significant deviance resulting from unobserved factors that are scientifically unimportant simply because of the large numbers of cases involved.

Unfortunately, conclusions about the importance of individual explanatory variables in a model are strictly valid only if the model fitted is correct. In practice we will believe a model to be correct if it appears to fit reasonably well, i.e. if the residual deviance is not statistically significant. This raises the question of how to proceed if there is a degree of residual variation that we cannot explain.

In geographical studies it is quite likely that such variation will be due to unobserved variables that are spatially autocorrelated and in this case we can include appropriate terms in the model. Typically this is done for data in areal form using a conditional autoregression (CAR) model (Wakefield et al. 2000) while, for continuous data, Kelsall and Diggle (1998) use a generalised additive model (GAM) which effectively gives an extra term in the model estimating residual variation non-parametrically. These ideas are important but are somewhat beyond the scope of this chapter; for a good overview see Diggle (2000). We only remark that the issue may not always be as significant as some authors maintain. The deviances of the terms that are fitted in a model will still be a reliable indication of their importance unless they are confounded with the unobserved variables that are inflating the deviance; in this case fitting a spatial model merely tells us that this confounding has a spatial structure – it does not help us to identify the variable or determine its scientific importance.

8.4   Mapping Disease Risk

The mapping of disease risk is a central endeavour of geographical epidemiology: a map is as convenient for portraying such location-specific information as it is for indicating the geography of the land to which it relates. It is therefore no surprise to discover that mapping has a long history pre-dating any systematic development of the statistical principles that underlie it.

As with other areas of geographical epidemiology, many methods have been proposed. Broadly speaking, these can be divided into two classes, model-based and non-parametric. Methods in each of these classes can be applied to data in either areal or continuous form. It is important to appreciate, however, that, whatever method is applied, there is inevitably a degree of smoothing involved that is to some extent arbitrary and under the control of the investigator.

For example, the simplest form of map is the so-called *chloropleth* map, which uses a grey or colour scale to depict the risk of $\mathcal{D}$ in each of a number of areas, usually administratively defined so that denominators are easily available. Here the degree of smoothing is determined by the size of the areas A_i, since the process represents the risk as being the same for the whole of a given area. An example of a chloropleth map is given in Chap. I.3 of this handbook.

Similarly, data in continuous point form can be mapped using the methods described in Sect. 8.3.4 by plotting the RRF $\widehat{\theta}(x, y)$. Here the smoothing is determined by the degree of smoothing used in the estimation of the densities: it is a commonplace of this methodology that some smoothing parameter always has to be used, though there are data-driven methods for estimating the most appropriate smoothing parameter. For an early example of this method applied to small numbers of cases and controls, see Bithell (1990).

It may be noted that the method can easily be adapted to areal data by suitably modifying the customary density estimation methods (Bithell 1999).

Figure 8.1 depicts the incidence of childhood cancer in a 50 km square region of Oxfordshire using data from the UK National Registry of Childhood Tumours maintained by the NRCT in Oxford. They consist of 279 cases of childhood cancer (other than leukaemia and non-Hodgkin lymphoma) registered under the age of 15 years between 1966 and 1987. Each case was located in one of 150 electoral wards for which expected numbers of cases were calculated using similar methods to those for the leukaemia data described in Sect. 8.3.2. The point observations for the cases were used to construct a density estimate $\widehat{\psi}(x, y)$ using the *average shifted histogram* (ASH) method due to Scott (1992). For the controls the density estimate $\widehat{\pi}(x, y)$ was constructed by treating the centroids of the wards as point locations weighted by the expectations and using a version of ASH modified accordingly.

The basis of the ASH method is to count the numbers of cases in the cells of a square grid; these are then smoothed by slightly shifting the grid a number of times and averaging the resulting counts; this process effectively smoothes the surface by spreading out the contributions of the points through neighbouring grid squares.

The RRF was then obtained by dividing the density estimates for the cases and controls to give $\widehat{\theta}(x, y) = \widehat{\psi}(x, y) / \widehat{\pi}(x, y)$. This is depicted in Fig. 8.1 as a contour plot with a scale in km and an origin located in South-West Oxfordshire.

The methods sketched above may be regarded as empirical or non-parametric, in that there is nothing underlying them that is more sophisticated than the division of one number by another (specifically a count by a denominator or one density estimate by another). In particular, it is generally very difficult to see how to determine the appropriate degree of smoothing by any objective process, as distinct from using intuitively plausible and aesthetically pleasing values.

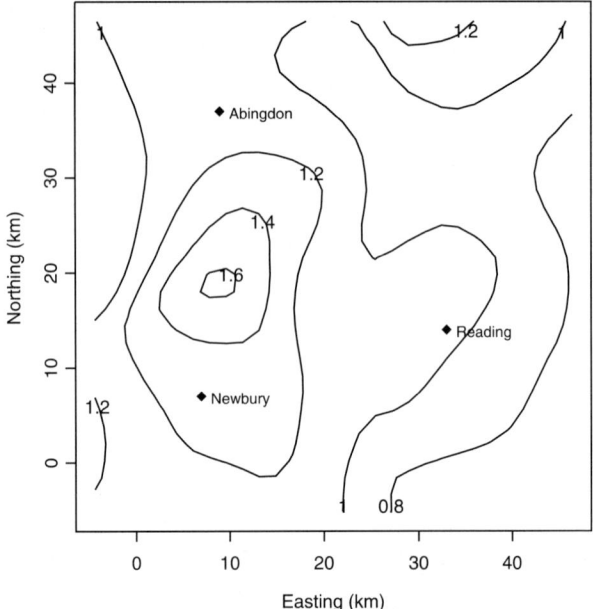

Figure 8.1. Relative Risk Function for childhood cancer in a region of Oxfordshire, estimated from areal data. The three town centres are shown only approximately. The ASH smoothing parameter used was 8 (see Bithell (1999) for details)

The need for a degree of smoothing can easily be seen by considering a chloropleth map, for which we have areas A_i with small numbers of cases, either because we have chosen small areas or because $\mathcal{D}$ has low incidence. In this case the estimates of the risk in each A_i will be subject to large sampling error; our belief about the true risk in A_i will be determined in part by the observed rate, but it will also rely on information from the region as a whole, to the extent that we believe there will be some comparability between the areas.

This idea has led to the development of model-based approaches using Bayesian arguments to integrate area-specific information with information from the whole region, using a statistical model for the underlying variation of the true risk. In a classical treatment of this problem, Clayton and Kaldor (1987) suppose that the true risk θ_i in A_i is distributed over the areas as a whole according to a gamma distribution with mean μ and variance σ^2. It can then be shown that the posterior distribution of θ_i has mean

$$\tilde{\theta}_i = \frac{y_i + \mu^2/\sigma^2}{e_i + \mu/\sigma^2} \, ,$$

where y_i is the observed value of the count Y_i in A_i. This formula can be seen to be a form of average of the maximum likelihood estimate $\widehat{\theta}_i = y_i/e_i$ of each θ_i

and the overall mean μ, which can be estimated by $\sum y_i / \sum e_i$. The value of σ^2 can also be estimated from the data as a whole, though this requires an iterative method.

This method and variants of it provide *empirical Bayes* estimates, in that the prior distribution of the θ_i can be estimated from the data. The method is essentially non-spatial, in the sense that the true θ_i are supposed to vary independently. In practice, it is likely that rates in neighbouring areas will be consistently more similar to one another than those in more separated areas. If this were not so, it would be essentially fruitless to attempt to produce a smoothly varying map. The Bayesian methodology has been extended to permit the prior distribution of the θs to depend on the values in neighbouring areas. These more complicated models involve a greater number of arbitrary assumptions, however. They are gaining ground in popularity and appear to be used quite successfully. The reader is referred for more details and references to Clayton and Bernardinelli (1992).

Attractive though these ideas are, the maps they produce need careful interpretation, since they have imposed a degree of spatial auto-correlation and this process is capable of making adjacent areas look more similar than they really are. In a sense this is true of all mapping methods and is a feature as intrinsic as the implicit smoothing itself.

In a challenging paper, Gelman and Price (1999) discuss the issue and illustrate the phenomenon of induced spatial pattern by means of simple modelling paradigms. They point out that the probability that a particular area rate $\widehat{\theta}_i$ exceeds a given value increases with the population size, n_i, say. The effect of this is that high observed rates of disease tend to be observed predominantly in low population areas; since these tend to be spatially aggregated – i.e. low population areas are more likely to occur next to other such areas – observed rates also appear to be spatially related even when in fact no such relationship exists for the underlying risk.

They further demonstrate that plotting the posterior means from a Bayesian analysis produces observed rates that are likely to exceed a particular value with probabilities that are *decreasing* functions of n_i, so that such plots over-correct in some sense. Although scores exist – at least for continuous observations – that are not subject to these artefacts, they have no direct interpretation as estimates of the θ_i.

One is driven to the conclusion that disease maps are potentially misleading when used as anything except what Gelman and Price call "look-up tables", i.e. as a convenient way of depicting the rate in a given area *without reference to neighbouring areas*. It is the temptation to use the map to generalise about the spatial pattern of rates that can be misleading and it is probably better to formulate such questions within the context of a statistical model rather than to attempt to portray spatial relationship graphically. However, one suspects that this timely caution is unlikely to diminish the enthusiasm for constructing and over-interpreting disease maps.

The Detection
of Generalised Heterogeneity

8.5.1   The Assessment of Heterogeneity in Areal Data

Heterogeneity is the key to epidemiology, in the sense that a uniform risk in observed data gives no possibility for associating differences with factors that may have aetiological significance. We have already touched on the issue of modelling in Sect. 8.3.1 and our objective there is to find a model that appears to fit well in the sense that the residual deviance is not statistically significant – i.e. it is consistent with chance deviations from the predictions of the model.

As long as we have Poisson data with reasonably large means we can assess the residual deviance as if it had a chi-square distribution with a number of degrees of freedom (d.f.) determined by the model – specifically the number of units minus the number of parameters fitted. It is important to remember, however, that this is based on asymptotic theory which, roughly speaking, supposes that the total number of cases is large compared with the number of units – areal or otherwise – in the analysis. A rule of thumb suggests that the expectations of the counts in a Poisson regression should mostly be in excess of 5. When the average expectation falls below this, we should expect the distribution of the deviance in a correct model to depart progressively from a chi-square distribution, which of course means that a corresponding statistical test of goodness of fit of the model based on the chi-square distribution would not be valid.

In this situation, we can obtain an approximate assessment of the value of the deviance – and hence the goodness of fit of the model – by simulation. Typically we would generate, say, s new samples of data from Poisson distributions with means obtained from the model $\mathcal{M}_{\text{fitted}}$ fitted to the actual data. For each simulated sample, we would re-fit the same model and compute the residual deviance. The s values of the deviance thus obtained provide an estimate of the distribution of the deviance. This in turn provides a means of calibrating the deviance observed for our actual data. A formal test of goodness of fit would only be approximate since we are simulating from $\mathcal{M}_{\text{fitted}}$ rather than the true model with the true (unknown) parameter values. This situation is typical of "bootstrapping" and the theory of this subject could in principle lead to better approximations. For an account of bootstrapping see, for example, Efron and Tibshirani (1993).

8.5.2   Detecting Heterogeneity in Poisson Data

A special case arises when we have expectations, provided, for example, by some prior analysis or by simple calculation from population data and we merely wish to detect whether the Poisson distribution fits well with the assumed e_i, without reference to any model fitting. This is sometimes seen as a problem of detecting "clustering", though there are qualifications to this interpretation that we discuss below: for the moment we prefer to regard this as the problem of assessing heterogeneity, i.e. variations in risk between areas without reference to a possible geographical origin for the phenomenon.

Relating this to the deviance of a Poisson model suggests that the deviance of the observations, defined in (8.1), Sect. 8.3.2, would be a sensible test statistic. The fact that this test is a likelihood ratio test means that it is *asymptotically* fully efficient – i.e. its power approaches that of the best possible test against a Poisson alternative in which the relative risks are different from unity.

Popular alternative contenders include Pearson's chi-square statistic

$$X^2 = \sum (Y_i - e_i)^2 / e_i,$$

and the Potthoff–Whittinghill statistic (Potthoff and Whittinghill 1966)

$$PW = \sum Y_i(Y_i - 1)/e_i,$$

which is regarded by some authors as a test of clustering. The former is, at least in simple cases, asymptotically equivalent to the deviance but is easier to compute and to study analytically. The asymptotic requirement, however, implies that the expectations should be large and the theoretical properties give rather little guidance on which test is best for small expectations.

Table 8.2 shows the results of a simulation study, designed to provide such guidance, in which the expected significance level (ESL) of each test has been estimated in each of three conditions. (The ESL is a convenient alternative criterion to power (Dempster and Schatzoff 1965): a smaller ESL corresponds to a more powerful test.) In each case the ESLs were estimated from 10,000 simulations performed under varying conditions. These were chosen to produce values in a critical range corresponding to situations where the test would be quite likely to lead to different conclusions at conventional significance levels. In each case, a specific number k of wards were supposed to have the same expectations e under the null hypothesis, while under the alternative hypothesis these expectations were multiplied by a set of RR factors θ_i sampled from a gamma distribution with mean one and variance σ^2.

Table 8.2. Expected significance levels (ESL) % and their standard errors for Pearson's X^2, the deviance and the Potthoff–Whittinghill tests: k wards each with expectation e under H_0 and an alternative expectation dispersion with variance σ^2

e	σ^2	k		Pearson	Deviance	Potthoff
5.0	0.05	200	ESL	6.6	3.5	44.5
			s.e.	0.22	0.18	0.50
1.0	0.2	500	ESL	3.5	2.7	6.3
			s.e.	0.18	0.16	0.24
0.2	1.0	1000	ESL	14.2	23.8	3.3
			s.e.	0.35	0.43	0.20

In interpreting this table, we suppose that the key parameter is the size of the expectation e. Because the test statistic will be roughly proportional to the number of wards k, this latter parameter represents the amount of information and was chosen to bring the ESLs into an interesting range; it would not be expected to change the relative ordering of the three tests. The variance σ^2 represents the distance between the null and alternative hypotheses and the values were chosen to be typical of the sort of discrepancy that one could reasonably expect to detect in practical situations. It could conceivably affect the relative properties of the different tests but is less likely to do so than e.

It will be seen that, with an expectation of $e = 5$, the deviance is indeed the best test, while the Potthoff–Whittinghill test trails behind Pearson's chi-square test. The difference between X^2 and D becomes marginal around $e = 1$ while, for smaller expectations, the ordering is reversed and the Potthoff–Whittinghill test appears to be superior. These results suggest that it would be wise to carry out simulations in particular marginal cases to determine the best test to use. It should also be emphasised that one should evaluate the significance of the chosen statistic using simulation when the e_i are small, since the Pearson and deviance statistics are then likely to have distributions markedly different from the chi-square.

8.5.3   Spatial and Non-spatial Analyses

A test of heterogeneity in areal data of the kind described above provides only a non-spatial test of the heterogeneity of our observations. Whether this is appropriate depends on whether or not the areal units are defined by essentially geographical criteria. If, for example, they are defined by simply dividing our region $\mathcal{R}$ into urban and rural areas, then a factor associated with the degree of urbanisation could be expected to induce heterogeneity into the areas irrespective of their spatial positions.

More frequently, however, areas are merely convenient administrative subdivisions of $\mathcal{R}$. In this case we might expect a factor that raises the incidence in one area to do so in adjoining areas also. Then, a test that takes no account of the spatial relationship of the areas will be less powerful than one that does.

To take a simple hypothetical example, suppose that $\mathcal{R}$ consists of two subregions: $\mathcal{R}_1$ with n areas each having expectation $e_i = 9$ and $\mathcal{R}_2$ with n areas each having expectation $e_i = 11$. A dispersion test based on Pearson's chi-square statistic would use the variance of the observations to test the null hypothesis H_0 that all the expectations are the same:

$$X^2_{2n-1} = \sum_{i=1}^{2n}(Y_i - e)^2/e,$$

where $e = \sum_1^{2n} Y_i/n$ is the (estimated) expected count based on all $2n$ observations. To a good approximation, this statistic would have a chi-square distribution with $2n - 1$ degrees of freedom under H_0. If, however, we knew which areas belonged to

$\mathcal{R}_1$ and which to $\mathcal{R}_2$, we would base the test on the equivalent statistic for testing the difference between the totals for the two sub-regions:

$$X_1^2 = \frac{\left(\sum_1^n Y_i - ne\right)^2 + \left(\sum_{n+1}^{2n} Y_i - ne\right)^2}{ne}$$

and it is fairly obvious that this would be a much more powerful test of H_0. This idealised situation is analogous to isolating sources of variation in an analysis of variance.

In practice, of course, we will almost certainly not be in a position to divide $\mathcal{R}$ into high and low risk areas *a priori*, but this example does suggest that the detection of non-uniformity of risk should take account of the spatial structure of the data. A classical account of tests of spatial autocorrelation is given by Cliff and Ord (1981), who establish some theoretical properties of their sampling distributions, particularly in the case of normally distributed observations. In one of the few comparative studies published, Walter (1993) examines the power empirically for three of the most popular tests against a variety of geographically plausible alternatives. The three considered were

— the I statistic of Moran (1948), which is analogous to a correlation coefficient and is defined by:

$$I = \frac{n \sum_{ij} w_{ij}(x_i - \bar{x})(x_j - \bar{x})}{\sum_{ij} w_{ij} \sum_i (x_i - \bar{x})^2} \ .$$

— the c statistic of Geary (1954), which is similar to I and
— a non-parametric test statistic which uses only the ranks of the observations.

The first two statistics used as observations $x_i = y_i/e_i$, the standardised incidence ratios for the different areas, and spatial weights w_{ij} chosen to be one if A_i and A_j are adjacent and zero otherwise. Walter's Table II shows that, in each of the situations he considered, Moran's I had the highest power of the three and it would seem that this should be the method of choice, at least for detecting generalized spatial relationship as opposed to isolated peaks in the risk. The question of whether higher power could be achieved by using more sophisticated weighting than a simple adjacency matrix, or by weighting the pairs of observations according to the amount of information they contain (in terms of sample size, for example), has not been much considered. Walter concludes that "the precise type of spatial pattern involved may have a major impact on the spatial power of the analysis" and that "more experience is needed to better understand the potential of these methods, and their limitations". Nevertheless this study was a useful contribution and the use of Moran's I to detect spatial autocorrelation is probably a good choice.

8.5.4   Heterogeneity Tests Based on the Risk Surface

If we have continuous data – i.e. observations at the individual level – we can base a test of uniformity on the RRF $\widehat{\theta}(x, y)$ as estimated by the methods described in Sect. 8.3.4. We may regard a test statistic as being defined by a functional of $\widehat{\theta}(x, y)$ and there are various possibilities.

A natural choice is the weighted variance of $\widehat{\theta}(x, y)$:

$$T_{\text{var}} = \iint_{\mathcal{R}} \pi(x, y)\{\widehat{\theta}(x, y) - 1\}^2 \mathrm{d}x\mathrm{d}y \, .$$

In the absence of any reliable theory it is necessary to resort to Monte Carlo methods to test the statistic. For case-control data, we use a permutation method that is straightforward though laborious:

1. construct a map of the risk function $\theta(x, y)$ by a suitable method, using a degree of smoothing which is determined as a function of the data;
2. evaluate the chosen test statistic for the observed data t_{obs};
3. choose a new sample of "cases" by choosing at random n points from the set of $m + n$ cases and controls combined;
4. compute the value of the statistic t_1, say, for the simulated data, using the same procedure as in Step 1;
5. repeat Steps 3 and 4 $s - 1$ times so that there are s simulated values altogether;
6. reject at level $\alpha = m/(s + 1)$ the null hypothesis of uniformity of cases if t_{obs} is greater than all but $m - 1$ of the simulated observations;
7. or alternatively estimate the p-value of the test as the number of $\{t_i \geq t_{\text{obs}}\}/s$.

This general Monte Carlo procedure is applicable in very general circumstances and it is especially useful in the analysis of spatial data, where construction of suitable models is difficult. We must remember, however, that a hypothesis test is, by itself, of very little inferential value without some idea of how probable the observed results would be under a plausible alternative.

The method can easily be adapted to a test based on a risk surface constructed from areal data as described in Sect. 8.4. The simulation would take the form of sampling areal counts from Poisson distributions with expectations e_i and computing the variance over a square grid as before. In either the continuous or areal data case the degree of smoothing used in the density estimation process determines the scale of aggregation for which the test is most sensitive and is analogous to the choice of weights w_{ij} in Moran's statistics.

The use of tests of this sort is still in its infancy, but the underlying philosophy is attractive and increasing computing power is making them more practicable even for large data sets.

Clustering 8.6

Closely related to the idea of heterogeneity is the concept of clustering, with which much of geographical epidemiology is preoccupied. There is a large literature on the subject, not all of which is very clear on the issue of what we actually mean by the words "cluster" and "clustering". We may conveniently define a cluster as a localised aggregation of disease cases greater than can easily be explained by chance. Clustering may be regarded as the tendency to form clusters or, more generally, as any departure from the assumptions of uniform risk and independence of case occurrences as discussed in Sect. 8.2.1. We will continue to use the word heterogeneity to refer to a departure from uniformity and reserve the word clustering as far as possible to refer to mechanisms in which case occurrences are not independent. This kind of clustering may be supposed to act locally, whereas heterogeneity is more likely to be observed throughout $\mathcal{R}$ and is sometimes referred to as "generalised clustering". For further discussion of the issues the reader is referred to a useful paper by Diggle (2000).

We can give here only the briefest of accounts. We will distinguish between methods based on increased levels of risk and methods based on the proximity of neighbours. First, however, we make two general points about clustering.

In the first place, it is a well accepted fact of spatial statistics that it is not possible to distinguish on the basis of a single realisation of observed data from a spatial process whether any non-uniformity of the distribution of points (relative to an expected population distribution) is due to a variation of underlying risk, with cases occurring independently (i.e. points generated by a non-homogeneous Poisson process or its equivalent), or to a mechanism in which existing cases induce others nearby, such as would happen in a contagious process. Secondly, we remark that, from an abstract point of view, clustering may take place in any continuum and, in the geographical context, we may observe clustering in space, time or the "product-space" of time and geographical space. This mathematical commonality means that tests can be adapted from one problem to another, with very fruitful consequences.

Methods Based on the RRF 8.6.1

Clustering is likely to be observed as an increase in risk in some locality and it follows that we can use the estimated risk surface $\widehat{\theta}(x, y)$ to provide an appropriate test. What functional of $\widehat{\theta}(x, y)$ we use will depend on the alternative we have in mind or, equivalently, the pattern we would most like to detect. If, for example, we are content to demonstrate a single cluster or aggregation of cases we could choose as our test statistic the maximum of the $\widehat{\theta}(x, y)$ over the whole region $\mathcal{R}$:

$$T_{\max} = \max_{x,y \in \mathcal{R}} \{\widehat{\theta}(x, y)\}.$$

This does not, of course, preclude the possibility that we would detect multiple clusters, but it is likely that our test would be most powerful in the situation where there are in fact very few. We could of course extend the statistic to consider, for example, the mean of the r largest peaks in $\widehat{\theta}(x, y)$ but it is unlikely that we would have good *a priori* grounds for fixing r. Tests based on peaks of incidence must also be expected to be quite sensitive to the scale of the clustering phenomenon and to the degree of smoothing we employ in constructing $\widehat{\theta}(x, y)$.

A statistic likely to have similar properties to T_{max} is based on a scanning window, typically a square that moves over $\mathscr{R}$. At each point of a fine grid the observed number of cases is compared with its expectation; the test statistic is defined as the maximum discrepancy using a suitable criterion such as the incidence ratio. Here the size of the window plays the role of a smoothing parameter; the main difference from T_{max} is that a peak incidence is weighted according to its radial extent; it seems likely that it behaves in a similar manner to T_{max} for suitably chosen smoothing parameters. Anderson and Titterington (1995) describe a version of this method that varies the window size to keep constant the expected number of cases under the null hypothesis.

In fact the scanning window is a two-dimensional version of an approach originally used for detecting clustering in time; even this one-dimensional version is notoriously intractable analytically and simulations or other numerical methods would seem to be unavoidable.

8.6.2   Knox's Test

The use of what we may call pairing methods is historically older than the methods based on the risk surface discussed above; they have the attraction of being very simple to describe and understand.

The earliest such test is due to Knox (1964), who counted the number, Z, of pairs of children with leukaemia diagnosed within sixty days and one kilometre of each other in Northumberland and Durham, two counties in the North-East of England (see Table 8.3, taken from Knox (1964)). The study used local registration and hospital records as well as death certificates to ascertain 185 children with an onset of leukaemia under 15 years of age between the years 1951 to 1960 inclusive. However, certain cases were excluded and Table 8.3 refers just to children under the age of six, a restriction that needs to be borne in mind when interpreting the results; in fact older children showed no effect.

Table 8.3. Pairs of cases of childhood leukaemia classified according their closeness in space and time (see text)

		Distance apart (km)		
		0–1	Over 1	Total
Time apart	0–59	5	147	152
(days)	60–3651	20	4388	4408

The rationale for this test is explicitly related to the non-independence of the cases, namely that a contagious mechanism passing a disease from one individual to another would be likely to lead to cases that are closer to one another in space and time than would be expected by chance. This in turn leads to the idea of considering pairs of cases.

Knox refers this statistic to its expectation calculated on the assumption that the spatial locations and times of occurrence of the disease are independent. This is given by

$$\mathbf{E}[Z] = \frac{N_T N_S}{\binom{n}{2}},$$

where N_T, N_S are the numbers of pairs of cases close in time and close in space respectively and the denominator is the total number of pairs out of the n cases.

In effect this becomes a test of the independence of these two variables and it uses their *marginal* distributions to determine the null distribution of Z. Knox conjectures that Z should follow a Poisson distribution approximately; this is shown to be true in certain circumstances in work reported by David and Barton (1966), who give a formula for the variance of Z. It is wise to calculate this or to use a Monte Carlo test in which the times of occurrence of the cases are randomly permuted relative to the space coordinates and the statistic Z is re-computed a large number of times. For Knox's data, the value of $\mathbf{E}[Z]$ is 0.83, for which $Z = 5$ has a p-value of 0.0017 when tested as a Poisson observation. David and Barton report an early simulation experiment for Knox's data carried out by M.C. Pike; the latter finds $Z \geq 5$ in 4 out of 2000 simulations. This leads to an estimated significance level of 0.002 which is very close to that based on the Poisson approximation.

The choice of the critical distance and time separation is of course crucial. It determines the scale of clustering likely to be detected and it should ideally be fixed in advance for the formal validity of the testing procedure. In particular, it is certainly not formally valid to test at a large number of different critical distances and times and then select the most significant result without allowance for this selection. If we really have no idea of the time and distance scales that would be appropriate, we need to use a data-driven method of identifying the most promising values (see Sect. 8.6.6).

Other Space-Time Clustering Methods 8.6.3

An alternative test based on the proximity in space and time of pairs of cases is proposed by Jacquez (1996). This is based on the number out of the l nearest neighbours in space of a given case that are also among the l nearest neighbours in time. Like the Knox test it can be adapted to provide a test of space-only clustering. Jacquez claimed superior power to that of the Knox test, though in practice this is likely to depend on the alternative being considered. Here the parameter l serves as a kind of scale parameter since it determines how far we look for association between cases.

Knox's very elegant idea permits us to dispense with the need to estimate the marginal distributions, though only under the assumption that space and time are in fact independently distributed in the population. This assumption applies of course to Jacquez' test also. It will clearly be violated by population drift, i.e. a change of population distribution with time. Kulldorf and Hjalmars (1999) examine the size of this effect and conclude that it can be "a considerable problem". They recommend that space-time clustering should be tested using the joint space-time distribution of the population size but this is of course rather hard to obtain with good accuracy and resolution. It seems likely that the use of the interaction tests will remain popular.

8.6.4   Case-Only Clustering

Knox's idea of counting pairs has been very fruitful and has been adapted to a number of related situations, including the use of a sample of controls to provide a reference distribution when testing for space-only clustering (Pike and Smith 1974). The essential idea here is to regard the controls as being similar to the cases, except that they are considered to have occurred at different "pseudo-times", while the cases are considered to have occurred simultaneously. The statistic computed is then the number of pairs of cases that are close in space, and it is not hard to see that this is formally equivalent to Z, with identical distributional statistical properties.

8.6.5   Population Distance

A kind of dual approach is proposed, also for case-control data, by Cuzick and Edwards (1990). This is based on the count of the number of individuals among the l nearest neighbours of each case that are also cases (as opposed to controls). The quantity l in the Cuzick–Edwards test serves as a determinant of the scale of clustering to be detected in this method. It is given in terms of the number of individuals likely to be within a region of contagion, rather than a distance.

This may be seen as more relevant for some, though not for all, mechanisms of disease spread. Indeed, for any given pair we can think of closeness in terms of distance or in terms of the number of other members of the population residing between the two members of the pair. The choice between these two metrics is crucial, though which is the more appropriate will presumably depend on the supposed aetiology of the disease.

The idea of a population distance lies behind another method of testing, due to Besag and Newell (1991), who consider each case in turn and aggregate the areas around it that are necessary to include the rth nearest case. The expectation for the aggregate of these areas is then compared with r in the usual way. This can be regarded as a kind of inverse sampling and again the number of cases considered, r, is a parameter that determines the scale of clustering to which the procedure is sensitive.

Choosing Scale Parameters 8.6.6

Every clustering phenomenon has an implied scale of the clustering effect and it is clearly desirable to have some idea of this before attempting to detect it. When we have no idea the temptation to perform multiple testing arises and it is important to make allowance for this. A method for testing a range of distances and times in the Knox test is proposed by Abe (1973); effectively this examines a multi-way table for association between space and time, making due allowance for the non-independence of the pairs. This statistic is sensitive to association over the whole range of distances and times rather than attempting to identify the most interesting scale. To identify the scale of maximal clustering effect we can use a general data driven procedure that can be constructed along the following lines:

1. Test the data at each of a number of critical space and time distance pairs.
2. Form a single test statistic, either using some aggregate over different values of the scale parameters or using some measure of the maximum degree of clustering; call this statistic t_{obs}.
3. Simulate further data sets under the null hypothesis: for Poisson data this will probably involve sampling Poisson–distributed counts, while for case-control data it may involve pooling all the cases and controls and randomly selecting a subset to serve as simulated "cases".
4. Rank the simulated values of the statistic $t_1, t_2, \ldots, t_s$ and compare the ranked values with t_{obs}.

This Monte Carlo procedure is of general applicability and provides a way of getting round the problem of unknown scale. It does of course sacrifice power by comparison with a test that correctly focuses on the true degree of clustering, so that the more carefully alternative hypotheses can be framed *a priori* the better.

Faced with this wide variety of tests it is difficult for the researcher to know which to use. Each new test published typically is claimed to be more powerful than previously existing tests, but there is a wide variety of alternatives to uniformity of risk that could be considered and it is certain that no one test is uniformly most powerful against all alternatives. In principle it is open to the researcher to examine competing tests to see which would be best for the data and the alternative hypothesis in question, but this can be an arduous exercise. This is an area where we badly need more insight into which tests are preferable.

Pre-defined Sources of Risk 8.7

One of the epidemiological questions most often asked in a geographical context is whether there appears to be an aggregation of cases around a putative source of risk s such as an industrial plant. For example, there has been much interest in the UK, as in other countries, in the possibility of elevated risk of childhood leukaemia around nuclear power stations. This results in part from the finding of an unusually large aggregation of cases near the nuclear reprocessing plant at Sellafield, which is situated on the coast of Cumbria in the North-West of England. In fact ordinary nuclear generating stations have little in common with the reprocessing plant and the experimental reactor at Sellafield; nor is there evidence of significant releases of radioactivity into the environment from generating stations. Nevertheless, public anxiety persists about the safety of the plants, partly perhaps because of the difficulty in comprehending the nature of nuclear power and partly because of sensational reporting in the news media. In fact, there is little evidence of a general increase in risk (Bithell et al. 1994), but it is highly desirable that the best statistical procedures are used to test the data that come under scrutiny. The public may not have a very sophisticated understanding of statistics, but it is obvious even to the uninitiated that some of the procedures used in the past have not been well-chosen from the point of view of maximising the chance of detecting a real effect.

Aggregations around $\mathcal{S}$ are sometimes referred to as "clusters", but it is not generally supposed that the cases involved are related, only that the risk to individuals in the vicinity of $\mathcal{S}$ is elevated. Analyses could therefore proceed using the methods described in Sect. 8.3.1, with the obvious qualification that geographical variables clearly represent spatial relationship to $\mathcal{S}$. In practice this nearly always means using distance from $\mathcal{S}$ or some function of it, so that the analysis is implicitly one-dimensional. Moreover, analyses are often required in situations where the number of cases is very small and in this situation the fitting of GLM's tends to be unstable and to lead to parameter estimates with large standard errors and unknown distributional properties.

8.7.1   Tests for Concentration of Risk

In this situation it is probably better to rely on a formal significance test and the issue then becomes that of selecting the most powerful test against a suitable hypothesis or range of hypotheses. The resulting analyses are likely not to be very powerful in any case, but choosing the most powerful test at least increases the chance that a significant result can be attributed to a genuine departure from the null hypothesis of uniform risk.

The method of early investigators of simply comparing the risk in the area around $\mathcal{S}$ with a reference or "control" rate outside the area defines a test procedure that is in fact powerful only against an alternative hypothesis that prescribes a uniform excess risk within the area which drops to zero on the boundary. This is clearly implausible and critically dependent on the size of the area chosen; one inevitably concludes that a better test would be one designed for some systematic relationship between the risk and the distance from $\mathcal{S}$. We may reasonably suppose that this relationship is monotonic, but the rate of decay and the shape of the RRF (expressed now as a function of distance) will determine the power of the test.

An ingenious class of tests designed to be powerful against general monotonic alternatives was proposed by Stone (1988). His "MLR test" compares the ratio of the maximum of the likelihood under the null hypothesis of uniform risk against the likelihood of the observations maximised subject to the restriction that the risk is a non-increasing function of distance from $\mathcal{S}$, i.e

$$H_1 : \theta_1 \geq \theta_2 \geq \ldots \geq \theta_k \quad (\geq 1), \qquad (8.2)$$

where θ_i is the relative risk in the ith area in order of increasing distance from $\mathcal{S}$. Stone's test has become very popular in the UK epidemiological literature, though it is now known that it is never the most powerful test against a specific hypothesis, this being provided by a *linear risk score* (LRS) test of the form

$$T = \sum_j \ln \left(\theta \left(d_j \right) \right),$$

where d_j is the distance of the jth case from $\mathcal{S}$ and $\theta(d)$ is the risk at a distance d from $\mathcal{S}$ as specified by the alternative hypothesis (Bithell 1995).

Unfortunately, knowing the most powerful test against a specific alternative hypothesis does not greatly help if we do not know what that alternative is. However, it provides a bench-mark against which we can judge other tests and, in particular it enables us to determine the sensitivity of the power to variation in the alternative. It turns out that statistics of the form

$$T = \sum_j 1/\phi \left(d_j \right),$$

for monotonic functions $\phi(\cdot)$ define a class of *canonical* tests which can come to close to optimal power in many circumstances. In particular,

$$\phi \left(d_j \right) = \text{rank} \left(d_j \right) \text{ and } \phi \left(d_j \right) = \sqrt{d_j}$$

behave well in areas with a reasonably uniform population distribution. However, the latter affects quite strongly which of the canonical tests actually is most powerful and it is wise to check the performances of the competing tests in each different area using a simulation study.

Because the LRS test statistics are sums, they should in principle have an approximately normal distribution and it is easy to compute their moments. In small samples this asymptotic normal approximation will not necessarily apply and it is advisable to use simulation also to carry out the tests, i.e. to carry out Monte Carlo tests. In doing so, it is easy to see that the way the samples are drawn can be either to fix the total number of cases and use the multinomial distribution or to use unconstrained Poisson distributions to determine the counts in the areas A_i. Which of these two sampling schemes is used is very important and will typically affect the results quite substantially. The first method defines a conditional test which might be appropriate if the expectations e_i for the rates in the different areas are unreliable in absolute terms (though possibly still all right relatively); it is important to note though that, if the expectations are correct, the null hypothesis could be rejected because of a deficit of cases near the boundary of the region rather than an excess near $\mathcal{S}$. The second, unconditional, test is appropriate if the rates are reliable and in this case the test statistic combines the evidence from the overall relative risk in the area as well as from the spatial distribution. In this case, the appropriate form of Stone's test should also include the last inequality in (8.2) above.

8.7.2   Summary of Recommendations

In summary, this is an area of geographical epidemiology where some progress has been made in identifying efficient procedures, perhaps because the problem is essentially one-dimensional. Because data sets are usually small it is especially important to use tests of maximum power and this criterion seems to be sensitive to the population distribution as well as the precise alternative considered. It is recommended that a study should be guided by the following considerations:

1. First and foremost, thought should be given to the patterns of risk that it is desired to detect; these can be expressed in terms of the RRF and may reasonably be supposed to be monotonic decreasing unless special circumstances prevail. The more specifically this can be linked to a biological hypothesis, the more convincing a positive result will be.
2. Next, a circular region of radius R around δ should be chosen and the observed and expected numbers of cases in the areas A_i obtained. There is no great advantage for testing purposes in calculating the numbers within fixed distance bands from δ. The magnitude of R is important since, if it is much greater than the distance of any conceivable risk, the analysis will inevitably lose power. As a guideline, it would seem sensible to choose the radius R so that the excess relative risk might reasonably be supposed to have declined to half its value at distance $R/2$.
3. The choice between a conditional and an unconditional test should be made, this depending largely on the perceived reliability of the expectations and whether it is desired to detect an overall excess in the area as well as spatial pattern.
4. One or more alternative hypotheses should be identified and the average power or the ESL of each of a number of tests should estimated by simulation, using the population data specific to the area being studied.
5. The analysis should then proceed using the test identified as best, using simulation to perform a Monte Carlo test unless the expectations are quite large.

8.7.3   Example: Childhood Leukaemia Around UK Nuclear Installations

The tests described above were developed partly in conjunction with analyses of the distribution of childhood leukaemia around nuclear installations. An analysis of all major sites in England and Wales is described by Bithell et al. (1994) using the data on leukaemia and non-Hodgkin lymphoma described in Sect. 8.3.2. At

Table 8.4. Average power of five tests and significance levels achieved for the 80 wards within 25 km of Hinkley Point, in which there were 57 cases observed against 57.2 expected

Test	MLR	Pmax	1/rank	1/distance	$\sqrt{1/\text{distance}}$
Power	0.359	0.204	0.421	0.649	0.630
p-value	0.150	0.020	0.108	0.357	0.341

the time of these analyses Stone's test was popular and was used as the principal test statistic in this study, with the LRS test based on distance rank calculated for corroboration. As remarked above, the results were largely negative.

However, public interest in the possibility of a raised risk persists and updated analyses are in progress. These have been carried out in line with the above recommendations and in particular tests were selected individually to be most powerful at each site. Experience of these analyses suggests that the power does indeed depend on the population distribution, but it has been found that, for the majority of test sites the most powerful test against the alternatives considered was the LRS test based on $1/\sqrt{\text{distance}}$.

Table 8.4 shows the average power averaged over 75 alternative hypotheses and the significance levels achieved by each of five tests for one of the datasets from the 1994 analysis. It will be noticed that the smallest *p*-value was the Poisson maximum (often known as "Pmax"); this is in effect the maximum value of the cumulative relative risk as we move out from $\mathcal{S}$. The most powerful test, on the other hand, gives a non-significant result. This analysis is a timely warning against judging a test by the significance level achieved in a real dataset. More details and discussion of this analysis are given in Bithell (2003).

Conclusions

In this chapter we have attempted to give a simple but unifying overview of the statistical methods that underlie geographical epidemiology. We have been able to refer to only a small proportion of the very large number of methods that have been proposed for different aspects of the subject. For further reading we refer to edited volumes by Elliott et al. (1992), Lawson et al. (1999) and Elliott et al. (2000) and to the Encyclopedia of Biostatistics edited by Armitage and Colton (1998), for example the review article by Bithell (1998).

It will be clear that the rational choice of method is not an easy matter. Although the classical theory of statistics provides a number of principles leading to optimal procedures, there are areas of geographical epidemiology where they do not apply. In the first place, they apply essentially to the frequentist paradigm: the increasingly popular Bayesian methods raise essentially new optimality issues that are not easy to resolve. Secondly, many optimal results are asymptotic: when observations are effectively widely distributed throughout two-dimensional space asymptotic results are less likely to be applicable even in moderately large data-sets. Thirdly, many methods are essentially non-parametric and the classical optimality theory applies less directly to these. Lastly, the theoretical results apply mostly to situations where there is a large degree of independence in the structure of the data; they are therefore less applicable to models for the contagious processes needed to model alternatives to the null hypotheses in studies on clustering.

It follows that evaluating the relative merits of different methods has in practice to proceed by largely empirical methods, making extensive use of simulation. This makes appraisal difficult because of the large number of parameters that can be varied in the simulation experiments. It is important that any general principles suggested by the underlying theory are used to direct the empirical investigations, as for example, exemplified by the discussion of methods for pre-defined sources of risk in Sect. 8.7. We conclude that geographical epidemiology, despite its practical limitations, can in principle provide useful pointers to the aetiology of disease, but that the methodology would be much more convincing if we knew more about its behaviour in various plausible situations.

References

Abe O (1973) A note on the methodology of Knox's tests of "Time and Space Interaction". Biometrics 29:67–77

Anderson NH, Titterington DM (1995) Some methods for investigating spatial clustering, with epidemiological applications. Journal of the Royal Statistical Society Series A 160:87–105

Antó JM, Sunyer J (1992) Soya bean as a risk factor for epidemic asthma. In: Elliott P, Cuzick J, English D, Stern R (eds) Geographical environmental epidemiology: Methods for small-area studies. Oxford University Press for World Health Organization, Oxford, pp 323–341

Armitage P, Colton T (eds) (1998) Encyclopedia of biostatistics. Wiley, Chichester

Baris YI, Simonato L, Saracci R, Winkelmann R (1992) The epidemic of respiratory cancer associated with erionite fibres in the Cappadocian region of Turkey. In: Elliott P, Cuzick J, English D, Stern R (eds) Geographical environmental epidemiology: Methods for small-area studies. Oxford University Press for World Health Organization, Oxford, pp 310–322

Besag J, Newell J (1991) The detection of clusters in rare diseases. Journal of the Royal Statistical Society Series A 154:143–155

Bithell JF (1990) An application of density estimation to geographical epidemiology. Statistics in Medicine 9:691–701

Bithell JF (1995) The choice of test for detecting raised disease risk near a point source. Statistics in Medicine 14:2309–2322

Bithell JF (1998) Geographical analysis. In: Armitage P, Colton T (eds) Encyclopedia of biostatistics. Wiley, Chichester, pp 1701–1716

Bithell JF (1999) Disease mapping using the relative risk function estimated from areal data. In: Lawson AB, Biggeri A, Böhning D, Lesaffre E, Viel J-F, Bertollini R (eds) Disease mapping and risk assessment for public health decision making. Wiley, Chichester, pp 247–255

Bithell JF (2003) Selecting a powerful test for detecting risk near point sources. Bulletin of the International Statistical Institute 54th Session, pp 97–98

Bithell JF, Dutton SJ, Draper GJ, Neary NM (1994) Distribution of childhood leukaemias and non-Hodgkin's lymphomas near nuclear installations in England and Wales. British Medical Journal 309, 6953:501–505

Bithell JF, Dutton SJ, Neary NM, Vincent TJ (1995) Use of regression methods for control of socio-economic confounding. Journal of Epidemiology and Community Health 49, Suppl 2:S15–S19

Clayton D, Bernardinelli L (1992) Bayesian methods for mapping disease risk. In: Elliott P, Cuzick J, English D, Stern R (eds) Geographical environmental epidemiology: Methods for small-area studies. Oxford University Press for World Health Organization, Oxford, pp 205–220

Clayton D, Kaldor J (1987) Empirical Bayes estimates of age-standardized relative risks for use in disease mapping. Biometrics 43:671–682

Cliff AD, Ord JK (1981) Spatial processes: Models and applications. Pion, London

Cook DG, Pocock SJ (1983) Multiple regression in geographical mortality studies, with allowance for spatially correlated errors. Biometrics 39:361–372

Cox DR, Snell EJ (1984) The analysis of binary data, 2nd edn. Chapman and Hall, London

Cuzick J, Edwards R (1990) Spatial clustering for inhomogeneous populations (with discussion). Journal of the Royal Statistical Society, Series B 52:73–104

David FN, Barton DE (1966) Two space-time interaction tests for epidemicity. British Journal of Preventive and Social Medicine 20:44–48

Dempster AP, Schatzoff M (1965) Expected significance levels as a sensitivity index for test statistics. Journal of the American Statistical Association 60:420–436

Diggle PJ (2000) Overview of methods for disease mapping and its relationship to cluster detection. In: Elliott P, Wakefield JC, Best NG, Briggs DJ (eds) Spatial epidemiology: Methods and applications. Oxford University Press, Oxford, pp 87–103

Diggle PJ, Rowlingson BS (1994) A conditional approach to point process modelling of elevated risk. Journal of the Royal Statistical Society Series A 157:433 440

Efron B, Tibshirani R (1993) An introduction to the bootstrap. Chapman and Hall, New York

Elliott P, Cuzick J, English D, Stern R (eds) (1992) Geographical environmental epidemiology: Methods for small-area studies. Oxford University Press for World Health Organization, Oxford, pp 323–341

Elliott P, Wakefield JC, Best NG, Briggs DJ (eds) (2000) Spatial epidemiology: methods and applications. Oxford University Press, Oxford, pp 87–103

Geary RC (1954) The contiguity ratio and statistical mapping. The Incorporated Statistician 5:115–145

Gelman A, Price PN (1999) All maps of parameter estimates are misleading. Statistics in Medicine 18:3221–3234

Jacquez GM (1996) A k nearest neighbour test for space-time interaction. Statistics in Medicine 15:1935–1949

Kelsall JE, Diggle PJ (1998) Spatial variation in risk: a nonparametric binary regression approach. Applied Statistics 47:559–573

Knox EG (1964) The detection of space-time interactions. Applied Statistics 13:25–29

Kulldorf M, Hjalmars U (1999) The Knox method and other tests for space-time interaction. Biometrics: 55:544–552

Lawson AB, Biggeri A, Böhning D, Lesaffre E, Viel J-F, Bertollini R (eds) (1999) Disease mapping and risk assessment for public health decision making. Wiley, Chichester

McCullagh P, Nelder JA (1989) Generalized linear models, 2nd edn. Chapman and Hall, London

Moran PAP (1948) The interpretation of statistical maps. Journal of the Royal Statistical Society, Series 10:243–251

Pike MC, Smith PG (1974) A note on a 'close pairs' test for space clustering. British Journal of Preventive and Social Medicine 28:63–64

Potthoff RF, Whittinghill M (1966) Testing for homogeneity II. The Poisson distribution. Biometrika 53:183–190

Scott DW (1992) Multivariate density estimation. Wiley, London

Silverman BW (1986) Density estimation for statistics and data analysis. Chapman and Hall, London

Snow J (1855) On the mode of communication of cholera, 2nd edn. Churchill, London

Stone RA (1988) Investigations of excess environmental risks around putative sources: statistical problems and a proposed test. Statistics in Medicine 7:649–660

Wakefield JC, Best NG, Waller L (2000) Bayesian approaches to disease mapping. In: Elliott P, Wakefield JC, Best NG, Briggs DJ (eds) Spatial epidemiology: Methods and applications. Oxford University Press, Oxford, pp 87–103

Walter SD (1993) Assessing spatial patterns in disease rates. Statistics in Medicine 12: 1885–1894

Part III
Applications of Epidemiology

Social Epidemiology

Tarani Chandola, Michael Marmot

1.1   Introduction

Social epidemiology has been defined as the branch of epidemiology that studies the social distribution and social determinants of health (Berkman and Kawachi 2000). As all aspects of human life are inextricably bound within the context of social relations, every conceivable epidemiological exposure is related to social factors. In this broad sense, all epidemiology is social epidemiology (Kaufman and Cooper 1999) with perhaps the latter discipline making explicit the analysis of the social determinants of health.

The idea that social conditions influence health is not new. Chadwick (Flinn 1965) wrote about the insanitary conditions of the working classes and how over-crowding, damp and filth contributed to their lower life expectancy. Durkheim (1966) wrote about how social norms and conditions affect risks of suicide in the population. Social epidemiology builds and expands on this literature by posing new research questions, utilising new research methods and influencing govern-ment policy agenda. The rest of this chapter will discuss each of these three developments in social epidemiology.

1.2   Research Questions

1.2.1   The Social Determinants of Health

If the social environment is an important cause of health, this is likely to be manifested as social inequalities in health. People from better social environments with greater access to socio-economic resources are likely to have better health.

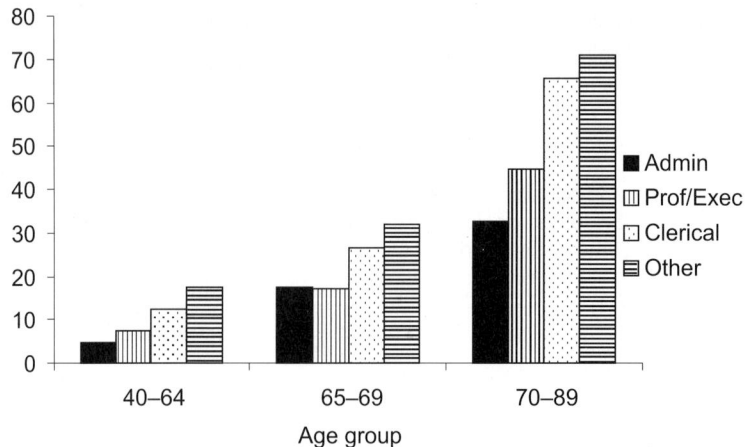

Figure 1.1. All cause mortality per 1000 person years by employment grade: Whitehall men, 25 year follow up (from Marmot and Shipley 1996)

Supporting this view, social inequalities in health have been documented for most countries, for most causes of deaths and diseases, and in most age-groups. People from lower socio-economic backgrounds are more likely to be unhealthier and have lower life expectancies, even in the richest countries. In Fig. 1.1, from the first Whitehall study on the health of civil servants in the United Kingdom (Marmot and Shipley 1996), men in the lowest, office support employment grades have mortality rates four times that of men in the highest administrative grades in the youngest age-group. This difference in mortality between hierarchies in the civil service remains even after retirement among men in the oldest age group. What remains unclear are the pathways leading from the social structure to health- or the social determinants of health.

There have been a number of attempts to delineate the pathways underlying the social determinants of health. One such example is illustrated in Fig. 1.2 (from Marmot and Wilkinson 1999). Social structure, top left of Fig. 1.2, influences well-being and health, at the bottom right. The influences of the social structure operate

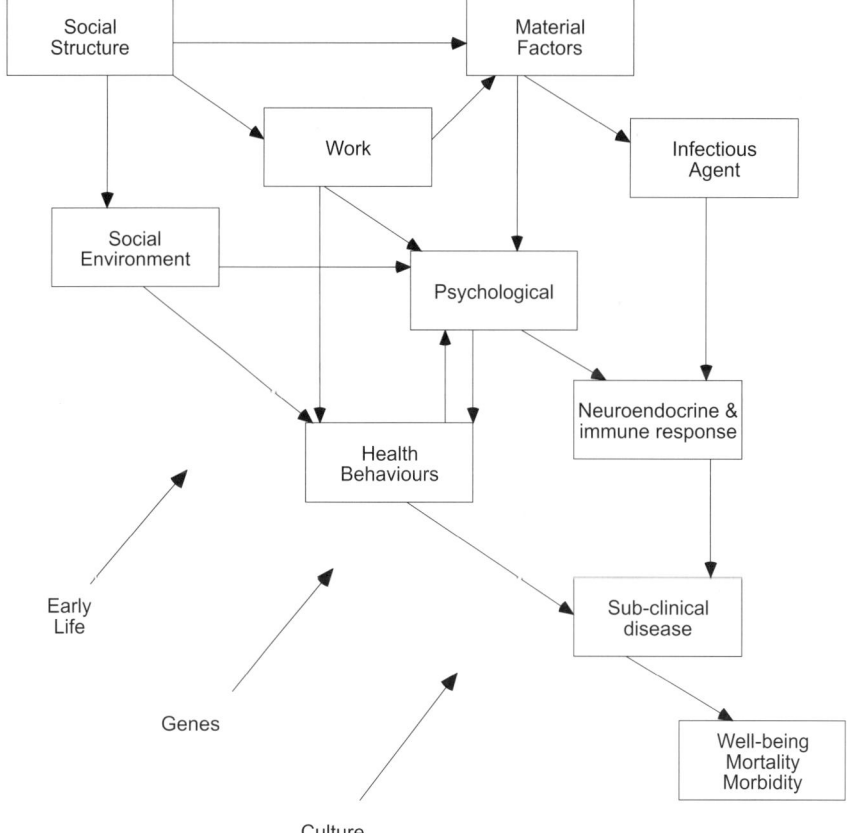

Figure 1.2. The social determinants of health

via three main pathways- material factors, work and the social environment. While material factors such as poverty and unhygienic circumstances may be directly related to disease through infectious agents, the social and work environments may affect health through psychological and behavioural pathways, which in turn have biological consequences for well-being, morbidity and mortality. Work environments may also affect health through hazardous material working conditions such as radiation or chemical/biological hazards. There has been relatively little testing of the pathways between social structure and health, primarily because to date, there have been few data available to test these pathways. However, a few studies have examined some of these pathways and their contribution towards understanding social inequalities in health. The rest of this section of the book chapter will highlight some of the research on the search for the social determinants of health.

1.2.2   Health Behaviours

People from lower socio-economic groups are more likely to smoke, drink alcohol excessively, have less physical exercise and unhealthier diets. It is likely that such unhealthy behaviours form part of the pathways underlying social inequalities in health. Poor people in the UK are less likely than those who are well off to eat a good diet, more likely to have a sedentary lifestyle, more likely to be obese, and more likely to be regularly drunk (Fig. 1.3, from Colhoun and Prescott-Clarke 1996). Some studies have analysed the contribution of such health behaviours to explaining the social gradient in health and have found that a substantial social gradient in health still remains even after adjusting for such (un)healthy lifestyles

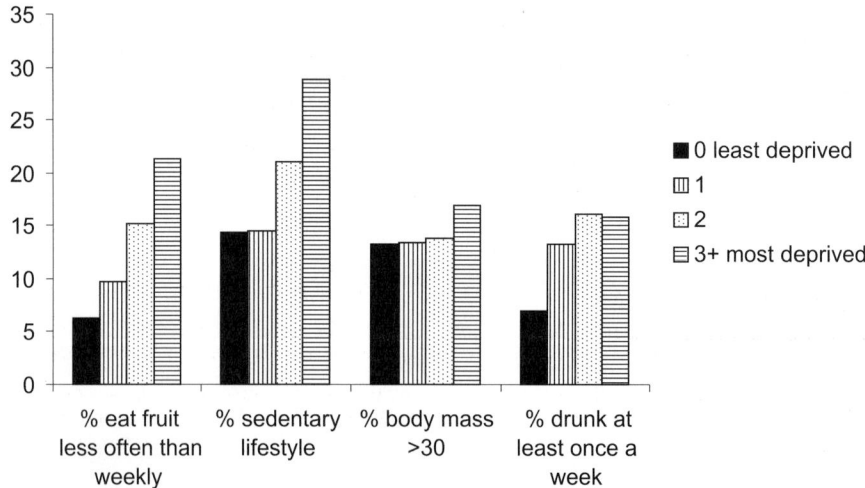

Figure 1.3. Distribution of some health behaviours among men by level of socio-economic deprivation (from Colhoun and Prescott-Clarke 1996)

(Marmot et al. 1978). So there may be other social determinants of health not directly related to health behaviours, as suggested by the pathways through work and material factors in Fig. 1.2. Some evidence of these other pathways is discussed in Sects. 1.2.3 to 1.2.7.

Lynch et al. (1997) argue that we still need to understand why poor people behave poorly. Without some understanding of how the social environment influences behaviour (through, for example, social norms or environments which may be health damaging or health promoting such as workplace restrictions on smoking or stressful environments for which smoking may be an effective, albeit temporary coping strategy), interventions to modify behavioural risk factors may not be successful.

Material, Economic and Political Determinants of Health   1.2.3

The link between health and material or socio-economic circumstances has been observed at least since mid 19th century Britain, if not earlier. Chadwick (Flinn 1965) wrote about how overcrowding, damp and filthy living conditions contributed to the lower life expectancy of working class men. In 1848, partly through fear of cholera and partly through pressure from Chadwick, the British parliament passed the first Public Health Act. This, in addition to the pioneering work of the epidemiologist John Snow (1855), set in motion the public health movement in 19th century Britain which saw improvements in housing, sewage and drainage, water supply and contagious diseases and provided Britain with the most extensive public health system in the world.

It has also been argued that much of the decrease in the mortality rate in the 19th and early 20th century was primarily due to better nutrition in the population which led to increased host resistance to opportunistic infections (McKeown 1979). The driver behind better diets in the general population can be traced to economic growth which made nutritious foods more easily affordable by most of the population. Others, like Szreter (1988), argue that the public health movement of the mid 19th century in the UK also played an important role in combating deaths due to infectious disease. It is likely that a combination of macro-economic factors (economic growth) and public policies (public health measures) led to the overall decreases in mortality rates due to infectious diseases and increases in life expectancy.

In 20th century industrialised societies, infectious diseases played an increasingly smaller role in causing deaths while chronic diseases such as heart disease and cancers caused the majority of deaths. Although people from poorer social classes are more susceptible to such chronic diseases (repeating the patterns of infectious diseases like cholera in 19th century Britain), the mechanisms underlying this social patterning of chronic diseases are not easy to specify. A single infectious agent such as a bacterial agent which thrives in unhygienic circumstances is unlikely to account for why poorer, less advantaged people have more heart attacks.

Some authors argue that, even today, economic and political processes are the fundamental determinants of health and disease (Coburn 2000; Navarro and Shi

2001). Determinants of health can be analysed in terms of who benefits from specific government policies and practices. Economic and political institutions and decisions that create, enforce and perpetuate social inequality also create and maintain social inequalities in health. For example, neo-liberal (market oriented) policies which favour the dismantling of the welfare state may help to widen existing social inequalities in health. Navarro and Shi (2001) found that countries with more economic and social redistributive policies (Sweden, Finland, Norway, Denmark and Austria) were more successful in improving the health of their populations (reducing their infant mortality rate). In contrast, neo-liberal countries (Canada, United States, United Kingdom, Ireland) where the market reigns supreme and the welfare state is the weakest had the lowest rates of improvements in the infant mortality rates. The substantial decline in life expectancy in Russia in the 1990s has been linked to its transition to a neo-liberal economy (Walberg et al. 1998).

1.2.4   Life Course

The idea that a person's experiences over a life time can have cumulative effects on their health is a central idea within social epidemiology. The study of long term effects of physical and social exposures during gestation, childhood, adolescence, young adulthood and later adult life on the risk of chronic disease has been defined as a life course approach to chronic disease epidemiology (Ben-Shlomo and Kuh 2002). Such studies include biological, behavioural and psychosocial pathways that operate over an individual's life course, as well as across generations, to influence the course of chronic disease. However, it is only in fairly recent years that adequate data and appropriate statistical methods have been made available to test the hypotheses associated with a developmental and life course perspective.

There are three different ways in which factors from early life might influence subsequent disease risk (Power and Hertzman 1997). The first is a latency model of early life experiences which hypothesises that experiences in utero and early life affect cardiovascular disease in adulthood (Barker 1991, 1997). Barker found evidence that birthweight and other indicators of fetal growth in the newborn are related to fibrinogen and insulin resistance fifty years later. He also found that birthweight is related to functioning of the hypothalamic-pituitary-adrenal axis. Low birthweight is associated with poorer childhood health which some researchers have linked to lower social position in adulthood (Illsley 1986). This evidence suggests that a short term exposure in utero can have a long latency period with adverse health and social consequences in adulthood.

Another theory of the life course suggests that the accumulation of social advantage and disadvantage throughout the life course affects adult health (Ross and Wu 1995). Studies that have examined social circumstances in childhood and beyond do show an effect of social advantage throughout the lifetime (in childhood, early adulthood and later adulthood) on blood pressure, obesity (Wadsworth 1997) and measures of health status. A third life-course pathway is one in which childhood circumstances may not affect adult risk of ill health and disease directly. It is possible that parental social class and educational qualifications are important because they help to determine the social circumstances in which the offspring lives and works in adult life, and it is these circumstances that give rise to social inequalities in disease. Some studies have found the relationship of education on adult health can be explained in terms of occupational class and income (Dahl 1994, Davey Smith et al. 1998). Although other studies have found the relationship of education to health remains strong even after controlling for occupational class and income (Winkleby et al. 1992).

Social Biology   1.2.5

Human beings are both social and biological, and understanding the interaction between the two is crucial to understanding the social determinants of health. The biological processes that underlie the social determinants of health makes explicit the pathways from psychosocial factors to biological responses. Psychosocial factors may affect health in two distinct ways – they may directly cause biological changes which predispose to disease, or they may, indirectly, influence behaviours such as smoking and diet, which in turn affects health (Brunner 2000).

The direct effect of psychosocial factors on biology may be through the experience of chronic stresses which in turn modify neuroendocrine and physiological functioning (Selye 1956). Humans are adapted to meet the challenge of short-term threats. However, frequent and prolonged activation of the fight-or-flight response or defence reaction appears to be maladapted (Sapolsky 1993). The main axes of the neuroendocrine response appears to be the sympatho-adrenal and hypothalamic-pituitary-adrenal (HPA) systems (Brunner 2000). The former, the sympatho-adrenal system is characterised by the rapid release of adrenaline from the adrenal medulla and noradrenaline from the sympathetic nerve endings, which produces among other things, cognitive arousal, raised blood pressure and glucose mobilisation. There is evidence of wide variations between individuals in the size and duration of these endocrine responses attributed to individual differences in psychological coping resources (Grossman 1991). The HPA system involves cortisol release from the adrenal cortex. Like the sympatho-adrenal system, functioning of the HPA axis also appears to be conditioned by psychosocial factors (Hellhammer et al. 1997). Lower social position is associated with prolonged elevations or cortisol release or blunted responses from a raised baseline (Suomi 1997). These patterns of cortisol secretion differ from the normal sharp response and rapid return to a low baseline. A comparison of Swedish and Lithuanian men given a stress test revealed higher morning cortisols and blunted reactivity among the low-income group drawn from the higher coronary risk Lithuanian population (Kristenson et al. 1998).

There is some evidence for the hypothesis that psychosocial factors directly affect neuroendocrine mechanisms which result in social inequalities in coronary heart disease. Hostility and anxiety have been linked with reduced heart rate variability (HRV) which refers to the beat-to-beat alterations in heart rate (Hemingway et al. 1998). HRV appears to be sensitive and responsive to acute stress as well as a marker of cumulative wear and tear. HRV has been shown to decline with the aging process which has been attributed to a decrease in efferent vagal tone and reduced beta-adrenergic responsiveness. By contrast, regular physical activity (which slows down the aging process) has been shown to raise HRV, presumably by increasing vagal tone.

The metabolic syndrome is a well-known precursor state to coronary heart disease (CHD) and is linked with increased risk of type-2 diabetes. The main components of the metabolic syndrome are impaired glucose tolerance, insulin resistance, and disturbances of lipoprotein metabolism characterised by raised serum triglycerides and low HDL cholesterol (Folsom et al. 1989; Seidell et al. 1990). Although the link between the metabolic syndrome and CHD is well-established, the association between psychosocial factors and the metabolic syndrome is less certain. Central obesity and other components of the metabolic syndrome are consistently related to low socio-economic position in industrialised countries (Brunner et al. 1993; Kaplan and Keil 1993) It is possible that chronic psychosocial stresses result (directly) in the metabolic syndrome pattern of abnormalities through the activation of the HPA axis. Increased HPA activity results in redistribution of body fat leading to central obesity, hypertension and type-2 diabetes as found in Cushing's syndrome (Howlet et al. 1985). The alternative explanation is that psychosocial stresses lead to unhealthy behaviours (smoking, inappropriate diets). However, in the Whitehall II cohort, adjusting for health behaviours did not change the social gradient in the metabolic syndrome, suggesting a direct neuroendocrine effect (Brunner et al. 1997).

Infectious disease may also contribute to social differences in morbidity. Helicobater pylori infection, acquired in childhood, is linked with deprivation and over-crowded housing, and may produce long-term low level systemic inflammatory responses which enhance atherogenesis. In Whitehall II, employment grade and chronic low control at work are linked to raised fibrinogen (Brunner et al. 1995) raising the possibility that inflammatory processes may mediate the effect of psychosocial circumstances on CHD.

1.2.6   Ecological Perspectives

In the UK and elsewhere, there are marked differences in health between areas. People living in areas with higher levels of poverty have poorer health on average and lower average life expectancy. However, explanations for these area differences in health remain debatable. Some argue that excess mortality in deprived areas can be wholly explained by the concentration of poorer people in those areas (Slogett and Joshi 1994; Duncan et al. 1993). In other words, the compositional or aggregate effect of poor individuals (each of whom has lower than average life expectancy) in an area explains the lower average life expectancy for the area. Others argue that such compositional effects cannot entirely explain area differences in health (Diez-Roux et al. 1997). They point out that even after adjusting for the composition of individuals living in an area (such as their income and wealth levels), significant area differences in health remain. They argue that there may be contextual or ecological reasons for area differences in health. There may be particular characteristics of an area such as its pollution levels or its lack of medical services which may have an impact on the health of everyone living in that area (Macintyre et al. 1993). Research from the United States has found that states with lower levels of trust have higher rates of violent crime, including homicide (Kawachi et al. 1999a). Such contextual effects may also interact with an individual's characteristics and this combined interaction may alter their risk of disease. For example, the lack of medical services may have a greater impact on the health of poor people living in an area compared to richer people who may have the resources to travel or access medical services outside their local area. Such ecological or contextual characteristics clearly form part of the social determinants of health and may play some role in explaining social inequalities in (individual) health.

Ecological approaches were disfavoured for many years in social epidemiology (Macintyre and Ellaway 2000). Although public health practioners in the 19th and early 20th centuries focused on dealing with health damaging and promoting environments such as sewage, clean water, housing and physical working conditions, the decline in infectious diseases led to less emphasis being placed on such ecological factors. The rediscovery of social inequalities in health towards the end of the 20th century focussed primarily on the role of individual health-risk factors such as behaviours, low income, lack of employment and education and a relative neglect of contextual or environmental determinants of health. This neglect has been explicitly addressed in the most recent literature with multilevel analyses that explicitly take into account compositional and contextual social factors that affect health (Macintyre and Ellaway 2000).

General Susceptibility to Disease   1.2.7

According to the general susceptibility hypothesis (Syme and Berkman 1976), social factors influence disease by creating a vulnerability or susceptibility to disease in general rather than to any specific disorder. This idea was built on the observation that many social conditions are linked to a broad range of diseases. While behavioural, environmental, biological and genetic factors influence specific diseases, these factors may interact with socially stressful conditions in the development of these diseases resulting in illness and early mortality.

As discussed above, research from social biology shows that some stressful experiences activate multiple hormones, affecting multiple systems and potentially producing wide-ranging organ damage. The cumulative experience of stress may affect a variety of chronic and infectious diseases through neuroendocrine-mediated biological pathways. There are a number of different sources of stressful experiences, some of which are discussed below. The linking of such stressful experiences (often measured using psychological concepts) to wider social circumstances has been called a psychosocial approach to understanding the social determinants of health.

Social Support

The effect of social support and social networks on health has been researched (at least) since the late 19th century when Durkheim investigated the links between social integration and suicide. He explained suicide in terms of social dynamics, arguing that suicide is not an isolated individual tragedy but a reflection of social conditions such as the lack of attachment and regulation in society. Attachment is also a core concept for Bowlby (1969) who argued that marriage is the adult equivalent of childhood attachment between mother and child. Secure attachment, whether in terms of parent-child or marital relationships, provides for successful and healthy development. Men who have never married or have recently divorced have a significantly greater risk of dying from both cardiovascular and non-cardiovascular diseases than married men (Ebrahim et al. 1995). Married women are generally healthier than unmarried women as well, although the health benefits of marriage may not be particularly strong for employed women (Waldron et al. 1996).

Throughout the 1970s and 1980s, a series of studies appeared which consistently showed that the lack of social ties or social networks predicted mortality from almost every cause of death (Berkman 1995). Social ties and networks were measured in terms of numbers of close friends and relatives, marital status, and membership in religious or voluntary associations. Since then, studies have gone on to focus on the provision of social support rather than on the elaboration of the structural aspects of social networks. Not all social ties or networks are supportive and there is variation in the type, frequency and extent of support provided. Social support, in theory, can be divided into emotional support (usually provided by a confidant or intimate other), instrumental support (or help in kind, money or labour), appraisal support (help in decision making) and informational support (provision of advice or information). Lack of emotional support has been linked to early cardiovascular disease mortality among both men and women, younger and older people (Berkman et al. 1992). Other studies have found that social integration, particularly operating though emotional support, influence recovery from strokes (Berkman and Glass 2000).

Social Disorganisation

Social scientists have puzzled over why some societies seem to prosper, possess effective political institutions and have better health outcomes compared to other societies. One of the hypotheses that has been proposed to explain this difference between societies is the amount of social capital or cohesion (and its converse-social disorganisation) in a particular society (Coleman 1988, Putnam 2000). Social cohesion refers to the extent of connectedness and solidarity among groups in society. A cohesive society has greater amounts of social capital (higher levels of interpersonal trust, reciprocity and mutual aid) than a disorganised society. There is emerging evidence that greater social capital is linked to lower mortality rates as well as better self-rated health (Kawachi and Berkman 2000). As mentioned in Sect. 1.2.6, states in the United States with lower levels of trust have higher homicide rates (Kawachi et al. 1999a). Even after adjusting for individual risk factors for poor self-rated health (e.g. low income, low education, smoking, obesity, lack of access to health care), individuals living in US states with low social capital were at increased risk of poor self-rated health (Kawachi et al. 1999b). Such results suggest that there are contextual explanations for area differences in health as discussed in the section on ecological perspectives.

Social capital may be linked to health through a number of different mechanisms. We have already discussed two types of explanations for understanding area differences in health- compositional and contextual explanations. Socially isolated individuals (not having contacts with friends or relatives, not belonging to any groups) are more likely to be living in communities with lower social capital so the association between social capital and health may be the compositional effect of the aggregation of socially isolated individuals. However, there may be other pathways by which social capital affects health (Kawachi and Berkman 2000):

1. Through health related behaviours. Social capital may influence the health behaviours of neighbourhood residents by exerting social control over deviant behaviours such as adolescent smoking, drinking and drug abuse.
2. Through access to services. Socially cohesive neighbourhoods are more successful at organisation access to services such as transport, health services and recreational facilities
3. Through psychosocial processes. Socially disorganised neighbourhoods with low social capital could have higher levels of fear of crime and other stressors which could negatively impact on the residents' health.

Work Stress

One of the more established results in epidemiology has been the link between physical working conditions and health. Reports on occupational health have highlighted the link between emphysema and other lung disease with coal mining, musculoskeletal disorders and accidents with certain types of manual work. In recent years, there has been increased research on work related stress and how that affects both physical and mental health.

There are two dominant models of work stress in the literature. The first, the job strain model is based on the concepts of job control and demands (Karasek et al. 1981). Workers with low levels of job control and high levels of demand are said to have high levels of job strain (or work stress). Job control (or decision latitude) consists of whether or not workers are able to utilise and develop skills (skill discretion) and their authority over decisions. Job demands consist of qualitative emotional demands as well as quantitative demands specifying output per unit of time. Prolonged and repeated exposure to job strain is hypothesised to increase sympathadrenal arousal and decrease the body's ability to restore and repair tissues which in turn affects health. Civil servants in the UK with greater exposure to job strain and lower job control have higher levels of fibrinogen (Brunner et al. 1996), which may result in their higher risks of coronary heart disease (Bosma et al. 1997).

The other model of work stress, the effort-reward imbalance model (Siegrist 1996), hypothesises that the degree to which workers are rewarded for their efforts is crucial for their health. When a high degree of effort does not meet a high degree of reward, emotional tensions arise and the risk of illness increases. Effort is the individual's response to their job demands and this response may be extrinsic effort (referring to the individual's effort to cope with external job demands) and intrinsic effort (referring to the individual's drive to fulfil their goals). Reward can be measured through financial rewards, self-esteem and social control. While there is some overlap between the job strain and effort reward imbalance models, the former is entirely focussed on the organisation of the structure of work while the latter includes the individual's way or coping methods of handling difficulties (through the concept of intrinsic effort).

There is some evidence that both models of work stress contribute independently of one another to predicting coronary heart disease events (Bosma et al. 1998). The cumulative adverse health impact of low job control and effort-reward imbalance indicates that both job stress factors provide supplementary information on the relevant stressors in the psychosocial work environment.

Unemployment and Job Loss

There has been considerable research into the effects of unemployment and job loss on health. However, this is an area of research that is particularly sensitive to the claims of "health selection", that the reason why unemployment is associated with ill health is because ill health selects people out of employment. The reverse argument is that a disadvantaged socio-economic position has an effect on a stable job career (and the risk of unemployment) as well as health. It is therefore important to disentangle the causal narrative in studies about unemployment and health and find out which comes first.

The evidence on unemployment and health supports both the social causation and health selection interpretations. In a review of the effect of unemployment on health, Kasl and Jones (2000) summarised the evidence as follows:

1. Unemployment is associated with a 20%–30% excess in all cause mortality in most studies
2. There is some evidence of the impact of unemployment on physical morbidity but with results that are more difficult to interpret
3. Unemployment is linked to biological indicators of stress reactivity
4. Unemployment is associated with behavioural and lifestyle risk factors although the direction of causality is hard to disentangle
5. Unemployment clearly increases psychological distress
6. Threatened job loss (job insecurity) is associated with physical and psychological morbidity and cardiovascular risk. The anticipation of job loss affects health even before changes in employment status (Ferrie et al. 1995).

Depression and Affective States

Depression is one of the most common psychiatric problems and is also common in patients with chronic medical conditions. Some depressive episodes are brought upon by physical illness, but many depressive patients have depressive episodes long before they develop any physical symptoms of illness. Furthermore, depression may alter the course and outcome of physical illness (Carney and Feedland 2000).

Depression has been associated with immunological dysfunction. Patients with major depression have been found to have blunted natural killer cell activity (Maes et al. 1994) increasing their risk for many acute and chronic illnesses. There is also some evidence that depression may play a causal role in the development of heart disease. There is some evidence of a social gradient in depression in a healthy, working population – it appears to be more common among those from poorer, more disadvantaged social positions (Stansfeld et al. 1998) and may originate from their lower control over aspects of their work and home environment (Griffin et al. 2002).

Another set of psychological pathways by which social conditions may affect health is through emotions and the physiological, cognitive and behavioural responses they evoke. Emotions may be transitory states brought on by specific situations, or traits, i.e. stable and general dispositions to experience particular emotions (Spielberger and Krasner 1988). Much of the research on emotion and health has carried out in relation to coronary heart disease. Much of this literature has focussed on type A behaviour, (which includes a free-floating but well rationalised hostility, hyperaggressiveness and a sense of time urgency), chronic anger and hostility, anxiety and a mixture of emotions associated with depression including hopelessness, loneliness, guilt and shame (Kubzansky and Kawachi 2000).

There is some evidence of a social patterning of emotions (Bradburn 1969; Mroczek and Kolarz 1998). Kemper (1993) suggests that many emotions are responses to power and status differentials embedded within social situations. Potentially stressful events can be associated with a variety of different emotions. Emotions can be considered as products of stress as well as mediators of its effects thus representing a crucial link in the chain of causation from social stressors to individual biological responses (Spielberger and Krasner 1988). Evidence from animal studies suggest that additional to hypothalamic control of the stress response, areas of the brain involved with emotional or affective responses such as the limbic system also play a major role in stress responses (Menzhaghi et al. 1993) and adaptation to the stress response (Sapolsky et al. 1986).

Research Methods   1.3

Applying a Population Perspective   1.3.1

Rose (1992) proposed that an individual's risk of illness cannot be considered in isolation from the risk of disease of the population to which they belong. For example, the distribution of cholesterol levels in the Finnish population is shifted to the right of the Japanese distribution – on average, Finnish people have higher cholesterol levels than Japanese people. The level of "normal" cholesterol for the Finnish population would be "abnormal" for the Japanese population and would be a risk factor for CHD in the latter population. Applying the population perspective into epidemiological research means asking "why does this population have this particular distribution of risk factors", in addition to asking "why did a particular individual get sick?" (Berkman and Kawachi 2000). Answering the second question has been the focus of clinical medicine while answering the first question is the key to the largest improvements in the health of the population as it focuses attention on the majority of cases of illness within the bulk of the population. Medical care can prolong survival after some serious diseases, but the social and economic conditions that affect whether people become ill are more important for health gains in the population as a whole.

1.3.2   Better Measures of Exposures

There is no simple relationship between social-structural conditions such as income distribution and welfare state regimes on the one hand and health inequalities in the population on the other. The different pathways by which different social factors can have an effect on different health outcomes implies that there is no single measure of social factors, health outcomes or single pathway between the two that can adequately represent the complexity of the associations between the social structure and health. One of the ways of advancing our knowledge of the social determinants of health is by utilising better measures of the social structure, the health outcomes as well as the pathways that link exposures and outcomes. One of the defining characteristics of research in social epidemiology has been the constant refinement of such measures and improvements in the methodology of measuring complex concepts and associations.

In the UK, the standard epidemiological measure of social class since the start of the 20th century has been the Registrar General's social class (RGSC). However, the RGSC as been heavily criticised by being atheoretical – the basis for classifying people into different social classes has never been made explicit (Szreter 1984). The changeover to a more theoretically based measure of social class – the National Statistics Socio-Economic Classification – based on differences in employment relations and conditions, was prompted in part by research in social epidemiology which found that the RGSC was not useful in understanding the social determinants of health (Bartley et al. 1996). Other research (Chandola 2001) has similarly argued that the standard epidemiological technique of controlling for social class does not have much meaning, especially when the measure of social class does not adequately represent the different dimensions of the social structure that affect health (such as housing and neighbourhood conditions, labour market conditions, employment relations, household income and social status). In attempting to understand the social determinants of health, research into social epidemiology has pioneered the use of better measures of the social structure.

Better Measures of Health   1.3.3

The concept of health is multidimensional (the WHO definition states that health is a state of complete physical, mental and social well-being), including hard to measure concepts like quality of life. Research in social epidemiology does not just focus on clinically measured disease outcomes because the absence of disease is not sufficient for health. Rather, one of the main focuses of social epidemiological research is the use of health related quality of life measures as valid measures of health outcomes (Fitzpatrick et al. 1992). Population mortality statistics tell us little about the health of general populations in developed countries. The use of standardised health related quality of life measures in different countries (Ware and Gandek 1998) enable international comparisons of physical, mental and social well-being.

Subjective health status covers a wide variety of areas, including role functioning (e.g. the ability to perform domestic and work tasks), the degree of social and community interaction, psychological well being, pain, tiredness and satisfaction with life (Bowling 1997). Health related quality of life has come to mean a combination of subjectively assessed measures of health, including physical function, social function, emotional or mental state, burden of symptoms and sense of well being (Coulter 1995). The development and use of such subjective measures of health status and health related quality of life, have been one of the defining aspects of social epidemiology.

Better Measures of the Association
Between the Social Structure and Health   1.3.4

As different measures of the social structure may have different pathways to different health outcomes, the reduction of such differences into a single regression model may obscure rather than elucidate the pathways underlying the social determinants of health. Furthermore, different dimensions of the social structure may influence people's health at different time points of the life-course. For example, in industrialised societies, the period of the life-course when compulsory education is completed may be a crucial time for the health of the population, not because young adults are at a particular high risk of disease or illness at that stage in life, but because educational qualifications are a strong determinant of social position in later adult life which in turn appear to be strongly linked to health outcomes later on in life. It is important to take account of the temporal and causal ordering of the various measures of social position and use methods that make explicit the various underlying causal pathways between different measures of social position and health. There are a number of such causal modelling methods being used in social epidemiological research (Greenland and Brumback 2002). Failure to take account of the different pathways between the social structure and health outcomes could result in biased results (Singh-Manoux et al. 2002).

Analysing Population Surveys, Birth Cohorts

One of the defining characteristics of research methods in social epidemiology is the use of population representative sample surveys in analysing the social determinants of health. Research in social epidemiology tends to use non-experimental observational studies, both cross sectional and longitudinal. All observational studies suffer from problems of causality – it is hard to determine and separate out cause from effect (cf. Chap. I.1 and I.9 of this handbook). This drawback has necessitated the use and development of complex study designs and analytical methods to disentangle the causal pathways underlying the social determinants of health.

Studies with good methodological designs (for example, Ferri et al. 2003) in social epidemiology tend to rely on data from large scale population representative sample surveys because of the complexity of the social structure and the different pathways to health. The representativeness of data is crucial in order to apply a population perspective in social epidemiological research. Smaller scale samples may not be representative of the broader population.

Birth cohort studies are a special type of such large scale population representative samples which incorporates a life course approach to epidemiology. The UK has taken a prominent role in the development of such longitudinal studies. The British Birth Cohort Studies of those born in one week of 1946, 1958 and 1970 link data from one part of the life course (from birth onwards) to another (childhood, adolescence, adulthood) for a large number of individuals. Comparisons between different birth cohort studies enable the disentangling of age, period and cohort effects, which could be problematic when analysing most cross-sectional and even longitudinal sample surveys. For example, in the book, "Changing Lives, Changing Britain" (Ferri et al. 2003), *cohort* effects that might be attributed to socio-economic change impacting differentially on people born at different times, can be differentiated from *age* differences reflecting the different changes between the stages of life, which in turn can be differentiated from the prevailing socio-economic context at the time of data collection – the *period* effect. Such analyses of this unique set of longitudinal data, incorporating a life-course perspective, is very promising for future research into social epidemiology.

Setting Government Policy Agenda

One of the goals of epidemiology has always been to use what we learn to improve public health. The science of social epidemiology has repeatedly shown evidence that social conditions are a major determinant of health. However, the translation of the research findings of social epidemiology into public policy has not been straightforward. Unlike results from some branches of epidemiology which can be more easily implemented into government guidelines (such as recommended alcohol intake) or public policy (reduction in smoking prevalence), programs to implement findings from social epidemiology need to take into the account the complexity of the pathways from the social structure to health.

Some authors argue that policy interventions are most effective when they are closest to the root causes of disease (Rothmane et al. 1998). Interventions at the upstream, social level may not be as efficient as interventions closer to disease occurrence. So, for example, policy interventions on reducing the social gap in smoking-related diseases, should focus on interventions on smoking cessation rather than interventions on the social causes of smoking. Others argue (such as Coburn (2000), mentioned in the Sect. 1.2.3) that interventions need to be upstream, at the societal and macro-economic level, in order to successfully reduce health inequalities.

The Black and Acheson Reports   1.4.1

The Black report (DHSS 1980) into inequalities in health in the UK had a number of wide-ranging policy recommendations for reducing such inequalities. However, the lack of implementation of these policies by the British government in the 1980s and early 1990s was due, in part, to a lack of political will and the high cost of these policy recommendations.

The change in government in Britain in 1996 (from Conservative to Labour) paved the way for the publication of the Acheson Report (Acheson 1998) on inequalities in health in 1998 with another list of recommendations for reducing health inequalities. What makes this publication unique is the acceptance by the UK government that some action was needed to reduce inequalities in health. For example, the UK government department of health has subsequently adopted targets on reducing inequalities in health (such as closing the social class gap in infant mortality rates). Here is some evidence that research in social epidemiology is being translated into government policy.

However, the policies that have been developed to reduce such health inequalities focus on reducing social inequalities in general (through income redistribution policies for example). The very fact that social epidemiology deals with the social structure necessitates policies aimed at changing the social structure. Such policies are not always easy to specify and detail. Furthermore, the diffuse ownership of such policies between government departments (such as education, health and treasury departments) makes their implementation harder. In recognition of the complexities of policies aimed at reducing health inequalities, the UK government set up a cross cutting spending review (across various government departments) on tackling health inequalities. This report (Department of Health 2002) explicitly acknowledges that policies on reducing health inequalities need to be co-ordinated across a wide range of government departments and bodies (not just the national health service), including local government and health organisations and sets in process the institutional framework for such co-ordination.

1.4.2   Collating Evidence for Policies Through Intervention Studies and Cross National Comparative Studies

One of the ways of ensuring appropriate policies for reducing inequalities in health are implemented is by studying the results from intervention studies. However, social epidemiological research does not easily lend itself to intervention studies, mainly because the complexity of the social structure makes it hard to disentangle the pathways to reductions in health inequalities. For example, it is hard to disentangle changes from behavioural change interventions from secular trends in society (Susser 1995). It is also difficult to separate out the influence of secondary support (from support groups organised around behavioural interventions) from the intended influence of the behavioural intervention (Spiegel et al. 1989). Social support interventions have had mixed results partly because as relationships develop and change slowly, the benefits of support interventions may be missed in the short-term (Glass 2000).

Another method of analysing policy recommendations for health inequalities is through international and longitudinal comparisons of health inequalities. Changes in taxation and income redistribution policies within a country may be hypothesised to have an effect on health inequalities. Furthermore, cross national longitudinal comparisons of different tax policies and their effect on health inequalities may be another way of analysing the effect of policies on health inequalities (Navarro and Shi 2001). However, to date, there has been little research in this area which means that current policies on reducing inequalities in health may not be entirely appropriate or well targeted.

1.5   Conclusions

Perhaps, the major contribution of social epidemiology to epidemiology in general has been in rediscovering and analysing the role of social factors in producing health and illness. This has primarily come about by the literature on social inequalities in health and consequently, research into the social determinants of health. The search for the pathways between the social structure and health has led to innovations in longitudinal research methodology. While social epidemiology shares common epidemiological problems of reliance on observational studies and problems in interpreting causality, the incorporation of a life-course perspective by analysing and comparing birth-cohort studies holds great promise for future studies. Research into social epidemiology has influenced wide ranging government social policies, because of the macro-societal level interventions that are needed to reduce inequalities in health.

Although there is some debate over the usefulness of the specialisation of social epidemiology within the medical sciences (Zielhus and Kiemeney 2001), others have argued that the overall contribution of social epidemiology towards understanding current and changing distributions of population health have been striking (Krieger 2001, Muntaner 2001). The interdisciplinary nature of social epidemiology has led to the incorporation of research questions, methods and policy agendas that have enriched our understanding of the social determinants of health.

Acknowledgements. Tarani Chandola is supported by a grant to the Whitehall II study by the Medical Research Council. Michael Marmot is supported by a Medical Research Council Research Professorship

References

Bowling A (1997) Measuring health: A review of quality of life measurement scales. Open University Press, Milton Keynes

Acheson D (1998) Inequalities in health: Report of an independent inquiry. HMSO, London

Barker DJP (1991) The foetal and infant origins of inequalities in health in Britain. Journal of Public Health Medicine 12:64–68

Barker DJP (1997) Fetal nutrition and cardiovascular disease in later life. British Medical Bulletin 53:96–108

Bartley M, Carpenter L, Dunnell K, Fitzpatrick R (1996) Measuring inequalities in health: An analysis of mortality patterns from two social classifications. Sociology of Health and Illness 18:455–475

Ben-Shlomo Y, Kuh D (2002) A life course approach to chronic disease epidemiology: Conceptual models, empirical challenges, and interdisciplinary perspectives. International Journal of Epidemiology 31:285–293

Berkman LF (1995) The role of social relations in health promotion. Psychosomatic Medicine 57:245–254

Berkman LF, Glass T (2000) Social integration, networks and health. In: Berkman LF, Kawachi I (eds) Social epidemiology. Oxford University Press, New York, pp 137–173

Berkman LF, Kawachi I (2000) A historical framework for social epidemiology. In: Berkman LF, Kawachi I (eds) Social epidemiology. Oxford University Press, New York, pp 3–12

Berkman LF, Leo-Summers L, Horwitz RI (1992) Emotional support and survival after myocardial infarction. A prospective, population-based study of the elderly. Annals of Internal Medicine 117:1003–1009

Bosma H, Marmot MG, Hemingway H, Nicholson A, Brunner EJ, Stansfeld S (1997) Low job control and risk of coronary heart disease in the Whitehall II (prospective cohort) study. British Medical Journal 314:558–565

Bosma H, Peter R, Siegrist J, Marmot MG (1998) Two alternative job stress models and the risk of coronary heart disease. American Journal of Public Health 88:68–74

Bowlby J (1969) Attachment and loss vol. 1 Attachment. Hogarth Press, London

Bradburn NM (1969) The structure of psychological well-being. ALDINE, Chicago

Brunner EJ (2000) Toward a new social biology. In: Berkman LF, Kawachi I (eds) Social epidemiology. Oxford University Press, New York, pp 306–331

Brunner EJ, Davey Smith G, Marmot MG, Canner R, Beksinska M, O'Brien J (1996) Childhood social circumstances and psychosocial and behavioural factors as determinants of plasma fibrinogen, Lancet 347:1008–1013

Brunner EJ, Marmot MG, Nanchahal K, Shipley MJ, Stansfeld SA, Juneja M, Alberti KGMM (1997) Social inequality in coronary risk: Central obesity and the metabolic syndrome. Evidence from the WII study. Diabetologia 40:1341–1349

Brunner EJ, Mendall MA, Marmot MG (1995) Past or present Helicobacter pylori infection and fibrinogen – a possible link between social class and coronary risk? Journal of Epidemiology and Community Health 49:545

Brunner EJ, Nicholson A, Marmot MG (1993) Trends in central obesity and insulin resistance across employment grades: The WII Study. Journal of Epidemiology and Community Health 47:404–405

Carney RM, Feedland KE (2000) Depression and mental illness. In: Berkman LF, Kawachi I (eds) Social epidemiology. Oxford University Press, New York, pp 191–212

Chandola T (2001) Ethnic and class differences in health in relation to British South Asians: Using the new National Statistics Socio-Economic Classification. Social Science and Medicine 52:1285–1296

Coburn D (2000) Income inequality, social cohesion and the health status of populations: The role of neo-liberalism. Social Science and Medicine 51:135–146

Coleman JS (1988) Social capital in the creation of human capital. American Journal of Sociology 94:S95–S120

Colhoun H, Prescott-Clarke P (1996) Health survey for England 1994. HMSO, London

Coulter A (1995) Measuring quality of life. In: Jones R, Kinmouth A (eds) Critical reading for primary care. Oxford University Press, Oxford, pp 203–210

Dahl E (1994) Social inequalities in ill health: The significance of occupational status, education and income – results from a Norwegian survey. Sociology of Health and Illness 16:644–667

Davey Smith G, Hart CL, Hole DJ, MacKinnon P, Gillis C, Watt G, Blane D, Hawthorne VM (1998) Education and occupational social class: Which is the more important indicator of mortality risk? Journal of Epidemiology and Community Health 52:153–160

Department of Health (2002) Tackling health inequalities: Summary of the 2002 cross cutting review. Department of Health, London

DHSS (1980) Inequalities in Health: Report of a Research Working Group, Chaired by Sir Douglass Black, DHSS

Diez-Roux AV, Nieto FJ, Muntaner C, Tyroler HA, Comstock GW, Shahar E, Cooper LS, Watson RL, Szklo M (1997) Neighborhood environments and coronary heart disease: A multilevel analysis. American Journal of Epidemiology 146:48–63

Duncan C, Jones K, Moon G (1993) Do places matter: A multilevel analysis of regional variations in health related behaviour in Britain. Social Science and Medicine 42:817–830

Durkheim E (1966) Suicide. Free Press, New York

Ebrahim S, Wannamethee G, McCallum A, Walker M, Shaper A (1995) Marital status, change in marital status, and mortality in middle-aged British men. American Journal of Epidemiology 142:834–842

Ferri E, Brynner J, Wadsworth M (2003) Changing Britain, changing lives. Education Press, London

Ferrie JE, Shipley MJ, Marmot MG, Stansfeld S, Davey Smith G (1995) Health effects of anticipation of job change and non-employment: Longitudinal data from the Whitehall II study. British Medical Journal 311:1264–1269

Fitzpatrick R, Fletcher A, Gore S, Jones D, Speigelhalter D, Cox D (1992) Quality of life measures in health care. I: Applications and issues in assessment. British Medical Journal 305:1074–1077

Flinn MW (1965) Chadwick, Edwin. Report on the sanitary condition of the labouring population of Great Britain. 1842 Ed. & Intro., Edinburgh

Folsom AR, Burke GL, Ballew C, Jacobs DR, Haskell WL, Donahue RP (1989) Relation of body fatness and its distribution to cardiovascular risk factors in young blacks and whites. American Journal of Epidemiology 130:911–924

Glass TA (2000) Psychosocial intervention. In: Berkman LF, Kawachi I (eds) Social epidemiology. Oxford University Press, New York, pp 267–305

Greenland S, Brumback B (2002) An overview of relations among causal modelling methods. International Journal of Epidemiology 31:1030–1037

Griffin J, Fuhrer R, Stansfeld SA, Marmot MG (2002) The importance of low control at work and home on depression and anxiety: Do these effects vary by gender and social class? Social Science and Medicine 54:738–798

Grossman AB (1991) Regulation of human pituitary responses to stress. In: Brown MB, Koob GF, Rivier C (eds) Stress: Neurobiology and neuroendocrinology. Marcel Dekker, New York, pp 151–171

Hellhammer DH, Buchtal J, Gutberlet I, Kirschbaum C (1997) Social hierarchy and adrenocortical stress reactivity in men. Psychoneuroendocrinology 22:643–650

Hemingway H, Shipley MJ, Christie D, Marmot M (1998) Cardiothoracic ratio and relative heart volume as predictors of coronary heart disease mortality: The Whitehall study 25 year follow up. European Heart Journal 19: 859–869

Howlet T, Rees L, Besser G (1985) Cushing's syndrome. Clinics in Endocrinology and Metabolism 14:911–945

Illsley R (1986) Occupational class, selection and the production of inequalities in health. The Quarterly Journal of Social Affairs 2:151–165

Kaplan GA, Keil JE (1993) Socioeconomic factors and cardiovascular disease: A review of the literature. Circulation 88:1973–1998

Karasek R, Baker D, Marxer F, Ahlbom A, Theorell T (1981) Job decision latitude, job demands and cardiovascular disease: A prospective study of Swedish men. American Journal of Public Health 71:694–705

Kasl SV, Jones BA (2000) The impact of job loss and retirement on health. In: Berkman LF, Kawachi I (eds) Social epidemiology. Oxford University Press, New York, pp 118–136

Kaufman JS, Cooper RS (1999) Seeking causal explanations in social epidemiology. American Journal of Epidemiology 150:113–120

Kawachi I, Berkman LA (2000) Social cohesion, social capital and health. In: Berkman LF, Kawachi I (eds) Social epidemiology. Oxford University Press, New York, pp 174–190

Kawachi I, Kennedy B, Wilkinson R (1999a) Crime: Social disorganization and relative deprivation. Social Science and Medicine 48:719–731

Kawachi I, Kennedy BP, Glass R (1999b) Social capital and self-rated health: A contextual analysis. American Journal of Public Health 89:1187–1193

Kemper TD (1993) Sociological models in the explanation of emotions. In: Lewis M, Haviland JM (eds) Handbook of emotions. The Guildford Press, New York, pp 41–52

Krieger N (2001) Commentary: Society, biology and the logic of social epidemiology. International Journal of Epidemiology 30:44–46

Kristenson M, Orth-Gomer K, Kucinskiene Z, Bergdahl B, Calkauskas H, Balinkyiene I, Olsson AG (1998) Attenuated cortisol response to a standardised stress test in Lithuanian vs. Swedish men. International Journal of Behavioural Medicine 5:17–30

Kubzansky LD, Kawachi I (2000) Affective states and health. In: Berkman LF, Kawachi I (eds) Social epidemiology. Oxford University Press, New York, pp 213–241

Lynch JW, Kaplan GA, Salonen JT (1997) Why do poor people behave badly? Variation in adult health behaviours and psychosocial characteristics by stages of the socioeconomic lifecourse. Social Science and Medicine 44:809–819

Macintyre S, Ellaway A (2000) Ecological apporaches: Rediscovering the role of the physical and social environment. In: Berkman LF, Kawachi I (eds) Social epidemiology. Oxford University Press, New York, pp 332–348

Macintyre S, Maciver S, Sooman A (1993) Area, class and health: Should we be focusing on places or people? Journal of Social Policy 22:213–234

Maes M, Meltzer H, Stevens W, Calabrese J, Cosyns P (1994) Immuendocrine aspects of major depression. Relationships between plasma interleukin-1 and soluble interleukin-2 receptor, prolactin and cortisol. Progress in Neuro-Psychopharmacology and Biological Psychiatry 18:717–730

Marmot MG, Rose G, Shipley M, Hamilton PJS (1978) Employment grade and coronary heart disease in British civil servants. Journal of Epidemiology and Community Health 32:244–249

Marmot MG, Shipley MJ (1996) Do socioeconomic differences in mortality persist after retirement? 25 year follow up of civil servants from the first Whitehall study. British Medical Journal 313:1177–1180

Marmot MG, Wilkinson RG (1999) Social determinants of health. Oxford University Press, Oxford

McKeown T (1979) The role of medicine: Dream, mirage or nemesis? Basil Blackwell, Oxford

Menzhaghi F, Heinrichs S, Pich E, Weiss F, Koob G (1993) The role of limbic and hypothalamic corticotropin releasing factor in behavioural response to stress. Annals of the New York Academy of Sciences 697:142–154

Mroczek D, Kolarz C (1998) The effect of age on positive and negative affect: A developmental perspective on happiness. Journal of Personality and Social Psychology 75:1333–1349

Muntaner C (2001) Social epidemiology: No way back. A response to Zielhus and Kiemeney. International Journal of Epidemiology 30:625–626

Navarro V, Shi L (2001) The political context of social inequalities in health. Social Science and Medicine 52:481–491

Power C, Hertzman C (1997) Social and biological pathways linking early life and adult disease. In: Marmot M, Wadsworth MEJ (eds) Fetal and early childhood environment: Long-term health implications. British Medical Bulletin 53, Royal Society of Medicine Press Limited, London, pp 210–222

Putnam R (2000) Bowling alone: The collapse and revival of American community. Simon and Schuster, New York

Rose G (1992) The strategy of preventive medicine. Oxford University Press, Oxford

Ross C, Wu C (1995) The links between education and health. American Sociological Review 60:719–745

Rothman K, Adami H, Trichopoulos D (1998) Should the mission of epidemiology include the eradication of poverty? Lancet 352:810–813

Sapolsky R, Krey L, McEwen B (1986) The neuroendocrinology of stress and aging: The glucocorticoid cascade hypothesis. Endocrine Reviews 3:301

Sapolsky RM (1993) Endocrinology alfresco: Psychoendocrine studies of wild baboons. Recent Progress in Hormore Research 48:437–468

Seidell JC, Bjorntorp P, Sjostrom L, Kvist H, Sannerstedt R (1990) Visceral fat accumulation in men is positively associated with insulin, glucose, and C-peptide levels, but negatively with testosterone levels. Metabolism 39: 897–901

Selye H (1956) The stress of life. McGraw-Hill, New York

Siegrist J (1996) Adverse health effects of high-effort/low-reward conditions. Journal of Occupational Health Psychology 1:27–41

Singh-Manoux A, Clarke P, Marmot M (2002) Multiple measures of socioeconomic position and psychosocial health: Proximal and distal effects. International Journal of Epidemiology 31:1192–1199

Slogett A, Joshi H (1994) Higher mortality in deprived areas: Community or personal disadvantage? British Medical Journal 309:1470–1474

Snow J (1855) On the mode of communication of cholera. Churchill, London

Spiegel D, Bloom J, Kraemer H, Gottheil E (1989) Effect of psychosocial treatment on survival of patients with metastatic breast cancer. Lancet 14:888–891

Spielberger CD, Krasner SS (1988) The assessment of state and trait anxiety In: Noyes RJr, Roth M, Burrows GD (eds) Enological factors and associated disturbances. Elsevier Science Publishers B.V., Holland, pp 31–50

Stansfeld SA, Head J, Marmot MG (1998) Explaining social class differences in depression and well-being. Social Psychiatry and Psychiatric Epidemiology 33:1–9

Suomi SJ (1997) Early determinants of behaviour: Evidence from primate studies. British Medical Bulletin 53:170–184

Susser M (1995) The tribulations of trials-interventions in communities. American Journal of Public Health 85:156–158

Syme SL, Berkman LF (1976) Social class, susceptibility, and sickness. American Journal of Epidemiology 104:1–8

Szreter S (1988) The importance of social intervention in Britain's mortality decline c.1850–1914: A re-interpretation of the role of public health. Social History of Medicine 1:1–37

Szreter SRS (1984) The genesis of the Registrar-General's social classification of occupations. British Journal of Sociology 35:522–545

Wadsworth MEJ (1997) Changing social factors and their long-term implications for health. In: Marmot M, Wadsworth MEJ (eds) Fetal and early childhood environment: Long-term health implications. British Medical Bulletin 53, Royal Society of Medicine Press Limited, London, pp 198–209

Walberg P, McKee M, Shkolnikov V, Chenet L, Leon D (1998) Economic change, crime and mortality crisis in Russia: Regional analysis. British Medical Journal 317:312–318

Waldron I, Hughes M, Brooks T (1996) Marriage protection and marriage selection – Prospective evidence for reciprocal effects of marital status and health. Social Science and Medicine 43:113–123

Ware J, Gandek B (1998) Overview of the SF-36 Health Survey and the International Quality of Life (IQOLA) Project. Journal of Clinical Epidemiology 51:900–912

Winkleby MA, Jatulis DE, Frank E, Fortmann SP (1992) Socioeconomic status and health: How education, income, and occupation contribute to risk factors for cardiovascular disease. American Journal of Public Health 82:1–6

Zielhus GA, Kiemeney LA (2001) Social epidemiology? No way. International Journal of Epidemiology 30:43–44

Occupational Epidemiology

III.2

Franco Merletti, Dario Mirabelli, Lorenzo Richiardi

Introduction

Occupational epidemiology has the same main goal as the broad field of epidemiology: to identify the causes of disease in a population in order to intervene to remove them. Occupational epidemiology is an exposure-oriented discipline; it is thus the systematic study of illnesses and injuries related to the workplace environment (Checkoway et al. 2004).

The first concern about occupational causes of disease may have been that of Hippocrates, who wrote about the lifestyle habits and environment of populations and patients. Nevertheless, it was the Italian physician Bernardino Ramazzini who recommended that doctors add questions about occupation to those recommended by Hippocrates, and it was Ramazzini who made the first systematic description of occupational diseases and their causes in his book *De Morbis Artificum* (Ramazzini 1713). His descriptions included different characteristics of skin ulceration in freshwater and sea fishermen, silicosis among stonemasons, ocular disorders among glass-blowers, and neurological toxicity among tradesmen exposed to mercury. It is noteworthy that he not only described the diseases but was also deeply concerned about the ethics of harmful work practices and the need for preventive measures, such as good ventilation and protective clothing.

Classic historical reports, such as those about scurvy in sailors in 1753, scrotal cancer in chimney sweeps in 1775, respiratory cancers in underground metal miners in 1879 and bladder cancer in dye workers in 1895, are clear examples of the importance of reports of case series by clinicians and by the workers themselves (Carter 2000). New occupational hazards came to light incidentally even in the mid-1900s, when the methodological landmark of the historical cohort study was designed (Doll 1952, 1955; Case et al. 1954) and occupational epidemiology developed as a discipline. Indeed, Case and co-authors suspected that rubber workers would have an elevated risk for bladder cancer while conducting a study on the high incidence of bladder tumours among dye manufacturers (Doll 1975). While reviewing hospital records of bladder cancer patients in Birmingham, England, chosen as a control area because it did not have a dye industry, they noticed that many workers had been employed in a rubber factory. Subsequent investigation confirmed the association with rubber production and showed that it resulted from exposure to an anti-oxidant containing the carcinogen 2-naphthylamine (Case and Hosker 1954; Coggon 2000).

Occupational epidemiology has contributed to the development of both study designs (such as the historical cohort study) and analytical methods that are now part of the broader field of epidemiology and of other exposure-oriented disciplines. For instance, quantitative and qualitative methods for assessing exposure, such as job-exposure matrices and job-specific questionnaire modules for assessment by experts, were developed by occupational epidemiologists and industrial hygienists. They have now been adapted and used in other disciplines, such as nutritional and environmental epidemiology, and are central to ensuring the validity and informativeness of epidemiological research in general.

Prevention is the final goal of all epidemiological research and findings. Occupational exposure was one of the first causes to be identified of diseases such as cancer and pulmonary illness, and epidemiological study of such exposures often led to the identification of specific causal agents. Occupational hazards are known causes of disease that are amenable to regulatory control, and thus especially suitable for prevention. This is in contrast to aspects of lifestyle, such as smoking and dietary habits, for which control requires modification of cultural and personal behaviour patterns. Free choice may contribute to some diseases attributable to environmental causes; for instance, the large majority of cases of lung cancer are attributable to tobacco smoking and can be prevented by avoiding the habit. The reason for interest in preventing occupational hazards is more subtle: as personal choice plays little or no role in occupational exposure, the protection of workers warrants special attention. Furthermore, while industrial effluents and products might cause illness in the general population, exposed workers are likely to be the first and most severely affected. Prevention at the level of the working environment will by the same token result in prevention in the general population.

This chapter will address issues in study designs and epidemiological methods as applied in the specific field of occupational epidemiology. They will include dose-response analysis, healthy worker effect and exposure assessment. Finally, how occupational epidemiology can help to evaluate the need and effectiveness of primary prevention interventions and policies will be described using the example of occupational cancer.

Study Designs   2.2

Classic epidemiological studies, such as cross-sectional (see Chap. I.3 of this handbook), case-control (see Chap. I.6) and cohort studies (see Chap. I.5), are commonly carried out in occupational settings. The principles of study design and data analysis are derived from general epidemiological methods; however, some specific aspects are worth addressing.

Cross-Sectional Studies   2.2.1

Cross-sectional studies are generally used to investigate non-fatal diseases, such as muscoloskeletal disorders, and symptoms or physiological functions, such as wheezing and forced expiratory volume in one second (FEV_1). They measure prevalences. Therefore, associations between exposure and disease are difficult to interpret, as they could depend either on an increased incidence or on a longer duration of disease among a subgroup of cases. For this reason and for problems of reverse causality arising from measuring exposures and diseases at the same time, the causal nature of an association can be weakly addressed using a cross-sectional approach.

Cross-sectional studies are vulnerable to the effect of non-response, particularly when they are carried out with the main aim of estimating the prevalence of diseases or their symptoms. Diseased workers may participate in the study differently from those who are not diseased, and their willingness to participate may depend on their exposure status. Occupational studies of fertility and sperm quality are an example of studies in which non-response is a critical problem. Since the observation of the toxic effects of 2,3-dibromo-3-chloropropane on testicular germ cells (Potashnik et al. 1978), the fertility of exposed male workers has been investigated in several studies. In one study, groups of traditional and organic farmers were selected randomly from the database of the Danish Ministry of Agriculture in 1995–96 and invited to participate in a study on semen, including total sperm count, sperm concentration, other indexes and serum concentrations of sex hormones (Larsen et al. 1999). A questionnaire eliciting information on previous exposure to pesticides was posted to 1124 farmers, of whom 86% answered and 256 provided semen samples. This low participation proportion was not unexpected, as the examination required by the study was somewhat demanding.

A further limitation of cross-sectional studies, which is specific to occupational epidemiology, is that only active workers are usually investigated, because the study base is defined as workers employed in a specific industry or exposed to a specific occupational factor. It follows that workers who have terminated their employment cannot be included in the study.

Let us consider the example of the cross-sectional studies on the health effects of exposure to diesel fumes (US Environmental Protection Agency 2002). Acute respiratory effects were investigated in several studies by measuring FEV_1 and other indicators of pulmonary function twice, at the beginning and at the end of a work shift, in workers employed in mines and garages. Chronic respiratory effects were studied through a single survey and a medical examination in workers with different levels of cumulative occupational exposure to diesel exhausts. Individuals who are susceptible to diesel exhaust exposure tend to move from jobs with a high level of exposure. Therefore, a cross-sectional study on the acute effects of exposure is presumably carried out among a selected group of workers, resulting in a possible underestimate of the effects. Regarding chronic effects, which are manifest a long period after the exposure has occurred, there is an underestimate of the association between exposure and disease, if the termination of employment is determined by the disease or its early symptoms.

2.2.2   Cohort Studies

The cohort study is a valid, but sometimes expensive and time-consuming design. Nevertheless, the availability of employment records and trade union registries often permits straightforward identification of past occupational cohorts. It is therefore not surprising that historical cohort studies have long been the method of choice in occupational epidemiology, and they have contributed significantly to the identification of occupational hazards.

Researchers usually identify a factory in which the exposure of interest occurs – to specific chemicals and substances or specific working conditions and job tasks – and select the members of the cohort from registries available at the factory. Alternatively, a study population can be identified from similar departments in different factories. Thus, when a single facility does not provide a sufficient number of workers or the time of follow-up is not long enough, a collaborative study can be conducted in similar factories in several centres. The cohort study of workers employed in the man-made vitreous fibre (MMVF) industry in Europe, coordinated by the International Agency for Research on Cancer (IARC) (Boffetta et al. 1997, 1999; Sali et al. 1999), is an example of such collaboration. The cohort was assembled in 1977 and consisted of approximately 22,000 workers who had ever been employed in 13 factories producing at least one of three types of MMVF, namely glass wool, continuous filaments of glass fibre and rock- or slag-wool, at any time between the year of starting production of MMVF and 1977. The follow-up ended between 1990 and 1995 in different factories, depending on subsequent updating.

Exposure was assessed on the basis of individual work histories, obtained from employment registries in 1977. It was known that important technological changes had taken place in the production of MMVF over the study period, so that the period of MMVF production was divided into three 'technological phases': early, intermediate and late. As the ambient levels of exposure to MMVF were estimated to have decreased with evolving production processes, the year in which each of the three phases began in each factory was assessed. Information on possible concomitant exposure to other agents, such as asbestos and bitumen, was also obtained for each factory. The researchers thus knew the duration of employment for each worker, by factory, technological phase and job task.

National mortality rates were used to calculate standardized mortality ratios (SMRs) (cf. Chaps. I.2 or I.3 of this handbook) for neoplastic and non-neoplastic causes of death, and cancer-specific standardized incidence ratios (SIRs) were estimated for the subcohorts in countries where cancer incidence rates are available from cancer registries. The effect of duration of employment was estimated in internal comparisons within the cohort, the reference group including workers employed for less than 5 years. Data were also analysed according to type of MMVF, job task, technological phase and time since first employment. Data on workers who had been employed for less than 1 year were analysed separately, as short-term workers might be high-risk individuals with particular lifestyles or occupational exposure to agents other than MMVF (see also Sect. 2.4.2).

In general, MMVF production workers did not have an excess risk of mortality or cancer incidence, although a small excess risk for lung cancer was found among rock- and slag-wool workers and increased mortality from heart diseases and non-malignant renal diseases was suggested. It is important to note that no information on lifestyle factors was available, which is a limitation of almost all historical cohort studies.

In countries where good, computerized population registries with a long history of registration exist, large occupational cohort studies can be carried out by linkage of information on occupational status from censuses with individual data on, e.g., mortality, cancer incidence and hospital discharges. The strength of record-linkage studies is the very large sample size. An occupational record linkage study of cancer incidence was conducted in the Nordic countries among persons aged 25–64 years who were listed in the 1970 censuses (Andersen et al. 1999). Overall, about 10 million persons were included in the study, and more than 500,000 incident cases of cancer cases occurred during the follow-up period, which ended between 1987 and 1990, depending on the country. Occupational exposure was evaluated for 54 occupational groups. Many cancer-specific associations were estimated, and they cannot be discussed here; however, the general finding was that risk of cancer is associated with occupation.

This record linkage study shows clearly that cohort studies can provide risk estimates for many outcomes and some of the findings might be unexpected. For instance, in a historical cohort study of 8226 workers employed in an aircraft manufacturing factory in northern Italy between 1954 and 1981, an unexpected excess of melanomas was found (6 observed, 1.02 expected cases) (Costa et al. 1989). When an unexpected association is found, the characteristics of the cases, including age, sex, period of employment, factory and job task, should be explored carefully, in order to identify any clusters of jobs or operations that suggest a common exposure. In the example of melanoma, the characteristics of the six cases were described in detail but no cluster could be identified.

There are two major limitations to the use of data from existing records rather then from ad-hoc questionnaires and environmental or biological measurements: lack of detailed information on exposure and lack of information on possible relevant confounders.

With regard to exposure, maximum cooperation between researchers and management, trade unions, occupational physicians and industrial hygienists is crucial to obtain information on the nature of both industrial processes and working environments. Basic information on the exposure of each worker should include the starting and ending dates of employment at the factory. Unfortunately, important information, such as the job task of each worker and changes in industrial processes over time, is often missing. Even when the job task is recorded, one would like to evaluate also the variability of exposure levels among workers carrying out the same job. The general lack of information may reduce the quality of the data on exposure, whatever approach is used to assess exposure, and finally bias the results of the study because of misclassification. Although it is theoretically possible to measure factory-specific levels of exposure at the time a study is conceived, strong assumptions should hold for a reliable imputation of past exposures.

In some studies, plant-specific ambient measurements had been recorded over time and were available for assessing exposure. A historical cohort of more than 74,000 workers employed between 1972 and 1987 in 672 factories in jobs that entailed exposure to benzene was assembled in China (Hayes et al. 1997). The cohort was followed-up for death from all causes and for incidence of haematological tumours, with an analogous cohort of approximately 36,000 unexposed workers for comparison. For the purposes of assessing exposure, information on the factory and department of employment and on the starting and ending dates of each job was obtained, for each worker, from employment records available at the factories (Dosemeci et al. 1994b). Moreover, information on production activities and changes in processes over time was obtained at each factory and for each job type. Importantly, the results of all past air monitoring (more than 8400 measurements) for benzene and other solvents were also obtained. Therefore, whenever possible, the exposure level was assigned to each worker on the basis of monitoring results either for specific combinations of job task, department and calendar period, or for adjacent calendar periods or similar job tasks.

Detailed information on exposure and confounders can obviously be obtained in concurrent cohort studies, which can be efficiently carried out when the induction period between exposure and disease is short. If the cohort is followed-up prospectively, temporal variations in exposure can be ascertained either at individual level, from questionnaires, personal dosimetry data or use of biomarkers of exposure, or at aggregate level, from environmental measurements and monitoring of changes in industrial processes.

Case-Control Studies 2.2.3

Nested case-control studies (see Chap. I.7 of this handbook) might solve some of the limitations inherent in the cohort design. As a nested case-control study covers fewer persons than a cohort study, the nested approach is efficient when the exposure assessment is not straightforward, as, for instance, when it is based on experts' judgement. The nested approach is also more efficient when worker-specific levels of exposure are estimated from biological samples or by direct interview with the workers or their next-of-kin. Measurement of biomarkers can result in accurate assessments of current exposure, but assumptions must be made about past exposure. Conversely, interviews allow detailed reconstructions of working histories and provide information on possible confounders. Information on actual exposure levels may nevertheless be rather imprecise, and the subjects are difficult to trace, especially when the follow up period is long.

The historical cohort study of workers employed in MMVF production coordinated by the IARC, described above, includes a clear example of a nested case-control design (Boffetta et al. 1997). The analyses of the cohort revealed a small excess risk for lung cancer among rock- and slag-wool production workers, but no information was available on possible confounders; furthermore, occupational histories were available up to 1977 only, and were limited to the information in the employment registries. The researchers therefore conducted a case-control study of 196 cases of lung cancer and 1715 matched controls nested in the cohort (Kjaerheim et al. 2002). The index subjects or their next-of-kin were traced and interviewed to obtain information on lifetime smoking habits, residential history and lifetime occupational history, both within and outside the MMVF industry. As anticipated by the study design, the proportion of completed interviews with the selected subjects was low: 68% for cases and 35% for controls. Two industrial hygienists evaluated the individual occupational histories for exposure to each of several occupational agents known or suspected to be associated with lung cancer. Moreover, an expert panel was formed to evaluate individual cumulative exposure to MMVF on the basis of the new information obtained at the interview. The smoking-adjusted estimates and the analyses by quartiles of cumulative level of exposure in the nested study did not support an association between exposure to rock- or slag-wool and lung cancer risk.

Quite often, a nested case-control design increases the efficiency of the computerization, cleaning and handling of data, even though information on exposure is available. Grayson (1996), for example, conducted a case-control study on brain cancer nested in a cohort of approximately 880,000 US Air Force members to evaluate the effect of occupational exposure to electromagnetic fields. The workers had to have been employed between 1970 and 1989. At the end of the follow-up period, 230 incident cases of brain cancer were found, and four controls for each case were randomly selected among cohort members. Information on past exposure to electromagnetic fields was obtained from several sources, including employment records, records of events exceeding existing limits and some personal dosimetry data. The final analysis was based on 1150 persons instead of more than 800,000 in the original cohort.

Population- or hospital-based case-control studies have frequently been used to investigate the health effects of occupational exposures. In the early 1980s, a multicentre case-control study was carried out to investigate the associations between laryngeal and hypopharyngeal cancer and smoking, alcohol, dietary habits and occupational factors (Tuyns et al. 1988). The study, coordinated by IARC, was population-based and included six centres in northern Italy, France, Spain and Switzerland. Information on occupational history and lifestyle factors was obtained by face-to-face interviews with cases and controls. Specifically, each person was asked to report all jobs held for at least one year since 1945, specifying their starting and ending years, a short description of specific tasks, the name of the company, the company's activity and the specific products of the department in which the interviewed person had worked. The occupational histories of 1010 interviewed cases and 2176 interviewed controls were coded, without knowledge of case or control status, according to standard international classifications of occupations and industries. Then, smoking- and alcohol-adjusted odds ratios for occupational factors were obtained by two approaches. First, an exploratory analysis was carried out on 156 occupations and 70 industrial activities in which at least nine individuals had been ever employed (Boffetta et al. 2003). Second, a working group created a job-exposure matrix (JEM) to categorize each combination of job and activity in terms of levels of probability, intensity and frequency of exposure to 16 occupational agents for which there was some a-priori evidence of an association with laryngeal cancer risk (Berrino et al. 2003). The agents investigated included asbestos, solvents, formaldehyde and polycyclic aromatic hydrocarbons. The JEM was used and evaluated in ad-hoc studies (Merletti et al. 1991; Ahrens et al. 1993; Luce et al. 1993; Orlowski et al. 1993; Stengel et al. 1993; Stucker et al. 1993). An account of its validation, based on a comparison between the results of the JEM and the experts' evaluation of the jobs as described in the questionnaires, is given in Table 2.1. Generally, the specificity and sensitivity of the JEM was agent-specific. The first analytical approach, based on job titles and industrial activities, provided risk estimates for several occupations, an advantage facilitated by the heterogeneity of the study subjects' working histories due to the multicentre design. Conversely, the second approach directly tested aetiological hypotheses. In both instances, the case-control design made it possible to control for the confounding effects of smoking, alcohol drinking and diet.

Table 2.1. Validation of the job exposure matrix (JEM) of the IARC case-control study on laryngeal and hypopharyngeal cancer: proportion of jobs not entailing an exposure to specific agents according to an expert's assessment compared with the results from the JEM

Agent[a]	JEM categories of intensity/probability of exposure[b]							
	No. of job periods	1	2	3a	3b	3c	4	5
Asbestos	3220	96	83	79	73		68[c]	
Solvents (1)	2712	96	92	89	70	47	58	16
Solvents (2)	929	87	83	62	67	35	37	9
Formaldehyde	884	75	90	59	47	50	29	–[d]
Wood dust	863	95	–[d]	50	50	–[d]	8	0
PAH	2571	98	68	88	85	98	74	39

[a] Agents were evaluated in the following studies: asbestos, Orlowski et al. (1993); solvents (1 = bladder cancer study; 2 = glomerulonephritis study), Stengel et al. (1993); formaldehyde and wood dust, Luce et al. (1993); PAH (polycyclic aromatic hydrocarbons), Stucker et al. (1993)
[b] Categories: 1. Job-related exposure is not higher than for the general population; 2. Job entails or may entail a cumulative exposure slightly higher than for the general population; 3. Job may entail exposure definitely higher than for the general population, but the coded information is not sufficient to discriminate between exposed and not exposed workers (3a: few workers are thought to be exposed, 3b: some workers are thought to be exposed, 3c: the majority of workers are thought to be exposed); 4. Job entails exposure to the specific agent at definitely higher level than the general population; 5. Job entails exposure to the specific agent and there are instances in which the exposure is known to be particularly high
[c] Categories 3c, 4, 5 were considered jointly
[d] Category with no jobs according to the JEM

Case-control studies can be used efficiently to investigate ubiquitous occupational exposures, which cannot be localized to a specific industry. This study design also permits the researcher to focus on minorities and on subgroups of the population that have often been poorly investigated. For example, at the first international conference on occupational cancer in women, in 1993, it was recognized that most of the information on occupational hazards had been obtained from studies on men: a survey showed that less than 10% of published epidemiological studies included and reported detailed results on women (Zahm et al. 1994). Although this picture has changed, efforts to study the effects of occupational exposures on women are still needed (Zahm and Blair 2003).

A case-control approach is often used in occupational epidemiology for exploratory studies. As in the study on laryngeal and hypopharyngeal cancer described above, an occupational history may be classified by several groups of job titles and industrial activities. As multiple comparisons are made, a Bayesian approach with semi-Bayes or empirical-Bayes adjustments might help to decrease the impact of false-positive results (Greenland and Poole 1994). For a formal explanation and practical examples of Bayesian approaches in occupational epidemiology, see Greenland and Poole (1994) and Steenland et al. (2000).

Mortality odds ratio studies have a case-control design and are a valid alternative to proportionate mortality studies, which have been widely used in occupational epidemiology (Miettinen and Wang 1981; Boyd et al. 1970). In proportionate mortality studies, the frequency of death for the diseases under study among exposed workers is compared with the corresponding figure calculated for a reference population (proportionate mortality ratio, PMR). PMRs are limited by the fact that they must add up to unity; therefore, elevated PMRs for some diseases are, by definition, counterbalanced by decreased PMRs for other diseases. Moreover, PMRs are biased if ascertainment of deaths is incomplete in a different proportion among exposed than unexposed subjects. These drawbacks are overcome in mortality odds ratio studies where the case-control approach is applied. In such studies the cases comprise deaths from the specific cause of interest, both exposed and unexposed, while the controls are other deaths selected on the basis of a presumed lack of association with the exposure. The principle of selecting the control causes of death for inclusion in the study is therefore the same as selecting a control series for any case-control study: controls are selected independently of exposure and with the aim of representing the proportion of exposure in the study base (Rothman and Greenland 1998).

2.3   Exposure Assessment

Exposure assessment (see Chap. I.11 of this handbook), a critical step in any epidemiological study, is central in occupational epidemiology. The most recent developments in the design of both cohort and case-control studies of work-related diseases rely on identification of exposure to specific agents, such as chemicals, rather than on the use of surrogates of exposures, such as being employed in a given industrial activity or holding a certain job. Furthermore, an attempt is often made to compute some measure of dose, such as cumulative exposure or average exposure, which in turn requires estimation of the level (intensity) of exposure and its variation over time.

2.3.1   Statistical and Deterministic Modelling

Two general strategies, statistical and deterministic modelling (Kauppinen et al. 1994), are available to assess exposure on the basis of the primary information collected in a study. Such information usually does not include satisfactory measures of exposure to the agent(s) of interest, and is sometimes limited to a description of the work setting, the operations performed by workers and the materials they handled. More accurate methods of estimating exposure are based on stochastic (statistical) modelling, in which missing data are calculated from a model fitted to the results of past industrial hygiene measurements, that are assumed to follow the log-normal distribution among groups of workers defined by plant, job title and work area (Kauppinen et al. 1994). When statistical modelling is applied to industry-based studies, such as cohort, cross-sectional and nested case-control studies, workers are classified into 'homogeneous' groups on the basis of combinations of plant, work area, job title and period. Then, the available industrial hygiene measurement series are broken down into the same groups.

The main limitations of the statistical approach are that: (1) any trends in exposure over time are often unknown, either because measurements were not made for previous processes and working conditions or because of difficulties in the interpretation of historical measurements; and (2) the inter-individual variation of exposure within a homogeneous group can be wider than that between groups. With respect to the latter, the difficulty of identifying groups with homogeneous exposure, without extensive measurements based on carefully planned strategies, has been documented (Kromhout et al. 1993).

In historical cohort studies, the availability and quality of industrial hygiene data are often different for the various settings included in the work histories of the study subjects; good data may exist for some periods and not for others. In these circumstances, the maximum achievable goal is a semi-quantitative approach in which jobs are compared according to materials handled and tasks performed. The jobs are then ordered in terms of assessed exposure, which is placed onto a semi-quantitative scale (e.g. high, intermediate, low).

Because comprehensive data on exposure are rarely available, less accurate methods have thus to be used. If the factors that determine the level of exposure can be identified, they can be used to construct a deterministic model (Kauppinen et al. 1994). In deterministic modelling in industry-based studies, the most significant factors that affect exposure intensity, such as type of plant and machinery, presence of local exhausts and workers proximity to sources, are identified. Their relative importance is then assessed, on the basis of either available past industrial hygiene data or, in their absence, a theoretical evaluation of how different tasks, operations and procedures could have affected exposure. A further possibility is experimental reconstitution of past working conditions and their measurement. It has been shown that complex industry-specific exposure matrices can be built on the basis of detailed knowledge of plant-, job-, and time-specific factors (Kauppinen and Partanen 1988). Semi-quantitative exposure levels can then be established for each study subject applying the matrix to the information on the jobs they held and the tasks they performed.

The main limitations of the deterministic approach are that: (1) the relative importance of the various determinants may prove difficult to assess, and agreement among experts may be poor; and (2) the quality of information on the determinants may be highly variable across study subjects; for some, the tasks involved in their job might have been recorded, while for others barely the job title is known.

In some recent multi-centre or pooled industry-based studies, considerable advances have been made in statistical modelling of exposure determinants, building industry-specific exposure matrices and collecting and using individual job histories (Burstyn et al. 2000, 2003; Mannetje et al. 2002; Harber et al. 2003). Current standards of practice imply that when good industrial hygiene data are available, at least for some historical periods, and the relative influences of changes in plant, process and activity can be evaluated, exposure can be assessed quantitatively and extrapolated to periods or plants for which no original quantitative information was available. With this method, quantitative data on a given job, in a given industrial activity and during a given period provide a baseline estimate of both the average exposure and its variation. Known differences in the presence and characteristics of determinants provide multiplicative weighting factors to be applied to the baseline estimate. Few validation studies of industry-specific exposure matrices are, however, available (Dosemeci et al. 1994a, 1996).

2.3.2   Job-exposure Matrices and Job-specific Modules

In population- and hospital-based case-control studies, statistical modelling has been used to set up job-exposure matrices (JEM) (Hoar et al. 1980; Macaluso et al. 1983). A JEM can be defined as a cross-classification of a list of job titles with a list of agents to which the workers performing the jobs might be exposed (Kauppinen and Partanen 1988). Deterministic modelling has been used in the interpretation and assessment of job histories by industrial hygiene experts when occupational questionnaires including job-specific modules (JSM) were developed to obtain the detailed information necessary for the experts' judgement (Siemiatycki et al. 1981; Macaluso et al. 1983; Ahrens et al. 1993). Researchers at the US National Cancer Institute showed that a deterministic approach can be used not only in expert- and JSM-based assessment but also to create and use more detailed, improved JEMs that might allow semi-quantitative or even quantitative exposure assessments (Dosemeci et al. 1990a). More recently, the same group suggested that the JEM-based assessment strategy should be abandoned in favour of the JSM-based expert assessment (Stewart et al. 1996). Use of JEMs has been reported to result in loss of both sensitivity and specificity in exposure assessment, in comparison with the use of a JSM-based individual assessment (Rybicki et al. 1997). Simulation studies suggested that use of JEMs may lead to loss of precision in odds ratio estimates, whereas expert-based assessment resulted in relatively low levels of misclassification (Bouyer et al. 1995).

Although it is somewhat difficult to assess the validity of expert-based exposure assessment in the field, some studies suggest that the agreement within and between experts might be satisfactory when experienced teams of raters are available (Siemiatycki et al. 1997; Fritschi et al. 2003). Two studies addressed the issue of expert-based exposure assessment validation by means of an objective index of past exposure to asbestos.

The first study (Pairon et al. 1994) comprised 131 cases of mesothelioma. The probability, level and frequency of exposure were assessed by using qualitative ordinal classifications of the job in which each person had maximum exposure. Combinations of assessed probability, level, and frequency were summarised in four classes: (1) unexposed or possibly exposed, (2) probable or definite exposure at low level, (3) probable or definite exposure at levels higher than low, with sporadic frequency, (4) probable or definite exposure at levels higher than low, with more than sporadic frequency. No attempt to build up a cumulative dose index was made. A limited correlation between the exposure assessment and objective indices of exposure to asbestos was observed, particularly with counts of asbestos bodies per gram of dried tissue. This study suffered from some shortcomings. Intensity and frequency were not used to compute a combined dose estimate, which prevented the calculation of a cumulative dose index. Frequency was used to discriminate between the third and the fourth summary class, but variations in frequency might actually be less important than those in intensity to determine the average exposure level. Only the highest exposure job was used in the assessment, so that other possible exposures have not been taken into account. The sensitivity of objective indexes of asbestos exposure in mesothelioma cases may be low.

In the second study (Takahashi et al. 1994), 42 cancer cases for whom necropsy material was available were assessed for exposure from a JSM-based questionnaire and by analysis of lung tissue fibres. A good correlation was found between the JSM-based exposure assessment and asbestos fibre counts, although some cases were found to have had exposure but had no asbestos in the lung. The main shortcomings of this study are its rather limited dimension and a potential necropsy selection bias; the heterogeneous nature of the cases as to their cancer site makes it difficult to extrapolate its results to a mesothelioma series.

Expert-based assessment with deterministic modelling in the hands of experienced raters has resulted in quantitative assessments in some population- and hospital-based case-control studies (Iwatsubo et al. 1998, Brüske-Hohlfeld et al. 2000, Rödelsperger et al. 2001).

Consequences of Errors in Exposure Assessment   2.3.3

The consequences of errors in exposure assessment are discussed extensively in the chapters on exposure assessment (Chap. I.11) and measurement error (Chap. II.5) in this handbook. When exposure is measured as a continuous variable at the individual level, random, non-differential errors in assessment, such as those deriving from errors in measurement, generally lead to attenuation of the exposure-disease association and diminish the goodness-of-fit of regression models (Armstrong 1998). When measurements are constrained by a lower limit, such as a detection limit, however, inflation of the exposure-response association can occur under certain circumstances (Richardson and Ciampi 2003). When exposure is measured as a continuous variable, but at group level, a rather different situation occurs:

The exposure level is the average for a sample of individuals in the group, and all individuals are assigned this average exposure. This leads to what is referred to as 'Berkson error'. In a 'classical' error, an individual is assigned a measured exposure, affected by random variability. In Berkson error, the group average exposure is affected by a considerably smaller random error, but the actual exposure of each individual in the group will be different from the average. The exposure-response association will not be biased by Berkson error (Armstrong 1998).

In many, probably most, study designs, exposure is scaled as a discrete variable on a dichotomous or a polytomous scale. When the exposure variable is dichotomised, non-differential misclassification will always bias the effect measure towards the null; however, when the exposure variable is polytomous, non-differential misclassification will bias the effect measure towards the null only if misclassification occurs between adjacent exposure categories. When it involves non-adjacent categories, bias away from the null may also occur (Armstrong 1998; Dosemeci et al 1990b).

Quantitatively, misclassification is a function of: (a) the sensitivity of the assessment method, i.e. the proportion of all truly exposed subjects correctly classified as exposed, and (b) its specificity, i.e. the proportion of all truly non-exposed subjects correctly classified as non-exposed. The relative importance of sensitivity and specificity in overall misclassification bias depends on exposure prevalence: when exposures are rare, like most occupational exposures in population- and hospital-based case-control studies, even small losses in specificity may strongly bias the relative risk estimate toward the null. Such effect is clearly depicted in Fig. 2.1, where a true relative risk of 4.0, sensitivity in exposure assessment of 0.9, and a range of commonly found exposure prevalences (from 0.001 up to 0.2) are assumed. The estimated relative risk is plotted against different specificities in exposure assessment.

This consideration does not of course imply that sensitivity is not important: When exposures are rare low sensitivity in exposure assessment causes loss in power, and requires substantial increases in sample size to compensate for it.

Special Issues in Occupational Epidemiology

2.4

2.4.1   Confounding

A general discussion of confounding is given in Chap. I.9 of this handbook. Information on several known possible confounders and on other occupational and non-occupational exposures of interest is almost always lacking for historical occupational cohorts. Methods to deal with confounding in historical cohorts include use of internal comparison groups, with general characteristics assumed to be similar to those of the exposed subjects, and use of available statistics on the

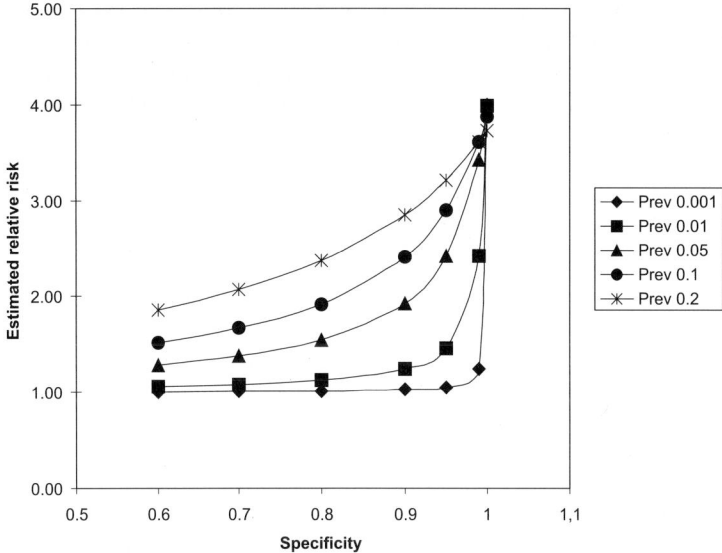

Figure 2.1. Bias toward the null of estimated relative risk due to loss in specificity in exposure assessment. True relative risk = 4 and exposure assessment sensitivity 0.9 are assumed. Estimated relative risk is plotted against different levels of specificity of exposure assessment, for exposure with prevalences (Prev) ranging from 0.001 to 0.2 (modified from Ahrens 1999)

distribution of confounders in the population from which the cohort originated. The first approach is commonplace in occupational epidemiology, although it is seldom possible to verify whether the comparison group has the assumed characteristics. Internal comparisons have the advantage of controlling part of the bias introduced by the 'healthy worker effect', that is discussed below. In a historical cohort study conducted in the Nordic countries to investigate the risks for cancer among airplane pilots (Pukkala et al. 2002), national cancer registry data were used to calculate standardized incidence ratios (SIRs). Since airplane pilots belong to a higher social class than the general population, however, the SIRs were possibly biased. In this study, cosmic radiation was the main exposure of interest; therefore, a cumulative dose of radiation experienced by each member of the cohort was calculated. This made it possible to check the main findings from the external comparison by analysing the effect of the exposure, using pilots with the lowest cumulative dose as the reference group. Such a comparison is unlikely to be confounded by social class.

The second approach, the use of available population statistics, was applied in the Norwegian part of the occupational record-linkage study in the Nordic countries, described in Sect. 2.2.2, with occupation-, sex- and birth cohort-specific information on smoking habits in the population obtained from external surveys (Haldorsen et al. 2004). The Norwegian study evaluated 42 occupational groups for risk of lung cancer in comparison with 12 other occupational groups assumed to be without exposure to occupational lung carcinogens. The magnitude of the associations of proportion of current and former smokers, and amount of cigarettes smoked with lung cancer risk was estimated among the 12 reference groups, using data from the external surveys. Then, the smoking-adjusted SIRs for the 42 occupational groups were calculated, and compared with the non-adjusted estimates. Limitations of this approach are that: (1) the quality of the information on the confounder depends on the quality of the surveys, and (2) the magnitude of the association between confounder and disease is not directly estimated at an individual level. The magnitude of the association can be either obtained from the best available studies, or from ad-hoc studies conducted in the same population, or estimated, as in the Norwegian study, using aggregate data.

When a study is conducted to determine whether an occupational exposure is associated with a disease, with no specific interest in the dose-response relationship, and when the estimate of the association is large, adjusted and unadjusted estimates are often similar. This has been shown in studies of occupational lung cancer risk, for which smoking is a strong potential confounder. In particular, using an indirect approach that is a type of sensitivity analysis, Axelson calculated that the confounding effect of smoking can hardly explain relative risks greater than 1.5 or below 0.7 when national rates are used for comparison (Axelson 1978; Axelson and Steenland 1988). He made sound assumptions about the proportions of moderate smokers (40%) and heavy smokers (10%) in the population used for calculating the number of expected cases, and also about the effects of moderate smoking (relative risk, 10) and of heavy smoking (relative risk, 20) on lung cancer risk. Then, the adjusted relative risks were calculated for different scenarios of association between smoking and being employed in specific occupations (Table 2.2). Axelson's suggestion that, under common circumstances, strong risk factors have weak confounding effects was investigated further and supported (Gail et al. 1988; Siemiatycki et al. 1988; Flanders and Khoury 1990).

In developing a protocol for a case-control study on the risk of female breast cancer associated with occupational exposure to magnetic fields, a simulation study was carried out to evaluate the potential confounding effects of several risk factors (Goodman et al, 2002). Twelve potential confounders, including a family history of breast cancer, country of birth, age at menopause and obesity, were selected on the basis of recent reviews on breast cancer epidemiology and evaluated both in univariable analyses and with combinations of two to five risk factors. Estimates of the strength of the associations between the risk factors and breast cancer risk and the prevalences of the risk factors in the general population were obtained from the literature. The aim was to identify confounders that, under different scenarios of their prevalence among cases, could increase a true odds ratio of 1 up to a distorted value of 1.5. In the univariable analysis, no risk factor was a strong confounder, unless an unrealistic increase in its prevalence among occupationally exposed women was assumed. Interestingly, the scenario in which the prevalences of several risk factors were increased also did not have a strong confounding effect. For instance, a twofold increase among exposed women in the prevalence of first-degree relatives with breast cancer, a history of cancer in one breast, benign

Table 2.2. Risk ratios for lung cancer in relation to the fraction of smokers in various hypothetical populations (source: Axelson 1978; Axelson and Steenland 1988)

Non smokers (risk of 1)	Type of smokers in the population (percentages)		Rate ratio
	Moderate smokers (risk of 10)	Heavy smokers (risk of 20)	
100	–	–	0.15
80	20	–	0.43
70	30	–	0.57
60	35	5	0.78
50[a]	40[a]	10[a]	1.00[a]
40	45	15	1.22
30	50	20	1.43
20	55	25	1.65
10	60	30	1.86
–	–	100	3.08

[a] Compared to reference population with 50% nonsmokers, 40% moderate smokers, and 10% heavy smokers

proliferative breast disease, obesity and consumption of at least two drinks per day inflated the odds ratio from unity to 1.38.

The similarity between adjusted and unadjusted estimates has also been shown empirically, in both cohort and case-control studies. SMRs of cancers of the lung, bladder and intestine, unadjusted for smoking, strongly correlated with smoking-adjusted estimates in analyses of occupational factors in a cohort of US veterans (Blair et al. 1985). Analogously, smoking was found to be a weak confounder in a review of several occupational case-control studies on lung cancer (Simonato et al. 1988). When selecting the final model for analysing a case-control study on occupational factors and lung cancer risk in two areas of Italy in 1990–1992 (Richiardi et al. 2004), we evaluated several models for addressing smoking as a confounder. Table 2.3 shows the results of an evaluation for two occupational categories, one positively associated and the other negatively associated with smoking. The evaluation showed that a simple model in which smokers are classified as current, former and never can accommodate for most of the potential confounding effect.

Healthy Worker Effect 2.4.2

Workers are not a random sample of the general population as the employment status is positively associated with the health status. First, relatively healthier people are more likely to seek a job and to be hired. Second, as sick people tend to leave their jobs, healthier workers remain employed longer. The two health-related selection forces cause a well-known selection bias in occupational epidemiology, known as the 'healthy worker effect' (Fox and Collier 1976; McMichael 1976). The

Table 2.3. Odds ratio, and 95% confidence intervals, of lung cancer for two selected job titles, obtained using seven different methods to model smoking in an Italian case-control study on lung cancer (source of data: Richiardi et al. 2004)

Model	Retail trade salesmen (54 exposed cases) OR (95% CI)[b]	Mail distribution clerks (58 exposed cases) OR (95% CI)
1	1.56 (1.04–2.35)	1.47 (1.00–2.17)
2	1.41 (0.93–2.15)	1.62 (1.07–2.45)
3	1.30 (0.85–2.01)	1.65 (1.08–2.52)
4	1.30 (0.84–2.03)	1.63 (1.06–2.51)
5	1.26 (0.81–1.95)	1.70 (1.10–2.61)
6	1.28 (0.82–2.00)	1.70 (1.10–2.63)
7	1.26 (0.81–1.98)	1.70 (1.10–2.65)

[a] All models were adjusted for age and study area. Model 1: no smoking variables; Model 2: smoking status categorized as ever/never smoker; Model 3: smoking status categorized as current/former (since at least 2 years)/never smoker; Model 4: same as model 3 with three levels for current smokers: 1–9, 10–19, 20+ packyears; Model 5: same as model 3 with number of packyears introduced as a continuous variable; Model 6: same as model 5 with 4 levels for time since cessation: 2–5, 6–10, 11–15, 16+ years; Model 7: same as model 6, using b-spline cubic regression with knots at 10, 20, 30, and 40 packyears to model the cumulative number of cigarettes smoked

[b] OR, odds ratio adjusted for age, study area; CI, confidence interval

first phenomenon is known as the 'healthy hire effect', whereas the second, associated with duration of employment, is known as the 'healthy worker survivor effect' (Arrighi and Hertz-Picciotto 1994). The magnitude of the phenomena depends on the type of work, general social conditions (e.g. unemployment rate), the disease under study (e.g. studies of cancer are generally less biased than studies of diseases with shorter induction period) and the study design (Choi 1992). The healthy worker effect is also seen as a traditional confounding problem, as employment status is associated at the same time with the health status of workers and disease risk (Checkoway et al. 2004). Because of the healthy worker effect, cohorts of workers may have lower mortality rates than the general population. Negative results in occupational epidemiological studies may therefore hide harmful exposures. Moreover, an increase in risk of a disease may artificially plateau at the highest level of cumulative exposure, at which workers have the longest duration of employment (Stayner et al. 2003).

A logical approach for controlling, or at least decreasing, the bias introduced by the healthy worker effect is to use an appropriate internal or external comparison group, namely a group of unexposed workers who possibly underwent similar health-related selection at the time of employment. Use of such a comparison group does not, however, imply unbiased estimates, as the healthy worker survivor effect may still persist. Indeed, as reviewed by Checkoway and colleagues (Checkoway et al. 2004), four time-related factors should be considered: age at first employment, duration of employment, length of follow-up (members of a cohort can be followed-up also after they have left the job) and age at risk. Arrighi and Hertz-Picciotto (1996) evaluated four suggested methods for controlling the healthy worker effect: (1) restricting analyses to long-term survivors; (2) excluding recent exposures, introducing a lag of 10–20 years; (3) introducing current employment status as a confounder in the models; and (4) modelling employment status simultaneously as a confounder (the same as in the third approach), and as an intermediate time-dependent variable (if the risk factor for the disease under study is also a determinant of job termination, and, therefore, of change in employment status). The latter technique uses the so-called G-method as suggested by Robins and colleagues (Robins 1986; Robins et al. 1992). This approach has the strongest theoretical support and was considered the most appropriate after empirical evaluation, although there are difficulties in its implementation. Lagging exposure is a valid, straightforward alternative, that can be implemented when the induction period between exposure and disease is not short.

Case-control and cross-sectional studies are not free from the healthy worker effect. In case-control studies, it can result in differential sampling of controls from the exposed and the unexposed population. For instance, if controls are selected from hospitalised patients and individuals with a particular occupational exposure tend to be healthier, then the proportion of exposed controls is artificially decreased. The odds ratio would, therefore, be overestimated, a bias that reverses the usual underestimation of SMRs introduced by the healthy worker effect in cohort studies.

In a cross-sectional study, workers with higher exposure may have a paradoxically lower prevalence of diseases or symptoms known to be associated with exposure, because diseased workers would tend to leave jobs entailing the exposure.

Dose-Response Analysis 2.4.3

As discussed in Chap. I.11, the dose is the level of the risk factor at the target organ, while exposure refers to the level of the risk factor in the external environment. Although the dose is the biologically relevant measure, the amount of exposure, as a surrogate of the dose, is usually the only available information in occupational studies, so that a dose-response analysis is in fact an exposure-response analysis. In some studies the actual dose can be estimated from measurements of exposure and knowledge of the specific agent uptake and clearance (US Environmental Protection Agency 2002).

Exposure can be measured using different metrics, namely duration, intensity and cumulative level (cf. Chap. I.11). The selection of the metric should be based on the – often unknown – mechanism of disease development and on the nature of the exposure itself. Importantly, the choice of the metric influences the magnitude of the estimates and the shape of the dose-response (Blair and Stewart 1992). Cumulative exposure, i.e. the product of intensity and duration, is a correct metric for several types of diseases where risk is directly proportional to dose. Duration of employment is a valid surrogate for cumulative exposure when intensity of exposure has been relatively constant over time, through working areas of the plant and across tenures (Checkoway 1986). Peak exposure is more important than duration in the study of diseases for which a threshold exists, such as back pain or acute toxicity.

A dose-response analysis is commonly carried out in occupational epidemiology for at least three main reasons. First, occupational exposures are time- and place-specific, implying that assessment of an association between an occupational exposure and a disease necessarily takes the level of exposure into account. Second, a dose-response relation is one of the well-known Bradford Hill's criteria for establishing causality (Hill 1965). When the risk for a disease increases continuously with increasing exposure, whatever the shape of the trend, the likelihood of a causal association is higher. However, on the one hand, a dose-response relation does not prove causality; on the other hand, the lack of such a relation does not imply lack of a causal association, as clearly demonstrated by threshold phenomena. Third, the dose-response analysis is one of the steps in risk assessment, which aims at quantifying the health effects of environmental and occupational exposures that can be modified by new policies and technologies. Risk assessment comprises: (1) hazard identification, on the basis of evaluation of the available evidence on the health effects of the agent; (2) exposure assessment, identifying the nature of the exposure in the population, the characteristics of the exposed individuals and the behaviour of the agent in humans; (3) identification of the exposure-risk model, which implies a dose-response assessment; and (4) risk characterization, determining the exposure level-specific health effects in the population (Nurminem et al. 1999; Checkoway et al. 2004).

Often, data on exposure in occupational epidemiology are summarized as qualitative, or semi-quantitative indices. For instance, JEMs usually produce indices of intensity and probability of exposure on an ordinal scale. Such information offers little basis for a dose-response analysis. In other instances, if quantitative information is available, cumulative exposure can be estimated for each study subject; it must be born in mind, however, that quantitative estimates are affected by measurement errors, falling in the two broad categories of classical and Berkson error already discussed in Sect. 2.3.3. Among many possible examples, we cite here the dose-response analysis carried out by Steenland and colleagues (1998) on occupational exposure to diesel exhaust in the trucking industry and the risk for lung cancer, which was used for quantitative risk assessment by the Health Effects Institute (1999). Steenland and colleagues conducted a case-control study, obtaining information on lifetime work histories from interviews with the study subjects' next-of-kin and from retirement registries. Then, for the purpose of exposure assessment, workers were assigned to the category in which they had been employed the longest. Contemporaneously, an industrial hygiene survey was conducted to measure levels of exposure to elemental carbon (a marker of exposure to diesel exhaust, which is a complex mixture of gases and particulates) in the main job categories within the trucking industry (Zaebst et al. 1991). Combining the lifetime work histories with the results of the survey and making several assumptions, in particular with regard to past exposure, the cumulative exposure of each worker was estimated. Although quantitative data were obtained, the level of misclassification of exposure was still presumably high, albeit non-differential. In particular, each subject's true exposure in each job category was a random variation of the exposure level that was assigned to that job based on the industrial hygiene survey.

There are several approaches to dose-response analysis, including simple parametric models, categorical analysis, biological-based models, polynomial regression, spline regression and nonparametric models, such as generalized additive models (cf. Chaps. II.2 and II.3 of this handbook). We will not describe and compare these techniques, but we highlight some aspects that are specific to occupational epidemiology. Interested readers may refer to the above chapters or one of the several available thematic textbooks (Härdle 1990; Hastie and Tibshirani 1990).

Categorical analysis, in which the exposure variable is subdivided into a certain number of categories on the basis of cut-points chosen a priori, is usually the starting point for a dose-response assessment, as it allows researchers to observe the shape of the dose-response relationship. The shape is obviously strongly influenced by the choice and number of the cut-points, that can be decided upon according to biological considerations, if available, or other criteria, including established standards or the percentile method. Evidence that an association is limited to the highest exposure levels should not lead to disregard causality without careful consideration of the possibility of a threshold for the effect of interest.

When the exposure variable is continuous, the simplest approach consists in fitting a regression model with a term for the exposure (e.g. cumulative exposure). This implies assuming a priori a shape of the dose-response curve, that seldom reflects biological knowledge, if any is available. When the exposure variable is not transformed, the assumed shape is usually log-linear or logistic. In occupational epidemiology, a levelling off in the increasing trend in risk for chronic diseases is often observed at the highest levels of exposure (Stayner et al. 2003). The explanations for this levelling off can be either biological (e.g. saturation phenomena, depletion of susceptible individuals) or methodological (e.g. misclassification of exposure, healthy worker effect), and a log transformation of the cumulative exposure variable is an option to consider.

Among the more complex alternatives, spline regression and its variants (b-splines and loess among the most popular) can be implemented quite easily with common software packages. It is therefore being used increasingly in occupational and environmental epidemiology (Greenland et al. 2000; Steenland et al. 2001; Thurston et al. 2002; Steenland and Deddens 2004). Spline regression, that is based on piecewise polynomials, has the advantage of providing a smoothed dose–response curve, although it does not always produce easily interpretable estimates (Harrell et al. 1988; Greenland 1995). Figure 2.2 shows an example of a dose-response analysis of data from men included in a case-control study on occupational factors and lung cancer risk that we carried out in two areas of northern Italy in 1990–1992 (Richiardi et al. 2004). The odds ratio (plotted on the log scale) of lung cancer increased with duration of employment until 10–15 years and slightly decreased after that. Estimates for the durations of employment above

30 years are not interpretable because of few observations and consequent large confidence intervals. This shape in dose-response is not entirely unexpected when duration of exposure is used in the analysis, as subjects with longer duration of employment may be those with lower intensity of exposure and better health status.

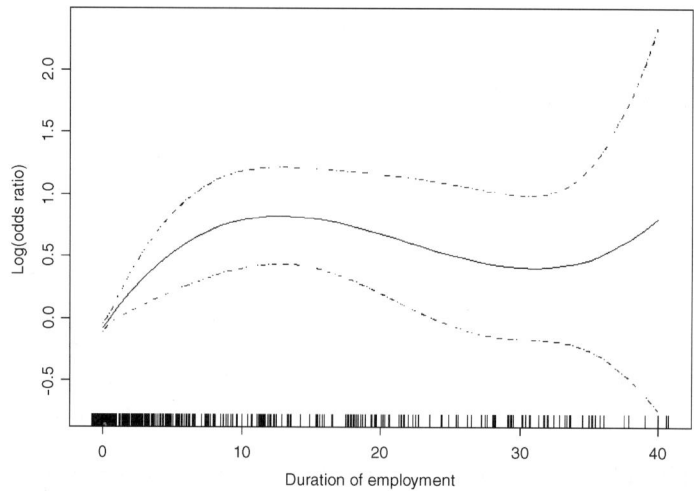

Figure 2.2. Association between duration of employment in occupations known to entail exposure to lung carcinogens and risk of lung cancer modelled using a generalized additive model with cubic b-splines (four degrees of freedom), adjusted for study area, age, and cigarette smoking (current/former/never smokers) (source of data: Richiardi et al. 2004)

Primary Prevention

How can occupational epidemiology help evaluate the need and effectiveness of primary prevention interventions and policies?

Sound epidemiological studies are typically needed to produce evidence of toxicity for occupational agents when long-term effects are present such as in occupational cancer that we use here as an example (Merletti and Mirabelli 2004). Complex mixtures entailing occupational exposures were among the first causes of cancer to be identified and finally led to the identification of specific causal agents. Thus the study of occupational cancers offered precious insights and paradigms for occupational epidemiology at large.

Agents currently established as causes of occupational cancer and occupations with sufficient evidence of increased cancer risk according to the International Agency for Research on Cancer can be found in this textbook (see Chap. IV.3 of this handbook; IARC 2004).

In appraising the body of evidence on occupational hazards and its relevance for control of occupational exposures, consideration must be given to the problem of who should bear the burden of proof, and what the proof should consist of: whether evidence of benefit from intervention or evidence of harm from exposure. Occupational exposures are imposed upon individuals who have little, if any, personal choice, freedom, and responsibility in accepting or avoiding them. Furthermore, they often lack the basic necessary knowledge. As consequence, the burden of proof is on the employer, to demonstrate that the production process is safe. Evidence that exposure may be harmful is sufficient to require intervention to eliminate it.

Primary prevention, in the field of exposure to carcinogens as well as of other chemical and physical hazards at work, is based on the application of basic industrial hygiene strategies at the industry level: (1) substitution with agents intended not to be as dangerous, (2) fully enclosed processing, (3) strict control of exposure by reduction of amounts used, by local exhaust, by personal protection, by cleaning practices, etc. This means to reduce the number of potentially exposed workers and their exposure level. Exposure control is better implemented by embedding it in the project of plants and processes, aiming to workers' protection as well as to that of neighbouring communities.

At the community and country level, primary prevention entails adopting regulations intended to favour preventive measures or to enforce them. The first country to forbid the manufacture of certain chemicals because of their carcinogenicity was the United Kingdom, with the Carcinogenic Substances Regulations in 1967, prohibiting beta-naphtylamine, benzidine, 4-aminobiphenyl and 4-nitrobiphenyl (UK 1967). The EC regulation on carcinogens at work has been developed starting with the 90/394/EEC Directive, but still today the only carcinogenic agents whose production and use is forbidden, apart from asbestos, are the same four as in the UK Carcinogenic Substances Regulations. In the USA no formal ban has been put on any carcinogenic agent, production, or process on grounds of workers' protection. Permissible exposure levels (PELs) have been established by OSHA largely on the basis of the 1987 list of the American Conference of Governmental Industrial Hygienists (ACGIH) threshold limit values (TLVs), with the result that: (1) the TLVs list has been updated and expanded by ACGIH, but the list of PELs is unchanged, (2) certain agents are commonly recognized carcinogens but their PELs were established without taking their cancer causing properties into account (Smith and Mendeloff 1999).

Despite these limitations, OSHA and EPA in the USA, and the EC in its regulation on classification, labelling and packaging of dangerous substances publish lists of substances officially recognized as carcinogens. The availability of lists of carcinogenic, and in general of toxic, chemicals is a useful tool for hazard identification, even if limited to intentionally used agents.

Workers' information on their exposures and on the risks entailed by them is a fundamental issue. It is the first step in their empowerment to verify that appropriate measures have been taken. The EC regulation requires that specific information is given to exposed workers, including special instructions on how to deal with accidents and emergencies.

Provided local regulations have been adopted, like all EC Member States should have done, law enforcement through technical public services specialized in inspecting workplaces is another key issue. Further, workers should be able to stand in courts not only when they are affected by work-related conditions, but just because they are exposed, and their cases should be fairly settled, which does not seem to occur currently even in large EC Member States (Editorial 2003).

It may be surprising that systematic reviews on the effectiveness of interventions and/or implementation activities aimed at exposure control are generally lacking. In the area of occupational cancer an exception may be the review by Kogevinas and coworkers in 1998 on the rubber industry (Kogevinas et al. 1998), where some changes in overall technology and chemistry were considered along with evidence on the persistence of previously observed cancer risks. This review is useful to point out the many and different difficulties we are confronted with while trying to gather evidence of effectiveness in occupational cancer prevention:

1. The long induction period of most human cancers prevents driving conclusions from early observations after changes are introduced, since workers first employed after intervention are not yet at risk, or fully at risk, of developing the disease.

2. Longer term observations, however, are difficult to carry out; they are also difficult to interpret because of changing patterns of incidence/mortality in the disease of interest, and of possible complex interactions with other exposures.

3. Often the exposure characteristics are not well understood and recorded, so it may become impossible to assess the quantitative relationship between exposure level and disease occurrence, which is precisely what is needed when exposure levels are reduced but the agent is not completely eliminated.

   a. Sometimes the nature of the relevant exposure is not understood, so that a carcinogenic agent may be withdrawn but its substitutes may be as dangerous, or almost as dangerous.

   b. Both industry-based and community-based epidemiological studies have major limits in exposure assessment, due to lack of suitable exposure data, and this is the origin of major uncertainties and controversies in the interpretation of epidemiological evidence.

This picture explains why it is difficult to obtain evidence of cancer risk reduction following the adoption of control measures, and why reports of this kind of evidence are rare.

Within the limits of the above mentioned uncertainties, some widespread occupational cancer risks (Cruickshank and Squire 1950) seem to have disappeared from industrial and agricultural settings in Europe and in the USA. Furthermore, some carcinogenic exposures also disappeared, or have been reduced to lower levels. Results in terms of reduction of the fraction of cancers attributable to occupation cannot be estimated currently and have to be the object of future scientific investigations.

Some contradictory experiences occurred either: Agents have been substituted with others now seemingly entailing the same risks, carcinogenic contaminants have been eliminated from agents used in certain industries only to be introduced in agents used in other processes, only partial elimination of risk has been achieved when relevant exposures were to complex mixtures rather than to simple chemicals (Evanoff et al 1993). Therefore, workers' exposure to carcinogens in industrialized countries is still not controlled as completely as it should be, given our current knowledge of the carcinogenic properties of chemical and physical agents. The most critical point, however, is continuation of productions and processes entailing exposure to carcinogens in developing countries, often lacking experience in the management of industrial hazards and power to enforce sound control strategies (Jeyaratnam 1994).

Conclusions 2.6

Attempts have been made to estimate the global burden of disease and injury due to occupational factors (Leigh et al. 1997, 1999; Ezzati et al. 2002). Although such global statistics are of difficult interpretation given, the very large number of assumptions underlying them, two major conclusions can be drawn: (1) the problem is still an important one throughout the world, including developed regions; (2) the burden is shifting to the developing world, which accounts to 70% of the world's work-force and where the globalization of industry is resulting in increased exposure to occupational agents. The situation is exacerbated by unsafe technology, transfer of hazardous industries and wastes from developed to developing countries, use of agents banned or restricted elsewhere, poor health and nutritional status of the work-force and ineffective legislation on occupational safety and health. Although prevention of exposure to occupational hazards will come from political and economic changes in the world, just as political and economic interests are the determinants of the present situation, much can still achieved, even in the current international situation (Pearce et al. 1994).

The applications of occupational epidemiology in public health decision-making are broadening, providing inputs to risk assessment, evaluation of occupational guidelines and extrapolation of findings from occupational settings to communities with the aim of setting policies at population level. These multiple applications mean increasing responsibility to ensure ethical scientific conduct and clear, thorough communication of the assumptions, limitations and uncertainties of the results of research and of risk assessment (Kriebel and Tickner 2001).

Recent discoveries in molecular biology and genetics have made it possible for researchers to examine how genetic characteristics affect responses to occupational and environmental exposures. The use of genetic biomarkers in epidemiology has provided potential understanding of the underlying mechanisms of disease and therefore ultimately contribute to Public Health. Despite the potential benefits of genetic information, its collection in epidemiological studies, particularly in occupational settings, presents ethical, legal and social challenges. Clarifying gene-environment interactions will have implications for difficult regulatory questions, such as protecting the most susceptible members of the population and its subgroups, but in the case of workers, genetic information could be used to discriminate them (Christiani et al. 2001). The challenge of identifying and applying genetic information in the study of human diseases in instances in which it will make a difference to prevention and public health (Millikan 2002; Merikangas and Risch 2003; Schulte 2004) may well also apply to occupational epidemiology.

Acknowledgements. This work was partially supported by the Italian Association for Cancer Research and the Special Project Oncology, Compagnia San Paolo. We thank Francesco Barone Adesi for useful comments.

References

Ahrens W, Jöckel KH, Brochard P, Bolm-Audorff U, Grossgarten K, Iwatsubo Y, Orlowski E, Pohlabeln H, Berrino F (1993) Retrospective assessment of asbestos exposure–I. Case-control analysis in a study of lung cancer: efficiency of job-specific questionnaires and job exposure matrices. Int J Epidemiol S2: 83–95

Ahrens W (1999) Retrospective assessment of occupational exposure in case-control studies. Ecomed, Landsberg

Andersen A, Barlow L, Engeland A, Kjaerheim K, Lynge E, Pukkala E (1999) Work-related cancer in the Nordic countries. Scand J Work Environ Health 25:1–116

Armstrong BG (1998) Effects of measurement error on epidemiological studies of environmental and occupational exposures. Occup Environ Med 55:651–656

Arrighi HM, Hertz-Picciotto I (1994) The evolving concept of the healthy worker effect. Epidemiology 5:189–196

Arrighi HM, Hertz-Picciotto I (1996) Controlling the healthy worker survivor effect: an example of arsenic exposure and respiratory cancer. Occup Environ Med 53:455–462

Axelson O (1978) Aspects of confounding in occupational health epidemiology. Scand J Work Environ Health 4:85–89

Axelson O, Steenland K (1988) Indirect methods of assessing the effects of tobacco use in occupational studies. Am J Ind Med 13:105–118

Berrino F, Richiardi L, Boffetta P, Esteve J, Belletti I, Raymond L, Troschel L, Pisani P, Zubiri L, Ascunce N, Guberan E, Tuyns A, Terracini B, Merletti F, Milan JEM Working Group (2003) Occupation and larynx and hypopharynx cancer: a job-exposure matrix approach in an international case-control study in France, Italy, Spain and Switzerland. Cancer Causes Control 14: 213–223

Blair A, Stewart PA (1992) Do quantitative exposure assessments improve risk estimates in occupational studies of cancer? Am J Ind Med 21:53–63

Blair A, Hoar SK, Walrath J (1985) Comparison of crude and smoking-adjusted standardized mortality ratios. J Occup Med 27:881–884

Boffetta P, Saracci R, Andersen A, Bertazzi PA, Chang-Claude J, Cherrie J, Ferro G, Frentzel-Beyme R, Hansen J, Olsen J, Plato N, Teppo L, Westernholm P, Winter PD, Zocchetti C (1997) Cancer mortality among man-made vitreous fiber production workers. Epidemiology 8:259–268

Boffetta P, Andersen A, Hansen J, Olsen J, Plato N, Teppo L, Westernholm P, Saracci R (1999) Cancer incidence among European man-made vitreous fiber production workers. Scand J Environ Health 25:222–226

Boffetta P, Richiardi L, Berrino F, Esteve J, Pisani P, Crosignani P, Raymond L, Zubiri L, Del Moral A, Lehmann W, Donato F, Terracini B, Tuyns A, Merletti F (2003) Occupation and larynx and hypopharynx cancer: an international case-control study in France, Italy, Spain, and Switzerland. Cancer Causes Control 14:203–212

Bouyer J, Dardenne J, Hemon D (1995) Performance of odds ratios obtained with a job-exposure matrix and individual exposure assessment with special reference to misclassification errors. Scand J Work Environ Health 21:265–271

Boyd JT, Doll R, Faulds JS, Leiper J (1970) Cancer of the lung in iron (haematite) miners. Br J Industr Med 27:97–105

Brüske-Hohlfeld I, Möhner M, Pohlabeln H, Ahrens W, Bolm-Audorff U, Kreienbrock L, Kreuzer M, Jahn I, Wichmann HE, Jöckel KH (2000) Occupational lung cancer risk for men in Germany: results from a pooled case-control study. Am J Epidemiol 151:384–395

Burstyn I, Kromhout H, Kauppinen T, Heikkala P, Boffetta P (2000) Statistical modelling of the determinants of historical exposure to bitumen and polycyclic aromatic hydrocarbons among paving workers. Ann Occ Hyg 44:43–56

Burstyn I, Boffetta P, Kauppinen T, Heikkala P, Svane O, Partanen T, Stucker I, Frentzel-Beyme R, Ahrens W, Merzenich H, Heederik D, Hooiveld M, Langard S, Randem BG, Jarvholm B, Bergdahl I, Shaham J, Ribak J, Kromhout H (2003) Estimating exposures in the asphalt industry for an international epidemiological cohort study of cancer risk. Am J Ind Med 43:3–17

Carter T (2000) Diseases of occupations – a short history of their recognition and prevention. In: Baxter PJ, Adams PH, Tar-Ching Aw, Cockcroft A, Harrington JM (eds) Hunter's diseases of occupations. Arnold, London, pp 917–925

Case RAM, Hosker ME (1954) Tumours of the urinary bladder as an occupational disease in the rubber industry in England and Wales. Br J Prev Soc Med 8:39–50

Case RAM, Hosker ME, McDonald DB (1954) Tumours of the urinary bladder in workmen engaged in the manufacture and use of certain dyestuff intermediates in the British chemical industry. Br J Ind Med 11:75–104

Checkoway H (1986) Methods of treatment of exposure data in occupational epidemiology. Med Lav 77:48–73

Checkoway H, Pearce N, Kriebel D (2004) Research methods in occupational epidemiology. Oxford University Press, Oxford

Choi BCK (1992) Definition, sources, magnitude, effect modifiers, and strategies of reduction of the healthy worker effect. J Occup Med 34:979–988

Christiani DC, Sharp RR, Collman GW, Suk WA (2001). Applying genomic technologies in environmental health research: challenges and opportunities. J Occup Environ Med 43:526–533

Coggon D (2000) Estimating the extent of occupational injuries and disease. In: Baxter PJ, Adams PH, Tar-Ching Aw, Cockcroft A, Harrington JM (eds) Hunter's diseases of occupations. Arnold, London, pp 27–35

Costa G, Merletti F, Segnan N (1989) A mortality cohort study in a north Italian aircraft factory. Br J Ind Med 46:738–743

Cruiskshank CND, Squire JR (1950) Skin cancer in the engineering industry from the use of mineral oil. Brit J Ind Med 7:1–11

Doll R (1952) The causes of death among gas-workers with special reference to cancer of the lung. Br J Ind Med 9:180–185

Doll R (1955) Mortality from lung cancer in asbestos workers. Br J Ind Med 12:81–86

Doll R (1975) Pott and the prospects for prevention. Br J Cancer 32:263–74

Dosemeci M, Stewart PA, Blair A (1990a) Three proposals for retrospective, semi-quantitative exposure assessments and their comparison with other assessment methods. Appl Occup Environ Hyg 5:52–59

Dosemeci M, Wacholder S, Lubin JH (1990b) Does nondifferential misclassification of exposure always bias a true effect toward the null value? Am J Epidemiol 132:746–748

Dosemeci M, McLaughlin JK, Chen JQ, Hearl F, McCrawley M, Wu Z, Chen RG, Peng KL, Chen AL, Rexing SH (1994a) Indirect validation of a retrospective method of exposure assessment used in a nested case-control study of lung cancer and silica exposure. Occup Environ Med 51:136–138

Dosemeci M, Li GL, Hayes RB, Yin SN, Linet M, Chow WH, Wang YZ, Jiang ZL, Dai TR, Zhang WU, Chao XJ, Ye PZ, Kou QR, Fan YH, Zhang XC, Lin XF, Meng JF, Zho JS, Wacholder S, Kneller R, Blot WJ (1994b) Cohort study among workers exposed to benzene in China: II. Exposure assessment. Am J Ind Med 26:401–411

Dosemeci M, Yin SN, Linet M, Wacholder S, Rothman N, Li GL, Chow WH, Wang YZ, Jiang ZL, Dai TR, Zhang WU, Chao XJ, Ye PZ, Kou QR, Fan YH, Zhang XC, Lin XF, Meng JF, Zho JS, Blot WJ, Hayes RB (1996) Indirect validation of benzene exposure assessment by association with benzene poisoning. Environ Health Perspect S6:1343–1347

Editorial (2003) Who will take responsibility for corporate killing? Lancet 361:1921

Evanoff BA, Gustavsson P, Hogstedt C (1993). Mortality and incidence of cancer in a cohort of Swedish chimney sweeps: an extended follow-up study. Brit J Ind Med 50:450–459

Ezzati M, Lopez AD, Rodgers A, Vander Hoorn S, Murray CJ, Comparative Risk Assessment Collaborating Group (2002). Selected major risk factors and global and regional burden of disease. Lancet 360:1347–1360

Flanders WD, Khoury MJ (1990) Indirect assessment of confounding: graphic description and limits on effect of adjusting for covariates. Epidemiology 1:239–246

Fox AJ, Collier PF (1976) Low mortality rates in industrial cohort studies due to selection for work and survival in the industry. Br J Prev Soc Med 30:225–230

Fritschi L, Nadon L, Benke G, Lakhani R, Latreille B, Parent ME, Siemiatycki J (2003) Validation of expert assessment of occupational exposures. Am J Ind Med 43:519–522

Gail MH, Wacholder S, Lubin JH (1988) Indirect corrections for confounding under multiplicative and additive risk models. Am J Ind Med 13:119–130

Goodman M, Kelsh M, Ebi K, Iannuzzi J, Langholz B (2002) Evaluation of potential confounders in planning a study of occupational magnetic field exposure and female breast cancer. Epidemiology 13:50–58

Grayson JK (1996) Radiation exposure, socioeconomic status, and brain tumor risk in the US Air Force: a nested case-control study. Am J Epidemiol 143:480–486

Greenland S, Poole C (1994) Empirical-Bayes and semi-Bayes approaches to occupational and environmental hazard surveillance. Arch Environ Health 49:9–16

Greenland S (1995) Dose-response and trend analysis in epidemiology: alternatives to categorical analysis. Epidemiology 6:356–365

Greenland S, Sheppard AR, Kaune WT, Poole C, Kelsh MA (2000) A pooled analysis of magnetic fields, wire codes, and childhood leukemia. Childhood Leukemia-EMF Study Group. Epidemiology 11:624–634

Haldorsen T, Andersen A, Boffetta P (2004) Smoking-adjusted incidence of lung cancer by occupation among Norwegian men. Cancer Causes Control 15:139–147

Harber P, Muranko H, Shvartsblat S, Solis S, Torossian A, Oren T (2003) A triangulation approach to historical exposure assessment for the carbon black industry. J Occup Environ Med 45:131–143

Härdle W (1990) Applied nonparametric regression. Cambridge University Press, Cambridge, New York

Harrell FE Jr, Lee KL, Pollock BG (1988) Regression models in clinical studies: determining relationships between predictors and response. J Natl Cancer Inst 80:1198–1202

Hastie T, Tibshirani R (1990) Generalized additive models. Chapman and Hall, London

Hayes RB, Yin SN, Dosemeci M, Li GL, Wacholder S, Travis LB, Li CY, Rothman N, Hoover RN, Linet MS (1997) Benzene and the dose-related incidence of Hematologic Neoplasms in China. J Natl Cancer Inst 89:1065–1071

Health Effects Institute (1999) Diesel emissions and lung cancer: Epidemiology and quantitative risk assessment. A Special Report of the Institute's Diesel Epidemiology Expert Panel. Flagship Press, Andover, MA

Hill AB (1965) The environment and disease: association or causation. Proc R Soc Med 58:295–300

Hoar SK, Morrison AS, Cole P, Silverman DT (1980) An occupational exposure linking system for the study of occupational carcinogenesis. J Occup Med 22:722–726

IARC (2004) List of IARC evaluations (http://monographs.iarc.fr/monoeval/grlist.html) Accessed June 03, 2004

Iwatsubo Y, Pairon JC, Boutin C, Menard O, Massin N, Caillaud D, Orlowski E, Galateau Salle F, Bignon J, Brochard P (1998) Pleural mesothelioma: dose-response relation at low levels of asbestos exposure in a French population-based case-control study. Am J Epidemiol 148:133–142

Jeyaratnam J (1994). Transfer of hazardous industries. In: Pearce N, Matos E, Vainio H, Boffetta P, Kogevinas M (eds) Occupational cancer in developing countries. International Agency for Research on Cancer, Lyon, pp 23–29

Kauppinen T, Partanen T (1988) Use of plant- and period-specific job-exposure-matrices in studies on occupational cancer. Scand J Work Environ Health 14:161–167

Kauppinen TP, Pannet B, Marlow DA, Kogevinas M (1994) Retrospective assessment of exposure through modelling in a study on cancer risks among workers exposed to phenoxy herbicides, chlorophenols and dioxins. Scand J Work Environ Health 20:262–271

Kjaerheim K, Boffetta P, Hansen J, Cherrie J, Chang-Claude J, Eilber U, Ferro G, Guldner K, Olsen JH, Plato N, Proud L, Saracci R, Westerholm P, Andersen A (2002) Lung cancer among rock and slag wool production workers. Epidemiology 13:445–553

Kogevinas M, Sala M, Boffetta P, Kazerouni N, Kromhout H, Hoar-Zahm S (1998). Cancer risk in the rubber industry: a review of the recent epidemiological evidence. Occup Environ Med 55:1–12

Kriebel D, Tickner J (2001). Reenergizing public health through precaution. Am J Public Health 91:1351–1355

Kromhout H, Symanski E, Rappaport SM (1993) A comprehensive evaluation of within- and between-workers components of occupational exposure to chemical agents. Ann Occup Hyg 37:253–270

Larsen SB, Spano M, Giwercman A, Bonde JP (1999) Semen quality and sex hormones among organic and traditional Danish farmers. ASCLEPIOS Study Group. Occup Environ Med 56:139–144

Leigh JP, Marcowitz SB, Fahs M, Shin C, Landrigan PJ (1997) Occupational injury and illness in the United States. Arch Int Med 157:1557–1568

Leigh J, Macaskill P, Kuosma E, Mandryk J (1999) Global burden of disease and injury due to occupational factors. Epidemiology 10:626–631

Luce D, Gerin M, Berrino F, Pisani P, Leclerc A (1993) Sources of discrepancies between a job exposure matrix and a case by case expert assessment for occupational exposure to formaldehyde and wood-dust. Int J Epidemiol S2:113–120

Macaluso M, Vineis P, Continenza D, Ferrario F, Pisani P, Audisio R (1983) Job exposure matrices: experience in Italy. In: Acheson ED (ed) Job exposure matrices: proceedings of a conference held in April 1982 the University of Southampton. MRC-EEU Scientific Report no.2, Southampton General Hospital

Mannetje A, Steenland K, Checkoway H, Koskela RS, Koponen M, Attfield M. Chen J, Hnizdo E, DeKlerk N, Dosemeci M (2002) Development of quantitative exposure data for a pooled exposure-response analysis of 10 silica cohorts. Am J Ind Med 42:73–86

McMichael AJ (1976) Standardized mortality ratios and the "healthy worker effect": Scratching beneath the surface. Occup Med 18:165–168

Merikangas KR, Risch N (2003) Genomic priorities and public health. Science 302:599–601

Merletti F, Mirabelli D (2004) Occupational exposures. In: Evidence-based cancer prevention: Strategies for NGOs. A UICC handbook for Europe. International Union Against Cancer, Geneva (in press)

Merletti F, Boffetta P, Ferro G, Pisani P, Terracini B (1991) Occupation and cancer of the oral cavity/oropharynx in Turin, Italy. Scand J Work Environ Health 17:248–254

Miettinen OS, Wang JD (1981) An alternative to the proportionate mortality ratio. Am J Epidemiol 114:144–1488

Millikan R (2002) The changing face of epidemiology in the genomics era. Epidemiology 13:472–480

Nurminem M, Nurminem T, Corvalàn CF (1999) Methodologic issues in epidemiologic risk assessment epidemiology 10:585–593

Orlowski E, Pohlabeln H, Berrino F, Ahrens W, Bolm-Audorff U, Grossgarten K, Iwatsubo Y, Jöckel KH, Brochard P (1993) Retrospective assessment of asbestos exposure–II. At the job level: complementarity of job-specific questionnaire and job exposure matrices. Int J Epidemiol S2:96–105

Pairon JC, Orlowski E, Iwatsubo Y, Billon-Gailland MA, Dufour G, Chamming's S, Archambault C, Bignon J, Brochard P (1994) Pleural mesothelioma and exposure to asbestos: evaluation from work histories and analysis of asbestos bodies in bronchoalveolar lavage fluid or lung tissue in 131 patients. Occup Environ Med 51:244–249

Pearce N, Matos E, Vainio H, Boffetta P, Kogevinas M (eds) (1994) Occupational cancer in developing countries. International Agency for Research on Cancer, Lyon, pp 23–29

Potashnik G, Ben-Aderet N, Israeli R, Yanai-Inbar I, Sober I (1978) Suppressive effect of 1,2-dibromo-3-chloropropane on human spermatogenesis. Fertil Steril 30:444–447

Pukkala E, Aspholm R, Auvinen A, Eliasch H, Gundestrup M, Haldorsen T, Hammar N, Hrafnkelsson J, Kyyronen P, Linnersjo A, Rafnsson V, Storm H, Tveten U (2002) Incidence of cancer among Nordic airline pilots over five decades: occupational cohort study. BMJ 325:567–569

Ramazzini B (1964) Diseases of workers. [Translation of De Morbis Artificium 1713 text.] Hafner, New York

Richardson DB, Ciampi A (2003) Effects of measurement error when an exposure variable is constrained by a lower limit. Am J Epidemiol 157:355–363

Richiardi L, Boffetta P, Simonato L, Forastiere F, Zambon P, Fortes C, Gaboricau V, Merletti F (2004) Occupational risk factors for lung cancer in men and women: a population-based case-control study in Italy. Cancer Causes Control 15:285–294

Robins JM (1986) A new approach to causal inference in mortality studies with sustained exposure period: application to control of the healthy worker survivor effect. Math Model 7:1393–1512

Robins JM, Blevins D, Ritter G, Wulfson M (1992) G-estimation of the effect of prophylaxis therapy for Pneumocystis carinii pneumonia on the survival of AIDS patients. Epidemiology 3:319–336

Rödelsperger K, Jöckel KH, Pohlabeln H, Romer W, Woitowitz HJ (2001) Asbestos and man-made vitreous fibers as risk factors for diffuse malignant mesothelioma: results from a German hospital-based case-control study. Am J Ind Med 39:262–275

Rybicki BA, Cole Johnson C, Peterson EL, Kortsha GX, Gorell JM (1997) Comparability of different methods of retrospective exposure assessment of metals in manufacturing industries. Am J Ind Med 31:36–43

RothmanKJ, Greenland S (eds) (1998) Modern epidemiology, 2nd edn. Lippincott-Raven Publishers, Philadelphia

Sali D, Boffetta P, Andersen A, Cherrie JW, Claude JC, Hansen J, Olsen JH, Pesatori AC, Plato N, Teppo L, Westerholm P, Winter P, Saracci R (1999) Nonneoplastic mortality of European workers who produce man made vitreous fibres. Occup Environ Med 56:612–617

Schulte PA (2004) Some implications of genetic biomarkers in occupational epidemiology and practice. Scand J Work Environ Health 30:71–79

Siemiatycki J, Day N, Fabry J, Cooper J (1981) Discovering carcinogens in the occupational environment: a novel epidemiologic approach. J Natl Cancer Inst 66:217–225

Siemiatycki J, Wacholder S, Dewar R, Cardis E, Greenwood C, Richardson L (1988) Degree of confounding bias related to smoking, ethnic group, and socioeconomic status in estimates of the associations between occupation and cancer. J Occup Med 30:617–625

Siemiatycki J, Fritschi L, Nadon L, Gerin M (1997) Reliability of an expert rating procedure for retrospective assessment of occupational exposures in community-based case-control studies. Am J Ind Med 31:280–286

Simonato L, Vineis P, Fletcher AC (1988) Estimates of the proportion of lung cancer attributable to occupational exposure. Carcinogenesis 9:1159–1165

Smith JS, Mendeloff JM (1999) A quantitative analysis of factors affecting PELs and TLVs for carcinogens. Risk Anal 19:1223–1234

Stayner L, Steenland K, Dosemeci M, Hertz-Picciotto I (2003) Attenuation of exposure-response curves in occupational cohort studies at high exposure levels. Scand J Work Environ Health 29:317–324

Steenland K, Deddens JA (2004) Practical guide to dose-response analyses and risk assessment in occupational epidemiology. Epidemiology 15:63–70

Steenland K, Deddens JA, Stayner L (1998) Diesel exhaust and lung cancer in the trucking industry: exposure-response analyses and risk assessment. Am J Ind Med 34:220–228

Steenland K, Bray I, Greenland S, Boffetta P (2000a) Empirical Bayes adjustments for multiple results in hypothesis-generating or surveillance studies. Cancer Epidemiol Biomarkers Prev 9:895–903

Steenland K, Deddens JA, Zhao S (2000b) Biases in estimating the effect of cumulative exposure in log-linear models when estimated exposure levels are assigned. Scand J Work Environ Health 26:37–43

Steenland K, Mannetje A, Boffetta P, Stayner L, Attfield M, Chen J, Dosemeci M, DeKlerk N, Hnizdo E, Koskela R, Checkoway H, International Agency for Research on Cancer (2001) Pooled exposure-response analyses and risk assessment for lung cancer in 10 cohorts of silica-exposed workers: an IARC multicentre study. Cancer Causes Control 12:773–784

Stengel B, Pisani P, Limasset JC, Bouyer J, Berrino F, Helmon D (1993) Retrospective evaluation of occupational exposure to organic solvents: questionnaire and job exposure matrix. Int J Epidemiol S2:72–82

Stewart P, Stewart W, Heineman EF, Dosemeci M, Linet M, Inskip PD (1996) A novel approach to data collection in a case-control study of cancer and occupational exposures. Int J Epidemiol 25:744–752

Stucker I, Boyer J, Mandereau L, Hemon D (1993) Retrospective evaluation of the exposure to polycyclic aromatic hydrocarbons: comparative assessments with a job exposure matrix and by experts in industrial hygiene. Int J Epidemiol S2:106–112

Takahashi K, Case BW, Dufresne A, Fraser R, Higashi T, Siemiatycki J (1994) Relation between lung asbestos fibre burden and exposure indices based on job history. Occup Environ Med 51:461–469

Thurston SW, Eisen EA, Schwartz J (2002) Smoothing in survival models: an application to workers exposed to metalworking fluids. Epidemiology 13:685–692

Tuyns AJ, Esteve J, Raymond L, Berrino F, Benhamou E, Blanchet F, Boffetta P, Crosignani P, Del Moral A, Lehmann W, Merletti F, Péquignot G, Riboli E, Sancho-Garnier H, Terracini G, Zubiri A, Zubiri L (1988) Cancer of the larynx/hypopharynx, tobacco and alcohol: IARC international case-control study in Turin and Varese (Italy), Zaragoza and Navarra (Spain), Geneva (Switzerland) and Calvados (France). Int J Cancer 41:483–491

UK (1967) Carcinogenic Substances Regulations – Statutory Instrument No. 487

US Environmental Protection Agency (EPA) (2002) Noncancer health effects of diesel exhaust. In: Health assessment document for diesel engine exhaust. Prepared by the National Center for Environmental Assessment, Washington, DC, for the Office of Transportation and Air Quality. EPA/600/8-90/057F pp 5.2–5.23

Zaebst DD, Clapp DE, Blade LM, Marlow DA, Steenland K, Hornung RW, Scheutzle D, Butler J (1991) Quantitative determination of trucking industry workers' exposures to diesel exhaust particles. Am Ind Hyg Assoc J 52:529–541

Zahm SH, Blair A (2003) Occupational cancer among women: where have we been and where are we going? Am J Ind Med 44:565–575

Zahm SH, Pottern LM, Lewis DR, Ward MH, White DW (1994) Inclusion of women and minorities in occupational cancer epidemiologic research. J Occup Med 36:842–847

Environmental Epidemiology

III.3

Lothar Kreienbrock

3.1 **Introduction**

3.1.1 **Issues of Environmental Epidemiology**

The human environment – "the aggregate of surrounding things, conditions, or influences especially as affecting the existence or development of someone or something" (Webster's Encyclopedic Unabridged Dictionary of the English Language 1989) – is a topic of ever increasing public awareness. Concern about the safety of the environment has stimulated controversial debates both in the general public as well as in the scientific community. Environmental safety has to meet defined standards for the protection of public health and epidemiological knowledge has to be gathered on the impact of risk factors on human health.

Environmental epidemiology may be defined as "the study of the effect on human health of physical, biological, and chemical factors in the external environment. By examining specific populations or communities exposed to different ambient environments, environmental epidemiology seeks to clarify the relation between physical, biological, and chemical factors and human health" (NRC 1991).

Although this is a modern definition of the relation between environmental hazards and humans, the ideas of environmental epidemiology are linked to medical history. Environmental hazards were observed in ancient times. For example, Locher and Unschuld (1999) cite the antique scripts of Hippokrates "De aere aquis locis" or Aristoteles, recommending that cities have to be located in a healthy environment, and that air and water should be clean so as not to impair human well-being.

Another example of an environmental issue is the radon problem, which was first addressed in 1492 by Paulus Niavis in his essay, "Ludicium Iovis" oder "Das Gericht der Götter über den Bergbau":

"Wie man vom Schneeberge und von den Gruben zu sprechen hat: Die arbeiten darin, und die Luft im Berge, die sehr ungesund ist, nimmt ihnen die natürliche Farbe, sehr oft geschieht es auch, dass sie frühzeitig mit Tod abgehen." (cited by Schüttmann 1992).

More than 500 years ago, the very first observations were made of a possible relationship between "the air within the mine" (*die Luft im Berge*) and symptoms of disease and early mortality in the area of ancient ore mining around the village of Schneeberg in Saxony, Germany. Writings by famous early modern physicians like Agricola, *Bermannus oder über den Bergbau.* (1555), *De Re Metallica.* (1556), or Paracelsus, *Von der Bergsucht und anderen Bergkrankheiten* (1567), report cases of a special disease and describe disease clusters in Schneeberg, Joachimstal, and in other villages in this area. The disease was thus called Schneeberg's Lung Disease (*Schneeberger Lungenkrankheit*) (Schüttmann 1992).

Agricola and Paracelsus did not know the real cause of the disease; it was more than 300 years until the *Schneeberger Lungenkrankheit* was identified as lung cancer in the year 1879. With this the occupational causality was stated, but the real source of exposure was not known until the processes of radiation were discovered at the beginning of the 20th century. In 1909 the mines around Schneeberg were investigated and radioactivity was measured. Based on this, a director of the mines formulated in 1913 the hypothesis of an exposure-effect relationship between the "Radium Emanation" radon and lung cancer. Although the real nature of the dose-effect relationship was not known, the *Schneeberger Lungenkrankheit* was officially recognized in 1925 as an occupational disease in Germany in cases of diseased workers that had been extensively exposed in the mines. These observations led to the question of whether radon is a common risk. Due to the ubiquitous presence of the gas it can extrapolated that radon constitutes an environmental hazard in the general population (Schüttmann 1992).

Another classical example of environmental epidemiology is the famous risk map of John Snow, who reported cases of cholera in Soho, London, in the middle of the 19th century (Fig 3.1).

The increasing number of cholera cases in London in 1849 and 1853/54 caused a great awareness of the real reasons for the epidemic. John Snow's map can be considered as one of the initial steps in spatial statistics and spatial epidemiology (cf. Chap. II.8 of this handbook). It identified the source of the epidemic in the contaminated water of the Broad Street Pump. Additional research was carried

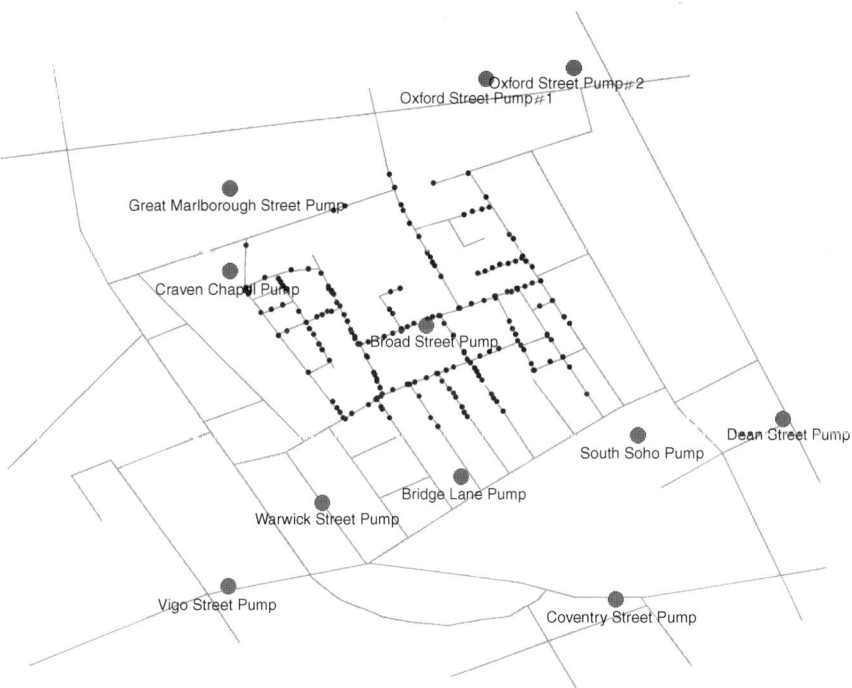

Figure 3.1. John Snow's map of cholera cases in Soho, London (figure modified from EpiInfo[TM] 2000)

out and it was discovered that cholera incidence differed substantially in the water supply areas of the Lambeth water company and the Southwark and Vauxhall water companies. While in "Lambeth's Area" 461 cases were observed in a population of 173,748, 4093 cases occurred in a population of 266,516 in the "Southwark and Vauxhall Area". The risk ratio of 5.8 indicated a serious problem with water contamination in the "Southwark and Vauxhall Area".

These classical examples illustrate that the impact of the environment on human health was realized very early and that this impact depends on the social and political situation of a population. Nowadays there are different environmental health concerns in the developed and the developing countries. With the foundation of modern epidemiology by Sir Richard Doll and others in the middle of the 20th century, the general focus of public and scientific concern was first on risk factors like smoking, occupation, and nutrition, and their association with cancer and cardiovascular diseases. Many methods of modern epidemiology were developed as applications on these associations. In the developed world, environmental issues of public and scientific concern are ambient air pollution, environmental tobacco smoke (ETS), or special agents known as hazardous from occupational exposures like lead and mercury and their impact on human health. In contrast, in the developing world the major concerns are pure air, sanitation, and clean water. Infectious diseases (cf. Chap. IV.1 of this handbook) in particular are of major interest, although severe exposures to chemical agents may occur in the developing world, as well.

Incomplete understanding of causes of many common diseases in both developed and developing countries focuses interest on identifying environmental hazards and incorporating this knowledge in strategies of risk management.

Concepts of Environmental Epidemiology and Toxicology

3.1.2

The concept of common risk analysis has been suggested as an approach to gaining basic comprehension of all processes necessary to understand and manage risks on human health (cf. e.g. Graham 1997). Risk analysis could be defined as a three-stage process including risk assessment, risk management, and risk communication. Risk assessment may be understood as a purely scientific process, in which information is collected to describe risk factors and their impact on human health, while risk management and risk communication describe the political and social process to put this information into population-relevant actions, rules, and laws.

The general principles of a scientific environmental risk assessment may be described as a four-step process:
— hazard identification, i.e.
   does the agent have the potential to cause an adverse effect?
— exposure assessment, i.e.
   what exposures are experienced or anticipated under relevant conditions?

— exposure-outcome assessment, i.e.
what is the relation between exposure and outcome in humans?
— risk characterization, i.e.
what is the estimated incidence and severity of an adverse effect in a given population?

The basic scientific methodologies to deal with environmental risks and to answer the questions of risk assessment are environmental epidemiology and environmental toxicology. Both concepts should be recognized as partners within a common risk assessment.

The risk assessment process in environmental toxicology usually comprises several steps of in vitro and animal experiments over a broad range of exposure intensities, leading to a NOEL (no observed effect level) in a sensitive animal species and the ADI (acceptable daily intake) that incorporates an appropriate safety factor, usually 100 or higher. This process of risk assessment to protect humans works well for numerous compounds, but it also has a number of shortcomings.

First, many agents like cancerogenic, genotoxic, and allergenic chemicals are not considered to have a threshold exposure level and may induce cancer or an allergic reaction at extremely low exposures. Second, usually single compounds are tested, although we are exposed to numerous agents simultaneously. The possibility of both synergistic and antagonistic interactions between agents greatly complicates the risk assessment process. Of particular importance are synergistic reactions that have been demonstrated in vitro and in experimental animals in some instances. Here, a single agent does not induce any – or only minor – adverse effects, while the simultaneous administration of two agents elicits a strong toxicological effect. Obviously, the NOEL-ADI approach using single agent administration does not incorporate the possibility of agent interactions. Therefore, additional methods must be developed to approach this problem. Third, the current concept does not take previous exposure into account. That is of special relevance for persistent bioaccumulative compounds like heavy metals. For these compounds the ADI should be based on estimation of human body burdens and body burden-response relationships.

Another problem is the difficulty of extrapolation to very low doses. The restriction in the number of animals per group that can be used and the paucity of data on the mechanistic action of agents are the main reasons for these difficulties. Much effort is being spent and more should be on the development of alternative methods in risk assessment to reduce the use of experimental animals. A number of cell and organ cultures of animal and human origin have been developed. The relative simplicity of these systems in comparison to whole animal models can be both advantageous and disadvantageous. However, few in vitro systems available at present are accepted as alternatives to whole animal models both in the scientific community and in regulatory agencies. It is clear that in vitro systems cannot reflect the entire organism and thus can reduce and refine, but not entirely replace animal experiments. However, in vitro systems can be of enormous help to understand the mechanisms of toxic action.

These limitations of in vitro and animal experiments in toxicology call for human data from observational epidemiological studies. In general, epidemiological investigations of environmental hazards have to be conducted with the same care as in other fields, but in environmental studies some special features have to be considered.

On the one hand, an environmental risk factor may cause severe diseases such as cancer or strong respiratory symptoms; on the other hand, these outcomes are also induced by many other risk factors; therefore the relative impact of the environmental agent is small. This is true for many environmental problems, as for example the effects of air pollution on respiratory health, the effects of water contaminated with heavy metals and subsequent permanent damage to children's intellectual potential, or the effects of residues in food on human health. Furthermore, there are only a few situations in which high concentrations of an environmental agent affect a large part of the population. These cases may be related to "special sources" and often result from an accident like the Chernobyl disaster, or from exposure of a population within a restricted area as a consequence of chronic pollution of the soil, e.g. by an industrial plant.

Investigation of small risks is one of the main characteristics of environmental epidemiology. At this point it has to be noted that a small relative risk does not mean that the risk is not important. Many environmental risk factors are ubiquitous, and large proportions of a population can be exposed. This may cause population-attributable risks that cannot be neglected, and results in an important task for risk management.

> "For example, the risk of death in males aged 45–74 years with a diastolic blood pressure of 95 mm Hg in the Framingham study was only about 1.15 times the risk in those with a diastolic blood pressure of 85 mm Hg, yet the amount of disease that could be prevented in the population by reducing diastolic pressures to 85 mm Hg would be substantial. Increased use of hypertension medication, along with improvements in diet and exercise, is thought to be responsible for some part of the substantial decline in cardiovascular mortality in the last 20 years" (NRC 1997).

But addressing small risks for multifactorial diseases leads to several problems in conducting an epidemiological investigation. First, all possible risk factors linked to a disease outcome should be incorporated into a study to avoid bias due to confounding and to study the possible interactions among all risk factors. This in turn requires that a large number of parameters be incorporated into a risk model. Therefore, large sample sizes are necessary to provide sufficient statistical power. Besides financial constraints, the logistic requirements are a major issue of the field work in an environmental epidemiological investigation.

Second, the overall power of an investigation will be influenced by the definition of exposure itself. For example "air pollution" is a mixture of hundreds of agents. If for this purpose an exposure-disease relationship has to be detected, the definition of exposure has to be clarified in advance. There are many different possibilities to assess the exposure and to conduct measurements, and each of them may contribute to the real exposure-disease relationship. As a consequence, a proper exposure assessment is of substantial importance and much effort has to be made to conduct a powerful investigation.

Therefore special methodological issues have to be taken into account in environmental epidemiology. Before these are described, special research situations need to be addressed in more detail as typical examples.

Examples of Research Fields in Environmental Epidemiology 3.2

There are numerous exposures and disease outcomes in environmental epidemiology, and there are many bibliographies, dictionaries and structured data bases with detailed information on the risks of environmental exposures. Only a few of them can be discussed further here.

Outdoor Air Pollution 3.2.1

From the earliest times, the impact of air pollution has been a major public health issue of interest in environmental epidemiology. For example, as early as 1294, the mayor of Venice is reported to have given orders to manufacturers of metals like mercury or tin to change the company's location to avoid exposing the population to "un-healthy smoke" (Locher and Unschuld 1999).

Industrial air pollution, coal burnt in domestic hearths, and traffic in combination with special weather conditions were the reasons for the London smog episode in early December, 1952. Smoke and sulphur dioxide pollution increased dramatically during this time. The visibility in central London dropped to a few meters and there was an up to 10-fold increase of ambient air concentrations of sulphur dioxide. Traffic and general public life were strongly restricted. More than 4000 deaths were attributed to the air pollution during that time, and mortality increased upon the average even in the months after this environmental disaster.

The London smog episode may be considered the beginning of quantitative risk assessment of the effects of air pollution on human health; it continues to influence the ideas and methods of environmental epidemiology today, as is shown for example by reanalysis of the 1952 data (e.g. Bell et al. 2004). As a political and social consequence, the British government introduced its first "Clean Air Act" in 1956 to reduce air pollution. As a scientific consequence air pollution was first defined by the level of sulphur dioxide and the concentration of particulate matter. Afterwards it was possible to make a more detailed analysis of the relationship between air pollution and human health by looking more closely at the diameter of particles, nitric (di)oxide, ozone, and other constituents.

The outcome of concern during the London smog was daily mortality, which was approximately four times above the average daily mortality during December.

The deaths attributed to the smog were primarily linked to pneumonia, bronchitis, tuberculosis, and cardiovascular failures. This caused a controversy on whether these deaths occurred only among people with previous severe illness or whether the smog caused additional deaths. Another problem is the aggregation of cause-specific mortality rates by day. In such aggregated data, there may be perfect correlation between the exposure in question and other health risks like smoking which might confound the association. Individual-based studies are better suited for the investigation of multifactorial diseases, because perfect correlation between variables is very unlikely and it is thus feasible to separate their effects.

Since then, many studies have been conducted to resolve this debate. One of the most famous is the "Six City Study" conducted as follow-up study by the Harvard School of Public Health in the U.S. cities Watertown, Massachusetts; Portage, Wisconsin; Topeka, Kansas; Kingston/Harriman, Tennessee; St. Louis, Missouri; and Steubenville, Ohio. In this concurrent cohort study with a 14-to-16-year mortality follow-up, the effects of air pollution on mortality were estimated, and individual risk factors were monitored for 8111 adults. The Harvard group found that higher levels of fine particles and sulphate were associated with an increase in mortality by 26% (95% confidence interval: 8% to 47%), when the most polluted city was compared to the least polluted city. A positive association of mortality with concentrations of fine particles was found for cardiopulmonary disease. The authors therefore concluded: "Although the effects of other, unmeasured risk factors cannot be excluded with certainty, these results suggest that fine-particulate air pollution, or a more complex pollution mixture associated with fine particulate matter, contributes to excess mortality in certain U.S. cities" (Dockery et al. 1993).

Other studies corroborated the finding that long-term residence in cities with elevated ambient levels of air pollution is associated with an increase in mortality (e.g. Pope et al. 1995; Anderson et al. 1996; Katsouyanni et al. 1997; Samet et al. 2000; Vedal et al. 2003), but many questions still remain open. For example, a re-analysis of the "Six City Study" suggested that there is a modifying effect of education on the relationship between air quality and mortality (Krewski et al. 2004).

The epidemiology of air pollution is a highly complex and grave public health issue: On the one hand, mortality is only the endpoint of one possible health outcome; respiratory and cardiovascular disease or cancer are other serious issues. On the other hand, additional agents may be identified as characterizing parts of air pollution. Not surprisingly, the number of epidemiological studies of the impact of air pollution on human health is overwhelming (cf. WHO 2000; Brunekreef and Holgate 2002).

3.2.2   Residential Radon

A major issue of epidemiological research during the last 60 years has been the development of exposure-risk functions between radiation and different (cancer) outcomes. The main sources of the average annual radiation exposure in industrialized countries are medical examinations and therapies, inhalation of radon and its progeny, ingestion of natural radiation sources, and cosmic and terrestrial radiation (UNSCEAR 2000). Other sources, like the fallout from nuclear weapon experiments, the Chernobyl disaster, or the occupational exposure of workers in the nuclear industry, are low or affect only a very small part of the general population.

Worldwide the average annual effective dose from radon and its decay products is estimated at 1.15 mSv (UNSCEAR 2000). Therefore, natural radon seems to be an environmental risk factor of great interest. Its harmful character was recognized very soon after the discovery of radiation at the beginning of the 20th century and its identification as the real cause of the *Schneeberger Lungenkrankheit* (cf. Sect. 3.1.1).

In the history of radiation research many (animal) experiments and measurements have been undertaken, with the usual uncertainties in extrapolating the results to humans. However, in the middle of the 20th century, cohort studies in (uranium) miners were started to investigate the true exposure-disease relationship between radon and lung cancer. These studies confirmed that exposure to the radioactive gas radon (^{222}Rn) and its progeny increases the risk of lung cancer among workers in the uranium and other mining industries (Lubin et al. 1994; NRC 1999; IARC 2001; Table 3.1).

Table 3.1. Individual and pooled results of 11 cohort studies in miners on radon exposure and lung cancer (Lubin et al. 1994)

Study	# Cases	(ERR/WLM)%	CI
China	980	0.16	0.1–0.2
Czechoslovakia	661	0.34	0.2–0.6
Colorado	294	0.42	0.3–0.7
Ontario	291	0.89	0.5–1.5
Newfoundland	118	0.76	0.4–1.3
Sweden	79	0.95	0.1–4.1
New Mexico	69	1.72	0.6–6.7
Beaverlodge	65	2.21	0.9–5.6
Port Radium	57	0.19	0.1–0.6
Radium Hill	54	5.06	1.0–12.2
France	45	0.36	0.0–1.3
Pooled	**2701**	**0.49**	**0.2–1.0**

ERR = Excess Relative Risk
WLM = Working Level Month as a measure of cumulative radiation exposure
CI = 95% Confidence Interval

The study results in Table 3.1 are reported with exposures in Working Level Month (WLM). This cumulative measure was developed historically with the idea of there being a safe threshold for radiation exposure of workers. This was defined as 1 Working Level (WL) and was stated as 100 pCi/l, which in today's SI units is equivalent to 3.7 kBq m^{-3} (1 Bq m^{-3} is 1 radioactive decay per second in 1 m^3 air). With an average time of occupation of 170 h per month this cumulates to 1 WLM.

Overall a strong exposure-effect relationship was observed. When the occupational-related exposure scale is transformed from WLM in usual $Bq\,m^{-3}$ (for details on the assumptions and calculations of the transformation cf. e.g. NRC 1999), the overall estimate of the excess relative risk per WLM was estimated as 0.49 (Table 3.1). As 1 WLM corresponds to $170 \times 3.7\,kBq\,m^{-3}$ we get an estimate of $0.49/(170 \times 3.7) = 0.08$ per $100\,Bq\,m^{-3}$, i.e. per additional average exposure of $100\,Bq\,m^{-3}$ the lung cancer risk will increase by 8%. This exposure-effect relationship is further influenced by the time since exposure (TSE), the age at exposure, and by other risk factors like the exposure to arsenic or other dusts, and the smoking habits of the workers. These factors were not investigated deeply within the cohorts and therefore uncertainties remain about the dose-response relationship.

The public health concern about major radioactive exposure, however, is the long-term exposure of the general population to the much smaller concentrations of radon in homes. When the exposure-effect relationship from the miner studies is extrapolated to the level of radon exposure in homes, an average population-attributable risk of lung cancer of 5 to 15% can be estimated in industrialized countries (Lubin and Steindorf 1995; Steindorf et al. 1995; Darby et al. 2001). If this extrapolation is true, exposure to residential radon is the most hazardous environmental risk factor for cancer in the general population, and risk management strategies need to be developed.

However, a direct transfer of the risk estimates derived from miner studies or animal experiments to residential environments may not be appropriate due to substantial differences in the levels of radon exposure; other physical factors such as breathing rate; the distribution of aerosol particles size; the unattached fraction of radon progeny; confounding factors such as smoking, asbestos and other occupational risks; nutrition; leisure time activities; social conditions; genetic susceptibility; and age, gender, and regional circumstances.

In the past decade a series of well-conducted epidemiological studies investigated the risk of lung cancer in relation to indoor radon exposure in the general population via case-control studies (Schoenberg et al. 1990; Blot et al. 1990; Pershagen et al. 1992, 1994; Létourneau et al. 1994; Alavanja et al. 1994, 1999; Ruosteenoja et al. 1996; Auvinen et al. 1996; Darby et al. 1998; Field et al. 2000; Kreienbrock et al. 2001; Lagarde et al. 2001; Tomášek et al. 2001; Oberaigner et al. 2002; Wang et al. 2002; Barros-Dios et al. 2002; Kreuzer et al. 2003). Some of them found a statistically significant increased lung cancer risk, others not. It has been suggested that detection of an underlying association of lung cancer and indoor radon exposure, if present, has been impeded by uncertainty in assessment of exposure, low statistical power, and a limited range of radon concentrations (Lubin et al. 1995).

3.2.3   Non-ionizing Radiation

Exposure to electric and magnetic fields (EMF) in the occupational as well as in the residential environment is a matter of major public concern in the developed world. The debate on health consequences is widespread, and there is speculation on possible effects of exposure ranging from the development of cancer to headaches, depressions, or general malaise.

A first investigation of Wertheimer and Leeper (1979) brought EMF and childhood leukemia to the special attention of the public. The authors conducted a case-control study with 155 cases and the same number of controls, and found a risk ratio of around three. So-called "wire-codes" of distances to electric power lines were introduced as a measure of exposure to EMF.

Further studies followed. Greenland et al. (2000) and Ahlbom et al. (2000) summarized the results of these studies by pooling them into two joint analyses in the U.S. and in Europe (Fig. 3.2).

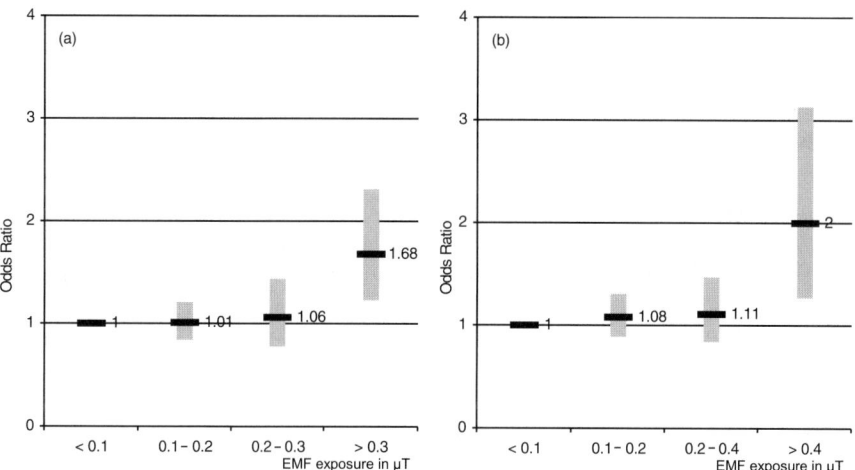

Figure 3.2. Leukemia risk in children due to EMF exposure: odds ratios and 95% confidence intervals by EMF exposure in µT from pooling studies (a) in the U.S. (Greenland et al. 2000) and (b) in Europe (Ahlbom et al. 2000)

Figure 3.2 suggests a similar risk pattern in the U. S. and in Europe, with an overall statistical significance in the highest exposure group. However, the discussion on EMF risks is ongoing, primarily due to limitations of exposure assessment for the use of wire codes as well as for recent techniques of (personal) measurements and exposure assessment.

Habash et al. (2003a) therefore stated: "Currently, the evidence in support of an association between EMF and childhood cancer is limited, although this issue warrants further investigation. Evidence of an association between EMF exposure and adult cancers, derived largely from occupational settings, is inconsistent, precluding clear conclusions. There is little evidence of an association between EMF and noncancer health effects. … Further research is needed to clarify the ambiguous findings from present studies and to determine if EMF exposure poses a health risk."

Special Methodological Issues in Environmental Epidemiology

Although there is great variation in study designs and in measurement techniques, methods of exposure assessment and statistical analyses used in environmental epidemiology share common features that will be summarized in the following.

3.3.1   Principles of Study Design

As mentioned above one of the major problems in studying an environmental risk factor is often the low risk associated with it. Therefore the overall power of a study has to be large to increase the chance of identifying health hazards. The proper choice of the study design is thus a basic step in conducting an investigation in environmental epidemiology.

Standardization of Study Designs

The power of an epidemiological study is related to two major components, namely the sample size and the precision of all instruments. The number of available cases and the financial budget are constraints that determine the limitations of every investigation. Therefore, it is desirable to standardize study designs to increase the precision of the results and to establish a basis for comparisons between different studies.

For example, the designs of studies of the impact of residential radon developed gradually over time. In a very first step ecologic studies were performed to investigate the numerical correlation between radon concentration and lung cancer mortality with aggregated data, e.g. on the basis of administrative districts (Stidley and Samet 1993). This type of study design is very popular in environmental epidemiology, but is strongly influenced by different types of biases, especially confounding bias (cf. Chap. I.3 of this handbook). Figure 3.3 shows an example of an ecologic analysis for radon data in West Germany.

Figure 3.3 shows a typical problem which occurs in ecologic studies in environmental epidemiology when the environmental risk factor is associated with a low risk and the disease is influenced by a strong risk factor that is itself associated with the risk factor under study. On the one hand, in Germany – as in other industrialized countries – smoking is much more popular in cities and urban areas (e.g. the major cities Berlin, Hamburg, Düsseldorf, Bremen) than in rural areas (e.g. the rural districts Niederbayern, Oberpfalz, Tübingen in the south of Germany). In addition, smoking prevalences decrease from north to south. On the other hand, radon concentration is low in cities and urban areas, while higher measurements are much more likely in rural areas. This pattern causes a "protective radon effect" if the smoking habits are neglected.

This type of misleading findings in ecologic studies is known as the ecologic fallacy and can be observed in many studies on radon (Cohen 1993, 1997) as well as

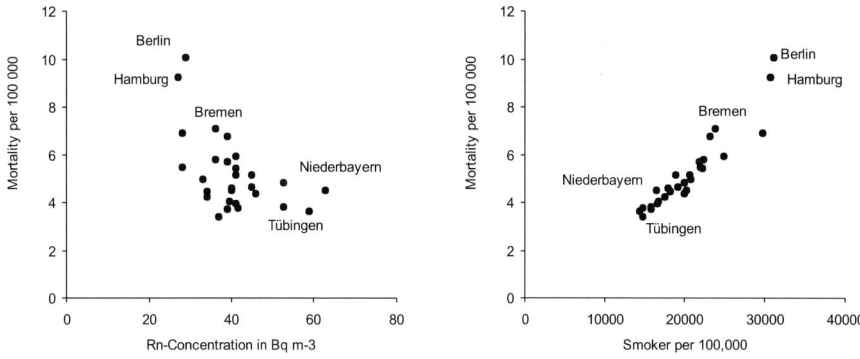

Figure 3.3. Lung cancer and radon in West Germany; (**a**) lung cancer mortality in women by average radon concentration in West German districts (*Regierungsbezirke*); (**b**) lung cancer mortality in women by average smoking prevalence among females in West German districts (Kreienbrock and Schach 2000, modified)

on other environmental risk factors. Therefore ecologic studies are only reasonable as a starting point for discussion. Causal relationships could not be concluded from this type of study design.

Study designs based on individuals are necessary to investigate the causal role of environmental risk factors. For studies on the radon-related lung cancer risk in the general population, Pershagen (1993; personal communication) described three generations of studies following the ecologic studies (see Table 3.2).

The studies from the first and second generations were very small and therefore did not have the power to detect the radon-related lung cancer risk, which is expected to be low. Thus in 1989, 1991, and 1993, workshops were organized

Table 3.2. Three generations of radon studies with individuals (Pershagen 1993; personal communication)

Generation	Characterization
I	– conducted in the early 1980s
	– small sample sizes
	– no or crude Rn measurements
	– no or only small control for confounding
II	– conducted in the late 1980s
	– small sample sizes
	– Rn measurements in one house
	– some control for confounding
III	– conducted in the 1990s
	– big sample sizes
	– Rn measurements in all homes
	– control for confounding

with all principal investigators of ongoing studies during that time to develop "Guidelines for Conducting Radon Studies" (Samet et al. 1991). These workshops led to a standardization of study protocols and formed a basis for future pooling of studies.

Although this process of standardization cannot be established as a general rule in environmental epidemiology, it should be recognized as a strategy that may enhance the overall power of investigations.

Because the risk ratio of an environmental risk factor is usually low and many of the diseases under study are not frequent, a case-control study is the type of study design that is most appropriate to investigate an environmental risk factor within the common population. This is usually done for studies on radon and lung cancer as well as for most of the studies investigating the impact of environmental agents on cancer. For example, of the 20 studies on residential radon mentioned in Sect. 3.2.2, only the Czech study was conducted as a cohort study in which a case-control study is nested (Tomášek et al. 2001).

In contrast, at first glance cohort studies seem to be rare in environmental epidemiology due to the extensive efforts they require. Nevertheless, there are well-known examples of this study design, such as the "Six City Study" on indoor air pollution and mortality (Dockery et al. 1993, cf. Sect.3.2.1), and other longitudinal designs, studying long-term effects of the relation between air pollution exposure and public health (Brunekreef 2003). Therefore the use of cohorts is increasing in different fields of environmental interest. For example, cohorts are now being used in investigations on the impact of nutrition on human health, like the EPIC project (European Prospective Investigation into Cancer and Nutrition), which studies more than 500,000 participants in ten European countries (Slimani et al. 2002).

Selection of Study Participants and Choice of the Study Area

The first step in planning an investigation in environmental epidemiology is the choice of the study area. For this purpose, monitoring data of measurements is very helpful to find out whether the risk factor is present within a defined region and which variation it shows. This is necessary to distinguish between exposed and non-exposed populations or to evaluate an exposure-effect relationship for a common range of possible exposures.

However, areas with high average concentrations or with a greater proportion of elevated values do not by definition guarantee a proper environmental study. If the risk factor is distributed equally, cases and controls of the study region will be exposed to a similar degree and no effect of the risk factor can be observed in the study. This problem is known as "overmatching on the exposure factor". It can be avoided by separating areas with different levels of the risk factor. This problem is commonly discussed in studies on the possible impact of outdoor air pollution as a risk factor (e.g. Dockery et al. 1993; Pope et al. 1995; Heinrich et al. 2000; Hoek et al. 2000).

A different problem occurs in studies on the indoor environment: The concentration in homes is influenced by outdoor air, geology, or other factors related to the outside environment, but will be modified by the type of house and the (ventilation) habits of the inhabitants. This may result in low measurements even in areas with a great impact of outdoor air or geology on increased concentrations of the agent under study. Taking into account the fact that measurements are only one component of the exposure assessment (see below), it is possible that both cases and controls will be exposed at a very low level. This effect was observed for example in many radon studies, for instance in the study in Winnipeg, Canada (Létourneau et al. 1994) or the study in West Germany (Kreienbrock et al. 2001), where measurement programs showed areas with high radon concentrations on average, while exposures of study participants were low. This was mainly due to the mobility of the population that resulted in low average exposures of individuals (Warner et al. 1996).

Therefore the choice of the study area has to be influenced both by the presence of a monitoring program indicating areas with elevated concentrations of the risk factor and by a population density that yields a sufficient number of study participants.

The selection of cases within the study area is dependent on the health system within this area. If national or regional registers are available, cases will usually be recruited from these registers; if not, case recruitment from hospitals will be the usual sampling strategy. The problem of a proper selection of a group of cases is similar in all kinds of epidemiological applications, but if measurements on environmental agents have to be conducted, this causes additional problems, especially if the cases are to be recruited in hospitals and the measurement campaign is (technically) complicated. This will decrease the response proportion in the case group and the rates may be differential by disease stage, and thus may cause a selection bias. On the other hand even in studies with registers this type of problem is present, especially if next-of-kin interviews have to be conducted instead of interviews of cases.

Similar problems due to selection procedures and exposure assessment may be present for the control group in environmental studies. As in any other epidemiological study the different types of bias may occur, but these may be strongly influenced by the type of measurement to be conducted. This problem can be observed mainly in "special circumstances studies", where recent environmental problems of great public interest are studied. This may cause different response proportions among subgroups within the general population, which may introduce a severe selection bias and impair comparability between subgroups.

An example of a special circumstances situation was described by Oberaigner et al. (2002) for radon epidemiology. In 1989, high lung cancer mortality rates were reported for the District of Imst, Tyrol, Austria, in an alpine region without any industry. First investigations in this district (Ennemoser et al. 1994a,b) identified one village with extremely high radon concentrations; the highest concentrations measured in residences were above 100,000 Bq m^{-3}. In the meantime detailed cross-sectional investigations have examined both the radon gas concentrations and the geology. In fact, only half of the village was affected, and about 40 residences were identified with concentrations above 1000 Bq m^{-3}. There were only few and isolated high concentrations in the other villages of this region. In fact the scientific interest in this area was linked to population's interest and response. While in the beginning the whole population was interested, in cross-sectional measurement programs there was a gradual decrease in response proportions, linked, unfortunately, with increasing exposure.

Decreasing response proportions were also observed during the 90s after the re-unification of Germany, when many environmental measurement programs identified numerous areas with elevated levels of environmental agents of scientific interest in the former German Democratic Republic (Heinrich et al. 2002; Frye et al. 2001). One may call this effect a possible bias due to "over-examination".

These examples indicate that selection bias is of special interest in environmental epidemiology and special efforts have to be undertaken during field work to avoid possible selection effects. Besides an exact definition of inclusion and exclusion criteria of study participants, selection effects are mainly dependent on a proper documentation of the reasons for response and non-response combined with an additional investigation on the non-responders. Moreover, it is necessary to make corrections for selection bias.

Sampling Procedures and Correction for Non-response Bias

Usually the recruitment of study participants is described as a process of selecting a study population from a target population by means of a defined sampling scheme. If the study population is a representative sample of the target population, the study results should be unbiased; otherwise a selection bias may occur which will have to be discussed. For studies in environmental epidemiology these biases may be described from two different perspectives.

On the one hand, different selection procedures for the exposed and the non-exposed populations are possible, as observed in many environmental studies. Heinrich et al. (2002) described studies on air pollution and respiratory health and allergies in the former German Democratic Republic, where response proportion decreased with increasing exposure. On the other hand, response proportions may differ between cases and controls of a study. This effect is often due to the fact that controls are less motivated so that their response proportions are lower than that of the cases who want to know whether environmental hazards are responsible for their disease.

Investigation of the non-response patterns seems to be necessary to investigate these processes and to establish a basis for an adjustment for possible selection effects caused by non-response. The general principle of a non-response investigation was initially outlined by Hansen and Hurwitz (1946) and is illustrated in Fig. 3.4. It may be assumed that study response is a characteristic of the members of the target population that partitions the population in two strata, N_1 responders and N_2 non-responders. An epidemiological study of study size n may be interpreted as a stratified random sample from the target population, i.e. a stratified sample of real responders n_1 and non-responders n_2. This process can be interpreted as a first phase of a sampling plan. In a second phase a real sample of size n_2^* is drawn from the n_2 non-responders, and all efforts are made to get information

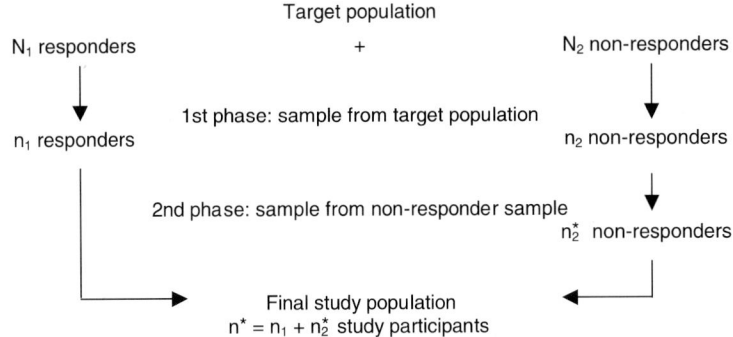

Figure 3.4. Two-phase sampling scheme for collecting sampling information on non-responders

from this second-phase subsample of size n_2^*, e.g. by conducting additional telephone interviews etc. The final study population n^* will be calculated as the sum of these subsample sizes.

If a non-responder investigation is conducted, adjustment for non-response will be possible in a straightforward way. For simple linear statistics like prevalences or means (of exposures), an adjusted estimator can be computed as a simple weighted mean of the two strata means of responders, denoted as $\bar{y}_1$, and non-responders, say $\bar{y}_2$, i.e.

$$\bar{y}_{adj} = \frac{n_1}{n^*} \cdot \bar{y}_1 + \frac{n_2^*}{n^*} \cdot \bar{y}_2 \qquad (3.1)$$

This type of adjustment (3.1) is useful in environmental epidemiology, especially if diseases or exposures under study are rare and therefore prevalences are low. Figure 3.5 displays the impact of selection bias due to non-response on the estimation of a prevalence of five percent by comparing the adjusted estimator from (3.1) with the usual estimator, namely the average $\bar{y}_1$, that is calculated without adjustment for non-response. This situation may occur for example in a cross-sectional study investigating the impact of air pollution on respiratory symptoms like asthma in boys. It can be shown that selection bias increases with increasing non-response, depending on the magnitude of the difference of the exposure prevalences between responders and non-responders.

A linear adjustment is not suitable for estimating ratios, and the strata of responders and non-responders have to be split up into the exposed and the non-exposed sub-populations. Kleinbaum et al. (1982) therefore introduced the 2×2 table of an epidemiological study as the selected outcome from the target population that results in a 2×2 table of selection probabilities for subjects from the entire target population (Table 3.3).

If selection of study participants is outlined as in Table 3.3 an epidemiological study to estimate a population odds ratio is unbiased if the odds ratio of the selection probabilities $W = \left(W_{DE}W_{\overline{D}\,\overline{E}}\right)/\left(W_{D\overline{E}}W_{\overline{D}E}\right)$ is equal to unity. If W is

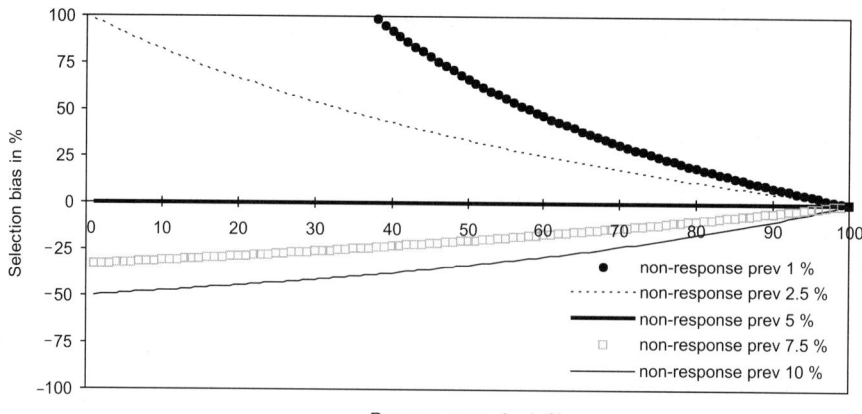

Figure 3.5. Selection bias in % due to non-response for estimating a prevalence in the target population of 5% for varying exposure prevalences among non-responders

Table 3.3. Realization of study subjects n_{ij} as sample with probability W_{ij} from the members N_{ij} of the target population, $i = D$ for diseased and $\overline{D}$ for non-diseased subjects, $j = E$ for exposed and $\overline{E}$ for exposed and non-exposed subjects

	Exposed	Non-exposed
Diseased	$n_{DE} = W_{DE}N_{DE}$	$n_{D\overline{E}} = W_{D\overline{E}}N_{D\overline{E}}$
Non-diseased	$n_{\overline{D}E} = W_{\overline{D}E}N_{\overline{D}E}$	$n_{\overline{D}\,\overline{E}} = W_{\overline{D}\,\overline{E}}N_{\overline{D}\,\overline{E}}$

greater than unity, the study will be biased away from the null, else the bias is towards the null.

Investigations in environmental epidemiology may be very sensitive to selection bias. The odds ratio of the selection probabilities W may be used both for a quantitative and a qualitative assessment of the possible bias. If, based on the study design and the sampling techniques applied, the sampling probabilities can be computed, and a quantitative adjustment for selection bias will be possible by multiplying the study odds ratio with the inverse W^{-1}.

If sampling probabilities are not available, a qualification of the direction of selection bias is possible. Examples for a qualitative assessment of the bias can be adopted from cross-sectional studies of the impact of air pollution on respiratory health. Here, the motivation of the study subjects may be influenced by the disease and by the exposure situation. In contrast, subjects who are not ill and who are not exposed may not be motivated to participate. This will decrease the selection probability $W_{\overline{D}\,\overline{E}}$, hence $W < 1$ and the study odds ratio will be biased towards the null.

In contrast, if the same study is conducted in a "special circumstances area", the effect may be vice versa if the healthy exposed population is unwilling to participate. This will decrease the selection probability $W_{\overline{D}E}$, hence $W > 1$ and the study odds ratio will biased away from the null.

Measurements and Exposure Assessment   3.3.2

The measurement of an environmental agent such as the risk factor under study is the primary issue of an investigation in environmental epidemiology. Such measurements can be used directly or as a basis of an exposure assessment. The main problems to be addressed in any investigation in environmental epidemiology are an appropriate choice of the measurement technique, the method of exposure assessment, and the statistical evaluation to model the exposure-effect relationship.

Numerous types of exposures may be distinguished in environmental epidemiology. One useful categorization is to distinguish between short-term and long-term exposures and between short-term and long-term effects. The time interval between exposure and effect is often called time since exposure (TSE). Table 3.4 shows typical examples that may occur in environmental epidemiology within these categories.

Table 3.4. Examples of short-term and long-term exposure-effect relationships in environmental epidemiology

Exposure-effect relationship	Example
short-term exposure/short-term effect	traffic-related agents – acute respiratory symptoms smog episodes – mortality
short-term exposure/long-term effect	fallout from nuclear weapon tests – cancer incidence contaminated food – new variant of Creutzfeldt-Jacob disease
long-term exposure/long-term effect	environmental tobacco smoke – lung cancer residential radon exposure – lung cancer

The relationship of short-term exposures to short-term effects as well as the relationship of long-term exposures to long-term effects may be postulated as the typical situations under study in environmental epidemiology, while the situation in which a short-term (single) exposure causes a long-term effect seems to be rare. It may be argued that it is much more complicated to assess long term-exposures and that short-term exposures may be described by the measurement itself. However, this is not a general rule.

For radon and for many other agents, residential exposure is a long-term exposure starting at birth and ending with the study recruitment, e.g. by the index date of diagnosis or the date of a standardized personal interview. The outcome under study is lung cancer as a long-term effect. Taking into account the fact that residential exposure is characteristic of the homes a study participant has lived in during his or her life, the overall exposure can be outlined as in Fig. 3.6.

The exposure pattern depicted in Fig. 3.6 seems to be typical for a long-term exposure to an environmental agent, i.e. that individuals are exposed to different

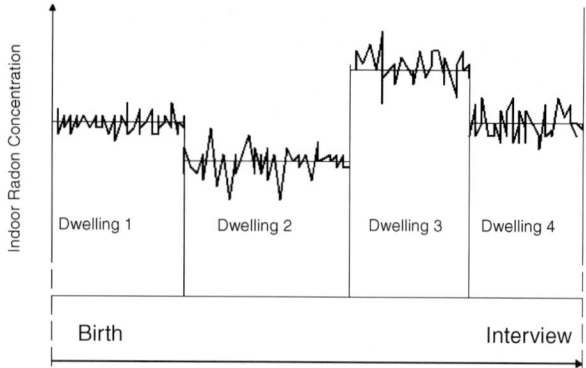

Figure 3.6. Residential radon exposure during a participant's life (fictitious participant's biography) (Wichmann et al. 1998, modified)

average levels with varying intensities around these levels in different time windows over their lifetimes. In the radon example, different levels of exposure are related to different dwellings the study participants have lived in during their lives. Each of the resulting time windows cover many years, a typical situation in many studies where the exposure conditions are linked to locations and these exposures are more or less constant over time. Additional examples for this situation are found in all studies investigating the impact of indoor or outdoor residential exposures on human health like the different agents responsible for air or soil pollution.

Sometimes the time windows of different exposure levels may be subdivided if there is additional knowledge about external circumstances and about the habits of the participants. For the radon example these modifications of exposure can be summarized as follows. It is known that radon concentrations in homes differ due to temperature and air pressure, resulting in different concentrations over the seasons (on average, the concentration in winter is twice as high as in summer) as well as over the day (higher concentrations during the night than in the daytime). From this point of view time windows on a monthly or even on a hourly basis have to be considered. But the living habits of the participants will also influence the exposure pattern. For example, the time spent indoors during the day as well as during the year will be an important factor for an individual's exposure. In addition, exposure will be modified by living habits like ventilation behavior, by the existence and pattern of utilization of different rooms within the homes, and by other individual habits.

The combination of both dimensions of exposure windows due to the external circumstances and to the habits of the participants may provide a sophisticated structure of the exposure windows, which on the one hand will decrease the variation of exposure around an average exposure within a time window. On the other hand the process to obtain proper information and measurements within these time windows will be much more complicated and difficult.

Different strategies to model an exposure-disease relationship are suitable in environmental epidemiology. As a very rough strategy the real exposure may be extrapolated by means of a (categorical) variable that is used as a surrogate. Such variables and scores are widely used because no measurements have to be made and information can often be collected easily by means of a questionnaire or even by simple observation. Thus, classical categorization into exposed and non-exposed groups can be used, e.g. by definition of areas with high or low industrialization or by geology. For example, early studies of the impact of radon on cancer tried to assess the exposure by categorizing the type of house as a surrogate.

Such scores are insufficient to assess an exposure pattern as in Fig. 3.6, and measurements of the agent under study should be carried out. Besides technical and financial restrictions, for epidemiological purposes it has to be clarified whether these measurements are suitable for a population-based study. Continuous measurement of the agents under study for every study subject will be rare, and the most frequently applied technique uses short-term or cumulative passive samplers. For example, for radon exposure assessment, passive sampling techniques were utilized by applying an information and measurement sampling scheme as outlined in Fig. 3.7.

Measurement	no	yes	yes	yes
Information from new tenant	no	yes	yes	not applicable
Information from study subject	few	yes	yes	exhaustive
Recent tenant	new tenant	new tenant	new tenant	study subject
Residential history	dwelling 1	dwelling 2	dwelling 3	dwelling 4

Period of interest for exposure assessment

Birth   Interview

Figure 3.7. Information and measurement sampling scheme for a residential radon exposure (fictitious participant's biography) (Wichmann et al. 1998, modified)

The information and measurement sampling scheme given in Fig. 3.7 was used in modified versions in many studies investigating the impact of residential radon on the general population. In a personal interview with trained interviewers the following information was recorded using a standardized questionnaire for each dwelling inhabited over a given period relevant for exposure assessment (e.g. 30 years before date of interview):

- average time spent in each room per day, ascertained separately for each dwelling inhabited during the exposure assessment period,

- average periods of regular absence from the residence in each residence period, such as holiday, weekly absence due to occupation, etc.,
- persistent characteristics such as type of house, year of construction, type of construction, and type of basement,
- changeable characteristics such as insulation of basement and windows, heating system, and ventilation habits,
- calendar years of residence periods in each dwelling inhabited, and
- calendar years of alterations of building characteristics within a residence period.

This information was not collected in detail for dwellings outside the period relevant for exposure assessment. Measurements of radon concentrations were carried out by means of so-called alpha track detectors placed both in the living room and in the bedroom of the present and former dwellings of the participants. The relevant information gathered from the participants and the subsequent tenants of the former dwellings were recorded according to their periods of residence.

These data provide the basis for different methods of exposure assessment. The most popular one integrates the several measurements as a time-weighted average exposure representative of the period of exposure assessment. In addition the exposure assessment has to adjust the current measurements for alterations of living habits and for occupancy times in the present and previous residences as well as for seasonal effects if the measurement took place in a non-typical season.

In the first approach the exposure has to be calculated as a usual linear weighted average in the same scale in which measurements are reported. For radon concentrations this is in $Bq\,m^{-3}$. The second approach considers the cumulative exposure for a defined period before the interview. This exposure window should be the most relevant time interval with respect to the disease under study. For the lung cancer risk due to radon, time windows from 5 to 15 up to 5 to 30 years prior to diagnosis are under discussion (ICRP 1993; Lubin et al. 1994). Here, the measurements in the present homes are supplemented by measurements in the previous homes, corrected by changes due to reconstruction of the house or different ventilation habits of the study subjects and the present inhabitants and by seasonal adjustment. This cumulative exposure can be expressed in $Bq\,m^{-3}$ per year.

To evaluate corrections of measurements due to changes between subjects and present inhabitants in all rooms measured (e.g. living room and bedroom), a bivariate version of a multiplicative model of the following type can be assumed

$$rn = \mu \times \beta_1 \times \beta_2 \times \beta_3 \times \ldots \times \beta_J \times \exp(\varepsilon), \tag{3.2}$$

where rn denotes the observed radon concentration, μ is an overall baseline radon concentrations, $\beta_1, \beta_2, \beta_3, \ldots, \beta_J$ are J categorized effect parameters corresponding to the factors of house characteristics, ventilation habits, reconstructions and so on, and ε is an error term from a normal distribution with zero mean.

The univariate version of (3.2) is well established in the context of radon surveys (Gunby et al. 1993; Kreienbrock and Siehl 1996). It is based both on the physical model that changing habits will lead to an exchange of a specific fraction of indoor and outdoor air and on the usual figure that indoor radon concentrations have been found to follow a log-normal distribution (Bäverstam and Swedjemark 1991; Gunby et al. 1993; Miles 1994; Lubin et al. 1995).

The log transformation of (3.2) leads to a bivariate normal distribution of the transformed radon measurements both in the living room and bedroom, which is required for standard MANOVA (multivariate analysis of variance, Anderson 1984). An additive model can be computed which estimates final model effects $\beta_{jk}^{(i)}$, for each category k of a factor j in room i, with $k = 1, \ldots, K_j$, number of categories of factor $j, j = 1, \ldots, J$, factors in the model, and $i = 1, 2$ rooms.

With $K = 1$ as the reference category for each factor j, correction factors for the measured radon concentrations of present inhabitants can be defined as

$$\text{Correction}_j^{(i)} = \frac{\exp\left(\beta_{jk_j}^{(i)}\right)}{\exp\left(\beta_{j\ell_j}^{(i)}\right)}, \quad j = 1, \ldots, J, \quad i = 1, 2, \tag{3.3}$$

where the participant's category is k_j and present inhabitant's category is ℓ_j relating to factor $j, j = 1, \ldots, J$ (cf. Gerken et al. 2000). These factors may be estimated from the above linear model by an ordinary least square algorithm, and are then used for calculating the corrected average cumulative radon exposure per year and individual.

A correction for all measurements has to be applied to evaluate adjustments of measurements for seasonal effects. It can be assumed that the logarithm of the radon concentration in a given house follows a sine-cosine curve over one year. Then, the cumulative measurement obtained from the alpha track detector involves a time integral over the sine-cosine curve, i.e.

$$\ln\left(rn_i\right) = \mu_i + 1 \Big/ \left(t_{i2} - t_{i1}\right) \int_{t_{i1}}^{t_{i2}} s_t dt + \varepsilon_i \tag{3.4}$$

with rn_i being the observed radon concentration, μ_i the mean radon concentration in room i over the entire year, t_{i1} and t_{i2} the first and last day of measurement, ε_i an error term, and s_t the sine-cosine curve given as

$$s_t = \alpha_1 \cdot \cos\left(2\pi/365 \cdot t\right) + \alpha_2 \cdot \sin\left(2\pi/365 \cdot t\right) \quad \text{for } t = 1, \ldots, 365, \tag{3.5}$$

where α_1 and α_2 are parameters that can be estimated from the data within the framework of a standard linear model (Pinel et al. 1994; Oberaigner et al. 2002; Baysson et al. 2003). A result of an adjustment process like (3.4) and (3.5) is outlined in Fig. 3.8 for a radon study in Austria, where the maximum radon concentration was reached in mid-February (2.62 times the mean concentration), and the minimum concentration in mid-August (0.38 times the mean concentration).

Overall the exposure assessment may be summarized as a weighted cumulation of several stages of information based on measurements, questionnaire data and modeling (see Fig. 3.9).

This process of exposure assessment can be considered as a very typical situation in environmental and in other fields of epidemiology. Additional examples of the calculation of cumulative exposures are the concept of working level month as a cumulative measure of the exposure to ionizing radiation among workers in the uranium mining industry (cf. Sect. 3.2.2; NRC 1999), the concept of fibreyears for the cumulative exposure to asbestos (cf. Chap. III.3 of this handbook), or the packyear concept that summarizes all cigarettes smoked during lifetime (1 packyear = 1 pack of 20 cigarettes a day for 1 year = 7300 cigarettes).

Although these concepts are very popular, and sophisticated solutions of integrating exposures are available, a cumulative exposure quantification may lead to substantial problems in evaluating a risk model. These strategies need retrospective information and may therefore be influenced by information bias. This is especially true if information is based on interviews and participants' memory. As a famous example, the British Doctors' Study showed that there was a large gap between the initial reporting of the smoking habits of study participants and the same subjects' answers' to the same questions on his or her past habits some years later (Doll and Peto 1976).

Besides this general problem the real nature of an exposure-risk relationship may not be well described for an agent if integrated exposures are used. It is known that the risk may differ in different exposure patterns even if cumulative exposure is constant. These effects are sometimes addressed as the inverse dose-rate effect that results in higher risks if the same cumulative exposure is reached with a low dose-rate in contrast to the same cumulative exposure reached by a high dose-rate over a shorter time interval. This effect was reported in cancer epidemiology for smoking as well as for exposure to asbestos or ionizing radiation. To evaluate such effects this has to be taken into account by the risk model used.

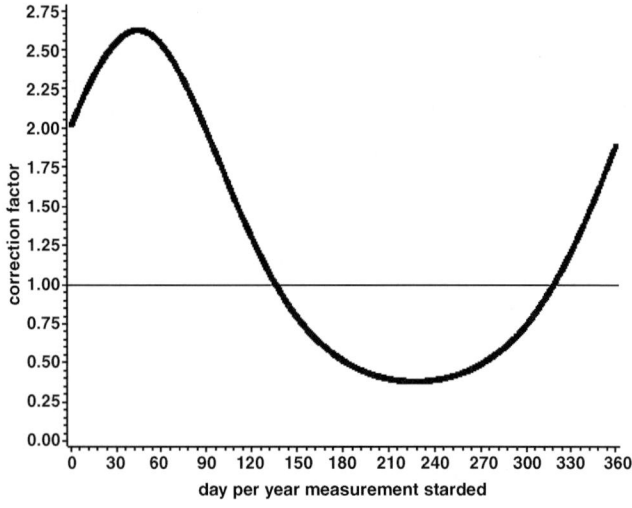

Figure 3.8. Seasonal correction of radon measurements (Oberaigner et al. 2002, modified)

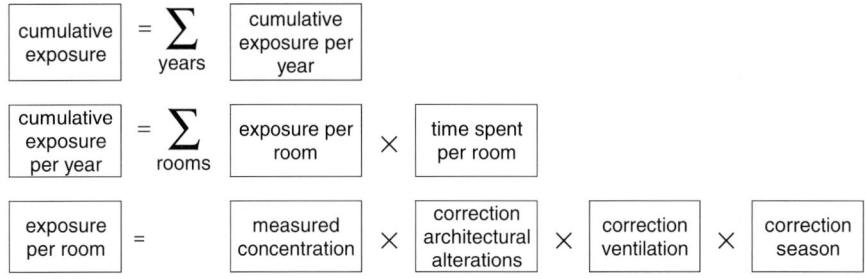

Figure 3.9. Assessment of residential radon exposure

Influenced by studies of the effect of a single exposure in a very short time interval, studies of the impact of environmental agents make use of the concept of time since exposure (TSE) that generally leads to the effect that risk decreases or even disappears if TSE is increased. This effect is able to modify the response to a cumulative exposure. If a single point in time is indicated when an exposure occurs, TSE can be well defined. This is possible for several studies when a point in time is well defined, e.g. studies of the health impact of the exposures to the atomic bombs of Hiroshima and Nagasaki, for many occupational exposures, or for exposure due to medical examinations.

However, for most of the exposures in environmental research, as for radon exposure, the concept of a single point in time is not applicable, since continuous exposures have to be taken into account (see Fig. 3.6). Therefore additional strategies on modeling exposure have to be used.

Finkelstein's approach makes direct use of the time window structure to better understand the influence of a special risk factor over time (cf. Finkelstein 1991). This exploratory method can be described as a series of risk models that include total cumulative exposure and an additional covariate for exposure received during a fixed time interval. Characteristics of the fitted models provide insight into the influence of exposure increments on disease risk at different points in time.

Let Y_i denote the disease status of individual i ($i = 1, \ldots, n$), and let $x_i(t)$ denote the exposure of the ith individual at time t before interview ($t \in [0, T]$), where T depends on the length of collected exposure histories. Additional covariates $z_i = (z_{1i}, \ldots, z_{mi})$ are used to adjust for confounding.

Then a time window approach sequentially fits models that include cumulative exposure to attained age, A, and cumulative exposure received over a time interval of fixed width k as covariates. Intervals of various width k can be considered. For the time window centered at time c before interview, where $c \in [k/2, T - k/2]$, a model M_c of the form

$$\text{logit} \Pr\left(Y_i = 1 | z_i, ; x_i(t), t \in [0; T]\right) = \alpha_0 + \alpha' z_i + \beta_1 \int_0^{A_i} x_i(t)\mathrm{d}t + \beta_2 \int_{c-k/2}^{c+k/2} x_i(t)\mathrm{d}t$$

$$(3.6)$$

may be fitted, and the likelihood ratio test statistic can be computed as

$$\text{LR}_c = -2 \log \frac{\max_{\alpha,\beta} L\left(M_c | \beta_2 = 0\right)}{\max_{\alpha,\beta} L\left(M_c\right)}, \tag{3.7}$$

which compares model (3.6) with the corresponding "null" model without the time window exposure variable, i.e. $\beta_2 = 0$. The value of c is then varied over its range. For fixed c, the parameter β_1 represents the increase in the log odds ratio per unit exposure, while β_2 represents the additive effect on a log scale of a unit exposure that occurred during the specific time window of length k centered at time c. The likelihood ratios between the models with and without the time window, LR_c, can be compared to assess the significance of the additional exposure variable. In this way, a continuous weighting of the impact of the exposure over time is possible (see Fig. 3.10; Hauptmann et al. 2000 a,b).

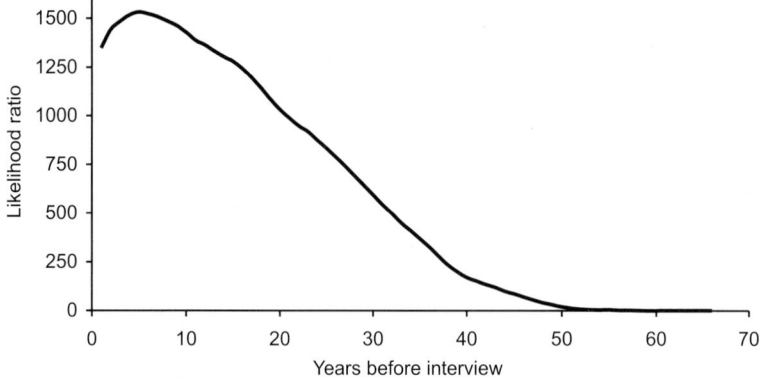

Figure 3.10. Continuous time-weighting of exposure and its impact on risk (modified from Hauptmann et al. 2000a)

Overall it may be stated that the process of sampling information and measurements to conduct an exposure assessment is the major issue in an investigation of the impact of an environmental agent on human health. Besides technical and financial constraints several types of information bias and uncertainty influence this process, and uncertainty of exposure measurements still remains, even if detailed descriptions of the exposures are available. This should be considered during the statistical analysis of a study.

3.3.3   Statistical Analysis

As in all other fields of epidemiology classical concepts of risk models like the categorical analyses of (stratified) contingency tables or modeling approaches like logistic regression or Cox' proportional hazards models are used in the study of the risk of environmental agents on human health to describe the relationship between exposure and disease (cf. Chap. II.3 of this handbook). In general, low risks, the problem of strong confounding with other major risk factors, the problem of proper exposure assessment, and the basic assumption of the nature of the exposure-disease relationship lead to additional strategies for statistical modeling that are of special importance for environmental epidemiology.

Modeling the Exposure-Disease Function

One basic issue in the study of environmental risks is the choice of an exposure-disease function to describe the real nature of the response of an environmental hazard on human health. Two main strategies may be distinguished. If, based on former studies, on animal experiments, or on general toxicological considerations, a class of functions between exposure and disease can be specified, then a parametric version of a risk model will be suitable. This strategy may be appropriate if exposure is measured on a continuous scale, as in studies on the risks of ionizing or non-ionizing radiation, or in air pollution studies. The functional type specified will be related to the preliminary considerations, but linear and log-linear parameterizations of the risk ratio are very popular in environmental studies, at least as a starting point.

The linear (excess) relative risk model may be introduced as

$$\frac{p}{1-p} = \mu \cdot (1 + \beta x) , \tag{3.8}$$

where p is the risk of an interesting disease under study, μ is a multiplicative intercept, x specifies the exposure quantity, and β is the excess odds ratio, i.e. the increase of the odds ratio in percent. In model (3.8) the true odds ratio equals $1 + \beta x$.

In contrast the log-linear model may be stated as

$$\ln\left(\frac{p}{1-p}\right) = \alpha + \gamma \cdot x , \tag{3.9}$$

where p is the risk, α is an intercept, γ is the log odds ratio and x the exposure. Model (3.9) corresponds to the usual logistic regression model where the odds ratio is given as $\exp(\gamma \cdot x)$.

Both models (3.8) and (3.9) are very popular in environmental epidemiology for reasons of easy interpretation as well as for an easy model fit in statistical and epidemiological software packages. Likelihood based confidence intervals as well as tests on statistical hypotheses on the parameters can be computed straightforwardly.

However, based on the range of possible exposures in the human environment, both models have to be considered very carefully. For very small exposures x it holds that $\exp(x) \approx 1 + x$ and therefore (3.8) and (3.9) yield similar results for large parts of a general population. The risk models (3.8) and (3.9) will differ substantially for the part of a population which is exposed to a higher degree. This is demonstrated in Fig. 3.11 for the risk of residential radon und lung cancer as an example.

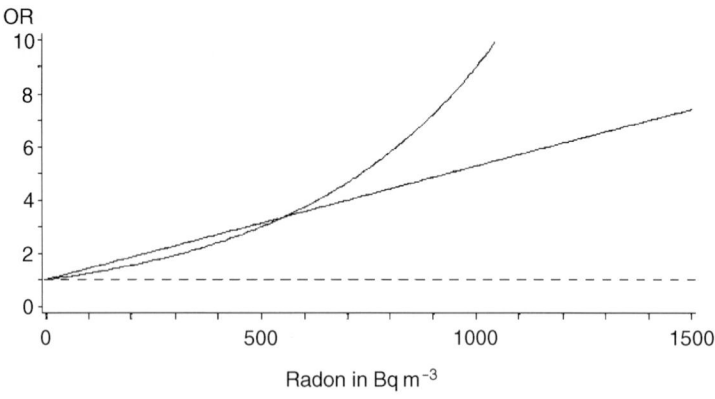

Figure 3.11. Lung cancer risk due to residential radon; comparison of linear and log-linear risk (modified from Oberaigner et al. 2002)

As an example let us come back to radon exposure. It can be assumed that the exposure to radon is low for large parts of the population and that concentrations above 500 Bq m^{-3} are unusual in the residential environment. Within this lower range both models, the linear and the log-linear approaches, yield a similar magnitude of risk. For exposures above 500 Bq m^{-3}, the two models will give different results that may lead to different consequences for risk management.

Therefore, nonparametric approaches are applied, namely risk models based on categorical exposures using ordinary contingency tables, especially if the real nature of relationship is not known. There are numerous examples of this strategy, even in situations in which exposure assessment was conducted on a continuous scale and categories of exposure were defined afterwards. Studies on EMF-related risks are a typical example of the use of this type of model. Figure 3.12 shows the results of a study on this topic conducted in Germany (Schüz et al. 2001).

Studies on EMF risks are usually influenced by many factors, and exposure assessment has to be conducted carefully. According to Fig. 3.12 the advantages of a model fit using categories instead of a continuous exposure assessment are obvious. While Fig. 3.12a suggests a strong increase in risk in the upper exposure category, Fig. 3.12b shows a smoother increase from one exposure category to the next. Thus, models using exposure categories increase the degrees of freedom, and any kind of exposure-disease relationship may be estimated. But this strategy is fully data-driven, and exposure-disease relationships may occur which are not plausible in any situation. For example, Ahlbom et al. (2000) reported results from a meta-analysis on EMF exposures with the same exposure categories as in Fig. 3.12. Albom et al. (2000) reported odds ratios of 1.58, 0.79, and 2.13 for the categories 0.1 to 0.2 μT, 0.2 to 0.4 μT, and more than 0.4 μT, respectively, compared to the reference category of less than 0.1 μT. These results do not agree with a monotonous exposure-disease relationship, and evidence for its true nature will be hard to obtain. However, the general strategy of using nonparametric

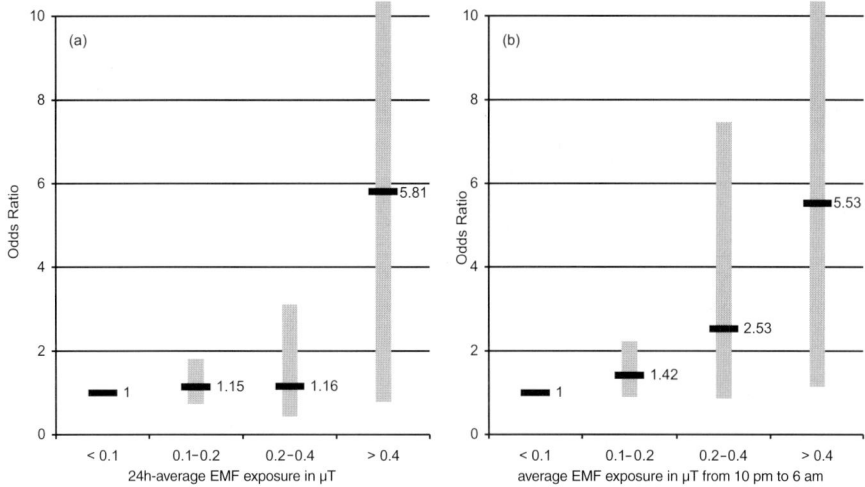

Figure 3.12. Leukemia risk due to EMF exposure in Germany; odds ratios and 95% confidence intervals by EMF exposure in µT; (**a**) average exposure during 24h; (**b**) average exposure during the night from 10 pm to 6 am (Schüz et al. 2001)

approaches is well established in all kinds of epidemiological studies and can be considered as a basic tool for estimating risk coefficients in environmental studies.

Confounding and Interaction and their Impact on Low Risks

Selecting the type of statistical model for investigations in environmental epidemiology is also influenced by further risk factors that may confound or modify the association under study. Given that most environmental risk factors will cause a low risk, these potentially distorting influences need careful scrutiny to avoid biases and misinterpretations of the results.

The influence of smoking in relation to the effects of environmental exposures on respiratory health may be used as a classical example. The smoking-related relative risk (RR) of lung cancer is reported to be in the order of ten or more, in contrast to the RR of residential radon or indoor air pollution, with RRs of less than two (Pershagen et al. 1994; Boffetta et al. 1998; Kreienbrock et al. 2001). The effect of smoking on respiratory symptoms like strong cough or obstructive bronchitis is in the range of around two to three, but only in the order of 1.3 for the comparison of areas that are polluted differently (Dockery et al 1993; Pope et al. 1995; Wolf-Ostermann et al. 1995). On the one hand, these examples suggest that it is necessary to incorporate these strong risk factors into a common risk model. On the other hand, these risk factors may dominate the model, requiring the development of proper strategies for the process of model and variable selection.

Following Greenland (1989) the selection of variables in epidemiological studies is based on two concepts: classical selection procedures such as backward or forward selection in regression models (cf. Chap. II.3 of this handbook); and a sophisticated analysis of the associations and interacting mechanisms of the variables under study made in advance.

These in-advance analyses have to be conducted carefully. Sensitivity analyses can be considered as an appropriate way to deal with this problem. Here, sensitivity analyses have to be carried out of both the disease variable as well as the different risk factors under study.

Studies on respiratory health and air pollution may serve as a typical example. First, respiratory health has to be defined precisely. Often very different definitions are possible. The definition of asthma is a classical example: The U.S. National Heart, Lung, and Blood Institute defines asthma as "a chronic inflammatory disorder of the airways [that] causes recurrent episodes of wheezing, breathlessness, chest tightness and coughing, particularly at night or in the early morning, usually associated with widespread but variable airflow obstruction that is often reversible, either spontaneously or with treatment." In contrast the American Lung Association defines asthma as "a chronic disease of the lungs in which the airways overreact to certain factors by becoming inflamed or obstructed, making it difficult to breathe comfortably." (JHSM 2004).

This shows that varying definitions of a disease may result in a large variety of measures that will influence prevalence and incidence measures and also affect the dependent variable under study in a regression model. Therefore it is helpful to calculate the same risk models for different definitions of the outcome to compare the patterns of the exposure-disease relationship.

If, as in most cancer studies, a symptom is defined in a clear and unequivocal way, sensitivity analyses of (concurrent) risk factors are worthwhile. Risk models can be calculated by systematically omitting one of the risk factors to assess the influence of the omitted factor by comparing the reduced model with the full model. This type of sensitivity analysis is a basic method in meta-analysis to assess the impact of each single study (cf. Chap. II.7 of this handbook).

If a large number of risk factors and/or strong and weak risk factors are incorporated simultaneously into one model, this may yield cross-classifications with only small numbers of observations, even if the overall sample size of the study is large. This causes a reduced statistical power due to a loss of precision, as can be demonstrated by studies on the interaction of smoking and residential radon, like the Swedish nationwide study conducted by Pershagen et al. (1994) (Table 3.5).

This substantial study included 1281 cases and 2576 controls. Assigning these subjects to the exposure categories and especially dividing them into sub-strata related to both smoking and environmental exposure yield small sample sizes in special sub-classes. For example, the number of subjects is small in the highest exposure category (more than $400 \, \mathrm{Bq \, m^{-3}}$). Stratifying this group into subgroups by smoking status results in small numbers and leads to less precision in estimating the related effects, as is reflected by the wide confidence intervals shown in Table 3.5.

Sensitivity analyses of all possible risk factors have to be a combination of an exploratory process of exposure assessment and of the analyses of the association, confounding, and interaction mechanisms between these factors. The etiology

Table 3.5. Lung cancer risk due to smoking and residential radon in Sweden: number of cases and controls (subj.), odds ratios (OR) and 95% confidence intervals (CI) (Pershagen et al. 1994)

Smoking status	Radon exposure in Bq m^{-3}									
	< 50		50–80		80–140		140–400		> 400	
	subj.	OR (CI)	subj.	OR (CI)	subj.	OR (CI)	subj.	OR (CI)	subj.	OR (CI)
Never smoked	64 / 443	1 / –	36 / 240	1.1 (0.7–1.7)	35 / 252	1.0 (0.6–1.5)	38 / 198	1.5 (1.0–2.3)	5 / 31	1.2 (0.4–3.1)
Ex-smoker	35 / 105	2.6 (1.6–4.2)	21 / 69	2.4 (1.3–4.3)	24 / 63	3.2 (1.8–5.6)	27 / 48	4.5 (2.6–8.0)	1 / 8	1.1 (0.1–9.0)
Current < 10 cig. a day	103 / 128	6.2 (4.2–9.2)	60 / 79	6.0 (3.8–9.4)	62 / 79	6.1 (3.9–9.5)	53 / 59	7.3 (4.5–11.7)	12 / 4	25.1 (7.7–82.4)
Current > 10 cig. a day	168 / 102	12.6 (8.7–18.4)	85 / 63	11.6 (7.4–18.0)	94 / 71	11.8 (7.7–18.2)	83 / 42	15.0 (9.4–24.0)	16 / 4	32.5 (10.3–102.1)
Unknown	82 / 174	4.7 (2.9–7.7)	66 / 110	5.9 (3.5–10.0)	57 / 103	5.3 (3.1–9.2)	45 / 89	5.4 (3.1–9.5)	9 / 12	8.8 (3.3–23.7)

of pediatric asthma may serve as a consolidated example of this processes as summarized by Johnson et al. (2002) (see Fig. 3.13).

The outcome of persistent (pediatric) atopic asthma has to be recognized as a complicated process involving different steps of development of the disease and common and interacting influences by different risk factors. Environmental agents may play a role as independent risk factors or as interacting and confounding variables. For example, most of the possible risk factors in the areas "residence" and "environmental hygiene" in Fig 3.13 are more or less associated, and confounding bias may be present if this is not adequately described or modeled in an epidemiological investigation. Some studies report such associations (Weiland et al. 1994; Ponsonby et al. 2000), although the majority of studies do not support a strong relationship between air pollution and atopic asthma.

The Committee on the Assessment of Asthma and Indoor Air, Division of Health Promotion and Disease Prevention, Institute of Medicine concluded that there is sufficient evidence for a causal relationship between exposure to allergens produced by cats, cockroaches, and house dust mites and exacerbations of asthma in sensitized individuals; and between environmental tobacco smoke exposure and exacerbations of asthma in pre-school-aged children. Besides these findings it was suggested that there is sufficient evidence of associations between several exposures and exacerbations of asthma, like the exposure to biological allergens produced by dogs, fungi, molds, and rhinovirus, and to chemicals such as high levels of NO_2 and NO_x. Limited evidence of an association was suggested for exposures of children and adults to the biological allergens domestic birds, *Chlamydia pneumoniae, Mycoplasma pneumoniae*, or Respiratory Syncytial Virus RSV, or to the chemicals environmental tobacco smoke, formaldehyde, or fragrances (IOM 2000).

The evaluations of the Institute of Medicine are a synopsis of hundreds of studies on this topic. But the overall evidence of a single risk factor is influenced by a "network of associations of risk factors", from which some are identified as causal and some as associated. For example, allergens related to pets like cats and dogs may be measured and separated as factors. However, strong associations of behaviors in pet holding have to be taken into account, and it is difficult to separate them from the exposure factors above, especially if there is a large association between factors.

Therefore powerful studies are needed both in terms of sample sizes as well as in terms of high quality in exposure assessment. Synopses like the asthma studies mentioned above, systematic reviews, meta-analyses, and pooling of studies may be useful to avoid biased conclusions about the effect of weak risk factors in environmental epidemiology.

Correction for Errors in Exposure Assessment

As outlined in Sect. 3.3.2 one major problem of an investigation in environmental epidemiology is the categorical or the continuous assessment of an environmental exposure. The statistical inference on this risk factor is linked to the problem of

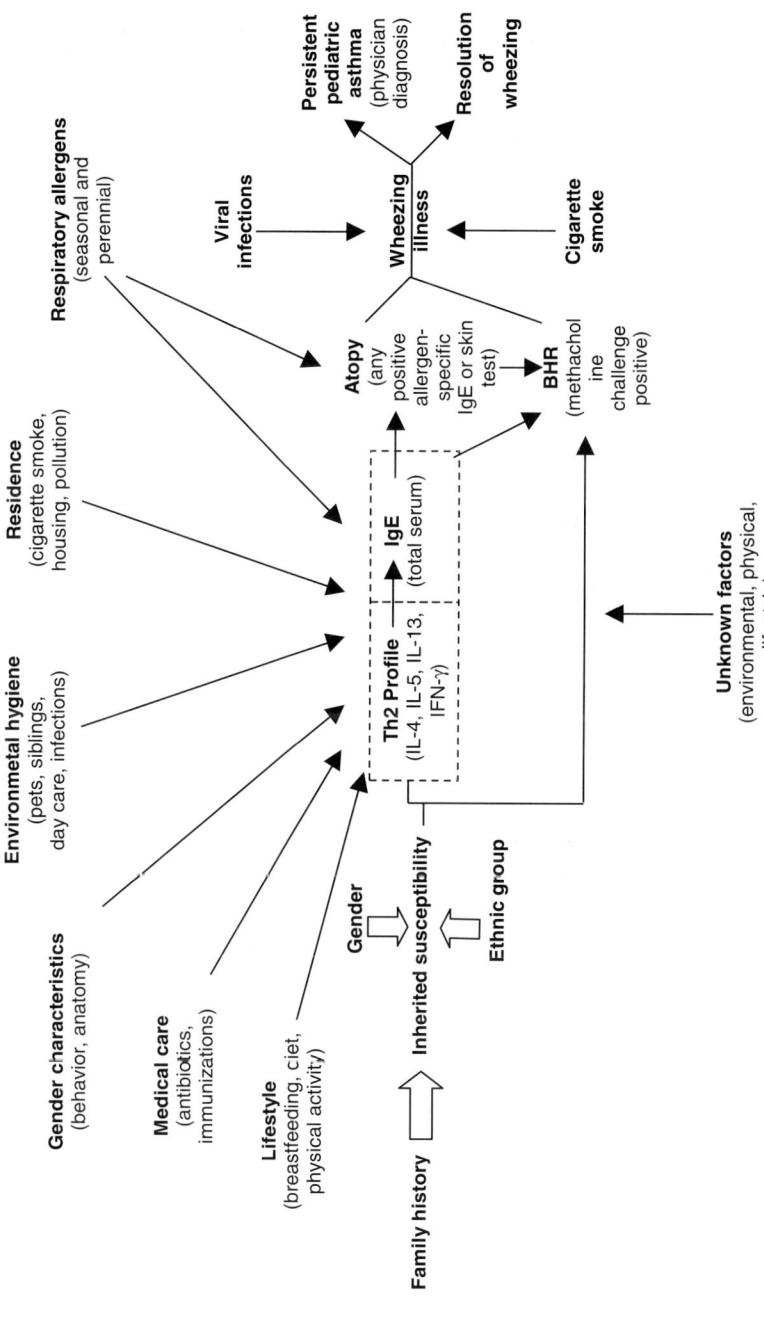

Figure 3.13. Factors and markers potentially associated with the development of persistent pediatric atopic asthma; TH, T-helper cell; Ig, immunoglobulin; IL, interleukin; IFN-γ, interferon gamma; BHR, bronchial hyperactivity (modified from Johnson et al. 2002)

information bias if misclassification (for categorical exposures) or uncertainty (for continuous exposures) in the exposure assessment occurs.

There exist numerous examples for information biases due to misclassification in exposure assessment. Misclassification is often due to recall bias, that is typical in case-control studies. It may occur if cases report environmental exposures more often than controls, who do not care so much about environmental exposures because they are not diseased. In this situation a bias away from the null is introduced and variables may be erroneously identified as risk factors. The same direction of bias may result if interviewers tend to ask more detailed questions on exposures in cases than in controls.

Biases due to misclassification should be avoided by the design of a study and during data collection, e.g. by standardization of interview techniques (cf. Chap. I.10 of this handbook). Under certain assumptions they may be corrected by appropriate methods of adjustment for misclassification. This is usually done by estimating the sensitivity and the specificity of the categorical exposure assessment and adjusting the observed measures of disease by these estimators (cf. Chap. II.5 of this handbook).

But even the continuous measurement of environmental exposures may lead to uncertainty in the exposure assessment. The sources of error are numerous, like the accuracy of the detectors, the laboratory procedures, the positioning of the measurement devices, extrapolations to past exposure, or gaps in the exposure history.

These errors have to be incorporated into the statistical models used to estimate risk coefficients similar to the procedures of adjustment for misclassification. Statistical models that take uncertainty in exposure assessment into account are related to special computational efforts and therefore different techniques were developed especially during the 90s thanks to the overall availability of high-capacity computers (cf. also Tosteson et al. 1989; Armstrong 1990, 1998; Carroll et al. 1995; Michels 2001). Often the development of these techniques was motivated by examples from environmental epidemiology. Here, the exposure assessment is based on measurements and the ordinary assumption of a continuous risk factor with uncertainty is fulfilled. For example, Thomas et al. (1993) applied special techniques for studies of the impact of EMF on childhood leukemia. Lagarde et al. (1997), Reeves et al. (1998), and Heid et al. (2002) investigated models for proper incorporation of the uncertainty of radon exposures, and its impact on lung cancer risk. Zeger et al. (2000) and Dominici et al. (2000) examined the impact of errors in the particulate matter on mortality.

These studies show that the impact of information bias tends to increase the impact of usual random error. It is therefore of major importance to incorporate the error in the exposure assessment into the risk model. Correction for errors in exposure generally requires several models (cf. Chap. II.5): the model for the true exposure, the true exposure-disease model linking true exposure and disease, and the error model linking true exposure and measured exposure. Given these models, the exposure-disease model accounting for errors in exposure measurement can be derived by linking measured exposure and disease (Fig. 3.14).

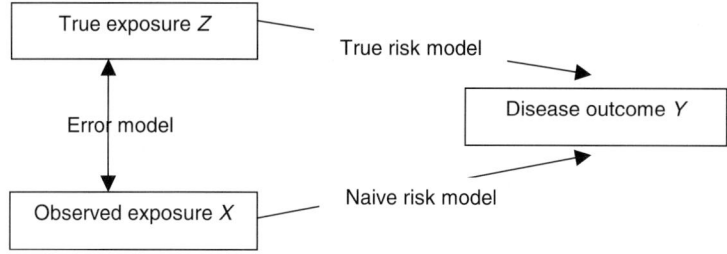

Figure 3.14. True exposure Z and observed exposure X and their relationship to the disease outcome Y

As a general strategy the variable X, which represents the observed result of an exposure assessment (cf. Sect. 3.3.2) is not fixed, but has an error structure. The variable X has to be contrasted with the true value Z of the exposure. Following Heid (2002) in describing the deviation between X and Z, five classifying characteristics of error models may be considered: (1) random vs. systematic error, (2) non-differential vs. differential error, (3) homoscedastic vs. heteroscedastic error, (4) additive vs. multiplicative error, and (5) classical vs. Berkson error.

A random error is generally considered as a measurement error. It is characterized by an unsystematic deviations below or above the true value that average to zero. Usually all laboratory devices used in environmental measurements are prone to this error. In contrast, systematic errors lead to an overestimation or an underestimation of all individual measurements and do not average to zero. This problem may occur, if measurements were conducted on different technical levels, which is a special problem in multi-center studies or in meta-analyses. Here, intercomparison exercises of the different methods will give a deeper insight into the problem (Hollander et al. 1990; Kreienbrock et al. 1999; Wellmann et al. 2001; Bochicchio et al. 2002; Janssens 2004).

Similar to the effect of non-differential misclassification of categorical exposures, it can be assumed that error in the exposure assessment will attenuate the true exposure-disease relationship as long as this error is non-differential. A non-differential misclassification of the exposure is present if the error has the same magnitude and direction among diseased and non-diseased study participants. Otherwise (differential error) the direction of bias is not obvious in advance and any direction is possible (cf. Chap. II.5 of this handbook). Figure 3.15 shows the effect on non-differential error for studies of lung cancer risk due to residential radon in the UK and in Sweden, where the reported excess relative risk increases by approximately 50% after adjustment for measurement error. This situation may be considered as typical in environmental epidemiology.

The problem of homoscedastic vs. heteroscedastic errors as well as the problem of additive or multiplicative errors are related to the nature of the statistical distributions which are stated for the measurements or for the exposure in general. For an additive error, the spread of the true exposure given the measured exposure is constant for the full range of the exposure. In this situation a normal

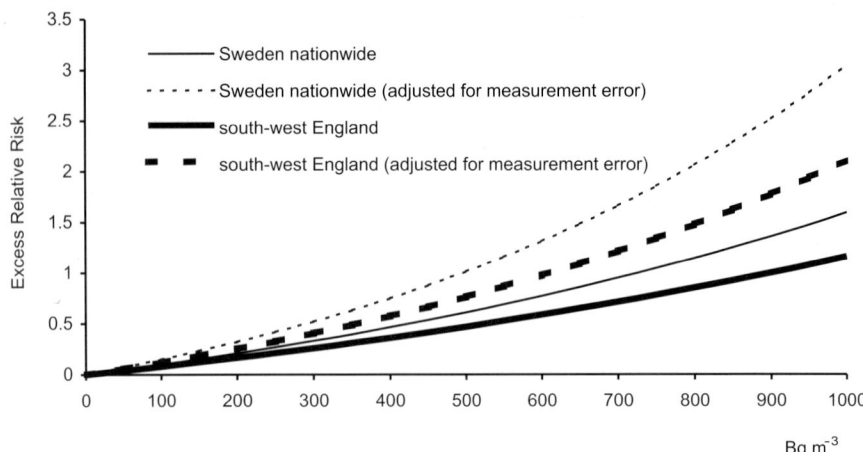

Figure 3.15. Excess relative risk due to residential radon in the UK and in Sweden; results of classical log-linear models and adjustment for measurement error (Darby et al. 1998; Lagarde et al. 1997)

distribution is often appropriate. In contrast, for a multiplicative error the spread increases proportional to increasing exposure. Therefore multiplicative errors usually are assumed to be log-normal, which often is evaluated by measurement and monitoring programmes on the population level. This is more or less true for many environmental agents like radon (Bäverstam and Swedjemark 1991; Gunby et al. 1993; Miles 1994; Lubin et al. 1995), classical pollutants of outdoor air (Ebelt et al. 2001, Wallace et al. 2003), endotoxin levels (Park et al. 2000), and many more.

Finally, errors of the classical type arise, if a quantity X is based on measurements by some device and repeated measurements would vary around the true value Z. This situation can be assumed for all kinds of laboratory devices, for which a measurement error is reported.

In contrast, error of the Berkson type occurs if the exposure, which is assigned to each individual, is derived from an overall group characteristic. The same approximate exposure value (proxi) X is used for all members of the group, and the true exposure Z varies randomly around this proxi with mean equal to it. This type of error may occur in a study on the effects of air pollution on respiratory health, if all study participants of a defined region are assigned to the same proxi X, e.g. the result of a single measurement station. Thus, Berkson error may occur if exposure is measured via (locally) fixed monitors instead of personal detectors, or if exposures have to be approximated due to missing values in the measurements. (cf. Chap. II.5 of this handbook; Lagarde et al. 1997; Armstrong 1998; Reeves et al. 1998).

An overwhelming variety of models exists to estimate the effects of uncertainty of exposure assessment. Regression calibration is one of these (cf. Chap. II.5; Rosner et al. 1989; Carroll et al. 1995). The main advantage of regression calibration is that it can be used in rather complicated measurement error models. The method includes three steps: first find a mean (calibration) model for the true regressors Z depending on the exposure assessment X, and second fit the main model by plugging in the estimates from the calibration model. The third step is the correction of the variance estimation of the main model. Although this method was developed for multiple logistic regression accounting for errors in more than one variable, application is usually restricted to account for errors of the primary risk factor of interest. The error model, i.e. the mathematical formulation of the deviation of the measured exposure X from the true exposure Z, is the most important model assumption, upon which all of the correction methods rely. In fact, assumptions about the error model are a particular source of concern regarding correction of measurement error (Michels 2001).

Therefore, substantial effort was devoted to evaluate these assumptions about the different model characteristics as well as in the different fields of applications. This was done by theoretical considerations, by simulation studies as well as by applying different techniques on selected studies (Armstrong et al. 1990; Thomas et al. 1993; Ibibarren et al. 1996; Lagarde et al. 1997; Reeves et al. 1998; Carrothers and Evans 2000; Dominici et al. 2000; Zeger et al. 2000; Heid et al. 2002; Field et al. 2002; Heid et al. 2004).

In conclusion, a clear distinction between the components of classical and Berkson error is essential in the assessment of error sources and for establishing an error model. This differentiation is crucial due to the different impact of these two error types. The classical error is able to induce severe bias on the risk estimate; multiplicative classical error may even distort the dose-response curve. This bias can be reduced by using the mean of multiple measurements in the analysis that require internal replicate measurements for each individual, or it can be corrected for by using the information from (internal or external) replicate measurements of a subgroup. Also the spuriously narrow confidence intervals for uncorrected risk estimates in the presence of classical error can be adjusted. Therefore it can be recommended that more internal repeated measurements in future epidemiological studies should be conducted, for example by using more than one detector per study participant.

At first glance, the Berkson error is less problematic in environmental epidemiology, since usually it does not induce notable bias of the risk estimates. However, Berkson error weakens the precision of the estimates, and therefore leads to a loss of power that should be avoided, e.g. by a proper individual exposure assessment. This will, however, introduce the classical error which may be reduced by replicate measurements, but this does not hold for the Berkson error. Simplified, classical error is related to the measurement process, whereas Berkson error is often a matter of defining the exposure groups. Using stationary monitors (e.g. using the distance of a home to the next emitter of an environmental agent instead of individual measurements), or using a person's affiliation to a group in order to use the exposure assigned to this group (e.g. using job-environment-exposure matrices instead of personal monitors) is a question of how to define the exposure group; this induces Berkson error.

The general statement that non-differential, random and homoscedastic errors attenuate regression coefficients applies only to the classical error. To assume the sum of both error type's sizes as known and to vary the percentage of the Berkson error is one option (cf. Mallick et al. 2002). An additional option is a two-dimensional view to the measurement error, i.e. a classical type dimension and a Berkson type dimension, where the size of each dimension needs to be studied separately. The full error is represented in the continuum of a two-dimensional space (cf. Zeger et al. 2000). Exposure assessment should therefore not only aim to be as accurate and precise as possible, but should also provide a model of the measurement errors that unavoidably remain even with clear differentiation of classical and Berkson components.

3.4   Conclusions

By definition, environmental epidemiology focuses on health problems due to the environment where individuals live rather than due to their personal characteristics or lifestyles. During the past centuries, there has been a remarkable discourse on environmental health and environmental epidemiology, and a huge number of individual studies as well as pooling of individual studies and meta-analyses have contributed to a large overall knowledge base on environmental hazards. As a consequence, many public health issues have been addressed by reducing contamination of air, water, soil, and food to the benefit of many parts of the world's population.

However, many multifactorial diseases are not yet fully understood, and the scientific focus has changed during the last decade, as developments in epidemiology have kept up with those in molecular biology and genetics.

A typical example is the discussion on the health impact of air pollution on respiratory diseases. One such issue is atopic asthma, and studies were conducted to find a relationship between air pollution and the incidence of the disease. But the studies failed, or observed only little environmental influence. Therefore, the focus was shifted to the nature of allergic disease itself, and techniques of molecular biology and genetics have now been widely used to deepen our knowledge on this topic (cf. Johnson et al. 2002).

Therefore, the study of gene-environment interactions has been and will continue to be a major subject of epidemiological investigations, e.g. for asthma, for cancer and for other diseases for which molecular and genetic markers and methods of molecular biology and genetics are available. A serious disadvantage of all these studies is that investigations in molecular and genetic epidemiology tend to be very expensive, so that study sizes have to be restricted. For example, Kalayci et al. (2004) compared plasma levels of MCP-4 in 30 patients who presented for emergent treatment of asthma with levels in 90 subjects with chronic-stable asthma matched for age, gender, and ethnicity within an entire cohort of 596 subjects.

Thus, there is a contradiction between the original idea of an environmental study with large sample sizes and a study in molecular and genetic epidemiology with small sample sizes. Small studies may fail to find interactions due a lack of power. In addition the informativeness of studies on gene-environment interactions is often limited because of their insufficient ability to account for confounding.

This situation may be called the "small sample size problem" in the analysis of gene-environment interactions. Two major ways may be identified for further research on this topic. To increase power, all possible measures have to be taken to improve the precision of molecular and genetic techniques and the assessment of exposures (cf. Sects. 3.3.2 and 3.3.3, and Chaps. III.7 and III.8 of this handbook). For example, first studies on the impact of environmental tobacco smoke (ETS) on respiratory diseases used urinary cotinine concentrations as a biomarker (Ehrlich et al. 1992). However, cotinine levels in the urine reflect only recent exposures and can therefore not replace exposure histories from questionnaires that give a good estimate of the long-term cumulative exposure.

The second approach to cope with the "small sample size problem" is directly linked to the design and the statistical analysis of the investigation. In practice it is often impossible to detect an effect of a single agent because the various exposures are strongly correlated and the exposure that has been measured may actually act as a surrogate the whole mixture of agents. Therefore it is necessary to find statistical models which make use of the correlation of all possible independent risk factors, as well as all modifying and confounding variables. For example, in a study on the health impact of toxic substances ingested with food, strong correlations have to be made explicit that are due to nutritional habits, like the consumption of special types of seafood etc. Therefore this has to be addressed in detail during the phase of constructing a final risk model, and by appropriate specification of statistical methods (cf. Chap. II.3 of this handbook).

The development of these models, besides the molecular and genetic view on a special health issue, is ordinarily linked to the personal exposures of an individual recruited for the study. On the other hand, many environmental exposures act on an aggregated level. For example, outdoor air pollution is the same, drinking water is the same, or contaminated soil often is the same for major parts of a population, e.g. all inhabitants of a particular area. From the statistical point of view this yields a Berkson-type error, and a correlation of the exposures between the study participants, or even more extremely, it yields sub-classes of participants exposed in the exact same way. On the one hand, classes of hierarchical models may be used to find a proper risk model in this situation. On the other hand, the extraordinarily large number of possible environmental hazards may even force epidemiologists to conduct ecological studies to find rough estimates of risk.

In regard to the complex nature of possible environmental hazards, Pekkanen and Pearce (2001) pointed out that increasing emphasis on individual exposures, susceptibility and disease mechanisms, puts environmental epidemiologists in danger of losing their population perspective of disease causation and prevention. To avoid this and to continue the successful work of environmental epidemiology and public health, environmental health problems should be approached on four different levels: the molecular, the individual, the population, and the ecosystem level. Within and between these levels research and development of new methods is needed, but it will be crucially important to choose the most appropriate level of research for a particular environmental problem. For example, the health impact of climate change will be one of the most important health problems of the future requiring research, but ordinary designs and exposure assessments may not be adequate to give answers to the underlying questions.

This may initiate new methodological concepts in study designs, in biological and genetic markers, in exposure assessment, as well as in the statistical analysis of studies in environmental epidemiology. In the past decade new analytical methods in molecular biology and genetics have enriched designs and techniques in epidemiological investigations on environmental hazards. The challenge for further work is to exploit these new areas of scientific cooperation.

Summarizing, it must be determined whether there is
— sufficient evidence of an association,
— limited or suggestive evidence of an association,
— inadequate or insufficient evidence to determine whether or not an association is present,
— limited or suggestive evidence of no association, or
— evidence of no association.

This judgment should be combined with an evaluation of the public health impact of an environmental problem. For this purpose, assessment of the etiologic fraction due to the exposure in question may give an important input.

Acknowledgements.   The author likes to thank Michael Gerken, Michael Hauptmann, Iris Heid, Michaela Kreuzer, Wilhelm Oberaigner, Angelika Schaffrath Rosario, H.-Erich Wichmann and Jürgen Wellmann for their substantial help in preparing this manuscript, and Judith McAlister-Hermann for her work in reviewing. A very special gratitude for their help and patience has to be offered to the editors of this handbook, Wolfgang Ahrens and Iris Pigeot.

References

Ahlbom A, Day N, Feychting M, Roman E, Skinner J, Dockerty J, Linet M, McBride M, Michaelis J, Olsen JH, Tynes T, Verkasalo PK (2000) A pooled analysis of magnetic fields and childhood leukaemia. Br J Cancer 83:692–698

Alavanja MCR, Brownson RC, Lubin JH, Berger E, Chang J, Boice JD Jr (1994) Residential radon exposure and lung cancer among nonsmoking women. J Natl Cancer Inst 86:1829–1837

Alavanja MC, Lubin JH, Mahaffey JA, Brownson RC (1999) Residential radon exposure and risk of lung cancer in Missouri. Am J Public Health 89:1042–1048

Anderson TW (1984) An introduction to multivariate statistical analysis, 2nd edn. Wiley, New York

Anderson HR, deLeon AP, Bland M, Bower JS, Strachan DP (1996) Air pollution and daily mortality in London: 1987–1992. Br Med J 312:665–669

Armstrong BG (1990) The effects of measurement errors on relative risk regression. Am J Epi 132:1176–1184

Armstrong BG (1998) Effect of measurement error on epidemiological studies of environmental and occupational exposures. Occup Environ Med 55:651–656

Auvinen A, Mäkeläinen I, Hakama M, Castrén O, Pukkala E, Reisbacka H, Rytömaa T (1996) Indoor radon exposure and risk of lung cancer: a nested case-control study in Finland. J Natl Cancer Inst 88:966–972, Erratum. J Natl Cancer Inst (1998) 90:401–402

Bäverstam U, Swedjemark G-A (1991) Where are the errors when we estimate Radon exposure in retrospect? Radiation Protection Dosimetry 36:107–112

Barros-Dios JM, Barreiro MA, Ruano-Ravina A, Figueiras A (2002) Exposure to residential radon and lung cancer in Spain: a population-based case-control study. Am J Epi 156:548–555

Baysson H, Billon S, Laurier D, Rogel A, Tirmarche M (2003) Seasonal correction factors for estimating radon exposure in dwellings in France. Radiat Prot Dosimetry 104:245–252

Bell ML, Davis DL, Fletcher T (2004) A retrospective assessment of mortality from the London smog episode of 1952: The role of influenza and pollution. Environ Health Perspect 112:6–8

Blot WJ, Xu Z-Y, Boice JD, Zhao D-Z, Stone BJ, Sun J, Jing LB, Fraumeni JF (1990) Indoor radon and lung cancer in China. J Natl Cancer Inst 82:10–25

Bochicchio F, McLaughlin JP, Walsh C(2002) Comparison of radon exposure assessment results: ^{210}Po surface activity on glass objects vs contemporary air radon concentration. Radiat Meas 36:211–215

Boffetta P, Agudo A, Ahrens W, Benhamou E, Benhamou S, Darby SC, Ferro G, Fortes C, Gonzalez CA, Jöckel KH, Krauss M, Kreienbrock L, Kreuzer M, Mendes A, Merletti F, Nyberg F, Pershagen G, Pohlabeln H, Riboli E, Schmid G, Simonato L, Tredaniel J, Whitley E, Wichmann HE, Winck C, Zambon P, Saracci R (1998) Multicenter case-control study of exposure to environmental tobacco smoke and lung cancer in Europe. J Natl Cancer Inst 90:1440–1450

Brunekreef B (2003) Design of cohort studies for air pollution health effects. J Toxicol Environ Health A 66:1731–1734

Brunekreef B, Holgate ST (2002) Air pollution and health. Lancet 360:1233–1242

Carroll RJ, Ruppert D, Stefanski LA (1995) Measurement error in nonlinear models. Chapman and Hall, London

Carrothers TJ, Evans JS (2000) Assessing the impact of differential measurement error on estimates of fine particle mortality. J Air Waste Manag Assoc 50:65–74

Cohen BL (1993) Relationship between exposure to radon and various types of cancer. Health Physics 65:529–531

Cohen BL (1997) Problems in the radon vs lung cancer test of the linear no-threshold theory and a procedure for resolving them. Health Physics 72:623–628

Darby SC, Whitley E, Silcocks P, Tharkar B, Green M, Lomas P, Miles J, Reeves G, Fearn T, Doll R (1998) Risk of lung cancer associated with residential radon exposure in south-west England: a case-control study. British Journal of Cancer 78:394–408

Darby SC, Hill D, Doll R (2001) Radon: A likely carcinogen at all exposures. Ann Oncol 12:1341–1351

Dockery DW, Pope CA, Xu X, Spengler JD, Ware JH, Fay ME, Ferris BG, Speizer FE (1993) An association between air pollution and mortality in six U.S. cities. N Engl J Med 329:1753–1759

Doll R, Peto R (1976) Mortality in relation to smoking: 20 years' observations on male British doctors. BMJ 25:1525–1536

Dominici F, Zeger SL, Samet JM (2000) A measurement error model for time-series studies of air pollution and mortality. Biostatistics 1:157–175

Ebelt S, Brauer M, Cyrys J, Tuch T, Kreyling WG, Wichmann HE, Heinrich J (2001) Air Quality in Postunification Erfurt, East Germany: Associating Changes in Pollutant Concentrations with Changes in Emissions. Environ Health Perspect 109:325–333

Ehrlich R, Kattan M, Godbold J, Saltzberg DS, Grimm KT, Landrigan PJ, Lilienfeld DE (1992) Childhood asthma and passive smoking. Urinary cotinine as a biomarker of exposure. Am Rev Respir Dis 145:594–599

Ennemoser O, Ambach W, Auer T, Brunner P, Schneider P, Oberaigner W Purtscheller F, Sting V (1994a) High indoor radon concentrations in an alpine region of western Tyrol. Health Physics 67:151–154

Ennemoser O, Ambach W, Brunner P, Schneider P, Oberaigner W, Purtscheller F, Stingl V, Keller G (1994b) Unusually high indoor radon concentrations from a giant rock slide. Sci Total Environ 151:235–240

EpiInfo™ (2000) A database and statistics program for public health professionals using Windows® 95, 98, NT, and 2000 computers

Field RW, Steck DJ, Smith BJ, Brus CP, Fisher EL, Neuberger JS, Platz CE, Robinson RA, Woolson RF, Lynch CF (2000): Residential radon gas exposure and lung cancer: the Iowa Radon Lung Cancer Study. Am J Epi 151:1091–1102

Field RW, Smith BJ, Steck DJ, Lynch CF (2002) Residential radon exposure and lung cancer: variation in risk estimates using alternative exposure scenarios. J Expo Anal Environ Epidemiol 12:197–203

Finkelstein MM (1991) Use of time windows to investigate lung cancer latency intervals at an Ontario steel plant. American Journal of Industrial Medicine 19:229–235

Frye C, Heinrich J, Wjst M, Wichmann HE; Bitterfeld Study Group (2001) Increasing prevalence of bronchial hyperresponsiveness in three selected areas in East Germany. Eur Respir J 18:451–458

Gerken M, Kreienbrock L, Wellmann J, Kreuzer M, Wichmann HE (2000) Models for retrospective quantification of indoor radon exposure in case-control studies. Health Physics 78:268–278

Graham JD (1997) The role of epidemiology in regulatory risk assessment. Elsevier, Amsterdam

Greenland S (1989) Modeling and variable selection in epidemiologic analysis. American Journal of Public Health 79:340–349

Greenland S, Sheppard AR, Kaune WT, Poole C, Kelsh MA (2000) A pooled analysis of magnetic fields, wire codes, and childhood leukemia. Childhood Leukemia-EMF Study Group. Epidemiology 11:624–634

Gunby JA, Darby, SC, Miles, JC, Green, BM, Cox DR (1993) Factors affecting indoor radon concentration in the United Kingdom. Health Physics 64:2–12

Habash RW, Brodsky LM, Leiss W, Krewski D, Repacholi M (2003a) Health risks of electromagnetic fields, part I: Evaluation and assessment of electric and magnetic fields. Crit Rev Biomed Eng 31:141–195

Habash RW, Brodsky LM, Leiss W, Krewski D, Repacholi M (2003b) Health risks of electromagnetic fields, part II: Evaluation and assessment of radio frequency radiation. Crit Rev Biomed Eng. 31:197–254

Hansen MH, Hurwitz WN (1946) The problem of non-response in sample surveys. JASA 41:517–529

Hauptmann M, Lubin JH, Rosenberg PS, Wellmann J, Kreienbrock L (2000a) The use of sliding time windows for the exploratory analysis of temporal effects of smoking histories on lung cancer risk. Stat Med 19:2185–2194

Hauptmann M, Wellmann J, Lubin JH, Rosenberg PS, Kreienbrock L (2000b) Analysis of exposure-time-response relationships using a spline weight function. Biometrics 56:1105–1108

Heid IM (2002) Measurement error in exposure assessment: An error model and its impact on studies on lung cancer and residential radon exposure in Germany. Doctoral Thesis Ludwig-Maximilians-Universität München

Heid IM, Küchenhoff H, Wellmann J, Gerken M, Kreienbrock L, Wichmann HE (2002) On the potential of measurement error to induce differential bias on odds ratio estimates: an example from radon epidemiology. Stat Med 21:3261–3278

Heid IM, Schaffrath Rosario A, Kreienbrock L, Küchenhoff H, Wichmann HE (2004) The impact of measurement error on studies on lung cancer and residential radon exposure in Germany. J Tox Env Health, in press

Heinrich J, Hoelscher B, Wichmann HE (2000) Decline of ambient air pollution and respiratory symptoms in children. Am J Respir Crit Care Med 161:1930–1936

Heinrich J, Hoelscher B, Frye C, Meyer I, Wjst M, Wichmann HE (2002) Trends in prevalence of atopic diseases and allergic sensitization in children in Eastern Germany. Eur Respir J 19:1040–1046

Hoek G, Brunekreef B, Verhoeff A, van Wijnen J, Fischer P (2000) Daily mortality and air pollution in The Netherlands. J Air Waste Manag Assoc 50:1380–1389

Hollander W, Morawietz G, Bake D, Laskus L, van Elzakker BG, van der Meulen A, Zierock KH (1990) A field intercomparison and fundamental characterization of various dust samplers with a reference sampler. J Air Waste Manag Assoc 40:881–886

IARC, International Agency on Research on Cancer (2001) Ionizing radiation, part 2: Some internally deposited radionuclides. IARC monographs on the evaluation of carcinogenic risks to humans, vol 78. International Agency on Research on Cancer, Lyon

Ibibarren C, Sharp D, Burchfield CM, Ping S, Dwyer JH (1996) Association of serum total cholesterol with coronary disease and all-cause mortality: Multivariate correction for bias due to measurement error. Am J Epi 143:463–471

ICRP, International Commission on Radiological Protection (1993) Protection against radon 222 at home and at work. ICRP Publication 65. Annals of the ICRP, vol 23, No 2. Didcot, Oxon

IOM, Institute of Medicine (2000) Clearing the Air: Asthma and Indoor Air Exposures. National Academic Press, Washington D.C.

Janssens A (2004) Environmental radiation protection: philosophy, monitoring and standards. J Environ Radioact 72:65–73

JHSM, Division of Pulmonary and Critical Care Medicine, Johns Hopkins School of Medicine (2004) (http://www.hopkins-lungs.org/programs/asthma/) Accessed May 8, 2004

Johnson CC, Ownby DR, Zoratti EM, Hensley Alford S, Williams LK, Joseph CLM (2002) Environmental epidemiology of pediatric asthma and allergy. Epidemiologic Reviews 24:154–175

Kalayci O, Sonna LA, Woodruff PG, Camargo CA Jr, Luster AD, Lilly CM (2004) Monocyte chemotactic protein-4 (MCP-4; CCL-13): a biomarker of asthma. J Asthma 41:27–33

Katsouyanni K, Touloumi G, Spix C, Schwartz J, Balducci F, Medina S, Rossi G, Wojtyniak B, Sunyer J, Bacharova L, Schouten JP, Ponka A, Anderson HR (1997) Short-term effects of ambient sulphur dioxide and particulate matter on mortality in 12 European cities: results from time series data from the APHEA project. Air pollution and health: A European approach. Br Med J 314:1658–1663

Kleinbaum DG, Kupper LL, Morgenstern H (1982) Epidemiologic research. Van Nostrand Reinhold, New York

Kreienbrock L, Schach S (2000) Epidemiologische Methoden, 3rd ed. (in German). Spektrum, Heidelberg

Kreienbrock L, Siehl A (1996) Multiple statistische Analyse von Radon-Erhebungsmessungen in der Bundesrepublik Deutschland. In: Siehl A (ed). Umweltradiaoaktivität – Geologie und Ökologie im Kontext. Ernst & Sohn, VCH, Berlin, pp 299–310

Kreienbrock L, Poffijn A, Tirmarche M, Feider M, Kies A, Darby SC (1999) Intercomparison of passive Rn-detectors under field conditions in epidemiological studies. Health Physics 76:558–563

Kreienbrock L, Kreuzer M, Gerken M, Dingerkus G, Wellmann J, Keller G, Wichmann HE (2001) Case-control study on lung cancer and residential radon in West Germany. Am J Epi 153:42–52

Kreuzer M, Heinrich J, Wölke G, Schaffrath Rosario A, Gerken M, Wellmann J, Keller G, Kreienbrock L, Wichmann HE (2003) Residential radon and risk of lung cancer in Eastern Germany. Epidemiology 14:1–10

Krewski D, Burnett RT, Goldberg MS, Hoover K, Siemiatycki J, Abrahamowicz M, White WH (2004) Validation of the Harvard Six Cities Study of particulate air pollution and mortality. N Engl J Med 350:198–199

Lagarde F, Pershagen G, Akerblom G, Axelson O, Bäverstam U, Damber L, Enflo A, Svartengren M, Swedjemark GA (1997) Residential radon and lung cancer in Sweden: risk analysis accounting for random error in the exposure assessment. Health Physics 72:269–276

Lagarde F, Axelsson G, Damber L, Mellander H, Nyberg F, Pershagen G (2001) Residential radon and lung cancer among never-smokers in Sweden. Epidemiology 12:396–404

Létourneau EG, Krewski D, Choi NW, Goddard MJ, McGregor RG, Zielinski JM, Du J (1994) Case-control study of residential radon and lung cancer in Winnipeg, Manitoba, Canada. Am J Epi 140:310–322

Locher W, Unschuld PU (1999) Geschichtliches zur Umweltmedizin. In: Wichmann HE, Schlipköter HW, Fülgraff G (eds) Handbuch der Umweltmedizin. ecomed, Landsberg/Lech, pp II-1.1–II-1.12

Lubin JH (1988) Models for the analysis of radon-exposed populations. Yale Journal of Biology and Medicine 61:195–214

Lubin JH, Steindorf K (1995) Cigarette use and the estimation of lung cancer attributable to radon in the United States. Radiat Res 141:79–85

Lubin JH, Samet JM, Weinberg C (1990) Design issues in epidemiologic studies of indoor exposure to Rn and risk of lung cancer. Health Physics 59:807–817

Lubin JH, Boice JD, Edling CH, Hornung R, Howe G, Kunz E, Kusiak A, Morrison HI, Radford EP, Samet JM, Tirmarche M, Woodward A, Xiang YS, Pierce DA (1994) Radon and lung cancer risk: A joint analysis of 11 underground miners studies. US National Institutes of Health. NIH publication No 94–3644

Lubin JH, Boice JD Jr, Samet JM (1995) Errors in exposure assessment, statistical power and the interpretation of residential radon studies. Radiation Research 44:329–341

Mallick B, Hoffmann FO, Carroll RJ (2002) Semiparametric regression modeling with mixtures of Berkson and classical error, with application to fallout from the Nevada test site. Biometrics 58:13–20

Michels KB (2001) A renaissance for measurement error. Int J Epi 30:421–422

Miles JCH (1994) Mapping the proportion of the housing stock exceeding a radon reference level. Radiation Protection Dosimetry 56:207–210

NRC, National Research Council (1991) Environmental epidemiology: Public health and hazardous wastes. National Academy Press, Washington D.C.

NRC, National Research Council (1997) Environmental epidemiology, vol 2: Use of the gray literature and other data in environmental epidemiology. National Academy Press, Washington D.C.

NRC, National Research Council (1999) Health effects of exposure to radon, BEIR VI. Committee on health risks of exposure to radon. Board on Radiation Effects Research, Commission on Life Science. National Academy Press, Washington D.C.

Oberaigner W, Kreienbrock L, Schaffrath Rosario A, Kreuzer M, Wellmann J, Keller G, Gerken M, Langer B, Wichmann HE (2002) Radon und Lungenkrebs im Bezirk Imst/Österreich. Fortschritte in der Umweltmedizin. Ecomed Verlagsgesellschaft, Landsberg am Lech

Park JH, Spiegelman DL, Burge HA, Gold DR, Chew GL, Milton DK (2000) Longitudinal study of dust and airborne endotoxin in the home. Environ Health Perspect 108:1023–1028

Pekkanen J, Pearce N (2001) Environmental epidemiology: Challenges and opportunities. Environ Health Perspect 109:1–5

Pershagen G, Liang ZH, Hrubec Z, Svensson C, Boice JD (1992) Residential radon exposure and lung cancer in women. Health Physics 63:179–186

Pershagen G, Akerblom G, Axelson O, Clavensjö B, Damber L, Desai G, Enflo A, Lagarde F, Mellander H, Svartengren M, Swedjemark GA (1994) Residential radon exposure and lung cancer in Sweden. N Engl J Med 330:159–164

Pinel J, Fearn T, Darby SC, Miles JCH (1994) Seasonal correction factors for indoor radon measurements in the United Kingdom. Radiation Protection Dosimetry 58:127–132

Ponsonby AL, Couper D, Dwyer T, Carmichael A, Kemp A, Cochrane J (2000) The relation between infant indoor environment and subsequent asthma. Epidemiology 11:128–135

Pope CA 3rd, Thun MJ, Namboodiri MM, Dockery DW, Evans JS, Speizer FE, Heath CW Jr (1995) Particulate air pollution as a predictor of mortality in a prospective study of U.S. adults. Am J Respir Crit Care Med 151:669–674

Reeves GK, Cox DR, Darby SC, Whitley E (1998) Some aspects of measurement error in explanatory variables for continuous and binary regression models. Stat Med 17:2157–2177

Rosner B, Willett WC, Spiegelman D (1989) Correction of logistic regression relative risk estimates and confidence intervals for systematic within-person measurement error. Stat Med 8:1051–1069

Ruosteenoja E, Mäkeläinen I, Rytömaa T, Hakulinen T, Hakama M (1996) Radon and lung cancer in Finland. Health Physics 71:185–189

Samet JM, Stolwijk J, Rose S (1991) International workshop on residential radon-epidemiology. Health Physics 60:223–227

Samet JM, Zeger SL, Dominici F, Curriero F, Coursac I, Dockery DW, Schwartz J, Zanobetti A (2000) The national morbidity, mortality, and air pollution study, part II: Morbidity and mortality from air pollution in the United States. Res Rep Health Eff Inst 94:5–70; discussion 71–79

Schoenberg JB, Klotz JB, Wilcox HB, Nicholls GP, Gil-del-Real MT, Stemhagen A, Mason TJ (1990) Case-control study of residential radon and lung cancer among New Jersey women. Cancer Research 50:6250–6254

Schüttmann W (1992) Das Radonproblem im Bergbau und in Wohnungen – Historische Aspekte. In: Reiners C, Streffer C, Messerschmidt O (eds) Strahlenrisiko durch Radon. Gustac Fischer, Stuttgart, Jena, New York, pp 5–24

Schüz, J, Grigat JP, Brinkmann K, Michaelis J (2001) Residential magnetic fields as a risk factor for childhood acute leukemia: results from a German population based case-control study. Int J Cancer 91:728–735

Slimani N, Kaaks R, Ferrari P, Casagrande C, Clavel-Chapelon F, Lotze G, Kroke A, Trichopoulos D, Trichopoulou A, Lauria C, Bellegotti M, Ocke MC, Peeters PH, Engeset D, Lund E, Agudo A, Larranaga N, Mattisson I, Andren C, Johansson I, Davey G, Welch AA, Overvad K, Tjonneland A, Van Staveren WA, Saracci R, Riboli E (2002) European Prospective Investigation into Cancer and Nutrition (EPIC) calibration study: rationale, design and population characteristics. Public Health Nutr 5:1125–1145

Steindorf K, Lubin JH, Wichmann HE, Becher H (1995) Lung cancer deaths attributable to indoor radon exposure in West Germany. Int J Epi 24:485–492

Stidley AC, Samet JM (1993) A review of ecologic studies of lung cancer and indoor radon. Health Physics 65:234–251

Thomas D, Stram D, Dwyer J (1993) Exposure measurement error: Influence on exposure-disease relationships and methods of correction. Annual Review of Public Health 14:69–93

Tomášek L, Müller T, Kunz E, Heribanová A, Matzner J, Plaèek V, Burian I, Holeèek J (2001) Study of lung cancer and residential radon in the Czech Republic. Centr Eur J Publ Health 9:150–153

Tosteson TD, Stefanski LA, Schafer DW (1989) A measurement-error model for binary and ordinal regression. Stat Med 8:1139–1147

UNSCEAR, United Nations Scientific Committee on the Effects of Atomic Radiation (2000) Sources and effects of ionizing radiation. UNSCEAR 2000 Report to the General Assembly, with Scientific Annexes. Vol. I: Sources. United Nations, New York

Vedal S, Brauer M, White R, Petkau J (2003) Air pollution and daily mortality in a city with low levels of pollution. Environ Health Perspect 111:45–51

Wallace LA, Mitchell H, O'Connor GT, Neas L, Lippmann M, Kattan M, Koenig J, Stout JW, Vaughn BJ, Wallace D, Walter M, Adams K, Liu LJS (2003) Particle Concentrations in Inner-City Homes of Children with Asthma: The Effect of Smoking, Cooking, and Outdoor Pollution. Environ Health Perspect 111:1265–1272

Wang Z, Lubin JH, Wang L, Zhang S, Boice JD Jr, Cui H, Zhang S, Conrath S, Xia Y, Shang B, Brenner A, Lei S, Metayer C, Cao J, Chen KW, Lei S, Kleinerman RA (2002) Residential radon and lung cancer risk in a high-exposure area of Gansu Province, China. Am J Epi 155:554–564

Warner KE, Mendez D, Courant PN (1996) Toward a more realistic appraisal of the lung cancer risk from radon: The effects of residential mobility. American Journal of Public Health 86:1222–1227

Webster's Encyclopedic Unabridged Dictionary of the English Language (1989) Portland House, New York

Weiland SK, Mundt KA, Ruckmann A, Keil U (1994) Self-reported wheezing and allergic rhinitis in children and traffic density on street of residence. Ann Epidemiol 4:243–247

Wellmann J, Miles J, Kreienbrock L (2001) Identification of outliers in an international radon intercomparison exercise. In: Kunert J, Trenkler G (eds) Mathematical statistics with applications in biometry. Festschrift in Honour of Prof. Dr. Siegfried Schach. Josel Eul, Lohmar/Köln, pp 253–262

Wertheimer N, Leeper E (1979) Electric wiring configurations and childhood cancer. Am J Epi 109: 273–284

WHO, World Health Organisation (2000) Air quality guidelines for Europe, 2nd edn. WHO Regional Publications, European Series No 91. WHO, Regional Office for Europe, Copenhagen

Wichmann HE, Kreienbrock L, Kreuzer M, Gerken M, Dingerkus G, Wellmann J, Keller G (1998) Lungenkrebsrisiko durch Radon in der Bundesrepublik Deutschland (West). ecomed, Landsberg/Lech

Wolf-Ostermann K, Luttmann H, Treiber-Klötzer C, Kreienbrock L, Wichmann HE (1995) Kohortenstudie zu Atemwegserkrankungen und Lungenfunktion bei Schulkindern in Südwestdeutschland – Teil 3: Einfluß von Rauchen und Passivrauchen. Zentralblatt für Hygiene und Umweltmedizin 197:459–488

Zeger SL, Thomas D, Dominici F, Samet JM, Schwartz J, Dockery D, Cohen A (2000) Exposure measurement error in time-series studies of air pollution: Concepts and consequences. Environ Health Perspect 108:419–426

Nutritional Epidemiology

III.4

Dorothy Mackerras, Barrie M. Margetts

Introduction

> The main objective of nutritional epidemiological research is to provide the best
> possible scientific evidence to support an understanding of the role of nutrition
> in the causes and prevention of ill-health.
>
> Margetts and Nelson (1997)

The tools and methodology of nutritional epidemiology have developed mostly
over the last 20 years. Over that time a number of texts and recent papers have
described the broad area, and it is not necessary to repeat details that can easily
be found elsewhere (Margetts and Nelson 1997; Willett 1998; Margetts et al. 2003;
Nelson and Beresford 2004). Nutritional epidemiological studies follow the general
principles of all epidemiological studies. There are really only two issues that must
be considered in all studies: how to develop a clear and testable research question;
and how to provide an unbiased answer to that question. These general issues are
covered elsewhere in this handbook (cf. Chaps. I.11–I.13 of this handbook). The
concerns with assessing outcomes are not specific to nutritional studies, and will
not be discussed in any detail in this chapter.

Nutritional epidemiology seeks to describe the distribution and variation in the
nutritional behaviour of individuals and groups and, primarily but not exclusively,
to relate that behaviour to some health outcome, to explore the causal relationship
between exposure and outcome. Exposure is a generic term which we use here to
describe different aspects of dietary and nutritional behaviour. In the past, health
outcomes have generally been confined to lack of health, but here we consider
health as a wider concept than the absence of illness.

Nutritional epidemiological studies can also be used for the purposes of identifying groups at risk and for monitoring and surveillance. They can provide
an evidence base for deciding plans of action; what actions (interventions) to
take and in whom, based on a comparison of the target population nutritional
behaviour/measure with some reference measure (amount of fruit and vegetables
consumed in the poorest compared with a dietary guideline, or calcium intake
compared to a reference nutrient intake, or % of children above a weight for height
centile standard).

Our aim in this chapter is to focus on those issues that affect nutritional studies
in particular. The main focus has been on how to assess nutritional exposure in
large groups of people with sufficient accuracy to provide a valid estimate of the
impact of variation in diet on health outcomes. The need to develop methods to
assess diet, and to understand the sources of errors associated with these methods,
has arisen because of the recognised importance of diet in the aetiology of the
major causes of death and morbidity around the world.

Poor nutrition has direct effects on growth and normal development, as well as
on the process of healthy ageing. For cancer, it has been estimated that between
40 and 70% of deaths can be attributed to poor nutrition (Willett 1995). Every

day about 15,000 children die from the effects of malnutrition. In resource poor countries the population is increasingly facing the burden of high rates of infectious diseases, as well as rising rates of chronic diseases. Prevention remains the only strategy for long term improvements. In order to understand the best approach to prevent nutrition related health problems it is necessary to understand the role of nutrition in the causes of these health problems. It is essential to have an evidence-based approach to decision making as to what are the most effective strategies to improving nutrition related health. The role of poor nutrition in many of the major causes of death is obvious, and the solution should be obvious. A lack, or excess, of energy will lead to wasting or obesity; lack of specific micronutrients will lead to specific clinical consequences, from impaired function to death. The effects of poor diet on chronic diseases is more complex, such as, for example, the role of micronutrients in maintaining optimal cell function and reducing the risk of cancer and cardiovascular disease. Foods contain more than nutrients, and the way foods are prepared may enhance or reduce their harmful or beneficial effects on health. While it is possible to establish in animal experiments exactly how much of a nutrient is required to avoid deficiency, it is more complex to assess how much is required to maintain optimal function throughout life, against a background of potentially changing demands. It is possible to define the level of vitamin C required to prevent scurvy, but it is more complex to define the optimal level of vitamin C (and other micronutrients) that may improve health. The optimal supply of the essential elements in foods is not static, but a function of the demands placed on the individual (which may be wider environmental and social and economic factors that affect the basic and underlying causes), to grow, to fight infections (or cope with the wider environmental stresses such as poor sanitation and water quality), to overcome the effects of smoking, and so on. It is because of this complexity that expertise in nutritional epidemiology is required. There is not one measure of nutritional exposure that will give the correct estimate of the relevant exposure in all situations; it is important to establish which approach is optimal to answer the particular research question being posed.

The following section of this chapter describes the measurement and definition of nutritional exposures; the third section covers adjustment for confounding by energy intake; the fourth section discusses the organisation and presentation of data, with consideration of the implications for meta-analyses and reviews; the fifth section discusses the role of nutritional epidemiology in public health, and the final section draws some conclusions from the chapter.

Measurement and Definition of Nutritional Exposures

4.2

It is important to be clear what is meant by the terms used: diet, food, nutrients, nutritional status are often incorrectly used. Food describes the individual items that make up a diet (or dietary pattern), nutrients are derived from an analysis of diet (occasionally nutrients are measured directly in foods, but most often are estimated through the use of the composition of food tables). Anthropometric measures are often incorrectly described as measures of nutritional status. Ideally a measure of nutritional status reflects the dynamic balance between dietary supply, body pools, and the metabolic demands. Simply measuring food intake does not represent status; at the same level of dietary intake a subject may be able to function well or poorly, depending on the demands being placed upon him/her. If an individual is growing or fighting an infection (and has diarrhoea for example or a fever) the dietary supply of a nutrient may or may not be adequate to enable and maintain optimal function. From a biological perspective the available substrates for function come from that which is eaten, plus body pools. Where there is competition for these metabolic substrates, one function may be compromised over another. In an epidemiological study, which can rarely measure true nutritional status, it is often assumed that a reported measure of intake reflects the true functional availability. Dietary intakes are used because they reflect what is eaten, and it is the impact that food supply has on the overall dynamic that needs to be understood if causal mechanisms, and preventive strategies can be understood.

Increasingly, epidemiological studies are exploring food intake to assess dietary/ food patterns, as well as the nutrient intakes derived from these dietary patterns. There has been a growing interest in approaches to summarise dietary patterns, either by using some sort of 'healthy eating' index, or to use a measure derived from a mathematical summary of the variation in the data such as by using principal components analysis. These food patterns, either derived from some a priori understanding of the way in which people eat foods, or based on a mathematical summary, should reflect the way foods are consumed and may provide a more useful insight than studying individual foods or nutrients. The assumption is that, for example, people who eat more of some foods will eat less of others, or if people eat wholegrain cereals, they may also be more likely to eat more fruits and vegetables, or grilled rather than fried meats etc. In terms of explaining health outcomes these patterns may be more informative because they describe the overall exposure and potential interaction between exposure that may enhance or reduce risk. In deriving nutrients from food intake data, although it is possible directly to analyse the nutrient content of foods, most often food composition tables are used. These tables are usually developed from the analysis of a relatively limited number of foods, either in their raw or cooked state. There is a great deal of potential for error in deriving nutrient intakes using these food tables. However, the most important source of error in assessing nutrient intakes comes from the incorrect assessment of food intake; if a subject does not accurately report what he/she eats or ate, it does not matter how accurate the food tables may be. A great deal of effort has gone into improving the food tables, but surprisingly less in to improving and understanding the errors associated with obtaining the original intake data.

A benefit of using food patterns, rather than nutrients, is that the patterns are not dependent on the accuracy of the food tables. Another benefit, of using food patterns is that people eat foods and foods contain a mix of nutrients (and other substances, such as phytochemicals, additives, etc), and by describing the patterns it may give a clearer insight into how these nutrients (or other substances) may interact to enhance or adversely affect function.

Irrespective of what measure is used (diet, food, nutrients), there are a number of considerations to deriving the relevant exposure in any study:

1. *Study type.* Ecological, cross-sectional, analytical and experimental studies require measurements made at different levels: national, community, household or individual (see Table 4.1).
2. *Time period.* Nutritional exposures can be chronic or acute in their effects. Deciding on the time at which to assess an exposure is critical to the purpose of the study. A cohort study that characterises nutritional status in terms of both dietary intakes and blood biochemistry may provide information relevant to the initiation of cancer but not necessarily to its progression.
3. *Point of measurement.* Relevant exposures can be measured in terms of food consumption, nutrient intake, blood and tissue levels of nutrient, functional consequences of nutrient action (including genetic interaction) and excretion.
4. *Type of measurement.* Examples of exposure measures that are direct (foods, nutrients), functional or metabolic (physiology, biochemistry), cumulative (anthropometry) or indirect (socio-demographic and cultural).

For nutritional studies the most complex issue is to be clear as to how to measure the relevant exposure, based on a consideration of the above four aspects, with the required level of accuracy. The study question and study design suitable to address that question will have an effect on the choice of approach to the best way to measure the relevant exposure. The skill is in balancing the theoretically optimal approach with that which is practical, while maintaining validity and avoiding bias.

Most, but not all, epidemiological studies are interested in exploring the causal relationship between usual long term diet and risk of some health outcome in individuals. In these studies, mostly cohort or case-control studies, the method of choice for measuring exposure will depend on what is the relevant exposure. Ideally exposure should be measured at the moment the exposure is believed to cause the outcome; this may rarely be possible to identify. For case-control studies the relevant exposure is recalled some time in the past, and it then must be assumed that that recalled exposure reflects the relevant exposure. For cohort studies, even though the exposure is measured before the outcome, it still may be measured some time after the relevant time period where the exposure initiated the disease process. In some case-control studies a measure of current diet is used as a proxy for past diet, assuming that current and past diet are similar. Cohort studies can measure diet in the present; the choices are most commonly either a food frequency questionnaire or a food record or recall. There are pros and cons for each method. The vast majority of cohort studies use a food frequency questionnaire, and ideally after that method has been validated by comparison with a more accurate measure of exposure.

Table 4.1. Methods of dietary assessment by type of epidemiological study (modified from Margetts et al. 2003)

Epidemiological study	Level of aggregation required; expression of information (comment)	Method (comment)
Population or household level		
Aggregate population/ecological	• Average per capita intake compared across countries or regions or households • Trends over time within a country or region or household	Food disappearance Food balance sheets Household budget surveys
Community experiment or intervention	Group level of analysis: Compare outcomes for different exposures	As above or Sentinel assessment of representative individuals
Individual level		
Cross-sectional (Prevalence survey)	Absolute level	Food records or recalls (multiple days to describe within-person variation; number depends on measure required) Biochemical (check dose response relationship with diet)
	Ranking	Food records (usually single days) 24 hour recall (single or multiple days) FFQ Biochemical markers
Case-control	Past exposure at time of initiation or as proxy for past; usually categorised, but may use continuous measure. (Absolute accuracy not required; assess misclassification and take into account)	FFQ of present or past diet Diet history
Cohort	Subjects intake at start of study ranked and categorised (expressed as exposed, not exposed), but may use continuous measure. (Absolute accuracy not required; assess misclassification and take into account, unless absolute risk to be described)	Food records 24 hour recall FFQ Biochemical markers (does it relate to diet in sensitive manner?)
Experimental study	Individual level (usually needs to be accurate at absolute level)	Food records (multiple days to assess within person variation) 24 hour recalls FFQ (for patterns or group level comparison) Diet quality indices Biochemical markers

FFQ = Food frequency questionnaire

When deriving a measure of exposure, the exposure will vary from the truth for a number of reasons: all methods of measuring diet are associated with both random and systematic errors, that operate both within, and between, subjects. Errors arise because of the methods, but also because of the difficulty of capturing true within subject variation in intake. Any measure of variance in a population will be a mix of these errors, which are theoretically identifiable, but in practice difficult to separate out. Random errors weaken our ability to identify the true causal relationship between exposure and outcome, whereas systematic errors may either exaggerate or diminish the apparent causal relationship. While we should try to minimise random errors, we should avoid systematic errors where known.

Here we will briefly summarise the key issues in assessing diet using a method that assesses current intake (such as a diet record) and in one that assesses usual intake (food frequency questionnaire). For any method it must be piloted before being used to check that it gives the required information in the study population; this should include assessing the validity of the measure in the population.

Food Frequency Questionnaire (FFQ)

The detail of the development of an FFQ can be found in Margetts and Nelson (1997) and Willet (1998). In developing an FFQ a number of decisions need to be made:

— which foods to include in the list that are relevant for the study aims and population (commonly now many studies assess all aspects of diet, even when there is a specific hypothesis, to enable the researcher to explore the effects of other aspects of diet).

— whether to take account of food preparation techniques: for example, do you need to differentiate between raw and cooked foods, or between different cooking and processing methods; does it matter if the foods are cooked from fresh or frozen? If you group similar foods (such as fruits, will you lose important information about differences in levels of nutrients in different fruits?). If you have a very long questionnaire, respondents may not complete it, but if you miss or compress foods into too few groups you may lose important information.

— over what period of time the 'usual' diet covers; this is often a month, but sometimes a whole year.

— whether to use usual portions of each food, or to give options as to number and size of each portion used.

— how to organise categories of consumption, ensuring that there are no gaps (ranging from never consume to once or more a day).

— whether the FFQ can be self-administered or whether it needs to be conducted by interview (if the population is illiterate there may be no option); consider the impact of the approach on response rate.

Once the data are collected what will be done with it? Is the aim to: describe the frequency of consumption, or assess amount of food eaten, or to derive nutrient intakes? If the aim is to derive nutrient intakes, how will the foods be converted to nutrients? Will food composition tables be used? If so, are these accurate and appropriate for the foods and nutrients of interest?

Food Record

One important advantage of an open ended method such as a record, is that the researcher does not have to make assumptions as to which foods to include. A potential disadvantage is that if the day of recording diet is unusual, or affected by the process of recording diet, what appears to be a more technically accurate measure, may actually be less accurate in terms of reflecting what people would eat if you could observe their behaviour unobtrusively. Another disadvantage of records/recalls is that they take a lot of time to process by the researcher once they have been collected. Most FFQs are self coded, some are even optically readable, and thus have minimal burden on researcher time (although it is always important to assess each questionnaire before coding to ensure that answers are clear and consistent).

Depending on how the data are to be analysed, single or multiple days of recording will be required. If the study aims to record group mean intake, and assuming the errors in the study sample are randomly distributed, a one day record will provide a reasonable estimate. Where the requirement is to measure an individual's dietary intake, then more days of recording will be required, depending on the extent of the within person variability of the nutrient of interest. Micro-nutrients that are found in large amounts in foods rarely eaten (vitamin A in organ meats) will require more days (perhaps up to 30 days) of recording to capture those days when the nutrient rich foods are eaten. Macro-nutrients are generally supplied from a wide range of foods, and an individual's usual intake can probably be derived from 3–4 days of recording. Nelson and Bingham (1997) have discussed these issues in more detail.

4.2.1 Validation of the Measure of Exposure

A measure is valid if it measures the truth (Fig. 4.1). Absolute validity of a dietary measure would imply that for every gram, for example, increase in true intake, the measured intake would increase by one gram. The biggest problem is how to define the truth as this cannot be known. The truth is usually estimated by reference to another method, and many researchers prefer to describe this as relative validity. Relative validity describes the agreement between a test measure (that being used in the study) and some other measure thought to be more accurate (reference measure). The assessment of validity should be under the same circumstances in which the test method will be used in the main study. The studies undertaken to assess this are often called comparison or calibration studies, in recognition of the difficulty of establishing the truth. Ideally every method used for gathering data should be validated before the main study begins. A great deal of research and effort has gone into trying to establish the validity of the methods used in nutritional epidemiological studies (Table 4.1). Different study designs use different methods to assess diet, often for reasons of cost, time and effort. Ideally, however, the best method should be used to answer the question. As each compromise that is taken moves the method away from the ideal, the researcher must be sure that this does not undermine the validity (fit for purpose) of the measure derived from the method. If a method has been validated for another purpose in a different population, it can not be assumed that the method will give the same degree of relative validity in the new study population.

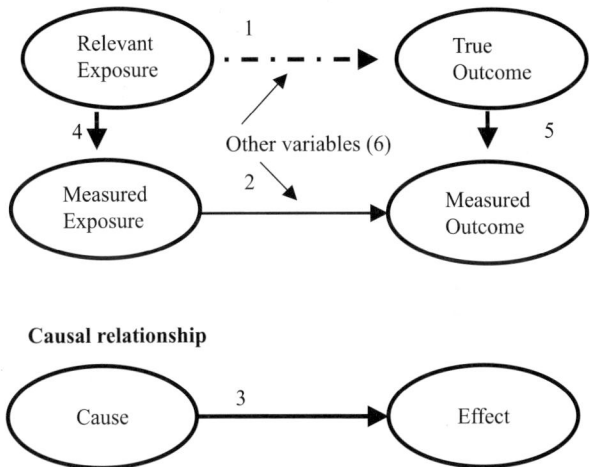

Causal relationship

Figure 4.1. Relationship between exposure and outcome, cause and effect. 1: This represents the true relationship between relevant exposure and outcome. 2: This represents the observed relationship between measured exposure and outcome. 3: This represents the true causal pathway. The cause must precede the effect. 1 and 3 are the same if other variables[6] (confounders) are either absent (no residual confounding) or taken account of (by stratification or mathematical adjustment). 4: This represents the relationship between relevant exposure and measured exposure. 5: This represents the relationship between true outcome and measured outcome. 6: Variables that should be measured and reported that may influence the relationship between exposure and outcome. The extent to which the measured exposure and outcome vary from the true and relevant measures should be described in a validation study that presents the measurement errors

It is important to establish a priori how the results of the validation study will be interpreted and used in the main study. The main issue is to establish what level of agreement is considered good enough to reduce measurement error to an acceptable level (that is, so that in the way the measure is to be used in the analysis of the main study data, the true underlying relationship between exposure and outcome can be seen, or, if the measure is used for assessing compliance with a quantitative target, how well the test method can identify whether people truly are above or below the target). It is important to establish the sample size required for a validation study; this will be a function of the level of agreement required and the variability of the exposure in the population. If a sample is too small this will inevitably lead to wider confidence intervals around the measures of association. As a result, differences between the reference and test measures which are large enough to be important may not be statistically significant. Perhaps paradoxically, a small validation study may lead to a falsely optimistic measure of the validity of the measure, if, for example, the comparison between test and reference measure is by comparing mean intakes and 95% confidence intervals. This can lead to the erroneous conclusion that the test measure is valid, because the confidence intervals overlap.

The purpose of the main study will determine the correct way to assess and express the measure of validity. If the main study uses a continuous measure of exposure then a continuous measure of exposure should be assessed in the validation study. If the exposure measure is categorical in the main study, then the validation study should assess how well the test measure can categorise the exposure compared with the reference measure. If the study aim is to assess the relative risk of one level of exposure with another, then the validation study should assess how well the test measure can do this compared with the reference measure. A particular concern is whether those who misreport their intake are different in other important characteristics from those that do not. Most work has been done on misreporting energy intake by level of body mass index and suggests that overweight people tend to under-report their fat intake. Recent work also suggests that fruit intake is over-reported by low consumers because they know they should eat more fruit but do not, particularly amongst more educated subjects (Amanatidis et al. 2001). If this tendency to differential over- or under-reporting is known before the study begins then it may be possible to take this into account in the design of the study; for example by excluding overweight people. This then, of course means, that the study results can not be generalised to the whole population, but if a study is not internally valid, it can never be externally valid. It is better to be aware of the factors affecting internal validity and to design and interpret the study accordingly.

Debate has centred on the best way to assess diet in large cohort studies. In summary, most large cohort studies use food frequency questionnaires (FFQ) where subjects describe their usual behaviour over a defined period of time (often a year, sometimes a month). Most validation studies compare the intake of nutrients (and, more recently, individual foods) derived from the FFQ (the test measure) with a reference measure derived from multiple days of recording of dietary intake. More recently biomarkers, or measures of energy expenditure (or proxies such as estimated basal metabolic rate) have been used as a second reference measure (Margetts and Nelson 1997), and described in more detail as the method of triads by Kaaks (1995). The thinking behind using a second reference method is that this gives a sense of how well the first reference measure may be measuring the underlying truth, if the reference measure is wrong, the comparison between the test and reference measure will be wrong. The problem, at present, is that there are few relevant and accurate potential second reference measures.

The term gold standard is not used anymore, to describe any reference measure as it gives false sense of accuracy. The nearest to a true gold standard is for the measurement of energy expenditure as a proxy for energy intake using doubly labelled water (DLW). DLW provides an integrated measure of components of energy expenditure, usually over 7–14 days. The technique involves ingestion of a small amount of water with hydrogen replaced by deuterium, and the both, the deuterium and the oxygen isotopically labelled. It is then possible to track these labelled tags through the body. The rate of loss of these labelled elements can then be used to provide an estimate of energy expenditure (Goran and Astrup 2002). Apart from DLW and urinary nitrogen there are few other robust independent measures that are relevant. If the aim is to validate a measure such as vitamin A intake, it might be tempting to assume that a blood measure of vitamin A would be the ideal reference measure. The assumption is that there is a clear linear dose response relationship between level of dietary intake (which is the relevant exposure) and blood level. Bates et al. (1997) have shown that this is rarely the case. It may be particularly important when there is a curvilinear relationship and where the study population distribution of intake is either at the lower or higher end of the distribution. If this is the case, the comparison of the dietary measure and the blood measure will show a poor agreement between the measures, and the incorrect decision may be made that the dietary assessment is poor. Ideally therefore before using any reference measure it is important to establish that it is an appropriate measure of true relevant exposure, and that variation in the level of the reference measure relates to true variation in the target population.

Evidence for the debate as to which is the best method to assess diet in cohort studies comes from validation studies using DLW as the reference measure for energy intake. These studies seem to suggest that there is no or little association between energy intake derived from the FFQ and energy expenditure derived from DLW, particularly in overweight or obese subjects. It seems that, based on DLW, many people under-report their intake (Subar et al. 2003). A further refinement is to express the energy intake as a function of the resting or basal metabolic rate (BMR); if energy intake is less than the BMR it would seem reasonable that subjects who are not losing weight are under-reporting as it would not be possible to survive on less energy than the body needs simply to maintain organ function. Usually a factor is added to the equation to allow for some level of physical activity (PAL), where PAL multiples of BMR of 1.2 to 1.5 are often used. In the national diet and nutrition surveys of British adults, using a seven day weighed record, about 40% of subjects under-report their intake, allowing for some degree of moderate activity (Black et al. 1991). However, under-reporting has been found across all levels of PAL, and it is thus not safe simply to exclude people with an energy intake below a certain BMR $*$ PAL level. Also, excluding 40% of subjects reduces the power of the study and may cause selection bias, but may be essential to avoid information bias.

It is more statistically powerful to maintain the exposure as a continuous measure and assess risk of outcome per unit change of exposure. However, most cohort studies convert continuous measures of exposure into categorical data, and express risk of the outcome in say the upper fifth of intake compared with the lowest fifth. Given that the point of assessing risk is so that the risk can be altered (to improve health), it is important that the correct measure of risk is obtained. Table 4.2 shows the proportion of people who are classified into the correct fifth by reference (or alternative) measures that have decreasing correlations with the reference (Walker and Blettner 1985). For a measure with a correlation of 0.5, only 32.1% of subjects are placed into the correct fifth, another 37.9% are only one fifth too high or low, but the remainder are two to four fifths wrong. The impact of this on the study is profound. Assuming a cohort study with a 'true' incidence of 2% in the lowest fifth and 6% in the highest (i.e. a relative risk of 3.0), using an alternative measure with a correlation of 0.5 with the reference exposure measure would lead to incidences of 3.1% and 4.9% in the lowest and highest fifths, a relative risk of 1.58. For these relative risks to be statistically significant, the cohort using the reference measure requires a sample of 2496 individuals whereas the cohort using the imperfect alternative requires a sample size of 12,192 individuals. Similar calculations for the equivalent case-control studies required sample sizes of 430 or 2046 respectively (Walker and Blettner 1985). Even if a validity study has not been done, the test-retest correlation (reliability) (Armstrong et al. 1994; cf. Chap. I.10 of this handbook) can provide a guide as to the minimum level for inflating the sample size to allow for imperfect validity, because a measure cannot be more highly associated with another measure than it is with itself. In other words, the correlation between the test and reference measures can not be greater than the correlation of repeat measures of the test measure (Walker and Blettner 1985).

Table 4.2. Probabilities of misclassification of a reference ranking in fifths using an imperfect alternative that has various correlations with the reference (from Walker and Blettner (1985))

Absolute difference in quintile ranks	correlation coefficient between the reference and alternative			
	0.9	0.7	0.5	0.3
0	0.573	0.403	0.321	0.263
1	0.378	0.400	0.379	0.355
2	0.047	0.156	0.203	0.225
3	0.002	0.037	0.081	0.118
4	0.000	0.003	0.017	0.038

4.2.2   Measuring Nutritional Exposures in Different Groups

The characteristics of the target population and the circumstances in which they live influence the approach that has to be taken in gathering information about nutritional exposures. It can not be assumed that an approach that works in one community, or sector of society, will work in another sector of society. It is more complex than whether the population is literate or not. We have found that people from different cultures have different ways of conceptualising and expressing what is important for themselves. For example, people who gather their food from the wild will often have very detailed names for all the edible foods, but often have only one name that describes all the other foods that they do not eat.

Concepts of time and distance may be quite different between urban and rural Indian women, who are illiterate. In a study assessing physical activity in rural women we could not ask how long women spent doing tasks, and how far in miles they walked; we had to develop an approach that used concepts that the women understood (Rao et al. 2003). It is therefore very important to test the approach that is believed to work in the target group before the study proper starts. Focus group discussions and qualitative research methods are very valuable tools and approaches that complement quantitative methods.

Defining Reference Categories and Cut-Points

4.2.3

In aetiological research into chronic diseases, nutrient or food intake data are commonly used in a categorical form rather than a continuous form in models. These are created by dividing the continuous data into thirds, fourths or fifths based on the tertiles, quartiles or quintiles, respectively, of the study population distribution. The categorical approach makes no assumptions about the underlying shape of the association between the nutrient and the outcome. Even if intakes are used in a continuous form, analyses based on categories should be done to check whether the assumptions assumed in the continuous approach is justified. For example, in logistic regression the assumption of linearity in the logit can be assessed by also examining the variable when entered in quantiles (Hosmer and Lemeshow 1989; cf. Chaps. II.2 and II.3 of this handbook). The reason why dietary data is more commonly entered in a categorical than a continuous form in studies of diet-disease relationships is not clear. Authors usually do not report whether they examined the association using both methods. One reason in favour of the categorical approach is that it allows results for dietary factors to be expressed in the same way. For example, population average intake by adults of thiamin is usually about 1.5–2 mg/day whereas the average calcium intake may be 600–1200 mg/day. If both were entered as continuous variables, then the resulting odds ratio, for example, would be the odds per mg increment. A 1 mg increment relates to quite a different change at the population level for these two nutrients. However, the odds ratio for the highest vs. lowest fifth can be directly compared to assess the relative impact in the population.

For categorised data, one group is selected to be the referent category for calculating odds ratios or relative risks for the other groups. If the study factor is cigarette smoking or an industrial exposure, then it is clear that the referent is the group with no exposure to the substance. However, in the area of nutrition, many variables of interest have no group with a zero level (for example, no one has a body weight of zero grams or could survive with a zero intake of any essential nutrient) or there may be reason to think that those with a zero level differ from the general population in too many respects to constitute the most appropriate referent group (e.g. teetotallers, vegans). There are some exceptions when a true zero group does exist, for example, when investigating food additives or accidental contaminants. There is no clear cut way to choose the referent group in the nutritional area and different authors make different decisions. Some choose the highest group, some the lowest group and some the intermediate group. If studies investigating the same topic have used different referents, then the results might look contradictory when in reality they are not.

Table 4.3 shows that the same data can be used to yield three different sets of odds ratios, depending on which group is chosen as the referent. Although the odds ratios are numerically different, the message given by the three sets is the same. There is a 3-fold difference in risk between the high and low intake groups. These results could be described in ways that would imply different findings. The results when the referent is the high intake group could be described as 'low intakes increased the risk' whereas when the referent is the low group the results could be described as 'high intakes reduce risk'. These two descriptions could be interpreted differently by the public. In the second case, it may be interpreted as suggesting that taking supplements would be beneficial. The general tendency in the literature is to set lowest diet intake group as the referent, possibly due to some sense that low is closest to unexposed. However in the case of diet, it could often be argued that the low intake group are 'exposed' to a risk and that the higher intake group is not exposed to risk. This thought leads some to set the referent at the end of the distribution that ensures that most odds ratios or relative risks for the other categories are above 1.0. This approach could lead to confusion if two nutrients with opposing effects were studied in the same report, for example fat and fibre intakes. Using the middle group as the referent category is not frequently done for dietary data. However, it makes sense for a characteristic such as body mass index or birthweight where both ends of the distributions have less favourable outcomes than a middle group and emphasising this fact is desired.

Table 4.3. Comparison of the odds ratio when different groups are chosen as the referent

| Intake category | cases | controls | Odds ratio when the referent group is the | | |
			high	medium	low
High	100	200	1.0	0.5	0.33
Medium	200	200	2.0	1.0	0.67
Low	300	200	3.0	1.5	1.0

The most important thing is for the reader to be aware that different referents can be chosen and to check approach each author has used. If a review is being conducted, it may be useful to recalculate some results so that they can be interpreted more easily.

Where data are collected and reported as continuous measures the risk is expressed in terms of per unit of exposure; if fruit intake is expressed in grams the reduction in risk associated with increased consumption will be per gram. At one level this is ideal, provided the reader knows what level of consumption is inferred. The study should always indicate what the average level of consumption is in the study population to give the reader a sense of whether the change in risk is relating to changes in intake from 200 to 300 grams, or 120 to 130 grams. In most studies data are categorised and risk is assessed in relation to a referent group, as described above. In interpreting and comparing results it is important to describe the range of exposure covered by the referent group (and in the whole population), as well as describing how the referent group was defined. The category boundaries tend to be based on a within-study distribution. As the goal is to compare the cases of disease with the underlying population, categorisation is generally, but not always, based on the entire population at baseline in a cohort study and the control distribution in a case-control study. However, this makes the comparison of results between studies somewhat problematical because the quantile cutpoints are different and the range of intake within each quantile and overall will generally vary between studies. For example, data from various different cohort studies was used to examine the effects of various foods on breast cancer (Missmer et al. 2002). The authors chose to divide each study into fifths using the distribution from that study. This meant that the relative risk for the top and bottom fifths for one study related to a difference of 35 grams red meat and, in another study, to a difference of 128 grams red meat. Clearly, if there were a continuous association between red meat intake and risk, the relative risk for the second study should be nearly four times as large as the relative risk in the first study. Despite this, the relative risks were combined to derive an overall figure which does not relate to any particular range of dietary intake and misses the opportunity of examining a much wider range of intakes than in usually available (Friedenreich 2002).

Using an external cutpoint might be an alternative to basing categories on the within-study distribution. For example, one might choose the level being recommended to the public such as 30% of energy from fat or 30 grams fibre. Even in this approach, one could define either the high or the low group as the referent. The drawback is that using these levels may obscure important new findings that should lead to changing the advice being given. In addition, this approach would generally allow only two categories to be defined and so dose-response relationships could not be defined unless each group was further divided and this leads back to the problem of comparing across studies. By contrast, dividing the study population evenly makes no assumptions about the 'best' intake and avoids the potential problem of results in a group with small numbers being overly influential. Ideally a number of different approaches should be explored before deciding on any one approach, although when there is no clear guidance about a critical level around which risk changes, it will be most efficient to divide the population evenly into thirds or fourths.

Methods for Analysis: Adjustment for Confounding by Energy Intake

4.3

People who eat a lot of food tend to have higher intakes of many or all nutrients. Hence, the question arises as to whether risks associated with high or low intakes of a single nutrient are actually due to confounding by total energy intake (or the intake of other nutrients). Persons may also have high energy intakes because they are very active, or because they are overweight.

The term 'energy adjustment' is used to describe both adjustment to remove the effects of confounding and also correction to remove the effects of under- or over-reporting of total food intake. In this section, energy adjustment only refers to control for confounding by energy intake. Some of these procedures have also been proposed as methods to deal with reporting bias but this is not necessarily successful in all circumstances, especially if there is differential reporting of food groups between subgroups of the population (Bellach and Kohlmeier 1998).

One of the problems with controlling for confounding in nutritional epidemiology studies arises because many nutrients travel together in foods resulting in high correlations between their intakes. High correlations make models unstable. For example, Slattery et al. (1988) noted that "because of the high correlation between calories, fat, and protein (r = approximately 0.9), we were unable to simultaneously adjust for calories, fat, and protein in the logistic regression models". The size of the correlations is determined by the proportion that each macronutrient contributes to energy and also the intercorrelations among the macronutrients (Gordon et al. 1984). High correlations between variables inflate their variance. This is quantified by $1/(1 - r^2)$. For a correlation of 0.9 between two variables, the variance inflation factor is 5.3 and the standard deviation of the coefficient for both variables is increased by the square-root, 2.3-fold. Until about 20 years ago, the problem of high correlations was managed by entering nutrients into the model as nutrient density (for macronutrients, density is the energy from the macronutrient expressed at the % of the total energy intake, for micronutrients, mg/1000 kJ or other multiple) rather than as absolute intakes. For many years, it was thought that calculating energy density would adjust for energy intake and so the term for energy itself was usually left out of the model. However, nutrient density has a low, but non-zero, correlation with energy and so residual confounding by energy intake remains if the energy term is not included. The nutrient density often has a correlation in the opposite direction from the parent nutrient. For example, Holbrook et al. (1988) reported that the correlation between calcium and energy was +0.6 but that the correlation between calcium density and energy was −0.3. This seems to be a general pattern for the vitamins and minerals but not necessarily for fat (Gordon et al. 1984). Thus if calcium density is used, it does not completely adjust for energy and reverses the direction of the confounding by energy, which is not always obvious, and makes it difficult to interpret the results.

4.3.1   How Many Independent Variables?

Datasets for investigating the relationship between macronutrients and chronic disease would generally have five columns of data – protein, fat, carbohydrate, alcohol and energy. Therefore it is tempting to think that there are five independent variables that can be used in analysis but this is not correct. Energy is derived from the macronutrients. There are only four independent variables because the fifth can be determined once any four are known. As a result, it is not possible to find five independent parameters (cf. Dorfman et al. 1985).

Macronutrients and Four Methods for Adjusting for Energy Intake 4.3.2

Many of the concepts in this section will be illustrated using data from a study in which one twin from each of 196 pairs kept a 4-day food record (Mackerras 1996).

In 1986, Willett and Stampfer (1986) proposed that the technique of residualising a variable should be applied to the nutrition area and this led to an extensive discussion about the relative merits and interpretation of the four different methods – the standard multiple, the residual, the partition and the density models – that could be used to adjust for total energy intake. It should be noted that some of this discussion comparing the methods was not actually related to control of confounding per se, but to the range of intake over which relative risks or odds ratios were calculated as a result of applying various methods.

The following discussion will be simplified by grouping the macronutrients as fat and non-fat (i.e. protein, carbohydrate and alcohol) and they will be expressed as kJ energy such that total kJ = fat kJ + non-fat kJ. The same models can be run entering fat and other macronutrients as grams but the different energy content of the various macronutrients needs to be remembered if trying to equate the effects. Dietary data collected using 4-day weighed food records from a study of adult twins (Tables 4.4 and 4.5) described elsewhere (Mackerras 1996) will be used to illustrate certain points. The general dietary patterns in this group are similar to those reported in other studies.

Table 4.4. Characteristics of the twin selected from each of 196 pairs (from Mackerras (1996))

Variable	Mean	Standard Deviation	Centile 12.5th	Centile 87.5th
Quetelet Index [BMI] (kg/m^2)	24.2	3.8	20.3	28.5
Energy (MJ)	8.7	2.8	5.7	11.9
EI/BMR[a]	1.4	0.5	0.9	2.0
Fat (g)	89.1	34.1	55.6	127.3
Fat residual[b] (g)	0.0	14.7	−13.9	13.6
Fat (% energy)	37.6	5.9	30.7	44.3
Vitamin C (mg)	86.8	56.4	30.8	141.2
Vitamin C residual[b] (mg)	0.0	54.7	−51.3	45.3
Vitamin C (mg/MJ)	10.8	8.0	4.0	18.0

[a] Ratio of the energy intake to the basal metabolic rate estimated using the age- and sex-specific Schofield equations for weight and height (Schofield et al. 1985)

[b] Residuals from regression equations containing the nutrient as the outcome variable and total energy intake as the predictor variable. For simplicity, logarithmic transformation was not used. The population mean has not been added to the residuals, although this is often done

Table 4.5. Correlations between nutrients and different modes of expressing nutrient, 196 twins (Mackerras (1996))

Energy or nutrient (units)	Nutrient (units)	Pearson's correlation coefficient
Energy (kJ)	fat (kJ or g)	0.90
	fat (% energy)	0.14
	fat (residual, kJ or g)	0.00
Non-fat (kJ)	energy (kJ)	0.95
	fat (kJ or g)	0.72
	fat (% energy)	−0.14
	fat (residual, kJ)	−0.31
Fat (% energy)	fat (kJ or g)	0.52
	fat (residual, kJ or g)	0.91
Fat (residual, kJ or g)	fat (kJ or g)	0.43
	non-fat (kJ)	1.00
Energy (kJ)	vitamin C (mg)	0.25
	vitamin C (mg/MJ)	−0.32
	vitamin C (residual, mg)	0.00
Vitamin C (mg/MJ)	vitamin C (mg)	0.72
	vitamin C (residual, mg)	0.82
Vitamin C (residual, mg)	vitamin C (mg)	0.97
Fat (kJ or g)	vitamin C (mg)	0.18
Fat (% energy)	vitamin C (mg/MJ)	−0.18
Fat (residual, kJ or g)	vitamin C (residual, mg)	−0.10

As found in most datasets, there is a strong correlation between fat and energy intake in the twins (Fig. 4.2, Table 4.5). Although there is a range of fat intakes at any energy intake, and vice versa, the strong correlation means that those with low energy intakes are unlikely to have very high fat intakes. Assuming that energy intake fulfils the other criteria for confounding, the usual way to deal with this would be to enter both fat and energy into a model:

$$\text{logit risk} = \alpha + \beta_1(\text{fat kJ}) + \gamma_1(\text{total kJ}) . \qquad (4.1)$$

Model (4.1) has become known as the standard multiple model and β_1 is the amount of risk associated with a 1 kJ increase in fat intake *given that total energy is held constant*. This can only occur if there is a simultaneous decrease of 1 kJ in non-fat energy sources. Therefore β_1 is not the risk for changing fat intake alone, it is the risk for the net effect of increasing fat intake and decreasing non-fat intake. The size of this relative risk will depend on both whether fat is associated with risk and whether any of the non-fat components are associated with risk (Brown et al. 1994).

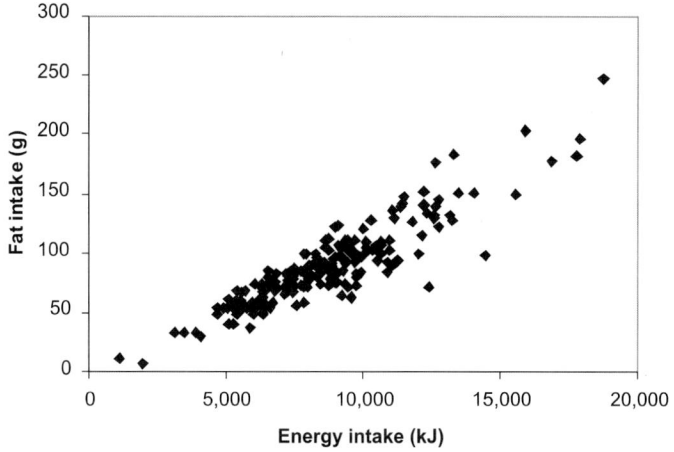

Figure 4.2. Scatterplot of average daily energy and fat intake; Twin study (Mackerras 1996)

By contrast, γ_1 is the risk associated with a 1 kJ increase in total energy *given that fat is held constant.* Thus γ_1 is not the risk for increasing total energy from any source; it is the risk for increasing non-fat kJ. Although total energy was entered into this model, the regression coefficient associated with it is for non-fat energy, not total energy. As described above, the variance of both these coefficients will be inflated owing to their high correlation.

An alternative model, to enter non-fat energy rather than total energy, has become known as the partition model:

$$\text{logit risk} = \alpha + \beta_2(\text{fat kJ}) + \gamma_2(\text{non-fat kJ}) . \tag{4.2}$$

It gives the relative risk for a change of 1 kJ in fat intake *given that intake of the other macronutrients is held constant* and the relative risk for a change of 1 kJ in non fat kJ *given that fat intake is held constant.* This model has some surprising results at first glance. Although different variables were entered into the models, γ_1 from Model (4.1) and γ_2 from Model (4.2) have the same value (Pike et al. 1992) because they represent the same thing – increasing energy from non-fat while holding fat intake constant. However β_1 from Model (4.1) and β_2 from Model (4.2) are not the same because in Model (4.2), fat kJ are added rather used to replace some of the non-fat kJ. The effect associated with holding total energy constant can be calculated from Model (4.2), but its standard error is less easy to calculate (Kipnis et al. 1993).

The previous models have adjusted for energy in the risk model. An alternative approach is to restructure the definition of fat intake to be energy-intake-specific before it is used in the risk model. For example, in the twin group, the average fat intake for those consuming 5 MJ and 8 MJ is 48.5 g and 81.5 g respectively. These values can also be expressed as the residuals from a model with fat kJ as the outcome variable and total energy the predictor variable. Thus individuals consuming 70 g fat and 5 MJ or 8 MJ would have new values of +21.5 g and −11.5 g respectively

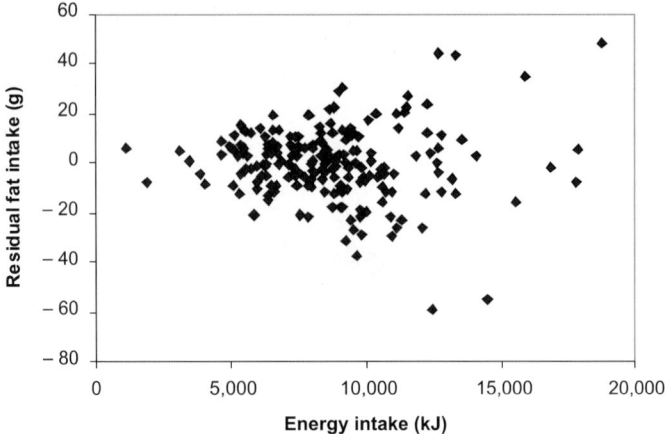

Figure 4.3. Scatterplot of average daily energy intake and energy-adjusted (residual) fat intake, twin study

(Table 4.4). By definition, this procedure removes the association between fat intake and energy intake (Fig. 4.3). The units are kJ of fat if fat was entered into the model as kJ. Next, each person's residual is used in the logistic model instead of the original measure of total fat intake:

$$\text{logit risk} = \alpha + \beta_3(\text{fat}_{\text{res}} \text{ kJ}) \qquad (4.3)$$

and β_3 will have the same value as β_1 from Model (4.1) providing that there is no threshold in the effect of fat on disease. Even though the correlation between fat and the fat residual is not high (Table 4.5), β_1 and β_3 are the same because the scaling among those with the same total energy intake has been preserved. Like in the standard multiple model, the risk for fat is the effect of a simultaneous change in both fat and non-fat sources of energy and depends on whether either or both of these substances have a risk. As there is a zero correlation between the fat residual and energy, the energy term is not needed as it cannot confound this relationship. However, if transformed nutrient data is being used, the correlation with an untransformed energy should be checked.

Some authors recommend that the population mean should be added to the residuals to remove the negative numbers. This does not affect the odds ratio or relative risk calculated in the risk models. Doing this is potentially misleading as it makes the residuals look like real population intakes and they are not – they are relative intakes.

The nutrient density method is an alternative way of expressing fat intake relative to energy intake:

$$\text{logit risk} = \alpha + \beta_4(\text{fat }\%) + \gamma_4(\text{total kJ}) . \qquad (4.4)$$

The fat residual and the fat % will rank individuals in a similar way because they are highly correlated (Table 4.5, Fig. 4.4) but the value of β_4 will be different from β_3 because their units are different. If the correlation between energy and nutrient density for fat is not zero (Table 4.5, Fig. 4.5) it should, technically, be included in the model to control for any remaining confounding. The low correlation means that the bias in the odds ratio for fat from omitting energy from the model may not be very serious, especially in studies where the correlation between energy and fat density is even lower than in the twin group (Shekelle et al. 1987; Willett and Stampfer 1987). As y_4 is the effect of energy while holding relative fat constant, it is the effect of increasing energy from all macronutrients in their relative proportions.

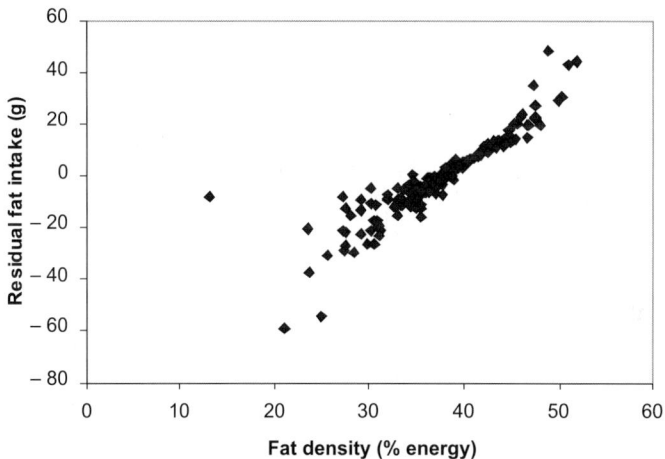

Figure 4.4. Scatterplot of energy-adjusted (residual) fat intake and fat density, twin study

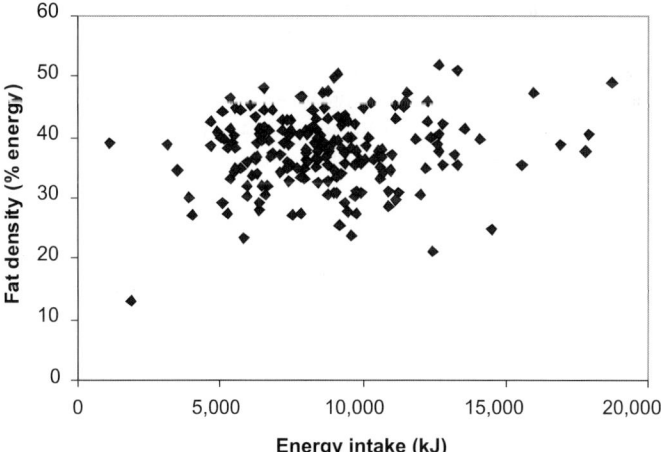

Figure 4.5. Scatterplot of average daily energy intake and fat density, twin study

The odds ratios or relative risks for fat intake yielded in the above four models are all adjusted for energy intake. However, at present in the literature, authors who give a result for 'energy-adjusted fat' generally mean that they have residualised the fat variable and different terms than 'energy-adjusted' are used if other methods were done.

The above discussion has considered fat as the prime focus. However, it is also possible to write an equivalent to Model (4.1) with carbohydrate, for example, as the focus:

$$\text{logit risk} = \alpha + \delta(\text{carbohydrate kJ}) + \gamma_5(\text{total kJ}) . \tag{4.5}$$

In this model, δ is the amount of risk associated with a 1 kJ increase in carbohydrate intake *given that total energy is held constant.* It is not the relative risk for changing carbohydrate alone but is the net effect of increasing carbohydrate intake and decreasing non-carbohydrate intake. If protein and alcohol are neutral, then β_1 from Model (4.1) will equal $-\delta$ from Model (4.5). In this event, the same changes in diet are modelled even though two different models appear to have been run. One wonders about the extent to which this explains results such as those of Francheschi et al. (1996) who reported that the odds ratios for breast cancer were 1.3 and 0.81 for the lowest vs. highest fifth of energy-adjusted (i.e. residualised) fat and available carbohydrate respectively.

In a similar vein, the following model could be considered:

$$\text{logit risk} = \alpha + \eta(\text{non-fat kJ}) + \gamma_6(\text{total kJ}) . \tag{4.6}$$

In this model, $\eta = -\beta_1$ from Model (4.1) for the reasons just explained and γ_6 equals β_2 from Model (4.2). The mathematical equivalences described in this section may not hold exactly if the variables need to be transformed.

It is worth reiterating that, because there are five different columns of data but only four independent variables, the same changes in diet will be modelled by more than one variable (Table 4.6). Just because different nutrients are entered into the model does not mean that the interpretation of the output will be different. The meaning of any model involving macronutrients must be thought through carefully and not interpreted at face value.

Table 4.6. Summary of the dietary changes modelled by various adjustment methods

Dietary change modelled	Coefficient in model				
	(4.1)	(4.2)	(4.3)	(4.4)	(4.6)
Substituting fat for non-fat energy	β_1		β_3	β_4	η
Adding energy as fat		β_2			γ_6
Adding energy as non-fat	γ_1	γ_2			
Adding energy from all macronutrients in current proportion				γ_4	

Depending on the hypothesis being tested, similar models can be constructed but their interpretation needs to be thought about. For example, Hu et al. (1999) entered the various types of fat and protein and energy into models, and as they noted, in this case total energy is only derived from carbohydrate. In this instance the standard multiple model is essentially the same as the partition model.

Macronutrients: Categorisation Affects the Range of the Relative Risk Estimate

4.3.3

When the nutrients are used as continuous variables in the model, the relative risk estimate will be per gram or per kilojoule or per % of energy. When the variables are categorised, the relative risk is for the comparison between quantiles. As noted above, some of the earlier discussion about the methods for controlling for confounding by energy related more to the range over which the risks were estimated than to the actual estimation of the relative risk itself. This arises when nutrient or food data are categorised because the results are generally described as 'for the highest vs. lowest fifth'. The results are especially cloudy if the authors fail to describe the absolute intake relating to each fifth. By contrast, if the data are used in a continuous form, tables of results are generally specific about the difference that the odds ratios or relative risks pertain to.

In the twins, the difference between the median values of the top and bottom fourths (i.e. the 12.5th and 87.5th percentiles), of fat intake is 71.7 g (Table 4.4) on the absolute scale but only 27.5 g when residualised. The reason for this is shown in Fig. 4.6. The horizontal lines show the quartile boundaries for fat on the absolute scale and the diagonal lines show the quartile boundaries of the residuals. In the twin group, a relative risk for the top vs. bottom fourth in the standard multiple and partition models relates to a 71.7 g fat difference but to a 27.5 g difference in the residual model. Although the standard multiple and residual models yield the same coefficients when fat is entered as a continuous variable, they will yield different results when fat intake is categorised. The much smaller range of the residualised (adjusted) fat intake than the absolute fat variable is not unique to the twins and would occur with any food component that is highly correlated with energy intake. As shown in Table 4.7, the range between the top and bottom group is much smaller for the energy-adjusted fat using the residual than the parent fat variable, but calculating the energy-adjusted intake does not reduce the range to the same extent for nutrients which have a lower correlation with energy such as cholesterol or fibre.

Although the residual and density models both express fat intake relative to total energy, they have different units and so, when used as continuous variables, the change in risk per unit will also be different. However, these two ways of expressing fat intake are highly correlated (Table 4.5, Fig. 4.4), they place virtually the same individuals in the various fourths (Table 4.8) and therefore will yield virtually identical relative risks when the fat intake data is categorised. Brown et al. (1994) discuss the conditions under which the coefficient for fat from the partition model will be higher or lower than the coefficient for fat from the standard multiple model.

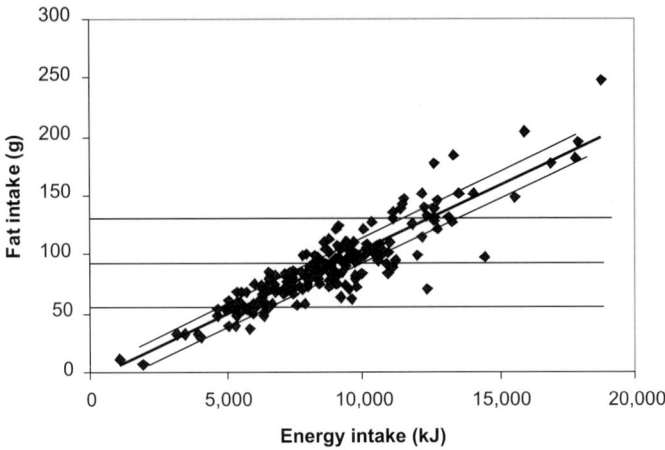

Figure 4.6. Scatterplot of average daily energy and fat intake showing boundaries for fourths of absolute fat intake (*horizontal lines*) and energy-adjusted (*residual*) fat intake (*diagonal lines*), twin study

4.3.4   Micronutrients

Only the standard multiple, residual and density models are relevant for non-energy providing nutrients and food components. However, the partition model may appear in a different context if micronutrients are subdivided. For example many studies of vitamin A and lung cancer divided vitamin A intakes into that derived from plants and preformed retinol to determine which of the two components was important (Shekelle et al. 1981). This is clearly another version of the partition model and it would be inappropriate to put total vitamin A intake into the model in addition to the subcomponents.

Most of the micronutrients are not highly correlated with energy intake (Table 4.5, Fig. 4.7). This means that the energy-specific range of intakes is similar to the total population range and so converting vitamin C intake to a residual or a density does not achieve much (Figs. 4.8 and 4.9). The difference between the 12.5th and 87.5th percentile for the absolute values and the residuals is 110.4 mg and 96.6 mg respectively (Table 4.4). The same is true for any component that is not highly correlated with energy intake. The fact that the range changes substantially for cholesterol but not fibre in Table 4.7 shows that cholesterol has a stronger correlation with energy intake than does fibre. When there is a low correlation with energy, relative risks or odds ratios will be very similar for categorical analyses from the standard multiple and residual models because the range over which they are calculated is similar.

4.3.5   Choosing a Model

In some respects, it would seem that there is little to choose among the models for macronutrients because the same relative risks for a particular difference in fat

Table 4.7. Data from other studies showing the range of intakes across fourths or fifths for different ways of expressing nutrient intakes

Author		Fifths			
Nutrient and method	Lowest	2	3	4	5
Willett et al. (1987) – data from 4 one-week diet records in 179 women					
Total fat					
Mean absolute (g)	47	59	68	75	98
Energy-adjusted (g)[a]	56	64	69	72	78
Mean % energy	32	36	39	41	44
Cholesterol					
Mean absolute (mg)	204	262	325	345	436
Mean energy-adjusted (mg)[a]	216	268	301	337	423
Mean mg/1000 kcal	136	166	188	212	276
Brisson et al. (1989) – data from a food frequency questionnaire					
Total fat					
Median absolute (g)	56	78	97	132	–
Median energy-adjusted (g)[a]	78	88	96	106	–
Median % energy	33	36	38	40	–
Cholesterol					
Median absolute (mg)	201	291	362	487	–
Median energy-adjusted (mg)[a]	249	312	357	442	–
Median mg/1000 kcal	127	144	157	181	–
Fibre					
Median absolute (g)	4.3	6.5	8.2	11.1	–
Median energy-adjusted (g)[a]	4.8	6.7	8.2	10.4	–

[a] Each person's residual has been added to the mean for the population for that nutrient

intake can be obtained, with more or less work, from Models (4.1), (4.2) and (4.3). As regards micronutrients, most have such low correlations with energy that there seems little reason to convert them to residuals or density. Clear, unambiguous expression of the range of intake to which the cited relative risk relates is paramount to allow others to use it.

As Kipnis et al. (1993) comment, the four models described in this section have slightly different meanings and, although their coefficients can be converted into each other, calculating the standard error is much easier if done in Model (4.1) and so deciding on the main focus of interest should be a primary consideration. There are several other factors that might influence the choice of model for macronutrients. There is a trade-off between the two sets of models – on the one hand, the standard multiple and partition models (set 1) examine a wider range of intakes which increases the power of a study while on the other hand, reducing the correlation between the variables in the model (as in set 2, the residual and density models) also increases the power of the study. Brown et al. (1994) show

Table 4.8. Cross classification of twins according to fourths of fat as % energy and fat as the residual, twin study (from Mackerras (1996))

| | | Residual | | |
Density	Low	2	3	High
High	–	–	1	48
3	–	2	46	1
2	6	41	2	–
Low	43	6	–	–

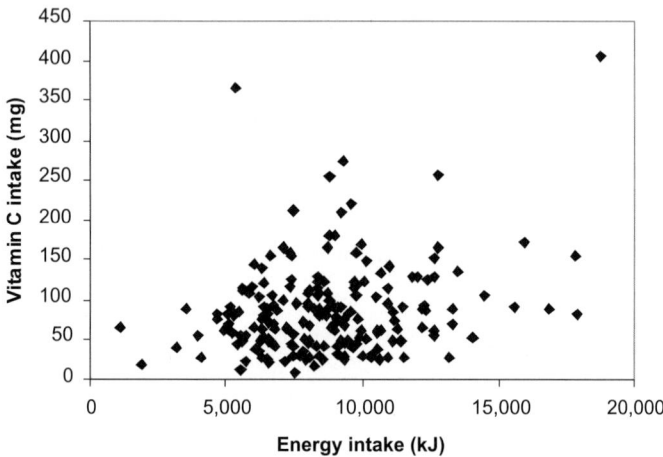

Figure 4.7. Scatterplot of average daily energy and vitamin C intake, twin study

that the gain in power from reducing the correlation, and thus the standard error, in the residual model is greater than the gain from the wider range of the standard multiple model. Hence a nutrient may not be significant in a standard multiple model when it is significant in the equivalent residual model both because the residual model requires fewer parameters to be estimated and also because the collinearity has been removed. The residual model is inconvenient, especially if transformations are required to obtain the residuals. There is little to choose between the residual and density models from the variance inflation point of view but they are on a different scale and this may be important. Although usually discussed in the context of energy adjustment, the partition model is open to misinterpretation as the relative risk for the primary nutrient variable is not energy independent but is the combined effect of increasing itself and energy on risk.

There is an important assumption underlying both the relative intake methods (residual and density). It is that there is no threshold of effect in the nutrient-disease risk relationship. If this cannot be assumed then both of these methods would be poor choices. As mentioned above, the reason for controlling for energy intake is to try to mimic the effects of an experiment when isoenergetic substitutions are made

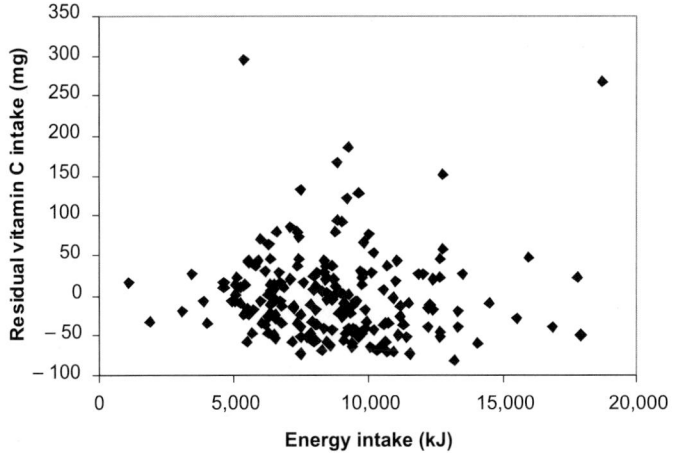

Figure 4.8. Scatterplot of average daily energy intake and energy-adjusted (*residual*) vitamin C intake, twin study

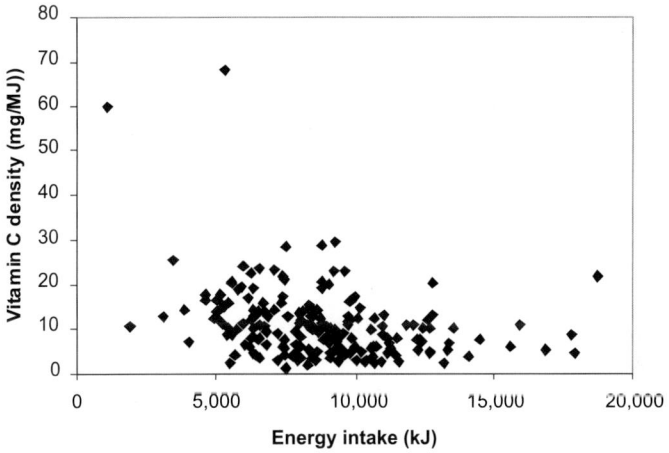

Figure 4.9. Scatterplot of average daily energy intake and vitamin C density, twin study

in the diet and so change in weight is prevented. However, change in weight can occur even when isoenergetic substitutions are made (Ballard-Barbash et al. 1999), and given the likely correlations in the errors of dietary variables, it is interesting to speculate on what other approaches to dealing with confounding from this source may arise in future. In addition, the above discussion has assumed that there is no error in the way that the nutrients are measured. Some studies indicate that reported energy intakes do not agree well with objective measures (Subar et al. 2003) and so this may have important impacts on the results obtained. For a general discussion of measurement errors see Chap. II.5 of this handbook.

Organisation and Presentation of Data: Implications for Meta-Analysis and Reviews

4.4

In a meta-analysis from literature (MAL), data that has been previously published is combined to form a summary estimate whereas in a pooled analysis, i.e. in a meta analysis with individual patient data (MAP), data are obtained from the authors and reanalysed (cf. Chap. II.7 of this handbook). In a drug study, authors are generally very specific about the dosages used and so those doing meta-analysis can easily determine if effects varied by dose and allow for this source of heterogeneity in the analysis. Owing to the propensity of dietary studies to present relative risks or odds ratios for categories rather than on a continuous scale, the difference in 'dose' is rarely apparent. This is an additional source of heterogeneity over and beyond others that may arise from using dietary tools with different validity and reliability, variations in which important dietary and non-dietary confounders were controlled for and other sources of bias that make meta-analysis of observational studies less robust than meta-analysis of randomised controlled trials.

The problem of using different categorisations can be quite severe. For example, Boyd et al. (1993) calculated a summary relative risk by combining the relative risk or odds ratio of the top vs. bottom quantile from 23 case-control and cohort studies of dietary fat and breast cancer. The categorisation in these studies was halves (1 study), thirds (4 studies), fourths (11 studies), fifths (5 studies). One study gave the odds ratio of the 90th vs. 10th centile, which are the medians of the top vs. bottom fifth and the final study presented the odds ratio of a difference of 24 g of fat. Even if the underlying dietary intakes and the association between the nutrient and breast cancer were exactly the same in all 23 studies, there would

Table 4.9. Median point of fat and vitamin C intakes when divided into different quantile groups, twin population data from 4-day weighed food records

Nutrient	Category division	Midpoint of the category					Range lowest-top category
		Lowest	2	3	4	5	
Fat	halves	69	103	–	–	–	34
(g/day)	thirds	59	84	111	–	–	52
	fourths	56	75	94	127	–	71
	fifths	54	72	84	99	132	78
Vitamin C	halves	49	108	–	–	–	59
(mg/day)	thirds	41	79	126	–	–	85
	fourths	31	64	90	140	–	109
	fifths	29	55	80	99	154	125

have been five different relative risks reported in these studies. To illustrate why, Table 4.9 shows the medians for these categories for fat and vitamin C intake in the twin group. (The means or medians show the range over which these five relative risks were typically calculated, but the median is less influenced by extreme values than the mean). The summary estimate in the meta-analysis would depend on the number of studies that had used each categorisation method, and the number of individuals in the study (if the inverse variance was used as the weighting factor in the meta-analysis). However, if the underlying studies in the meta-analysis have not reported the absolute intakes, then it is not possible to know what range of intake the final result from the meta-analysis relates to. If they are all similar populations, then it may be possible to make a guess from other information such as national surveys in these populations.

Choice of Adjustment Model Affects Interpretation of Results in Studies and Meta-Analyses

4.4.1

As there is no universal method to adjust for energy intake, and the most popular method has changed over time, reviews will inevitably include studies that controlled for confounding by energy using a variety of methods.

Kushi et al. (1992) examined the relationship between fat intake and breast cancer in their cohort study and found that the increment in risk between the highest and lowest fourth ranged from 13% to 38% depending on which energy adjustment method was used, although none were statistically significant (Table 4.10). From the foregoing discussion, it should be clear that these results are not surprising but follow the pattern that would be predicted from understanding the models. The range from the top and bottom fourths of absolute fat intake is about 70 g (Tables 4.4 and 4.7) in a Western population and this is the range over which the relative risks are calculated in the standard multiple model. However the range of residual fourths is only 30 g and so it is expected that the relative risk is much smaller in the residual model than the standard multiple model. As density and residuals categorise individuals in virtually the same way, the almost identical relative risks in these two models are expected. The fourths in the partition model have the same range as the standard multiple model, but the relative risk for fat is the combined effect of increasing energy and fat intakes whereas in the standard multiple model, the relative risk for fat is the effect of replacing non-fat energy with energy from fat. Whether these two relative risks would be different or the same cannot be predicted ahead of time as it depends on the effects of the other components of the diet.

Several different pooled analyses have been done examining the effect of fat on breast cancer. The one combining case-control studies found a positive association (Howe et al. 1990) and the one combining cohort studies found no association (Hunter et al. 1996). This difference could be attributed to the intrinsic differences in potential recall bias etc. between these two study designs, age groups included or to differences in the non-dietary factors that were adjusted for. However, the two

Table 4.10. Estimates of breast cancer risk for various nutrients and models for highest vs. lowest group of intake in postmenopausal women (from Kushi et al. 1992) (RR = relative risk; CI = confidence interval)

Method of adjusting fat intake For energy intake	RR for the highest vs. lowest fourth of total fat intake	95% CI
Standard multiple	1.38	0.86–2.21
Partition	1.26	0.87–1.84
Residual	1.16	0.87–1.55
Density	1.13	0.84–1.51

overviews adjusted for energy differently and it is worth considering how much this may have contributed to the difference in their findings.

Howe et al. (1990) used the standard multiple model with the nutrient intake data in a continuous form, but multiplied the odds ratios per gram/milligram by a factor of 100 g representing the range between the 10–90th centiles in the Canadian study in the analysis (Table 4.11). Therefore the odds ratio of 1.48 is for increasing fat intake by 100 g regardless of whether this is from 100 g to 200 g per day or from 23 g to 123 g per day. However the odds ratio of 1.48 cannot yet be used to calculate the benefit from a population-wide reduction in fat intake. First the likelihood of achieving a reduction in 100 g must be determined. As shown in Tables 4.4 and 4.7, it is impossible to reduce the population intake by an average of 100 g. The odds ratio of 1.48 may be correct, but it is irrelevant for policy needs. Of more interest would be the prevention perspective, e.g. an odds ratio relating to a 25 g reduction in total fat intake. This can be easily calculated, as the meta-analysis used nutrient data in a continuous form, and is 0.91 (from OR = 1.48 = e^{100x} where x is the risk associated with 1 g fat).

Table 4.11. Pooled analysis of 12 case-control studies investigating the risk of diet on breast cancer in post-menopausal women (Howe et al. 1990) (OR = odds ratio)

Nutrient	Unit for the OR	OR	*p*
Energy	8.4 MJ[a]	1.4	< 0.001
Total fat, g	100 g	1.48	< 0.001
Dietary fibre[b]	20 g	0.83	0.002
Vitamin C[b]	300 mg	0.63	< 0.001

[a] 8.4 MJ = 2000 kcal
[b] Controlled for total fat intake

If a 25 g decrease in average fat intake of women seems feasible in a population, then a 9% reduction in breast cancer incidence would be predicted. Citing the 32% reduction associated with the 100 g increment would be misleading if projecting the effect of a health promotion campaign. Note that the results of Howe et al.

(1990) can be quoted as showing that the odds ratio per 100 g increment is 1.48 or that the odds ratio per 25 g increment is 1.10. Both statements are correct and are consistent with each other. Apparent contradictions and confusions would arise if the units of the calculations were omitted from the statement.

The pooled analysis of Hunter et al. (1996) used residualised fat intakes in the analysis (Table 4.12) Although they do not report the fat intake data that relates to their fifths, the relative risk of 1.05 for the top vs. bottom fifth probably relates to a range of about 32 g (Tables 4.7 and 4.9). They also report the results from the same data analysed as continuous variables: a relative risk of 1.02 for an increment of 25 g fat intake. Thus it is clear that the difference between the results of the two pooled analyses (Tables 4.11 and 4.12) is more apparent than real. When converted to the same units – the relative risk for a difference of 25 g fat intake – much of the discrepancy disappears. Similarly the odds ratio of 1.4 for a difference of 2000 kcal (Howe et al. 1990, Table 4.11) reduces to 1.02 for a 100 kcal difference and this is much closer to the result of Hunter et al. (1996, Table 4.12). When describing studies for others, it is important to ensure that the range that a result relates to is clearly expressed, and if policy makers are the audience, that the range is relevant given the current intake of population.

Table 4.12. Pooled analysis of 7 cohort studies investigating the risk of diet on breast cancer (Hunter et al. 1996) (CI = confidence interval)

| | Fat intake (residualised) | | Energy intake | |
	Relative risk	95% CI	Relative risk	95% CI
As quintiles				
Lowest	referent	–	referent	–
2	1.01	0.89–1.14	1.01	0.91–1.12
3	1.12	1.01–1.25	1.13	1.02–1.25
4	1.07	0.96–1.19	1.04	0.92–1.17
Highest	1.05	0.94–1.16	1.11	0.99–1.25
Continuous data				
Per 25 g	1.02	0.94–1.11	–	–
Per 420 kJ (100 kcal)	–	–	1.01	0.99–1.02

Nutritional Epidemiology in Public Health Practice

4.5

The foregoing sections have focused on methods and their applications to research studies investigating the effects of dietary components on the risk of disease. In this section, we make some comments on the consequences of within-person variation in the context of using nutritional epidemiological methods for descriptive epidemiology and public health nutrition practice rather than research. In particular, we focus on national dietary surveys and the assessment of population intakes with respect to external references because there have been several important changes in methodological approach and terminology in recent years.

4.5.1 Assessing the Usual Intake of a Population

With the notable exception of the United Kingdom, countries that have conducted national surveys investigating dietary intake have generally collected one day of intake from participants, usually as a 24-hour recall but occasionally as a 1-day record. In the United Kingdom, 4–7 days of records have been collected in all national diet and nutrition surveys (recent cycle began in 1986 with adults, and has covered all age groups, up to repeating adults in 2002).

The external references (see below) used to assess diet are based on the assumption that usual intake has been assessed in the individuals participating in the survey. Hence, if national survey data which collected a single day of information from each individual are compared to the reference, the wrong prevalence will be obtained. If the interest is in describing the proportion of the population with low intakes, then using single day data will overestimate the true prevalence when the population average lies above the cut-off (cut-off A in Fig. 4.10) but will underestimate the true prevalence if the population average lies below the cut-off (cut-off B in Fig. 4.10). Conversely, if the interest is in describing the proportion with high intakes, then single day data will underestimate and overestimate the true prevalences respectively. The extent of the error will depend on the location of the cut-off with respect to the population average and also the ratio of the standard deviations of the single-day and usual intake distributions. This ratio is lower for those nutrients found in a wide range of foods which are eaten every day (e.g. macronutrients such as protein) and highest for those nutrients which are found in a small range of foods where the alternatives have different nutrient contents (e.g. the vitamin A content of vegetables varies enormously).

There are two alternative ways of dealing with this problem. One is to take the route used in the UK and obtain multiple days of intakes from all participants in a survey. This clearly has large consequences for the cost, logistical complexity and respondent burden associated with the survey. The second way is to obtain an estimate of the ratio of the standard deviations of the two distributions and to correct the distribution obtained on all participants using the ratio (Sempos et al. 1991). As dietary intakes and patterns vary with age and sex, it would be necessary to do this work on all important sub-groups in the population and not to obtain one ratio, in for example adults, to apply to all other groups. This method is obviously cheaper. Its main drawback is that it may limit some other uses of the data if the survey has multiple purposes.

One-way analysis of variance allowing for random effects and repeated measures can be used to separate the between-person variance (s_b) from the total variance (s_{total}) in the sub-sample with multiple measures (Mackerras 1998). Then the ratio

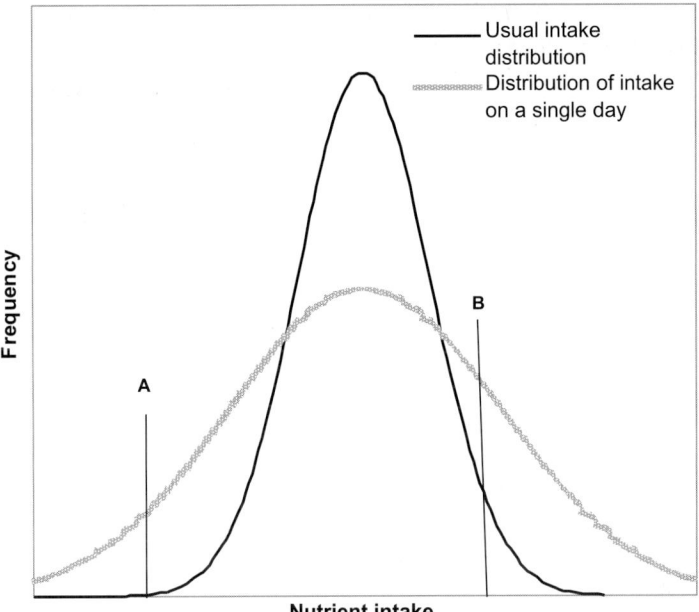

Figure 4.10. The distribution of the usual intake of individuals has a narrower standard deviation than the intake on a single day. When cut-offs (e.g. A or B) are based on the assumption that usual intake has been measured, the incorrect prevalence will be obtained if single day data is used

can be used to adjust each individual's single-day value (x_i) in the main survey relative to the sample mean $(\overline{X})$ (Sempos et al. 1991; Rutishauser 2000):

$$\text{adjusted value} = \overline{X} + \left(x_i - \overline{X}\right)\left(s_b/s_{\text{total}}\right) .$$

Depending on the nutrient, the 10–90th centile range of the corrected distribution could be as little as 66% of the 10–90th centile range of the uncorrected distribution. It is important to note that although the corrected population distribution was created by applying a factor to each individual's datapoint, the resulting values for each individual cannot be interpreted as each individual's true usual intake (Guenther et al. 1997; Murphy 2003). They are only correct on average and this is sufficient to generate the corrected population distribution. If an estimate of usual intake is desired for each individual (for addressing other purposes of the survey) then multiple days of intake data must be collected from each individual.

Just as nutrient intake varies from day to day, so too does the intake of foods and non-nutrient food components. Given various current recommendations to increase intake of foods such as fruit and vegetables it is important for dietary surveys that collected single-day data to correct the standard deviation of foods or food groups using the same approaches. Although there are a number of studies describing the extent of the variability of nutrient intakes (e.g. Beaton et al. 1979,

1983; Nelson et al. 1989), there are few reports supplying the same information for food intakes (Palaniappan et al. 2003).

References for Assessing Dietary Intake in Populations

For many years, 'recommended' intakes of nutrients have been promulgated by various national bodies. However, the correct use of these figures has never been very clear. This situation is probably partly related to a more general problem that diagnostic criteria for assessing individuals are often misinterpreted as indicators for population surveillance, or vice versa, when they are based on the same underlying measurements or data. A typical use of national dietary surveys is to compare the results to external references such as 'recommended intakes'.

Firstly, it is important to realise that all committees agree that the 'recommended' figures they produce are expressed as daily amounts for convenience only. All committees agree that it is long-term diet that is important and that the 'recommended' figures should never be compared to a single day of intake for either populations or individuals. As shown in Fig. 4.10, the incorrect prevalences will be found if they are compared to single-day data. The following discussion of the second problem assumes that usual intake distributions are available for the population.

Until about 10 years ago, most countries set only one type of dietary reference figure for each age-sex group for each nutrient. At present this figure is called the Reference Nutrient Intake (RNI) in the UK, the Population Reference Intake in the European Union, the Recommended Dietary Allowance in the USA and Canada and the Recommended Dietary Intake in Australia (Department of Health 1991; The Scientific Committee for Food 1993; Food and Nutrition Board 2000; Truswell et al. 1990) and will be referred to here as the RNI. The RNI is generally set well above the average requirement so that, if everyone ate this amount, there would be a low probability of deficiency in the population. Sometimes there was enough information to set the RNI at 2 standard deviations above the Estimated Average Requirement (EAR). Often the committees just added a large safety margin. As the margin added varied by nutrient, it was not possible to express the RNI amount as a constant multiple of the underlying average requirement.

The UK was the first country to set multiple values when it revised its dietary references (Department of Health 1991) and specified the location of the EAR. The European Union then followed suit, naming its equivalent figures Average Requirements (The Scientific Committee for Food 1993) and more recently the USA and Canada have also described the EAR that their recommended dietary allowances were derived from (Food and Nutrition Board 2000).

Advising individuals to have intakes that meet the RNI is sensible because this advice carries a low probability of suggesting inadequate intakes for that person. However, could the RNI be used to assess the adequacy of population intakes? In earlier times when the EAR was not specified, two methods were used quite commonly. They were to determine whether the mean intake is equal to or above the RNI or to determine the proportion falling below the RNI. Neither of these is satisfactory (Beaton 1999).

Because the standard deviation of the intake distribution is generally much wider than the standard deviation of the requirement distribution (Beaton 1999), many people might have intakes below their requirements when the median population intake lies on the RNI (RNI(a) in Scenario 1, Fig. 4.11). The extent to which this happens depends on how the RNIs were set in the past. If they were set by adding a safety margin that was larger than twice the $SD_{requirement}$, then the greater margin, the less the underestimation of the prevalence of inadequate intakes (RNI(b) in Scenario 1, Fig. 4.11). It is true that, if everyone has an intake above the RNI, the prevalence of inadequate intakes will be essentially 0 (Scenario 2, Fig. 4.11). However, many people will be consuming much more than their personal requirements. It is clear that there could be some overlap between the two distributions that is still

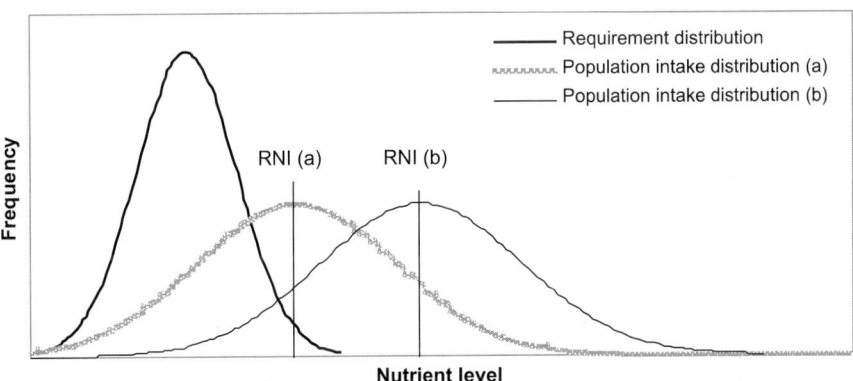

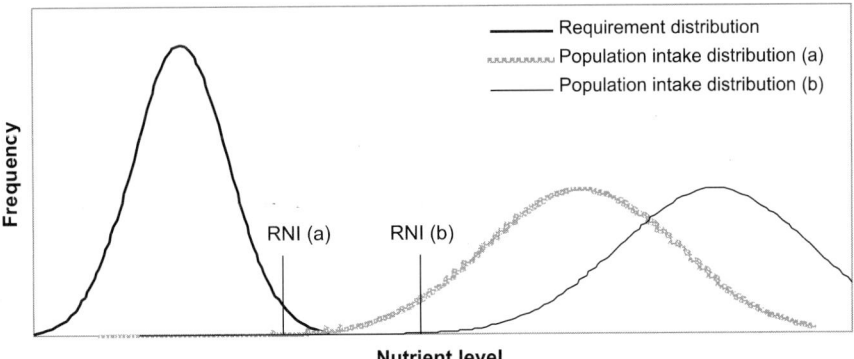

Figure 4.11. Illustration of how the RNI has been used in the past to assess population intakes, assuming two different RNIs that had been set in different ways (adapted from Beaton (1999))

consistent with a low probability of inadequate intakes. A third method that has been used in the past is to calculate the proportion of the population with intakes below 70% of the RNI on the assumption that the requirement distribution had a coefficient of variation of 20%. As this was rarely the case, this approach would overestimate the true prevalence for some nutrients and underestimate the true prevalence for other nutrients. Consequently, this approach would not necessarily reveal which nutrient is in shortest supply in the population. So the question is 'How much overlap can there be between the requirement and intake distributions before the prevalence of inadequate intakes is unacceptably high?'. A method for multiplying the two probability distributions was described in 1986 (Subcommittee on Criteria for Dietary Evaluation 1986) and the more powerful computers of today can do the calculations more easily. However, if the requirement distribution is symmetrical, and the intake distribution is approximately normal, then a short-cut method can be used: if the intake mean is at least EAR + 2 × SD_{intake} (with 2 being approximately the 97.5 quantile of a standard normal distribution) higher than the EAR, then the prevalence of inadequate intakes will be 2.5% or less (Fig. 4.12). In other words, if the assumptions are met, the proportion below the EAR is the proportion with inadequate intakes, although no definite statements can be made about which individuals have intakes below the EAR. Other multiples of the SD_{intake} could be used if other criteria are desired. Note that the standard deviation in this formula is for the intake distribution, not the requirement distribution and the reference point is the EAR and not the RNI. The details of this approach and further information on other situations, such as when the requirement distribution is asymmetrical, can be found elsewhere (Subcommittee on Criteria for Dietary Evaluation 1986; Beaton 1999; Food and Nutrition Board 2000).

As a final note, the illustration above has assumed that intake distributions are normal. If these must be transformed, then care needs to be taken to apply the

When the intake median=EAR+2SD$_{intake}$

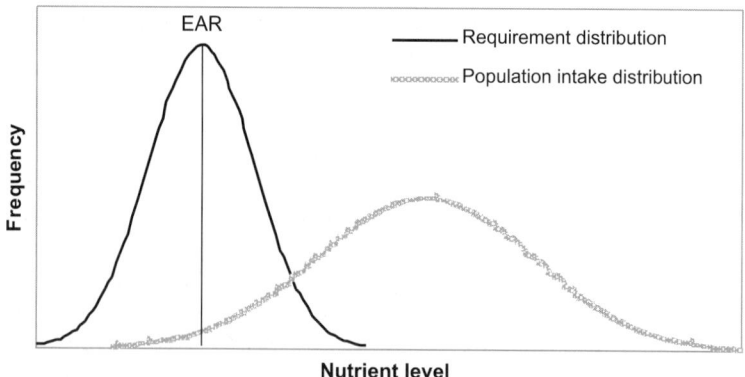

Figure 4.12. If the mean population intake is 2 × SD_{intake} above the EAR then the prevalence of inadequate intakes in the population is 2.5%

correction factors appropriately. The above comments about the RNI do not apply to energy, because the energy recommendations are set at the EAR and not at two SD above the EAR. It is also important to examine how words are used in each country, because the same word may be used to signify different concepts in different locations, and to realise that definitions might vary within a document. Values for the EAR and RNI may vary between countries, either because they have been based on different indicators of nutritional status or based on a different range of literature or because they have been determined as mg/kg and the mean weight of the population varies.

Impact of Under-Reporting of Intake 4.5.3

Because people tend to underestimate their intakes by most dietary methods (Black et al. 1991), the data collected in a national survey will tend to underestimate total intake. For example, when the criteria of Goldberg et al. (1991) for assessing a 24-hour intake were applied to the 1995 Australian survey, 11.9% of men and 20.6% of adult women had energy intakes that were implausible. Compared to the total population surveyed, those with plausible intakes had higher intakes of all nutrients (Table 4.13). Clearly leaving those with implausible intakes in the data can affect the results of the analysis, especially for some of the minerals. Therefore analyses of national surveys that have not excluded these individuals would tend to overestimate the prevalence of low intakes of most nutrients. However, one problem with simply excluding them is that people may underreport some foods differently from others. If energy containing foods are under-reported to a greater extent than low-energy foods such as fruit and vegetables, then excluding the implausible reporters may incorrectly inflate intakes of nutrients such as vitamins A and C, and to some extent folate and fibre. A further problem is that equivalent criteria for defining those with implausibly high reports is not available.

Consequences of Within-Person Variability in Other Areas of Public Health Nutrition Practice 4.5.4

As noted above, intra-individual variation in dietary measures is not due to the subjective nature of the measure. The error related to reporting or measurement occurs in addition to the underlying instability of the parameter being measured. Many 'objective' measures also vary every time they are measured. Blood pressure is a notable example – it can vary from minute to minute. Even biochemical measures also exhibit within-person variability. Some parameters have a regular variation (e.g. diurnal variation) in addition to random variation. The particular problems with dietary measures occur because the within-person variance is larger, generally much larger, than the between-person variance. However, the observed prevalence can be affected even for parameters where the within-person variance is smaller than the between-person variance. Looker et al. (1990) found that the prevalence of impaired iron status (based on mean corpuscular volume, transferrin saturation

Table 4.13. Comparison of median nutrient intakes in the total survey sample and persons with plausible EI/BMR ratios, adults 19 years and older, by sex. 1995 National Nutrition Survey, Australia (ABS & HEALTH 1998)

Nutrient	Men		Women	
	Total	Plausible[a]	Total	Plausible[a]
Energy (kJ)	10,377	10,997	7083	7824
Protein (g)	100.1	106.4	69.5	76.3
Total fat (g)	89.8	96.4	61.6	70.3
Dietary fibre (g)	23.8	25.1	18.9	20.5
Vitamin A (ug retinol equivalents)	941	1012.9	753.6	833.0
Thiamin (mg)	1.7	1.8	1.2	1.3
Riboflavin (mg)	2.0	2.2	1.6	1.7
Niacin equivalents (mg)	47.1	49.8	32.3	35.1
Folate (mg)	285.3	299.6	216.7	232.6
Vitamin C (mg)	102.9	110.2	85.4	92.2
Calcium (mg)	827.3	891.4	663.1	737.6
Magnesium (mg)	360.3	380.8	266.9	291.1
Iron (mg)	15.2	16.1	11.1	12.2
Zinc (mg)	12.8	13.6	8.7	9.6

[a] Plausible intakes: 24-hour intakes with an energy intake/basal metabolic rate ratio of 0.9 or greater are above the lower bound of the 95% confidence interval in a weight stable individual undertaking light activity (Goldberg et al. 1991)

and erythrocyte protoporphyrin) was 10% in a national survey using the single measure data. This was reduced to 4% when corrected for within-person variation.

The within-person variation is why many parameters are measured more than once before a diagnosis and treatment decision can be made in the clinical setting. Irwig et al. (1991) show that the interpretation of a single measure of cholesterol level in an client depends on knowing the underlying population distribution, and that single measures cannot be used to assess whether the client's true underlying average has changed since the previous measurement. These observations can be generalised to other characteristics as well.

Program evaluation is another area where taking a single measure may yield misleading results because of within-person variability and measurement error. People may be eligible to enter a program because their level of a characteristic is below a cut-off. In this case, the mean level of the characteristic in the eligible group will be higher when it is measured again than it was at baseline even if the program has no effect. Similarly, if people are selected because their characteristic is above a cut-off, then the group mean will be lower on the second occasion, even if the program is ineffective. In both cases, the mean value of the second measurement is closer to the mean in the total unselected population than was the mean of the first measurement. This effect occurs because of a statistical phenomenon called regression to the mean (Davis 1976; Newell and Simpson 1990;

Bland and Altman 1994). If the evaluation uses a randomised control design, then the effects of regression to the mean and other explanations such as seasonal or secular trends occur in the control group and so they can be excluded by comparing the follow-up level in the intervention group to the follow-up level in the control group instead of comparing the follow-up to the baseline levels in the intervention group. Because randomised studies are perceived as very complex, it may be tempting to do a non-randomised study and use ineligible people (i.e. those whose values did not meet the criterion for eligibility) as a control group but this will not allow the regression to the mean effect to be detected. Sometimes a specific sub-group is not selected at the outset but the total group may be divided up in the analyses and authors may report that those with the most extreme values at baseline benefited most from the intervention. If there is no randomised control arm, this sort of finding is a warning that the results being reported may be due to regression to the mean rather than the intervention (Vickers and Altman 2001).

Whether a national survey provides a useful source of information for studying diet disease relationships depends on exactly how it is carried out. Even though it may be possible to demonstrate associations, national surveys which assess dietary intake and outcome markers such as blood pressure, haemoglobin levels etc. are cross-sectional surveys, even if the information is collected over a few days, and this inevitably limits causal inference. It is not possible to determine the temporal direction between, for example, the concentration of blood fat or blood pressure and consumption of fat type or sodium. Sometimes, a population involved in a national survey may be followed up beyond the survey. Even though this converts a cross-sectional survey into a cohort study, the extent of the analysis would depend on the initial measurements obtained. If only a single 24-hour recall was obtained, then correlation and regression coefficients will be attenuated (Liu et al. 1978; Sempos et al. 1985) as previously described.

Conclusions
4.6

There are few health outcomes for which nutrition does not play either a direct or indirect role in causation, and therefore in disease prevention. Increasingly there are in all countries a complex mix of problems of over and undernutrition occurring, often stratified by education or economic group. Some of these nutrition related problems are clear, and simply require the political will and resources to be dealt with. Others are more complex and the correct way to solve the problem may not be known or obvious. This is where nutritional epidemiology has a critical role to play. In order to improve and maintain public health, it is important to have a strong evidence-base to guide action. This is particularly the case where there are vested interests that may not want the dietary patterns to change. In order to justify and support such changes it is essential that the evidence supports policy. The methods of nutritional epidemiology guide that evidence-base.

The major specific concerns in nutritional epidemiology are how to define and measure with required accuracy the relevant measure of exposure, free from bias. Because diet and other behaviours are complex and interrelated, it is important, both in the design and interpretation of studies, to understand how this complexity may affect the results of the study. These issues can not simply be resolved by statistical adjustment, it is essential to have an understanding of the underlying biology.

Because most studies are of limited statistical power there is a growing tendency to undertake meta-analyses using pooled data. Before data are pooled it is important to assess whether this is logical and a fair reflection of the underlying differences between studies. This is more than assessing the heterogeneity using a statistical technique. It is important to establish whether the differences in dietary assessment methods and ways of presenting data allow such pooling. The range of exposure in the referent category, the way data are sub-divided into thirds or fourths, will all affect the size of the estimate of risk in each study.

References

ABS & HEALTH (1998) National Nutrition Survey. Nutrient intakes and physical measurements Australia 1995. Catalogue No 4805.0. Australian Bureau of Statistics, Canberra

Amanatidis S, Mackerras D, Simpson JM (2001) Comparison of two frequency questionnaires for quantifying fruit and vegetable intake. Public Health Nutrition 4:233–239

Armstrong B, White E, Saracci R (1994) Principles of exposure measurement in epidemiology. Oxford University Press, Oxford

Ballard-Barbash R, Forman MR, Kipnis V (1999) Dietary fat, serum estrogen levels, and breast cancer risk: a multifaceted story. J Natl Cancer Inst 91:492–494

Bates CJ, Thurnham DI, Bingham SA, Margetts BM, Nelson M (1997) Biochemical markers of nutrient intake. In: Margetts BM, Nelson M (eds) Design concepts in nutritional epidemiology, 2nd edn. Oxford University Press, Oxford, pp 170–240

Beaton GH (1999) Recommended dietary intakes: individuals and populations. In: Shils ME, Olson JA, Shike M, Ross AC (eds) Modern nutrition in health and disease, 9th edn. Williams and Wilkins, Baltimore

Beaton GH, Milner J, Corey P, McGuire V, Cousins M, Stewart E, de Ramos M, Hewitt D, Grambsch PV, Kassim N, Little JA (1979) Sources of variance in 24-hour dietary recall data: implications for nutrition study design and interpretation. Am J Clin Nutr 32:2546–2549

Beaton GH, Milner J, McGuire V, Feather TE, Little JA (1983) Source of variance in 24-hour dietary recall data: implications for nutrition study design and interpretation. Carbohydrate sources, vitamins, and minerals. Am J Clin Nutr 37:986–995

Bellach B, Kohlmeier L (1998) Energy adjustment does not control for differential recall bias in nutritional epidemiology. J Clin Epidemiol 51:393–398

Black AE, Goldberg GR, Jebb SA, Livingstone MB, Cole TJ, Prentice AM (1991) Critical evaluation of energy intake data using fundamental principles of energy physiology: 2. Evaluating the results of published surveys. Eur J Clin Nutr 45:583–599

Bland JM, Altman DG (1994) Some examples of regression towards the mean. BMJ 309:780

Boyd NF, Martin LJ, Noffel M, Lockwood GA, Trichler DL (1993) A meta-analysis of studies of dietary fat and breast cancer risk. Br J Cancer 68:627–636

Brisson J, Verreault R, Morrison AS, Tennina S, Meyer F (1989) Diet, mammographic features of breast tissue, and breast cancer risk. Am J Epidemiol 130:14–24

Brown CC, Kipnis V, Freedman LS, Hartman AM, Schatzkin A, Wacholder S (1994) Energy adjustment methods for nutritional epidemiology: the effect of categorization. Am J Epidemiol 139:323–338

Davis CE (1976) The effect of regression to the mean in epidemiologic and clinical studies. Am J Epidemiol 104:493–498

Department of Health (1991) Report of Health and Social Subjects 41. Dietary reference values for food energy and nutrients for the United Kingdom. Report of the Panel on Dietary Reference Values of the Committee on Medical Aspects of Food Policy. HMSO, London

Dorfman A, Kimball AW, Friedman LA (1985) Regression modeling of consumption or exposure variables classified by type. Am J Epidemiol 122:1096–1107

Food and Nutrition Board, Institute of Medicine (2000) Dietary Reference Intakes: Applications in dietary assessment. National Academy Press, Washington DC (http://www.nap.edu/catalog/9956.html) Accessed April 29, 2004

Franceschi S, Favero A, Decarli A, Negri E, La Vecchia C, Ferraroni M, Russo A, Salvini S, Amadori D, Conti E, Montella M, Giacosa A (1996) Intake of macronutrients and risk of breast cancer. Lancet 347:1351–1356

Friedenreich CM (2002) Commentary: improving pooled analyses in epidemiology. Int J Epidemiol 31:86–87

Goldberg GR, Black AE, Jebb SA, Cole TJ, Murgatroyd PR, Coward WA, Prentice AM (1991) Critical evaluation of energy intake data using fundamental principles of energy physiology: 1. Derivation of cut-off limits to identify under-recording. Eur J Clin Nutr 45:569–581

Goran MI, Astrup A (2002) Energy metabolism. In: Gibney MJ, Vorster HH, Kok FJ (eds) Introduction to human nutrition. Blackwell Publishing, Oxford

Gordon T, Fisher M, Rifkind BM (1984) Some difficulties inherent in the interpretation of dietary data from free-living populations. Am J Clin Nutr 39:152–156

Guenther PM, Kott PS, Carriquiry AL (1997) Development of an approach for estimating usual nutrient intake distributions at the population level. J Nutr 127:1106–1112

Holbrook TL, Barrett-Connor E, Wingard DL (1988) Dietary calcium and risk of hip fracture: 14-year prospective population study. Lancet II:1046–1049

Hosmer DW, Lemeshow S (1989) Applied logistic regression. John Wiley and Sons, New York

Howe GR, Hirohata T, Hislop TG, Iscovich JM, Yuan JM, Katsouyanni K, Lubin F, Marubini E, Modan B, Rohan T, Toniolo P, Shunzhang Y (1990) Dietary factors and risk of breast cancer: combined analysis of 12 case-control studies. J Natl Cancer Inst 82:561–569

Hunter DJ, Spiegelman D, Adami HO, Beeson L, van den Brandt PA, Folsom AR, Fraser GE, Goldbohm RA, Graham S, Howe GR, Kushi LH, Marshall JR, McDermott A, Miller AB, Speizer FE, Wolk A, Yaun SS, Willett W (1996) Cohort studies of fat intake and the risk of breast cancer – a pooled analysis. N Engl J Med 334:356–361

Hu FB, Stampfer MJ, Rimm E, Ascherio A, Rosner BA, Spiegelman D, Willett WC (1999) Dietary fat and coronary heart disease: a comparison of approaches for adjusting for total energy intake and modeling repeated dietary measurements. Am J Epidemiol 149:531–540

Irwig L, Glasziou P, Wilson A, Macaskill P (1991) Estimating an individual's true cholesterol level and response to intervention. JAMA 266:1678–1685

Kaaks R, Riboli E, van Staveren W (1995) Calibration of dietary intake measurements in prospective cohort studies. Am J Epidemiol 142:548–556

Kipnis V, Freedman LS, Brown CC, Hartman AM, Schatzkin A, Wacholder S (1993) Interpretation of energy adjustment methods for nutritional epidemiology. Am J Epidemiol 137:1376–1380

Kushi LH, Sellers TA, Potter JD, Nelson CL, Munger RG, Kaye SA, Folsom AR (1992) Dietary fat and postmenopausal breast cancer. J Natl Cancer Inst 84:1092–1099

Liu K, Stamler J, Dyer A, McKeever J, McKeever P (1978) Statistical methods to assess and minimize the role of intra-individual variability in obscuring the relationship between dietary lipids and serum cholesterol. J Chronic Dis 31:399–418

Looker AC, Sempos CT, Liu KA, Johnson CL, Gunter EW (1990) Within-person variance in biochemical indicators of iron status: effects on prevalence estimates. Am J Clin Nutr 52:541–547

Mackerras D (1996) Energy adjustment: the concepts underlying the debate. J Clin Epidemiol 49:957–962

Mackerras D (1998) Within- and between-subject variability. In: Kerr CB, Taylor R, Heard G (eds) Handbook of public health methods. McGraw-Hill, Sydney

Margetts BM, Nelson M (eds) (1997) Design concepts in nutritional epidemiology, 2nd edn.. Oxford University Press, Oxford

Margetts BM, Vorster HH, Venter CS (2003) Evidence based nutrition: the impact of information and selection bias on the interpretation of individual studies. SAJCN 16:79–87

Missmer SA, Smith-Warner SA, Spiegelman D, Yaun SS, Adami HO, Beeson WL, van den Brandt PA, Fraser GE, Freudenheim JL, Goldbohm RA, Graham S, Kushi LH, Miller AB, Potter JD, Rohan TE, Speizer FE, Toniolo P, Willett WC, Wolk A, Zeleniuch-Jacquotte A, Hunter DJ (2002) Meat and dairy food consumption and breast cancer: a pooled analysis of cohort studies. Int J Epidemiol 31:78–85

Murphy SP (2003) Collection and analysis of intake data from the integrated survey. J Nutr 133:585S–589S

Nelson M, Black AE, Morris JA, Cole TJ (1989) Between- and within-subject variation in nutrient intake from infancy to old age: estimating the number of days required to rank dietary intakes with desired precision. Am J Clin Nutr 50:155–167

Nelson M, Beresford S (2004) Nutritional epidemiology. In: Gibney MH, Margetts BM, Arab L, Kearney J (eds) Public health nutrition. Blackwell Publishing, Oxford

Newell D, Simpson J (1990) Regression to the mean. Med J Aust 153:166–168

Palaniappan U, Cue RI, Payette H, Gray-Donald K (2003) Implications of day-to-day variability on measurements of usual food and nutrient intakes. J Nutr 133:232–235

Pike MC, Bernstein L, Peters RK (1992) Re: "Dietary fat and postmenopausal breast cancer." J Natl Cancer Inst 84:1666–1667

Rao S, Kanade A, Margetts BM, Yajnik CS, Lubree H, Rege S, Desai B, Jackson AA, Fall CHD (2003) Maternal activity in relation to birth size in rural India: The Pune maternal nutrition study. Eur J Clin Nutr 57:531–542

Rutishauser IHE (2000) Getting it right: how to use the data from the 1995 National Nutrition Survey. Commonwealth Department of Health and Aged Care, Canberra (http://www.sph.uq.edu.au/NUTRITION/monitoring/p3.htm) Accessed April 29, 2004

Schofield WN, Schofield C, James WPT (1985) Basal metabolic rate – review and prediction together with annotated bibliography of source material. Human Nutrition: Clinical Nutrition 39C Suppl 1:1–96

Sempos CT, Johnson NE, Smith EL, Gilligan C (1985) Effects of intraindividual and interindividual variation in repeated dietary records. Am J Epidemiol 121:120–130

Sempos CT, Looker AC, Johnson CL, Woteki CE (1991) The importance of within-person variability in estimating prevalence. In: Macdonald I (ed) Monitoring dietary intakes. Springer-Verlag, Berlin

Shekelle RB, Lepper M, Liu S, Maliza C, Raynor WJ, Rossof AH (1981) Dietary vitamin A and risk of cancer in the Western Electric Study. Lancet II:1186–1190

Shekelle RB, Nichaman MZ, Raynor WJ (1987) Re: "Total energy intake: implications for epidemiologic analyses."(Letter) Am J Epidemiol 126:980

Slattery ML, Schumacher MC, Smith KR, West DW, Abd-Elghany N (1988) Physical activity, diet, and risk of colon cancer in Utah. Am J Epidemiol 128:989–999

Subar AF, Kipnis V, Troiano RP, Midthune D, Schoeller DA, Bingham S, Sharbaugh CO, Trabulsi J, Runswick S, Ballard-Barbash R, Sunshine J, Schatzkin A (2003) Using intake biomarkers to evaluate the extent of dietary misreporting in a large sample of adults: the OPEN study. Am J Epidemiol 158:1–13

Subcommittee on Criteria for Dietary Evaluation (1986) Nutrient adequacy: Assessment using food consumption surveys. National Academy Press, Washington DC (http://www.nap.edu/books/0309036348/html) Accessed April 29, 2004

The Scientific Committee for Food (1993) Nutrient and energy intakes for the European Community. Thirty-first series: Food – science and techniques series. Office for Official Publications of the European Communities, Luxembourg (http://europa.eu.int/comm/food/fs/sc/scf/reports_en.html) Accessed April 30, 2004

Truswell AS, Dreosti IE, English RM, Palmer N, Rutishauser IHE (eds) (1990) Recommended nutrient intakes. Australian papers. Australian Professional Publications, Mosman

Vickers AJ, Altman DG (2001) Analysing controlled trials with baseline and follow-up measurements. BMJ 323:1123–1124

Walker AM, Blettner M (1985) Comparing imperfect measures of exposure. Am J Epidemiol 121:783–790

Willett WC (1995) Diet, nutrition, and avoidable cancer. Environ Health Perspect 103(suppl 8):165–170

Willett WC (1998) Nutritional epidemiology. Oxford University Press, New York

Willett WC, Stampfer MJ (1986) Total energy intake: implications for epidemiologic analyses. Am J Epidemiol 124:17–27

Willett WC, Stampfer MJ (1987) The authors reply. (Letter) Am J Epidemiol 126:982–983

Willett WC, Stampfer MJ, Colditz GA, Rosner BA, Hennekens CH, Speizer FE (1987) Dietary fat and the risk of breast cancer. N Engl J Med 316:22–28

Reproductive Epidemiology   III.5

Jørn Olsen, Olga Basso

Introduction

Reproductive Epidemiology: Reading Instructions

In writing this chapter we assumed that the reader is familiar with the basic concepts in epidemiology. You will not find any overview of different designs, measure of disease occurrence, standardisations, other ways of adjusting for confounders, or any general discussion on bias, confounding or on measuring effects. If you are not familiar with these topics you should start by reading other parts of the book or turn to one of the many fine available textbooks.

Our intent is to point out the problems and methods that are of particular interest in reproductive epidemiology and the areas that are perhaps peculiar to this field of epidemiology.

We focus upon methodology and, for the most part, we avoid reporting on any 'state of the art' overview on what is known about specific exposures or endpoints. Such reviews are soon outdated and, furthermore, space does not permit them.

By focusing upon some of the aspects that set reproductive epidemiology somewhat apart from other areas of epidemiology, we hope to alert readers to the problems and options that this field presents and to illustrate how important it is to develop a highly critical outlook. Research in reproductive epidemiology, like research in general, is not to prove or confirm anything, but rather to question and make critical appraises.

We use references to illustrate specific problems of methodological interest. We use more of our own work than could ever be justified on the basis of our modest contribution to the field. Our excuse is that these references reflect our source of information for learning about the many problems inherent to reproductive epidemiology. We cannot rule out that they also reflect our inflated egos. Most of the references we have selected present information of methodological relevance. We also provide references to full textbooks in reproductive epidemiology.

We do not in any way claim to provide a complete list of problems, which you should be aware of as a student of reproductive epidemiology. We do not know all these problems ourselves: some are yet to be described and some have not yet caught our attention. Even describing all the specific problems that we are aware of would require more space than you, the reader, would like us to have. What we have tried to do is to describe the most important problems as we see them. Our choice is a subjective one, reflecting our experience.

Reproductive health was defined by the WHO at the Cairo conference in 1994 as:

> … a state of complete physical, mental and social well-being and not merely the absence of disease or infirmity, in all matters relating to the reproductive system and its functions and processes.
>
> Reproductive Health, therefore, implies that people are able to have a satisfying and safe sex life and that they have the capability to reproduce and the

freedom to decide if, when, and how often to do so. It also includes sexual health, the purpose of which is the enhancement of life and personal relationships, and not merely counselling and care related to reproductive and sexually transmitted diseases.

We do not intend to cover all the possible topics related to this definition, nor do we intend to provide research methods for studying well-being or even happiness. We will limit our focus to the more traditional domain of epidemiology, namely to the studies of determinants of diseases directly related to reproduction, as long as these studies can be applied to human populations. Although many diseases will have an effect on procreation through biological, psychological or social mechanisms, we will restrict ourselves to studies dealing with fecundity, pregnancy, birth, and early markers of child health. Many of the diseases we describe only manifest themselves in the time period of reproduction; such as subfecundity, pre-eclampsia and, of course, all the diseases related to the child.

Our experience mainly stems from research in Europe and the USA, and we do not cover research problems of particular relevance to developing countries. Since reproductive health problems are usually larger in these countries, we are aware that this is a major shortcoming, and our only excuse is our limited experience in this field. We do want to stress, however, that research in developing parts of the world should also be based upon sound methods. We do not believe in low quality research anywhere, but we accept that circumstances may set limitations for what can be done.

Many diseases of the reproductive organs, like cancer or infections, may have an effect on reproduction if the diseases appear before or during reproductive age. In most cases, studying the determinants of these diseases will be similar to studying determinants of other diseases and, as such, they are not pertinent to the analysis in this chapter.

Our aim is not to provide a cookbook for research in reproductive health. Our aim is only to make the reader aware of the aspects he or she should be concerned about. Associations come in many shapes, and they are not always what they pretend to be. 'Be careful' is the main (and perhaps the only) message we want to convey, and if you are happy with that you could stop here – if you want to know why you should be careful, please go on reading. We expect you to disagree on several occasions. Remember, you may be right and we may be wrong.

Reproductive Health – Specific Epidemiologic Research Problems

5.1.2

Unlike epidemiologists studying cancer and chronic diseases, reproductive epidemiologists deal with an area that has been shaped by evolution. Selective forces operate before and during pregnancy, even in the highly medicalized industrialized world; keeping this feature in mind when dealing with reproductive epidemiology is important when trying to understand events that occur in pregnancy.

Most epidemiologists deal with identifying determinants of diseases, which might operate over time spans of varying length. The induction periods may be very short (e.g. is a migraine attack triggered by a given nutritional component?) or may span many years (e.g. does prenatal exposure to smoking affect semen quality?) In reproductive health we study determinants of factors that play a role for successful reproduction. Sometimes this involves studies that span generations, and many studies address couples, or families, rather than individuals. Unlike other fields of epidemiology, the individuals studied in reproductive epidemiology are often not ill in the common meaning of the word. Women who have repeated abortions or give birth to dead or severely malformed children are usually healthy themselves, and so are their partners. Similarly, even women who become severely ill during pregnancy, for instance with pre-eclampsia, often fully recover if the pregnancy has been interrupted in time. Their risk of experiencing pre-eclampsia in their next pregnancy is, however, relatively high.

In many cases, reproductive epidemiology deals with hidden phenomena that may represent serious disorders, which, however, may never come to light if a woman does not become pregnant. Furthermore, many women experience several pregnancies in their lifetime, so that a pregnancy rather than an individual will be the unit of analysis. All these elements intrinsic to reproduction provide interesting design options and challenging methodological problems, and they set reproductive epidemiology somewhat apart from other areas of epidemiology.

Successful reproduction in evolutionary terms means that the parents' genes are transferred to viable offspring, who will, eventually, produce offspring of their own. Part of this process is subject to epidemiologic observation. Although the maternal and paternal evolutionary interests are similar as far as gene transmission is concerned, the mother plays an additional role. She provides not only half of the foetal genes, but also the environment in which the foetus develops and is nourished over the duration of pregnancy and, in many cases, also for a period of time after birth (through breastfeeding). Pregnancy can be life threatening for the mother, and it is estimated that in Africa the lifetime risk for a woman to die of pregnancy-related causes is 1 in 16, while in more developed countries this figure is 1 in 1800 or even lower (AbouZahr 1998). Situations may thus occur when a pregnancy, which is too costly, is interrupted for the sake of the mother's chance of reproducing again (Haig 1993). The uterine environment's role is therefore of great importance, but it is often difficult to disentangle its effects from those that are genetically mediated by the mother. Sometimes it is the interaction between foetal and maternal genes that may trigger adverse outcomes, such as recurrent spontaneous abortions. Reproductive epidemiology has acquired a powerful tool with the new genetic technologies. Using these tools will, hopefully, provide new important clues on the complex events taking place from conception to birth and onwards.

Most of the time, we can only obtain data on deliveries or abortions (and usually only on abortions of clinically recognised pregnancies, thus missing the early ones) and most of the processes leading to these events are hidden or altogether absent from the data we have access to. We thus have to take into consideration what potentials for errors this entails.

The time period of reproduction is short within a life span in most countries, and it is under intensive surveillance. What we are able to study is often the causal links that remain after health care providers have tried to prevent negative outcomes. Data on births and, sometimes, spontaneous abortions are routinely collected in several countries at national levels following standardised procedures, therefore allowing comparisons over time and place on some occasions. In some countries, at least part of the data are computerised and thus of relatively easy access to epidemiologists. Most countries produce reports of some indicators of reproductive health at regular intervals.

Reproductive health, at least the part associated with pregnancy and childbirth, covers events that are often frequent and serious, such as infertility, spontaneous abortions, preterm birth, and pre-eclampsia. Events that we would rather prevent than treat, and most are willing to accept that prevention must be based upon research of good quality. We not only need to identify determinants of reproductive failures connected to lifestyle, occupation, environment, diet, or medication, but also to find out how antenatal care (ANC) can be best organized. Antenatal care is, in many countries, the most expensive part of preventive care within the health care system. At present, only a limited part of ANC is evidence-based and much more research is still needed, especially in countries where resources are sparse. Much of this documentation has to be time- and place-specific. Evidence on health care technology cannot just be transferred from one country to another. But many of the findings related to causation will apply to most populations. Treatment effects may also be non-particularistic in some situations.

By developing more and more efficient contraceptive methods and, especially, by producing more and more sophisticated methods for treating infertility, we are increasingly interfering with the forces of evolution. We should make it one of the priorities of reproductive epidemiology to study whether and to what extent these factors will affect future generations. Reproduction is, in many ways, a playground for new technologies that are being introduced without much concern for the long-term consequences. Children of in vitro fertilization (IVF) are still too young for us to study whether they may suffer any long-term health consequence associated with the mode of their conception. Interventions like intracytoplasmic sperm injection (ICSI) may undermine the very core of the natural selective forces behind reproduction. At present we do not know if ICSI is a safe assisted reproductive technology (Ludwig and Diedrich 2002), although early reports are reassuring to some extent.

Trying to solve health problems for some may introduce health problems for others, especially in reproductive health related to treatment of infertility. Some of those health problems may never come to the attention of the treating physician and must be disentangled by research. In relation to this and many other technologies, epidemiologists have an important role to play in monitoring disease data over time in the population. Reproductive health should be an important part of any health surveillance system.

It is peculiar to reproduction that during pregnancy the mother provides most of the exposures that may influence the future health of the unborn child. The foetus is only partly protected by the placental barrier. Many toxic substances pass this barrier and the developing foetus will often be less able than the mother to metabolise these substances, especially early in pregnancy. This is e.g. the case with alcohol, caffeine, and several drugs.

Thus, another important feature of reproductive epidemiology is that not just one individual is involved in the process under study, but three: the mother, the father (through foetal genes and, possibly, substances carried by semen) (Savitz et al. 1994), and the foetus itself through its continuing interaction with the mother during the pregnancy period. When studying reproductive outcomes it is, in many cases, insufficient to focus only on the mother, although she usually represents the most accessible player.

It is now known that during pregnancy and delivery there is a two-way traffic of cells between the mother and the foetus, and that these cells can persist in the bloodstream for decades (Bianchi et al. 1996). This phenomenon, called 'microchimerism', is a quickly developing area of research, as it is suspected that these cells may interfere with the immune system and thus contribute to the aetiology of several diseases, especially those of autoimmune origin (Bianchi 2000; Whitacre et al. 1999). That pregnancy itself, or phenomena related to pregnancy, might have something to do with the aetiology of these diseases is suggested by the fact that females are more subject to autoimmune diseases than males, although these differences may also depend on immunological, hormonal, or other factors that are related to sex but not specifically to pregnancy (Whitacre et al. 1999; Whitacre 2001). Changes in physiological status during pregnancy may have health implications for the mother as well as for the child, and the growing foetus totally depends upon maternal supply of nutrition and oxygen. Changes in this supply may 'reprogramme' organ development with possible long-term health consequences (Barker 1994).

Pregnancies as Repeated Events: Problems and Design Options

5.1.3

Each pregnancy provides a new set of observations and, in populations with a high fertility, a woman may be subject to repeated studies of exposures of interest for the outcome of each pregnancy. A pregnancy is a new event that, at the same time, is correlated with the previous pregnancy/ies. Most reproductive failures (such as spontaneous abortions, preterm delivery, pre-eclampsia, etc.) have a tendency to repeat themselves because time-stable causes (e.g. genes or part of the maternal environment) are present during all events. However, it is not clear how this aspect should be taken into consideration when analysing data.

In animal studies, the variance within a litter and between litters is dealt with separately, probably even successfully, in the statistical analysis, but the situation is different for humans. Human births are usually sequential, except for multifoetal pregnancies, which, however, are relatively rare and often not comparable to single pregnancies. Methods have been developed to take into account the statistical dependence resulting from women contributing more than one pregnancy (Hoffman et al. 2001), but we have limited confidence in these methods (Olsen and Andersen 1998).

Each new pregnancy has a number of features in common with the previous pregnancy, and a number of features that are unique to it. In some situations, each new pregnancy is an independent event and should be treated as such, but the contrary argument can be made as well. However, even if the dependency between pregnancies were to be modelled in the analysis, it is not clear whether doing this would produce a different type of bias, because the statistical model will not take selective change in behaviours related to pregnancy history into consideration. Pregnancies are, in many cases, planned as a function of the outcome of a previous pregnancy, and this aspect can hardly be addressed by methods aimed at accounting for the statistical dependency between pregnancies. An unwanted abortion or a stillbirth may be replaced very shortly with a new pregnancy in order to have the desired child. A surviving child with severe handicaps may delay or stop further childbearing, while parents of a child that dies with the same handicap may attempt a new pregnancy soon. Some exposures will be avoided as a result of how previous pregnancy ended. A mother who is a heavy smoker and had a child with a very low birth weight may well give up smoking when she becomes pregnant again, even in situations where smoking was not the only or even the major cause of the low birth weight. If smoking was not the only cause of low birth weight, she may then become a non-smoking pregnant woman with a high a-priori risk of getting a child with a low birth weight. How should that be addressed in the statistical analysis? Or how would we be able to design a proper counterfactual comparison? This type of confounding by the risk that triggers a change in exposure is very difficult to rule out, and it is a common and often neglected problem. A valid analytical solution may be to study first pregnancies only (Olsen 1994), but this approach may prove to be too conservative in the sense that it removes available information and will thus reduce statistical power. Furthermore, there is heterogeneity on outcomes depending on parity, some of which may be due to selection (not all women will be able – or want – to have a new pregnancy), others probably depend on physiology or on changes in the uterine environment brought about by the previous pregnancy/ies. A first pregnancy modifies the uterine arteries in such a way that placentation is facilitated in the successive pregnancies.

When studying the effect of a given determinant on an adverse reproductive outcome, one may be tempted to stratify on (or adjust for) a previous occurrence of that outcome (e.g. spontaneous abortion). Such a temptation should be resisted if the intent is to study aetiology, since adjustment for any factor that is caused in part by the exposure under study and is also correlated with the outcome will likely bias the estimate (Weinberg 1993). If the intent is purely descriptive, however, this approach is acceptable.

Beyond the difficulties and traps caused by the fact that women have more than one pregnancy, however, this feature also provides reproductive epidemiologists with a powerful tool that is unique to this discipline. Many reproductive outcomes tend to recur in different pregnancies of the same woman, and this provides the opportunity to examine whether some putative factors play a role in the aetiology of a given event by studying women who had the outcome in question in a pregnancy and estimating whether their recurrence risk changes accordingly as a function of a change in a given factor in between the two pregnancies (Olsen et al. 1997). This design, which we called 'the computerized square dance design', makes it possible to estimate whether the paternal genome plays a role by studying maternal half siblings. It can be applied to reproductive failures as well as disorders occurring in early childhood, such as febrile seizures (Vestergaard et al. 2002). One of the advantages of this approach is that a great deal of confounding is adjusted for by using the woman as her own control. One aspect that has to be taken into consideration is that time plays a role, and thus the interval between pregnancies may have to be taken into account, especially when studying the effect of changing partners, since women who change partner tend to have a much longer interpregnancy interval (Basso et al. 2001; Skjaerven et al. 2002).

The Problem of Incomplete Denominators

Ideally, we would like to be able to study the outcome of all conceptions that take place in a given population in a given time period, in order to be able to observe how many end in very early losses, how was the karyotype of the lost foetuses, their sex ratio, etc. Less ideally, we would like to be able to obtain information on all conceptions surviving the first 8 weeks of gestation, because missing them may lead to serious bias in studies examining specific exposures. In many instances, reproductive epidemiologists work with incomplete denominators.

Spontaneous Abortions

A frequent outcome of a pregnancy, spontaneous abortion, is probably to a large extent part of nature's own quality control system (Quenby et al. 2002). Some spontaneous abortions are, however, man-made and could in principle be avoided if their causes were identified. Some abortions occur in the pre-clinical phase, before the pregnancy is recognised, while others occur after the pregnancy is recognised. The timing of observation thus becomes of crucial importance.

The best approach would be to start observation before conception, but this requires access to women who plan their pregnancies (Wilcox et al. 1988). Pregnancy planners are likely to include an excess of subfecund women (women with a low probability per cycle of conceiving), as women who become pregnant as a result of contraceptive failures are less often subfecund. Participating women may thus be at higher risk of a number of adverse outcomes, since subfecundity is correlated with several reproductive failures (Basso et al. 2003).

Currently, few investigators have attempted to detect pregnancies by using biomarkers (usually hCG, human chorionic gonadotropin). These studies (Wilcox et al. 1988; Bonde et al. 1998a, b) do not tell us how frequent abortions really are, but they suggest that at least 30% of conceptions end as spontaneous abortions and that a little more than half of these occur in the pre-clinical phase.

An exposure that only delays abortions without increasing their incidence would appear as a risk factor in a study based exclusively upon recognised pregnancies. Such an exposure may move an abortion from the preclinical phase to the detectable phase. Exposures that advance the time of abortions would appear to prevent the occurrence of abortions. Such an exposure would produce a low abortion rate because abortions now would occur in the pre-clinical phase. For this reason, the timing of pregnancy diagnosing is important. If women who take a long time to become pregnant seek earlier confirmation of pregnancy (compared to women who have not waited a long time), they will also be aware of early losses that would not be detected by women who were not aware that they were pregnant. This type of bias may be partly responsible for the association between subfecundity and spontaneous abortion, where good quality data on early conceptions are available (Baird et al. 1993). The use of early pregnancy tests may play a role in analysing and interpreting data from studies based upon pregnancy planners. Such studies are difficult and expensive to conduct and require a very cooperative study population.

If you study environmental determinants of abortions, you may like to exclude 'habitual aborters' – women who will abort any pregnancy no matter what. Such women will not provide information related to risk following the exposure (Gladen 1986; Weinberg et al. 1994b). The problem is that these habitual aborters can only be identified by their abortion history and thus cannot be identified at all if they have no pregnancy history at all. Stratifying results on pregnancy number can distort associations, since only some of the women with many abortions will be habitual aborters. Some will abort due to chance and some will abort due to the exposure under study.

Measuring Infertility

When we are interested in measuring the biological component of fertility, called fecundity, we are often able to ask pregnant couples how long it took them to become pregnant. While doing that we also need to identify planned pregnancies, which may be difficult since planning is often not a well defined concept. We also need to find a way to deal with couples who had not planned their pregnancy as well as with those who became pregnant despite using contraception. Their underlying fecundity may differ from that of couples who plan a pregnancy. We would also like to have information on all couples that conceived and had an early pregnancy loss (Jensen et al. 1998) or failed to conceive because they were sterile or gave up trying for any reason. When studying time to pregnancy in samples of pregnant women, one must be reasonably confident that giving up a pregnancy attempt is completely independent of the putative risk factors under study, a condition similar to what we encounter when working with censored data in general (Basso et al. 2001).

Congenital Malformations

Congenital malformations are relatively frequent and they constitute a major cause of infant mortality and morbidity. They are also a very stressful event for the involved families, making it difficult to get comparable information in a case-control study addressing determinants of congenital malformation.

It is now well accepted that congenital malformations are usually measured as a prevalence at the time of birth. The incidence of congenital malformations is normally not available for study, given that it is a function of new events since time of conception. Congenital malformations that occur in utero and end as abortions, some as very early abortions, are usually not detected. Some exposures may simultaneously increase the incidence of some congenital malformations while at the same time reducing the survival rate of the affected foetuses (or embryos) in utero, thus decreasing the prevalence at birth. Monitoring systems of congenital malformations with no data on spontaneous abortions could therefore miss important teratogens and even wrongly conclude that a given factor is protective. Many of the established monitoring systems on the possible teratogenic effects of medicines taken during pregnancy are based only on data on prevalence at birth. When dealing with spontaneous abortions and congenital malformations, missing early losses may lead us to biased effects measures. Many of the routine monitoring systems are furthermore of poor quality, partly because only some of the congenital malformations are visible at birth. Heart defects may e.g. only produce symptoms – and thus first surface to clinical detection – under extreme physical strain late in life (Knox et al. 1984).

Time Matters

If you were a student of mortality you would know that the question is not *if* people die, but *when* they die. Mortality rates (MR) reflect this time function, as 1/MR is the life expectancy in the same time unit as the rate is measured, given that a number of conditions are fulfilled. All estimates of risks come with a time tag. The estimate depends upon the length of time it represents. Time is underlying all occurrence research, even when it is not explicitly mentioned. All events happen in time. If you do not wake up in the morning (or later), it is because you are dead. You ran out of time.

In reproductive health, time is important from several points of view, not only as the time from exposure to the endpoint of interest. The timing of exposure itself is more important in this area than in most others. Specific windows of vulnerability open and close over the time of gestation. The time of organogenesis and organ development plays a crucial role. The time periods of interest may even date back generations. Not only may malformations of genital organs impair reproduction, but also the number of Sertoli cells is at least partly determined in foetal life and this has implications for sperm production lasting decades into adult life (Sharpe and Skakkebaek 1993; Wilcox et al. 1995). Organ development is under the influence of hormonal factors that operate at certain time periods. Fetotoxic exposures may have different outcomes as a function of the timing of exposure, and growth-determining factors may only play a role during a time period of rapid foetal growth.

The time period of spermatogenesis and ovulation may be under the influence of external exposures and genetic factors. Factors that reduce the sexual libido affect quality of life at any time but have consequences for reproduction only if present during the time window of procreation.

Soon after conception, the risk of abortion is high, but we know very little about the determinants of early abortions. Avoidable abortions probably depend to a great extent on the timing of the exposure that causes the abortion, but this time period may be difficult to identify, partly because foetal death need not coincide with the expulsion of foetal tissue. Fever could e.g. appear to be a cause of spontaneous abortion (Andersen et al. 2002), because fever may be induced by dead foetal tissue. In that case, the association would be from foetal death to fever and not from fever to foetal death (reverse causation). However, Andersen et al. did not find that fever was associated with spontaneous abortions.

It is a point of fact that the period at risk for teratogenic actions (usually the second and third months of gestation) is almost over when antenatal care (ANC) begins. All legal actions taken to reduce e.g. occupational exposures during pregnancy are usually put into operation too late. Some types of prevention (like the use of folic acid to prevent neural tube defects) need to be activated even before the pregnancy is planned. If a given toxicant (such as lead) is stored in the maternal tissue over a long period of time, its mobilization during pregnancy may affect the mother or the embryo many years after the exposure took place (Rothenberg et al. 2002).

It is possible, perhaps even likely, that relevant exposure windows for specific effects are only open during short time periods. Exposure to influenza virus has e.g. been associated with schizophrenia in the offspring, but only for infections during the second trimester of pregnancy (Mednick et al. 1994). On the other hand, neurotoxic exposures may influence brain development, if they operate at the time of the vulnerable structural changes that take place throughout foetal life and in early childhood. It is possible that diseases like ADHD (Attention Deficit and Hyperactive Disorders), autism or Tourette's syndrome have a pre- or perinatal aetiology (Linnet et al. 2004).

The nutritional demand of the foetus is at its maximum in late gestation, when foetal growth is rapid. Smoking in this period is much more closely associated with low birth weight than smoking early in pregnancy (Smoking or Health 1977).

The Dutch famine study indicated that the timing of under-nutrition during gestation played an important role for later health outcomes (Susser and Stein 1994). Being exposed to undernutrition in the last trimester was associated with obesity later in life (Ravelli et al. 1976).

Most side effects of drugs taken during pregnancy depend heavily on the timing of the drug intake within the gestational period. This is true not only for teratogenic effects. Drugs are particularly difficult to study as an exposure, because the effect of the drugs may not always be easily discerned from the effect of the indication for taking the drug in the first place (what is usually termed 'confounding by indication') (Olsen et al. 2002). If two or more drugs with the same indication but different active molecules are available and are prescribed to pregnant women independently of the severity of the indication, this may provide useful options for better characterizing the effects related to one of these drugs.

The foetal alcohol syndrome (FAS) is characterised by specific facial characteristics, low birth weight, and cognitive impairment. It is likely that these impairments are the result of time specific exposures and, if so, binge drinking may be of concern, even binge drinking among low or moderate alcohol drinkers. Still, no studies in humans have shown that binge drinking alone causes cognitive impairments or any other important FAS characteristics, perhaps because all studies have been too small. If the exposure window is short, then only a small fraction of binge drinkers will be at risk and small studies will thus have no power to detect an effect unless all the study subjects are exposed at the right gestational time. FAS is seen in children of some women, who drink large amounts of alcohol every day. A high daily intake leads to exposure during the time periods of vulnerability, regardless of their duration.

Exposure to mercury, determined on the basis of amounts found in umbilical cord blood at birth, has been associated with impaired cognitive functions (Grandjean et al. 1997). An umbilical cord measurement reflects an average exposure throughout gestation and, as such, it does not indicate whether certain time periods are more vulnerable than others.

Hormonal factors play a profound role in foetal life. Sexual hormones are e.g. needed for a foetus to develop a male phenotype. It is furthermore believed that hormonal factors influence the probability of developing some diseases in adult life. For example, it has been suggested that a high intrauterine oestrogen level may modify breast cancer risk (Trichopoulos 1990) and reduce the number of Sertoli cells, thus subsequently reducing semen production and increase the risk of undescended testis, hypospadia and testis cancer. This latter hypothesis is, however, not corroborated by epidemiologic findings in general and it probably has to be modified to fit existing data (Strohsnitter et al. 2001). There is, on the other hand, clear evidence of an association between some of these diseases. Patients with testis cancer have a higher frequency of undescended testis and apparently a lower fecundity before the cancer is diagnosed (Jacobsen et al. 2000) Macro-epidemiologic (ecologic) studies furthermore show that the geographical variation in e.g. testis cancer is often followed by similar geographical variations in low sperm counts and a high prevalence of malformations of the male genitalia. The link between testis cancer and undescended testis is considered established, although most studies have been based upon self-report of undescended testis, often reported retrospectively. Many undescended testis descend spontaneously shortly after birth or at puberty. More recent studies based upon recording at birth show a weaker association between testis cancer and undescended testis (Stang et al. 2001; Sabroe and Olsen 1998). It is possible that only persistent undescended testis correlate with the risk of testis cancer. It is unclear whether descent through treatment eliminates the risk or whether the risk is caused by the underlying reasons of the displacement itself. If the risk is a function of underlying hormonal disturbances at the time period of organogenesis, treatment is not expected to affect cancer risk.

Single peak exposures to drugs are seen in pregnant women who try to commit suicide by taking an overdose of medicine. In principle, these studies provide unique data for studying the fetotoxic effects of these drugs, since they often bypass confounding by indication (unless the study concerns anti-depressant drugs). Many of these studies, however, have not taken abortions (induced or spontaneous) into consideration and have often been too small to detect teratogenic effects, since such studies must focus upon suicide attempts in specific and short time periods. Furthermore, many women terminate their pregnancy after a suicide attempt because of fear of a fetotoxic effect or because of their inability to cope with a pregnancy. Newborn children available for this type of study are thus few and, to some extent, selected. Most of the findings from these studies have been reassuring, indicating that healthy babies are often born after a single exposure to some specific drug (Flint et al. 2002).

Although it is generally accepted that timing is of crucial importance for most outcomes of pregnancy, many studies rely on exposures where the timing is not specified. Many studies that make use of retrospective data from pregnancies and exposures are thus difficult to place in time, when they took place months or years before reporting. Large cohort studies have been started or are being planned in order to provide researchers with prospective data on exposures (Olsen et al. 2001).

5.2   The Case-Parent-Triad Design

There are several design options for studying genetic risk factors. Most of these are described in Chaps. I.7, III.6 and III.7 of this handbook. One of these designs is, however, of particular interest in reproductive epidemiology, namely the case-parent-triad design. The idea is to use parents of affected children to serve as genetic controls. Case-control studies may easily be confounded by genetic factors when they are applied to populations with a mixture of different ethnic groups. The parents are by definition ethnically matched to the case, and they are furthermore usually motivated to take part in the study. The two non-transmitted parental alleles can be compared to the two transmitted alleles, and since this Mendelian transmission occurs at random the observed allele structure can be compared with the expected values. If the parents e.g. both have the allele structure Aa, the children will under Mendelian transmission be AA, Aa, Aa or aa with equal probabilities; 25% probability of AA and aa, respectively, and 50% of Aa.

If the genotype is associated with the disease under study, affected children will have an allele distribution that deviates from these expected values. All this may be analysed using well-known log-linear models (Weinberg et al. 1998). The main limitation in using this design for diseases with an adult onset is that the assumption of non-selective survival of the parents to the time of the study is a strong assumption, at least for severe diseases. For diseases with an early onset the assumption will usually be fulfilled. Using this design in e.g. studying genetic causes of congenital malformations is an attractive option. The parents will be available, motivated, and present in a setting where a blood sample can easily be taken at any time.

Infertility and Subfecundity

5.3

Measures Used to Describe Fertility

5.3.1

The fertility rate is defined as the number of live births a woman has during her reproductive life. A fertility rate of 1.3 means that in a population of 100 women there will be, on average, 130 liveborn children – not enough to replace their parents. A fertility rate of more than 2.0 is needed to bring the population into a steady state. How much more depends upon the life expectancy and the sex ratio of the newborn children in the population. On average, one woman should produce one girl who survives until her reproduction age in order to bring the population to a steady state if life expectancy is stable over time.

Fertility is determined by both a biological capacity to reproduce (fecundity) and the desire for a given family size, which may be under the influence of social and cultural conditions broadly defined, and methods available for family planning play, of course, a crucial role. Fertility is a term used by demographers to describe the actual production of live children, whereas infertility is used by the medical profession to describe a reduced biological capacity to reproduce. This dual use of the same terminology is confusing. The best would be to let fertility (and infertility) be reserved for demographers to indicate de facto reproduction.

We suggest the term fecundity to be used as a broad term to describe the biological capacity to reproduce, and fecundability (the probability of conceiving within a given menstrual cycle) to be a quantitative estimate of fecundity. Unlike Cramer and Goldman (1994), we propose to let the more specific details of the terms be defined in the actual study in order not to have too many words describing rather similar conditions. Reproduction, in its historical form, requires sexual contact, fertilisation, implantation, and survival until the age of reproduction. Now alternative methods exist.

Most studies use a recognised pregnancy (or birth) as the endpoint, and recognition of pregnancy usually depends upon clinical or biochemical measures. Fecundity could therefore, depending on the specific study, describe the ability to obtain a biochemically detected pregnancy (by means of hCG), a clinically recognised pregnancy, or a pregnancy that led to a liveborn child. Fecundity can thus be used to describe the capacity to achieve any of these endpoints, which may be confusing. On the other hand, having a specific term for each of these situations would complicate communication to an even larger extent. The fact that we use the term fecundity to refer to a variety of situations has to be kept in mind.

Childlessness can be voluntary or involuntary, and the latter may be subject to epidemiologic research. Subfecundity is a frequent problem, and treatment for subfecundity is a rapidly growing sector of many health care systems. Research that can potentially lead to prevention of subfecundity is therefore receiving increasing attention, and epidemiology plays an important part in this research. Subfecundity is a measure for a couple and is defined on the basis of unsuccessful attempts for a given length of time (usually 6, 12, or 24 months). In many industrialised countries, about 15% of all couples that try to become pregnant will experience subfecundity, if this is defined as a waiting time of 12 months (Juul et al. 1999). The term infertility usually describes an unsuccessful waiting time of 12 or 24 months. Often the cut-point of 12 months is used in affluent societies and 24 months in countries with limited health care resources.

Sterility is defined as an absent capacity to reproduce – a fecundability of 0. Since most couples' probability of conceiving is very rarely 0, many women will eventually become pregnant, if they keep trying, even when on an ineffective treatment.

Time to Pregnancy

If a normal fecundability is 0.25, then 3% of normal couples will not succeed within 12 months of trying $((1-0.25)^{12})$ just because of bad luck. These couples need no treatment, but may (and some will) be treated nonetheless, usually with an 'excellent prognosis' (25% success rate for each cycle). The remaining 12% would be the proper candidates for treatment. If all couples who wait unsuccessfully for 12 months or more to become pregnant receive treatment, then any treatment will to some degree be a success. Some couples will have normal fecundity, and some will have subnormal fecundity without being sterile. An effective treatment has to demonstrate better performance than chance alone would produce.

If a couple is defined as subfecund after an unsuccessful waiting time of 24 months, then only about 0.1% of 'normal' couples will meet the definition, and those targeted for treatment will include 99.9% of actually subfecund couples. For this reason, less affluent societies do not start infertility treatment until couples have tried for at least 24 months.

Since fecundability is related to the duration of a waiting time to pregnancy (TTP), TTP is a frequently used measure in subfecundity research. The measure was first used by demographers when they examined the time from marriage to the first liveborn child; in this context, TTP is a measure that only has biological relevance in societies where procreation starts with marriage and contraception is not practiced.

In societies with a higher degree of family planning, TTP (now defined as the number of cycles that a couple take from the moment they first start trying to when they actually conceive a clinically recognised pregnancy) becomes a useful tool in the study of determinants of subfecundity. It has been used in epidemiology since the early 1980s (Rachootin and Olsen 1982, 1983; Olsen et al. 1983; Baird et al. 1986). It appears that women are able to recall with sufficient accuracy how long they took to conceive, even after several years (Joffe et al. 1993; 1995). Time to pregnancy is easy to use and, perhaps for this very reason, has undoubtedly been used too frequently without proper concern for its shortcomings and pitfalls.

Design Options in Studies of TTP   5.3.2

The best option is to study TTP in a longitudinal design that starts when couples stop using contraception in order to conceive (starting time). Exposures of interest can then be recorded independently of the length of TTP and at the relevant point in time. They can also be registered for attempts that do not lead to a pregnancy. Studies that rely on exposures recorded at the time of pregnancy rather than the starting time may produce biased results, especially for exposures suspected to cause infertility. If smokers stop smoking after having tried in vain to become pregnant for a certain time period, but not if they conceive quickly, smoking recorded during pregnancy will correlate with a short waiting time, as if smoking prevented subfecundity. In fact, almost all evidence points towards the opposite assessment: smoking impairs fecundity, especially in women (Rachootin and Olsen 1983; Baird and Wilcox 1985; Bolumar et al. 1996; Alderete et al. 1995).

The proportion of couples that become pregnant during the 1st cycle is an estimate of the fecundability rate in the population. The entire TTP distribution will, however, normally be used in the analysis, e.g. in a discrete Cox model. Such a study need not last 12 or 24 months. Even a study with a follow-up time of only one cycle could provide evidence that smoking women have, on average, a fecundability that is approximately 20% lower than that of non-smoking women. We would then e.g. expect 30 out of 100 non-smoking women to be pregnant within the first cycle versus 24 out of 100 smoking women. Exclusion criteria may be used to get rid of non-informative couples in the study of environmental causes of sub-fecundity. Sexual activity could be recorded and taken into consideration in the analysis as well as time of pregnancy detection. Such a study is straightforward to design and to analyse, but extremely difficult and expensive to carry out, unless it is based upon couples that are seeking treatment for infertility, like IVF patients. Results from infertility patients are, however, hampered by limited generalizability to the population at large, partly because the couples are highly selected, partly because of the forces of clinical selection that are being used. Spermatozoa, eggs, and fertilised eggs are selected by the health personnel according to criteria quite different from the 'natural' selection. A longitudinal study on pregnancy planners may also provide other related endpoints, such as information on early abortions or semen quality.

Epidemiologists have looked for less expensive designs than the concurrent follow-up of pregnancy planners. These designs have mainly been population based cross-sectional studies or designs based upon samples from pregnant women, both of which are prone to a number of problems.

Cross-sectional surveys rest upon the assumption that women recall their TTP with some accuracy even a long time after the event. In a survey, the selected women will try to record attempts to become pregnant, exposures of relevance – often from the same time period – infertility treatment, and TTP (or time waited in unsuccessful pregnancy attempts). Population studies of this type are relatively inexpensive and they usually rest on random sampling principles. The main problem is accurate recall, especially of exposures at the relevant point in time (the starting time), and the ability to obtain response rates that do not introduce selection bias. Analysing data may be simple, although TTPs usually have to be recorded in quite broad categories, and often referring to months rather than to cycles. Women may be able to recall if they had to wait for 6, 12 or more months to become pregnant, but usually they will not be able to remember if they became pregnant after 5, 6 or 7 months of waiting time when that waiting time took place several years ago. (They will probably remember if they became pregnant in the first month of trying.) Digit preference also has to be taken into consideration, as clusters of reporting will be seen at specific waiting times (such as 6 or 12 months).

Using pregnant women in data collections has, for obvious reasons, been a convenient design. In most countries, pregnant women are easy to locate and to contact. They are usually more willing to take part in studies than other women, and they are usually able to accurately report their TTP if the pregnancy was planned. They usually remember when planning started, and may be able to recall the exposures around the starting time, at least if the planning did not start too long ago, or if the exposure refers to the occupation they held at the time, or whether they were smoking or not. Since pregnancy is a condition for participation in the study, this design is unable to pick up an all-or-none effect of an exposure. An exposure that causes sterility will not be identified in a sample of pregnant women. Fortunately, most exposures that we know of are not of this type, and the exposures that reduce fecundability will show a longer TTP in a pregnancy-based study. The qualitative effect measure that comes from a study of this kind is, however, not a measure of fecundability in itself (Olsen and Andersen 1999), although it will correlate with fecundability under a number of conditions. The most important, and often neglected, of these conditions is the persistency in trying to become pregnant. This persistency should not be related to the exposure under study, because, if so, the exposure may falsely appear to increase fecundity (Basso et al. 2000b). The timing of diagnosing a pregnancy also plays a role. If couples wait very long to have a pregnancy verified, then an early abortion may count as waiting time. Had they used a sensitive pregnancy test early, the event would have been recognized as a TTP of a given length followed by an abortion. The length of the waiting time may influence the timing of detecting, thus potentially producing bias (Baird et al. 1993). Since socio-cultural factors may influence the couples' behaviour, this could pose a problem, especially if the exposure of interest is an occupational one that correlates with social and cultural conditions.

Exposures that cause irregular or long cycles may also interfere with the timing of pregnancy recognition as well as with the ability to report the starting time on the TTP.

The use of family planning methods should be taken into consideration. Couples who use unsafe contraceptive methods without getting pregnant will, over time, include an increasing fraction of couples with a low fecundability. Couples who know how to time sexual intercourse around the time of ovulation have shorter waiting times than other couples, all other factors being equal. Couples who, in the past, have experienced subfecundity may have modified their exposures or their sexual behaviour in a way that may severely distort our ability to find a proper reference group.

It has also been suggested to calculate a standardized fertility ratio (Starr and Levine 1983). The idea is to compare the observed fertility with the expected fertility for couples of the same age and from the same region. Such a standardized fertility ratio can then be calculated before and after an exposure of interest – if the exposure impairs fecundity the fertility ratio after start of exposure is less than one, other things being equal. The observed number of liveborns before exposure may be close to expected values based upon age and calendar time specific rates in the population at large. The exposure may then reduce this observed/expected ratio. Although this method was able to detect the fecundity reducing effect of dibromochloropropane (DBCP), it rests upon strong assumptions, and it only works when examining exposures that have a specific (and known) starting point in time.

In addition to the problems mentioned, there are other sources of bias in time to pregnancy studies (Weinberg et al. 1994a; Weinberg and Wilcox 1998; Baird et al. 1994). It is not an easy task to develop a monitoring design sensitive enough to pick up subtle changes in fecundity over time (Olsen and Rachootin 2003). Studies that aim at detecting determinants of fecundity are probably less vulnerable to bias.

Only about half or less of those who experience infertility seek medical help, making treated patients a poor measure of the problem of subfecundity in the population (Olsen et al. 1998a, b). Infertile couples in infertility treatment are therefore a selected part of all couples in the population, which should be considered when using infertility patients in epidemiology studies.

If the forces of selection are correlated with the exposure under study, then a case-control study with a population-based definition of the source population is not a valid option for an analytic study. We expect these forces of selection to treatment to be related to several factors, such as cultural background of the population, age, parity, education, social status, and availability of treatment facilities. Some of these conditions may well correlate with life-style factors, dietary factors, infections or other putative causes of subfecundity.

Given these conditions the source population has to be defined by the case series. The source population could be defined by all those who would come to our treatment centre if they had a similar infertility problem as our cases had in the time period of study. The source population is then defined by all potential cases (and, of course, by the enrolled cases as well). Had we known the source population, we could have sampled controls from this group at the time the cases came to be detected. Candidates for controls selection would then be couples who have planned a pregnancy and who would be cases if they had a waiting time of 12 months or longer. We could then compare exposures at starting time, or before, and estimate the relative risk of being infertile as a function of the exposures under study. The problem in this design is that we do not know the source population and it may be impossible, even in principle, to identify it along with its exposure experience. A viable option may be to take advantage of the fact that infertility is a couple phenomenon. Infertility is sometimes caused by exposures mediated through female factors, sometimes through male factors, and sometimes through both male and female factors. If we e.g. take an interest in exposures to prenatal tobacco smoking as a cause of 'male infertility' we may then compare the frequency of this exposure for males in couples that had a male problem (e.g. poor sperm quality) with the exposure frequency in males for couples where the female was identified as having the problem. Both sets of couples sought help and therefore belong to the source population. Since couples where both members have a fecundity problem belong to both the case and the control group, they do not provide useful information for the question under study and can be excluded.

If the exposure is more frequent in cases than in controls, it suggests that the exposure is a risk factor for the disease, although it may be impossible to calculate proper quantitative effect estimate from this type of a case/non-case study (Olsen and Basso 2001). This type of design may furthermore produce estimates that are too conservative if the studied exposures affect both male and female fecundity, especially if the exposures cluster in couples, like some lifestyle and occupational factors will.

Alternative design options for monitoring fecundity have been proposed like using dizygotic twinning rates as a surrogate for fecundity (Tong et al. 1997), but one of the problems is to exclude twins that are a result of infertility treatment.

Studies on semen quality may also be used as a surrogate measure of fecundity. Much of the concern for a declining fecundity stems from studies on semen (Carlsen et al. 1992).

The main problems related to using measures of semen quality in epidemiologic studies relate to low participation rates in most studies and difficulties with obtaining comparable conditions of the analyses. Time since last ejaculation has to be taken into consideration, the conditions related to the ejaculation itself, time from ejaculation to analysis, the technical conditions for the analysis, the season of sampling (higher sperm counts in winter than summer periods in temperate climates) as well as recording of potential confounders. Specific diseases may interfere with sperm production, together with external exposures.

5.4   Twins

Since twinning can be the result of infertility treatment, it is difficult to say what the 'natural' incidence is. It also varies in different ethnic groups – but the 'natural' incidence in Caucasian populations is probably around 1 in 80 births. Dizygotic twins may be seen as a sign of a high male and female fecundity, since they require two eggs to be fertilised by two sperms within a short time period.

Twins may also be seen as an anomaly, since twinning is associated with a higher risk of perinatal morbidity, including possibly congenital malformations. Twins, however, may not only be seen as a gift to their parents, but to epidemiologists as well, since they provide a very interesting source of data concerning the nature-nurture discussion in disease occurrence. Twin studies have been the basic epidemiologic design to disentangle the effect of genes and the environment.

Genetic disorders are expected to have higher correlation (concordance) in monozygotic (MZ) twins than in dizygotic (DZ) twins. MZ twins are genetically identical (although some minor genetic differences have been found to exist and have even been used to identify a genetic cause of a congenital malfunction (Kondo et al. 2002)) and DZ twins share genes like ordinary sisters/brothers. Compared to the latter, however, DZ twins share the same uterine environment as well as more similar conditions in early childhood and these factors considerably reduce the confounding that would arise by comparing ordinary siblings. Although the twin model is definitely of interest, the situation is clearly more complicated. MZ twins have the same gene map but need not have the same functional genetic expression. Since females are mosaics where a random X chromosome is inactivated in each cell line, female twins are not functionally genetically identical, and genetic imprinting may differ. Furthermore, MZ twins' intrauterine conditions are not the same, as inferred by the – often large – variation in foetal growth between babies in a pair. Furthermore, both twins have to survive to be part of a twin study and twin mortality is higher than what we see for singletons, most likely from the time of conception.

It is well documented that some singletons started as twins but one foetus did not survive, and it has been suggested that the surviving twin is at increased risk of e.g. cerebral palsy (Pharoah and Adi 2000).

Twins are often excluded from epidemiologic studies on possible fetotoxic hazards, since they often cannot be grouped together with singletons in a meaningful analysis due to their higher risk of low birth weight, preterm birth, and congenital abnormalities. In most studies, there are too few twins to provide an informative subgroup for analysis, which is unfortunate. It would often be of interest to study the effect of fetotoxic exposures on twins only.

Twin pregnancies have been used as a model to study the effect of hormone exposure during pregnancy. The oestrogen level is high in all twin pregnancies and twins of different sex also offer unique intrauterine exposure conditions (Storgaard et al. 2002).

Measuring Reproductive Failures

5.5

Estimating the frequency of reproductive failures is, in many ways, similar to estimating the frequency of any disease in populations. Frequencies are measured by means of rates or proportions (and many proportions are unfortunately called rates). Measurements address new events over time as incident events or existing states at a given point in time, prevalence.

Rates are used to present reproductive failures as a function of observation time, e.g. the incidence of cervix cancer in Danish women in 1997 was 11.42 per 100,000 years of observation in women.

The cumulative risk is estimated by the proportion of people who contract the disease over a given time span. The estimation can be done directly in a population where follow-up is complete, e.g. the cumulative risk of stillbirth can be estimated if a given number of pregnant women can be followed from their 24th week of gestation until they give birth (if 24 weeks define the separation of abortions and births for terminated pregnancies). If complete follow-up is not possible, as for longer follow-up periods, the risk may be estimated by connecting incidence rates (IR) to risk (CI) according to the formula $CI = 1 - e^{-IR}$ (cf. Chap. I.2 of this handbook). This calculation from rates to risk requires stable incidence rates over the time period during which they are measured. Rates describe occurrence of events per time unit, like new respiratory syncytial virus (RSV) cases per 1000 observation months in children less than 1 year in a given region and a given time period. Rates are thus for populations. Risks indicate the probability of a given event in a given time period and for an average member of the population in question. In a population with complete follow-up, the risk of e.g. 2nd trimester abortions in 500 pregnant women who are followed until the start of the 3rd trimester is estimated as 0.02 if 10 of the 500 women abort in these 3 months.

Incidence rates and cumulative risks are based upon data from a population at risk, that is, a population at risk of getting the disease but without having the disease at the time when the observation starts. Prevalence proportions are estimated as the number of people with the disease in question at a given point in time divided by all in the population at that time, regardless of their disease status. If 500 women are pregnant in a population of 50,000, the pregnancy prevalence proportion is 0.01 (500/50,000). Since prevalence (P) is a function of incidence (I) and duration (D), the incidence of new pregnancies in a steady state population would be 500/8, if the average duration of a pregnancy is set at 8 months, taking abortions into consideration, that is 62.5 pregnant women per month in the population of 50,000, or 750 per year.

Measuring reproductive failures during pregnancy is often complicated by the fact that the time of conception is unknown. When the pregnancy is planned, the time from the start of the pregnancy planning to a recognised pregnancy and to the end of the pregnancy may be known. Estimating the incidence rate of spontaneous abortions requires registration of time from conception to the abortion in question or to gestational week 24. At best, the time of conception may be identified by means of biochemical measures at a very early stage, but in most cases a pregnancy diagnosis is not established until 3–4 weeks after conception at the earliest, and then it is retrospectively estimated by means of last menstrual period data (LMP) or – later – by using growth measures based upon ultrasound examination. Observation time for calculating rates of spontaneous abortions, therefore, often starts at different time periods in gestation, and in studies we have to take this delayed entry into consideration to obtain meaningful results when we try e.g. to identify determinants of spontaneous abortions (Baird et al. 1993).

The Measures Used to Describe Mortality 5.5.1

The World Health Organization (WHO) defines live births, foetal deaths and induced abortions in the following way:

> The definition of a *live birth* is the complete expulsion or extraction from the mother of a product of human conception, irrespective of the duration of pregnancy which, after such expulsion or extraction, breathes or shows any other evidence of life, such as beating of the heart, pulsation of the umbilical cord, or definite movement of voluntary muscles whether or not the umbilical cord has been cut or the placenta is attached.
>
> *Foetal death* is defined as death prior to the complete expulsion or extraction from the mother of a product of human conception, foetus and placenta, irrespective of the duration of pregnancy: the death is indicated by the fact that, after such expulsion or extraction, the foetus does not breathe or show any other evidence of life, such as beating of the heart, pulsation of the umbilical cord, or definite movement of voluntary muscles. Heartbeats are to be distinguished from transient cardiac contractions; respiration is to be distinguished from fleeting respiratory efforts or gasps.

This definition excludes induced terminations of pregnancy.

Induced termination of pregnancy is defined as the purposeful interruption of an intrauterine pregnancy with the intention other than to produce a liveborn infant, and which does not result in a live birth. This definition excludes management of prolonged retention of productions of conception following foetal death.

Induced Termination of Pregnancy Rate (Conceptions). This measure uses live births, induced terminations of pregnancy, and foetal deaths in the denominator.

$$
\begin{array}{l}
\text{Induced Termination} \\
\text{of Pregnancy Rate} \\
\text{(conceptions)}
\end{array}
=
\frac{
\begin{array}{l}
\text{Number of induced terminations occuring} \\
\text{during a specific time period}
\end{array}
}{
\begin{array}{l}
\text{Number of induced terminations} + \\
\text{live births} + \\
\text{reported foetal deaths during the same} \\
\text{time period}
\end{array}
} \times 1000
$$

Induced Termination of Pregnancy Rate (Population). This is the probability that women of reproductive age will have an induced termination of pregnancy within a given time period.

$$
\begin{array}{l}
\text{Induced Termination} \\
\text{of Pregnancy Rate} \\
\text{(population)}
\end{array}
=
\frac{
\begin{array}{l}
\text{Number of induced terminations occurring} \\
\text{during a specific time period}
\end{array}
}{
\text{Female population aged 15 through 44 years}
} \times 1000
$$

$$
\text{Foetal Death Rate} =
\frac{
\begin{array}{l}
\text{Number of foetal deaths} \\
\text{during a specific time period}
\end{array}
}{
\begin{array}{l}
\text{Number of foetal deaths + number of live births} \\
\text{during the same time period}
\end{array}
} \times 1000
$$

$$
\text{Foetal Death Ratio} =
\frac{
\begin{array}{l}
\text{Number of foetal deaths} \\
\text{during a specific time period}
\end{array}
}{
\text{Number of live births during the same time period}
} \times 1000
$$

Maternal mortality ratio is the number of deaths attributed to maternal conditions in a given time period divided with a number of live births during the same time period.

WHO recommends including maternal deaths that occur within 42 days of the end of the pregnancy. Some countries use other time periods (i.e., within one year).

Although international comparisons are difficult to make because of variable reporting practices, we know that wide differences in maternal mortality exist worldwide (AbouZahr 1998).

The *perinatal mortality ratio* is the number of foetal deaths (> 24 weeks of gestation) and deaths during the first 7 days of life divided by the number of stillbirths and liveborn children in the same period. Stillbirths are births of foetus that show no sign of life at births that occur after 24 weeks of gestation.

Recent results indicate that this definition should be separated into stillbirths and death during the first weeks of life. Stillbirths should furthermore be divided into death before labour and death during labour. In the past, foetal death and early death after birth often had asphyxia as the common cause. Congenital malformations are now a much more common cause of death around the time of birth (Kramer et al. 2002).

> *Infant mortality* is computed as the number of deaths, usually during the first year of life, divided by the number of live births during the same time period. Instant mortality rates vary between 5‰ to 10% in the poorest countries in the world.

Many of these measures are difficult to record in a comparable way over time and between countries. Live births are well registered in many countries, but that is not the case with stillbirths, partly because the gestational age that separates abortions from births differs between countries, partly because stillbirths do not count in population statistics (Gourbin and Masuy-Stroobant 1995).

In some countries, the threshold of 24 weeks is used to distinguish birth from an abortion. Other cut offs have been 28 weeks or 27 weeks. The complicating issue is, however, that birth with a liveborn child is a birth, regardless of the time of delivery. This may also be applied for children, who did not survive but showed signs of life. Any study that makes use of routine registration systems to identify births and where both live- and stillbirths are of interest, should make sure that the time at risk for the outcome of interest is comparable (e.g. including in the analysis only babies born from the 28th week onward, if that is the threshold for defining a stillbirth). It is often very difficult to identify the cause of death for stillbirths (Winbo et al. 1997) or the time of death, which may be of importance in a monitoring system. It has e.g. been suggested that foetal death during labour is a better indicator of the quality of obstetric care than foetal death before labour (Kiely et al. 1985).

Foetal and Infant Death 5.6

When we study mortality we usually estimate mortality rates, the number of people who die as a function of the size of the underlying population, and the period of time during which this population was under observation. Since mortality rates strongly depend upon age (and sex), we usually calculate age (and sex) specific mortality rates. The mortality rate for people of 90 years of age will be the number of 90-year-olds who die within a year divided by the number of observation years we have for 90-year-olds in that population. We will count observation time from their 90th birthday until they turn 91, die or leave the population for other reasons.

In perinatal epidemiology, age is even more important, but the problem is that age may be counted from either the time of conception or the time of birth. We expect mortality to be high shortly after conception and we also expect mortality to be high when the foetus leaves the intrauterine environment. We would prefer to present mortality as a function of observation time in the population at risk from conception, which is difficult for early foetal deaths (abortions) because we usually do not know how many have conceived in the source population. We have to start our observation when the pregnancy is diagnosed and that often varies. Sometimes the pregnancy is first diagnosed by the occurrence of a spontaneous abortion, and sometimes a conception ends in a spontaneous abortion without the woman ever realizing that she was pregnant. Moreover, since some women bleed early in pregnancy this may cause problems in the attribution of gestational age (Gjessing et al. 1999).

An additional problem is that the timing of foetal death is often not known, and only the time of expulsion is. In early gestation these two points in time may differ by several days or even weeks (missed abortions), and some dead foetuses may even be absorbed rather than aborted. Later in gestation we expect a stillbirth to be closer to the time of death. When signs of life disappear most women in affluent societies will seek medical assistance. The foetal death will be diagnosed and an abortion induced. For multiple pregnancies where only one twin dies the situation may be different.

Some studies on foetal death use survival methods that take delayed entry and gestational age into consideration, or they use the ratio of all abortions to births as the endpoint. In any case, caution is called for. If exposures cause very early (pre-clinical) spontaneous abortions these will not be detected. Exposures that move clinical abortions to the pre-clinical stage will appear as if they prevented abortion for both measures, regardless of whether they are based upon rates or cumulative risk.

The time in which a pregnancy is diagnosed depends upon a number of known and unknown factors. It is reasonable to expect a planned pregnancy to be detected earlier than an unplanned pregnancy. On average, women with regular menstrual cycles probably become aware of the pregnancy earlier than women with irregular cycles. A woman who has been pregnant before may detect symptoms of a pregnancy earlier than a woman who is pregnant for the first time. Availability and sensitivity of pregnancy tests will also play a role for the starting point of observation.

Assume that we base our study upon a cohort of pregnant women. Assume furthermore that we take an interest in an exposure that, for some reason, correlates with how early the pregnancy is recognized. The exposed women would then enter the cohort at a later (or earlier) gestational age than the unexposed women. Since the risk of abortion decreases with gestational age, their ratio of spontaneous abortions to birth would be lower (or higher) than that of the unexposed group and the results would thus be biased. Comparison of gestational age-specific abortion rates should, however, be unbiased – provided that the exposure does not modify the time period from foetal death to expulsion.

If an exposure changes only the timing of pregnancy detection, gestational week specific abortion rates remain valid. If the exposure changes the timing of abortions around the threshold for their detection, all the possible abortion measures may be biased.

Studying spontaneous abortions may also be complicated for other reasons. Since the risk of spontaneous abortions varies largely with gestational age, it is important to use valid data for gestational age in the model that is left truncated at the time of entry. Unfortunately, precise data on gestational ages are difficult to obtain, even if ultrasound measures were done. A foetus with a poor survival destiny may show early growth patterns that deviate from standard values, possibly making ultrasound estimates invalid. Furthermore, the exposure of interest may correlate with the validity of estimates of gestational age, which may make it impossible to obtain unbiased comparisons even when doing the proper statistical analyses. Furthermore, the start of observation time need not coincide with the time of exposure. If the exposure causes abortion after a short exposure time, the susceptible pregnancies may be removed from our study for those who had been exposed before start of observation time, leaving a selected group available for study. This selection could attenuate or eliminate an effect of the exposure on the risk of spontaneous abortion.

Using a case-control approach to study causes of spontaneous abortions may be prone to bias in some situations. Controls should (using the principles of incidence density sampling, see Chap. I.6 of this handbook) be selected at the time of foetal death (which is often unknown) and not at the time of abortion. Furthermore, hormonal measures at the time of abortion that change over gestational time may be poor indicators of the cause of foetal death, even in situations where they are the cause of death, rather than a consequence of it.

Dietary habits (such as coffee consumption during pregnancy) may change when nausea disappears, and since a foetal death would reduce nausea, cases may then have a higher intake of coffee than controls, not because coffee killed the foetus, but because nausea and aversion against coffee disappeared when the foetus died. The exposure frequency is then high in the time from death to abortion, but was not so at the time of death. The high coffee intake is a consequence of foetal death, not a cause of death.

When the child is born, an entirely new time schedule starts. Preterm or very preterm children will start this time clock before their foetal maturation has come to its natural end. Babies born in week 35 will start their extrauterine life 5 weeks before a baby born at term. Diseases that originated in utero with a fixed induction time will have an onset that perhaps should have been counted from conception time rather than the time of birth. Childhood colic is perhaps a disease that peaks at a given time from conception, independently of the time of birth (Sondergaard et al. 2000).

Measures that use births as the denominator rather than the population at risk in the proper time intervals apply a practice that deviates from the practice that normal age specific rates usually rest upon. Foetal death rates would, in normal practice, be seen as death within a given gestational time period divided by the observation time for foetuses at that gestational age, just as infant mortality is estimated as death during the first year of life divided by observation time for children less than 1 year of age in that population.

Rather than using survival principles in studying determinants of abortion, many use the ratio of spontaneous abortions to birth, or spontaneous abortions/ (induced abortions + spontaneous abortions + births). The latter presents a proportion of spontaneous abortions among all who terminate their pregnancy with either a birth or an abortion. The first measure will overestimate the cumulative risk of spontaneous abortions, as it does not take induced abortions into consideration (some of which would have ended in a spontaneous abortion). The latter estimate will attenuate the cumulative risk since some of the induced abortions would have contributed to the numerator had they not been induced. The frequency of induced abortion and the timing of induced abortion thus becomes a source of bias in these studies (Olsen 1984), unless data are analysed by means of survival techniques.

The risk of ending a pregnancy with a spontaneous abortion is high, especially if the mother is more than 35 years of age (Andersen et al. 2000). How high abortion rates are from the time of conception is not known because we only have data on conception for very specific in vitro fertilization (IVF) conceptions, which do not represent the general population. Kline et al. (1989) estimated that 50% of all conceptions end as spontaneous abortions; 40% of pregnancies that could be detected by hCG measures and 10%–15% among clinically recognized pregnancies. These figures probably do not need much adjustment today, although a new cohort study among pregnancy planners found a slightly lower abortion rate in the pre-clinic, but detectable, phase of pregnancy of about 25%–30% (Hjollund et al. 2000), close to what Wilcox found in his study of pregnancy planners (Wilcox et al. 1988). No biological measure is at present able to pick up the very early foetal life.

Many abortions have chromosomal aberrations, especially among the very early losses (Macklon et al. 2002). Chromosomal aberrations, or more specific genetic defects, may be used to perform more detailed analyses of cause-specific mortality. If all spontaneous abortions were grouped together, the measure would represent a general mortality endpoint and, since most exposures are expected to be specific in their causal action, a general mortality measure may in many situations be too imprecise for meaningful research. The problem is, however, that obtaining and genotyping foetal tissue when an abortion occurs is neither easy nor inexpensive in an epidemiologic study that often includes large numbers of participants.

When studying a specific exposure that is not believed to cause chromosomal aberrations, it would be wise to restrict the outcome to abortions without such defects, if possible. Chromosomal analysis may, in some situations, be used to distinguish between consequences of foetal death from causes of the death itself. If e.g. coffee intake is a result of foetal death rather than the cause of it, one should expect to see coffee equally associated with abortion with and without chromosomal aberrations. If coffee drinking is causally related to the foetal death, it will probably operate either via chromosomal aberrations or through another fetotoxic mechanism independently of the chromosomal aberrations. These analytical principles were to some extent used in a study by Cnattingius et al. (2000).

Some reproductive failures correlate (Basso et al. 1998a) and they often have a tendency to repeat themselves (Basso et al. 1999). It may be necessary to take this into consideration when designing a study.

Perinatal Mortality and Health Care

It is obviously desirable to reduce foetal and early childhood deaths as much as possible, at best by removing or reducing the underlying causes of death, especially if these causes also lead to long-term health problems for those who survive. Still, the main investments in most affluent societies have been spent on improving treatment. In some situations effective treatment will not only save the life of the foetus but also lead to a better potential for a normal and healthy life. In other situations, treatment may increase the incidence of diseases (by keeping alive babies (often very preterm) that may be severely impaired).

A number of mortality measures, especially perinatal mortality rates, have been used to monitor how part of the health care system performs. Perinatal mortality has declined over time in most countries and is reaching very low values in many affluent societies.

It has been suggested to stratify perinatal mortality by birth weight in order to obtain a better monitoring instrument for the quality of treatment. The idea is that advanced treatment would especially show its effect on children born with a low birth weight; the babies having the highest risk of not surviving the early extra uterine life.

When the method of stratifying mortality rates according to birth weight (and sex) became widespread, a number of so-called paradoxes appeared. The offspring of smoking mothers had lower mortality at low birth weights than the offspring of non-smoking mothers with the same low birth weight. The same was seen for populations living at high altitudes and for African Americans compared with European Americans in the US (Adams et al. 1991). These paradoxes could be seen as a result of confounding by the underlying causes of impaired foetal growth. Smoking may, for example, be a less harmful way of reducing foetal growth than whatever caused the growth retardation among those not being exposed to intrauterine tobacco smoke, although smoking in general increases perinatal mortality.

Another explanation of the paradoxes was given by Russell and Wilcox (1991) and Wilcox (2001), who showed that the strongest predictor of perinatal mortality in a population is not the proportion of newborns with a low birth weight, but the proportion of newborns with a birth weight that falls outside the population specific Gaussian birth weight distribution (the residual). Birth weight usually follows a normal distribution with a small 'bump' in the left side tail, mainly representing pre-term births. The size of the residual (usually reported in percent of the total) is a stronger predictor of the perinatal mortality for the population than the proportion of newborns with a low birth weight ($< 2500\,\text{g}$), which is the present indicator used in monitoring systems. If we follow Allen Wilcox's thinking, the aim should not be to change the birth weight distribution for the population, but to reduce the residual portion of the distribution, i.e. the proportion falling outside the Gaussian distribution. This translates mainly into preventing pre-term birth rather than increasing birth weight. Most reproductive epidemiologists would probably agree on this strategy. The present obesity epidemic in many countries is e.g. expected to increase birth weight in the coming years, but not to decrease perinatal mortality; in fact, we may observe the opposite.

Stratifying perinatal mortality according to birth weight ranks (or a z-score) for the particular distribution rather than the absolute birth weight also eliminates the paradox of crossing mortality risk in most situations, indicating that birth weight in itself may be an inappropriate indicator of mortality risk.

Birth weight has been used because it is available in most countries. Data on gestational age are less often available and the quality may be poor. Still, uncritical use of birth weights as an 'exposure' or endpoint in reproductive epidemiology is not appropriate.

5.7   Foetal Growth and Birth Weight

If a woman is exposed to agents that reduce foetal growth, growth may be reduced proportionally or disproportionally. If mainly fat tissue is reduced, as seen in smoking women, the newborn baby may have normal height but a reduced birth weight. The ponderal index is a measure that attempts to distinguish between thin and normal body proportions. The index is calculated as the newborn's weight divided by height raised to the third power. Readers, who are familiar with the Body Mass Index (BMI), will know that the ponderal index deviates from BMI only by raising height to the power of 3 rather than to the power of 2. The only reason for this difference is to obtain a more symmetrical distribution of the ponderal index in newborns. How well this index actually reflects body composition among newborn children is, however, not well known.

There are of course other anthropometric measures of interest than birth weight or birth length. Head circumference is one such measure. Abdominal circumference may also be of interest. Most of these measures are probably measured with less precision than birth weight, at least in countries that use standard weighing conditions (like time since birth) and well-calibrated electronic weights. It is also more difficult to measure the length of a baby, or a circumference. It is e.g. likely that babies born vaginally will present a molding of the cranial plates that will modify their head circumference compared to babies born with a caesarean section. Also, it is possible that some of these additional measurements would not be taken if a baby were ill at birth, so that excluding babies because not all measures were taken may produce selection bias.

Since birth weight is a function of both pregnancy duration and foetal growth, pregnancy duration is usually taken into consideration when analysing birth weight. The simplest procedure is to stratify results on preterm and term birth, but this may not fully adjust for confounding related to gestational age. Another option is to estimate small for gestational age (SGA), which implies identifying the, say, 10% with the lowest birth weight among children born during each given gestational week. Since the birth weight distribution is population specific, it is wise to use an internal reference rather than an external reference if the study is large enough. Using SGA measures has the disadvantage that they do not make use of the birth weight distribution. The SGA term should furthermore not be taken as a measure of intrauterine Growth Retardation (IUGR) since the term SGA is purely descriptive. The term IUGR should be restricted to situations where it is known that the foetus is growth retarded. Such a measure would in principle require a documented deviance from the foetal natural growth curve.

Gestational age could also be included in the statistical model to adjust for gestational age confounding. In order to account for non-linearity in confounding, it may be preferred to include gestational age plus gestational age squared, or to include several categories of gestational age as dummy variables (for an introduction to regression models see Chap. II.3 of this handbook).

The drawback of adjusting for gestational age one way or the other (or to use SGA measures) is mainly related to the often poor quality of data for gestational age. Birth weight is measured more accurately than gestational age and, by using an endpoint like small for gestational age (SGA), good data may be turned into bad data by making use of a composite measure that includes a variable that is imprecise at best and possibly even biased. An exposure with no effect on foetal growth that causes irregularities in the menstrual cycle could show a biased effect on SGA, if gestational age was based upon LMP data, or a biased effect if gestational age is measured by ultrasound and the exposure correlates with early foetal growth.

The term 'small for gestational age' is misleading, since it is a purely descriptive population concept: the baby is among the smallest in this particular population. Usually, we would like to know if the baby is small because it is growth retarded. A baby that has achieved its full genetic growth potential could be an SGA baby just because it is genetically small. We expect such a baby to be at low risk for all complications and diseases that may be related to poor foetal growth.

Our interest in birth weight from a health perspective should focus upon a deviation from the genetic growth potential rather than on the absolute birth weight. The soundness of this approach was elegantly demonstrated by our Norwegian colleagues, who compared observed birth weights with the expected birth weight estimated from their sibling's (and mother's) birth weight. A birth weight lower than expected was the most important risk factor for perinatal mortality all over the birth weight distribution – not only for newborn children with a low birth weight (Skjaerven et al. 2000).

Unfortunately, however, we do not know the genetic programming of the foetus and we often have to rely upon indirect estimates that could lead to severe misclassification.

Given the fact that birth weight has been used for convenience – too extensively and during too long a period – a group of scientists (Adams et al. 2003) met in June 2002 in Denmark to announce the so-called Sostrup Statement (named after the residency where the meeting took place). These statements concluded that:

1. In population studies, 'percent low birth weight' (LBW) is a poor research tool for detecting factors or conditions that damage perinatal health.
2. 'Percent LBW' is a poor index of population perinatal health.

3. Adjustment for absolute birth weight is rarely justifiable in looking for effects of specific exposures on infant or perinatal mortality.
4. Some exposures or conditions may compromise foetuses without causing preterm delivery or impaired foetal growth.

It is, however, difficult to propose another indicator than LBW that is easy to obtain and subject to a small degree of error, especially if we want such an indicator to be applicable in less affluent countries. The best alternative for a single indicator is probably preterm birth, although that may be subject to a higher degree of misclassification.

5.7.1   Optimal Birth Weight

The concept of an 'optimal birth weight' has been used in the literature mainly to indicate the birth weight with the lowest perinatal mortality in specific populations. We do not recommend the concept to be used broadly since an optimal birth weight depends upon what the birth weight has to 'optimise'; mortality, immune defence, cognitive development, etc. Studies on 'optional birth weight' in the context of mortality have, nonetheless, shown interesting results. The 'optimal birth weight' is higher than the average birth weight, which may reflect a trade-off between the mother's and the child's interests (Haig 1993). The foetus will try to take as much of the nutritional supply as possible, while the mother needs to reserve some for herself to continue her (reproductive) life. According to Haig, during the course of evolution genes have been shaped to balance these two aims. Data furthermore show that the 'optimal birth weight' is population specific but is correlated with the average birth weight in the specific population (Graafmans et al. 2002). According to the evolutionary theories, it is to be expected that the 'optimal birth weight' is, in fact, a given birth weight for a given individual.

5.8   Gestational Age: Pre- and Post Term Delivery

A pregnancy of course starts at conception but, since the time of conception is usually unknown, the starting point is often taken from the first day of the last menstrual period (LMP), which is usually around 2 weeks prior to conception. A pregnancy is expected to last 40 weeks or 280 days, according to this calculation.

In most countries, Naegele's rule is still applied to estimate gestational age from using LMP data. The expected day of birth is calculated starting from the first day of LMP, then 3 months are subtracted and one week is added.

This rule works well for women who remember their menstrual periods and whose periods are regular (and close to 28 days of duration). The Naegele rule also works best in non-leap years at the population level (Basso et al. 2000a). With the easy access to electronic calendars, one would expect to see more electronic devices that simply add 280 days to LMP, taking leap years into account.

In affluent societies, ultrasounds (US) are more and more often used as a way of estimating gestational age, even in normal pregnancies with a certain LMP date. The idea behind the estimate is that certain structures, like the biparietal diameter (BPD), grows linearly and similarly for all in the beginning of the pregnancy.

A given diameter is compared with a growth standard and the gestational week is based upon the measure read from the standard growth curve – 16 weeks in the example above (cf. Fig. 5.1).

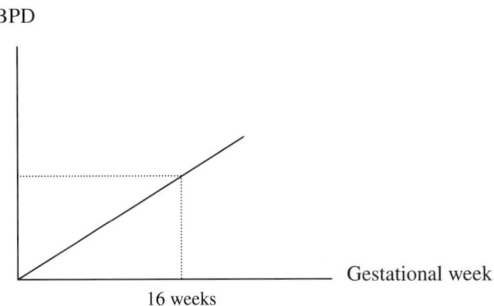

Figure 5.1. BPD according to time since conception

Experience has shown that ultrasound estimates are more precise than LMP measures and for this reason they are more precise in clinical predictions of the date of delivery. They need not always be better for research, however. If you study exposures that impair early foetal growth, then an ultrasound measure may cause bias. The bias is probably too small to be of relevance for clinical practice, but it may be of concern in research. There may be research projects that are better off with an unbiased estimate with a low precision (like LMP) than with a biased estimate with a high precision. It has been shown that smoking, for example, may impair even early foetal growth (Henriksen et al. 1995) and, if this is the case, then

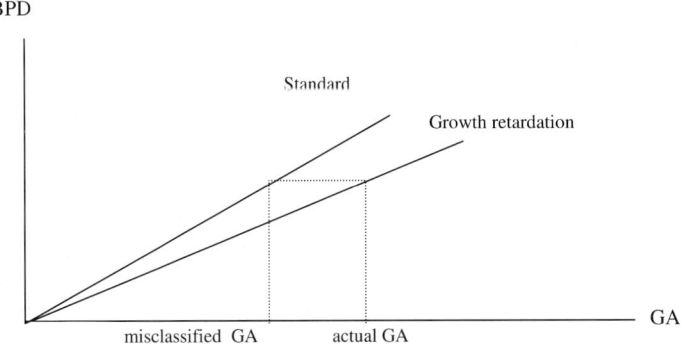

Figure 5.2. Actual and standard BPD growth curves

smokers would systematically be misclassified with an earlier gestation than their actual one because the growth function will be lower than the standard, as shown in Fig. 5.2. Assume that the difference between the actual and estimated GA is two days. If the woman gives birth shortly after 37 weeks of gestation, she would – in error – be defined as giving birth preterm.

If an inappropriate standard is used at the population level indicating a more rapid growth than for the population, gestational age will then be biased towards a low value, which will lead to a higher frequency of preterm birth. Using an inappropriate standard for the population under study will thus have impact on the estimated proportions of preterm and post-term birth for the population.

Gestational age is counted in days or in completed weeks. Preterm birth is a birth occurring before the woman has reached week 37, while post-term birth is defined as a birth taking place after completion of the 42nd week. The term prematurity was sometimes used in the past for newborns with a birth weight of less than 2500 g. This term should be avoided, because we do not know if newborns with a birth weight of less than 2500 g are premature; some will not be. Preterm is a better factual description, and sometimes it will be useful to study very preterm as well. Very preterm has been defined as birth before 34, 33, or 32 weeks (Berkowitz and Papiernik 1993). We prefer not to have a fixed definition for very preterm but to let it be defined in the study. The best definition may depend not only on the hypothesis you want to examine, but also on the available sample size.

The frequency of preterm and post-term births depends upon precision and validity of the estimates of gestational age. If the central tendency of two measures (ultrasound and LMP) are the same, but one is measured with larger measurement errors (like LMP), then the imprecise measure will lead to more pre- and post-term births, provided that the central tendency is the same. In a study of pre- or post-term delivery it is therefore important that gestational age is at least measured using the same methods in the groups to be compared. If studies are based upon routine registrations of gestational age, it may not be known how it was measured. If the exposure under study correlates with early foetal growth, LMP should be applied. If the exposure correlates with menstrual irregularities, then ultrasound is preferable. In order to detect a given difference in gestational age between two compared groups, a larger sample size is usually needed if gestational age is estimated by LMP compared with ultrasound estimates.

An example of the latter case may occur when studying whether a long time to pregnancy leads to preterm delivery. If only LMP measures are available, one may find that women with irregular or long menstrual periods have a longer TTP, as many women with subfecundity may have irregular cycles. The measure of time to pregnancy itself will be affected by this irregularity, since time to pregnancy, although sometimes reported in months, should – however – reflect the number of cycles that a couple takes to achieve a clinically detectable pregnancy. In such cases, not only imprecision but also bias can affect the effect measures, and the burden to estimate how much the observed effect can be ascribed to these problems falls on the researcher. If ultrasound measurements are not available, one way to assess whether the association may be due to bias caused by differential misclassification of gestational age could be to use birth weight as a support measure to corroborate the finding. Since birth weight is less subject to error and its accuracy is less, if at all, dependent on correlates of the exposure, this may provide reassurance for the finding – or grounds for rejecting it. If there is no difference in the birth weight distribution according to time to pregnancy before adjustment for gestational age, this suggests that most of, or all, the observed effect is due to differential measurement error of gestational age. If, on the other hand, the birth weight of children born to women with a long time to pregnancy is lower than that of women with a short time to pregnancy, this is an indication that there is at least some effect of time to pregnancy on gestational duration, if there are no residual confounders that can reduce birth weight that are more common in women with long time to pregnancy. (This would be a problem if, for instance, short women – who have lighter babies – also had a longer time to pregnancy than tall women, but a gestation of the same duration). A long time to pregnancy may have an effect on foetal growth as well as on gestational age, and one could thus estimate this by adjusting for gestational age when examining birth weight as a function of time to pregnancy.

Another example of a factor affecting the accuracy of gestational age selectively in exposed and non-exposed women may occur when examining the effect of short interpregnancy intervals (the time between the previous birth and the next conception) on the gestational age of the subsequent pregnancy. Women who have short intervals are likely to have less accurate estimate of gestational age, because cycles resume some time after a pregnancy, and they may be irregular at first. Therefore, women with very short intervals may have systematically inaccurate measures of gestational age. Again, by checking with birth weight one can try to assess whether there is evidence of this phenomenon. Although short interpregnancy intervals have been associated with both preterm delivery and low birth weight, in a study among Danish women (Basso et al. 1998b) only the association with preterm delivery was observed, while the one with low birth weight disappeared entirely after adjustment for preterm delivery.

As stated previously, being born pre- or post-term may have stronger health impacts than deviates from a 'normal' birth weight. Using e.g. the proportion of preterm births as an indicator in a monitoring programme is therefore of interest. In the past, such a measure was based upon LMP data. Now it would often be partly LMP and partly ultrasound based, or based upon ultrasound measures only. From a monitoring point of view this raises issues of concern related to comparability over time. The standard used to estimate gestational age based upon BPD should be appropriate and that means both time- and population-specific. It should be a standard for the population it is applied to, and it should be changed over time if foetal growth in the population changes over time. Many countries face increasing obesity problems, which may influence not only birth weights but also early foetal growth. If so, BPD standards need frequent adjustments for an ultrasound-based monitoring system of preterm births to be unbiased.

No matter how gestational ages are calculated, you will sometimes find implausible gestational ages based upon the newborn children's birth weight or maturity. We prefer to code such data as missing rather than use some of the methods that have been proposed to clean gestation age data (Parker and Schoendorf 2002). For estimating gestational age at abortion, the LMP method is to be recommended in most cases, even if ultrasound was used. A foetus that does not survive might have been severely growth-retarded.

The pregnancy period is, in many countries, under intense monitoring by health care personnel. The effects of any exposure under study reflect only the effect remaining after health care intervention. This limitation is always true, but it is especially important to keep in mind when studying pregnancy duration, especially post-term birth. A birth may be induced when the clinicians believe the child is better off outside the uterus, or perhaps just because they believe the child is sufficiently mature to be born, or if the mother's health is at risk if the pregnancy is continued. A pregnancy may then be terminated by a caesarean section, by medically induced labour, or by other means. In any case, a substantial number of pregnancies are not carried to a 'natural' end, and these observations are censored in the life table terminology. Since the censoring, in many cases, will be associated with the risk of pregnancy or birth complications, we cannot study e.g. the risk associated with post-term birth per se. The only option is to study what remains of risk after health care intervention. In like manner, one cannot study determinants of post-term delivery, only determinants for pregnancies that are allowed to continue after 42 weeks of gestation. Although these limitations are self-evident, they are often not mentioned in scientific reports – perhaps because they are self-evident. In our experience they may be self-evident but are often 'forgotten', even among experienced epidemiologists. In any case, the necessary precautionary warnings are often omitted from the discussion, and the results could thus mislead the public.

The risk associated with being born at an early or late gestational age may reflect a risk associated with gestational time itself or the underlying conditions leading to early or late birth. Only occasionally will it be possible to distinguish between these two possibilities.

Preterm birth is a frequent and strong risk factor for child health. Our ability to prevent preterm birth is limited by our sparse knowledge of avoidable causes of the condition. A number of social, environmental and dietary factors may play a role. Much of the present research effort is devoted to determining the role of infections, but it remains true that preterm birth is one of the important hazards where our preventive efforts have had limited success. In many countries, preterm birth remains a frequent determinant of perinatal morbidity and mortality. It is furthermore a frequent problem affecting 4%–6% of all births or even more. The best-known predictor of preterm birth is having had a previous preterm birth. Low social status and smoking, which are well recognized in predicting a poor birth weight outcome, are not strong determinants of preterm delivery.

There are, however, many types of preterm delivery, since births can be induced early in mothers at risk (pre-eclampsia is the most frequent cause of iatrogenic preterm birth, for example), so some authors prefer to consider only rupture of the membranes and disregard other types of preterm births, such as induced deliveries. This approach will provide a 'purer' set of cases, which might share a more homogeneous aetiology than the totality of preterm births.

Congenital Malformations

Congenital malformations have been subject to numerous epidemiologic studies and monitoring systems because they are very serious for the affected children, their families, and society in general. Researchers dealing with studies of teratogenic or fetotoxic effects prefer to include a wider range of abnormalities than structural malformations. Some prefer to use the broader term congenital anomalies (CA) that will include genetic disorders and some functional impairment as well. CA will be present in 2%–7% of all newborn children, depending upon the definition and upon the level of diagnostic procedures that have been applied. Many anomalies will not be diagnosed until childhood or even later, and a number of defects (such as some heart malformations) may go undetected for many years. Effectiveness of prenatal screening followed by induced abortion of affected foetuses also plays a role for the prevalence of congenital anomalies at birth.

If congenital anomalies are taken to be all structural or functional defects or deviations that are present at birth (whether or not they are detected at the time), their frequency could be defined to cover many more. Many functional defects may be present at birth in a form that is not yet detectable with the diagnostic means we have at present, like cognitive defects, other brain defects, mutations of importance for cancers like childhood leukaemia, or testis cancer. Foetal organ programming of organ functioning could, in principle, also be seen as congenital anomalies in the sense that programming may increase susceptibility to many diseases, like insulin resistance and all the diseases it may lead to. Clearly, using such a broad approach makes congenital abnormalities an impracticable or even impossible endpoint for studies or monitoring. Most studies and monitoring systems will restrict the endpoint to what is described in official disease classifications, such as Chap. 17 in the International Classification of Diseases (ICD10).

Monitoring systems of congenital malformations have been, and are still being, used in order to detect changes in the prevalence of malformations over time. Many of these systems have their root in the Thalidomide disaster. Thalidomide was released on the market in the 1950s to treat nausea and insomnia and was regularly used by pregnant women. The drug was teratogenic, as reported by Lenz and MacBride in 1961 (Diggle 2001), in about 40% of the pregnant women who used the drug during organogenesis (mainly in the 2nd and 3rd gestational months), and the most common defect produced at birth was phocomelia, a syndrome where the extremities were severely underdeveloped. The drug is not teratogenic in all experimental animals and, since pregnant women are never included in premarketing randomised trials, pregnant women in the population are often the first to experience potential side effects of new drugs. It is therefore important to set up programmes that fully utilise the information generated by pregnant women using new drugs. At present, we are short of such information systems (Olsen et al. 2002).

It is currently hoped, somewhat naïvely, that the monitoring systems will pick up new teratogenic drugs, even at an early phase and that such an effect will be detected by the reporting of side effects. Most drugs, especially new ones, are, however, only used by few pregnant women, and should they cause only one (or a few) specific congenital malformations they will not be detectable in a general monitoring system or in a side effect register, since the person who prescribes the drug is usually not the same as the person who diagnoses a congenital malformation. A monitoring system of congenital malformations would, on the other hand, be of importance for setting up specific studies, because good quality data on congenital malformations are often lacking in routine medical records.

The technology available to detect congenital malformations at an early stage in gestation is continuously improving with the use of ultrasound or biochemical and genetic methods. Clearly, measuring prevalence at birth may become a questionable endpoint if prenatal diagnosis is not used in exactly the same way in the groups to be compared.

Since specific malformations are rare, most studies on determinants of congenital malformations will be based upon large routinely collected data sources covering many thousands, possibly hundreds of thousands, of pregnant women, or by using a case-control approach. The main advantage with the case-control is having the possibility to collect valid exposure information concerning the pregnancy (often very early pregnancy) by means of interviews. These data may, however, be difficult or even impossible to obtain for exposures that are difficult to recall. The recall easily leads to bias related to a lack in symmetry of the information obtained from a woman who had a child with a severe handicap when compared to the information provided by a woman who had a healthy child. Using another set of patient controls (e.g. another type of congenital malformation than the one under study) may be a possible solution, although it is not without problems. When using patient controls as a surrogate for representative source population samples, the "control" disease should neither be caused nor prevented by the exposure under study, and, since we know so little about the causes of most malformations, this might be a hazardous decision to make. However, interviewing women who all had a child with congenital malformations should render the quality of information more comparable, thus reducing the potential for bias (Swan et al. 1992). There is indication of a more accurate recall of medicine intake in mothers who had a child with a congenital malformation than in mothers, who had a healthy child (Rockenbauer et al. 2001). Furthermore, it has been shown that the way questions on medicine intake are phrased plays an important role (Mitchell et al. 1986).

Using a case-crossover design (Maclure 1991) might be an option to overcome biased reporting (and confounding by personal characteristics). Since only exposures at a given time period may be of relevance for the malformations under study, another time interval during gestation before or after the index exposure may be selected as a reference. The relative prevalence ratio for the case in question can be estimated by dividing mothers who were exposed in the exposure window but not in the reference window and vice versa, given that these windows have the same duration. The rest of the exposure combinations do not provide any information to the study concerning the associations between drug intake and the specific malformations.

A case-control approach will allow specific diagnostic classification of the cases. By setting up specific diagnostic standards it is possible to make sure that only the individuals with the malformation in question enter as cases (high specificity) although some with the disease may not meet the criteria (sensitivity < 1). As long as specificity is high, however, a relative effect measure will not be biased by a low sensitivity, but the study power will be reduced. The following example illustrates why this is the case.

Imagine that the underlying source population has the following structure:

Exp	Cases	All births
+	2000	100,000
−	1000	100,000

$$RP = \frac{2000/100,000}{1000/100,000} = 2.0$$

Now assume that only half of the time cases will be diagnosed. The display of data would then be:

Exp	Cases	All births
+	1000	100,000
−	500	100,000

$$RP = \frac{1000/100,000}{500/100,000} = 2.0$$

The relative prevalence ratio (RP) is still 2, simply because there are still twice as many diagnosed children with malformations among the exposed compared with the non-exposed. The low diagnostic sensitivity did not change this. It is easy to design a case-control study to replicate these results. It is just a matter of proper sampling from the source population.

A case-control sampling using all cases and a sample from the base from any of the two above situations would produce an unbiased estimate of the RP. A 1 : 5 case-control sampling would, in the first case, give:

Exp	Cases	Controls
+	2000	7500
−	1000	7500
All	3000	15,000

$$OR = \frac{2000/1000}{7500/7500} = 2.0$$

and in the second case:

Exp	Cases	Controls
+	1000	3750
–	500	3750
All	1500	7500

$$\text{OR} = \frac{1000/500}{37,500/3750} = 2.0$$

The power would be less in the second example, as is reflected by a larger variance. The variance of the OR is 0.0018 and 0.0035 in the first and second study, respectively.

Pregnancy Complications

Operational Definition

During pregnancy almost all maternal physiological systems are subjected to major changes. Cardiac output increases by 30%–50% and thus the kidneys have to filter a much higher amount of blood. The space taken up by the enlarging uterus changes the way the lungs and digestive systems work. The major changes are, however, hormonal, and the placenta produces a large amount of hormones that help maintain the pregnancy. The immune system is also affected, as pregnancy is a mildly immuno-depressed state. Also, there are indications that pregnancy requires a shift in the type of immune response from Th1 (pro-inflammatory) to Th2 (antibody-mediated), modifying the maternal type of immune response as well.

Because of these major changes, there are a number of pre-existing diseases (such as diabetes, kidney disease, affections of the thyroid, heart failure, autoimmune diseases) that may be exacerbated by pregnancy and harm the woman or the foetus. Some autoimmune diseases improve in pregnancy; others relapse or worsen, or present a cluster of onsets immediately following a pregnancy.

Pregnancy complications are defined in the Medical Subject Headings as the co-occurrence of pregnancy and a disease. The disease may have started before conception or after. This definition is rather general and not in line with what most people would think of as being a pregnancy complication. A puerperal depression is considered as triggered by the birth and not just a depression that happens to occur shortly after delivery, although it may be difficult to distinguish a depression triggered by birth from a depression that would have occurred in any case. In these paragraphs we will, therefore, deal with some aspects of complications that are only seen during pregnancy, or which are only defined as such during a pregnancy. We will briefly deal with some common pregnancy complications (such as hyperemesis and placenta previa), reserving a particular emphasis to gestational diabetes and pre-eclampsia, the former because it is a clear example of some of the problems facing epidemiologists who deal with pregnancy complications. Pre-eclampsia is relatively common and a serious complication of pregnancy, and it is also one of the most fascinating mysteries of reproduction.

Other chronic diseases pose a risk to the mother and to the foetus. It is likely that most of them will be seen among pregnant women, but with a lower prevalence than in the general population, especially if they are severely debilitating for the woman in her reproductive years. The 'healthy pregnancy effect' is analogous to the better known 'healthy worker effect' and is due to the fact that a reasonably good health is required to conceive and carry a pregnancy to term. This "effect" need not cause bias if properly addressed in the design of the study. The 'healthy pregnancy effect' only underlines the fact that many diseases will be less frequent among parous women if these diseases interfere with actual fertility.

Methodological Challenges 5.10.2

Defining a Disease: Choosing a Cut-Point

A general problem in studying pregnancy complications is due to the fact that many such conditions are defined as an extreme of events that occur in the course of a normal pregnancy. Thus, a disease that represents an extreme value of the distribution of a given trait rather than a qualitatively different entity will be more problematic to study. In this case, the distinction between normal and pathological becomes relatively blurred, and very often the challenge faced by clinicians is that of defining a cut-point beyond which a condition is declared a disease (as in obesity, diabetes, hypertension, and pre-eclampsia) and below which the same condition is considered within the norm. It is immediately evident that definitions of this type are susceptible to many problems, as is the case with all diseases defined this way, because any arbitrary threshold will introduce some degree of misclassification, especially since pregnancy is a condition under intensive medical surveillance, which will then make pregnant women a population in which virtually the entirety of its members will be screened for severe diseases one way or the other and, in most cases, more than once in the course of pregnancy. It is well-known that even a test with a high specificity will produce a large number of false positives in a population with a low prevalence of a disease, and this leads to women being unnecessarily treated and subjected to the stress of being diagnosed with a disease they may not have. On the other hand, missing women with a given disease by moving the cut-point towards more extreme values will result in a low sensitivity that will lead to missing cases with consequences that may be very serious for the mother and the baby. The extent of these problems depends not only on the criteria for defining a disease but also on the approach adopted by the care providers, the access to prenatal care, and the frequency with which pregnant women are monitored. The more frequently women are seen and their blood glucose, blood pressure, or proteinuria are measured, the more likely it will be that they can be wrongly classified as having a given disorder, especially if these measures fluctuate over time. Conversely, women that are not screened often or do not comply with prenatal care may be under-diagnosed in these circumstances. Factors related to monitoring, such as insurance coverage, distance from antenatal care centres, etc., can thus produce bias, especially – but not only – if risk factors for the disease are also part of the reasons why women comply less with prenatal care (smoking may, in some circumstances, fulfil these criteria). In some cases, modelling the number of ANC visits or other factors affecting the access to ANC (distance, social class, insurance plan when applicable) might provide a clue about whether a problem of this type has occurred, but this will not necessarily be sufficient to correct for the bias.

Even if women comply equally with prenatal care, problems may arise if the exposures under study correlate to some degree with the probability of being diagnosed, as health care personnel may differentially screen women according to their risk profiles.

Furthermore, the consensus on the cut-points usually changes in time and is often not even geographically homogeneous at the same point in time. Comparisons over time and between different areas thus become difficult to perform and of questionable value depending on the level of prenatal care and definition of the disorder. Often researchers do not have the crude values of what is actually measured but only the clinical diagnosis, which makes virtually every study susceptible to well founded criticism because the uncertainty and potential inaccuracy of the diagnosis may well depend on the putative risk factors under study. Random errors will also tend to dilute associations, often conspiring towards this end with the number of false positives that will be included in most case series. We are thus left with studying the phenotype that clinicians in that particular region and at a given point in time call a disease, which may not be the best classification from an etiological point of view.

ROC curves

Most readers will be familiar with the concepts of sensitivity and specificity. In the presence of a 'gold standard' diagnosis that is the 'truth' about whether a patient has a disease or not, the sensitivity of a given test is calculated as the number of subjects who test positive among the diseased divided by the total number of diseased. A test has a sensitivity of 1 when all with the disease are identified by the test. The specificity of a test, on the other hand, is calculated as the total number of subjects who test negative among the non-diseased divided by the total number of all non-diseased (cf. Chap. III.10 of this handbook). A test with a specificity of 1 will correctly identify as negatives all truly negative (no disease). There is probably no single test that will have both a sensitivity and a specificity of 1, so researchers have to live with a margin of error, even when several tests are used in a sequence or in parallel. The use of the concepts of sensitivity and specificity relies on a rather strong and often forgotten assumption: that the process in question (the disease) is inherently dichotomous (that is, of the yes/no type). Although we often think of a disease as either present or absent and, for practical purposes, that is the way clinicians often treat them, this concept is a construct that depends on the definition of the disease, its severity and on the stage of the disease and does not necessarily reflect the underlying physiology – especially when we use a single marker to determine presence or absence of the disease. However, with this *caveat* in mind, the concepts of sensitivity and specificity can be useful. Associated with these are the concepts of positive and negative predictive values, which are the fractions that will be truly positive (or negative) given that they had tested positive (or negative). A test performed in a population with a high prevalence will, in general, perform fairly well in terms of negative and positive predictive values as long as sensitivity and specificity are high. In a large population with a low prevalence (say 1/1000), however, even a test with unrealistically high values of sensitivity and specificity for a clinical test (say, a sensitivity of 0.99 and a specificity of 0.98) will yield a large fraction of false positives among all those who test positive (with the above values, of the 21 that would be classified as positive in a population of 1000, 20 would be false positives). This misclassification will pose a serious problem to any epidemiologic study by diluting the case series.

In a situation where a given marker is distributed differently between diseased and non diseased subjects and where a cut-point is chosen to screen the population, a situation analogous to the one depicted in Fig. 5.3 will appear.

In the fictitious example given in Fig. 5.3, the population represented by the distribution on the left represents people without the disease under study, and the blood marker that is measured has a Gaussian distribution with a mean of 1.25 and a standard deviation of 0.12. The population on the right has the disease, and the same marker has a mean value of 1.55, with a standard deviation of 0.13. The two populations do not need to have the same absolute size, as what is represented in the figure are the relative proportions (in %) of each category of values. It appears from the figure that a large fraction of the diseased and of the non-diseased overlap as far as the marker value is concerned. A test that uses such a marker to discriminate between healthy and diseased subjects will either miss a large number of the diseased or include many false positives. In other situations there will be less (or more) overlap, but the same argument holds.

To establish a cut-point for a test (serological, or a blood pressure measurement) in order to define diseased and non-diseased subjects, 'Receiver Operating Curves' (ROC) has been used as a method to evaluate a test (Metz 1978). Each chosen cut-point would result in a certain proportion of subjects, who fail to be classified as diseased, being diseased (false negatives) and in a certain proportion of subjects, who would test positive, being in truth negative (false positives). To build a ROC curve the test is performed by progressively moving the cut-point from a lax one (in which a great number of false positives would be included) to a strict one (in which a high proportion of false negatives would be included; see also Chap. III.10 of this handbook). In the figure, a cut-off point of about 1.19 would produce

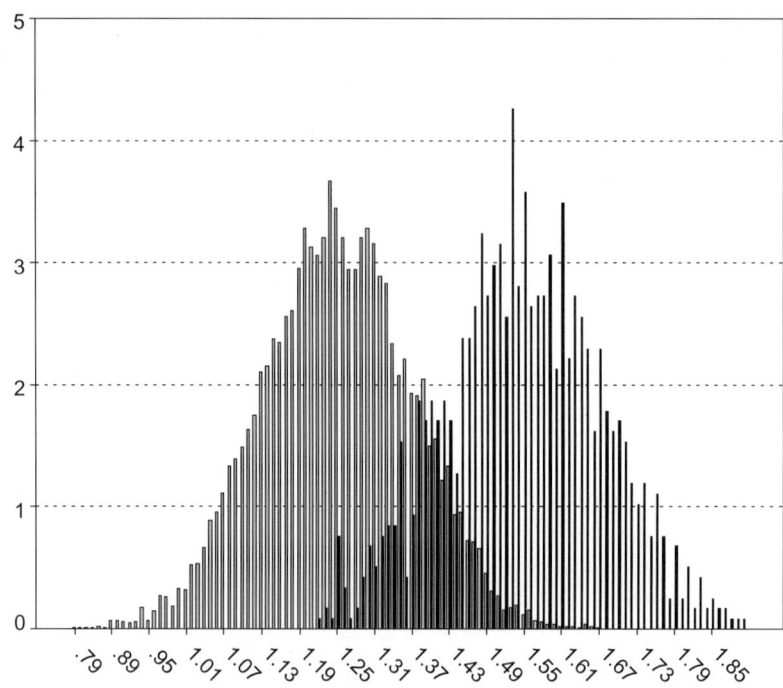

Figure 5.3. Hypothetical distribution of a blood marker in two populations, with (*left*) and without (*right*) a given illness. The *area of overlap* reflects the misclassification encountered when a given threshold is used to determine the disease status

a sensitivity close to 1, and a cut-off at 1.67 a specificity close to 1. When the measurement is not quantitative but is based – for instance – on radiographic results, the observer is asked to classify several times the same subject using a different rating for classifying disease: *very likely positive/likely positive/unlikely positive/very unlikely positive*. Of course, the 'true status' of the subjects has to be known with a degree of 'certainty' from a different source when building ROC curves. ROC curves are used to find the cut-point that maximizes benefits and minimizes side effects (taking into consideration the cost of missing a true positive and that of having a number of false positives).

The curve is built by plotting on the *x*-axis the proportion of FP (False Positives; 1-specificity) and on the *y*-axis the fraction of TP (True Positives; sensitivity).

When selecting the subjects for the experiment conducted in order to build a ROC curve, an adequate spectrum of the manifestations of the disease should be selected for the test to be applicable to the target population.

If prevalence is low, then the FP fraction must be kept low, unless it is of vital importance that all positives are identified. A combination of two tests could then be used (one very sensitive on all subjects, followed by a very specific test on the positive ones: this is applied, for example, in screening for HIV, where an Elisa test (very sensitive) is followed by a Western Blot (highly specific)). The higher and the more to the left a curve is, the better is, in general, its performance.

In case there is no overlapping between diseased and non-diseased for the studied variable, the area underneath the curve is 1 and the curve passes through $y = 1$ and is parallel to the x-axis. When the assessment is totally random, the curve is the diagonal for the first quadrant, and the area is 0.5. An area of 0.8 means that a random diseased subject has a higher value of the test than a random non-diseased subject 80% of the time (Zweig and Campbell 1993).

Design Strategies

In general, i.e. if the exposure prevalence is low, relative effect measures, such as the relative risk or the odds ratio, are more profoundly affected by low specificity than by low sensitivity. A possible strategy when dealing with diseases that have been classified on the basis of a definition determined by exceeding a given cut-point is to limit the number of false positives by restricting the study to the more severe cases (which will, most likely, be identified with a lesser degree of error), if the possibility to do so exists. However, this will often have the consequence of substantially reducing the power of the study when dealing with disorders that, in general, are quite rare to start with.

Ad hoc studies (made for the specific purpose of investigating a given disease in a defined population) with access to medical records are an important option, which, however, will be more costly than studies based on routine information and will, once again, raise the issue of how many cases will be available for the study.

In some cases, combining the clinical diagnosis of the disease of interest with a feature that should be concomitantly present if the disease is actually present may increase the quality of the data for the study.

For example, placenta previa is a relatively rare pregnancy complication, where the placenta is wrongly positioned to partly cover the opening to the birth canal. In early pregnancy, however, the placenta will relatively often appear to be wrongly positioned but will in many cases spontaneously reposition itself during the course of pregnancy (Dashe et al. 2002). If a study is based on all diagnoses, even those made in early pregnancy, cases may include a number of these early cases, which represent a rather harmless condition. However, if placenta previa persists, the common practice is that of performing a caesarean section to deliver the baby and thus, by including only the women diagnosed with placenta previa who were later delivered by caesarean, one will probably be limiting the analysis to the more severe or, at least, the more persistent cases. This has been done, for example, in studies investigating whether pregnancies with placenta previa presented a higher male to female ratio (Wen et al. 2000; Ananth et al. 2001). Whether this type of approach should be used or not has to be evaluated depending on the specific aim of the study.

The significance of the same symptom may also change across the duration of pregnancy, and it may be a cause or a consequence of another condition also depending on the timing. This is probably the case, for example, of bleeding during pregnancy, which, in the last trimester, is probably a consequence of placenta previa or placental abruption, while it may be an entirely different entity in the first two trimesters (such as threatened abortion). Hyperemesis, severe vomiting in pregnancy, is another example of a normal condition becoming pathological when presenting itself in an extreme fashion. Several studies investigated foetal outcome among women who had hyperemesis, with conflicting results (Depue et al. 1987; Kallen 1987; Godsey and Newman 1991; Hallak et al. 1996; Gross et al. 1989). Yet, a recent review states that severe vomiting does not have a negative effect on perinatal outcome (Eliakim et al. 2000). However, if the definition of the case series is based on a hospital diagnosis without taking severity into consideration, then the cases may include a number of women with a relatively mild disease that is not really distinct from the 'normal' nausea and vomiting of pregnancy. Restricting cases to those where some objective biomarkers, such as severe ketosis or serum electrolyte disturbance, can be measured may then provide a more purely defined case series, which might be one of the reasons for the inconsistent findings.

Timing of the disease may also be of relevance, as in two studies investigating the association between hyperemesis and female sex of the baby it was noted that the association was strong only for hospitalised cases of hyperemesis occurring in the first trimester of pregnancy (Askling et al. 1999; Basso et al. 2001). Hyperemesis occurs more frequently in women carrying multiple foetuses, as well as in women (carrying singletons) who will later be diagnosed with pre-eclampsia (Zhang and Cai 1991). These observations suggest that there might be multiple causal paths leading to hyperemesis and that, in some women, a large placenta (with a high hormone production) may be the cause of the disease, while in others hyperemesis may be a sign of some other pathological process under way. In any circumstance, whenever etiologic heterogeneity exists in a process, and signs and symptoms are the same as that of another process (so that they are considered the same disorder), it is always very difficult to disentangle what is being studied. If only a small fraction of the case population represents a different etiologic entity, even a moderately strong predictor will likely appear not to be associated with the mixed entity and it will be repeatedly missed. If the fraction is large, then a predictor will be called a risk factor for both entities, and perhaps this uncertainty contributes to some of the failures of epidemiology to encourage changes in people's habits and in policies. When these conditions occur in pregnancy, it may, in some cases, be possible to discriminate to some extent between different entities by paying particular attention to the timing in which events occur.

5.10.3   Gestational Diabetes

As many other metabolic functions, the metabolism of carbohydrates is altered in normal pregnancies. The fasting blood glucose level decreases early in pregnancy until the 12th week, and it usually remains at this lower level until the end of pregnancy. Insulin, by contrast, remains stable during the 1st and 2nd trimesters, but increases during the 3rd. Outside pregnancy, on the other hand, the blood glucose level returns rapidly to fasting levels after a meal, and in pregnancy both glucose and insulin levels reach higher peaks than they would after a similar meal in the non-pregnant state. This level is furthermore maintained for a longer time. Human placental lactogen (hPL) is the hormone that is believed to be responsible for these changes in the metabolism (Haig 1993). In general, pregnancy is a state of mild insulin resistance, and some women develop gestational diabetes. As an adaptation, insulin production is increased at the same time that the mother is becoming insulin-resistant. Haig (1993) proposes an interesting hypothesis about why this change may occur within his evolutionary theory about the genetic conflicts of pregnancy. Glucose is an important nutrient for the growing foetus, but it is also important for the mother's survival that not too many of her resources are depleted by the foetus, which may happen if foetal demands went unopposed: the decline in blood glucose early in pregnancy could thus represent a maternal attempt to limit foetal uptake. In addition, after every meal there will be a competition between the mother and the foetus over the respective share. The longer it takes the mother to reduce her blood sugar, the higher the share taken by the foetus, hence the insulin resistance, according to Haig. At the beginning of pregnancy, the foetus has limited growing demands and limited 'power', which is why the mother succeeds in 'hiding' her blood glucose. During the third trimester, however, the foetus has very high growing demands and it is strong enough to take the upper hand in the competition with the mother. When seen in the light of how to optimise survival probabilities, this is an attractive hypothesis, although hard to test.

Barker (1995, 1998) has a different hypothesis, suggesting that insulin resistance is a consequence of limited nutrient supply. Clearly, however, glucose metabolism is crucial in pregnancy, and a mechanism has evolved that creates a delicate balance between the maternal and foetal needs. Diabetes during pregnancy is a complex problem and requires a very careful management to prevent damages to the foetus and to the mother. The consequences of gestational diabetes may be dire for the foetus; as with gestational diabetes there is an increased risk of stillbirth and macrosomia (Schmidt et al. 2001; Johnstone et al. 1990). Macrosomia is the most frequent outcome in diabetic mothers, and this can complicate delivery to the point that a caesarean section is required. Women who have had gestational diabetes are at increased risk of having it again in a subsequent pregnancy and are also at risk of developing diabetes (Dornhorst and Beard 1993), especially type 2, later in life. Gestational diabetes, as well as other types of diabetes, is also a risk factor for pre-eclampsia (Schmidt et al. 2001), another potentially severe pregnancy complication. Obesity is a predisposing factor (with insulin resistance the underlying condition), as is advanced maternal age or having a family history of diabetes.

The definition of gestational diabetes is problematic and the subject of many a controversy (Dornhorst and Beard 1993; Martin et al. 1995; Gabbe 1998; Bonomo et al. 1998; Schmidt et al. 2000). The discussion extends to whether there should be universal screening for all pregnant women. In 1996, the American Diabetes Association concluded that universal screening should be done, but these recommendations were then revised in 1997 and 1998 to selective screening of women satisfying at least one criterion among (1) age above 25, (2) age below 25 and a body mass index above 27, (3) a family history of diabetes, and (4) belonging to ethnic groups with a known higher predisposition to diabetes. There is no agreement over the 'gold standard' test for women who are screened positive. The oral glucose tolerance test is the norm, but the load (the dose of administered glucose) varies geographically. There is also discussion about which cut-off limits should be used, as the prevalence of gestational diabetes would change depending upon the threshold, and the risk would be to either define too many women who are not diabetic as such or to miss too many women who are diabetic and at risk of having an adverse pregnancy or health outcome. There is no clear distinction between normal and pathological values, which hampers any diagnostic criterion. Often, epidemiologists do not deal with the actual values of glucose level but with the clinical diagnosis collected over several hospitals, without guarantee of uniformity in the criteria used for screening and diagnosis. The diagnosis will also depend on whether glucose is measured or not and, since gestational diabetes is mostly asymptomatic, this is an added complication. Researchers planning studies requiring an accurate diagnosis of gestational diabetes should thus be aware of the medical attitude towards screening in pregnancy in the locations where they plan to collect their data and of the tools and cut-off levels in use, as well as of the criteria that govern which women are screened and which are not. At best, studies are based upon follow-up of cohorts that are all subject to testing within the same protocol.

Geographical variations in the definition and incidence, as well as changes in definition and screening attitudes over time are also to be taken into consideration when making comparisons between places and periods. Long-term as well as short term consequences for the foetus have been identified, and in some countries the focus of the diagnosis of gestational diabetes has now shifted from the likelihood of progression to later chronic diabetes in the mother to the outcome of pregnancy; a shift that also has consequences on the diagnostic criteria. Since obesity is associated with a highly increased risk of type-2 diabetes as well as gestational diabetes, a number of women would only be diagnosed during pregnancy and the two types of diabetes would then be confused. However, since both types of diabetes increase the risk of pregnancy complications (such as pre-eclampsia) and of adverse foetal outcome, this may not be a major problem, depending on the specific purpose of the study. When studying pre-eclampsia, for instance, there are situations where it would be advisable to exclude women with pre-existing diabetes but not those with gestational diabetes (which shares with pre-eclampsia obesity as a risk factor and, possibly, other predictors) and this may prove to be difficult to do accurately. If and how much of an impact this could have on the estimates will once again depend on the specific situation and will in many cases be hard to evaluate.

5.10.4   Pregnancy-Induced Hypertension and Pre-Eclampsia

Definition and Diagnosis

In the first trimester of pregnancy, blood pressure is usually reduced from normal values. In many women, however, blood pressure increases around mid-pregnancy to above normal values. A modest degree of hypertension is thus a rather common condition of pregnancy and has not been consistently associated with unfavourable outcomes.

Pre-eclampsia is, on the other hand, one of the most common and potentially severe complications of pregnancy. In pre-eclampsia, the maternal blood pressure can increase dramatically and heart, brain, and kidneys may be severely damaged. If the mother survives, the affected organs usually return to normality shortly after delivery, but pre-eclampsia can also be fatal. If seizures occur, the disease is called eclampsia (a very rare occurrence in countries with well-functioning health care systems) and the risk for both the mother and the foetus is then much higher. While eclampsia is a dramatic event that is probably rarely misclassified, pre-eclampsia is, by definition, much more elusive. In most countries, it is currently defined as the concurrent presence of hypertension and proteinuria. Gestational hypertension is defined as either a persistent rise of 25 mm Hg in systolic blood pressure during pregnancy compared to pre-pregnant values (if the pre-pregnant values are not known, a systolic blood pressure of 140 mm Hg or higher), or as a rise of 15 in diastolic blood pressure (DBP) (or as a DBP above 90). The definitions of gestational hypertension do, however, vary geographically. For the disorder to be called pre-eclampsia hypertension must be accompanied by a certain minimum level of proteinuria. The degree of severity depends on the values of blood pressure and the amount of protein loss, as well as additional signs and symptoms, often including oedema. Previously, pre-eclampsia was defined by the concomitant presence of two out of three symptoms (hypertension, proteinuria, and oedema), but the definition has changed to be restricted to cases where both hypertension and proteinuria are present at the same time, as oedema appeared to be too unspecific. The problem with this definition is, however, that a mild state of hypertension is common in pregnancy and, often, the pre-pregnant values are not known. What is termed moderate preeclampsia may thus, in some cases, be nothing more than a change in values of blood pressure and proteinuria within the norm. Sometimes, changes in these values may be severe enough to qualify for the diagnosis, but they will escape detection. Furthermore, some women become nervous when their blood pressure is taken in a clinical setting, and thus they would be classified as hypertensive while they are not ('white coat' hypertension). On the other hand, a number of cases may be missed by applying this definition, either because of ignorance of the baseline pre-pregnancy values, or because the women do not have their blood pressure measured at the moment of the increase and, if there are no severe symptoms, the diagnosis will never be made. In severe cases, women become very sick and there is little doubt about the diagnosis, but these cases are the minority.

The reported incidence of pre-eclampsia appears to vary widely across places, from an estimated 2% to approximately 8%. This variation may reflect real variations in susceptibility and determinants across populations, but it almost certainly also depends on the sources of information for the diagnosis as well as on the access to prenatal care and the problems mentioned above.

The only known 'cure' for pre-eclampsia is to end the pregnancy, as the placenta appears to be the organ that causes the disease, and pre-eclampsia is therefore the major cause of iatrogenic preterm delivery.

Pathophysiology of Pre-Eclampsia

In normal pregnancy, the maternal spiral arteries are modified and penetrate deeply into the decidua (first trophoblastic invasion) and, around the 16th to 18th week, into the myometrium (second trophoblastic invasion). The invasive trophoblast enlarges the vessels from within, and a fibrin substance that renders them flaccid and unresponsive to maternal vasoconstriction replaces the vessels' internal lining. In pre-eclampsia often, but not always, the second trophoblastic invasion does not occur, or occurs only to a very modest degree (Salas 1999; Roberts and Lain 2002), resulting in placental perfusion being severely compromised because the arteries are narrow and with a high resistance instead of being wide, low-resistance vessels, as they would be if the invasion had proceeded normally.

Haig (1993) expresses the view that hypertension in pregnancy is a foetal adaptive mechanism. Because of the structure of the spiral arteries and the fact that sympathetic nerves disappear from the placental site during pregnancy, the maternal control of the blood flow to the placenta is limited and the placental site is characterized by low resistance to blood flow. Due to these characteristics, for any given resistance of the placental unit, a compensatory rise in the maternal peripheral blood pressure will increase the blood flow to the placenta. According to Haig, this may be a sign of a feto-maternal conflict, where the growing foetus is able – by some unknown mechanism – to increase maternal blood pressure and thus increase the placental blood flow. Drug-induced reduction of mean arterial pressure may be associated with a reduction in foetal growth (von Dadelszen et al. 2000)

Pre-eclampsia is not, however, always accompanied by defective placentation, and is, most likely, a common syndrome resulting from heterogeneous causes (Ness and Roberts 1996). It is believed that large placental mass (as seen in multiple pregnancies) and endothelial disease (as seen in diabetics) are mechanisms that can also produce placental hypoperfusion and start the cascade of events that leads to pre-eclampsia (Salas 1999).

Known Predictors of Pre-Eclampsia

The aetiology of pre-eclampsia is mostly unknown, and this disorder is one of the most tantalizing mysteries of reproductive epidemiology. The best-known predictors are nulliparity, obesity, and multi-foetal pregnancies, while smoking is protective for reasons unknown, although several hypotheses have been raised to explain this association (Condé-Agudelo et al. 1999). Africans and African-Americans appear to be at a higher risk, possibly because susceptibility to pre-eclampsia is related to susceptibility to cardiovascular disease (Roberts and Lain 2002). Recent evidence suggests that only women giving birth with pre-eclampsia preterm are at a higher risk of later death for cardiovascular disease, while women giving birth with pre-eclampsia at term have no increased risk compared to non pre-eclamptic women (Irgens et al. 2001).

Several trials have addressed the association between pre-eclampsia and dietary factors, mostly calcium, magnesium, antioxidants, and fish oil. Unfortunately, no clear answer has emerged from these studies, except for the finding that calcium appears to be protective among women with a very low baseline intake or for women with a very high risk of pre-eclampsia (Villar and Belizan 2000). In general, however, the attempts to prevent pre-eclampsia through dietary supplements or aspirin have been overall disappointing (Sibai 1998; Dekker and Sibai 2001).

It is well accepted that a genetic component to pre-eclampsia exists, since children born of pre-eclamptic pregnancies are themselves at a higher risk of having children born of pregnancies with pre-eclampsia (Esplin et al. 2001). Also, males whose partner had pre-eclampsia have almost twice the risk of having their subsequent partner developing pre-eclampsia compared to males whose partner had not developed it (Lie et al. 1998).

A large number of biomarkers and genetic factors have also been explored as predisposing to pre-eclampsia (Broughton Pipkin 1999; Roberts and Cooper 2001). Genetic studies on pre-eclampsia have not consistently revealed a specific genotype associated with pre-eclampsia, although women with pre-eclampsia are more likely to have a heterozygous factor V Leiden mutation and other thrombophiliac mutations (Alfirevic et al. 2002). Not all researchers agree on the role of thrombophiliac mutations (Livingston et al. 2001), however.

Methodological Challenges in Studies of Pre-Eclampsia

Although pre-eclampsia is probably the most studied among all pregnancy complications and keeps fascinating researchers from many areas of medicine, several difficulties face the investigators, mainly because of the difficulty of accurately identifying cases in sufficient numbers, without incurring selection problems. Research based upon nationwide hospital registries can provide population-based data that may, however, be of limited quality if the only available information is the code according to the International Classification of Diseases. The advantages of these studies are that women are most likely unselected and that the numbers will be large enough to allow studying even relatively rare predictors or outcomes. In some cases, these studies might be the only viable option. If, to improve the quality of the data, researchers restrict their case series to severe pre-eclampsia only, then the numbers will be dramatically reduced but, possibly, fewer false positives will be included.

On the other hand, studies of the case-control type where medical charts are available would provide a much better case series if proper diagnostic procedures can be applied to document the disease, whereas problems may exist in recruiting a sufficient number of controls retaining a sufficient confidence that self-selection will not bias the study. If the women who accept to enter the study as controls do so according to the exposure under study, this will produce biased estimates to an extent that is often impossible to judge. Since pregnant women are invited to lead a healthy lifestyle for the sake of the baby if not their own, it is likely that some women whose pregnancy went well but whose habits were not beyond reproach would be relatively unwilling to take part in a study where such habits would be questioned. On the other hand, women who had a negative experience may be less reluctant to having their behaviour under scrutiny, because they want to know what went wrong. However, problems in studying pre-eclampsia go well beyond the objective difficulties of appropriately defining cases or of finding unselected study populations.

Pre-eclampsia is a cause of preterm delivery, mostly iatrogenic. This fact complicates the interpretation of studies attempting to evaluate whether pre-eclampsia is associated with conditions that are more common in babies that are born preterm, such as e.g. cerebral palsy. Some studies have reported that babies of pre-eclamptic pregnancies were protected from cerebral palsy when the risk was examined by gestational week at birth (Gray et al. 1998; Murphy et al. 1995). Is this a protection conferred by pre-eclampsia, or is it an artefact due to the fact that the causes of preterm delivery in pre-eclamptic pregnancies differ from those of other preterm deliveries, where the causal factors may include those of cerebral palsy? Because babies born preterm for causes other than pre-eclampsia have other pathological mechanisms that advanced birth, disentangling the effects of preterm birth from its causes is a major challenge, and so is examining the various causal paths leading to preterm birth that may very well be implicated in the diseases 'associated' with preterm birth. Also, many cases of pre-eclampsia are delivered by emergency caesarean section, and the delivery complications due to caesarean section are generally different from those arising from vaginal deliveries, as many preterm deliveries will be. If complications that can arise from vaginal delivery are associated with cerebral palsy (e.g. anoxia), then comparing pre-eclamptic women with non pre-eclamptic will result in a biased comparison.

Another problem is that of studying pre-eclampsia in connection with other conditions or factors that are associated with preterm delivery. If a given factor causes preterm delivery, it may also appear to be protective of pre-eclampsia simply because women with a shortened pregnancy have had less opportunity of developing it, since pre-eclampsia often occurs after the 36th week of gestation, but being pregnant (or just delivered) is a necessary condition for being diagnosed. If the date when pre-eclampsia was first diagnosed is known, data may be analysed through Cox regression or survival methods to overcome this problem (for a general introduction to survival analysis see Chap. II.4 of this handbook).

If an important confounder is systematically omitted when studying a given disease, this will lead to the potential establishment of a wrong conclusion (cf. Chap. I.9 of this handbook). For example, a currently accepted hypothesis about the aetiology of pre-eclampsia proposes that a maternal immune reaction to paternal antigens may be a cause of the failed trophoblastic invasion. This hypothesis was mainly based on the observation that pre-eclampsia is more frequent in first pregnancies. Among multiparous, women who had changed their partner from the previous pregnancy had an increased risk (Dekker et al. 1998; Dekker 1999; Trupin et al. 1996; Lie et al. 1998; Li and Wi 2000). Also, women with a long period of sexual cohabitation prior to a pregnancy and women using oral contraceptives appeared to be at a lower risk of the disease than women with a short cohabitation period or those using barrier contraceptive methods (Robillard et al. 1994; Dekker et al. 1998). This suggested that a prolonged exposure to the partner's sperm may have constituted a protection that would reduce the risk of pre-eclampsia, thus leading to the expression that 'primipaternity' was a risk factor for pre-eclampsia. For some researchers (including the authors of this chapter), however, this hypothesis has lost some attraction since three studies (two based on the Norwegian Birth Registry (Skjaerven et al. 2002; Trogstad et al. 2001), and one based on a sample from the Danish Birth Registry (Basso et al. 2001)) independently reported that this increased risk with change of partner disappeared if the interval between births was adjusted for. Women who change partner have, on average, a much longer interval between births: if any factor correlated with time has an impact on the risk of pre-eclampsia, then women waiting a longer time will have an increased risk, regardless of whether they change partner. This was found to be true in the above-mentioned studies, even after maternal age was controlled for. This finding prompted a further study where time to pregnancy was investigated in association with pre-eclampsia, as a fraction of the women waiting a long time between pregnancies may be subfecund. Time to pregnancy, as previously mentioned, is a proxy for the couple's fecundity and thus a relatively crude marker, since it reflects a multitude of disorders. It is, however, interesting that an association between long time to pregnancy and pre-eclampsia could be found despite these limitations (Basso et al. 2003), and this evidence may lead to further research for identifying a subgroup of infertile women with a specific disorder that relates to pre-eclampsia.

Pre-eclampsia is most likely the result of an interaction between the maternal and the foetal systems, but its diagnosis relies exclusively on symptoms that are observed in the mother. It is perhaps for this reason that, so far, pre-eclampsia has eluded most attempts to clarify its aetiology.

Delivery Complications   5.11

Delivery complications may arise before or during delivery and present a risk for the mother and/or the baby. Some have to do with the foetus's presentation or its inability to pass through the birth canal. Until less than a century ago impacted births were the major cause of foetal and maternal morbidity and mortality. Because of malnutrition, many women had under-developed pelvises and the baby's head would remain trapped in the birth canal. Nowadays, foetal or maternal death because of this is a very rare event in industrialized countries but still a major problem in developing countries, where most babies are delivered at home and hospitals are far away and are perhaps lacking adequate resources. The three major causes of maternal mortality in developing countries are haemorrhage and sepsis, as well as hypertensive disorders, and the first two usually result from delivery complications.

Beyond foetal presentation (and position), and foeto-pelvic disproportion, delivery complications also include weak contractions, prolonged labour (of any of the three stages), prolapse of the umbilical cord, perineal or vaginal tears, foetal asphyxia, retention of the placenta, haemorrhage, etc. Caesarean sections, which account for between 15% and 30% of all births, depending on countries, constitute perhaps the major difficulties when studying delivery complications. Caesarean sections can be planned or acute, and the latter could be started before delivery or during delivery. Emergency caesarean sections, themselves considered a 'delivery complication', are triggered by complications arising in the mother or the foetus.

In the case of delivery complications even more than in other cases, researchers have to study what is left after physicians have acted. Therefore, only babies being born vaginally will be at risk of getting the umbilical cord wrapped around their neck, or of having any other accident during their descent through the birth canal that may affect the supply of oxygen to the brain. This would not be a problem if the decision of delivering a woman by caesarean section were independent of any factors that may put the baby at higher risk of encountering such mishaps, but – usually – this is not the case. Since the relative size of the mother and the baby or signs of foetal distress may well trigger the decision of performing a caesarean section, it is likely that babies born vaginally and those born by caesarean are not comparable before delivery, which will complicate any interpretation of findings associated with a given delivery complication. This will also complicate any study trying to evaluate the 'effects' of any given intervention during delivery, as it will be difficult to separate the effects of the intervention from the causes that provoked it, which may also be the causes of the outcome of interest. Even restricting to planned caesareans may not be sufficient to solve the problem, as caesareans are planned for a reason, and one likely reason is that a complication is foreseen and a caesarean section may prevent it from occurring. Experience in previous pregnancies will also affect the mode of delivery. A woman who has previously had a caesarean section will, in many cases, have one also for her next delivery, especially if the two pregnancies are close in time. Since many events tend to repeat themselves in one woman's reproductive life, it will be hard to decide what to do with such a woman, especially if the cause for her previous caesarean is not known.

A caesarean section is the preferred choice of delivery mode for an increasing number of women and immediate risks appear to be few. Only little is, however, known about long-term effects and recent results suggest that the risk of asthma may be increased (Kero et al. 2002), although these findings have to be examined cautiously.

Obstetric complications have been associated with schizophrenia (Geddes and Lawrie 1995; Verdoux et al. 1997), and hypoxia correlates with cerebral palsy (Blair and Stanley 1993). Anoxia or hypoxia will most likely cause cerebral damage and it is reasonable to assume a causal link. But it may also be argued that a baby who had brain damage (which will later cause cerebral palsy) prior to birth will be more likely to have a complicated delivery and suffer from anoxia.

In general, if one wishes to study a delivery complication that may, in some cases, lead to a caesarean section (or to induction of delivery), it will be necessary to have information on why the caesarean section was performed. Practice of caesarean section, induction of delivery, instrumental birth, etc., change between geographical areas and in time, and dealing with these variations may prove a daunting and perhaps impossible task. Usually, many elements are used in the decision to treat, and it may just be impossible to identify all these elements and control for them in the analysis. Confounding by indication is one of the strongest arguments for evaluating treatments in randomised trials, which, however, will often be difficult to carry out in this context.

Since the practice of inducing birth (also by other means than a caesarean section) is now widespread, with criteria for induction that often differ from one hospital to the other, it will always be complicated to study either the induction itself or phenomena such as post-term delivery or macrosomia, even when good information about the causes of the induction are present.

If preterm babies are at a higher risk of incurring delivery complications, it may be this latter fact rather than the timing of birth that makes them at higher risk of several diseases. On the other hand, if some babies who are born preterm are born preterm because of some damage that will later cause the disease and makes them at higher risk of delivery complications, then delivery complications will spuriously appear to cause the disease.

Foetal Origins of Adult Diseases   5.12

Most reproductive epidemiology has been related to the time period from pregnancy planning to the early time period of a new life. In the future, many diseases will be seen as trajectories that start at the time of conception during pregnancy or in early childhood. Obviously, studying exposures with an induction and latency time of causation spanning several decades raises severe problems of being able to control for intervening factors. Without longitudinal readings of the occurrence of possible confounding factors, such studies may often provide confounded results.

It is not unexpected (or not even questionable) news that exposures during foetal life may have lasting effects. What is new is that prenatal exposures may cause diseases that manifest themselves long after birth, perhaps even as late as in following generations. Foetal programming is the name that has been used to describe what could happen if a stimulus or insult at a critical period of organ development interferes with cell division and thus with the function of the affected organ. Permanent changes of organ function could, in principle, lead to many diseases (Olsen 2000), but best documented are the associations between origins of disproportional foetal growth and cardiovascular diseases, perhaps through insulin resistance (Barker 1994, 1995, 1998).

Although the brain growth seems to be less vulnerable to undernutrition, specific nutritional factors, stress, medicine, etc., may influence brain function. Studying determinants of brain function and brain pathology in foetal life should be a high priority research area.

Hormonal factors during foetal life may not only affect the reproductive organs but could also be associated with other diseases, such as cancer of the breast, prostate, and testis. As early as 1990, Trichopoulus suggested that breast cancer might originate in utero. It was suggested that oestrogen could play a role and, since oestrogen correlates with foetal growth, it is expected that rapid foetal growth could be associated with a higher risk of breast cancer five or more decades later. The hypothesis has, to some extent, been corroborated (McCormack et al. 2003).

5.13   Sources of Data

As in other subgroups of epidemiology, the data come from different sources; secondary routine data or ad hoc data based upon self-reported information, information from clinical measures, or information extracted from biological samples; blood, urine, placenta tissue, etc. (Longnecker et al. 2001).

More secondary data are available in reproductive health than in most other epidemiologic areas. Most pregnant women and most newborn children are carefully monitored and data are stored in medical records or even in computerized birth registers that may include not only birth data, but also exposure data such as smoking, medical treatment, etc. (Ericson et al. 1999).

The data that usually have to be collected for research are data that describe putative causes of reproductive failures. Many of these exposures have to be collected prospectively, since they are often forgotten and cannot be reconstructed in an unbiased way back in time, once the outcome of the pregnancy is known. This is often true for dietary factors, medical treatments, occupational exposures, etc. Data on infections, occupational exposures, life-style factors, dietary factors etc., cannot be recalled for more than a few weeks or perhaps months. Usually, the mother is, not unexpectedly, a better source for data on pregnancy and birth than the father (Coughlin et al. 1998).

For these and other reasons, it seems justified to set up large cohort studies, starting shortly after conception and with the aim of collecting exposure information during pregnancy. It is also necessary to establish cohorts that can be followed over long time periods, the best case scenario being from conception to death, including information on their offspring. These cohorts need to be large to provide sufficient information for rare outcomes. Large cohorts of this type were set up in the past, and the best known is probably the National Collaborative Perinatal Project from the USA, started in the late 1950s, where more than 50,000 pregnant women were enrolled. The cohort aimed at studying obstetrical complications and the risk of cerebral palsy and other neurological disorders, although the cohort has served many other research purposes since then.

The Danish National Birth Cohort (DNBC) enrolled 100,000 pregnant women from 1996 to 2002 (Olsen et al. 2001) and included data from interviews, registers, and self-administered questionnaires together with blood from the mother and child stored in a biobank (www.bsmb.dk). Similar studies are in progress in Norway, the USA, and several other countries.

Conclusions

In this chapter we have tried to highlight some of the main features of reproductive epidemiology as we see them. In particular, the fact that reproduction, even in our medicalised world, is a direct result of selective processes, which are still active. In addition, most of the events that we study in this area are what is left after main selection has taken place: selection of couples where a conception takes place, and further selection of those conceptions that will progress to clinical recognition and medical intervention, which may lead to anticipated delivery or a termination of pregnancy, or to treatment of a disorder. For this reason, denominators are usually unknown. Furthermore, the processes that occur during a pregnancy that ends in a birth are usually also hidden, and therefore we do not really know what has happened to the foetus during the most delicate phases of development.

Any event in reproduction generally concerns three individuals rather than one. In many instances pregnancies are voluntary events and many women have several, although the decision to have further pregnancies (and their outcomes) often depends to some extent on the outcome of the previous ones. Time is also of crucial importance when dealing with reproductive epidemiology, but its dimension is generally different from the time involved in the development of, say, cancer after exposure to a given mutagenic substance. The types of bias that can occur in this area are, in many cases, peculiar to this discipline, and they have to be taken into consideration.

We expect genetic and functional genetic studies to be important in future research. Although we may not be able to answer the big questions like how the entire process of organ development is coordinated, finding answers to less broad questions will also be of interest. We need to know much more about genetic and gene-environment interaction, not only in the development of congenital malformations and childhood cancers, but also for long-term organ programming (for an introduction to genetic epidemiology see Chap. III.7 of this handbook). Using information on genetic factors in e.g. metabolism of environmental exposures, like alcohol, may even be of help in examining confounding. How much of the association between e.g. alcohol and reproductive failures is due to confounding cannot be examined in a randomized trial, but the genetic factors that modify alcohol metabolism may follow 'Mendelian randomization' and thus provide a design for comparison that bypasses some of the problems associated with the intercorrelation between lifestyle factors (Smith and Ebrahim 2003).

The peculiarities of reproductive epidemiology offer a number of opportunities to researchers willing to exploit them. We have tried to introduce readers to a number of the features that make this area of epidemiology exciting, vibrating, and fairly unique.

References

AbouZahr C (1998) Maternal mortality overview. In: Murray CJL, Lopez AD (eds) Health dimensions of sex and reproduction. Harvard University Press, Boston, USA, p 144

Adams M, Nybo Andersen AM, Andersen PK, Haig D, Henriksen TB, Hertz-Picciotto I, Lie RT, Olsen J, Skjaerven R, Wilcox A (2003) Sostrup statement on low birth weight (LBW). Int J Epidemiol 32(5):884–885. (Letter to the editor)

Adams MM, Berg CJ, Rhodes PH, McCarthy BJ (1991) Another look at the black-white gap in gestation-specific perinatal mortality. Int J Epidemiol 20(4):950–957

Alderete E, Eskenazi B, Sholtz R (1995) Effect of cigarette smoking and coffee drinking on time to conception. Epidemiology 6(4):403–408

Alfirevic Z, Roberts D, Martlew V (2002) How strong is the association between maternal thrombophilia and adverse pregnancy outcome? A systematic review. Eur J Obstet Gynecol Reprod Biol 101(1):6–14

Ananth CV, Demissie K, Smulian JC, Vintzileos AM (2001) Relationship among placenta previa, fetal growth restriction, and preterm delivery: a population-based study. Obstet Gynecol 98(2):299–306

Andersen AM, Vastrup P, Wohlfahrt J, Andersen PK, Olsen J, Melbye M (2002) Fever in pregnancy and risk of fetal death: a cohort study. Lancet 360(9345):1552–1556

Askling J, Erlandsson G, Kaijser M, Akre O, Ekbom A (1999) Sickness in pregnancy and sex of child. Lancet 354(9195):2053

Baird DD, Ragan BN, Wilcox AJ, Weinberg CR (1993) The relationship between reduced fecundability and subsequent foetal loss. In: Gray R, Leridon H, Spira A (eds) Biomedical and demographic determinants of reproduction. Clarendon Press, Oxford, pp 329–341

Baird DD, Weinberg CR, Schwingl P, Wilcox AJ (1994) Selection bias associated with contraceptive practice in time-to-pregnancy studies. Ann N Y Acad Sci 709:156–164

Baird DD, Wilcox AJ (1985) Cigarette smoking associated with delayed conception. JAMA 253(20):2979–2983

Baird DD, Wilcox AJ, Weinberg CR (1986) Use of time to pregnancy to study environmental exposures. Am J Epidemiol 124(3):470–480

Barker DJ (1994) Mothers, babies and disease in later life. BMJ publishing Group, London

Barker DJ (1995) Fetal origins of coronary heart disease. BMJ 311(6998):171–174

Barker DJ (1998) Mothers, babies and health later in life, 2nd edn. Churchill Livingstone, Edinburgh

Basso O, Christensen K, Olsen J (2001) Higher risk of pre-eclampsia after change of partner. An effect of longer interpregnancy intervals? Epidemiology 12(6):624–629

Basso O, Fonager K, Olsen J (2000a) Are pregnancies shorter in leap years? Epidemiology 11(6):736–737

Basso O, Juul S, Olsen J (2000b) Time to pregnancy as a correlate of fecundity: differential persistence in trying to become pregnant as a source of bias. Int J Epidemiol 29(5):856–861

Basso O, Olsen J, Christensen K (1998a) Risk of preterm delivery, low birthweight and growth retardation following spontaneous abortion: a registry-based study in Denmark. Int J Epidemiol 27(4):642–646

Basso O, Olsen J, Christensen K (1999) Low birthweight and prematurity in relation to paternal factors: a study of recurrence. Int J Epidemiol 28(4):695–700

Basso O, Olsen J, Knudsen LB, Christensen K (1998b) Low birth weight and preterm birth after short interpregnancy intervals. Am J Obstet Gynecol 178(2):259–263

Basso O, Weinberg CR, Baird DD, Wilcox AJ, Olsen J (2003) Subfecundity as a correlate of preeclampsia: a study within the Danish National Birth Cohort. Am J Epidemiol 157(3):195–202

Berkowitz GS, Papiernik E (1993): Epidemiology of preterm birth. Epidemiol Rev 15(2):414–443

Bianchi DW (2000) Fetomaternal cell trafficking: a new cause of disease? Am J Med Genet 91(1):22–28

Bianchi DW, Zickwolf GK, Weil GJ, Sylvester S, DeMaria MA (1996) Male fetal progenitor cells persist in maternal blood for as long as 27 years postpartum. Proc Natl Acad Sci USA 93(2):705–708

Blair E, Stanley F (1993) When can cerebral palsy be prevented? The generation of causal hypotheses by multivariate analysis of a case-control study. Paediatr Perinat Epidemiol 7(3):272–301

Bolumar F, Olsen J, Boldsen J (1996) Smoking reduces fecundity: a European multicenter study on infertility and subfecundity. The European Study Group on Infertility and Subfecundity. Am J Epidemiol 143(6):578–587

Bonde JP, Ernst E, Jensen TK, Hjollund NHI, Kolstad H, Henriksen TB, Scheike T, Givercman A, Olsen J, Skakkebaek NE (1998a) Relation between semen quality and fertility, a population-based study of 430 first-pregnancy planners. Lancet 352(9135):1172–1177

Bonde JP, Hjollund NHI, Jensen TK, Ernst E, Kolstad H, Henriksen TB, Givercman A, Skakkebaek NE, Andersen AM Olsen J (1998b) A follow-up study of environmental and biologic determinants of fertility among 430 Danish first-pregnancy planners: design and methods. Reprod Toxicol 12(1):19–27

Bonomo M, Gandini ML, Mastropasqua A, Begher C, Valentini U, Faden D, Morabito A (1998) Which cutoff level should be used in screening for glucose intolerance in pregnancy? Definition of Screening Methods for Gestational Diabetes Study Group of the Lombardy Section of the Italian Society of Diabetology. Am J Obstet Gynecol 179(1):179–185

Broughton Pipkin F (1999) What is the place of genetics in the pathogenesis of pre-eclampsia? Biol Neonate 76(6):325–330

Carlsen E, Giwercman A, Keiding N, Skakkebaek NE (1992) Evidence for decreasing quality of semen during past 50 years. BMJ 305(6854):609–613

Cnattingius S, Signorello LB, Anneren G, Clausson B, Ekbom A, Ljunger E, Blot WJ, McLaughlin JK, Petersson G, Rane A, Granath F (2000) Caffeine intake and the risk of first-trimester spontaneous abortion. N Engl J Med 343(25):1839–1845

Condé-Agudelo A, Althabe F, Belizan JM, Kafury-Goeta AC (1999) Cigarette smoking during pregnancy and risk of preeclampsia: a systematic review. Am J Obstet Gynecol 181(4):1026–1035

Coughlin MT, LaPorte RE, O'Leary LA, Lee PA (1998) How accurate is male recall of reproductive information? Am J Epidemiol 148(8):806–809

Cramer DW, Goldman MB (guest eds) (1994) Infertility and reproductive medicine. Study designs and statistics for infertility research. Clinics of North America vol 5(2). W. B. Saunders Company, Philadelphia, USA

Dashe JS, McIntire DD, Ramus RM, Santos-Ramos R, Twickler DM (2002) Persistence of placenta previa according to gestational age at ultrasound detection. Obstet Gynecol 99(5 Pt 1):692–697

Dekker G, Sibai B (2001) Primary, secondary, and tertiary prevention of pre-eclampsia. Lancet 357(9251):209–215

Dekker GA (1999) Risk factors for pre-eclampsia. Clin Obstet Gynecol 42(3):422–435

Dekker GA, Robillard PY, Hulsey TC (1998) Immune maladaptation in the etiology of preeclampsia: a review of corroborative epidemiologic studies. Obstet Gynecol Surv 53(6):377–382

Diggle GE (2001) Thalidomide: 40 years on. Int J Clin Pract 55(9):627–631

Depue RH, Bernstein L, Ross RK, Judd HL, Henderson BE (1987) Hyperemesis gravidarum in relation to estradiol levels, pregnancy outcome, and other maternal factors: a seroepidemiologic study. Am J Obstet Gynecol 156(5):1137–1141

Dornhorst A, Beard RW (1993) Gestational diabetes: a challenge for the future. Diabet Med 10(10):897–905

Eliakim R, Abulafia O, Sherer DM (2000) Hyperemesis gravidarum: a current review. Am J Perinatol 17(4):207–218

Ericson A, Kallen B, Wiholm B (1999) Delivery outcome after the use of antidepressants in early pregnancy. Eur J Clin Pharmacol 55(7):503–508

Esplin MS, Fausett MB, Fraser A (2001) Paternal and maternal components of the predisposition to preeclampsia. N Engl J Med 344(12):867–872

Flint C, Larsen H, Nielsen GL, Olsen J, Sorensen HT (2002) Pregnancy outcome after suicide attempt by drug use: a Danish population-based study. Acta Obstet Gynecol Scand 81(6):516–522

Gabbe SG (1998) The gestational diabetes mellitus conferences. Three are history: focus on the fourth. Diabetes Care 21 Suppl 2:B1–2

Geddes JR, Lawrie SM (1995) Obstetric complications and schizophrenia: a meta-analysis. Br J Psychiatry 167(6):786–793

Gjessing HK, Skjaerven R, Wilcox AJ (1999) Errors in gestational age: evidence of bleeding early in pregnancy. Am J Public Health 89(2):213–218

Gladen BC (1986) On the role of "habitual aborters" in the analysis of spontaneous abortion. Stat Med 5(6):557–564

Godsey RK, Newman RB (1991) Hyperemesis gravidarum. A comparison of single and multiple admissions. J Reprod Med 36(4):287–290

Gourbin G, Masuy-Stroobant G (1995) Registration of vital data: are live births and stillbirths comparable all over Europe? Bull World Health Organ 73(4):449–460

Graafmans WC, Richardus JH, Borsboom GJ, Bakketeig L, Langhoff-Roos J, Bergsjo P, Macfarlane A, Verloove-Vanhorick SP, Mackenbach JP, EuroNatal working group (2002) Birth weight and perinatal mortality, a comparison of "optimal" birth weight in seven Western European countries. Epidemiology 13(5):569–574

Grandjean P, Weihe P, White RF, Debes F, Araki S, Yokoyama K, Murata K, Sorensen N, Dahl R, Jorgensen PJ (1997) Cognitive deficit in 7-year-old children with prenatal exposure to methylmercury. Neurotoxicol Teratol 19(6):417–428

Gray PH, O'Callaghan MJ, Mohay HA, Burns YR, King JF (1998) Maternal hypertension and neurodevelopmental outcome in very preterm infants. Arch Dis Child Fetal Neonatal Ed 79(2):F88–93

Gross S, Librach C, Cecutti A (1989) Maternal weight loss associated with hyperemesis gravidarum: a predictor of fetal outcome. Am J Obstet Gynecol 160(4):906–909

Haig D (1993) Genetic conflicts in human pregnancy. Q Rev Biol 68(4):495–532

Hallak M, Tsalamandris K, Dombrowski MP, Isada NB, Pryde PG, Evans MI (1996) Hyperemesis gravidarum. Effects on fetal outcome. J Reprod Med 41(11):871–874

Henriksen TB, Wilcox AJ, Hedegaard M, Secher NJ (1995) Bias in studies of preterm and postterm delivery due to ultrasound assessment of gestational age. Epidemiology 6(5):533–537

Hjollund NH, Jensen TK, Bonde JP, Henriksen TB, Andersson AM, Kolstad HA, Ernst E, Giwercman A, Skakkebaek NE, Olsen J (2000) Spontaneous abortion and physical strain around implantation, a follow-up study of first-pregnancy planners. Epidemiology 11(1):18–23

Hoffman EB, Sen PK, Weinberg CR (2001) Within-cluster resampling. Biometrika 88(4):1121–1134

Irgens HU, Reisaeter L, Irgens LM, Lie RT (2001) Long term mortality of mothers and fathers after pre-eclampsia: population based cohort study. BMJ 323(7323):1213–1217

Jacobsen R, Bostofte E, Engholm G, Hansen J, Olsen JH, Skakkebaek NE, Moller H. (2000) Risk of testicular cancer in men with abnormal semen characteristics: cohort study. BMJ 321(7264):789–792

Jensen TK, Henriksen TB, Hjollund NHI, Scheike T, Kolstad H, Giwercman A, Ernst E, Bonde JP, Skakkebaek NE, Olsen J (1998) Caffeine intake and fecundability. A follow-up study among 430 Danish couples planning their first pregnancy. Reprod Toxicol 12(3):289–295

Joffe M, Villard L, Li Z, Plowman R, Vessey M (1993) Long-term recall of time-to-pregnancy. Fertil Steril 60(1):99–104

Joffe M, Villard L, Li Z, Plowman R, Vessey M (1995) A time to pregnancy questionnaire designed for long term recall: validity in Oxford, England. J Epidemiol Community Health 49(3):314–319

Johnstone FD, Nasrat AA, Prescott RJ (1990) The effect of established and gestational diabetes on pregnancy outcome. Br J Obstet Gynaecol 97(11):1009–1015

Juul S, Karmaus W, Olsen J (1999) Regional differences in waiting time to pregnancy: pregnancy-based surveys form Denmark, France, Germany, Italy and Sweden. The European Infertility and Subfecundity Study Group. Hum Reprod 14(5):1250–1254

Kallen B (1987) Hyperemesis during pregnancy and delivery outcome: a registry study. Eur J Obstet Gynecol Reprod Biol 26(4):291–302

Kero J, Gissler M, Gronlund MM, Kero P, Koskinen P, Hemminki E, Isolauri E (2002) Mode of delivery and asthma – is there a connection? Pediatr Res 52(1):6–11

Kiely JL, Paneth N, Susser M (1985) Fetal death during labor: an epidemiologic indicator of level of obstetric care. Am J Obst Gynecol 153(7):721–727

Kline J, Stein Z, Susser M (1989) Conception to birth – epidemiology of prenatal development. Monographs in Epidemiology and Biostatistics vol 14. Oxford University Press, New York

Knox EG, Armstrong EH, Lancashire R (1984) The quality of notification of congenital malformations. J Epidemiol Community Health 38(4):296–305

Kondo S, Schutte BC, Richardson RJ, Bjork BC, Knight AS, Watanabe Y, Howard E, de Lima RL, Daack-Hirsch S, Sander A, McDonald-McGinn DM, Zackai EH, Lammer EJ, Aylsworth AS, Ardinger HH, Lidral AC, Pober BR, Moreno L, Arcos-Burgos M, Valencia C, Houdayer C, Bahuau M, Moretti-Ferreira D, Richieri-Costa A, Dixon MJ, Murray JC (2002) Mutations in IRF6 cause Van der Woude and popliteal pterygium syndromes. Nat Genet 32(2):285–289

Kramer MS, Liu S, Luo Z, Yuan H, Platt RW, Joseph KS (2002) Analysis of perinatal mortality and its components: time for a change? Am J Epidemiol 156(6):493–497

Li DK, Wi S (2000) Changing paternity and the risk of preeclampsia/eclampsia in the subsequent pregnancy. Am J Epidemiol 151(1):57–62

Lie RT, Rasmussen S, Brunborg H, Gjessing HK, Lie-Nielsen E, Irgens LM (1998) Fetal and maternal contributions to risk of pre-eclampsia: population based study. BMJ 316(7141):1343–1347

Linnet KM, Dalsgaard S, Obel C, Wisborg K, Henriksen TB, Rodriguez A, Kotimaa A, Moilanen I, Tomsen PH, Olsen J, Jarvelin MR (2003) Maternal lifestyle factors in pregnancy risk of attention deficit hyperactivity disorder and assiocated behaviors: review of the current evidence. Am J Psychatry 160(6):1028–1040

Livingston JC, Barton JR, Park V, Haddad B, Phillips O, Sibai BM (2001) Maternal and fetal inherited thrombophilias are not related to the development of severe preeclampsia. Am J Obstet Gynecol 185(1):153–157

Longnecker MP, Klebanoff MA, Zhou H, Brock JW (2001) Association between maternal serum concentration of the DDT metabolite DDE and preterm and small-for-gestational-age babies at birth. Lancet 358(9276):110–114

Ludwig M, Diedrich K (2002) Follow-up of children born after assisted reproductive technologies. Reprod Biomed Online 5(3):317–322

Macklon NS, Geraedts JP, Fauser BC (2002) Conception to ongoing pregnancy: the 'black box' of early pregnancy loss. Hum Reprod Update 8(4):333–343

Maclure M (1991) The case-crossover design: a method for studying transient effects on the risk of acute events. Am J Epidemiol 133(2):144–153

Martin FI, Ratnaike S, Wootton A, Condos P, Suter PE (1995) The 75 g oral glucose tolerance in pregnancy. Diabetes Res Clin Pract 27(2):147–151

McCormack VA, dos Santos Silva I, De Stavola BL, Mohsen R, Leon DA, Lithell HO (2003) Fetal growth and subsequent risk of breast cancer: results from long term follow up of Swedish cohort. BMJ 326(7383):248

Mednick SA, Huttunen MO, Machon RA (1994) Prenatal influenza infections and adult schizophrenia. Schizophr Bull 20(2):263–267

Metz CE (1978) Basic principles of ROC analysis. Semin Nucl Med 8(4):283–298

Mitchell AA, Cottler LB, Shapiro S (1986) Effect of questionniare design on recall of drug exposure in pregnancy. Am J Epidemiol 123(4):670–676

Murphy DJ, Sellers S, MacKenzie IZ, Yudkin PL, Johnson AM (1995) Case-control study of antenatal and intrapartum risk factors for cerebral palsy in very preterm singleton babies. Lancet 346(8988):1449–1454

Ness RB, Roberts JM (1996) Heterogeneous causes constituting the single syndrome of preeclampsia: a hypothesis and its implications. Am J Obstet Gynecol 175(5):1365–1370

Nybo Andersen A-M, Wohlfahrt J, Christens P, Olsen J, Melbye M (2000) Maternal age and fetal loss: population based register linkage study. BMJ 320(7251):1708–1712

Olsen J (1984) Calculating risk ratios for spontaneous abortions: the problem of induced abortions. Int J Epidemiol 13(3):347–350

Olsen J (1994) Options in making use of pregnancy history in planning and analysing studies of reproductive failure. J Epidemiol Community Health 48(2):171–174

Olsen J (2000) Prenatal exposures and long-term health effects. Epidemiol Rev 22(1):76–81

Olsen J, Andersen PK (1998) Accounting for pregnancy dependence in epidemiologic studies of pregnancy outcomes. Epidemiology 9(3):363–364

Olsen J, Andersen PK (1999) We should monitor human fecundity, but how? A suggestion for a new method that may also be used to identify determinants of low fecundity. Epidemiology 10(4):419–421

Olsen J, Basso O (2001) Study design. In: Olsen J, Saracci R, Trichopoulos D (eds) Teaching epidemiology. A guide for teachers in epidemiology, public health and clinical medicine, 2 edn. Oxford University Press, New York, pp 41–52

Olsen J, Basso O, Spinelli A, Küppers-Chinnow M and the European Study Group on Infertility and Subfecundity (1998a) Correlates of care seeking for infertility treatment in Europe. Eur J Public Health 8(1):15–20

Olsen J, Czeizel A, Sorensen HT, Nielsen GL, de Jong van den Berg LT, Irgens LM, Olesen C, Pedersen L, Larsen H, Lie RT, de Vries CS, Bergman U (2002) How do we best detect toxic effects of drugs taken during pregnancy? A EuroMap paper. Drug Saf 25(1):21–32

Olsen J, Juul S, Basso O (1998b) Measuring time to pregnancy. Methodological issues to consider. Hum Reprod 13(7):1751–1753

Olsen J, Melbye M, Olsen SF, Sorensen TI, Aaby P, Andersen AM, Taxbol D, Hansen KD, Juhl M, Schow TB, Sorensen HT, Andresen J, Mortensen EL, Olesen AW, Sondergaard C (2001) The Danish National Birth Cohort – its background, structure and aim. Scand J Public Health 29(4):300–307

Olsen J, Rachootin P, Schiodt AV, Damsbo N (1983) Tobacco use, alcohol consumption and infertility. Int J Epidemiol 12(2):179–184

Olsen J, Rachootin P (2003) Invited commentary: monitoring fecundity over time – if we do it, then let's do it right. Am J Epidemiol 157(2):94–97

Olsen J, Schmidt MM, Christensen K (1997) Evaluation of nature-nurture impact on reproductive health using half-siblings. Epidemiol 8(1):6–11

Parker JD, Schoendorf KC (2002) Implications of cleaning gestational age data. Paediatr Perinat Epidemiol 16(2):181–187

Pharoah PO, Adi Y (2000) Consequences of in-utero death in a twin pregnancy. Lancet 355(9215):1597–1602

Quenby S, Vince G, Farquharson R, Aplin J (2002) Opinion. Recurrent miscarriage: a defect in nature's quality control? Human Reprod 17(8):1959–1963

Rachootin P, Olsen J (1982) Prevalence and socioeconomic correlates of subfecundity and spontaneous abortion in Denmark. Int J Epidemiol 11(3):245–249

Rachootin P, Olsen J (1983) The risk of infertility and delayed conception associated with exposure in the Danish workplace. J Occup Med 25(5):394–402

Ravelli GP, Stein ZA, Susser MW (1976) Obesity in young men after famine exposure in utero and early infancy. N Engl J Med 295(7):349–353

Roberts JM, Cooper DW (2001) Pathogenesis and genetics of pre-eclampsia. Lancet 357(9249):53–56

Roberts JM, Lain KY (2002) Recent insights into the pathogenesis of pre-eclampsia. Placenta 23(5):359–372

Robillard PY, Hulsey TC, Perianin J, Janky E, Miri EH, Papiernik E (1994) Association of pregnancy-induced hypertension with duration of sexual cohabitation before conception. Lancet 344(8928):973–975

Rockenbauer M, Olsen J, Czeizel AE, Pedersen L, Sorensen HT (2001) Recall bias in a case-control surveillance system on the use of medicine during pregnancy. Epidemiology 12(4):461–466

Rothenberg SJ, Kondrashov V, Manalo M, Jiang J, Cuellar R, Garcia M, Reynoso B, Reyes S, Diaz M, Todd AC (2002) Increases in hypertension and blood pressure during pregnancy with increased bone lead levels. Am J Epidemiol 156(12):1079–1087

Russell IT, Wilcox AJ (1991) A criterion for low birthweight. Int J Epidemiol 20(4):1145

Sabroe S, Olsen J (1998) Perinatal correlates of specific histological types of testicular cancer in patients below 35 years of age: a case-cohort study based on midwives' records in Denmark. Int J Cancer 78(2):140–143

Salas SP (1999) What causes pre-eclampsia? Baillieres Best Pract Res Clin Obstet Gynaecol 13(1):41–57

Savitz DA, Sonnenfeld NL, Olshan AF (1994) Review of epidemiologic studies of paternal occupational exposure and spontaneous abortion. Am J Ind Med 25(3):361–383

Schmidt MI, Duncan BB, Reichelt AJ, Branchtein L, Matos MC, Costa e Forti A, Spichler ER, Pousada JM, Teixeira MM, Yamashita T (2001) Gestational diabetes mellitus diagnosed with a 2-h 75-g oral glucose tolerance test and adverse pregnancy outcomes. Diabetes Care 24(7):1151–1155

Schmidt MI, Matos MC, Reichelt AJ, Forti AC, de Lima L, Duncan BB (2000) Prevalence of gestational diabetes mellitus – do the new WHO criteria make a difference? Brazilian Gestational Diabetes Study Group. Diabet Med 17(5):376–380

Sharpe RM, Skakkebaek NE (1993) Are oestrogens involved in falling sperm counts and disorders of the male reproductive tract? Lancet 341(8857):1392–1395

Sibai BM (1998) Prevention of preeclampsia: a big disappointment. Am J Obstet Gynecol 179(5):1275–1278

Skjaerven R, Gjessing HK, Bakketeig LS (2000) New standards for birth weight by gestational age using family data. Am J Obstet Gynecol 183(3):689–696

Skjaerven R, Wilcox AJ, Lie RT (2002) The interval between pregnancies and the risk of preeclampsia. N Engl J Med 346(1):33–38

Smith GD, Ebrahim S (2003) 'Mendelian randomization': can genetic epidemiology contribute to understanding environmental determinants of disease. 30th Thomas Francis Jr. Memorial Lecture, delivered by George Davey Smith at the University of Michigan, School of Public Health, 6 March 2003. Int J Epidemiol 32:1–22

Smoking or Health – the third Report from the Royal College of Physicians of London (1977) Pitman Medical Publishing, London

Sondergaard C, Skajaa E, Henriksen TB (2000) Fetal growth and infantile colic. Arch Dis Child Fetal Neonatal Ed 83(1):F44 47

Stang A, Ahrens W, Bromen K, Baumgardt-Elms C, Jahn I, Stegmaier C, Krege S, Jöckel KH (2001) Undescended testis and the risk of testicular cancer, importance of source and classification of exposure information. Int J Epidemiol 30(5):1050–1056

Starr T, Levine RJ (1983) Assessing effects of occupational exposure on fertility with indirect standardization. Am J Epidemiol 118(6):897–904

Storgaard L, Bonde JP, Ernst E, Andersen CY, Kyvik KO, Olsen J (2002) Effect of prenatal exposure to oestrogen on quality of semen: comparison of twins and singleton brothers. BMJ 325(7358):252–253

Strohsnitter WC, Noller KL, Hoover RN, Robboy SJ, Palmer JR, Titus-Ernstoff L, Kaufman RH, Adam E, Herbst AL, Hatch EE (2001) Cancer risk in men exposed in utero to diethylstilbestrol. J Natl Cancer Inst 93(7):545–551

Susser M, Stein Z (1994) Timing in prenatal nutrition: a reprise of the Dutch Famine Study. Nutr Rev 52(3):84–94

Swan SH, Shaw GM, Schulman J (1992) Reporting and selection bias in case-control studies of congenital malformations. Epidemiology 3(4):356–363

Tong S, Caddy D, Short RV (1997) Use of dizygotic to monozygotic twinning ratio as a measure of fertility. Lancet 349(9055):843–845

Trichopoulos D (1990) Hypothesis: does breast cancer originate in utero? Lancet 335(8695):939–940

Trogstad LI, Eskild A, Magnus P, Samuelsen SO, Nesheim BI (2001) Changing paternity and time since last pregnancy; the impact on pre-eclampsia risk. A study of 547,238 women with and without previous pre-eclampsia. Int J Epidemiol 30(6):1317–1322

Trupin LS, Simon LP, Eskenazi B (1996) Change in paternity: a risk factor for preeclampsia in multiparas. Epidemiology 7(3):240–244

Verdoux H, Geddes JR, Takei N, Lawrie SM, Bovet P, Eagles JM, Heun R, Mc-Creadie RG, McNeil TF, O'Callaghan E, Stober G, Willinger MU, Wright P, Murray RM (1997) Obstetric complications and age at onset in schizophrenia: an international collaborative meta-analysis of individual patient data. Am J Psychiatry 154(9):1220–1227

Vestergaard M, Basso O, Henriksen TB, Oestergaard JR, Olsen J (2002) Risk factors for febrile convulsions. Epidemiol 13(3):282–287

Villar J, Belizan JM (2000) Same nutrient, different hypotheses: disparities in trials of calcium supplementation during pregnancy. Am J Clin Nutr 71(5 Suppl):1375S–1379S

von Dadelszen P, Ornstein MP, Bull SB, Logan AG, Koren G, Magee LA (2000) Fall in mean arterial pressure and fetal growth restriction in pregnancy hypertension: a meta-analysis. Lancet 355(9198):87–92

Weinberg CR (1993) Toward a clearer definition of confounding. Am J Epidemiol 137(1):1–8

Weinberg CR, Baird DD, Wilcox AJ (1994a) Sources of bias in studies of time to pregnancy. Stat Med 13(5–7):671–681

Weinberg CR, Baird DD, Wilcox AJ (1994b) Bias in retrospective studies of spontaneous abortion based on the outcome of the most recent pregnancy. Ann N Y Acad Sci 18(709):280–286

Weinberg CR, Wilcox AJ (1998) Reproductive epidemiology. In: Rothman KJ, Greenland S (eds.) Modern epidemiology, 2nd edn. Lippincott-Raven, Philadelphia, USA

Weinberg CR, Wilcox AJ, Lie RT (1998) A log-linear approach to case-parent-triad data: assessing effects of disease genes that act either directly or through maternal effects and that may be subject to parental imprinting. Am J Hum Genet 62(4):969–978

Wen SW, Demissie K, Liu S, Marcoux S, Kramer MS (2000) Placenta praevia and male sex at birth: results from a population-based study. Paediatr Perinat Epidemiol 14(4):300–304

Whitacre CC (2001) Sex differences in autoimmune disease. Nat Immunol 2(9):777–780

Whitacre CC, Reingold SC, O'Looney PA (1999) A gender gap in autoimmunity. Science 283(5406):1277–1278

Wilcox AJ (2001) On the importance – and the unimportance – of birthweight. Int J Epidemiology 30(6):1233–1241

Wilcox AJ, Baird DD, Weinberg CR, Hornsby PP, Herbst AL (1995) Fertility in men exposed prenatally to diethylstilbestrol. N Engl J Med 332(21):1411–1416

Wilcox AJ, Weinberg CR, O'Connor JF, Baird DD, Schlatterer JP, Canfield RE, Armstrong EG, Nisula BC (1988) Incidence of early loss of pregnancy. N Engl J Med 319(4):189–194

Winbo IG, Serenius FH, Dahlquist GG, Kallen BA (1997) A computer-based method for cause of death classification in stillbirths and neonatal deaths. Int J Epidemiol 26(6):1298–1306

Zhang J, Cai WW (1991) Severe vomiting during pregnancy: antenatal correlates and fetal outcomes. Epidemiol 2(6):454–457

Zweig MH, Campbell G (1993) Receiver-operating characteristic (ROC) plots: a fundamental evaluation tool in clinical medicine. Clin Chem 39(4):561–577

Textbooks in Reproductive Epidemiology

Bracken MB (ed) (1984) Perinatal epidemiology. Oxford University Press, New York

Kallen B (1988) Epidemiology of human reproduction. CRC Press, Boca Raton

Keith LG, Papiernik E, Keith DM, Luke B (eds) (1995) Multiple pregnancy: epidemiology, gestation and perinatal outcome, 1st edn. Parthenon Publishing Group, New York

Kiely M (ed) (1991) Reproductive and perinatal epidemiology. CRC Press, Boca Raton

Kline J, Stein Z, Susser M (1989) Conception to birth – epidemiology of prenatal development. Monographs in Epidemiology and Biostatistics vol 14. Oxford University Press, New York

McDowall ME (1985) Occupational reproductive epidemiology: the use of routinely collected statistics in England and Wales, 1980–82. Her Majesty's Stationery Office, London

Murray CJL, Lopez AD (eds) (1988) Health dimensions of sex and reproduction. In: Global Burden of Disease and Injury Series, Vol III, 1998. WHO, Geneva

Molecular Epidemiology

Paolo Vineis, Giuseppe Matullo, Marianne Berwick

6.1 Introduction

Molecular epidemiology can be defined simply as the application of the techniques of molecular biology to the study of populations, with a particular focus on the investigation of disease. Molecular investigations, as we will see, have several aims and can contribute to the elucidation of disease causation.

The most critical issues in molecular epidemiology include an appropriate *study design*, careful attention to sources of *bias and confounding*, and the development of *markers* that can be applied on a population scale. The study design is particularly important, because past research that applied laboratory methods to human populations was often based on "convenience samples" – i.e. groups of patients recruited in the most comfortable way without a proper design – that were frequently affected by bias.

This chapter mainly refers to chronic diseases, and more specifically to cancer, but the methodological considerations have a general relevance.

Markers used in the molecular epidemiology of cancer are usually divided into the three categories: *markers of internal dose, markers of early response and markers of susceptibility* (Bartsch 2000; Schulte and Perera 1998; Toniolo et al. 1997). The underlying concept is that there is *continuity* between exposure to a toxic (carcinogenic) agent, metabolism (activation or deactivation), adduction to proteins or deoxyribonucleic acid (DNA) (i.e. formation of links by the active metabolite), DNA alterations like mutations or chromosome damage, and finally cancer onset. These concepts are schematically represented in Fig. 6.1.

In fact each category includes sub-categories. For example, protein adducts and DNA adducts are both markers of internal dose, but their biological meaning is different. *Adduct* is a word that refers to the binding of an external compound to a molecule such as a protein or DNA. While protein adducts are not repaired, i.e. they reflect external exposure more faithfully, DNA adducts are influenced by individual repair ability; in fact, if they are not eliminated by the DNA repair machinery, they may induce a mutation. Markers of early response are a heterogeneous category, that encompasses DNA mutations and gross chromosomal damage. The main advantage of early response markers is that they are more frequent than cancer itself and can be recognized earlier, thus allowing researchers to identify effects of potentially carcinogenic exposures earlier. Finally, markers of susceptibility include multiple sub-categories, in particular a type of genetic susceptibility that is related to the metabolism of carcinogenic substances (Vineis et al. 1999), and another type that is related to the repair of DNA (Berwick and Vineis 2000; Berwick et al. 2002) (see below).

Technical advances such as *high-throughput technologies* for the analysis of SNPs (single nucleotide polymorphisms) will make molecular epidemiology more powerful in the future, but will also bring new scientific and ethical challenges.

The purpose of this chapter is to give an overview of a rapidly developing field of epidemiological research, molecular epidemiology. The structure of the chapter includes an introduction on the meaning and the main features

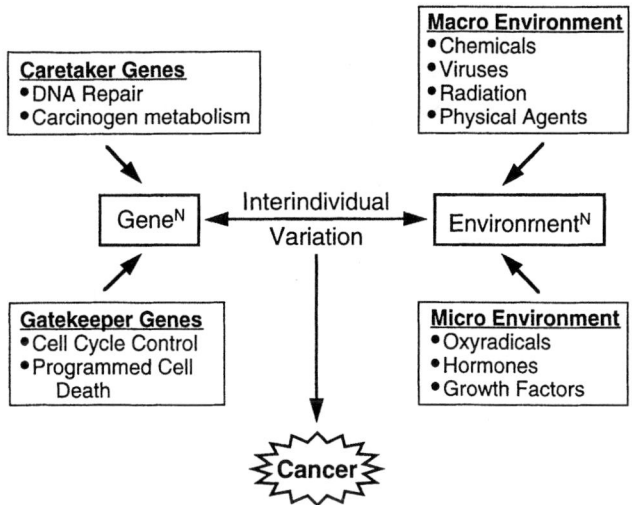

Figure 6.1. Many genes and environmental exposures contribute to the carcinogenic process. The effects can be additive or multiplicative, which are modifiable by interindividual variation in genetic function. We propose to include carcinogen metabolic activity and detoxification genes as caretaker genes involved in maintaining genomic integrity. (Reprinted with permission from the American Society of Clinical Oncology from Shields and Harris (2000))

of molecular epidemiology; a section aimed at training the reader to a critical analysis of molecular epidemiology papers; and three examples we have chosen from field research to illustrate the main metholodological problems that are encountered in the conduct and interpretation of a molecular epidemiology study.

Critical Analysis of Molecular Epidemiology Studies

6.2

The design of a study of molecular epidemiology does not differ substantially from other epidemiological study designs, and requires the same critical approach regarding selection or information bias, the comparability of groups that are recruited (cases and controls, exposed and unexposed), the presence of potential confounding and the issue of statistical power. However, there are also areas peculiar to molecular epidemiology, that we will describe through a few examples. While for bias in epidemiology in general we refer to other chapters in Part I of this handbook, the following are the most frequently encountered specific methodological issues (see also Box 1).

Box 1. Methodological problems that need to be addressed in molecular epidemiology studies

Transitional studies
Choice of design
    Case-control
    Cohort
    Case-control nested in a cohort or case-cohort
    Case only
    Other
Half-life of biomarker
Collection and storage of samples
Reproducibility and repeatability of laboratory tests
Heterogeneity of results and their sources
Confounding, e.g. population admixture
Publication bias
Biological interpretation of the test

Transitional Studies.   Transitional studies can be compared to Phase II studies in the development of new treatments. They do not have a "formal" design (for example Phase II studies are not necessarily randomized), and often have a small size. The main purpose is to validate biomarkers and to produce findings that assess the relevance of the marker for a certain disease. For example, transitional studies on bladder cancer consisted of case series in which $p53$ mutations or 4-ABP (4-aminobiphenyl)-DNA adducts were related to tobacco smoking without a case-control design. Smokers tended to have $p53$ mutations and 4-ABP adducts more frequently than non-smokers, thus suggesting the relevance of these markers for the etiologic pathways of bladder cancer.

Choice of the Design and Half-Life of Biomarkers.   In "traditional" epidemiology the case-control design is particularly valid when the disease is rare and exposure is frequent and easily identifiable. In molecular epidemiology of chronic diseases, in which a biomarker is measured, the case-control approach has serious limitations if the marker has a short half-life, i.e. it refers to exposures that took place a short time before the disease onset. In fact, in the study of cancer and other chronic diseases we are usually interested in events that took place many years before the disease onset. DNA adducts in white-blood cells have a half-life of months, and hemoglobin adducts have a half-life of weeks (Box 2). From this point of view, prospective studies are more meaningful, although they have the limitation of being usually based on a "one time" biological sample that is not necessarily representative of the usual exposure (thus introducing random misclassification).

> **Box 2. Half life of different markers: examples**
>
> Phenol (metabolite of benzene) in urine: 6 hours
>
> Carbon monoxide in blood: 5 hours
>
> Hemoglobin aromatic adducts: 120 days
>
> DNA aromatic adducts in lymphocytes: several months

Similar considerations apply to most early response markers, such as mutations in plasma DNA: in this case the case-control approach is clearly limited because the mutation is likely to express a marker of cancer itself rather than an intermediate event between exposure and disease. Concerning studies on genetic susceptibility, single nucleotide gene polymorphisms (SNP) are inherited and stable in time, so that they should not be affected by the elapsed time and thus either design, case-control or cohort, will be adequate. Unfortunately, this is not totally true since some SNPs affect survival so that surviving cases in a case-control design can represent a distorted subset as far as the role of SNPs in etiology is concerned. This problem can be avoided by restricting studies to incident cases. In general, it is believed that the most promising design for future studies of molecular epidemiology is the case-control study nested in a cohort.

Practical Issues (Collection and Storage of Samples).   Several types of samples can be collected in molecular epidemiology studies (see Box 3). Urines can be collected to measure metabolites (e.g. NNAL for NNK in smokers) or centrifuged to collect exfoliated bladder cells (to measure e.g. DNA adducts). Blood can be stored as such or centrifuged to collect red blood cells (RBC), plasma, serum or buffy coat (i.e. white blood cells, WBC). RBC are a source of hemoglobin which can be used for the measurement of adducts. The use of WBC for the measurement of adducts will be described later in an example. WBC are in general a source of DNA that can be used, for example, for the genotyping of subjects. Another important source is represented by buccal washes or buccal swabs that are relatively easy to obtain in epidemiological studies.

> **Box 3. Measures used in molecular epidemiologic studies for specific biological materials. It should be noted that this list will change over time**
>
> Biological Material: Measures
> 1. DNA
>   a. Genomic DNA
>   Single nucleotide polymorphisms (SNPs) (> 1% prevalence)

box to be continued

  b. Tumor DNA
      Mutations ($< 1\%$ prevalence)
  c. Mitochondrial DNA
      Insertions, deletions

2. RNA
    RT-PCR (reverse transcriptase polymerase chain reaction (PCR))
    Microarray chips for expression of RNA

3. WHOLE CELLS
    a. Lymphocytes
        Incorporation of damaged plasmid (host cell reactivation assay (HCRA))
        Comet assay
    b. Chromosomes (cytogenetic assays to assess mutagen sensitivity)
        Chromosome breaks and deletions
        Sister chromatid exchanges (SCEs)
    c. Shed cells
        (1) Exfoliated bladder cells
            Measures of damage and repair (Comet assay)
        (2) Oral buccal cells
            Measures of DNA adducts
        (3) Broncholavage
        (4) Micronuclei
    d. Adducts (i.e. exogenous chemicals bound to DNA)

4. PLASMA/SERUM
    Measurement of biochemicals, i.e. Vitamin E
    Tumor and genomic DNA in plasma and serum

5. RED BLOOD CELLS
    Hemoglobin, hemoglobin adducts, biochemical content, i.e. folate

6. URINE
    a. Urinary metabolites
        Biochemical assays
    b. Exfoliated bladder cells
        See above

7. HAIR
    Chemicals, i.e. arsenic

8. FINGERNAILS, TOENAILS
    Chemicals, i.e. mercury

The main problems with the collection of biosamples are (1) the information given to the subjects and the type of informed consent collected (see below, ethical issues); (b) how the samples are collected and stored, in relation to the stability of different components; (c) the amount that needs to be collected, depending on the test that we wish to perform.

Stability should be carefully considered. At $-20\,°C$ urine is stable; at $-70\,°C$ cell viability (if not cryopreserved) is limited although DNA is stable, serum is stable, most hormones are stable, most vitamins are stable; at $-120\,°C$ hormones, carotenoids and other nutients are stable.

In general, the goals of collection and storage procedures are:
— to ensure standardized procedures for all phases
— to ensure collection of biological material in ways that are acceptable to volunteers/patients
— to avoid loss of material (e.g. malfunctioning of freezers)
— to ensure optimal preservation of material for study purposes
— to ensure blinding in all phases
— to ensure easy access to the material when needed
— to ensure easy matching of biological material with individual identity
— to ensure respect for confidentiality
— to be prepared for emergencies.

Reproducibility and Repeatability of Laboratory Tests, and Other Technical Issues.   In spite of the large number of papers published using a certain laboratory test (like DNA adducts or a cytogenetic test), the reproducibility of some assays has not been carefully assessed. The experimental error in such assays may be larger than many epidemiologists would expect. For example, for DNA adducts measured by P^{32}-postlabelling the coefficient of variation is at least 30% (Phillips and Casteg-naro 1999).

Technical sensitivity is also matter of concern. It refers to the ability of detecting the relevant marker, e.g. DNA adducts, also in extremely low amounts. Box 4 reports several kinds of techniques for the measurement of DNA adducts and their main features. Box 5 gives examples of how different markers have been used in epidemiological studies.

Technical sensitivity is different from sensitivity in the usual epidemiological meaning, i.e. the proportion of correct positive results (although the two are clearly related). Box 6 gives sensitivity and specificity estimates for different genotyping methods, compared with a "consensus" panel. A BRCA1 polymorphism was initially typed by allele-specific oligonucleotide (ASO) hybridisation using radiolabelled oligos. Then it was evaluated with the PE Biosytems TaqMan technology, with the RsaI forced digest and with the Invader Cleavase technology (Third wave Inc). It can be seen that there is a noticeable variation among them that makes a decision on which one to use crucial.

Box 4. Different techniques for the measurement of DNA adducts

P^{32}-postlabeling	Very sensitive, small amounts of DNA required; laborious, not very reproducible
Immunoassay	Sensitive, easy to perform (specificity?)
GC-MS	Specific, quantitative; high cost
For certain adducts:	
Electrochemical methods	Easy, sensitive (specificity?)
Fluorescence	Easy, specific, large amounts of DNA required
Atomic absorption	Specific and sensitive

Box 5. Examples of markers of carcinogenic exposure

Type of marker	organ or tissue	meaning
Aflatoxin B1-DNA adducts	urine, liver	genetic damage from aflatoxin
PAH-DNA adducts	blood, lung, placenta	genetic damage from polycyclic aromatic hydrocarbons
4-aminobiphenyl-hemoglobin adducts	blood	active or passive exposure to tobacco smoke
Mutations in p53 gene	lung, liver, skin	pattern of mutation may reveal the type of carcinogenic exposure

Box 6. Sensitivity and specificity of different genotyping methods applied to genotyping of a BRCA1 polymorphism; nominators represent actual test results, denominators those of a "consensus" panel (from A Dunning, personal communication)

Method	Sensitivity	%	Specificity	%
ASO	836/864	97	753/836	90
TaqMan	826/864	96	812/826	98
RsaI digest	125/173	72	103/125	82
Invader	62/92	67	45/62	73

Finally, Box 7 describes several laboratory methods to screen for mutations or SNPs, to genotype, or to measure effects on whole cells. Advantages and disadvantages of such methods are described.

Box 7. Several laboratory methods for measuring susceptibility

	Screening Methods used to determine IF there is a mutation or SNP.	Genotyping Methods used to determine WHAT the SNP is.	Whole cells assays Methods used to measure effects on whole cells.
Method	(1) SSCP	(1) RFLP	(1) Chromosomal aberrations (mutagen sensitvity)
	(2) DHPLC	(2) Hybridization	(2) HCRA (lymphocyte incorporation of damaged plasmid)
		(3) OLA	(3) Comet assay (damage and repair)
		(4) Primer extension	
		(5) Nuclease cleavage	
Description	(1) Single-stranded DNAs are generated by denaturation of PCR products and separated on a nondenaturing polyacrylamide gel.	(1) PCR products are digested with restriction endonucleases specifically chosen for the base change at the SNP, leaving a "restriction cut" for one allele, but not the other.	(1) Chromosomal breaks and gaps are counted in mutagen-exposed lymphoctes from cases and controls for comparison.
	(2) Similar to SSCP, but the output is based on the melting characteristics of the DNA strand which is defined by the sequence, so that a SNP will look different from wildtype.	(2) Complementary oligonucleotide sequences are hybridized.	(2) The rate of repair of a damaged plasmid introduced into lymphocytes is measured.

box to be continued

	Screening	**Genotyping**	**Whole cells assays**
	Methods used to determine IF there is a mutation or SNP.	Methods used to determine WHAT the SNP is.	Methods used to measure effects on whole cells.
		(3) Two oligonucleotides adjacent to each other are ligated enzymatically by a DNA ligase when the bases next to the ligation position are complementary to the template.	(3) Cells are subjected to a damaging agent. The response minus the baseline damage is measured to calculate "damage". Repair is measured after a time for repair has elapsed. The measurement is based on the "tail moment" (length of the migrating DNA) and the density of DNA in the "head".
		(4) An oligonucleotide is hybridized NEXT to a SNP.	
		(5) Plain hybridization with the probe enzymatically degraded. A fluorescent dye and a florescent quencher are carried on the nucleotide probe.	
Advantages/ Disadvantages	(1) SSCP: Simple, inexpensive, intermediate throughput. Only short sequences (< 200 bp), no information on the position of the change.	(1) Simple, time consuming, low throughput and relatively expensive per SNP.	(1) Not automated. Time consuming. Gives a "whole" picture of specific individual's lymphocytes' response to DNA damage and ability to repair.
	(2) DHPLC: Simple, relatively inexpensive with relatively high throughput. Similar limitations as SSCP.	(2) Not as robust as methods that use hybridization PLUS enzymatic steps.	(2) Not automated although can be batched better than above assay. Has the advantage that the lymphocyte itself is not damaged.

box to be continued

Screening	Genotyping	Whole cells assays
Methods used to determine IF there is a mutation or SNP.	Methods used to determine WHAT the SNP is.	Methods used to measure effects on whole cells.
	(3) Can genotype large panels of informative markers. Difficult to optimize and multiplex highly GC-rich DNA regions.	(3) This assay is still in development. Critical that results present reproducibility of specific laboratory. Potential for automation in the future. Can measure both response to damage and repair kinetics.
	(4) Many versions.	
	(5) Many versions.	

Heterogeneity of Results. For several reasons, mostly unexplored, results of molecular epidemiology tend to be heterogeneous. For example, many studies on genetic polymorphisms and cancer give conflicting results. This may be due to the sum of several different problems, including measurement error, genuine inter-population and intra-population variability in response, and unpredictable interactions between environmental exposures and genetic susceptibility.

Confounding. Confunding can arise in unusual or unpredictable ways, since pathways can be extremely complex; for example, cruciferous vegetables both protect from lung cancer and induce Phase I or Phase II enzymes, i.e. markers of individual susceptibility. Phase I enzymes are those involved in activation of procarcinogens, Phase II enzymes are involved in detoxification. Therefore, the association between the phenotype for such an enzyme and lung cancer can simply reflect an indirect (i.e. confounded) relationship.

Population Stratification. The fact that a genetic variant is associated with ethnicity, which, in turn, can be an important determinant of several diseases, has been called the phenomenon of "population admixture" in studies of gene-environment interactions. This is nothing new for epidemiologists, being another example of confounding. However, this is a particularly important type of confounding in the era of the Genome project (i.e. the systematic sequencing of the human genome) and of extensive studies on genes and disease. In fact, if we do not stratify by ethnicity we risk attributing to genes a causal responsibility that is in fact related to other characteristics associated with ethnicity, such as other genetic traits or environmental exposures. For example, African-Americans tend to smoke more, to have a higher prevalence of hypertension, and also have a different distribution of many genetic polymorphisms in comparison with Caucasians. Therefore, in an unstratified study, in which "population admixture" occurs, one could find a spurious association between smoking-related diseases or hypertension and some polymorphisms. The association could disappear after stratification by ethnicity. In a pooled analysis of the studies on CYP1A1 polymorphisms and the risk of lung cancer (Vineis et al. 2003) we have observed the odds ratios for the CYP1A1*2 polymorphism shown in Table 6.1.

Table 6.1. Odds ratios (OR) and corresponding 95% confidence intervals (CI) for CYP1A1*2 polymorphism according to ethnicity and risk of lung cancer

	Heterozygotes	Homozygotes
All Ethnicities		
OR	0.88	0.88
95% CI	0.77–1.01	0.68–1.14
Caucasians		
OR	1.02	2.36
95% CI	0.84–1.24	1.16–4.81
Asians		
OR	1.06	1.14
95% CI	0.81–1.41	0.78–1.69

While mixing ethnicity conceals any relationship (odds ratios are lower than 1 and not statistically significant), it is clear that, when we consider Caucasians and Asians separately, there is a clear association at least with the homozygous genotype in Caucasians. This phenomenon is an example of confounding since Asians have a much higher frequency of the variant genotype in comparison with Caucasians and smoke less, thus fulfilling the criteria for confounding (in this case negative confounding since the association disappears when mixing the populations).

There is currently a debate whether bias from population stratification (the mixture of individuals from heterogeneous genetic backgrounds) undermines the credibility of epidemiologic studies designed to estimate the association between genotype and risk of disease. However, Wacholder et al. (2000) found only a small bias from stratification in a well-designed case-control study of genetic factors that ignored ethnicity among non-Hispanic, U.S. Caucasians of European origin. In general, there are good reasons to argue that population admixture only rarely can distort the estimates. First, in the example above, it is very unlikely that the investigators would have ignored the simple Caucasian/Asian stratification. Second, the greater the degree of admixture within a population, and the smaller the difference in allele frequency or baseline disease risk, the less likely that population stratification leads to confounding (Wacholder et al. 2000). Third, when important confounding caused by population stratification does occur, it should be controllable by the usual design and analytical features employed by epidemiologists.

Finally, genetic studies are becoming more and more sophisticated, and the genetic background of populations can be investigated in several ways, for example by stratifying by microsatellite polymorphisms as markers of genetic heterogeneity within a population. For further details on studies in genetic epidemiology see Chap. III.7 of this handbook.

Publication Bias.   It can be particularly important in molecular epidemiology, since many assays are time-consuming and expensive, with the consequence that most studies are small. Positive results may arise by chance – due to small size – but have greater probability of being published than negative results.

SNPs are relatively cheap to analyze on a large scale (in large samples) compared to other biomarkers, but to date little information is available as to the function of many SNPs. This means that the interpretation of findings is not straightforward, and many findings could be easily due to chance. Again, positive findings on SNPs will tend to be published more easily than negative findings, thus distorting the overall picture in the literature.

Biological Interpretation of the Test.   The fact that, for example, micronuclei in buccal cells are found in excess among smokers does not necessarily express a direct link between disease and chromosomal damage – as an intermediate event in the carcinogenic process –, since micronucleated cells are not viable.

Examples   6.3

Molecular epidemiology is not distinct from traditional epidemiology, but represents a development that aims at achieving specific scientific goals. To better illustrate how molecular epidemiology tries to achieve such goals, we have chosen a few examples that show: (1) a better characterization of exposures, particularly when levels of exposure are low (in one example, by the means of adduct measurement); (2) the study of gene-environment interactions (through the example of DNA repair polymorphisms); (3) the use of markers of early response (such as *p53* mutations) in order to overcome the main limitations of chronic disease epidemiology, i.e. the relatively low frequency of specific forms of disease and the long latency period between exposure and the onset of disease. Through the examples we also want to stress the limitations of molecular epidemiology: the complexity of many laboratory methods with partially unknown levels of measurement error or inter-laboratory variability; the scanty knowledge of the sources of bias and confounding; and the uncertain biological meaning of markers, like in the case of some types of adducts or some early response markers.

The examples given below are not meant to be exhaustive of issues surrounding molecular epidemiologic studies, but should be representative.

Example 1: Reliability of *p53* measurement   6.3.1

The measurement of any biomarker is subject to inter- and intra-individual variability. The extent of variability in measurements can be measured itself in several ways (Carmines and Zeller 1979; Fletcher et al. 1988). A general measure of the extent of variation for continuous measurements is the Coefficient of Variation (CV = standard deviation/mean, expressed as a percentage). A more useful measure is the ratio between CVb and CVw : CVw measures the extent of laboratory variation within the same sample in the same assay, CVb measures the between-subject variation, and the CVb/CVw ratio indicates the extent of the between-subject variation relative to the laboratory error. Large degrees of laboratory error can be tolerated if between-person differences in the parameter to be measured are large.

A frequently used measure of reliability for continuous measurements is the intraclass correlation coefficient (ICC), i.e. the between person variance divided by the total (between plus within-subject) variance. The intraclass coefficient is equal to 1.0 if there is exact agreement between the two measures on each subject (thus differing from the Pearson correlation coefficient that takes the value 1.0 when one measure is a linear combination of the other, not only when the two exactly agree). A coefficient of 1.0 occurs when within-subject variation is null, i.e. laboratory measurements are totally reliable.

The intraclass correlation coefficient can be used to estimate the extent of between-subject variability in relation to total variability. The latter includes variation due to different sources (reproducibility, repeatability, and sampling variation). To measure reproducibility, i.e. the ability of two laboratories to agree when measuring the same marker in the same sample, the mean difference between observers (and the corresponding confidence interval) has been proposed (Brennan and Silman 1992). Let us consider the example in Table 6.2: two pathologists interpreted the slides of 40 subjects with bladder cancer, in order to quantify $p53$ overexpression as measured by immunohistochemistry. Table 6.2 gives the percentage of positive staining cells according to each pathologist and the difference between the two observers for each patient. The proposed measure of inter-observer agreement is the mean difference (in this case 0.9) and the corresponding 95% confidence interval, which is comprised between -20.9 and $+22.7$. What we can conclude is that there is good average agreement between the two pathologists (mean difference = 0.9), but a large confidence interval indicating large overall variability. In the case of immunohistochemistry, a very important source of variation is due to sampling since pathologists usually do not read the same fields, i.e. the same cells, at the microscope.

We have considered reliability as a property of the assay in the hands of different readers (reproducibility) or at repeat measurements (repeatability). Let us consider now validity of assessment, i.e. correspondence with a standard. It is essential to bear in mind that two readers may show very high levels of agreement, as measured e.g. by Pearson correlation coefficient (i.e. $r = 0.9$), even if the first consistently records twice the value of the second observer. Or, alternatively (for example, when using the intraclass correlation coefficient), two readers could show high levels of agreement (e.g. $ICC = 0.9$) but poor validity if the same errors repeat themselves for both raters.

Table 6.2. Measurement of inter-observer variation: immunohistochemistry for the expression of the *p53* gene (percentage of positive cells) as measured by two different pathologists in the same samples (data kindly provided by Professor Renato Coda) (*n* = 40)

| | Pathologist | | |
	First	Second	Difference
1	16.00	20.00	−4.00
2	83.00	60.00	23.00
3	18.50	28.00	−9.50
4	19.40	19.40	0.00
5	96.40	72.80	23.60
6	4.90	4.50	0.40
7	–	3.20	–
8	21.00	16.20	4.80
9	11.40	5.40	6.00
10	13.00	26.00	−13.00
11	9.40	6.00	3.40
12	4.60	1.70	2.90
13	9.70	1.80	7.90
14	20.80	32.10	−11.30
15	43.50	49.00	−5.50
16	5.60	12.50	−6.90
17	40.10	28.00	12.10
18	11.50	7.00	4.50
19	14.60	13.50	1.10
20	–	27.00	–
21	7.50	2.80	4.70
22	7.40	21.00	−13.60
23	16.30	4.40	11.90
24	21.00	46.50	−25.50
25	2.90	0.90	2.00
26	29.80	34.00	−4.20
27	82.00	69.50	12.50
28	75.00	75.20	−0.20
29	7.00	24.00	−17.00
30	7.20	8.40	−1.20
31	5.70	0.50	5.20
32	15.00	6.10	8.90
33	0.50	1.00	−0.50
34	18.00	7.50	10.50
35	9.80	11.00	−1.20
36	4.20	10.50	−6.30
37	15.20	18.00	−2.80
38	9.30	22.00	−12.70
39	–	–	–
40	52.60	29.30	23.30

table to be continued

Table 6.2. (continued)

| N | Difference parameters: | | | |
	Mean	Std Dev	Minimum	Maximum
37	0.9	10.907	−25.5	23.6

(3 missing values)

95% range for agreement: mean $\pm 2 \times$ std dev (diff) = $0.9 \pm 2 \times 10.9$ = $[-20.9; +22.7]$

According to the definition of validity, we are interested in the correspondence of the measurement with a conceptual entity, i.e. accumulation of the p53 protein as a consequence of gene mutation (in fact, without a mutation the protein has a very short half-life and rapidly disappears from the cells). Table 6.3 shows data on the correspondence between immunohistochemistry and p53 mutations. Sensitivity of immunohistochemistry is estimated as 85%, i.e. false negatives are 15% of all samples containing mutations; specificity is estimated as 71%, i.e. 29% of samples not containing mutations are falsely positive at immunohistochemistry. A combined estimate of sensitivity and specificity is the area under the Receiver-Operating-Curve (ROC), i.e. a curve which represents graphically the relationship between sensitivity and (1-specificity) (Fig. 6.2). In the example shown in Fig. 6.2, the area under the ROC curve is 90.3% (Cordon-Carlo et al. 1994).

It is usually believed (Fletcher at al. 1988) that sensitivity and specificity indicate properties of a test irrespectively of the frequency of the condition to be detected. In the example of Table 6.3, the proportion of samples showing a mutation is high (32/73 = 44%); it would be much lower for example in patients with benign bladder conditions or in healthy subjects. A useful measure to predict how many subjects, among those testing positive, are really affected by the condition, we aim to detect is the positive predictive value. In the example, among 39 patients testing positive at immuno-histochemistry, 27 actually have mutations, i.e. immuno-histochemistry correctly predicts mutations in 69% of the positive cases. Let us suppose, however, that the prevalence of mutations is not 44%, but 4.4% (32/730). With the same sensitivity and specificity values (85% and 71%, respectively) we would have a positive predictive value of 11.8%, i.e. much lower. The predictive value is a very useful measure, because it indicates how many true positive cases we will obtain within a population of subjects who test positive with the assay we are applying. However, we must bear in our minds that the predictive value is strongly influenced by the prevalence of the condition: a very low predictive value may simply indicate that we are studying a population in which very few subjects actually have the condition we want to identify.

Table 6.4 shows another set of estimates of validity, based on the clinical outcome. In this case, the aim is to understand how useful p53 immunohistochemistry may be to predict the risk of metastases. While in the previous example the conceptual entity to predict by immunohistochemistry were p53 gene mutations, here the conceptual entity is the aggressiveness of malignancy, as expressed by the

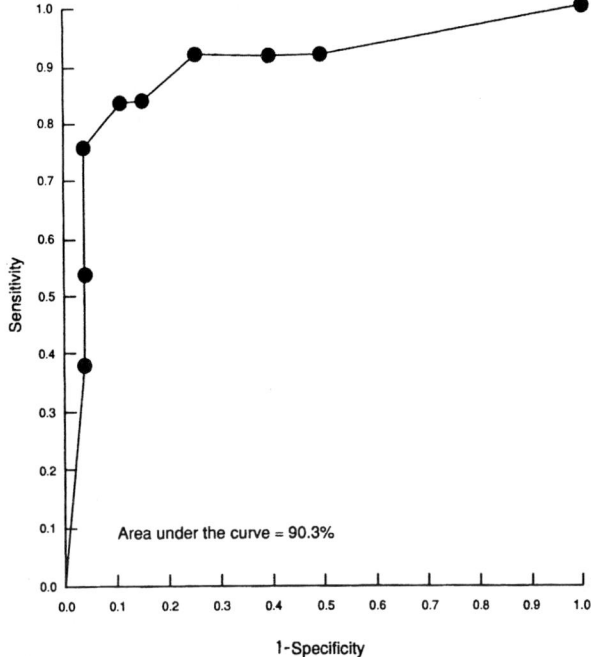

Figure 6.2. Receiver-operating-curve (ROC) statistical analysis of the sensitivity and specificity of immunohistochemistry as it relates to PCR-SSCP and sequencing results, representing identification of *p53* mutations. The area under the curve as a measure of diagnostic accuracy was estimated to be 90.3%. (Reprinted by permission of Wiley-Liss, Inc. from Cordon-Cardo et al. (1994))

occurrence of lymphnode invasion in the follow-up of patients who were tested for *p53* at diagnosis. In this case we are obviously interested in the positive predictive value, which, for example, is 60% at stage 1. However, we also want to establish whether immunohistochemistry is worth measuring, i.e. it adds something to what we know already from other clinical examinations. The best predictor of outcome is usually the clinical stage, based on the tumour size at diagnosis. We see that among stage 1 tumours, 7 out of 25 (28%) manifest lymph node metastases in the follow-up. The question is: does *p53* immunohistochemistry add any information to simple knowledge of the stage at diagnosis? A way to answer is to estimate the a posteriori probability of metastases after measurement of *p53* and compare it to the a priori probability (i.e. in the absence of *p53* measurement), which in this case is 28%. The a posteriori probability is computed by using the relationship: a posteriori odds = a priori odds × likelihood ratio. Table 6.4 shows that in stage 1 the measurement of *p53* allows the probability of metastases to increase from 28% (a priori) to 63% (a posteriori), while in stages 2 and 3 the contribution of *p53* measurement is totally insignificant.

Table 6.3. Validity of *p*53 immunohistochemistry as compared to mutations in the *p*53 gene (bladder cancer patients) (data from Esrig et al. 1994)

A*	*p*53 nuclear reactivity (immunohistochemistry)			
*p*53 mutations by SSCP	–	+	++	Total
No mutation	29	7	5	41
All mutations	5	8	19	32
Total	34	15	24	73

B** Theoretical distribution with prevalence of mutations = 4.4%			
Mutations	Immunohistochemistry		
	–	+/++	Total
Yes	5	27	32
No	496	202	698
Total	501	229	730

* sensitivity of immunohistochemistry (+ and ++) = 27/32 = 85%
* specificity = 29/41 = 71%
* positive predictive value = (8 + 19)/(15 + 24) = 27/39 = 69%
** sensitivity = 27/32 = 85%
** specificity = 496/698 = 71%
** positive predictive value = 27/229 = 11.7%

Table 6.4. Validity of *p*53 immunohistochemistry as compared to clinical outcome (occurrence of lymphnode metastases during the follow-up) (data kindly provided by Professor A. Fontana)

Stage 1	*p*53 immunohistochemistry		
	–	+	Total
Lymphnode invasion			
No	14	4	18
Yes	1	6	7
Total	15	10	25

positive predictive value = 6/10 = 60%
likelihood ratio = (6/7)/(4/18) = 3.9
a priori probability = 7/25 = 28%
a priori odds = a priori probability/(1− a priori probability) = 39%
a posteriori odds = a priori odds × likelihood ratio = 39% × 3.9 = 1.5

	A priori probability	A posteriori probability (when *p*53 is positive)
Stage 1	28%	63%
Stage 2	73%	80%
Stage 3	100%	–

Example 2: Sources of Heterogeneity for DNA Repair Polymorphisms

This example aims at illustrating the issue of heterogeneity of results, often interpretable in the light of the different study designs used.

Enzymes encoded by DNA repair genes constantly monitor the genome to repair damaged nucleotide residues resulting from environmental and endogenous exposures. Our example addresses issues related to the design of studies based on genotyping for polymorphisms in DNA repair genes and to the epidemiologic factors that affect the integrity and the generalizability of these studies. We will consider the following aspects of heterogeneity to explain variation in results:

— epidemiologic design
— laboratory methods
— strength of association
— consistency
— internal coherence
— time sequence
— confounding
— statistical considerations
— interactions
— biological sources of heterogeneity.

More details have been reported in an extensive review we have published (Berwick and Vineis 2000). More extensive and updated information can be found on the website http://perseus.isi.it/HuGe-Repair/HuGe-Repair.htm (ISI Foundation 2004).

Epidemiologic Design.   Most studies on DNA repair genotypes are case-control studies, and more specifically hospital-based studies. As described in Chap. I.6 of this handbook, such studies have several limitations. In particular, hospital-based studies often do not include all incident cases of a certain geographical area, so that selection bias can occur. Controls are chosen among patients with pathologies other than the one included in the case category. Such diseases can be related to the exposure/trait of interest. For example, we know rather little on the role of DNA repair enzymes in several different diseases, like atherosclerosis, to be sure that their inclusion in the control group will not alter the comparison with cases.

In the review we have published – see Berwick and Vineis (2000) – fourteen studies were hospital-based, seven were population-based case-control studies, one was a cohort study (nested case-control), one was a case-case study and five had a still different design. Concerning the choice of controls, they were extremely heterogeneous. It is noteworthy that one study compared Chinese cases living in the United States with Chinese controls living in China. One study used cadaveric transplant donors as controls, and one used friends of the cases. All these choices are debatable and may imply distortions in the results.

Several studies matched cases and controls for exposure because genes were the only variable of interest (typically, studies on lung cancer matched on smoking). However, in this way they prevented the study of gene-environment interactions. The response proportion was usually not reported by the published studies, although it may be used as an indicator of the degree of selection bias.

Laboratory Methods.   Few studies used a relatively *high-throughput* genetic technology (TaqMan or others), i.e. a highly automatized technique that allows large numbers of analyses. PCR-RFLP (a basic but robust method based on the identification of the length of DNA fragments after enzyme digestion) was the most frequently used method. Genotype-phenotype correlation and cancer status was sought in one study, with a comparison between HCRA (host cell reactivation assay) and genotyping for XPD – a specific DNA repair gene – in lung cancer patients. HCRA is a phenotypic test to evaluate the proficiency of DNA repair capacity in cells in culture, and it is expected to correlate with genetic polymorphisms of repair genes. Both cases and controls with the wild genotype had the most proficient DNA repair capacity as measured by the host cell reactivation assay. One study compared different genotyping techniques, namely PCR-RFLP and DHPLC (Denaturing High-Pressure Liquid Chromatography). The comparison of different techniques is extremely important to test the reliability of each.

Strength of Association.   Odds ratios (OR) tended to be moderately low (on the order of two or less), with the exception of oligoastrocytoma and ERCC1, with an OR of 4.6. Low OR are to be expected for low-penetrance genetic variants.

Consistency by Site and Genotype.   Twelve studies considered XRCC1 polymorphisms in ten different cancer sites (head and neck, colon-rectum, melanoma, breast, lung (three studies), bladder (two studies), stomach, esophagus, leukaemia). For bladder cancer, findings are inconsistent and based on relatively small numbers. Therefore, it was impossible to draw inferences on consistency of the findings. (For an update see the website http://perseus.isi.it/HuGe-Repair/HuGe-Repair.htm, ISI Foundation 2004.)

Internal Coherence.   One study compared two control groups (one population-based and one hospital-based) with very similar results. In general, large variation was found among ethnic groups, but this can be a genuine finding rather than an artifact. Also variation with age was noted. Auckley et al.'s results (Auckley et al. 2001) comparing DNA-PK activity (double-strand break repair) in peripheral lymphocytes with DNA-PK activity in lung tissue showed a strong correlation between the measurements. Whenever possible, a comparison between the proxy tissue, usually lymphocytes, with the target tissue should be made.

Time Sequence.   In studies on genotypes, the criterion of time sequence applies only if we suspect that the genotype influences survival. In this case, the recruitment of prevalent (not newly diagnosed) cases would lead to a bias in favor of the genotypes associated with longer survival. Apparently only one study included prevalent cases.

Genotype does not change with time, so that case-control studies using SNPs are not affected by the usual forms of bias that characterize the retrospective collection of information on exposures, unless, of course, survival is not affected by genotype, and gene-environment interactions are the focus of interest. In the latter instance, environmental data need to face the same rigorous scrutiny as in any epidemiologic study.

Bias

Confounding. Most studies have considered at least some potential confounders (e.g., age). The concept of confounding is related to the existence of a variable that is a risk factor for the disease and is associated with the genotype. If the prevalence of a certain genotype changes with age because of a survival effect, age is a confounder (since it is strongly predictive of cancer onset). Very often it is difficult to hypothesize which relevant confounders could exist in genotyping studies, other than population admixture. We found no evidence that population admixture could represent a problem in studies of DNA repair. For a more detailed description on confounding see Chap. I.9 of this handbook.

A Special Problem: Publication Bias. We mention here publication bias because it is a kind of bias, but not necessarily a source of heterogeneity, rather of homogeneity. Publication bias occurs when positive studies are preferentially published by scientific journals compared to negative studies, and particularly to small negative studies. In the genotyping studies we examined, all results (except one) were based on small or moderately small numbers. With the increasing recognition of this problem, more negative studies are being published.

Statistical Considerations (Sample Size, Power, Multiple Comparisons). The sample size is always a problem in this type of investigations. However, relatively common genotypes have been considered to date, so that statistical power is usually moderate. An important methodological problem is multiple comparisons: splitting the data into several subgroups increases the probability of finding statistically significant results.

Interactions. Most of the reported interactions in studies of DNA repair cannot be evaluated because of multiple comparisons and lack of formal statistical analyses for interaction. Interestingly, a few studies find an association between cancer and the relevant genotypes only among non-drinkers. Other examples are found in association between Helicobacter pylori-negative subjects and stomach cancer, and genotype influences on the basal-cell carcinoma risk among those with a family history of basal cell carcinoma. None of the studies, however, had a sufficient power to detect weak interactions. These studies are thus not possible to evaluate for true interaction effects. For a more detailed description on interaction see Chap. I.9 of this handbook.

Biological Sources of Heterogeneity.   Finally, a possible explanation for the heterogeneity of results could be that not only amino acid variants in different domains of a gene may affect different protein interactions, resulting in the expression of different phenotypes, but also the same allele could have divergent effects in different DNA repair pathways and on different types of DNA damage. Moreover, a certain variant could be in linkage with another responsible variant; in this case it is possible that different populations have different alleles in linkage disequilibrium with the responsible variant.

Perspectives.   Researchers are genotyping large samples of subjects as fast as new repair gene polymorphisms are discovered in order to conduct "association studies". However, information on the function and mechanistic interactions of these alterations is urgently needed. New technologies are being developed rapidly and they may be harnessed to answer the major question as to whether a small decrement in DNA repair capacity predisposes to cancer.

6.3.3   Example 3. Bulky DNA Adducts in Epidemiological Studies: Principles of Meta-Analysis

This example again concerns heterogeneity of results, which, in this case, can be tentatively attributed to measurement error or to genuine differences among the populations that have been studied. The test itself, in fact ("bulky" adducts) is affected by large coefficients of variation (at least 30%). In addition, through the example we will introduce some of the principles of meta-analysis.

"Bulky" DNA adducts represent an integrated marker of exposure to aromatic compounds. The level of bulky adducts in white blood cells (WBC) has been shown to correlate with external exposure to polycyclic aromatic hydrocarbons in a few investigations, while the association with tobacco smoke tended to be inconsistent. Their biological meaning for carcinogenesis has been illustrated in a few elegant experiments. For example, Denissenko and colleagues (Denissenko et al. 1998) have shown that the main metabolite of benzo(a)pyrene forms adducts in the same codon of the *p53* gene where characteristic mutations are found in the lungs of smokers.

Meta-Analysis.   Meta-analysis is a way to summarize the results from several different studies in order to provide a single summary estimate of association and to increase the overall power of the comparison (see also Chap. II.7 of this handbook). The following are the main methodological issues that should be addressed in preparing a meta-analysis, taken from a methodological paper (Egger et al. 1997):

"Meta-analysis should be as carefully planned as any other research project, with a detailed written protocol being prepared in advance. The a priori definition of eligibility criteria for studies to be included and comprehensive search for such studies are central to high quality meta-analysis. The graphical display of results from individual studies on a common scale is an important intermediate step, which allows a visual examination of the degree of heterogeneity between studies. Different statistical methods exist for combining the data, but there is no single 'correct' method. A thorough sensitivity analysis is essential to assess the robustness of combined estimates to different assumptions and inclusion criteria."

In general, a meta-analysis is extremely useful in identifying the main methodological problems in the studies that have been conducted on a certain scientific issue.

We have performed a meta-analysis to test the hypothesis that the presence of a high level of bulky DNA adducts in tissues is associated with an increased risk of cancer in humans (Veglia et al. 2003). The Medline database was searched for the

Study	Tumour n	mean(sd)	Control n	mean(sd)	WMD (95%CI Random)	Weight %	WMD (95%CI Random)
Popp 1993	20	0.57(0.80)	11	1.00(1.63)		8.4	-0.43[-1.46,0.60]
Tang 1995	52	2.08(1.83)	25	1.00(0.65)		14.2	1.08[0.52,1.64]
Hou 1999	35	1.00(0.84)	44	1.00(0.73)		17.2	0.00[-0.35,0.35]
Vulimiri 2000	34	2.11(0.37)	29	1.00(0.13)		19.5	1.11[0.98,1.24]
Peluso 2000	94	2.25(3.89)	27	1.00(1.43)		9.1	1.25[0.30,2.20]
Cheng 2000	38	2.59(1.62)	22	1.00(0.94)		12.9	1.59[0.94,2.24]
Tang 2001	36	1.96(0.72)	64	1.00(0.09)		18.6	0.96[0.72,1.20]
Total(95%CI)	309		222			100.0	0.83[0.44,1.22]

Test for heterogeneity chi-square=44.56 df=6 p<0.00001
Test for overall effect z=4.16 p=0.00003

Figure 6.3. Meta-analysis of studies on bulky DNA adducts and cancer. Random effect model. Current smokers only. *WMD* is the weighed mean difference between adducts in cases and adducts in controls (weight is given by study size); 95% confidence interval computed by the random effect model

Study	Tumour n	mean(sd)	Control n	mean(sd)	WMD (95%CI Random)	Weight %	WMD (95%CI Random)
Tang 1995	58	1.67(2.71)	34	1.00(0.98)		15.9	0.67[-0.10,1.44]
Hou 1999	54	1.10(1.02)	30	1.00(0.75)		43.1	0.10[-0.28,0.48]
Vulimiri 2000	6	2.18(5.34)	5	1.00(0.62)		0.6	1.18[-3.13,5.49]
Peluso 2000	42	0.66(0.54)	24	1.00(2.04)		14.0	-0.34[-1.17,0.49]
Tang 2001	35	0.72(0.86)	64	1.00(1.96)		26.4	-0.28[-0.84,0.28]
Total(95%CI)	195		157			100.0	0.04[-0.30,0.37]

Test for heterogeneity chi-square=4.99 df=4 p=0.29
Test for overall effect z=0.21 p=0.8

Figure 6.4. Meta-analysis of studies on bulky DNA adducts and cancer. Random effect model. Former smokers only. *WMD* is the weighed mean difference between adducts in cases and adducts in controls (weight is given by study size); 95% confidence interval computed by the random effect model

| Study | Tumour | | Control | | WMD | Weight | WMD |
	n	mean(sd)	n	mean(sd)	(95%CI Random)	%	(95%CI Random)
Popp 1993	3	1.54(1.25)	4	1.00(1.03)		9.2	0.54[-1.20,2.28]
Tang 1995	9	1.18(2.00)	39	1.00(1.36)		11.5	0.18[-1.19,1.55]
Hou 1999	82	1.00(0.88)	72	1.00(1.18)		18.8	0.00[-0.33,0.33]
Vulimiri 2000	3	0.16(0.04)	13	1.00(1.28)		16.6	-0.84[-1.54,-0.14]
Peluso 2000	22	3.42(3.51)	55	1.00(1.32)		10.6	2.42[0.91,3.93]
Cheng 2000	32	3.07(2.33)	11	1.00(0.53)		15.3	2.07[1.20,2.94]
Tang 2001	15	0.80(0.64)	30	1.00(1.05)		17.9	-0.20[-0.70,0.30]
Total(95%CI)	166		224			100.0	0.47[-0.26,1.19]

Test for heterogeneity chi-square=37.96 df=6 p<0.00001
Test for overall effect z=1.27 p=0.2

Figure 6.5. Meta-analysis of studies on bulky DNA adducts and cancer. Random effect model. Never smokers only. *WMD* is the weighed mean difference between adducts in cases and adducts in controls (weight is given by study size); 95% confidence interval computed by the random effect model

period between 1990 and March 2002, supplemented with manual bibliography review. We collected all the studies conforming to the following criteria:

1. case-control or cohort studies comparing bulky DNA adduct levels in cancer patients and control subjects;
2. separate comparisons for current, former and never-smokers.

We excluded specific adducts such as those formed by aflatoxin or cytostatic drugs.

The results of the meta-analysis are reported in Figs. 6.3–6.5 and in more detail elsewhere (Veglia et al. 2003). We will describe here some methodological issues we have considered.

Adduct Variability and Heterogeneity of Results

Average adduct levels differed markedly among studies, both in cases and controls, ranging from 0.4×10^{-8} to 7.9×10^{-8} in the WBC of controls. This may be due partially to inter-laboratory variability, partially to the different methods of blood collection and storing.

More standardized measurements are warranted in future investigations; an effort to compare and standardize laboratory procedures has been undertaken and published by a group of European researchers (Phillips and Castegnaro 1999).

To address heterogeneity, the results were standardized in the meta-analysis by dividing within each study all means and standard deviations by the average of the control groups. Therefore standardized control means were set to one in all studies. Studies were tested with Breslow-Day's test of heterogeneity (Breslow and Day 1980), and a random effect model was employed in the meta-analysis to account for inter-study variability (DerSimonian and Laird 1986). We have computed standardized, weighed mean differences (*WMD*) between cases and controls in each study, and the overall *WMD*. For each *WMD* we computed 95% confidence intervals.

As Figs. 6.3–6.5 show, the results vary according to smoking habits (current, former, never smoker). Current smokers (Fig. 6.3) show a statistically significant difference between cases and controls, with cases having 83% higher levels of adducts than controls. No association between adduct levels and the case status is observed in former smokers (Fig. 6.4), with complete consistency among investigations. Results on non-smokers (Fig. 6.5) are inconsistent; only two studies show a statistically significant positive difference between cases and controls. These observations are in accordance with the findings of the only prospective study available (Tang et al. 2001), which also found that DNA adduct levels measured in WBC were predictive of lung cancer occurrence only in current smokers.

Sensitivity Analysis. Sensitivity analysis is a way to assess the impact of methodological flaws on the results of a meta-analysis. A sensitivity analysis simply consists of examining whether the results (expressed as odds ratio or *WMD*) changes after exclusion of studies with methodological deficiencies. We assigned a qualitative score (from 0 to 3) to each study in the meta-analysis. If we exclude the papers with a quality score lower than 2, we still have in Fig. 6.3 three positive results out of 4. Another type of sensitivity analysis consists in including only studies on lung cancer and excluding an investigation that measured adducts in lung tissue. In this case the standardized difference for the Relative Adduct Level (RAL) is 0.79 (95% CI: 0.34–1.24) for current smokers, 0.10 (−0.29–0.49) for former smokers and −0.21 (−0.58–0.15) for non-smokers, a result similar to that obtained in the overall analysis.

In conclusion, the heterogeneity of results emerging from the meta-analysis in this case suggests three possible explanations: measurement error, which is high; differences related to the study design; or genuine biological differences, for example between smokers and non-smokers.

It should also be noted that WBC are not the target tissue (lung or bladder cancer), and that in case-control studies one could argue that the disease process itself may influence the adduct levels. Hence the superiority of prospective investigations becomes obvious.

Ethical Issues in Biomarker Research

6.4

In addition to the usual requirements for epidemiologic research, the recent developments of molecular – and in particular genetic – tests have induced more specific ethical considerations and led to the development of specific guidelines. To create a database of molecular epidemiology the following requirements should be met (Lowrance 2001):

1. follow respectful protocols in eliciting information (also on relatives)
2. secure broad and respectful informed consent
3. manage anonymisation of database interlinking
4. establish confidentiality and security safeguards
5. develop defensible responses to requests for personal data by various parties
6. devise sound data access, ownership, and intellectual property policies

7. be clear about whether and how individuals will be informed of findings that might be medically helpful for them

8. arrange supervision by research ethics and privacy protection bodies.

Clearly, each of these requirements would need extensive comments. In particular, how "broad" should the consent be (Point 2)? On one side, a broad consent (e.g. "the biological samples will be used for the identification of gene variants that may predispose to chronic diseases") implies a greater freedom for the researcher, who is not obliged to collect further consent forms each time a new gene is investigated. On the other side, such a generic informed consent form explains very little to the recruitees and does not even mention the basic distinction between highly-penetrant and low-penetrant genes. There is a broad agreement on the fact that low-penetrant variants (such as those of GSTM1 or NAT2), that are common in the general population and induce just a slight increase in the risk (interacting with environmental exposures) should not be subject to strict rules as far as ethical implications are concerned. In fact, knowledge of alleles involved in metabolic pathways neither allows the carrier to modify her risk profile substantially, nor allows the researcher to identify other members of the family, thus not violating confidentiality. For a more general discussion of ethical aspects see Chap. IV.7 of this handbook.

The case of highly-penetrant gene variants is different: first, the identification of the carrier of a rare mutation allows the researchers to identify other family members possibly affected, with potential detrimental effects (e.g. on insurance policies). Second, researchers should have a clear view of the practical implications of testing for the study subjects, and in particular what to do in each of these situations: no effective treatment is possible; treatment is available with close favourable/unfavourable effects balance; effective treatment is available with scarce unfavourable effects.

6.5   Conclusions

Conventional epidemiology, based on simple tools such as interviews and questionnaires, has achieved extremely important goals. Even a difficult issue such as the relationship between air pollution and chronic disease has been successfully dealt with by time-series analysis and other methods not based on the laboratory. Therefore, the use of molecular techniques coupled with an epidemiological design needs to be evaluated carefully.

As the examples we have provided demonstrate, molecular epidemiology is not distinct from traditional epidemiology, but represents a development that aims at achieving specific scientific goals: (1) a better characterization of exposures, particularly when levels of exposure are very low or different sources of exposure should be integrated in a single measure; (2) the study of gene-environment interactions; (3) the use of markers of early response, in order to overcome the main limitations of chronic disease epidemiology, i.e. the relatively low frequency of specific forms of disease and the long latency period between exposure and the onset of disease. Also limitations of molecular epidemiology should be acknowledged: the complexity of many laboratory methods, with partially unknown levels of measurement error or inter-laboratory variability; the scanty knowledge of the sources of bias and confounding; in some circumstances, the lower degree of accuracy (for example urinary nicotine compared to questionnaires on smoking habits); and the uncertain biological meaning of markers, like in the case of some types of adducts or some early response markers (typically, mutation spectra).

Acknowledgements. This work has been made possible by a grant of the Compagnia di San Paolo to the ISI Foundation and a grant from the European Union to P.V. for the project Gen-Air (QLK4-CT-1999-00927).

References

Auckley DH, Crowell RE, Heaphy ER, Stidley CA, Lechner JF, Gilliland FD, Belinsky SA (2001) Reduced DNA-dependent protein kinase activity is associated with lung cancer. Carcinogenesis 22(5):723–727

Bartsch H (2000) Studies on biomarkers in cancer etiology and prevention: a summary and challenge of 20 years of interdisciplinary research. Mutat Res 462(2–3):255–279

Berwick M, Vineis P (2000) Markers of DNA repair and susceptibility to cancer in humans: an epidemiologic review. JNCI 92(11):874–897

Berwick M, Matullo G, Vineis P (2002) Studies of DNA repair and human cancer: an update. In: Wilson SH, Suk WA (eds) Biomarkers of environmentally associated disease. Lewis Publishers, Boca Raton

Brennan P, Silman A (1992) Statistical methods for assessing observer variability in clinical measures. Br Med J 304:1491–1494

Breslow NE, Day NE (1980) Statistical methods in cancer research. Volume I – The analysis of case-control studies. IARC Scientific Publications No 32. International Agency for Research on Cancer, Lyon

Carmines EG, Zeller RA (1979) Reliability and validity assessment. Sage Publications, London

Cordon-Carlo C, Dalbagni G, Saez GT, Oliva MR, Zhang ZF, Rosai J, Reuter VE, Pellicer A (1994) p53 mutations in human bladder cancer: genotypic vs. phenotypic patterns. Int J Cancer 56:347–353

Denissenko MF, Pao A, Tang M, Pfeifer GP (1998) Preferential formation of benzo[a]pyrene adducts at lung cancer mutational hotspots in p53. Science 274(5286):430–432

DerSimonian R, Laird N (1986) Meta-analysis in clinical trials. Control Clin Trials 7:177–188

Egger M, Smith GD, Phillips AN (1997) Meta-analysis: principles and procedures. Br Med J 315(7121):1533–1537

Esrig D, Elmajian D, Groshen S, Freeman JA, Stein JP, Chen SC, Nichols PW, Skinner DG, Jones PA, Cote RJ (1994) Accumulation of nuclear *p53* and tumor progression in bladder cancer. N Engl J Med 331(19):1259–1264

Fletcher RH, Fletcher S, Wagner EH (1988) Clinical epidemiology – the essentials, 2nd edn. Williams and Wilkins, Baltimore

ISI Foundation (2004) DNA repair polymorphisms site. (http://perseus.isi.it/HuGe-Repair/HuGe-Repair.htm) Accessed June 18, 2004

Lowrance WW (2001) The promise of human genetic databases. Br Med J 322(7293):1009–1010

Phillips DH, Castegnaro M (1999) Standardization and validation of DNA adduct postlabelling methods: report of interlaboratory trials and production of recommended protocols. Mutagenesis 14(3):301–315

Schulte P, Perera FP (eds) (1998) Molecular epidemiology: Principles and practices. Academic Press, New York

Shields PG, Harris CC (2000) Cancer risk and low-penetrance susceptibility genes in gene-environment interactions. J Clin Oncol 18(11):2309–2315

Tang D, Phillips DH, Stampfer M, Mooney LA, Hsu Y, Cho S, Tsai WY, Ma J, Cole KJ, She MN, Perera FP (2001) Association between carcinogen-DNA adducts in white blood cells and lung cancer risk in the physicians health study. Cancer Res 61(18):6708–6712

Toniolo P, Boffetta P, Shuker D, Rothman N, Hulka B, Pearce N (1997) Application of biomarkers to cancer epidemiology. IARC Scientific Publications No 142. International Agency for Research on Cancer, Lyon

Veglia F, Matullo G, Vineis P (2003) Bulky DNA adducts and risk of cancer: a meta-analysis. Cancer Epidemiol Biomarkers Prev 12(2):157–160

Vineis P, Caporaso N, Cuzick J, Lang M, Malats N, Boffetta P (1999) Genetic susceptibility to cancer: metabolic polymorphisms. IARC Scientific Publication No 148. International Agency for Research on Cancer, Lyon

Vineis P, Veglia F, Benhamou Dorota Butkiewicz S, Cascorbi I, Clapper LM, Dolzan V, Haugen A, Hirvonen A, Ingelman-Sundberg M, Kihara M, Kiyohara C, Kremers P, Le Marchand L, Ohshima S, Pastorelli R, Rannug A, Romkes M, Schoket B, Shields P, Strange CR, Stucker I, Sugimura H, Garte S, Gaspari L, Taioli E (2003) CYP1A1 T^{3801}C polymorphism and lung cancer: a pooled analysis of 2451 cases and 3358 controls. Int J Cancer 104(5):650–657

Wacholder S, Rothman N, Caporaso N (2000) Population stratification in epidemiologic studies of common genetic variants and cancer: quantification of bias. J Natl Cancer Inst 92:1151–1158

Genetic Epidemiology

III.7

Heike Bickeböller

Introduction

Genetic epidemiology both emanates from and combines the scientific disciplines of human genetics and epidemiology as well as biometry. Strong interdisciplinary relationships exist among others with the fields of molecular genetics and medicine/medical care. Some overlap exists with molecular epidemiology (see Chap. III.6 of this handbook).

Genetic epidemiology is essential in the field of human genetics as it aims to detect the genetic origin of phenotypic variability in humans (Vogel 2000). In particular, genetic epidemiological studies unravel the genetic components that contribute to the development or the course of a disease, or in general terms to a *phenotype*, i.e. the observed trait.

Genetic epidemiology is the subdiscipline of epidemiology devoted to diseases/phenotypes with genetic components and to their respective genetic risk factors. The aims are (1) the description of genetically influenced phenotypes or diseases in populations and families, (2) the identification of genetic risk factors associated with the frequencies of phenotypes in the population and/or leading to familial aggregation, and (3) the modelling of the role of these genetic risk factors in populations and families (Khoury et al. 1993). Thus, both population-based and family designs are complementary and play a central role in genetic epidemiological studies. In contrast to classic epidemiology, the three main complications in genetic epidemiology are dependencies, use of indirect evidence and complex data sets: Genetic epidemiology is highly dependent on the direct incorporation of family structure and biology. The structure of families and chromosomes leads to major dependencies between the data and thus to customized models and tests. In many studies only indirect evidence can be used, since the disease-related gene, or more precisely the functionally relevant DNA variant of a gene, is not directly observable. In addition, the data sets to be analyzed can be very complex.

Genetic epidemiology is also a highly specialised subdiscipline of biometry and mathematical population genetics. The field has made major biometrical contributions to human genetics or, relying on earlier biometrical work (since the field was only recently endowed with the name) such as the description of the central Hardy–Weinberg equilibrium (HWE) (Hardy 1908; Weinberg 1908) and the development of statistical methods including segregation analysis, linkage analysis, association analysis, simulation methods and computer algorithms for all major study designs implemented.

The International Society of Genetic Epidemiology describes the field as a marriage between the disciplines of genetics and epidemiology (IGES 2003). It emphasises the need to join the fields. Genetics tends to focus on the genotype-phenotype correlation neglecting the environment. Epidemiology tends to focus on environmental risk factors as well as demographic factors (e.g. age, sex, ethnicity) and familial aggregation as a first step towards genetic risk factors. However, a full understanding of the etiology of complex traits may only be achieved by considering both, genetics and environment, and thereby explaining how genes are expressed in the presence of different environmental contexts. This chapter is solely devoted to methods dissecting the genotype-phenotype correlation with a binary phenotype (affected/unaffected). It is not covering the important subjects of quantitative phenotypes and gene-environment interaction.

Section 7.2 presents an overview of major study designs and types of analysis. Section 7.3 introduces the most important genetic models. Sections 7.4–7.6 will cover the three major types of analysis, i.e. segregation, linkage and association analysis.

Study Types 7.2

Genetic epidemiological investigations are usually triggered by epidemiological studies that demonstrate a *positive family history* as a risk factor for disease indicating putative genetic or shared environmental factors. Often the goal of initial studies is to estimate the *relative risk for relatives of affected individuals* in relation to the general population in order to support the genetic hypothesis.

To further investigate familial aggregation, a *segregation analysis* may be carried out in pedigrees. The aim of such an analysis is to determine whether a *major gene* is influencing a given phenotype in these families and if so to estimate the parameters of the underlying genetic model. All methods for segregation analysis are based on probability calculations for observed phenotypes conditional on hypothetical genetic model parameters and on family structure, i.e. *genealogies*. Parameter estimation is often based on likelihood-ratio tests in order to select the most plausible model nested within a hypothetical general model.

The primary cause of a so-called *monogenic disease* such as cystic fibrosis is a mutation within a single gene that segregates according to Mendelian laws (see below). The predisposing variants, i.e. the alleles carrying the risk, of this *major gene* are usually rare in the population. For *complex or multifactorial diseases*, Mendelian subforms such as the subform of breast cancer caused by the major gene BRCA1, genetic and non-genetic susceptibility factors, or risk modifying genes can exist. For rare monogenic diseases and rare Mendelian subforms of complex diseases, segregation analysis and subsequent further analyses perform well. However, complex diseases in general require more sophisticated methods of analysis than monogenic diseases. For example in Alzheimer's disease at least three major genes and several susceptibility genes confering moderate risk (*oligogenes*) exist. Oligogenes as genetic risk factors can be frequent in the population. *Polygenic* effects at many loci across the whole genome may contribute to disease, each with a minor effect.

If there is sufficient evidence for the existence of genetic factors contributing to a (complex) disease, the next step will be to locate or to identify susceptibility genes in order to quantify the genetic influence and to understand the underlying genetic model and pathway to the phenotype. For this purpose, measures of correlation between a *genetic marker* and the (unknown) *disease locus* are used. A genetic marker is a DNA segment with multiple alleles for which the localisation on the chromosome is known and the alleles can be determined. In general, methods assume Mendelian segregation of the marker (see Sect. 7.3.2). The most frequently used markers are multiallelic *restriction fragment length polymorphisms (RFLPs)* or *microsatellites* and biallelic *single nucleotide polymorphisms (SNPs)*. Usually the frequency of the most common variant must be less than 99% before a marker is termed a *polymorphism*.

For the analysis of complex diseases with genetic marker data we can distinguish two major approaches. Both investigate the genotype-phenotype correlation. Depending on the context, either the first or the second approach is more efficient (Clerget-Darpoux and Bonaïti-Pellié 1992). The first approach is a *genome scan*, i.e. the systematic coarse grid search of the whole genome with a map of genetic markers, with the objective to locate a region harbouring a susceptibility gene. A typical study would investigate approximately 350 markers with an average distance of 10cM (centiMorgan, see Sect. 7.3.3.) along the genome in families. The other approach is to investigate *candidate genes* (or candidate gene regions). Thereby, the focus is set on genes for which their function on the pathway to the phenotype can evidently be assumed. The most prominent example of a candidate gene system is the HLA (human leucocyte antigen) complex on chromosome 6. HLA is involved in immune resistance and is thus a natural candidate gene region for all autoimmune diseases.

The aims of a candidate gene investigation are to find evidence of any contribution of the candidate gene to the disease and to model its influence on the disease. The genotypes of the relevant functional component of the candidate genes are not always observed. We therefore need to use the information on genetic markers that lie in close proximity to the candidate gene in question. In general, nonparametric approaches are to be preferred, since they need fewer assumptions about the underlying genetic model.

There are two types of information that describe the correlation between a genetic marker and the susceptibility locus of a disease. (The correlation is maximized, when the genetic marker is identical to the functional variant for susceptibility):

- *Linkage (cosegregation at the family level)*: The common segregation of a marker and a disease is investigated. Inheritance is characterised by the transmissions of DNA segments from parents to offspring. If the transmissions at the marker locus and at the disease locus from one parent to a child are not independent, then this is denoted as linkage. Under linkage relatives with a similar disease status (e.g. both affected) are more similar at the marker locus than to be expected under independence.

- *Linkage disequilibrium (association at the population level)*: Linkage disequilibrium (LD) is present, if the probability for the existence of a specific marker allele together with a specific disease allele in a population gamete differs from the product of individual probabilities. Certain marker alleles of affected individuals will be more frequent or less frequent than in a randomly selected individual from the population.

Linkage analysis in families uses the concept of linkage. *Association analysis* in populations or families uses the concept of linkage disequilibrium. Some designs and corresponding statistical methods are capable of integrating both types of information into the analysis.

Detailed information on diseases used as examples in this chapter may be found in the standard reference of human genetics of McKusick (1998) or its online version, Online Mendelian Inheritance in Man (OMIM 2000).

Genetic Models

7.3

Fundamental to all investigations regarding genetic hypotheses is the assumption or the development of the genetic model. In the context of the parametrization of genetic models, some necessary genetic terminology (Thompson 1986) will be introduced. Only binary phenotypes are considered here. Quantitative phenotypes including threshold models creating a binary phenotype from a latent quantitative phenotype will not be considered.

Terminology

7.3.1

The *genome* is the complete collection of an individual's genetic material present in every cell. This material consists of *chromosomes*, i.e. long strands of DNA. A *gene* is a piece of a chromosome coding for a function that can be seen as the inheritable unit. The *locus* is the position of a piece of a chromosome along the chromosome. Thus, the locus might denote the position of e.g. a gene, a gene complex or a marker. The different variants of a gene are called *alleles*. Often the term gene is also used for each single variant of a gene.

The human genome is *diploid*, i.e. chromosomes are all paired *(homologous chromosomes)* with the exception of the sex-linked chromosome in males. Each human somatic cell contains 22 *autosomal* chromosome pairs and 1 pair of sex chromosomes. The autosomal chromosomes of a pair contain the same gene with possibly different alleles at the same gene location. During *meiosis*, a diploid set of chromosomes is reduced to a *haploid* chromosome set of a germ cell, the *gamete*. In this chapter we will exclusively consider the analysis of autosomes.

A pair of alleles of an individual at a locus is called *genotype*. If the two alleles are identical, the individual is called *homozygous* at the locus, otherwise *heterozygous*. Two copies of a gene are called *identical by descent (IBD)* if both copies are the same allele *and* they are copies of the same gene in a common ancestor. An individual is *homozygous by descent (HBD)* when its gene pair is IBD. When considering several loci simultaneously, the multilocus alleles which are inherited from the same parent are called *haplotype*.

Mendelian Single Locus Model

Mendelian segregation (Mendel 1865) is the simplest and most applied model for the *mode of inheritance*. It applies to a single locus. An individual randomly and independently inherits one allele from father and mother respectively. Each parent randomly and independently passes on a copy of one of two alleles to each of his/her offspring (binomial distribution with probability 0.5). All segregation events from parents to offspring are independent. The segregation process implies that copies of some alleles are frequently present in offspring and other alleles are lost in subsequent generations (genetic drift).

Consider the phenotype affected/unaffected of a certain disease. Let S denote a susceptibility gene with n alleles $S_1, S_2, \ldots, S_n$. The distribution of allele frequencies $P(S_r)$ in the population is denoted by:

$$p_r = P(S_r), \quad r = 1, \ldots, n.$$

For *ordered genotypes* the origin of inheritance (father or mother) is distinguished, for *unordered genotypes* not. There are four possible ordered genotypes and three unordered genotypes. Usually unordered genotypes are used. Under Hardy–Weinberg equilibrium (HWE), the (unordered) genotype frequencies are given by

$$P\left(S_r S_s\right) = 2p_r p_s = p_r^2 \quad \text{for } r = s$$

$$P\left(S_r S_s\right) = 2p_r p_s \quad \text{for } r \neq s.$$

HWE assumes random mating. Thus the frequencies are yielded by independence of the corresponding allele frequencies, while combining two ordered genotypes for heterozygotes. The maintenance of HWE in a population can be derived by applying Mendelian segregation to each possible parental mating type (see e.g. Khoury et al. 1993).

The *penetrance* describes the relation between genotype and phenotype. It is the conditional probability that an individual with a given genotype will be affected:

$$f_{rs} = P(\text{affected}|S_r S_s), \quad r, s = 1, \ldots, n.$$

For classical monogenic diseases, the disease is caused by a single major gene. The penetrances of the different genotypes will only take on the values 0 or 1. Often a locus S is assumed to be *biallelic*, i.e. to have only two different alleles. Let S_1 denote the 'susceptibility' allele (mutation) and S_2 the 'normal' allele (wild type). For a classical *dominant disease* all carriers of the susceptibility allele will become affected such that $f_{11} = f_{12} = f_{21} = 1$ and $f_{22} = 0$. For a classical *recessive disease* only homozygous carriers of the susceptibility allele will become affected such that $f_{11} = 1$ and $f_{12} = f_{21} = f_{22} = 0$.

Many classical hereditary diseases follow a Mendelian mode of inheritance. Often the prevalence of classical Mendelian diseases is below 1 in 1000 live births. Prominent examples are Chorea Huntington (autosomal dominant gene, CFTR, on chromosome 4) and cystic fibrosis (autosomal recessive gene, Huntingtin, on chromosome 7). Many different mutations of the gene CFTR (cystic fibrosis transmembrane regulator) cause cystic fibrosis. The gene Huntingtin causing Chorea

Huntington contains a variable number of CAG trinucleotide repeats. This number is low for unaffected individuals and high for those affected. Thus both genes are characterized by allelic heterogeneity. However, the assumption of a biallelic locus with two groups of alleles (susceptibility, normal) worked well in identifying these two genes as causes of a Mendelian hereditary disease, even though it is clear that the true inheritance is much more complicated. The aim in statistical genetics is not to specify a completely correct model in the first place, but to address the scientific question adequately with a parsimoneous mathematical model. If this model is too simple then extended or new biologically motivated models need to be implemented.

The relation of genotype to phenotype is not straightforward for many diseases. Individuals with a susceptibility genotype can stay unaffected (*incomplete penetrance*) and individuals with a non susceptibility genotype can become affected (*phenocopies*). In general terms, given different genotypes, penetrances at a specific gene locus may all be different. It may often be assumed, that the origin (father or mother) of an allele has no influence on a disease, i.e. $f_{12} = f_{21}$. For the general single locus mode of inheritance with susceptibility allele S_1 we assume $1 \geq f_{11} \geq f_{12} = f_{21} \geq f_{22} \geq 0$. For a recessive mode of inheritance we assume $f_{12} = f_{21} = f_{22}$, and for a dominant mode of inheritance we assume $f_{11} = f_{12} = f_{21}$.

Linkage

7.3.3

For the joint inheritance at two loci, it may not generally be assumed that there is independent Mendelian segregation, owing to crossover events and recombinations. Gametes are formed during meiosis. In this process, homologous chromosomes are arranged next to each other and partly overlap. A chromosome breakage and a *crossover* (or *crossing over*), i.e. an exchange between homologous chromosome segments, can occur. A *recombination* between loci A and B occurs when a gamete will have a haplotype other than the combination genes that occurred in the parents, due to crossovers between the loci.

Consider the formation of gametes during meiosis displayed in Fig. 7.1. Between very distant loci A and B (see Fig. 7.1a) a crossover is likely to result in a recombination of the haplotypes $A_1 B_1$ and $A_2 B_2$ to give the new haplotypes $A_1 B_2$ and $A_2 B_1$. If the two loci A and B are very close (see Fig. 7.1b) this is very unlikely. In fact, the *map distance* is defined as the expected number of crossovers between two loci (Haldane 1919). Since the map distance is an expectation, this distance measure is additive. Thus, for three (ordered) loci A, B and C the map distance between A and C is given by the sum of the map distances between A and B and between B and C. The map unit is Morgan, M, named after T.H. Morgan, 1866–1945. Often centiMorgan, cM, are given. The total length of the human autosomal genome is approximately 35 M. Single chromosome lengths are between 0.5 M and 3 M. As a very rough guide 1 cM corresponds to 1 Million base pairs in the physical map.

By genotyping it is possible to observe recombinations between two loci, but not crossovers. Figure 7.1a shows recombination due to a single crossover. For a double

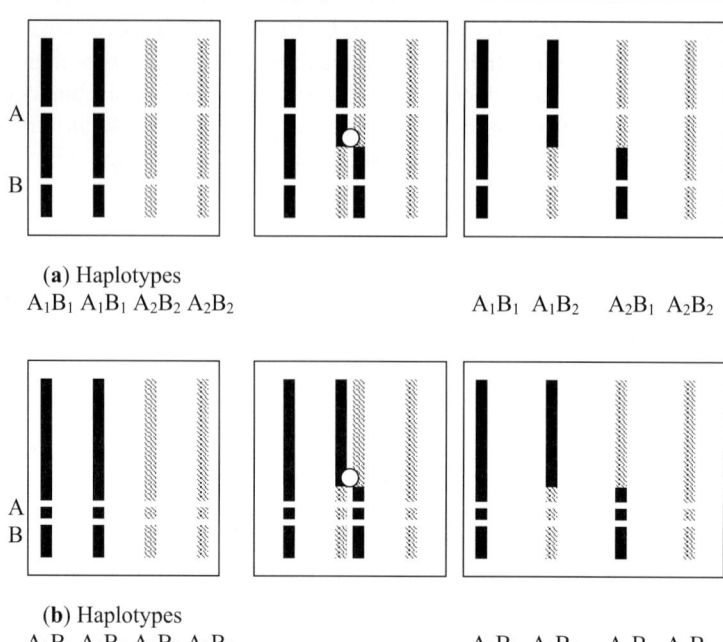

(a) Haplotypes
A_1B_1 A_1B_1 A_2B_2 A_2B_2 A_1B_1 A_1B_2 A_2B_1 A_2B_2

(b) Haplotypes
A_1B_1 A_1B_1 A_2B_2 A_2B_2 A_1B_1 A_2B_2 A_1B_1 A_2B_2

Figure 7.1. Formation of gametes during meiosis from one parental pair of chromosomes with a single crossover. *Left*: parental chromosome pair, *middle*: crossover event (crossover point denoted by the *circle*), *right*: gametes for offspring formation. At the two loci A and B the parent is double heterozygous A_1A_2 and B_1B_2. (a) The crossover occurred between locus A and B. The *two middle* gametes show recombination. (b) The crossover occurred above locus A and B, so that the gametes do not show recombination

crossover, i.e. two chromosomal exchanges between the loci A and B, no recombination would be observed. In mathematical terms a *recombination* between loci A and B can be defined as an uneven number of crossovers between them.

The *recombination rate* θ, i.e. the ratio of the number of recombinant gametes to the total number of gametes formed, is used as a measure of *genetic distance* between two loci. If loci are on different chromosomes or far away on the same chromosome they segregate independently during the formation of gametes. This results in $\theta = 0.5$, and the loci are designated unlinked. By definition there is *linkage* between the loci if $0 \le \theta < 0.5$ and no linkage if $\theta = 0.5$. If loci are closer to each other, recombination is less likely. Complete linkage, i.e. complete co-segregation, implies no recombination and thus $\theta = 0$.

In Fig. 7.2 a double heterozygous parent with haplotypes A_1B_1 and A_2B_2, and a double homozygous parent with haplotype A_3B_3 are considered. For the double heterozygous parent a meiosis can create the non-recombinant haplotypes A_1B_1 and A_2B_2 or the recombinant haplotypes A_1B_2 and A_2B_1. In order to determine recombination a parent homozygous even at one locus is not informative. Given that recombination is present, each of the two recombinant haplotypes occurs

Parents

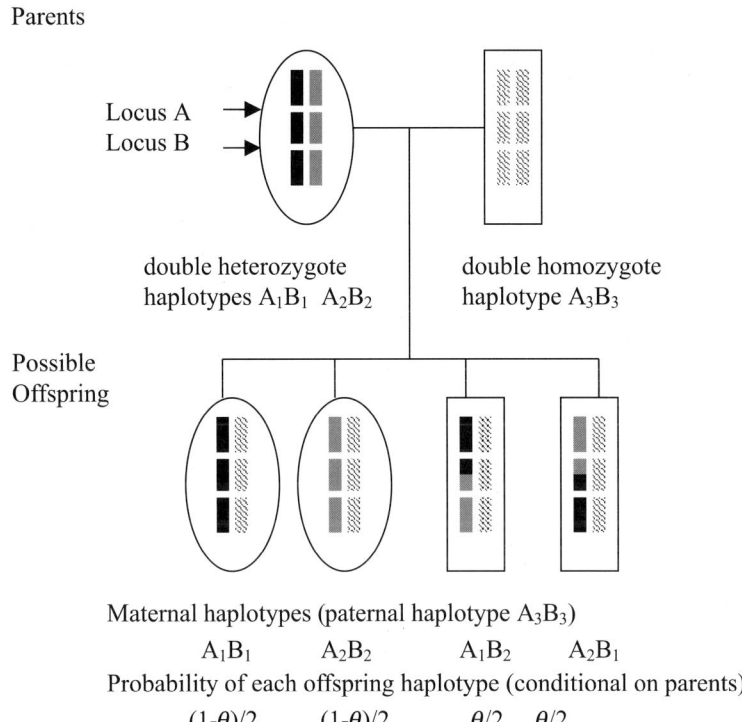

Locus A →
Locus B →

double heterozygote
haplotypes A_1B_1 A_2B_2

double homozygote
haplotype A_3B_3

Possible
Offspring

Maternal haplotypes (paternal haplotype A_3B_3)

| A_1B_1 | A_2B_2 | A_1B_2 | A_2B_1 |

Probability of each offspring haplotype (conditional on parents)

| $(1-\theta)/2$ | $(1-\theta)/2$ | $\theta/2$ | $\theta/2$ |

Figure 7.2. Formation of recombinant and non-recombinant haplotypes by meiosis

with probability 0.5. Given that no recombination is present, each of the two non-recombinant haplotypes occurs with probability 0.5. For $\theta = 0.5$ there is independent segregation so that all four possible haplotypes are equally likely.

If the distance between loci is small, i.e. $\theta \leq 0.1$, a recombination corresponds to a crossover. If three ordered close loci A, B and C are considered, $\theta_{AC} \approx \theta_{AB} + \theta_{BC}$. In contrary to the map distance in Morgan, recombination distances are not additive. A recombination between A and B and one between B and C corresponds to an even number of crossovers for the interval A to C and thus will not result in a recombination between A and C. With the help of so-called *mapping functions*, recombination distances can be translated into Morgans. In the majority of chromosomal regions recombination rates for women are higher than for men, which is most often neglected in genetic epidemiological studies.

To fully describe the segregation process in a (chromosomal) pedigree along a complete chromosome, it is sufficient to denote the paternal or maternal origin by 0 or 1 respectively for each meiosis in a pedigree along the whole chromosome (see Fig. 7.3). A crossover event is present at a particular position when the parental origin switches at a particular meiosis.

The potential informativity of a single marker chosen from an existing marker map (without consideration of the disease locus) is determined by its genetic

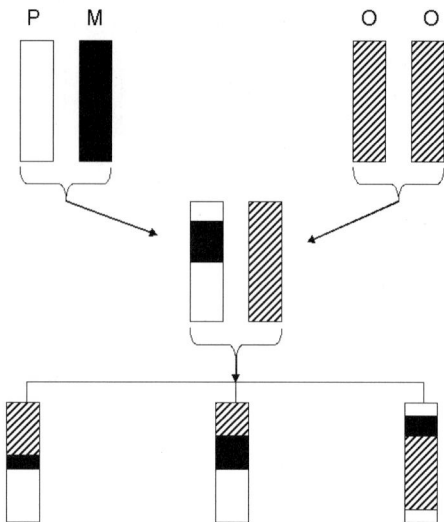

P   M   O   O

Figure 7.3. Three-generation chromosomal pedigree. The pedigree describes the grandparental inheritance of the haplotypes of three grandchildren which they inherited from the left grandparent. Consider the 'left' grandparent with its two chromosomes denoted by P (*white*) for paternal and M (*black*) for maternal. The segregation of these two chromosomes from the grandparent to its offspring (with a double crossover) and to its three grandchildren can be followed. For each meiosis the chromosomal segments are yielded by the crossover process. Chromosomal segments in the grandchildren are in part inherited from the chromosomes O (*dashed*) of the other grandparent. At each position along the chromosome and for each offspring chromosome, the paternal or maternal inheritance can be denoted by 0 or 1. This is true in the parent generation and in the child generation. Thus, the inheritance can be completely described by a vector of 0's and 1's with dimension equal to the number of meioses considered

variability, i.e. allele distribution, and by the relation of the marker's (laboratory) phenotype to its corresponding genotype. In this laboratory context, phenotype denotes the observed measure of the marker's true underlying genotype. An example of such an observed measure for a genotype is the length determined by a gel electrophoresis for an RFLP marker instead of the exact base sequence. Two measures of marker informativity are *heterozygosity H* and *polymorphism information content PIC* (Botstein et al. 1980). For a locus with n alleles, these are defined as follows:

$$H = \sum_{r \neq s}^{n} p_r p_s \,,$$

$$PIC = 1 - \sum_{r=1}^{n} p_r^2 - \sum_{r=1}^{n-1} \sum_{s=r+1}^{n} 2 p_r^2 p_s^2 = 2 \sum \sum p_r p_s (1 - p_r p_s) \,.$$

In HWE, the heterozygosity H equals the probability that a random individual is heterozygous. *PIC* denotes the probability that one of two randomly mating individuals is heterozygous and the other has a different genotype (Weiss 1993; Ott 1999).

Linkage Disequilibrium

Linkage and linkage disequilibrium (LD) are concepts that need to be distinguished. Linkage describes the co-inheritance at two loci and can only be observed in families. Linkage is independent of the specific alleles. LD describes the relation between alleles at two loci in a population.

Consider the frequencies of specific alleles at two loci S and M in a population. They can be in *linkage disequilibrium* (or gametic disequilibrium, LD). LD is present if the probability for the presence of specific S and M alleles in one gamete is not equal to the product of the individual probabilities at the single loci.

Let S denote the locus with n alleles $S_1, S_2, \ldots, S_n$ and allele frequencies

$$p_r = P(S_r), \quad r = 1, \ldots, n,$$

and M a locus with m alleles $M_1, M_2, \ldots, M_m$ and allele frequencies

$$q_i = P(M_i), \quad i = 1, \ldots, m.$$

A common measure of LD is the difference of the haplotype probability from its expectation under no association. For two biallelic loci it is denoted by D or δ. For multiallelic markers the parameter δ_{ir} is often used to define the linkage disequilibrium between M_i and S_r as

$$\delta_{ir} = P(M_i S_r) - P(S_r) P(M_i), \quad i = 1, \ldots, m; \quad r = 1, \ldots, n.$$

Linkage disequilibrium or LD is present if $\delta_{ir} \neq 0$ for at least one pair of alleles M_i, S_r.

Linkage equilibrium is present if

$$\delta_{ir} = 0 \quad \text{for all} \quad i = 1, \ldots, m; \quad r = 1, \ldots, n.$$

Under linkage equilibrium the allele distribution at locus M is independent of the specific S allele present.

Linkage disequilibrium can also be described by the coupling frequencies c_{ir} defined as

$$c_{ir} = P(M_i|S_r), \quad r = 1, \ldots, n; \quad i = 1, \ldots, m,$$

i.e. by the conditional probabilities that a gamete with S_r also has allele M_i. Other parametrizations of LD are also commonly used.

LD may also be considered between multiple loci. Of course the parametrization is more complicated in this case.

Linkage disequilibrium can have different origins (Suarez and Hampe 1994). At linked loci complete LD can be caused by a recent mutation at one locus. However, LD is also possible without linkage between the loci. In extreme cases the loci can even lie on different chromosomes. One important mechanism for the development of LD at unlinked loci is *population stratification*. This is often a result of the admixture of subpopulations (e.g. through immigration) with different allele distributions in the subpopulations. Non-random mating (e.g. by religion or social status) can also be such a cause.

The following formula describes a population genetics model for the degradation in generation time of an existing LD at generation time 0, δ_0, during g generations caused by recombination/linkage (Maynard Smith 1989):

$$\delta_g = (1 - \theta)^g \delta_0 \ .$$

An LD may not necessarily be caused by linkage (possible mechanisms given above), but in the presence of tight linkage it can stay strong during many generations. Without tight linkage LD will degrade rapidly. Thus LD provides indirect evidence for linkage.

As a conlusion of this section two additional widely used measures of LD for fine-scale mapping with biallelic marker data will be introduced (Devlin and Risch 1995).

Consider markers A and B, each with two alleles A_1, A_2 and B_1, B_2. In a haplotype, let the first position denote the allele at marker A, the second position the allele at marker B. The haplotype probabilities are listed in Table 7.1. Rows and columns portray the marginal probabilities. The LD as the difference of the haplotype probability from its expectation under no association can be calculated by

$$D = \pi_{11} - \pi_{1+}\pi_{+1} = \pi_{22} - \pi_{2+}\pi_{+2} = \pi_{11}\pi_{22} - \pi_{21}\pi_{12} \ .$$

D is an absolute measure of LD. Its value is 0 if marker A and marker B are not associated.

Table 7.1. Haplotype probabilities for two biallelic markers A and B

Marker A	Marker B		
	Allele B_1	Allele B_2	
Allele A_1	π_{11}	π_{12}	π_{1+}
Allele A_2	π_{21}	π_{22}	π_{2+}
	π_{+1}	π_{+2}	

Maximum and minimum possible values of D depend on the allele frequencies in the population. Thus, define D_{max} and D_{min} by

$$D_{max} = \min(\pi_{1+}\pi_{+2}, \pi_{+1}\pi_{2+})$$

$$D_{min} = \min(\pi_{1+}\pi_{+1}, \pi_{+2}\pi_{2+}) \ .$$

Rescaling D relative to its maximum and minimum results in the relative measure D' (Lewontin's D', Lewontin 1964):

$$D' = \begin{cases} \dfrac{D}{D_{\max}} = \dfrac{\pi_{11}\pi_{22} - \pi_{21}\pi_{12}}{\min\left(\pi_{1+}\pi_{+2}, \pi_{+1}\pi_{2+}\right)} & D > 0 \\[3ex] \dfrac{D}{D_{\min}} = \dfrac{\pi_{11}\pi_{22} - \pi_{21}\pi_{12}}{\min\left(\pi_{1+}\pi_{+1}, \pi_{+2}\pi_{2+}\right)} & D < 0 \,. \end{cases}$$

Since in essence LD is a correlation between the marker and the susceptibility gene in populations, the correlation coefficient can also be used as an LD measure (Hill and Robertson 1968), denoted by Δ:

$$\Delta = \frac{\pi_{11}\pi_{22} - \pi_{21}\pi_{12}}{\sqrt{(\pi_{1+}\pi_{2+}\pi_{+1}\pi_{+2})}} = \frac{D}{\sqrt{(\pi_{1+}\pi_{2+}\pi_{+1}\pi_{+2})}} \,.$$

Another LD measure based on odds ratios and motivated by the epidemiological measure 'attributable risk' (cf. Chap. I.2 of this handbook) is

$$\delta = \frac{\pi_{11}/\pi_{21} - \pi_{12}/\pi_{22}}{\pi_{11}/\pi_{21} + 1} = \frac{\pi_{11}\pi_{22} - \pi_{12}\pi_{21}}{\pi_{+1}\pi_{22}} = \frac{D}{\pi_{+1}\pi_{22}} \,.$$

Segregation Analysis 7.4

The aim of *segregation analysis* is to find evidence for the existence of a major gene for the phenotype under investigation and to estimate the corresponding mode of inheritance. Therefore, if possible, the pattern of inheritance over several generations within the structure of larger families is investigated. Sometimes segregation analysis has to be carried out on the basis of many small families.

Consider a Mendelian single locus model for a major gene with the susceptibility allele S_1 and the normal allele S_2. For classical Mendelian diseases the penetrances $P(\text{affected}|\text{genotype})$ take on only the values 0 and 1. For such diseases, the genotype-phenotype relation is so obvious that the discrete genotype translates into a discrete disease phenotype. Thus, families in which such a Mendelian disease gene segregates display very characteristic disease patterns. For example, in the case of autosomal dominant diseases generations should not be skipped by the disease, an affected individual married to an unaffected individual should produce an approximate 1 : 1 ratio of affected to unaffected offspring and the distribution of the trait among sexes should be almost equal (Tamarin 1986). Ratios like the above mentioned are called *segregation ratios*.

The simplest types of segregation analyses are based on tests for segregation ratios hypothesising a particular mode of inheritance. To illustrate the principle, consider first a rare autosomal dominant disease and a random sample of matings. Matings between an affected and an unaffected individual will usually be of the $S_1S_2 \times S_2S_2$ *mating type*. Since the susceptibility allele is rare,

$S_1S_1 \times S_2S_2$ matings for affected-unaffected couples can be neglected as a first approximation. Thus, for the moment consider only $S_1S_2 \times S_2S_2$ families and suppose that r of n offspring are affected. In the offspring generation the expected segregation ratio between affected and unaffected is 0.5. A test can be built on the binomial distribution, considering n as the number of trials, q as the probability for a single child to be affected, and r as the observed number of affected children. If the null hypothesis of $q = 0.5$ is not rejected, it may be concluded that the data are compatible (more precisely not inconsistent) with an autosomal dominant disease pattern. For further test procedures see e.g. Sham (1998).

More generally, the probability distribution of the six possible mating types $(S_1S_1 \times S_1S_1; S_1S_1 \times S_1S_2; S_1S_1 \times S_2S_2; S_1S_2 \times S_1S_2; S_1S_2 \times S_2S_2; S_2S_2 \times S_2S_2)$ can be formed according to the parental genotypes. For each given mating type, the distribution of genotypes and phenotypes in the offspring may be determined, on which tests can then be built. However, families are most often sampled according to recruitment criteria and not randomly, yielding an oversampling of families enriched for disease. Therefore, for a test procedure to be valid the probability distributions need to be corrected for *ascertainment bias*. Consider again the binomial distribution for the number of affected offspring in a sibship of a particular mating type. We assume ascertainment for families with 'at least one affected offspring'. The binomial distribution for the number of affected offspring could be corrected for ascertainment by considering a truncated binomial distribution assuming at least one affected offspring per family. Unfortunately, the ascertainment process could imply that families with more affected children have a higher chance of being part of the sample. Proper ascertainment correction maybe complicated and the ascertainment criteria should be known as precisely as possible. Moreover, mathematical assumptions must be made about the ascertainment sampling process in order to estimate genetic parameters or to test genetic models. In general, misspecification of the ascertainment process might cause serious bias in the estimation of genetic parameters (see e.g. Shute and Ewens 1988).

The ascertainment process is often parametrized by the *ascertainment probability*

$$\pi = P(\text{proband}|\text{affected}) ,$$

i.e. the probability that an individual will be part of the family data set given that the individual is affected. The following types of selection have been defined by the parameter π: If $\pi = 1$, this is called *truncate selection*. For truncate selection an individual will be recruited if he/she is affected. Families without affected members are not recruited. If $\pi \rightarrow 0$, we speak of *single selection*. In single selection families with r affected children are recruited with probability $r\pi$ and almost all families have only one affected child. Multiple selection is defined by $0 < \pi < 1$.

For *extended pedigrees* with many individuals and several generations a numerical procedure is needed for all probability calculations. Let L denote the likelihood for the observed phenotypes Y, given a genetic model M and the pedigree structure. L can be calculated by summing over all possible genotypic constellations $g_i, i = 1, \ldots, N$, where N denotes the number of individuals in the pedigree:

$$L(Y) = \sum_{g_1} \sum_{g_2} \cdots \sum_{g_N} P(Y|g_1 g_2 \cdots g_N) P(g_1 g_2 \cdots g_N) .$$

It is assumed that the phenotype of an individual is independent of the other pedigree members given its genotype.

Widely used in segregation analysis is the Elston–Stuart algorithm (Elston and Stuart 1971), a recursive formula for the computation of the likelihood L given as

$$L = \sum_{g_1} \sum_{g_2} \cdots \sum_{g_N} \prod_{j=1}^{N} f(g_j) \prod_{k=1}^{N_1} P(g_k) \prod_{m=1}^{N_2} \tau(g_m|g_{m1}g_{m2}) .$$

The notation for the formula is as follows: N denotes the number of individuals in the pedigree. N_1 denotes the number of *founder* individuals in the pedigree. Founders are individuals without specified parents in the pedigree. In general, these are the members of the oldest generation and married-in spouses. N_2 denotes the number of *non-founder* individuals in the pedigree, such that $N = N_1 + N_2$. $g_i, i = 1, \ldots, N$, denote the genotype of the ith individual of the pedigree. The parameters of the genetic model M fall into three groups: (1) The genotype distribution $P(g_k), k = 1, \ldots, N_1$, for the founders is determined by population parameters and often Hardy–Weinberg equilibrium is assumed. (2) The transmission probabilities for the transmission from parents to offspring $\tau(g_m|g_{m1}, g_{m2})$, where m_1 and m_2 are the parents of m, are needed for all non-founders in the pedigree. It is assumed that transmissions to different offspring are independent given the parental genotypes and that transmissions of one parent to an offspring are independent of the transmission of the other parent. Thus, transmission probabilities can be parametrized by the product of the individual transmissions. Under Mendelian segregation the transmission probabilities for parental transmission are $\tau(S_1|S_1 S_1) = 1$; $\tau(S_1|S_1 S_2) = 0.5$ *and* $\tau(S_1|S_2 S_2) = 0$. (3) The penetrances $f(g_i), i = 1, \ldots, N$, parametrise the genotype-phenotype correlation for each individual i.

This recursive formula works well on *simple pedigrees* of arbitrary size. Computations on *complex pedigrees*, i.e. pedigrees with marriage and inbreeding loops (such as consanguineous marriages) are often only possible with approximation methods.

Segregation analysis is a successful tool for monogenic diseases. Major problems in segregation analysis for complex diseases result in essence from the fact that the relationship of genotype to phenotype is not a straightforward 1 to 1 function or n to 1 function, i.e. the genotype does not unambiguously determine the phenotype. This unclear relationship is such a critical issue that some use this as a definition of complex diseases. Further, several genetic factors are assumed to have an influence on complex diseases. The penetrance can be incomplete and phenocopies can exist. In addition the penetrance can depend on other non-genetic factors such as age, gender and exposure factors for example.

For the definition of the phenotype, problems arise when specifying and applying diagnostic criteria. In addition, many complex diseases show a large phenotypic variation, which might be characterised by severity, by different diseases or by different co-occurrence of diseases.

Genetic heterogeneity is a further problem (Evans and Harris 1992). The same phenotype can be caused by different genes (locus heterogeneity). Different phenotypes can be caused by different alleles at the same locus (allelic heterogeneity). Owing to modifying factors different phenotypes can segregate within a family (intra-family heterogeneity). When different phenotypes segregate in different families, but the phenotype is constant within one family, this might indicate that a gene segregates in one family and not in the other (inter-family heterogeneity). In addition, there are further types of genetic heterogeneity such as genomic imprinting, where the penetrance of a heterozygous genotype depends on the (paternal oder maternal) origin of the susceptibility allele.

In the presence of heterogeneity the formation of homogeneous subgroups is a means to arrive at a clearer genotype-phenotype relation und thus, to identify a possible Mendelian subform of the disease. Homogeneous subgroups can be defined by e.g. clinical phenotypes, severity of the disease, age of onset of the disease, family history or ethnicity.

An example of a highly successful segregation analysis for a complex disease is breast cancer (Newman et al. 1988). The families were ascertained through a population-based large epidemiological programme in San Francisco and Detroit. The ascertainment criteria for index cases were women with breast cancer, Caucasian, diagnosis before the age of 55, histologically confirmed primary tumour, becoming incident in a specified period. No selection on positive family history was taken. The personal interview of the index case on her nuclear family, i.e. mothers and sisters, regarding breast cancer was considered sufficiently reliable. 1579 nuclear families were recruited and one large extended pedigree. This sample also included some rare cases of male breast cancer.

Complex segregation analysis was applied to these breast cancer families using the programme POINTER which is based on the so-called 'unified' model (Lalouel et al. 1984). This model is called 'unified', since it unifies the so-called 'mixed' model (Morton and MacLean 1974) and the concept of transmission probabilities mentioned above. The Mendelian 'mixed' model assumes an underlying normal distribution for each of the three genotypes S_1S_1, S_1S_2, S_2S_2, of the major factor which differ in their means. The disease status for breast cancer is considered as resulting from an underlying quantitative trait (as a mixture of the three normal distributions) by exceeding a certain threshold. In this threshold model, individuals affected with breast cancer have exceeded the threshold deterministic for disease, individuals not affected by breast cancer have a value for the quantitative trait below the threshold. Thus, for a predisposing genotype the mean is shifted in comparison to the distribution for the wildtype heterozygotes such that more individuals will exceed the threshold. In addition, this model assumes an additive effect of the major factor, a polygenic component and an environmental component. The following parameters have to be estimated for the mixed model: the allele frequency p of the susceptibility allele S_1, the displacement between the means for S_1S_1 and S_2S_2, the dominance parameter defined as the difference in the means for S_2S_2 and S_1S_2 and the heritability H, defined as the proportion of variance due to the polygenic component (see Sect. 7.2). Further parameters for the unified model are the transmission probabilities. In this case, the values 1, 0.5 and 0 for a Mendelian major gene as major factor should not be rejected. Evaluation of models with direct modelling (and estimation) of the transmission probabilities allows the identification of the major factor as a major Mendelian gene. In the above mentioned breast cancer study transmission probabilites were estimated close to the values required by Mendelian segregation and a model without a Mendelian inheritance factor could be rejected.

Several parameters need to be prespecified (as input parameters) for complex segregation analysis. For the breast cancer families the ascertainment probability was assumed within the bounds $\pi = 0.01$–0.27, the lower bound corresponding to almost single ascertainment and the upper bound corresponding to the mean proportion of breast cancer cases in the families. Liability classes for the population based liabilities were estimated from cumulative incidences in the general population of the regions under investigation. These are 0.0010 for women until age 15 and all men regardless of age, 0.0045 for women aged 16–40 years, 0.0283 for women aged 41–55 years and 0.0819 for women older than 55 years. These necessary parameters could be well estimated, since a large epidemiological study had been carried out in the region.

Complex segregation analysis requires many likelihood ratio comparisons between different assumed models for the estimation of parameters and the acceptance of a most parsimonious model. In the breast cancer study example the autosomal dominant major gene was postulated, since the general single locus model with three penetrance parameters and the dominant single locus model with only two penetrance parameters resulted in a comparable fit. In a first step we investigate whether the data are consistent with a major gene model and in a second step we consider with which mode of inheritance for the major gene the data are consistent. Important for the avoidance of false-positive results is the investigation into whether an identified major factor is really Mendelian by the use of transmission probabilities. In the breast cancer family data evidence for an autosomal dominant transmission was given both in the 1579 nuclear families and the one large extended family. These results were supported by the same qualitative results even under sensitivity analysis for the ascertainment probability and by the well-defined liability parameters based on prior studies. Thus, segregation analysis may be successful even for complex diseases. In the breast cancer example an autosomal dominant rare gene with high penetrance could be postulated for early onset breast cancer as a result of the segregation analysis.

If there are no major genes with high penetrances, but only a few genes with a moderate effect on the disease, segregation analysis will not be a valuable tool. It should be mentioned that many diseases are studied nowadays by linkage and association analyses without segregation analyses which normally would have been carried out prior to this.

7.5   Linkage Analysis

In *linkage analysis* the co-segregation between marker and disease is investigated in related individuals. The aim is to find evidence for linkage and often to estimate the recombination rate. Sometimes exclusion of linkage is possible.

The classical linkage analysis method is the *lod score method* (Morton 1955). This is a test for linkage between a susceptibility gene locus and a marker locus (null hypothesis $H_0 : \theta = 0.5$ versus alternative $H_1 : \theta < 0.5$) in combination with the estimation of the recombination rate. For a detailed description see Ott (1999).

For the lod score method, the mode of inheritance M_0, that is the parameter of the genetic model at the susceptibility locus, and the marker allele distribution, have to be known. The mode of inheritance may be estimated by segregation analysis. Let $L(\theta, M_0)$ denote the likelihood for the observed phenotypes at a particular value for θ conditional on M_0, on the marker allele distribution and on the given pedigrees. As in the usual notation, the underlying conditioning is sometimes left out. The lod score function ('log odds') is the log likelihood ratio

$$Z(\theta) = LOD(\theta) = \log_{10} \frac{L(\theta, M_0)}{L(0.5, M_0)}$$

as a function of θ. $Z(\theta)$ compares the likelihood under linkage with recombination rate θ with the likelihood under no linkage, i.e. $\theta = 0.5$. $Z(\theta)$ will be maximized over all possible values for θ, i.e. $0 \le \theta \le 0.5$. If $Z_{max} > 3$ then evidence for linkage exists. The recombination rate will be estimated by θ_{max}, the θ-value corresponding to Z_{max}. If $Z_{max} < -2$ linkage can be excluded. The limits 3 and -2 are based on a sequential Wald test, such that the a posteriori probability for linkage when rejecting the null hypothesis is 95% for a single alternative θ (Morton 1955). As logarithms of base 10 are used, the limits correspond to stopping limits of 1000 and 0.01 in the sequential testing procedure yielded by setting $\alpha = 0.001, \beta = 0.01$.

Let us determine the likelihood $L(\theta)$ for linkage between two loci A and B for a sibship of size n. The genotypes are observed directly. Thus, no underlying genetic model needs to be considered. The genotypes of the mother are $A_1 A_2$ and $B_1 B_2$ and the genotypes of the father are $A_1 A_1$ and $B_1 B_1$. Only the double heterozygous mother is informative for linkage. In general, it is not known which allele combinations of the mother are the result of the grandpaternal and the grandmaternal meiosis, i.e. which allele combinations form the haplotypes in the grandparental gametes. The so-called *phase* for the mother could be either composed of the haplotypes $A_1 B_1$ and $A_2 B_2$ (phase I with probability P_I) or by the haplotypes $A_1 B_2$ and $A_2 B_1$ (phase II with probability P_{II}).

Assume that the phase is known to be phase I, for example when the grandparents pass on this information. Let n_x and n_y denote the number of meioses from the mother to the n children, which are non-recombinants n_x or recombinants n_y, respectively. Then the likelihood $L(\theta)$ is

$$L(\theta) = \binom{n_x + n_y}{n_x} (1 - \theta)^{n_x} \theta^{n_y} .$$

For an unknown phase, phase I and phase II both have to be considered. If P_{II} is the true phase, then n_x children show recombination and n_y children show non-recombination. Under the assumption of linkage equilibrium phase I and phase II are both equally likely. Thus

$$L(\theta) = \binom{n_x + n_y}{n_x} \left[P_I(1 - \theta)^{n_x}\theta^{n_y} + P_{II}\theta^{n_x}(1 - \theta)^{n_y} \right]$$

$$= \binom{n_x + n_y}{n_x} \left[\frac{1}{2}(1 - \theta)^{n_x}\theta^{n_y} + \frac{1}{2}\theta^{n_x}(1 - \theta)^{n_y} \right].$$

For the sibship in Fig. 7.4 let us now determine the likelihood $L(\theta)$, the lod score function $Z(\theta)$, Z_{max} and θ_{max}. The notation in this pedigree is motivated by an autosomomal dominant susceptibility gene S with a rare susceptibility allele S_1 and a normal allele S_2. Thus, the affected father and all affected siblings have genotype $S_1 S_2$. In the pedigree the marker M is segregating with three alleles M_1, M_2 and M_3. The mother of the sibship of size 6 is homozygous and thus uninformative for linkage. She will not be considered further.

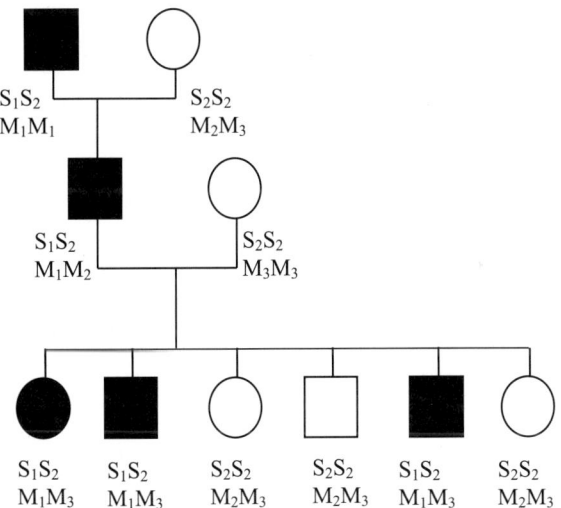

Figure 7.4. Pedigree with a sibship of size 6 with marker information and with genotype information concerning the susceptibility locus, owing to the clear-cut rare autosomal dominant mode of inheritance

As a result of the genotyped grandparents, the father's haplotypes are known: $S_1 M_1$ and $S_2 M_2$. Thus the phase is known and the likelihood is

$$L(\theta) = \binom{6}{0}(1 - \theta)^6\theta^0 = (1 - \theta)^6.$$

The lod score function is

$$Z(\theta) = LOD(\theta) = \log_{10} \frac{L(\theta)}{L(0.5)} = \log_{10} \frac{(1-\theta)^6}{(0.5)^6}$$

$$= 6\log_{10}(1-\theta) + 6\log_{10} 2$$

$$= 6\log_{10}(1-\theta) + C,$$

where C denotes a constant independent of θ. The maximum of the lod score function is $Z_{\max} = 1.8$ for $\theta_{\max} = 0$. This corresponds to complete linkage as supported by no observed recombinations.

Missing information on grandparental genotypes in Fig. 7.4 results in an unknown phase. Then the lod score function would be

$$Z(\theta) = LOD(\theta) = \log_{10} \frac{L(\theta)}{L(0.5)} = \log_{10} \frac{0.5\theta^6 + 0.5(1-\theta)^6}{(0.5)^6}$$

$$= \log_{10} \left(\theta^6 + (1-\theta)^6\right) + 5\log_{10} 2.$$

In this case, the maximum of the lod score function is $Z_{\max} = 1.5$ for $\theta_{\max} = 0$. Due to the uncertain phase, the maximum lod score is reduced. However, the estimate for the recombination rate stays at $\theta = 0$.

In Fig. 7.4, assume now that the second affected child has the genotype M_2M_3 (and the genotype S_1S_2). With the phase as indicated in the figure, one recombination needs to be taken into account now. Thus

$$Z(\theta) = LOD(\theta) = \log_{10} \frac{L(\theta)}{L(0.5)} = \log_{10} \frac{6\theta(1-\theta)^5}{6(0.5)^6}$$

$$= \log_{10} \theta + 5\log_{10}(1-\theta) + 6\log_{10} 2.$$

With one recombination the maximum of the lod score function is $Z_{\max} = 0.63$ for $\theta_{\max} = 1/6 = 0.17$. Now linkage is estimated as not complete and $Z_{\max}$ is markedly reduced.

If in Fig. 7.4 the genotypes of the father and his parents are unknown, the father's genotype can be inferred as either M_1M_1 or M_1M_2. If HWE can be assumed, the likelihood of the recombination rate $L(\theta)$ can be calculated as a function of the marker allele frequencies in offspring. A detailed calculation will show that in this case, a rare marker allele M_1 will result in a high lod score, a more common marker allele M_1 will result in a lower lod score.

The likelihood $L(\theta)$ can be computed for more complex pedigrees with the help of the Elston–Stuart algorithm (Elston and Stuart 1971):

$$L = \sum_{g_1} \sum_{g_2} \cdots \sum_{g_N} \prod_{j=1}^{N} f(g_j) \prod_{k=1}^{N_1} P(g_k) \prod_{m=1}^{N_2} \tau(g_m | g_{m1} g_{m2} \theta).$$

The notation is provided in the previous section with the extension that $g_j, j = 1, \ldots, N$, now refers to the haplo-genotypes, i.e. to the genotypes formed by the haplotypes of the underlying susceptibility locus S and the marker M. The recombination rate θ is now part of the transmission probabilities of the haplogenotypes, since they describe the formation of gametes as recombinants or non-recombinants.

Consider now a set of K families. Since the segregation process is independent in different families, the total likelihood is given by the product of the individual likelihoods. Thus, the logarithm of the total likelihood, $l(\theta)$, is given by the sum of the individual logarithms of the likelihood $l_i(\theta)$:

$$l(\theta) = \sum_{i=1}^{K} l_i(\theta) \,.$$

The lod score method and its extensions have been very successful in localizing major susceptibility genes, especially for rare monogenic diseases (e.g. cystic fibrosis). However, the analysis of complex diseases poses many difficulties (Lander and Schork 1994). Often the mode of inheritance is unclear. Hence, the preassumption of parameters for the mode of inheritance in the lod score analysis is very critical. Often several modes of inheritance are 'tried out' (Terwilliger and Ott 1994). A false model can lead to false negative tests, and thus the erroneous exclusion of chromosomal regions, which indeed harbour susceptibility loci. The use of LOD scores for exclusion mapping should be considered with caution. Maximizing LOD scores over several models or the whole range of recombination rates increases the *a posteriori* false positive rate (Risch 1991), i.e. linkage is inferred erroneously. False assumptions of marker allele frequencies can also lead to false positive results (Ott 1999). Where possible, marker allele frequencies should be estimated for a given study or population, since allele frequencies are often not well known and may differ from population to population. The estimation of the recombination fraction itself after concluding for linkage can be biased, i.e. the true location of the susceptibility gene might be many centi Morgans apart from the estimated location. Even a combined segregation and linkage analyses with parallel estimation of the necessary parameters does not lead to meaningful and significant results, owing to the flatness of the likelihood function.

The localization of the BRCA1 gene for breast cancer is an example of a successful lod score analysis (Hall et al. 1990), which was based on the segregation analysis described in the previous section (Newman et al. 1988). In this analysis, cumulative LOD scores were calculated by ascending average age-of-onset for breast cancer cases in the families. By this procedure, linkage could be demonstrated for early-onset families.

The difficulties in employing a parametric linkage analysis become more and more important with the degree of complexity of a disease. In order to avoid the necessity of critical assumptions about the underlying genetic model, so-called *non-parametric methods* or *model-free methods* have been developed. The aim of model-free methods is to provide evidence for linkage without specifying parameters of the underlying mode of inheritance and without estimating the recombination rate (Elston 1998; Lander and Schork 1994).

Many of these methods are based on the *identity-by-descent (IBD)* status. For example consider a patient and one of his/her siblings (Penrose 1953). Their *IBD* status can take on the values 0, 1 or 2, according to the number of marker alleles that have been transmitted to both siblings from exactly the same (grandpaternal or grandmaternal) copy of a parent's gene and are thus identical (see Fig. 7.5).

Allele sharing methods are based on the fact, that in the presence of linkage relatives with a similar disease status (e.g. both affected) are more frequently similar at the marker locus – in the sense of *IBD* – than to be expected under independent segregation. Relatives with a different disease status (e.g. discordant sibs: affected, unaffected) are less frequently similar at the marker than under no linkage. The aim of these methods is to provide evidence for linkage and not to estimate the recombination rate.

In the *affected-sib-pair* (ASP) *method* (Day and Simons 1976), affected sib pairs are classified according to the *IBD* status. The classical χ^2-test compares the observed number of (independent) sibling pairs with 0, 1 or 2 marker alleles *IBD* with the expected number assuming independent segregation. If marker and disease locus are unlinked, the probability for 0, 1, or 2 marker alleles *IBD* is 0.25, 0.5 or 0.25, respectively. If the observed *IBD* distribution significantly differs from the expected distribution, this indicates linkage. It is possible to use the χ^2-goodness-of-fit-test to test for a hypothesised genetic model, taking the derived numbers under the model as expected.

When considering only affected individuals, the method is robust towards incomplete penetrance. Other allele sharing methods also incorporate unaffected individuals in the analyses as well as different pairs of relatives other than siblings. The literature is extensive and more powerful methods than the original ASP method have been developed (e.g. Holmans 1993; Whittemore and Tu 1998).

The determination of the *IBD* status assumes that the marker is sufficiently polymorphic and that the parents are genotyped for the marker (or neighbouring loci and other relatives yield the missing information). If it is not possible to determine *IBD* unambiguously (see Fig. 7.5) it needs to be estimated. Sometimes the IBS status is used instead. IBS is the number of marker alleles that are identical in the pair of individuals (*"identity by state"*) without considering ancestry, taking

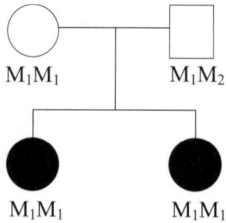

Figure 7.5. An affected sib-pair with parents. Marker genotypes are given. The IBS status is 2. The *IBD* status cannot be unambiguously determined, $P(IBD = 1) = P(IBD = 2) = 0.5$, since the mother transmits the grandpaternal allele M_1 or the grandmaternal allele M_1 with equal probability

on the values 0, 1, or 2. However, such methods are not robust towards imprecisions in the marker allele frequencies.

Association Analysis

The aim of *association studies* is to show evidence for association or linkage disequilibrium in a population. Linkage disequilibrium results in an association between marker alleles and alleles of a susceptibility gene, such that certain marker alleles will be present more often in affected individuals than in a random sample of individuals from the population.

In classic *case-control studies* marker allele frequencies or genotype frequencies in a group of unrelated affected individuals are compared to those in a group of unrelated unaffected individuals. Numerous associations have been identified with case-control studies, e.g. associations of autoimmune diseases (e.g. diabetes, multiple sclerosis) with the HLA system. A further example is the association of apolipoprotein E (APOE) allele $\varepsilon 4$ with Alzheimer's disease (Corder et al. 1993). The APOE $\varepsilon 4$ allele frequency is approximately 35% in Alzheimer's patients, but only approximately 15% in the older population not suffering from dementia. If a positively associated marker allele is frequent in a population, such as APOE $\varepsilon 4$, then it is by itself not a good predictor for disease status and the proportion of homozygotes for the allele is high. Linkage analysis methods are in general not very powerful in this situation.

Besides the usual limitations of classical case-control studies in epidemiology (cf. Chap. I.6 of this handbook), case-control studies to investigate linkage disequilibrium in genetic epidemiology must take a particular form of confounding into account, i.e. population stratification: cases and controls must originate from the same homogeneous (including ethnically homogeneous) source population. This is especially difficult to achieve, to assess or test for in genetic epidemiology. If individuals stem from subpopulations with different allele frequencies, and this is not taken into account, then linkage disequilibrium can be simulated. This means that stratified populations can evoke linkage disequilibrium without linkage. The detection of such linkage disequilibrium detracts from the identification of susceptibility genes. It must be considered as an annoyance to this aim and as such be evaluated as false positive. The technical term for such false positive results is *spurious association*.

If an association is found that is not considered spurious, this may have two causes (Lander and Schork 1994):
— The positively (or negatively) associated allele is the susceptibility allele itself. If so, this association is expected to occur in all populations harbouring this allele.
— The positively (or negatively) associated allele is in linkage disequilibrium with the susceptibility allele at the disease locus. If this is the case, then different associations can occur in different populations due to different haplotype frequencies of the allele combinations of both marker and susceptibility locus.

In the first case, both marker and disease locus are identical. Thus, $\theta = 0$ and linkage disequilibrium is complete. In the second case marker and disease locus are in general very close to each other. For this reason association studies are highly valuable for the investigation of candidate genes.

When an association is identified, it can be quantified with the help of odds ratios (Woolf 1955) (see also Chap. I.2 of this handbook). With rare diseases the odds ratio approximates the relative risk. In addition, parameters of the underlying genetic model may be estimated e.g. with the likelihood ratio method (Thomson 1983; Risch 1983).

As mentioned above, uncontrolled stratification of populations may result in spurious associations. For case-control studies, there are essentially two methods for taking the existence of subpopulations into account during statistical testing. Both methods require a set of additional markers along the genome to be genotyped. In the *genomic control* method (Devlin and Roeder 1999) a variance inflation factor is used to adjust the test statistic, taking into account correlations between individuals in subpopulations. The *structured association* method (Pritchard et al. 2000) initially aims at directly identifying the population structure and assigning individuals to a subgroup. Association is subsequently investigated by testing against the null hypothesis of independent association within subgroups.

Association studies with internal controls, or so-called *family based association studies*, are intended by design to avoid possible bias through inadequate controls and population stratification. The concept of *internal controls* was developed by Falk and Rubinstein (1987). For the original design nuclear families with at least one affected child have to be recruited. The two parental alleles not transmitted to the affected child are used as internal controls (Fig. 7.6).

This design has the important property that information is used on both, linkage and association between a marker and the susceptibility gene.

For a biallelic marker, the data resulting from this study design may be presented in different ways in a 2×2 contingency table (Table 7.2) and analysed with statistical tests (Terwilliger and Ott 1992; Schaid and Sommer 1994). All test procedures test for association ($H_0 : \delta = 0$ vs. $H_1 : \delta \neq 0$) and most for linkage as well. In principal, the tests investigate whether certain alleles are transmitted from the parents to an affected child more often than not.

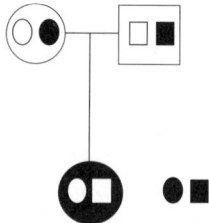

Figure 7.6. Nuclear family with one affected child. Alleles transmitted from the parents to the affected children are denoted in *white*. Alleles not transmitted from the parents to the affected child are denoted in *black*

The test procedures can be classified according to several criteria. Tests can be separated on the basis of whether genotypes or haplotypes are analysed. Haplotype-based analyses compare the transmitted allele with the non-transmitted allele. Genotype-based analyses compare the genotype transmitted to the affected child with the artifical genotype constructed from the two non-transmitted alleles. Another criterion is whether the tests are procedures for matched samples or not. The samples are indeed matched since one transmitted and one non-transmitted allele together describe the segregation from a single parent to an offspring.

Let M denote a biallelic marker with alleles M_1 and M_2; let M_1 be positively associated with the disease. Let genotypes, which are homozygous or heterozygous for M_1, be denoted with M_1 positive. Then, N families with an affected child can be presented in a 2×2 table as in Table 7.2. The traditional χ^2-test for independence can be applied to unmatched samples (Tables 7.2b and 7.2d) and the McNemar-test can be applied to matched samples (Tables 7.2a and 7.2c). The table for unmatched samples uses the marginal table of the corresponding table for matched samples.

The original *Haplotype Relative Risk* (HRR) *method* (Falk and Rubinstein 1987) is a genotype-based analysis for unmatched samples. The odds ratio in Table 7.2b, also called Haplotype Relative Risk (HRR), is a measure of association that is never more extreme, i.e. farther away from 1, than the estimator RR for the relative risk in a classic non-family based approach (Knapp et al. 1993). For $\theta = 0$, HRR = RR.

The most commonly used test is the *Transmission/Disequilibrium Test* (TDT) (Spielman et al. 1993). The TDT is a haplotype-based analysis of the matched sample (Table 7.2c). The test statistic is

$$TDT = (b - c)^2/(b + c) .$$

The TDT compares whether the M_1 allele is more often transmitted to an affected child (b) than the M_2 allele (c) from heterozygous parents, or visa versa. The test only considers $M_1 M_2$ parents, since homozygous parents are not informative for preferential transmission of either allele. This separation can be made due to the matched analysis. In addition matching reduces the variance of the test statistic, thereby yielding a higher power.

The literature on family-based association analysis is vast (see e.g. Whittaker and Morris 2001). Important extensions of the above methods allow the application to multiallelic markers, to tightly linked loci and to quantitative traits. In addition, the design also allows for other types of nuclear families, such as sibships with affected and unaffected individuals (Spielmann and Ewens 1998). If a particular mode of inheritance is suspected specialized versions of the TDT or related likelihood methods may yield higher power (Schaid 1999).

If a candidate gene is to be investigated in detail, then a haplotype analysis will be carried out considering several biallelic polymorphisms (SNPs) in the same gene. The first step in a haplotype analysis is the estimation of the haplotype frequency in a population or the estimation of the most probable haplogenotype (haplotype pair) in an individual. For cases and controls see Excoffier

Table 7.2. 2×2 contingency table for family-based association methods based on N families with one affected child and both parents. Consider a biallelic marker with alleles M_1, M_2 and let M_1 be positively associated with the disease. Genotypes, which are homozygous or heterozygous for M_1, are denoted with M_1 positive. Capital letters denote genotype counts, small letters denote allele counts. A, B, C and D are defined as in Table 2a. a, b, c and d are defined as in Table 2c. N and $2N$ denote the total number of transmitted genotypes and alleles, respectively, to the affected child from the $4N$ parental alleles

(a) Genotype-based analysis for matched samples

Transmitted genotype	Non-transmitted genotype		Total
	M_1 positive	M_1 negative	
M_1 positive	A	B	$A + B$
M_1 negative	C	D	$C + D$
Total	$A + C$	$B + D$	N

(b) Genotype-based analysis for unmatched samples (HRR method)

	M_1 positive	M_1 negative	Total
Transmitted genotype	$A + B$	$C + D$	N
Non-transmitted genotype	$A + C$	$B + D$	N
Total	$2A + B + C$	$2D + C + B$	$2N$

(c) Haplotype-based analysis for matched samples (TDT)

Transmitted allele	Non-transmitted allele		Total
	M_1	M_2	
M_1	a	b	$a + b$
M_2	c	d	$c + d$
Total	$a + c$	$b + d$	$2N$

(d) Haplotype-based analysis for unmatched samples

	M_1	M_2	Total
Transmitted allele	$a + b$	$c + d$	$2N$
Non-transmitted allele	$a + c$	$b + d$	$2N$
Total	$2a + b + c$	$2d + c + b$	$4N$

and Slatkin (1995), for family samples see Rhode and Fürst (2001) and Qian and Beckmann (2002). In the second step linkage disequilibrium is investigated on the basis of the estimated haplotypes or haplotype frequencies. Some of the implemented LD measures have already been described above (Devlin and Risch 1995).

Conclusions

This chapter could only introduce the basic methods of genetic epidemiological studies. Important topics had to be completely left out, such as quantitative phenotypes or gene-environment and gene-gene interaction. Others could only be mentioned, such as genome-wide linkage analysis. Some topics of general epidemiology interest are also not covered in this chapter, such as study designs appropriate for the discussed study types (cf. Chap. I.7 of this handbook), power, multiple testing and (genotyping) errors.

In addition, the area of genetic epidemiology is rapidly evolving. At the moment, most developments are made in the area of association analysis where the current technological need is highest. Initial progress has been made considering haplotype tagging SNPs as being representative for the genetic information in a LD block across a chromosomal region. Progress is needed in the area of genome wide scans using SNP chips in case-control samples as the corresponding technology is available and will be used.

References

Botstein D, White RL, Skolnick M, Davis RW (1980) Construction of a genetic linkage map in man using restriction fragment length polymorphisms. Am J Hum Genet 32:314–331

Clerget-Darpoux F, Bonaïti-Pellié C (1992) Strategies based on marker information for the study of human diseases. Ann Hum Genet 56:145–153

Corder EH, Saunders AM, Strittmatter WJ, Schmechel DE, Gaskell PC, Small GW, Roses AD, Haines JL, Pericak-Vance MA (1993) Genetic dose of apolipoprotein E type 4 allele and the risk of Alzheimer's disease in late-onset families. Science 261:921–923

Day NE, Simons MJ (1976) Disease susceptibility genes – their identification by multiple case family studies. Tissue Antigens 8:109–119

Devlin B, Risch N (1995) A comparison of linkage disequilibrium measures for fine-scale mapping. Genomics 29:311–322

Devlin B, Roeder K (1999) Genomic control for association studies. Biometrics 55:997–1004

Elston RC (1998) Methods of linkage analysis – and the assumptions underlying them. Am J Hum Genet 63:931–934

Elston RL, Stewart J (1971) A general model for genetic analysis of pedigree data. Hum Hered 21:523–542

Evans DGR, Harris R (1992) Heterogeneity in genetic conditions. Q J Med 84: 563–565

Excoffier L, Slatkin M (1995) Maximum-likelihood estimation of molecular haplotype frequencies in a diploid population. Mol Biol Evol 12:921–927

Falk CT, Rubinstein P (1987) Haplotype relative risks: an easy reliable way to construct a proper control sample for risk calculations. Ann Hum Genet 51:227–233

Haldane JBS (1919) The combination of linkage values and the calculation of distances between the loci of linked factors. J Genet 8:299–309

Hall JM, Lee MK, Newman B, Morrow JE, Anderson LA, Huey B, King MC (1990) Linkage of early-onset familial breast cancer to chromosome 17q21. Science 250:1684–1689

Hardy GH (1908) Mendelian proportions in mixed populations. Science 28:49–50

Hill WG, Robertson A (1968) Linkage disequilibrium in finite populations. Theor Appl Genet 38:226–231

Holmans P (1993) Asymptotic properties of affected-sib-pair linkage analysis. Am J Hum Genet 52:362–374

IGES (2003) International Genetic Epidemiology Society (http://www.biostat.wustl.edu/~genetics/iges/) Accessed June 03, 2004

Khoury MJ, Beaty TH, Cohen BH (1993) Fundamentals of genetic epidemiology. Oxford University Press, New York

Knapp M, Seuchter SA, Baur MP (1993) The haplotype-relative-risk (HRR) method for analysis of association in nuclear families. Am J Hum Genet 52:1085–1093

Lalouel JM, Rao DL, Morton NE, Elston RL (1984) A unified model for complex segregation analysis. Am J Hum Genet 26:484–603

Lander ES, Schork NJ (1994) Genetic dissection of complex traits. Science 265:2037–2048, Published erratum, Science 1994, 266:353

Lewontin RC (1964) The interaction of selection and linkage. I. General considerations; heterotic models. Genetics 49:49–67

Maynard Smith J (1989) Evolutionary genetics. Oxford University Press, New York

McKusick VA (1998) Mendelian inheritance in man. Catalogs of Human Genes and Genetic Disorders 12th edn. Johns Hopkins University Press, Baltimore

Mendel GJ (1865) Versuche über Pflanzenhybriden. Verhandlungen des Naturforschenden Vereins, Brünn

Morton NE (1955) Sequential tests for the detection of linkage. Am J Hum Genet 7:277–318

Morton NE, MacLean CL (1974) Analysis of familial resemblance. III. Complex segregation analysis of quantitative traits. Am J Hum Genet 26:484–503

Newman B, Austin MA, Lee M, King MC (1988) Inheritance of human breast cancer: evidence for autosomal dominant transmission in high-risk families. Proc Natl Acad Sci, USA 85:3044–3048

Online Mendelian Inheritance in Man, OMIM™(2000) McKusick-Nathans Institute for Genetic Medicine, Johns Hopkins University (Baltimore, MD) and National Center for Biotechnology Information, National Library of Medicine (Bethesda, MD) (http://www.ncbi.nlm.nih.gov/omim/) Accessed June 03, 2004

Ott J (1999) Analysis of human genetic linkage, 3rd edn. Johns Hopkins University Press, Baltimore

Penrose LS (1953) The general sib-pair linkage test. Annals of Eugenics 18:120–144

Pritchard JK, Stephens M, Rosenberg NA, Donnelly P (2000) Association mapping in structured populations. Am J Hum Genet 67:170–181

Qian D, Beckmann L (2002) Minimum-recombinant haplotyping in pedigrees. Am J Hum Genet 70:1434–1445

Rhode K, Fürst R (2001) Haplotyping and estimation of haplotype frequencies for closely linked biallelic multilocus genetic phenotypes including nuclear family information. Human Mutation 14:289–295

Risch N (1983) A general model for disease-marker association. Ann Hum Genet 47:245–252

Risch N (1991) A note on multiple testing procedures in linkage analysis. Am J Hum Genet 48:1058–1064

Schaid DJ (1999) Likelihoods and TDT for the case-parents design. Genet Epidemiol 16:250–260

Schaid DJ, Sommer SS (1994) Comparison of statistics for candidate-gene association studies using cases and parents. Am J Hum Genet 55:402–409

Sham P (1998) Statistics in human genetics. Wiley, New York

Shute NC, Ewens WJ (1988) A resolution of the ascertainment sampling problem. II. Generalizations and numerical results. Am J Hum Genet 43:374–386

Spielman RS, Ewens WJ (1998) A sibship test for linkage in the presence of association: The sib transmission/disequilibrium test. Am J Hum Genet 62:450–458

Spielman RS, McGinnis RE, Ewens JW (1993) Transmission test for linkage disequilibrium: the insulin gene region and insulin-dependent diabetes mellitus (IDDM). Am J Hum Genet 52:506–516

Suarez BK, Hampe CL (1994) Linkage and association. Am J Hum Genet 54:554–559

Tamarin RH (1986) Principles of genetics, 2nd edn. Prindle, Weber & Schmidt, Boston

Terwilliger JD, Ott J (1992) A haplotype-based 'haplotype relative risk' approach to detecting allelic association. Hum Hered 42:337–346

Terwilliger JD, Ott J (1994) Handbook of human genetic linkage. Johns Hopkins University Press, Baltimore

Thompson EA (1986) Genetic epidemiology: a review of the statistical basis. Statistics in Medicine 5:291–302

Thomson G (1983) Investigation of the mode of inheritance of the HLA associated diseases by the method of antigen genotype frequencies among diseased individuals. Tissue Antigens 21:81–104

Vogel W (2000) Genetische Epidemiologie oder zur Spezifität von Subdisziplinen der Humangenetik. Med Genet 4:395–399

Weinberg W (1908) über den Nachweis der Vererbung beim Menschen. Jahreshefte des Vereins für vaterländische Naturkunde in Württemberg 64:368–383

Weiss KM (1993) Genetic variation and human disease. Principles and evolutionary approaches. University Press, Cambridge

Whittaker JC, Morris AP (2001) Family-based tests of association and/or linkage. Ann Hum Genet 65:407–419

Whittemore AS, Tu IP (1998) Simple, robust linkage tests for affected sibs. Am J Hum Genet 62:1228–1242

Woolf B (1955) On estimating the relation between blood group and disease. Ann Hum Genet 19:251–253

Clinical Epidemiology

III.8

Holger J. Schünemann, Gordon H. Guyatt

8.1 Introduction

This chapter will begin with providing a brief overview of the history of clinical epidemiology and describe its relation with evidence based medicine. Clinical epidemiology differs from classical epidemiology in that clinical epidemiology supports other basic medical sciences such as biochemistry, anatomy and physiology because it facilitates their application in research through formulation of sound clinical research methods and, thus, puts these disciplines into clinical context. Therefore, clinical epidemiology goes beyond clinical trials. We will describe this concept in the following paragraphs (see Sect. 8.1.1 through 8.1.3). The following sections include case scenarios that facilitate the introduction of the key concepts about developing clinical questions, using diagnostic tests, evaluating therapy, appraising systematic reviews, developing guidelines and making clinical decisions.

8.1.1 Brief History of Clinical Epidemiology

Sackett provides an astute historical summary of the development of clinical epidemiology in his recent tribute in memory of Alvan Feinstein (Sackett 2002). Sackett's account gives John Paul credit for introducing the term clinical epidemiology describing it as the "new basic science for preventive medicine" (Paul 1938; Sackett 2002). Over the past 40 years, both Feinstein and Sackett himself made major contributions to the field of clinical epidemiology. Sackett founded, in 1966, the first clinical epidemiology research unit at the University at Buffalo, New York, USA, and in 1967 a department of clinical epidemiology and biostatistics at McMaster University in Hamilton, Canada, which he served as chair. The latter institution has trained numerous clinical epidemiologists, some of whom have taken on chair positions themselves. Today there are departments and units of clinical epidemiology throughout the world, though the development in some jurisdictions has been slower than in others. For example, it was in this millennium that the first department of clinical epidemiology was founded in the German speaking countries of Europe (Basel, Switzerland, H. Bucher, personal communication), although professorships of clinical epidemiology existed in these countries for some time.

8.1.2 A Definition of Clinical Epidemiology

Although seminal, Paul's simple description of clinical epidemiology was perhaps not sufficient in helping investigators and clinicians understand the principles underlying the term clinical epidemiology. Articles and textbooks have provided further definitions. Feinstein portrayed clinical epidemiology as investigating "the occurrence rates and geographic distribution of disease; the pattern of natural and post-therapeutic events that constitute varying clinical courses in the diverse spectrum of disease; and the clinical appraisal of therapy. The contemplation and investigation of these or allied topics constitute a medical domain that can be called clinical epidemiology" (Feinstein 1968; Sackett et al. 1991). Sackett defined clinical epidemiology as "the application, by a physician who provides direct patient care, of epidemiologic and biostatistical methods to the study of diagnostic and therapeutic processes in order to effect an improvement of health" (Sackett 1969, 2002; Sackett and Winkelstein 1967). Fletcher et al. (1996) described clinical epidemiology as the science of making predictions about individual patients by counting clinical events in similar patients, using strong scientific methods for studies of groups of patients to ensure that the predictions are accurate. Weiss (1996) defined clinical epidemiology as the study of variation in the outcome of illness and of the reasons for that variation. Despite the numerous definitions, one might argue that by providing the subheading "a basic science for Clinical Medicine" to their textbook "Clinical Epidemiology" Sackett and colleagues provided a pithy definition that not only turned the wheel back to John Paul, but widened it to all areas of clinical medicine by replacing *preventive medicine* with *clinical medicine* (Sackett et al. 2000).

Definitions are inevitably limited, and in depth understanding requires a more comprehensive discussion. We characterize clinical epidemiology by focusing on its purpose: to ensure that clinicians' practice and decision making is evidence-based. Clinical decision making requires answering questions about diagnosis, therapy, prevention and harm, providing estimates of prognosis and obtaining unbiased and precise estimates of intervention effects. Clinical epidemiology supports other basic medical sciences such as biochemistry, anatomy and physiology because it facilitates their application in research through formulation of sound clinical research methods and, thus, puts these disciplines into clinical context. Thus, clinical epidemiology provides the integrative force of medical science and medical practice.

Clinical Epidemiology and Evidence-based Medicine   8.1.3

When working optimally, clinical epidemiologists communicate results of investigations in ways that clinicians can readily apply in practice. Clinical epidemiology provides the evidence for management decisions resulting in more good than harm. Clinicians should use best evidence for clinical decision making. Thus, clinical epidemiology and evidence-based practice are closely linked. Clinical epidemiology grounds health care research in the mission to deliver optimal care to individual patients. As it turns out, clinicians optimally applying the evidence to their patient care must understand the basic concepts of clinical epidemiology (Guyatt et al. 2000). At the same time, while clinical epidemiology grounds the clinical investigators' viewpoint, evidence-based medicine (EBM) provides the framework for application of research findings in clinical practice. In the next sections of this discussion, we will describe the basics of clinical epidemiology methods and how insights from clinical practice may enlighten clinical epidemiologists.

The History and Philosophy of Evidence-based Medicine

When we first introduced the term evidence-based medicine (EBM) in an informal residency training program document, we described it as "an attitude of enlightened skepticism toward the application of diagnostic, therapeutic, and prognostic technologies in their day-to-day management of patients" (Guyatt 1991, 2002a, b). Through a series of articles published by the evidence-based medicine working group the term as well as the philosophy of EBM became well-known (Evidence-Based-Medicine-Working-Group 1992; Oxman et al. 1993). A Medline search revealed 7 citations including the term "Evidence Based Medicine" in 1993 and 2169 citations in 2002.

EBM evolved out of the efforts of clinicians with methodology training – that is, clinical epidemiologists – to apply their particular insights and approaches to solving clinical problems. In contrast to the traditional paradigm of clinical practice, EBM acknowledges that intuition, unsystematic clinical experience, and pathophysiologic rationale are not sufficient for making the best clinical decisions. Although it acknowledges the importance of clinical experience, EBM postulates that optimal clinical decision-making requires the integration of evidence from clinical research.

EBM places a lower value on authority than the traditional medical paradigm, and explicitly includes patients' and society's values in the clinical decision-making process. Patients or their proxies must always trade the benefits, harm, and costs associated with alternative treatment strategies, and in doing so must consider values and preferences.

To achieve the integration of research results in clinical practice, EBM proposes a formal set of rules to help clinicians interpret and apply evidence. Clinical epidemiologists have, by and large, developed these rules. These rules are characterized by a hierarchy of evidence (Fig. 8.1): confidence in research results is greatest if systematic error (bias) is lowest and increases if bias is more likely to play a role.

STUDY DESIGN

Randomized controlled trials

Controlled trials

Case-control studies and cohort studies

Cross-sectional studies

Case reports and case series

Likelihood of Bias

Figure 8.1. Depicts the hierarchy of quality of evidence. As the research design becomes more rigorous (moving from *bottom* to *top*) the quality of evidence increases and the likelihood of bias decreases

Although randomized and controlled study designs provide the highest quality of evidence, EBM is not a science of randomized controlled trials. Rather, because higher quality evidence often is not available, EBM acknowledges that a large body of highly relevant evidence comes from observational studies. That is, to answer clinical questions clinicians will often depend on observational studies in their evidence-based practice. Therefore, the practice and application of EBM requires an understanding and critical evaluation of all study designs. Clinical epidemiology provides the necessary toolbox for this evaluation. For example, clinical epidemiologists of the Cochrane Collaboration, an international organization dedicated to making up-to-date and accurate information about the effects of healthcare readily available worldwide, have provided important insights into the conduct of systematic reviews and meta-analysis that inform clinicians and patients choices. It produces and disseminates systematic reviews of healthcare interventions and promotes the search for evidence. It can be accessed at www.cochrane.org.

Case Scenario   8.2

Example 1.   Imagine you are the attending physician on ward rounds with your team. The senior resident presents the case of a 64 year old woman who came to the emergency room one early morning with left sided chest pain lasting for 15 minutes. The pain was severe enough to awaken her. She also had to sit up in her bed because of difficulties with getting her breath. Finally, her symptoms became so severe that she called an ambulance.

You immediately think that this woman has had an acute myocardial infarction. However, other diagnoses such as pulmonary embolism, pneumonia, pericarditis, asthma and a severe case of gastro-esophageal reflux disease also come to mind.

The resident continues with her presentation and tells you that the pain radiated to her left arm and you further hear that she had another episode of similar pain in the ambulance which was relieved within a few minutes by 0.4 mg nitroglycerin given under her tongue.

You feel that this information confirms your early intuition and that it makes a diagnosis of myocardial infarction more likely.

An EKG in the emergency room was unremarkable and cardiac enzymes drawn at arrival to the emergency room were borderline elevated (troponin I, a marker for myocardial injury, was 1.0 g/ml). Her chest X-ray was normal.

You now think that the diagnosis might be one of acute coronary syndrome, perhaps unstable angina or a myocardial infarction without EKG changes, and you continue to entertain pulmonary embolism, pneumonia and pericarditis as alternative – although less likely – diagnosis. The key decision you face is whether to admit the patient to hospital, possibly to a cardiac care unit, or to send her home with provision for subsequent investigation, perhaps an exercise test.

The patient's past medical history includes diabetes mellitus type 2. Her lipid profile is within the limits set by the National Cholesterol Education Program

Guidelines (NCEP 2001) and there is no significant family history of cardiovascular disease. She takes an oral hypoglycemic agent and 325 mg of aspirin daily as recommended by her physician. She has had similar chest pain over the past year when vacuuming her home. However, she did not mention these complaints to her physician because the discomfort always resolved after a few minutes of rest. The patient has no history of cough, wheezing, indigestion, heartburn or changes in her bowel habits. Physical examination shows an anxious patient, but there are no abnormal findings on physical examination.

Your team concludes that the probability that the presentation represents acute coronary syndrome is at least 50%. While you are discussing the patient and her further management, a second set of laboratory results shows that the troponin I is elevated at 4.1 g/l.

At this point you feel that a myocardial infarction without ST segment elevation on the EKG (a NSTEMI) is the most likely diagnosis and together with your team you consider further management.   ◆

8.3   Formulating a Clinical Question

Using research evidence to guide clinical practice requires formulating sensible clinical questions (McKibbon et al. 2002; Oxman et al. 1993; Richardson et al. 1995). For most questions the key components are the patients, the intervention or exposure, comparison interventions (or exposure) and the outcomes (Table 8.1).

Table 8.1. Formulating the clinical question

Component	Explanation
Population	Who are the relevant patients?
Interventions or exposures	What are the management strategies clinicians are interested in? For example: Diagnostic test, drugs, toxins, nutrients, surgical procedures, etc.
Comparison (or control) intervention or exposures	What is the comparison, control or alternative intervention clinicians are interested in? For questions about therapy or harm there will always be a comparison or control (including doing nothing, placebo, alternative active treatment or routine care). For questions about diagnosis there may be a comparison diagnostic strategy (for example troponin I compared to creatine kinase MB in the diagnosis of myocardial infarction).
Outcome	What are the patient-important consequences of the exposure clinicians are interested in?

The clinical scenario of an older diabetic women presenting with chest pain potentially generates several clinical questions (about her diagnosis, appropriate therapy, prevention of future events, prognosis). We will use some of these questions to demonstrate how clinical epidemiology helps solve clinical problems.

Diagnosis

Based on the framework for developing a clinical question, we will start with a question about diagnosis:

Population: In women with chest pain typical for angina pectoris
Intervention/exposure: What is the test performance of troponin I serum levels
Outcome: To predict myocardial infarction and associated adverse
                             outcomes (congestive heart failure, death, serious
                             arrhythmia or severe ischemic pain) in the next 72 hours.

The process of diagnosis is a complex cognitive task. There are different approaches to making a diagnosis, but pattern recognition, which is also known as the gestalt method, and logical reasoning play an important role (Glass 1996; Sackett et al. 1991; Sox et al. 1988). Clinicians always look for clues that help them establish a diagnosis, although with increasing clinical experience this process becomes increasingly subconscious. Some clues make a diagnosis more likely, other clues or the absence of certain clues make a diagnosis less likely (Ladenheim et al. 1987). In the scenario described at the beginning of this chapter, the first clue was the presence of left sided chest pain awaking the patient at night. This clue suggested that the patient might suffer from a cardiac problem. The presence of shortness of breath strengthened this suspicion, but brought other possible diagnosis into consideration (asthma, pneumonia and pulmonary embolus).

When clinicians use clues offered by clinical history, symptoms, signs or test results, they routinely, if often subconsciously, apply probabilities associated with these clues. For example, the presence of chest pain makes a heart attack more likely than no chest pain. Thus, a first step in making a diagnosis is to assign probabilities to the contemplated diagnoses. Clinicians then group the findings into coherent clusters, such as left sided (location) chest (heart or lungs) pain (symptom). These clusters inform the differential diagnoses. The differential diagnoses in the case scenario included acute myocardial infarction, pulmonary embolism, pneumonia, asthma or gastro-esophageal reflux disease. In the next step of making a diagnosis, the clinician incorporates new information, which lowers or increases the relative likelihood of the differential diagnoses. The process is therefore sequential. The presence of pain radiating to the left arm increased the probability of coronary heart disease and the absence of cough and gastrointestinal symptoms lowered the likelihood of pneumonia and gastrointestinal disease.

8.4.1 Establish the Framework for Bayesian Thinking for Diagnosis

As described above, the process of diagnosis can take place on a subconscious level where the clinician guesses the associated probabilities and relative likelihoods or it can employ explicit probabilities and relative likelihoods. For some clinical problems, such as diagnosing pulmonary embolism, clinicians intuition is good. The prospective investigation of pulmonary embolism diagnosis (PIOPED) study has shown this (PIOPED-Investigators 1990). Even when intuition is reasonably accurate, use of exact numbers generated by empirical studies can improve clinical decisions (Diamond and Forrester 1979; Diamond et al. 1980, 1981; Dolan et al. 1986). The latter approach of using explicit information is based on epidemiologic and biostatistical concepts, but both the intuitive and the explicit approaches are founded in Bayesian theory, because both approaches depend on probabilites that are altered by subsequent information (Bernardo and Adrian 1994; Berry 1996; Diamond 1999; Ledley and Lusted 1959; cf. Chap. I.1 of this handbook). Using the Bayesian approach in the diagnostic process the clinician starts with a certain probability (often called the pre-test probability) of a disease being present. Then, based on clues from the history, physical exam or test results, the clinician modifies this probability into another probability (often called the posttest probability).

8.4.2 Choosing the Right Test

The best test would be one that excludes or confirms a diagnosis beyond doubt. Using an ideal test, no patient would have the disease if the test is negative and all patients with a positive test would have the disease. For our example, were troponin I perfect, one could assume that a troponin I level $\geq$ 2 g/l proves beyond doubt that the patient has an acute myocardial infarction or will suffer a serious clinical event associated with acute coronary syndrome in the next 72 hours, and a level $<$ 2 g/l establishes that the patient does not have an acute myocardial infarction and will not suffer a serious event. Unfortunately, most information that clinicians obtain in clinical practice comes with uncertainty, and tests that definitively distinguish between disease and no disease are few and far between.

The typical cut-off value for troponin I in clinical practice is 2.0 g/l (Meier et al. 2002). However, astute clinicians would not dismiss a diagnosis of myocardial infarction in our scenario after the first troponin I level was $<$ 2.0 g/l, because both EKG and biomarkers may be what is typically defined as normal even when disease is present. Furthermore, they are aware that the troponin I may be normal early, and may rise subsequently. What clinicians expect of a good test is, that results change the probability sufficient to confirm or exclude a diagnosis. If a test result moves the probability below a threshold at which the disease is very unlikely and downsides associated with the treatment outweigh any anticipated benefit, then no further testing and no treatment are indicated. We call this probability the test threshold. If, on the other hand, the test result moves the probability of disease above a threshold at which one would not further test because disease is highly probable and one would start treatment we have found the treatment threshold. This scenario shows how a clinician can estimate the probability of disease and then compare disease probability to these two thresholds (Fig. 8.2).

In a clinical context in which the pre-test probability of a particular diagnosis is above the treatment threshold, further confirmatory testing that raises the probability further would not be helpful. On the other end of the scale, for a disease with a pre-test probability below the test threshold, further exclusionary testing lowering the probability would not be useful. When the probability is between the test and treatment thresholds testing will be diagnostically useful. Test results are of greatest value when they shift the probability across either threshold.

What determines our treatment thresholds? If adverse effects of treatment are frequent and severe, clinicians choose a higher treatment threshold. For example, because a diagnosis of pulmonary embolism involves long-term anticoagulation with appreciable bleeding risk, clinicians are very concerned about falsely labeling patients. The invasiveness of the next test will also impact on the threshold. If results from the next test (such as a ventilation-perfusion scan) are benign, clinicians are ready to choose a high treatment threshold. Clinicians are more reluctant to institute an invasive test associated with risks to the patient, such as a pulmonary angiogram, and this will drive their treatment threshold downward. That is, clinicians are more inclined to accept a risk of a false-positive diagnosis because a higher treatment threshold necessitates putting more patients through the risky test.

Accordingly, the more serious a missed diagnosis, the lower we will set our test threshold. Since a missed diagnosis of a pulmonary embolus could be fatal, clinicians are inclined to set their diagnostic threshold low. At the same time, the risks associated with the next test we are considering have an influence on where

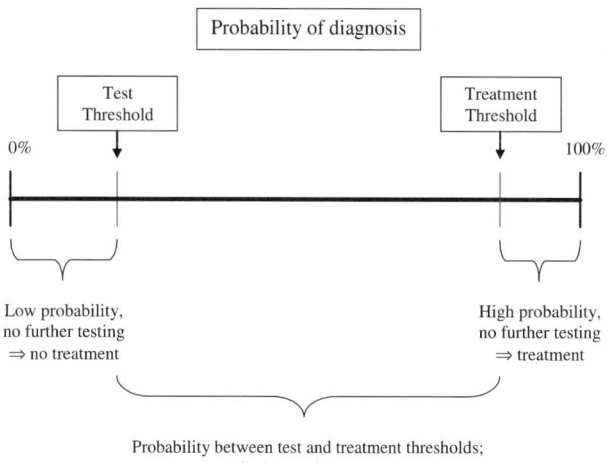

Probability of diagnosis

Test Threshold

Treatment Threshold

0%   100%

Low probability,
no further testing
⇒ no treatment

High probability,
no further testing
⇒ treatment

Probability between test and treatment thresholds;
⇒ further testing required

Figure 8.2. Test and treatment thresholds

to set the test threshold. If the risks are low, clinicians will be comfortable with a very low diagnostic threshold. The higher the risks, the more the threshold rises.

Likelihood Ratios

The center of any diagnostic process is a patient presenting with a constellation of symptoms and signs. Consider two patients with chest pain and shortness of breath in whom the clinician suspects a myocardial infarction without findings suggestive of pneumonia, airflow obstruction, pulmonary embolism or heart failure or other conditions. One patient is the 64-year-old woman described in the clinical scenario and the other is a 24-year-old man with a history of anxiety disorder. Clinicians would agree that the probability of myocardial infarction for these two patients – that is, their pre-test probabilities – are very different. In the woman described in the scenario, the probability is high; in the young man, it is low. Consequently, even if both patients had borderline elevated troponin I levels of 1.0 g/l at presentation, management is likely to differ between the two. An informed clinician might well treat the elderly woman immediately with aspirin and heparin but order further investigations in the young man.

One can draw two conclusions from these considerations. First, regardless of the results of the troponin I test, they do not definitively establish whether myocardial infarction is in fact the underlying disease, or whether the patient will suffer a serious event associated with an acute coronary syndrome. What they do accomplish is to alter the pre-test probability of the condition, yielding a new post-test probability. The direction and magnitude of this change from pre-test to post-test probability are determined by the test's properties. The test property of greatest value is the likelihood ratio.

Hill and colleagues (2003) investigated the diagnostic properties of troponin I as an early marker of acute myorcardial infarction or acute coronary syndrome with serious sequellae in the next 72 hours in patients who did not have definitively diagnostic EKG changes. The investigators found 20 individuals with a serious cardiac outcome by the reference standard and 332 individuals people who did not (Table 8.2). For all patients, troponin I tests were classified into four levels: < 0.5 g/l, 0.5 to < 2.0 g/l, 2.0 to < 10.0 g/l and ≥ 10.0 g/l). Several questions arise.

How likely is a substantially elevated (≥ 10 g/l) troponin I among people who suffered adverse outcomes? Table 8.2 illustrates that 3 of 20 (or approximately 15%) people with adverse outcomes had troponin I levels ≥ 10 g/l. How often is the same test result, a positive troponin I, found among patients in whom high risk acute coronary syndrome was suspected but ruled out? The answer is 4 out of 332 (or approximately 1.2%). The ratio of these two likelihoods is the likelihood ratio (LR); for a highly elevated troponin I test, it equals 0.15/0.012 (or 12.5). In other words, a highly elevated troponin I is 12.5 times as likely to occur in a patient with – in contrast to without – an ultimate adverse outcome.

In a similar fashion, one can calculate the likelihood ratios for troponin I values of ≤ 0.5 g/l, 0.5 to ≤ 2.0 g/l and 2.0 to ≤ 10.0 g/l. This calculation involves answering

Table 8.2. Test properties of early troponin I testing in myocardial infarction or ischemia-associated adverse outcomes (CI = confidence interval)

Test results	Myocardial infarction or other adverse outcomes				Likelihood ratio (95% CI)
	Present/proportion		Absent/proportion		
≥ 10.0 g/l	3	3/20 = 0.15	4	4/332 = 0.012	12.5 (3.0, 51.9)
2.0– < 10.0 g/l	2	2/20 = 0.10	5	5/332 = 0.015	6.6 (1.4, 32.1)
0.5– < 2.0 g/l	3	3/20 = 0.15	20	20/332 = 0.06	2.5 (0.8, 7.7)
< 0.5 g/l	12	12/20 = 0.60	303	303/332 = 0.910	0.7 (0.5, 0.9)
Total	20		332		

two questions: First, how likely it is to obtain a given test result (e.g., a troponin I < 0.5 g/l) among people with the target disorder (myocardial infarction)? Second, how likely it is to obtain the same test result (again, a troponin I < 0.5 g/l) among people without the target disorder? For this troponin I test result, the likelihoods are 12/20 (0.60) and 303/332 (0.91), respectively, and their ratio (the likelihood ratio) is 0.7.

Thus, the likelihood ratios indicate by how much a given diagnostic test result will raise or lower the pre-test probability of the target disorder. A likelihood ratio of 1 indicates that the post-test probability is identical to the pre-test probability. Likelihood ratios above 1.0 increase the probability that the target disorder is present, and the higher the likelihood ratio, the greater is this increase. Likelihood ratios below 1.0 decrease the probability of the target disorder, and the smaller the likelihood ratio, the greater is the decrease in probability and the smaller is its final value.

Users of likelihood ratios often ask "What are good likelihood ratios for a test?". The answer is that day-to-day clinical practice lets clinicians gain understanding and their own sense of interpretation, but one can consider the following as a guide:

- Likelihood ratios of > 10 or < 0.1 generate large and often conclusive changes from pre- to post-test probability
- Likelihood ratios of 5–10 and 0.1–0.2 generate moderate shifts in pre- to post-test probability
- Likelihood ratios of 2–5 and 0.5–0.2 generate small (but sometimes important) changes in probability
- Likelihood ratios of 1–2 and 0.5–1 alter probability to a small (and rarely important) degree.

How can clinicians use likelihood ratios to move from pre-test to post-test probability? Unfortunately, one cannot combine likelihoods directly, such as one can combine probabilities or percentages. Their formal use requires converting pre-test probability to odds, multiplying the result by the likelihood ratio, and then converting the post-test odds into a post-test probability. Although this calculation is relatively straightforward for an experienced user, it can be time consuming and, fortunately, there is an easier way.

Figure 8.3 shows a nomogram proposed by Fagan that performs the conversions and allows simple transition from pre- to post-test probability (Fagan 1975). The line on the left-hand side represents the pre-test probability, the middle line represents the likelihood ratio, and the line on the right-hand side depicts the resulting post-test probability. One can obtain the post-test probability by anchoring a straight line at the pre-test probability and rotating it until it lines up with the likelihood ratio of the relevant test result.

If we assumed a pre-test probability of 50% (see below) for the elderly woman with multiple risk factors and we applied the LR associated with a troponin I of 1.0 to the nomogram (connecting 0.5 or 50% on the left with a LR of approximately 2.5 on the middle line and extending it through the right line) we would obtain a post-test probability of approximately 70% (or 0.7). If we assumed a pre-test probability of 1 in 1000 or 0.1% for the young man and applied the same LR, the post-test probability remains very low at between 0.2 and 0.3%.

To further explain the application of LRs, let us assume the two patients had troponin levels of 0.3 g/l. Applying the associated LR (0.7) to the pre-test probability of 50% of the elderly women would result in a post-test probability of approximately

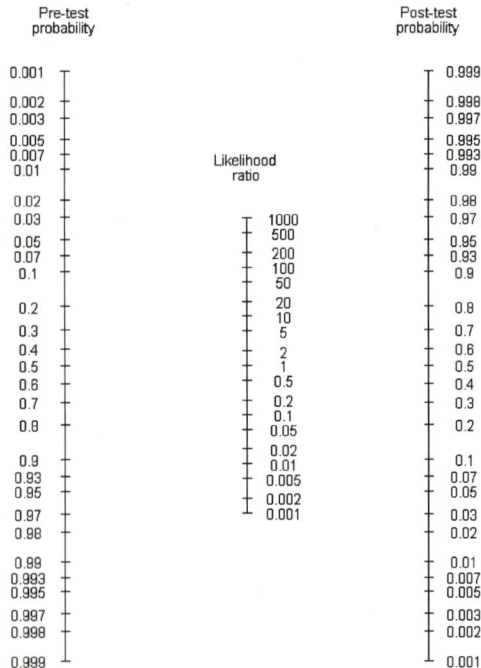

Figure 8.3. Likelihood ratio (Fagan) nomogram (Copyright 1975 Massachusetts Medical Society. All rights reserved. Reproduced with permission from the Massachusetts Medical Society)

45% (or 0.45). Applying this LR (0.7) to the pre-test probability of 0.1% of the young man results in a post-test probability of < 0.1%. It becomes evident from these latter two hypothetical examples that the test result has not altered the post-test probabilities to a large extent and further testing is necessary or that the clinician needs to make a decision on the basis of post-test probabilities that are similar to the pre-test probabilities. These strategies will differ between the two patients. Most clinicians would remain worried about the elderly women, but would safely discharge the young man.

Readers who are interested in the formula for converting pre-test probabilities to post-test probabilities, will note that it is based on Bayes theorem:

$$\text{Post-test odds} = \text{Pre-test odds} \times \text{Likelihood ratio}$$

Mathematically we can write this formula as:

$$O(D|R) = \big(O(D) \times P(R|D)\big) / P(R|\overline{D}),$$

where P is the probability of a specific test result R given the status of disease D = disease present, $\overline{D}$ = disease absent, $O(D)$ is the odds of disease to be calculated as $P(D)/[1 - P(D)]$.

Example 1. *(continued)*

Returning to our examples, for our elderly female patient with a test result of 1.0 µg/l and pre-test odds = 0.5/(1 − 0.5) = 1 this formula translates to:

$$\text{post-test odds of myocardial infarction} = 1 \times 0.15/0.06 = 2.5.$$

Post-test odds can be converted into post-test probabilities using the following formula:

$$\text{post-test probability} = \text{post-test odds}/(\text{post-test odds} + 1) = 2.5/(2.5 + 1)$$
$$= 71.4\%.$$

♦

This estimate is similar to the estimate on the Fagan Nomogram. In fact, had we been able to use the Nomogram as accurately as the calculator we would have obtained identical numbers. This probability moves us into the range of probability where most clinicians would treat patients without further testing because of the morbidity and mortality associated with myocardial infarction.

Example 1. *(continued)*

For the young male with a troponin of 1.0 this formula translates to:

$$\text{post-test odds of myocardial infarction} = \text{pre-test odds} \times 2.5.$$

We can derive the pre-test odds from the pre-test probability of 0.1% = 0.001/(1− 0.001) which is about 0.001.

Thus, it follows that the post-test odds can be calculated as

$$\text{post-test odds} = 0.001 \times 2.5 = 0.0025$$

and the post-test probability as

$$\text{post-test probability} = 0.0025/(0.0025 + 1)$$

which is approximately 0.25%.   ◆

Again, the estimate of 0.25% corresponds to the estimate using the Fagan Nomogram, but is the exact result of the application of Bayes theorem. Even a troponin I test associated with a LR greater than 1 and commonly considered elevated in the young man does not alter the probability for a myocardial infarction to a great extent.

8.4.4   How to Obtain Pre-Test Probabilities

We guessed at the pre-test probability of the two patients with chest discomfort. How do clinicians obtain valid pre-test probabilities? Intuitively, clinicians use their experience based on previous patients with similar presentations. However, the probabilities clinicians and in particular learners assume are prone to bias and error (Richardson 2002; Richardson et al. 2003).

Richardson has suggested that there are two different forms of clinical research that can guide clinicians estimates of pre-test probabilities (Richardson 2002). The first type are studies that yield disease probability based on representative patient cohorts with a defined clinical problem that carry out careful diagnostic evaluations and apply explicit diagnostic criteria. Examples include studies on causes of syncope (Soteriades et al. 2002) and cancer in involuntary weight loss (Hernandez et al. 2003). Control groups of randomized trials may serve for questions of prognosis. The study by Hill et al. (2003) that provided the estimates for the test properties of troponin I to obtain pre-test probabilities could also serve as example. The second type of studies are clinical decision rules. These studies assemble cohorts suspected of having the target disorder, apply standard reference tests and report the frequency of diagnoses in subgroups with identifying clinical features (McGinn et al. 2003). High quality studies that provide valid estimates of frequency are applicable to our patients and can provide precise estimates of pre-test probability. For example, Richardson et al. (2003) estimated in a consecutive patient series that for 78% (95% CI: (66%, 96%)) of clinical problems evidence of pre-test probabilities existed in the literature.

8.4.5   Sensitivity and Specificity

Likelihood ratios help users understand diagnostic tests. However, clinicians use two other descriptive terms for diagnostic tests. It is, therefore, helpful for those with interest in clinical epidemiology to understand these two other terms: sensitivity and specificity.

We could have described the test properties of the study by Hill and colleagues using the concepts of sensitivity and specificity defining normal and abnormal test results. We presented the four different interpretations of troponin I levels, each with the associated likelihood ratios. That classification allowed us to omit the terms normal and abnormal or positive and negative. However, this is not the way most investigators present their result. Investigators also often rely on concepts of sensitivity and specificity.

Sensitivity expresses the proportion of people with the target disorder in whom the test result is positive and specificity expresses the proportion of people without the target disorder in whom a test result is negative. Table 8.3 shows the general concept of sensitivity and specificity in a 2×2 table. We could transform the 4×2 table described above (Table 8.2) into three 2×2 tables, depending on what we call positive or negative. Let us assume that only troponin I values ≥ 10.0 g/l are positive (or abnormal).

To calculate sensitivity from the data in Table 8.2 for positive troponin I levels, we look at the number of people with proven myocardial infarction ($n = 20$) who were diagnosed as having the target disorder on troponin testing ($n = 3$) showing a sensitivity of 3/20, or approximately 15% ($a/(a + c)$). To calculate specificity, we use the number of people without the target disorder (332) whose troponin test results were classified as normal or < 0.5 g/l (303), yielding a specificity of 303/332, or 91% ($d/(b + d)$).

As indicated above, one can easily calculate LRs for different levels of quantitative test results while sensitivity and specificity require a definition of normal and

Table 8.3. Sensitivity and specificity of diagnostic tests ($a + b + c + d = 100\%$)

Test results	Disease or reference standard (proportion)	
	Present (positive)	Absent (negative)
Disease present (positive)	True Positive (a)	False Positive (b)
Disease absent (negative)	False Negative (c)	True Negative (d)
Sensitivity =	True positive/ positive reference standard $a/(a + c)$	
Specificity =		True negative/negative reference standard $d/(b + d)$
Likelihood ratio for positive test (LR+) =	Sensitivity/$(1 - $Specificity$) = (a/(a + c))/(1 - d/(b + d))$	
Likelihood ratio for negative test (LR-) =	$(1 - $Sensitivity$)/$Specificity $= (1 - (a/(a + c))/(d/(b + d)))$	

abnormal that is often arbitrary. In using sensitivity and specificity one has to either discard important information or recalculate sensitivity and specificity for every cut-point. Therefore, the likelihood ratio is much simpler and much more efficient when tests have more than two possible results, which is very often the case (Guyatt et al. 1990, 1992; Guyatt and Rennie 2002).

8.5 Therapy/Prevention

Example 1. *(continued)*

Returning to the clinical scenario and having treated the elderly woman with aspirin and heparin, the team questions what other therapeutic or preventive interventions may be of benefit. The resident points you to a study that aimed at maximizing platelet inhibition in patients with acute coronary syndrome, the Clopidogrel in Unstable Angina to Prevent Recurrent Events Trial (CURE) trial (CURE-Investigators 2001). You vaguely remember this study and that it is the only one you are aware of addressing this question in patients with acute coronary syndrome. You know that neurologists and cardiologists in your institution often use two antiplatelet agents to maximize platelet inhibition, but you wonder about the quality of the evidence supporting this conclusion and the magnitude of benefits and downsides. An electronic database search confirms that there is no additional evidence addressing this specific question in a randomized trial in patients with acute coronary syndrome. The CURE investigators addressed the question "In patients with acute coronary syndromes without ST-segment elevation, does early and long-term use of clopidogrel plus aspirin versus aspirin alone prevent cardiovascular events and is the combination safe?" You find that this question would be highly relevant to your patient in whom you want to prevent further cardiovascular events.

You decide to critically appraise this study together with your team. The resident retrieves the article through your library's online full text journal subscription and you evaluate the article with your team over lunch break.   ♦

The concepts of clinical epidemiology help clinicians appraise clinical research. We list the three commonly agreed on steps of critical appraisal for studies on therapy or prevention in Table 8.4 and describe how clinical epidemiology facilitates interpretation and evaluation of clinical research. This form addresses critical appraisal for most clinicians. Other important issues for experienced readers concern the appropriateness of the statistical methods.

The first factor that can influence confidence in research results is systematic error or bias. Bias is directly linked to the design and execution of a study. Therefore, the first step is an appraisal of whether results are valid and to what extend bias is present (Table 8.4 – Are the results valid?). The next step in the evaluation of research is the review of the results. Because clinicians often are unfamiliar with applying the magnitude of effects to patient care and because classical epidemiology applies research results in different contexts using different terminology, clinical epidemiologists can bring quantitative outcome measures closer to the clinician. This helps address the question "How large is the effect of an intervention and how large is the role of random error or chance (What are the results?)?". Finally, clinicians need to know whether the results are applicable to their patients. Therefore, clinicians need to appraise whether the results help with decision-making in individual practice circumstances (How can I apply the results to my patient care?). Clinicians must decide whether their patients are similar to those included in the studies from which they obtain the relevant evidence, but clinical epidemiologists can help them in the decision making process (see Sect. 8.8).

Critical appraisal (Table 8.4) of the CURE trial reveals that patients were randomized using a 24-hour computerized randomization service to conceal randomization. Control patients received placebos and investigators and outcome assessors were blinded to treatment assignment. While blinding refers to not being aware of treatment allocation when treatment has been assigned, concealment refers to avoiding biased allocation of patients because of prior knowledge of forthcoming treatment allocation. Investigators can achieve concealment through measures such as central (telephone) randomization and sealed envelopes. The more stringent the method for concealment the less likely are those allocating patients to temper with this important aspect of randomized controlled trials. Fulfilling these

Table 8.4. Critical appraisal of studies about therapy

Question	Therapy or prevention
Study design and execution – evaluation of bias	I. Are the results of the study valid? 1. Were patients randomized? 2. Was randomization concealed? 3. Were patients analyzed in the groups to which they were randomized? 4. Were patients in the treatment and control groups similar with respect to known prognostic factors? 5. Were patients aware of group allocation? 6. Were clinicians aware of group allocation? 7. Were outcome assessors aware of group allocation? 8. Was follow up complete?
Results and random error	II. What are the results? 1. How large was the treatment effect? 2. How precise was the estimate of the treatment effect?
Application and uptake	III. How can I apply the results to my patient care? 1. Were the study patients similar to my patients? 2. Were all clinically important outcomes considered? 3. Are the likely treatment benefits worth the potential harms and costs?

validity criteria protects against bias, because systematic reviews suggest that lack of blinding and concealment (see Table 8.4) may lead to systematic overestimation of treatment effects although the effects may differ by clinical specialty only (Balk et al. 2002; Moher et al. 1998).

The CURE investigators achieved a follow-up of greater than 99.9% (only 13 out of 12,562 patients were lost) and analyzed patients in the group they were assigned according to the intention to treat principle. The intention to treat principle refers to analysis of patient outcomes based on which group they were randomized regardless of whether they actually received the planned intervention. This analysis preserves the power of randomization, thus maintaining that important unknown factors that influence outcome are likely equally distributed in each comparison group.

The evaluation of clinical research results requires an understanding of measures of association or effect. As noted above clinical epidemiologists often use terms that are different from those of classical epidemiologists (see relative risk reduction and number needed to treat below in this section). Table 8.5 summarizes the measures we will now describe in more detail (cf. Chapter I.2 of this handbook).

Absolute Risk

The easiest measure of risk to understand in clinical epidemiology is the absolute risk. In the CURE trial, the main outcomes were a composite of death from cardiovascular causes, nonfatal myocardial infarction (MI), or stroke and a composite of death from cardiovascular causes, nonfatal MI, stroke, or refractory ischemia. Safety outcomes included major and minor bleeding. We will focus on the latter composite endpoint. The absolute risk for this combined primary endpoint was 16.5%, and the absolute risk for this outcome in the control group was 18.8% (Table 8.5). As described above, other terminology for the risk of an adverse outcome in the control group are baseline risk, absolute risk, or control event rate.

Absolute Risk Reduction

One can express treatment effects as the difference between the absolute risks in the experimental and control groups, the absolute risk reduction or the risk difference. This effect measure represents the proportion of patients spared from the unfavorable outcome if they receive the experimental therapy (clopidogrel), rather than the control therapy (placebo). In our example, the absolute risk reduction is 18.8% − 16.5% = 2.3 percentage points.

Relative Risk

The relative risk or risk ratio presents the proportion of the baseline risk in the control group that still is present when patients receive the experimental treatment (clopidogrel). The relative risk of the combined outcome after receiving clopidogrel is 1035/(1035 + 5224) divided by 1187/(1187 + 5116) (the risk in the control group), or 0.87. One could also say the risk of experiencing the combined outcome with clopidogrel and aspirin is approximately 87% of that with aspirin alone.

Table 8.5. Measures of association and effect

General 2 × 2 Table

	Outcome		Absolute risk of outcome:
	+	−	
Intervention (Y)	a	b	Intervention = $a/(a + b) = Y$
Control (X)	c	d	Control = $c/(c + d) = X$

2 × 2 Table for the Example from CURE et al. (CURE-Investigators 2001)

	Combined primary outcome		Absolute risk of outcome
	+	−	
Clopidogrel	1035	5224	Clopidogrel = $1035/(1035 + 5224)$
			= 16.5%
Placebo	1187	5116	Placebo = $1187/(1187 + 5116)$
			= 18.8%

Absolute risk reduction (ARR)
Definition: The difference in risk between the control group and the intervention group
ARR = $c/(c + d) - a/(a + b) = X - Y$
Example:
ARR = $1035/(1035 + 5224) - 1187/(1187 + 5116) = 2.3\%$

Relative risk or risk ratio (RR)
Definition: The ratio of risk in the intervention (Y) to the risk in the control group (X)
RR = Y/X
Example:
RR = $(1035/(1035 + 5224))/(1187/(1187 + 5116)) = 0.87$

Relative Risk Reduction (RRR)
Definition: The percent reduction in risk in the intervention compared to the control group
RRR = $1 - RR = (1 - X/Y) \times 100\%$ or
RRR = $[(X - Y)/X] \times 100\%$
Example:
RRR = $(1 - 0.87) \times 100\% = 13\%$

Number Needed to Treat (NNT)
Definition: Inverse of the ARR
NNT = $1/ARR = 1/(X - Y)$
Example:
NNT = $1/2.3\% = 44$

Relative Risk Reduction

The most commonly reported measure of dichotomous treatment effects is the complement of this relative risk, the relative risk reduction. One can obtain the relative risk reduction easily from the relative risk because it is the proportion of baseline risk that is removed by the experimental therapy and it is equivalent to 1.0 − relative risk. It can be expressed as a percent: (1 − relative risk) × 100 = (1 − 0.87) × 100 = 13% or 100% − 87% = 13% for this example. Alternatively, one may obtain the relative risk reduction by dividing the absolute risk reduction by the absolute risk in the control group. Therefore, the result is the same if it is calculated from 2.3% (the absolute risk reduction) divided by 18.8% (the risk in the control group) = 0.13 (13%). A relative risk reduction of 13% means that clopidogrel reduced the risk of combined outcome by 13% relative to that occurring among control patients. The greater the relative risk reduction, the more efficacious is the therapy. Investigators may compute the relative risk over a period of time, as in a survival analysis, and call it a hazard ratio, the weighted relative risk over the entire study (see Chap. II.4 of this handbook).

In fact, the CURE investigators calculated the hazard ratio which was slightly more in favor of clopidogrel (0.86). For practical purposes we use the relative risk for the CURE trial in our example. If we had used the hazard ratio for the calculation of the RR the RRR would have been 14%.

Odds Ratio

Instead of evaluating the risk of an event, one can estimate the odds of having an event compared with not having an event. Most individuals are familiar with odds in the context of sporting events, when sport reporters describe the odds of a team or player winning a particular event. When odds are used in the medical sciences it stands for the proportion of patients with the target outcome divided by the proportion without the target outcome. The odds in the control group of the example trial described are 1187 of 6303 divided by 5116 of 6303. Because the denominator is the same in both the numerator and the denominator, it is canceled out, leaving the number of patients with the event (1187) divided by the number of patients without the event (5116). The odds are 1187/5116 or 0.232. To convert from odds to risk, one divides the odds by 1 plus the odds. As the odds of the combined endpoint are 0.232, the risk is 0.232/(1 + 0.232), or 0.188 (18.8%), identical to the baseline risk reported in the CURE trial. Table 8.6 presents the link between risk and odds. The greater the risk, the greater is the divergence between the risk and odds. Odds and risk are about equal if the absolute risk is small.

In the CURE trial, the odds of the combined endpoint in the clopidgrel group are 1035 (those with the outcome) compared with 5224 (those without the outcome), or 1035/5224 = 0.198, and the odds of the combined endpoint in the placebo group are 0.232. Therefore, the ratio of these odds is (1035/5224)/(1187/5116), or 0.854. If one used a terminology parallel to risk (note, that epidemiologists call a ratio of risks in most instances a relative risk), one would call the ratio of odds relative odds. The commonly used term, however, is odds ratio (OR). Until recently the

Table 8.6. Relation between risks and odds

Risk	Risk (proportion)	Odds
80%	0.80	4.0000
60%	0.60	1.5000
50%	0.50	1.0000
40%	0.40	0.6667
33%	0.33	0.5000
25%	0.25	0.3333
20%	0.20	0.2500
10%	0.10	0.1111
5%	0.05	0.0526
1%	0.01	0.0101

odds ratio has been the most popular measure of association. The reason for the use of the odds ratio is that the odds ratio has a statistical advantage because it essentially is independent of the choice between a comparison of the risks of an event (such as death) or the analogous non-event (such as survival), which is not true of the relative risk.

However, clinicians do not easily understand a ratio of odds. Clinicians would like to be able to substitute the relative risk, because it is more intuitively understandable, for the odds ratio. As shown in Table 8.6, as the risk decreases, the odds and risk come closer together. For low event rates, the odds ratio and relative risk are very close. In fact, if the risk is below 25%, odds and risks are approximately equal and many authors calculate relative odds and then report the results as if they calculated relative risks. One can see from the example that the odds ratio of 0.85 is very similar to the relative risk of 0.87. Clinicians should be aware that if events are frequent in either the control group or experimental group, odds ratios can be a very inaccurate estimate of the relative risk. The RR and OR also will be more similar when the treatment effect is small (OR and relative risk are close to 1.0) than when the treatment effect is large. When considering RR, HR and OR, the RR is always closest to unity; the odds ratio is farthest away; and the HR is intermediate (Symons and Moore 2002). These differences can become large when effect sizes increase. When event rates are high and effect sizes are large, there are ways of converting the odds ratio to relative risk. Fortunately, clinicians will need to do this infrequently. One note of caution is that typical case control studies do not yield relative risks.

The Number Needed to Treat

Having seen that making a distinction between odds ratio and relative risk rarely will be important when evaluating clinical research, because high event rates are rare, one must give much more attention to distinguishing between the odds ratio or relative risk compared with the absolute risk reduction. Let us assume that the absolute risk of experiencing the combined outcome would be twice as high in both groups in the CURE trial. This could have happened if the investigators had conducted a study in patients at greater risk for the endpoint, for example by restricting the study population to older patients. In the clopidogrel group, the absolute risk would become 33% compared with 37.6% in the control group. Therefore, the absolute risk reduction would increase from 2.3% to 4.6% whereas the relative risk (and therefore the relative risk reduction) would remain identical at 33% divided by 37.6% = 0.87 (the relative risk reduction remains 13%). Therefore, the increase in the proportion of those experiencing the endpoint in both groups by a factor of 2 leaves the relative risk (and the relative risk reduction) unchanged, but increases the absolute risk reduction by a factor of 2.

A 13% reduction in the relative risk of the combined endpoint may not sound very impressive, however, its impact on patient groups and practice may be large. This notion is shown using the concept of the number needed to treat, the number of patients who must receive an intervention during a specific period to prevent one additional adverse outcome or produce one positive outcome (Laupacis et al. 1988). When discussing the number needed to treat, it is important to specify the treatment, its duration, and the outcome being prevented. The number needed to treat is the inverse of the absolute risk reduction, calculated as 1/absolute risk reduction. Therefore, in the example above with an absolute risk reduction of 4.6%, the number needed to treat would be 22 (1/4.6%) and it would be 44 (1/2.3%) in the CURE trial. Finally, imagine young patients with no additional risk factors for adverse outcomes. Such patients may carry a baseline risk of 4% for experiencing the endpoint and, therefore, the number needed to treat could increase to 192 [1/(0.13 × 4%)]. Given the duration, potential harms and cost of treatment with clopidogrel and the increased risk for bleeding, it could be reasonable to withhold therapy in that latter patient. Unfortunately, we do not know how best to present risk information to patients. Presenting the relative risk reduction alone is more persuasive for making actual or hypothetical medical decisions, because the actual benefit appears larger (Bucher et al. 1994; Edwards and Elwyn 1999; Edwards et al. 1999). Thus, direct to patient advertising and pharmaceutical industry detailing uses relative risk reduction as measure of effect to persuade clinicians and patients to use drug interventions. However, omitting the presentation of baseline risk or not informing those who receive this information that the baseline risk drives the absolute benefit is misleading.

How Clinicians Can Use Confidence Intervals

Until now we presented the results of the CURE trial as if they represented the true effect. The results of any experiment, however, represent only an estimate of the truth. The true effect of treatment actually may be somewhat smaller, or larger, than what researchers found. The confidence interval (CI) tells, within the bounds of plausibility, how much smaller or greater the true effect is likely to be. For each of the measures described, one can use statistical programs to calculate confidence intervals.

The point estimate within the confidence interval and the confidence interval itself help with two questions. First, what is the one value most likely to represent the true difference between treatment and control; and second, given the difference between treatment and control, what is the plausible range of differences within which the true effect might actually lie? The smaller the sample size or the number of events in an experiment, the wider the confidence interval. As the sample size gets very large and the number of events increases, investigators become increasingly certain that the truth is not far from the point estimate and, therefore, the confidence interval is narrower.

One can interpret the 95% confidence interval as "what is the range of values of probabilities within which, 95% of the time, the truth would lie?". If investigators or clinicians would not need to be so certain, one could ask about the range within which the true value would lie 90% of the time. This 90% confidence interval would be somewhat narrower.

How does the confidence interval facilitate interpretation of the results from the CURE trial? As described above, the confidence interval represents the range of values within the truth plausibly lies. Accordingly, one way to use confidence intervals is to look at the boundary of the interval that represents the lowest plausible treatment effect and decide whether the action or recommendation would change compared with when one assumes the point estimate represents the truth. Based on the numbers provided in the CURE trial, one can calculate a confidence interval around the point estimate of the relative risk reduction of 13% ranging from approximately 6 to 21%. Values progressively farther from 13% will be less and less likely. One can conclude that patients receiving clopidogrel are less likely to experience the combined endpoint – but the magnitude of the difference may be either quite small (and not outweigh the increased risk of bleeding) or quite large. This way of understanding the results avoids the yes/no dichotomy of testing a hypothesis. Because the lower limit of the CI is associated with a benefit, certainty about beneficial treatment effects from clopidogrel on the combined endpoint is relatively high. However, toxicity and expense will bear on the final treatment decision.

The chief toxicitiy of clopidogrel the authors of the CURE trial were concerned about was bleeding. They found that the absolute risk increase (ARI – conceptually similar to the absolute risk reduction but indicating an increase in risk from the investigational therapy) for major bleeding was 1 percentage point (an increase from 2.7% in the placebo group to 3.7% in the clopidogrel group). The investigators defined major bleeding as substantially disabling bleeding, intraocular bleeding or the loss of vision, or bleeding necessitating the transfusion of at least 2 units of blood. Similarly to the number needed to treat we can calculate the number of patients who must receive an intervention during a specific period to cause one additional harmful outcome. The number needed to harm (NNH) for major bleeding in the CURE trial is equal to 1/ARI or 1/0.01 = 100. The authors also provided the information for minor bleeding which they defined as hemorrhages that led to interruption of the study medication but did not qualify as major bleeding. The risk for minor bleeding was 5.1% in the clopidogrel group compared to 2.4% in the placebo group. Thus, the NNH for minor bleeding was 1/0.027 = 37. Clinicians should keep in mind that estimates of harm also come with uncertainty and, therefore, authors usually present confidence intervals around these harmful effects.

Use of Composite Endpoints

Investigators often use a composition of endpoints when they compare interventions. For example, the CURE trial investigators used a composite endpoint of death from cardiovascular causes, nonfatal MI, stroke, or refractory ischemia. Safety outcomes included major and minor bleeding with the definitions described in the foregoing paragraph. There are a number of reasons for combining several endpoints. First, investigators may believe that distinguishing between outcomes is unnecessary because the endpoints have the same consequences. For example, many investigators combine the outcome ischemic stroke with hemorrhagic stroke because they believe they may be similarly disabling (Lubsen and Kirwan 2002). Second, investigators may chose composite endpoints to avoid misleading conclusion when an intervention reduced an endpoint (usually less severe) by increasing another endpoint (usually more severe) that precludes patients from suffering the less severe endpoint. For example, surgery for cerebrovascular disease could reduce strokes by directly killing those at highest risk for stroke (those who die at surgery are no longer at risk for strokes) (van Walraven et al. 2002). Thus, the use of stroke alone as the endpoint would be misleading. To avoid an erroneous conclusion, an investigator facing this situation must combine the more and less serious outcomes, creating an endpoint such as "stroke or death". Third, investigators chose to combine endpoints because of the reduced sample size when event rates increase, as one would expect for a combined endpoint. The latter is the probably reason why the CURE investigators used a combined efficacy endpoint.

Using composite endpoints has a number of implications. The most obvious implication is that if these endpoints have different importance to patient (that is, patients have different underlying values and preferences for these outcomes) treating them as equally important is an oversimplification.

Using combined endpoints does not always support reaching conclusive results in clinical trials. Freemantle et al. (2003) reported on the use of composite endpoints in 167 trials published between 1997 and 2001 in 9 leading medical journals. The authors found that in 69 of these trials the difference between treatment arms in the CEP was not statistically significant. Investigators sometimes included component endpoints that reduced trial efficiency by diluting the treatment effect. For example, Freemantle and colleagues described that the CAPRICORN [CArvedilol Post-infaRct survIval COntRol in LV dysfunctioN] trial investigated the effects of carvedilol, a β-blocker, in 1959 patients with left ventricular dysfunction following myocardial infarction (The CAPRICORN Investigators 2001). Originally, the CAPRICORN investigators identified all-cause mortality as primary outcome in the trial protocol. However, while the study was ongoing, the data and safety monitoring board (whose assignment is to protect the patients in a trial) noted that the overall rate of mortality was lower than that predicted for the power analysis and sample size calculation. The board informed the CAPRICORN steering committee of the trial's insufficient power to identify the primary end point as significant (a preset level of significance α of 0.05). Taking the uncommon measure of altering the primary outcome, the steering committee defined a new composite outcome (all-cause mortality or cardiovascular hospital admissions). The steering committee assigned a critical level of significance of $\alpha = 0.045$ to this new composite outcome that they introduced while the trial was ongoing and reduced the significance level of the original primary outcome to achieve statistical significance to $\alpha = 0.005$. They reduced the level of α of the original primary outcome to penalize their retrospective action, but the board decided that if the p-value for either primary outcome achieved statistical significance at the new critical level, the study would be deemed positive.

At the end of the study, the original primary end point (all-cause mortality) achieved a p-value of 0.03 (ie, substantially larger than the new 0.005 allocated after consultation from the data safety and monitoring board, but smaller than the original critical level of significance), but the alternative primary outcome achieved a p-value of 0.30. Thus, the original primary outcome did not reach statistical significance at the new and more stringent level and neither did the new composite outcome. Although 12% of patients died in the carvedilol group, compared with 15% in the placebo group, 23% of patients in the carvedilol group and 22% of patients in the placebo group qualified for the composite outcome on the basis of hospitalizations alone, a result that undermined the relatively small reduction in mortality in the carvedilol group. Thus, CAPRICORN provides a neutral result, although the study would have been modestly statistically significant had the original primary outcome of all-cause mortality been maintained.

In summary, evaluating trials that use composite outcome requires scrutiny in regards to the underlying reasons for combining endpoints and its implications and has impact on medical decision making (see below in Sect. 8.8).

Systematic Reviews 8.6

The patient in our scenario took aspirin at a dose of 325 mg on admission. Aspirin use is associated with gastrointestinal bleeding and the risk for bleeding increases with the aspirin dose used (García Rodríguez et al. 2001; Weil et al. 1995). On the other hand, the beneficial effects of lower doses of aspirin on cardiovascular events likely does not differ from those of higher doses (Antithrombotic Trialists' Collaboration 2002). Taken together, studies comparing higher and lower doses of aspirin show similar effects. However, a clinician would ask the question "Which of the available studies should I trust and consider for decision making?". Even for clinicians trained in critical appraisal, evaluating all available studies would be a time-intensive solution.

Traditionally, clinicians – when they did not invest the time and resources to review individual studies – have relied on review articles by authorities in the field. However, experts may be unsystematic in their approach to summarizing the evidence. Unsystematic approaches to identification and collection of evidence risks biased ascertainment. That is, treatment effects may be underestimated or, more commonly, overestimated, and side effects may be exaggerated or ignored. Even if the evidence has been identified and collected in a systematic fashion, if reviewers are then unsystematic in the way they summarize the collected evidence, they run similar risks of bias. In one study, self-rated expertise was inversely related to the methodologic rigor of the review (Oxman and Guyatt 1993). One result of unsystematic approaches may be recommendations advocating harmful treatment; in other cases, there may be a failure to encourage effective therapy. For example, experts supported routine use of lidocaine for patients with acute myocardial infarction when available data suggested the intervention was ineffective and possibly even harmful, and they failed to recommend thrombolytic agents for the treatment of acute myocardial infarction when data showed patient benefit (Antman et al. 1992).

Systematic reviews deal with this problem by explicitly stating inclusion and exclusion criteria for evidence to be considered, conducting a comprehensive search for the evidence, and summarizing the results according to explicit rules that include examining how effects may vary in different patient subgroups. When a systematic review pools data across studies to provide a quantitative estimate of overall treatment effect, we call this summary a meta-analysis (cf. Chap. II.7 of this handbook). Systematic reviews provide strong evidence when the quality of the primary study design is high and sample sizes are large; they provide weaker evidence when study designs are poor and sample sizes are small. Because judgment is involved in many steps in a systematic review (including specifying inclusion and exclusion criteria, applying these criteria to potentially eligible studies, evaluating the methodologic quality of the primary studies, and selecting an approach to data analysis), systematic reviews are not immune to bias, for example publication bias.

Nevertheless, in their rigorous approach to identifying and summarizing data, systematic reviews reduce the likelihood of bias in estimating the causal links between management options and patient outcomes.

Over the past 10 to 15 years, the literature describing the methods used in systematic reviews, including studies that provide an empiric basis for guiding decisions about the methods used in summarizing evidence has rapidly expanded. Clinical epidemiologists have contributed significantly to this development (Egger et al. 2000).

Table 8.7 demonstrates the process of conducting systematic reviews.

As we described above for answering questions in clinical practice (see also Table 8.1), investigators who conduct a systematic review should begin by formulating a clinical question. This question formulation constitutes the essential specific selection criteria for deciding which studies to include in a review. These criteria define the population, the exposures or interventions, the comparison intervention, and the outcomes of interest. A systematic review will also restrict the included studies to those that meet minimal methodologic standards. For example, systematic reviews that address a question of therapy will often include only randomized controlled trials.

Table 8.7. The process of conducting systematic reviews

Define the question

— Specify inclusion and exclusion criteria
  — Population
  — Intervention or exposure (and comparison)
  — Outcome
  — Methodology

— Establish a priori hypotheses to explain heterogeneity

Conduct literature search

— Decide on information resources: databases, experts, funding agencies, pharmaceutical companies, hand-searching, personal files, registries, citation lists or retrieved articles
— Determine restrictions: time frame, unpublished data, language
— Identify titles and abstracts

Apply inclusion and exclusion criteria

— Apply inclusion and exclusion criteria to titles and abstracts
— Obtain full articles for eligible titles and abstracts
— Apply inclusion and exclusion criteria to full articles
— Select final eligible articles
— Assess agreement on study selection

Create data abstraction

— Data abstraction: participants, interventions, comparison interventions, study design
— Results
— Methodologic quality
— Assess agreement on validity assessment between data abstractors

Conduct analysis

— Determine method for pooling results
— Pool results (if appropriate)
— Decide on handling of missing data

Having evaluated the potential eligibility of titles and abstracts, and obtained the full text of potentially eligible studies, reviewers apply the selection criteria to the complete reports. Having completed the data collection process, they assess the methodologic quality of the eligible articles and abstract data from each study. Finally, they summarize the data, including, if appropriate, a quantitative synthesis or meta-analysis. The analysis includes an examination of differences among the included studies, an attempt to explain differences in results (exploring heterogeneity), a summary of the overall results, and an assessment of their precision and validity. Guidelines for assessing the validity of reviews and using the results correspond to this process and are available (Oxman et al. 2002).

Returning to our example, the question you want to address could be formulated as: "In patients with coronary artery disease does low dose aspirin (75 mg daily or less) compared with high dose aspirin (325 mg daily or more) confer similar mortality benefits". Keep in mind that gastrointestinal side effects are more likely with higher doses of aspirin.

A prudent clinician will look for a systematic review to answer this question. A recent systematic review by the Antithrombotic Trialists' Collaboration provides useful information to answer this question (Antithrombotic Trialists' Collaboration 2002). The investigators carefully evaluated 448 trials for inclusion and finally performed a meta-analysis of 195 trials of antiplatelet effects in cardiovascular disease. Overall they observed that aspirin markedly reduced the risk of recurrent events in patients with acute myocardial infarction (odds ratio 0.7) and patients with previous myocardial infarction (odds ratio 0.75). They identified three trials in patients at high risk for cardiovascular events that compared doses of aspirin of $\leq$ 75 mg daily to higher doses. Higher doses of aspirin conferred no additional benefit in preventing cardiovascular events when compared with lower doses. In fact the point estimate indicated a benefit of lower doses of aspirin (relative odds reduction 8%). However, these results were not statistically significant (95% CI ranging from approximately -12% indicating a slight benefit with higher doses to 28% indicating a benefit with lower doses). When the investigators compared the effects of low dose aspirin versus placebo and higher dose aspirin versus placebo the effects were similar. Although the evidence from direct comparisons is limited and the investigators included additional patient populations, such as patients with stroke, the systematic review and meta-analysis of all available trials provides additional indirect evidence for comparable effects of higher and low dose aspirin. Most clinicians would judge the biology for the role of aspirin in coronary artery disease and other cardiovascular disease to be sufficiently similar to have confidence in this extrapolation. Combining the available evidence in a properly conducted systematic review helps the clinician to obtain answers that are valid and based on methodological evaluation of the literature. Chapter II.7 of this handbook addresses methodological issues related to meta-analysis.

Having explained some of the benefits of systematic reviews we will explain how systematic reviews can be used to guide patient care. Available guidance on therapeutic or prevention goes beyond systematic reviews, because factors in addition to the quality of the evidence and treatment effects are important to make recommendations about treatment (Freemantle et al. 1999). However, systematic reviews should be conducted in the process of generating evidence-based guidelines that provide treatment recommendations.

8.7 Guidelines

Guidelines are systematically developed syntheses to support practitioners and patients in decision making about specific clinical circumstances. The key elements of each synthesis include the scope of the guidelines, the interventions and practices considered, the major recommendations and the and strength of the evidence and recommendations, and the underlying values and preferences (Guyatt et al. 2002a, 2004b; Schünemann et al. 2004). A list of guidelines maintained by the US Agency for Healthcare Research and Quality is available at the National Guidelines Clearinghouse (National-Guideline-Clearing-House 2004).

Organizations such as professional societies or governing boards, government agencies, academic or private institutions, typically develop guidelines by convening expert panels. Usually, guideline developers will define the topic of a guideline before evaluating the evidence for clinical sensible questions. Dialogue among clinicians, patients, and the prospective users of the guideline contribute to its refinement. Although it is possible to develop guidelines that are broad in scope, it requires considerable time and resources.

One method of defining and focusing the clinical questions of interest and also identifying the processes for which evidence needs to be collected and assessed is the construction of models or causal pathways (Woolf 1994). The causal pathway is a diagram showing the relation of the population, intervention(s) of interest and the intermediate, surrogate or definitive health outcomes (Shekelle et al. 1999). When designing the pathway, guideline developers should describe explicitly which outcomes (benefits and harms) they consider important and the associated values. This process reveals specific questions that the evidence must address and where high quality evidence is lacking, identifying areas for additional research.

While investigators have not tested alternative approaches to guideline development, one suggestion is to include all groups whose activities would be covered by the guidelines and any others with legitimate reasons for having input (Shekelle et al. 1999). A group size of six to 15 individuals with clearly identified roles, including group leader and members, specialist resource, technical support, and administrative support may be advisable (Shekelle et al. 1999). The group should comprise members proficient in the following areas: literature searching and retrieval, epidemiology, biostatistics, health services research, clinical area of interest (generalists and specialists), group process, writing, and editing.

A high-quality clinical practice guideline produced by such groups should consider the following steps (Schünemann et al. 2004):

1. Define explicit criteria to search for evidence. Similar to the clinical sensible questions identified above for searching the evidence and conducting systematic reviews, this step should include a clear definition of the population, the intervention and comparison intervention and the outcome of interest. The development of a clinical pathway helps in identifying the components of the clinical question and in identifying gaps.

2. Define explicit eligibility criteria for the identified evidence. Guideline development groups should define eligibility criteria for the evidence that they wish to include. Examples include restricting evidence to randomized controlled trials or studies that have used validated instruments for functional outcomes or assessed mortality.

3. Conduct or use comprehensive searches for evidence. A guideline development group should ensure that they conduct a complete evaluation of the evidence. The group may either use a high quality systematic review developed by others or conduct their own systematic review for each recommendation they make in their guideline.

4. Perform a standard consideration of study quality. If a systematic review is identified that answers the group's clinical question and may suffice for developing the guideline, the group should still consider an evaluation of the individual study quality. Should the group conduct a systematic review or update an existing review, the evaluation of study quality becomes an essential step in conducting a systematic review. Quality evaluation includes looking at the basic study design, the detailed study design and execution, and the directness of evidence. The directness of the evidence refers to reporting of surrogate outcomes, for example deep venous thrombosis by ultrasonography as risk factor for fatal events, versus outcomes such as mortality.

5. Summarize the evidence. Guideline development groups who use high quality systematic reviews often will find meta-analysis of studies included in the systematic review. The summaries help in obtaining estimates of intervention effects. It is important to note that summary estimates should be available for all important outcomes, both beneficial and harmful. Ideally the summary estimates also would be available for cost.

6. Acknowledge values and preferences underlying the group's recommendations. Many guideline reports take for granted that guideline developers adequately represent patients' interests. The latter is not necessarily correct and there is a risk that, for example, a specialty society may recommend procedures where the benefits may not outweigh the risks or costs (Woolf et al. 1999). For example, the American Urologic Society and the American Cancer Society recommend prostate cancer screening with prostate specific antigen (PSA) for men older then 50 while the American College of Preventive Medicine and the US Preventive Task Force Services (USPSTF) do not make this recommendation (American Urological Association 2000; Ferrini and Woolf 1998; Smith et al. 2003; USPSTF 2002). Thus, there should be clear statements about which principles, such as patient autonomy, nonmaleficence, or distributive justice, were given priority in guiding decisions about the value of alternative interventions to inform users of the guidelines (Shekelle et al. 1999). Guidelines should report whether it is intended to optimize values for individual patients, reimbursement agencies, or society as a whole. Groups that ensure representation by experts in research methodology, practicing generalists and specialists, and public representatives are more likely to have considered diverse views in their discussions than groups limited to content area experts.

7. Grade the strength of recommendations. Because clinicians are interested in the strength of a recommendation and the balance of benefits and risks, the next section is devoted to recommendations and the grading of the strength of recommendations.

Recommendations

Treatment decisions involve balancing likely benefits against harms and costs. Evidence-based guidelines and treatment recommendations are systematic syntheses of the best available evidence that provide clinicians with guidance for treating average patients in clinical practice. To integrate recommendations with their own clinical judgment, clinicians need to understand the basis for the clinical recommendations that experts offer them. A common systematic approach to grading the strength of treatment recommendations can minimize bias and aid interpretation.

As part of the first American College of Chest Physician (ACCP) Consensus Conference on Antithrombotic Treatment in 1986, Sackett suggested a formal rating scheme, derived from the Canadian Task Force on the Periodic Health Examination, for assessing levels of evidence (Canadian 1979; Sackett 1986). During the past 15 years, clinical epidemiologists from McMaster University have lead the evolution of these "rules of evidence" (Cook et al. 1992; Guyatt et al. 1995, 2001, 2002a, b), which experts have applied to generate grades of recommendations.

The strength of any recommendation depends on two factors: the trade-off between benefits and downsides and the quality of the methodology that leads to estimates of the treatment effect. The ACCP approach to grading of recommendations captures the magnitude of random error in the decision about the confidence in the tradeoff between benefits, harms and cost. The uncertainty associated with this tradeoff will determine the strength of recommendations. The grades that experts generate using the ACCP approach are 1A, 1C+, 1B, 1C, 2A, 2C+, 2B and 2C (Table 8.8). If experts are very certain that benefits do, or do not, outweigh harms and cost, they will make a strong recommendation – in the ACCP formulation, Grade 1. If they are less certain of the magnitude of the benefits and harms, and thus their relative impact, they must make a weaker Grade 2 recommendation. Grade 2 recommendations are those in which variation in patient values or individual physician values often will mandate different treatment choices, even among average or typical patients. The ACCP approach expresses the primacy of the benefit versus downxside judgment by placing it first in the grade of recommendation.

However, today a number of organizations other than the ACCP, including the US Preventive Services Task Force (Harris et al. 2001), the US Task Force on Community Preventive Services (Briss et al. 2000), Scottish Intercollegiate Guidelines Network (SIGN) (Harbour and Miller 2001), the National Institute for Clinical Excellence (NICE), and more than 100 other groups use various systems of codes to communicate grades of evidence and recommendations. All these organizations have definitions of varying length and detail for each letter or number code and a few use single words, such as "Strong" or "Weak", in addition to or in place of a code.

Health care practitioners, in particular learners, are often puzzled by the message the grade of these systems convey. For example, the administration of oral anticoagulation in patients with atrial fibrillation and rheumatic mitral valve dis-

Table 8.8. ACCP approach to grades of recommendations

Grade of recommendation	Clarity of risk/benefit	Methodologic strength of supporting evidence	Implications
1 A	Risk/benefit clear	RCTs without important limitations	Strong recommendation, can apply to most patients in most circumstances without reservation
1 C+	Risk/benefit clear	No RCTs but strong RCT results can be unequivocally extrapolated, or overwhelming evidence from observational studies	Strong recommendation, can apply to most patients in most circumstances
1 B	Risk/benefit clear	RCTs with important limitations (inconsistent results, methodological flaws)*	Strong recommendations, likely to apply to most patients
1 C	Risk/benefit clear	Observational studies	Intermediate strength recommendation; may change when stronger evidence available
2 A	Risk/benefit unclear	RCTs without important limitations	Intermediate strength recommendation, best action may differ depending on circumstances or patients' or societal values
2 C+	Risk/benefit unclear	No RCTs but strong RCT results can be unequivocally extrapolated, or overwhelming evidence from observational studies	Weak recommendation, best action may differ depending on circumstances or patients' or societal values
2 B	Risk/benefit unclear	RCTs with important limitations (inconsistent results, methodological flaws)*	Weak recommendation, alternative approaches likely to be better for some patients under some circumstances
2 C	Risk/benefit unclear	Observational studies	Very weak recommendations; other alternatives may be equally reasonable

* These situations include RCTs (randomized clinical trials) with both lack of blinding and subjective outcomes, where the risk of bias in measurement of outcomes is high, or RCTs with large loss to follow up.

Note: Since studies in categories B and C are flawed, it is likely that most recommendations in these classes will be level 2.

The following considerations will bear on whether the recommendation is Grade 1 or 2: the magnitude and precision of the treatment effect, patients' risk of the target event being prevented, the nature of the benefit, and the magnitude of the risk associated with treatment, variability in patient preferences, variability in regional resource availability and health care delivery practices, and cost considerations (see Table 8.2). Inevitably, weighing these considerations involves subjective judgment (reproduced with permission from Guyatt et al. (2004a).)

ease receives various grades of recommendation from different organizations. Oral anticoagulation in these patients is recommended as Class I based on level B evidence by the American Heart Association (ACC 2001), as a grade C recommendation based on level IV evidence by SIGN (http://www.guidelines.gov/) and as grade 1C+, where the 1 indicates the balance between benefit and downsides and C+ the methodological quality of the underlying evidence, by the American College of Chest Physicians (Albers et al. 2001). It is therefore possible that the different grading systems do not fulfill their intended function: to quickly and concisely communicate a clear message. In particular, if the same code, used by different systems, represents different meanings, bewilderment and incomprehension may result.

A group of guideline developers and clinical epidemiologists formed the Grades or Recommendation Assessment, Development and Evaluation (GRADE) Working Group with the hope of reaching agreement on a common, sensible approach to grading the quality of evidence and strength of recommendations (Atkins et al. 2004; Schünemann et al. 2003). The group has defined grade of evidence as indicating the extent to which one can be confident that an estimate of effect is correct and grades of recommendations as indicating the extent to which one can be confident that adherence to a recommendation will do more good than harm. The Grade group suggests that those developing recommendations should make sequential judgments about the quality of evidence for each important outcome, the overall quality of evidence across outcomes, and the recommendations. Judgments about the quality of evidence require consideration of study design, study quality, consistency and directness of the evidence. Additional considerations include reporting bias, sparse data and strength of associations. Judgments about recommendations require consideration of the balance between benefits and harms, the quality of the evidence, translation of the evidence into specific circumstances, and the certainty of the baseline risk. Recommendations should consider costs (resource utilization) as well as benefits and harms. The GRADE group further concludes that inconsistencies among systems for grading evidence and formulating recommendations reduce their potential to facilitate critical appraisal and improve communication of these judgments, and suggests a system that is new (though bears many similarities to the ACCP approach) that they hope will receive wide adoption.

Returning to our clinical scenario and applying the ACCP approach to grading of recommendation (ideally one will apply the GRADE approach when available), the use of clopidogrel in addition to aspirin would generate a 2A recommendation where the 2 indicates that the individual preferences and values influence the treatment decision and the A denomination indicates that evidence stems from one or more high-quality randomized controlled trials.

In the next section we will describe the importance of health related quality of life (HRQL) outcomes followed by a section on integrating patient preferences in decision making and how clinical epidemiology is key in obtaining patients' preferences and values.

Health Related Quality of Life Instruments and Their Application in Clinical Studies

8.8

Clinical journals have published trials in which HRQL instruments are the primary outcome measures. With the expanding importance of HRQL in evaluating new therapeutic interventions, investigators (and readers) are faced with a large array of instruments. Researchers have proposed different ways of categorizing these instruments, according to the purpose of their use, into instruments designed for screening, providing health profiles, measuring preference, and making clinical decisions (Osoba et al. 1991), or into discriminative and evaluative instruments.

We have also suggested a taxonomy based on the domains of HRQL which an instrument attempts to cover (Guyatt et al. 1989). According to this taxonomy, a HRQL instrument may be categorized, in a broad sense, as generic or specific. *Generic instruments* cover (or at least aim to cover) the complete spectrum of function, disability, and distress of the patient, and are applicable to a variety of populations. Within the framework of generic instruments, health profiles and utility measures provide two distinct approaches to measurement of global quality-of-life. *Specific instruments* are focused on disease or treatment issues specifically relevant to the question at hand.

8.8.1   Generic Instruments

Health Profiles

Health profiles are single instruments that measure multiple different aspects of quality-of-life. They usually provide a scoring system that allows aggregation of the results into a small number of scores and sometimes into a single score (in which case, it may be referred to as an index). As generic measures, their design allows their use in a wide variety of conditions. For example, one health profile, the Sickness Impact Profile (SIP) contains 12 "categories" which can be aggregated into two dimensions and five independent categories, and also into a single overall score (Bergner et al. 1981). The SIP has been used in studies of cardiac rehabilitation (Ott et al. 1983), total hip joint arthroplasty (Liang et al. 1985), and treatment of back pain (Deyo et al. 1986). In addition to the SIP, there are a number of other health profiles available: the Nottingham Health Profile (Hunt et al. 1980), the Duke-UNC Health Profile (Parkerson et al. 1981), and the McMaster Health Index Questionnaire (Sackett et al. 1977). Increasingly, a collection of related instruments from the Medical Outcomes Study (Tarlov et al. 1989), has become the most popular and widely-used generic instruments. Particularly popular is one version that includes 36 items, the SF-36 (Brook et al. 1979; Ware et al. 1995; Ware and Sherbourne 1992). The SF-36 is available in over 40 languages and normal values for the general population in many countries are available.

While each health profile attempts to measure all important aspects of HRQL, they may slice the HRQL pie quite differently. For example, the McMaster Health

Index Questionnaire follows the World Health Organization approach and identifies three dimensions: physical, emotional, and social. The Sickness Impact Profile includes a physical dimension (with categories of ambulation, mobility, body care, and movement), a psychosocial dimension (with categories including social interaction and emotional behavior), and five independent categories including eating, work, home management, sleep and rest, and recreations and pastimes.

General health profiles offer a number of advantages clinical investigators. Their reproducibility and validity have been established, often in a variety of populations. When using them for discriminative purposes, one can examine and establish areas of dysfunction affecting a particular population. Identification of these areas of dysfunction may guide investigators who are constructing disease-specific instruments to target areas of potentially greatest impact on the quality-of-life. Health Profiles, used as evaluative instruments, allow determination of the effects of an intervention on different aspects of quality-of-life, without necessitating the use of multiple instruments (and thus saving both the investigator's and the patient's time). Because health profiles are designed for a wide variety of conditions, one can potentially compare the effects on HRQL of different interventions in different diseases. Profiles that provide a single score can be used in a cost-effectiveness analysis, in which the cost of an intervention in dollars is related to its outcome in natural units.

The main limitation of health profiles is that they may not focus adequately on the aspects of quality-of-life specifically influenced by a particular intervention. This may result in an inability of the instrument to detect a real effect in the area of importance (i.e., lack of responsiveness). In fact, disease specific instrument offer greater responsiveness compared with generic instruments (Guyatt et al. 1999; Wiebe et al. 2003). We will return to this issue when we discuss the alternative approach, specific instruments.

Specific Instruments 8.8.2

An alternative approach to HRQL measurement is to focus on aspects of health status that are specific to the area of primary interest. The rationale for this approach lies in the increased responsiveness that may result from including only those aspects of HRQL that are relevant and important in a particular disease process or even in a particular patient situation. One could also focus an instrument only on the areas that are likely to be affected by a particular drug.

In other situations, the instrument may be specific to the disease (instruments for chronic lung disease, for rheumatoid arthritis, for cardiovascular diseases, for endocrine problems, etc.); specific to a population of patients (instruments designed to measure the HRQL of the frail elderly, who are afflicted with a wide variety of different diseases); specific to a certain function (questionnaires which examine emotional or sexual function); or specific to a given condition or problem (such as pain) which can be caused by a variety of underlying pathologies. Within a single condition, the instrument may differ depending on the intervention. For example, while success of a disease-modifying agent in rheumatoid arthritis should result in improved HRQL by enabling a patient to increase performance of physically stressful activities of daily living, occupational therapy may achieve improved HRQL by encouraging family members to take over activities formerly accomplished with difficulty by the patient. Appropriate disease-specific HRQL outcome measures should reflect this difference.

Specific instruments can be constructed to reflect the "single state" (how tired have you been: very tired, somewhat tired, full of energy) or a "transition" (how has your tiredness been: better, the same, worse) (MacKenzie and Charlson 1986). Theoretically, the same could be said of generic instruments, although none of the available generic instruments has used the transition approach. Specific measures can integrate aspects of morbidity, including events such as recurrent myocardial infarction (Olsson et al. 1986).

The disease-specific instruments may be used for discriminative purposes. They may aid, for example, in evaluating the extent to which a primary symptom (for example dyspnea) is related to the magnitude of physiological abnormality (for example exercise capacity) (Mahler et al. 1987). Disease-specific instruments can be applied for evaluative purposes to establish the impact of an intervention on a specific area of dysfunction, and hence aid in elucidating the mechanisms of drug action (Jaeschke et al. 1991). Guidelines provide structured approaches for constructing specific measures (Guyatt et al. 1986). Whatever approaches one takes to the construction of disease-specific measures, a number of head-to-head comparisons between generic and specific instruments suggests that the latter approach will fulfill its promise of enhancing an instrument's responsiveness, the ability to detect change in HRQL (Chang et al. 1991; Goldstein et al. 1994; Laupacis et al. 1991; Smith et al. 1993; Tandon et al. 1989; Tugwell et al. 1990).

In addition to the improved responsiveness, specific measures have the advantage of relating closely to areas routinely explored by the physician. For example, a disease-specific measure of quality-of-life in chronic lung disease focuses on dyspnea during day-to-day activities, fatigue, and areas of emotional dysfunction, including frustration and impatience (Guyatt et al. 1987). Specific measures may therefore appear clinically sensible to the clinician.

The disadvantages of specific measures are that they are (deliberately) not comprehensive, and cannot be used to compare across conditions or, at times, even across programs. This suggests that there is no one group of instruments that will achieve all the potential goals of HRQL measurement. Thus, investigators may choose to use multiple instruments. Some of these instruments are preferences or value instruments that can also be used for clinical decision making described in the next section.

Integrating Patient Preferences in the Decision Making Process and Resolution of the Clinical Scenario

8.9

In reviewing the data from the CURE trial, you conclude that if the patient before you remains untreated, the best estimate of the risk for recurrent myocardial infarction or any of the other endpoints summarized in the composite endpoint in the trial during the next year is 16.5%, and, further, that clopidogrel is likely to decrease this risk by approximately 13%, corresponding to absolute risk reductions (ARR) of 2.3% over a one-year period. As described above, this translates into a number needed to treat (NNT) for 1 year to prevent one of the endpoints summarized in the composite endpoint of approximately 44 for treatment with clopidogrel (Table 8.5).

Examining the likelihood of major bleeding, the CURE trial suggests an absolute risk increase of 1.0%. This estimate translates into a NNH of 100. In light of your knowledge that the patient before you is intelligent, conscientious, and very concerned about his health, you anticipate a high rate of adherence; in addition, you anticipate that the bleeding risk rate of 1% (or the NNT of 100) represents a good estimate for risk of the patient in front of you.

Considering these numbers, you are aware that the treatment decision may depend on the relative value the patient places on avoiding a recurrent myocardial infarction or any of the other endpoints summarized in the composite endpoint in the CURE trial and avoiding a major bleeding including those leading to vision loss. We have pointed out that since there are always advantages and disadvantages to an intervention, evidence alone cannot determine the best course of action. Patients, their proxies, or if a parental approach to decision making is desirable, the clinician as decision-maker, must always trade the benefits, harm, and costs associated with alternative treatment strategies, and values and preferences always bear on those trade-offs. Findings that patients vary greatly in the value they place on different outcomes will come as no surprise. Given this variability in patient's values, clinicians should proceed with great care; it is easy to assume that the patient's values are similar to one's own, yet this may be incorrect. For example, facing a decision concerning anticoagulation in atrial fibrillation, clinicians are more concerned about bleeding risk, and place less weight on the associated stroke reduction, than patients (Devereaux et al. 2001). Thus, a fundamental principle of EBM is the explicit inclusion of patients and society's values and clinical circumstances in the clinical decision-making process (Fig. 8.4) (Haynes et al. 2002). Clinical epidemiology can help identifying and applying the key issues in the decision making process.

Considering the model by Haynes et al. (2002) you are now faced with the problem of how to best incorporate the patient's values into the decision. Before resolving the scenario we will describe different ways to optimize decision making.

For many – perhaps most – of our clinical decisions, the tradeoff is sufficiently clear that clinicians need not concern themselves with variability in patient values. Previously healthy patients will all want antibiotics to treat their pneumonia or their urinary tract infection, anticoagulation to treat their pulmonary embolus, or aspirin to treat their myocardial infarction. Under such circumstances, a brief explanation of the rationale for treatment and the expected benefits and side effects will suffice.

When benefits and risks are balanced more delicately and the best choice may differ across patients, clinicians must attend to the variability in patients values (such as in a Grade 2A recommendation in the McMaster approach to grading recommendations). One fundamental strategy for integrating evidence with preferences involves communicating the benefits and risks to patients, thus permitting them to incorporate their own values and preferences in the decision. One advantage of this approach is that it avoids the vexing problem of measuring patients' values. Unfortunately, the problem of communicating the evidence to patients in a way that allows patients to clearly and unequivocally understand their choices is almost as vexing as the direct measurement of patient values.

A second basic strategy is to ascertain the relative value patients place on the key outcomes associated with the management options. One can then consider the likely outcomes of alternative courses of action and use the patient's values as the basis of trading off benefits and risks. When done in a fully quantitative way, this approach becomes a decision analysis using individual patient preferences (Guyatt et al. 2002a,b). A number of texts provide information on decision analysis and decision analyses are available for a number of topics, such as the prevention of

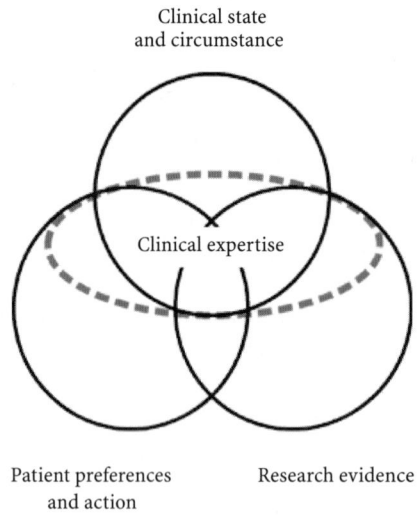

Figure 8.4. Model for Evidence-Based Decision Making. Reproduced with permission from Haynes et al. (2002)

ischemic stroke with warfarin in atrial fibrillation (Guyatt et al. 2002a,b; Petitti 1994; Thomson et al. 2000).

In addition, patients often have preferences not only about the outcomes, but about the decision-making process itself. These preferences can vary, and the patient's desired level of involvement should determine which approach the clinician takes (Degner et al. 1997; Stiggelbout and Kiebert 1997; Strull et al. 1984). Ethicists have characterized the alternative strategies (Emanuel and Emanuel 1992). At one end of the spectrum, the physician acts as a technician, providing the patient with information and taking no active part in the decision-making process. This corresponds to the first strategy for incorporating patient values, presenting patients with the likely benefits, risks, inconvenience and cost and then letting patients decide. At the opposite extreme, corresponding to the second strategy, ascertaining the patient's values and then making a recommendation in light of the likely advantages and disadvantages of alternative management approaches, the clinician takes a "paternalistic" approach and decides what is best for the patient in light of that patient's preferences.

However, intermediate approaches of shared decision making are generally more popular than those at either extreme. Shared decision making uses both of the two fundamental approaches to decision making presented above: The clinician typically shares the evidence, in some form, with the patient, while simultaneously attempting to understand the patient's values. Evidence that more active patient involvement in the process of health care delivery can improve outcomes and reported quality of life – and, possibly, reduce health care expenditures – provides empirical evidence in support of secular trends toward patient autonomy and away from paternalistic approaches (Greenfield et al. 1988; Stewart 1995; Szabo et al. 1997).

Clinicians should temper their enthusiasm for active patient involvement in decision making with an awareness that many patients prefer paternalistic approaches. For example, the results of a survey of 2472 patients suffering from chronic disease (hypertension, diabetes, heart failure, myocardial infarction, or depression) completed between 1986 and 1990 supported this approach (Arora and McHorney 2000). In response to the statement: "I prefer to leave decisions about my medical care up to my doctor", 17.1% strongly agreed, 45.5% agreed, 11.1% were uncertain, 22.5% disagreed, and only 4.8% strongly disagreed. In a more recent study of node-negative breast cancer patients considering adjuvant chemotherapy, 84% of 171 women preferred an independent or shared role in decision-making (Whelan et al. 2003). Increasing general levels of education, the advent of the Internet and the resulting access to medical information, and an increasingly litigious and consumerist environment have all contributed to patients wishing to play a more active role in decision-making and may explain a shift in patient preferences for decision making. Shared decision-making and patient-centeredness have become attractive approaches to resolving the profusion of challenging choices facing patients and clinicians (Charles et al. 1999a, b; Edwards and Elwyn 2001; Guyatt et al. 2004a).

Regardless of the decision-making approach chosen by the patient and clinician, integrating values and preferences and communicating options injects challenges into the process by insisting that clinicians consider quantitative estimates of benefits and risks, rather than just whether a treatment works or whether toxicity occurs. If clinicians leave the decisions to patients, they must effectively communicate the probabilities associated with the alternative outcomes to them. If they opt for taking responsibility for combining patient values with the evidence, they must quantify those values. A vague sense of the patient's preferences cannot fully satisfy the rigor of the optimal decision making approach.

We will now describe some of the specific strategies associated with two decision-making models: one in which the clinician presents the patient with the likely consequences of alternative management strategies and leaves the choice to the patient, and the other in which the clinician ascertains the patient's values and provides a recommendation.

Patient as Decision-Maker: Decision Aids

If the patient wishes to play the primary role in decision making, clinicians may use intuitive approaches to communicating concepts of risk and risk reduction that they have developed through clinical experience. They will answer the patient's questions and ultimately act on the patient's decision. Alternatively, if available for a particular decision, clinicians can use a decision aid that presents descriptive and probabilistic information about the disease, treatment options, and potential outcomes in a patient-friendly manner (Barry 2002; Holmes-Rovner et al. 2001; Levine et al. 1992; O'Connor 2001).

A well-constructed decision aid has two advantages. One is that someone has reviewed the literature and produced a rigorous summary of the probabilities. Clinicians who doubt that the summary of probabilities is rigorous can go back to the original literature on which those probabilities are based and determine their accuracy. A second advantage of a well-constructed decision aid is that it will offer a pre-tested and effective way of communicating the information to patients who may have little background in quantitative decision making. Most commonly, decision aids use visual props to present the outcome data in terms of the percentage of people with a certain condition who do well without intervention, compared to the percentage who do well with intervention. Decision aids will summarize the data regarding all outcomes of importance to patients.

Theoretically, decision aids present an attractive strategy for ensuring that patient values guide clinical decision making. What impact do decision aids actually have on clinical practice? O'Connor and colleagues conducted a systematic review, finding 17 randomized trials that used 11 different decision aids, for example the decision for or against hormone replacement therapy in women after menopause or decisions related to breast surgery in breast cancer (O'Connor et al. 2003, 2004). Of these 17 trials, decision aid impact on knowledge was evaluated in four. All four found greater knowledge in the decision aid group, with a pooled difference of 19 on a 100-point scale (95% CI: (14, 25)). Decision aids reduced decisional conflict using a validated decisional conflict scale in three of four trials in which investigators addressed this issue (mean effect: 0.3; 95% CI: (0.1; 0.4) on the 5-point scale decisional conflict scale). Three studies failed to show a difference in satisfaction with the decision made, although one of these three showed increased satisfaction with the decision-making process.

In summary, decision aids markedly increase patient knowledge and decrease discomfort with decision making as reflected in decisional conflict scores. The importance of the reduction in decisional conflict remains uncertain. Simple decision aids that clinicians can integrate into regular patient care could increase the extent to which patient values truly determine health care decisions.

Patient as Provider of Values

The second set of approaches all begin with, at minimum, establishing the relative value the patient places on the target outcomes. Doing so requires that the patient understand the nature of those outcomes. How, for instance, would a patient with atrial fibrillation facing a decision about using oral anticoagulation to prevent strokes imagine living with a stroke, or the experience of having a gastrointestinal bleeding episode as a side effect of the oral anticoagulation? Patients may find a written description of the health states (Table 8.9) useful in the process of describing their preferences (Devereaux et al. 2001).

Having made their best effort to ensure that patients understand the outcomes, clinicians can choose from among a number of ways of obtaining their values for those outcomes. They can gain a qualitative sense of their patients' preferences from a discussion without a formal structure. Alternatively, a direct comparison between outcomes may prove useful. For instance, with only two outcomes, the patient can make a direct comparative rating. The question may be: "How much worse would it be to have a stroke versus a gastrointestinal bleeding

Table 8.9. Sample descriptions of major stroke and gastrointestinal bleed

Major Stroke	Bleeding
You suddenly are dizzy and blackout	You feel unwell for two days then suddenly you vomit blood
You are unable to move one arm and one leg	
You cannot swallow or control bladder and bowel	You are admitted to hospital
	You stop taking warfarin
You are unable to understand what is being said	A doctor puts a tube down your throat to see where you are bleeding from
You are unable to talk	You receive sedation to ease the discomfort of the test
You feel no physical pain	
You are admitted to hospital	You do not need an operation
You cannot dress	You receive blood transfusions to replace the blood you lost
The nurse feeds you	
You cannot walk	You stay in hospital one week
After 1 month with physiotherapy, you are able to wiggle your toes and lift your arm off the bed	You feel well at the end of your hospital stay
	You need to take pills for the next six months to prevent further bleeding
You remain this way for the rest of your life	You do not take warfarin any more
Another illness will likely cause your death	After that you are back to normal

episode? Would it be equally bad? Twice as bad to have a stroke? Three times as bad?"

Using a somewhat more complex strategy, the clinician can ask the patient to place a mark on a visual analogue scale or "feeling thermometer", in which the extremes are anchored at dead and full health, to represent how the patient feels about the health states in question (Fig. 8.5).

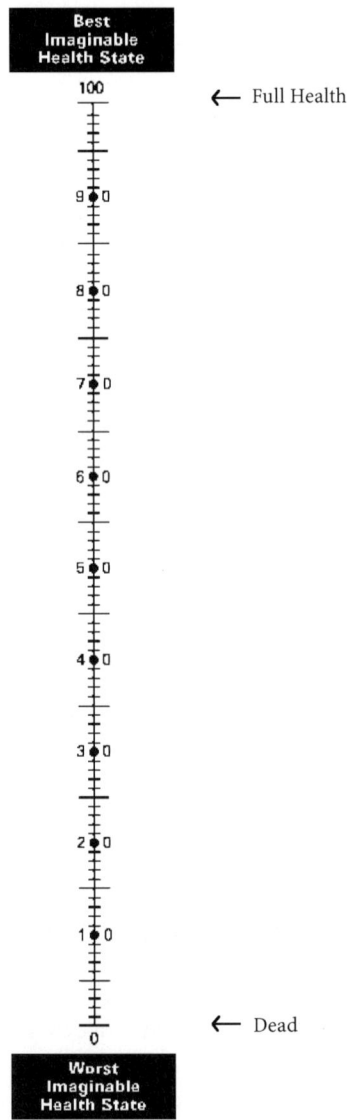

Figure 8.5. The feeling thermometer

When, as in the case of a gastrointestinal bleeding and a stroke, some health states are temporary and others are permanent, the clinician must ensure that patients incorporate the duration of the health state in their rating.

More sophisticated approaches include the time tradeoff and the standard gamble (Torrance 1986). In completing the time tradeoff, patients choose between a longer period in a state of impaired health (such as recovery from severe stroke) and a shorter period in a state of full health. With the standard gamble, by contrast, patients are asked to choose between living in a state of impaired health versus taking a gamble in which they may return to full health or die immediately. These latter approaches may come much closer to meeting assumptions that health economists argue are necessary for accurate ratings of the relative value of health states in the context of choice with uncertain outcomes.

Regardless of the strategy clinicians use to obtain patient values, they must somehow integrate these values with the likely outcomes of the alternative management strategies. Formal decision analysis provides the most rigorous method for making this integration. Practical software for plugging in the patients' values and conducting a patient-specific decision analysis for common clinical problems is being developed, although not yet available for routine use in daily clinical practice. Investigators have shown that, when patients' values are used in individualized decision analyses, their decisions about anticoagulation in atrial fibrillation differ from those suggested by existing guidelines (Protheroe et al. 2000). Whether the decisions would have differed had the patients been provided with the probabilities and asked to choose their preferred management strategy – as with a decision aid – remains unknown.

Even if the tools for individual decision analysis were widely available, application of the approach would depend on the availability of clinicians who could devote time to eliciting patient values. Such a process may be resource intensive, and issues of how much gain there is from the investment, or the intervention's cost-effectiveness, may become very important. Exactly the same considerations apply to the use of decision aids, in which the improvement of knowledge is clear but the impact on anxiety, or on the choices patients actually make, is not as obvious.

Another method of expressing information to patients that incorporates their values is the likelihood of being helped versus harmed (Sackett et al. 2000). Clinicians can apply the likelihood of being helped versus harmed to any clinical decision, and preliminary evidence suggests the approach may be useful on busy clinical services. The clinician begins by calculating the NNT and NNH for the average patients in a study or studies from which the data about treatment effectiveness and harm come. The clinician then adjusts the average NNT and NNH for the individual patient according to that patient's likelihood of suffering the target event that treatment is intended to prevent, and the risks it may precipitate, relative to the average patient. Having established the relative likelihood of help versus harm, the clinician explores the patient's values about the severity of adverse events that might be caused by the treatment relative to the severity of the target event that treatment helps prevent. The final adjustment of the likelihood of being helped versus harmed incorporates the patient's values without providing formal help by a decision aid.

Likelihood of Help Versus Harm

For sake of simplicity, we will assume that the patient in our scenario places a mean value on the composite endpoints cardiovascular disease (defined by the CURE investigators as death from cardiovascular causes, nonfatal MI, stroke, or refractory ischemia), major bleeding (substantially disabling bleeding, intraocular bleeding or the loss of vision, or bleeding necessitating the transfusion of at least 2 units of blood) and minor bleeding (any other bleeding leading to interruption of study medication), respectively. We will ignore other factors bearing on the decision, such as taking an additional pill daily.

During your discussion with the patient about the consequences of further cardiovascular disease and major bleeding you asked her to use the "feeling thermometer" (see Fig. 8.5) to estimate how she feels about each of the two combined outcomes. We will ignore minor bleeding episodes in this example, because your patient is not concerned at all about the risk and consequences of minor bleeding. However, she places a mean value of suffering additional consequences of cardiovascular disease at 0.2 and of living with a major bleed at 0.7. You use these on your handheld personal digital assistant to calculate her likelihood of being helped or harmed (LHH) from clopidogrel therapy versus placebo therapy.

Using the NNTs calculated in the scenario, the LHH for clopidogrel versus placebo becomes (Table 8.5):

$$LHH = (1/NNT) : (1/NNH) = (1/44) : (1/100) = 100/44 = 2.3 \,.$$

Note: we could also use (1/absolute risk reduction) : (1/absolute risk increase) but this uses decimal fractions and may increase the likelihood of arithmetic errors.

Therefore, you can tell the patient that clopidogrel is approximately twice as likely to help her as to harm her, when compared with placebo.

Incorporating her values that you elicited, the LHH becomes:

$$LHH = (1/NNT) \times (1 - \text{Uevent}) : (1/NNH) \times (1 - \text{Utoxicity})$$

$$= (1/44) \times (1 - 0.2) : (1/100) \times (1 - 0.7) = 6.1 \,,$$

where Uevent is the value of the outcome prevented (composite endpoint of death from cardiovascular causes, nonfatal MI, stroke, or refractory ischemia) and Utoxicity (Major bleeding) is the value of the side effect.

You can now inform the patient that clopidogrel is approximately six times as valuable to help her as to harm her. Including additional outcomes would increase the number of terms in the numerator (benefits) or denominator (adverse consequences).

Alternatively, a quicker way of incorporating the patient's values is to ask the patient to rate one event against another. For example, is the adverse effect about as severe as the event the treatment prevents – or 10 times as bad or only half as severe? This rating ("s") can then be used to adjust the LHH as:

$$LHH = (1/NNT) \times s : (1/NNH) \,.$$

Having ascertained the likely outcomes of the alternate courses of action, the clinician must either present patients with the options and outcomes and leave it for them to choose, try to discover the patient's values and having done so suggest a course of action to the patient (the paternalistic approach), or choose the middle course of shared decision making. The patient's preferred decision-making style will guide the clinician in this regard. However, communicating the nature of the outcomes and their probabilities in a way the patient will understand, or accurately ascertaining the patient's values regarding the outcomes, remains problematic.

The challenges of optimal clinical decision making should not obscure the realization that clinicians face these challenges in helping patients with every management decision. For each choice, clinicians guide patients with their best estimate of the likely outcomes. They then help patients balance these outcomes in making their ultimate decision. Finding better strategies to carry out these tasks remains a frontier for clinical epidemiology.

Semistructured Conversation and Resolution

Example 2. You discuss the option of clopidogrel therapy with your patient who is feeling better now and appears to have a good understanding of the information you are providing. You explain that – based on your assessment and the patients' values and preferences – benefit and harm of clopidogrel are finely balanced: for every 44 patients treated for one year in the CURE trial there was one less occurrence of the combined endpoint. However, for every 100 patients treated with clopidogrel for one year one additional patient suffered a major bleeding episode and for every 37 patients treated for one year there was one additional minor bleeding episode. You also explain that, because these are only estimates, the true effect might be somewhat smaller or larger for both the benefit and harms. Your patient states she would like to use clopidogrel.

Because the decision regarding taking clopidogrel depends on the patient's values and preferences regarding preventing the combined endpoint versus incurring additional risk of bleeding and you have the results of the calculation of the likelihood of being helped or harmed. You explain that the results of your calculation using the software on your personal digital assistant support her preference for taking clopidogrel. In terms of expense, you are uncertain about the cost of clopidogrel. Because you feel that this question will come up with additional patients and that you had wanted to address it for some time, you call the hospital pharmacist. She informs you that the cost for clopidogrel is approximately $90 per month and that at least one analysis has suggested the drug is not cost-effective (Gaspoz et al. 2002). The patient tells you that she has minimal co-pay for most medications and remains interested in taking the medication. Together, you decide that beginning clopidogrel treatment ultimately is in her best interest and you start the patient on a 300 mg loading dose of clopidogrel and continue with 75 mg daily. You also suggest reducing the dose of aspirin as lower doses of aspirin confer similar benefits and doses of 75 mg to 325 mg were given in the CURE trial together with Clopidogrel. ◆

8.10   **Conclusions**

We have presented several concepts of clinical epidemiology. Working through the clinical problems has implicitly highlighted some of clinical epidemiology's research challenges. The following makes explicit some of these challenges that clinical epidemiologists and other investigators need to tackle in future research. A number of important areas have been identified and we will list them here briefly. It is not clear what are the best ways to educate clinicians and students in the methodology of clinical epidemiology and educational researchers will have to focus on this aspect. The Cochrane Collaboration, other organizations and researchers will further elaborate the methodology of systematic reviews (e.g., of diagnostic studies, observational studies and health related quality of life outcomes). Obtaining further information about the most valid and informative ways of presenting statistical information and education of patients and clinicians about these issues is an important task for clinical epidemiologists. Research should also focus on improving the development of clinical practice guidelines and integrating cost information in guidelines and recommendations (Schünemann et al. 2004). Furthermore, research on implementing guidelines into clinical practice is an area of intensive research. It is clear that studies of guideline implementation should follow the same methodological rigor as other studies, but they are presented with different challenges, such as the need for large cluster randomized clinical trials. We described the integration of preferences and values in medical decision making as well as bedside decision making in particular above. Tools that facilitated this difficult task are in development. Health decision aids, in particular electronic decision aids promise to advance this science. Along with health decision aids, the integration of HRQL information into clinical practice and guidelines presents challenges that investigators need to resolve (Frost et al. 2003). Finally, conducting additional research of integrating electronic health (eHealth) (including multimedia decision aids) into clinical practice presents a fascinating but challenging outlook.

References

ACC (2001) ACC/AHA/ESC guidelines for the management of patients with atrial fibrillation. A report of the American College of Cardiology/American Heart Association Task Force on Practice Guidelines and the European Society of Cardiology Committee for Practice Guidelines and Policy Conferences. J Am Coll Cardiol 38:1231–1266

Albers G, Dalen JE, Laupacis A, Manning WJ, Petersen P, Singer DE (2001) Antithrombotic therapy in atrial fibrillation. Chest 119:194S–206S

American Urological Association (2000) Prostate-specific antigen (PSA) best practice policy. Oncology:267–286

Antithrombotic Trialists' Collaboration (2002) Collaborative metaanalysis of randomised trials of antiplatelet therapy for prevention of death, myocardial infarction, and stroke in high risk patients. BMJ 324:71–86

Antman EM, Lau J, Kupelnick B, Mosteller F, Chalmers TC (1992) A comparison of results of meta-analyses of randomized control trials and recommendations of clinical experts. Treatments for myocardial infarction. JAMA 268:240–248

Arora N, McHorney C (2000) Patient preferences for medical decision making: who really wants to participate? Med Care 38:335–341

Atkins D, Best D, Briss P, Eccles M, Falck-Ytter Y, Flottorp S, Guyatt GH, Harbour R, Haugh M, Henry D, Hill S, Jaeschke R, Leng G, Liberati A, Magrini N, Mason J, Middleton P, Mrukowicz J, O'Connell D, Oxman A, Phillips B, Schünemann H, Tan-Torres Edejer T, Varonen H, Vist G, Williams J, Zaza S (2004) Grading evidence and formulating recommendations. BMJ (in press)

Balk EM, Bonis PA, Moskowitz H, Schmid CH, Ioannidis JP, Wang C, Lau J (2002) Correlation of quality measures with estimates of treatment effect in meta-analyses of randomized controlled trials.[comment]. JAMA 287(22):2973–2982

Barry MJ (2002) Health decision aids to facilitate shared decision making in office practice. Ann Intern Med. Online 136(2):127–135

Bergner M, Bobbitt R, Carter W, Gilson B (1981) The Sickness Impact Profile: Development and final revision of a health status measure. Med Care 19:787–805

Bernardo JM, Adrian FM (1994) Bayesian theory. Smith Wiley, Chichester

Berry DA (1996) Statistics: A Bayesian perspective. Duxbury Press, Wadworth

Briss P, Zaza S, Pappaioanou M, Feilding J, Wright-de Aguero L, Truman BI, Hopkins DP, Mullen PD, Thompson RS, Woolf SH, Carande-Kulis VG, Anderson L, Hinman AR, MdQueen DV, Teutsch SM, Harris JR, The Task Force on Community Preventive Services (2000) Developing an evidence-based guide to community preventive services – methods. Am J Prev Med 18:35–43

Brook RH, Ware J, Davies-Avery A, Stewart A, Donald C, Williams KN, Johnston SA (1979) Overview of adult health status measures fielded in Rand's health insurance study. Med Care 17(Suppl 7):1–131

Bucher HC, Weinbacher M, Gyr K (1994) Influence of method of reporting study results on decision of physicians to prescribe drugs to lower cholesterol concentration. BMJ 309(6957):761–764

Canadian (1979) Task Force on the Periodic Health Examination. The periodic health examination. CMAJ 121:1193–1254

Chang S, Fine R, Siegel D, Chesney M, Black D, Hulley S (1991) The impact of diuretic therapy on reported sexual function. Arch Intern Med 151:2402–2408

Charles C, Gafni A, Whelan T (1999a) Decision-making in the physician-patient encounter: revisiting the shared treatment decision-making model. Soc Sci Med 49(5):651–661

Charles C, Whelan T, Gafni A (1999b) What do we mean by partnership in making decisions about treatment? BMJ 319(7212):780–782

Cook DJ GG, Laupacis A, Sackett DL (1992) Rules of evidence and clinical recommendations on the use of antithrombotic agents. Chest (102):305S–11S

CURE-Investigators (2001) Effects of Clopidogrel in addition to Aspirin in Patients with Acute Coronary Syndromes without ST-Segmen Elevation. N Engl J Med 345:494–502

Degner L, Kristjanson L, Bowman D, Sloan J, Carriere K, O'Neil J, Bilodeau B, Watson P, Mueller B (1997) Information needs and decisional preferences in women with breast cancer. JAMA 277:1485–1492

Devereaux PJ, Anderson DR, Gardner MJ, Putnam W, Flowerdew GJ, Brownell BF, Nagpal S, Cox JL (2001) Differences between perspectives of physicians and patients on anticoagulation in patients with atrial fibrillation: observational study. BMJ 323(7323):1218–1222

Deyo R, Diehl A, Rosenthal M (1986) How many days of bed rest for acute low back pain? a randomized clinical trial. N Engl J Med 315:1064–1070

Diamond GA (1999) The wizard of odds: Bayes theorem and diagnostic testing. Mayo Clin Proc 74(11):1179–1182

Diamond GA, Forrester JS (1979) Analysis of probability as an aid in the clinical diagnosis of coronary-artery disease. N Engl J Med 300(24):1350–1358

Diamond GA, Forrester JS, Hirsch M, Staniloff HM, Vas R, Berman DS, Swan HJ (1980) Application of conditional probability analysis to the clinical diagnosis of coronary artery disease. J Clin Invest 65(5):1210–1221

Diamond GA, Hirsch M, Forrester JS, Staniloff HM, Vas R, Halpern SW, Swan HJ (1981) Application of information theory to clinical diagnostic testing: the electrocardiographic stress test. Circulation 63:915–921

Dolan JG, Bordley DR, Mushlim AI (1986) An evaluation of clinicians' subjective prior probability estimates. Med Decis Making 6:216–223

Edwards A, Elwyn G (1999) How should effectiveness of risk communication to aid patients' decisions be judged? A review of the literature.[comment]. Med Dec Making 19(4):428–434

Edwards A, Elwyn G (2001) Evidence-based patient choice. Inevitable or impossible? Oxford University Press, New York

Edwards A, Elwyn G, Stott N (1999) Communicating risk reductions. Researchers should present results with both relative and absolute risks. BMJ 318(7183):603; author reply 603–604

Egger M, Davey Smith G, Altman D (2000) Meta-analysis in context. In: Egger M, Davey Smith G, Altman DG (eds) Systematic reviews in health care. BMJ Books, London

Emanuel E, Emanuel L (1992) Four models of the physician-patient relationship. JAMA 267:2221–2226

Evidence-Based-Medicine-Working-Group (1992) Evidence-based medicine. A new approach to teaching the practice of medicine. JAMA 268:2420–2425

Fagan T (1975) Nomogram for Bayes theorem. N Engl J Med 293:257

Feinstein A (1968) Clinical epidemiology I. The population experiments of nature and of man in human illness. Ann Intern Med 69:807–820

Ferrini R, Woolf SH (1998) American College of Preventive Medicine Practice Policy: screening for prostate cancer in American men. Am J Prev Med 15:81–84

Fletcher RH, Fletcher SW, Wagner EH (1996) Clinical epidemiology: The essentials, 3rd edn. Williams and Wilkins, Baltimore

Freemantle N, Mason J, Eccles M (1999) Deriving Treatment Recommendations from Evidence within Randomized Trials: The Role and Limitation of Meta-Analysis. Int J Technol Assess Health Care 15(2):304–315

Freemantle N, Calvert M, Wood J, Eastaugh J, Griffin C (2003) Composite outcomes in randomized trials: greater precision but with greater uncertainty? JAMA 289:2554–2559

Frost M, Bonomi A, Capelleri J, Schünemann H, Moynihan T, Aaronson N (2003) Applying quality of life data formally and systematically into clinical practice. Clin Ther 25:D10

García Rodríguez L, Hernández-Díaz S, deAbajo FJ (2001) Association between aspirin and upper gastrointestinal complications: Systematic review of epidemiologic studies. Br J Clin Pharmacol 52:563–571

Gaspoz JM, Coxson PG, Goldman PA, Williams LW, Kuntz KM, Hunink MG, Goldman L (2002) Cost effectiveness of aspirin, clopidogrel, or both for secondary prevention of coronary heart disease. N Engl J Med 346(23):1800–1806

Glass RD (1996) Diagnosis: A brief introduction. Oxford University Press, Melbourne

Goldstein R, Gort E, Guyatt GH, Stubbing D, Avendano M (1994) Prospective randomized controlled trial of respiratory rehabilitation. Lancet 344:1394–1397

Greenfield S, Kaplan SH, Ware JE, Jr., Yano EM, Frank HJ (1988) Patients' participation in medical care: effects on blood sugar control and quality of life in diabetes. J Gen Intern Med 3(5):448–457

Guyatt GH (1991) Evidence-based medicine. ACP J Club 114:A-16

Guyatt GH (2002a) Introduction. In: Guyatt GH, Rennie D (eds) Users' guide to the medical literature: A manual for evidence-based clinical practice. AMA Press, Chicago

Guyatt GH (2002b) Preface. In: Guyatt GH, Rennie D (eds) Users' guide to the medical literature: A manual for evidence-based clinical practice. AMA Press, Chicago

Guyatt GH, Rennie D (2002) Users' guide to the medical literature: A manual for evidence-based clinical practice. AMA Press, Chicago

Guyatt GH, Bombardier C, Tugwell P (1986) Measuring disease-specific quality-of-life in clinical trials. CMAJ 134:889–895

Guyatt GH, Walter S, Norman G (1987) Measuring change over time: assessing the usefulness of evaluative instruments. J Chronic Dis 40:171–178

Guyatt GH, Zanten SVV, Feeny D, Patrick D (1989) Measuring quality of life in clinical trials: a taxonomy and review. CMAJ 140:1441–1447

Guyatt GH, Patterson C, Ali M, Singer J, Levine M, Turpie I, Meyer R (1990) Diagnosis of iron-deficiency anemia in the elderly. Am J Med 88(3):205–209

Guyatt GH, Oxman AD, Ali M, Willan A, McIlroy W, Patterson C (1992) Laboratory diagnosis of iron-deficiency anemia: an overview. [erratum appears in J Gen Intern Med 1992 Jul-Aug;7(4):423]. J Gen Intern Med 7(2):145–153

Guyatt GH, Sackett D, Sinclair JC, Hayward R, Cook DJ, Cook RJ (1995) Users' guides to the medical literature IX. A method for grading health care recommendations. Evidence-based medicine working group. JAMA 274:1800–1804

Guyatt GH, King DR, Feeny DH, Stubbing D, Goldstein RS (1999) Generic and specific measurement of health-related quality of life in a clinical trial of respiratory rehabilitation. J Clin Epidemiol 52:187–192

Guyatt GH, Meade MO, Jaeschke RZ, Cook DJ, Haynes RB (2000) Practitioners of evidence based care. Not all clinicians need to appraise evidence from scratch but all need some skills. BMJ 320(7240):954–955

Guyatt GH, Schünemann H, Cook D, Pauker S, Sinclair J, Bucher H, Jaeschke R (2001) Grades of Recommendation for Antithrombotic Agents. Chest 119:3S-7S

Guyatt GH, Sinclair J, Cook D, Jaeschke R, Schünemann H (2002a) Moving from evidence to action. Grading recommendations – a qualitative approach. In: Guyatt GH, Rennie D (eds) Users' guides to the medical literature: A manual for evidence-based clinical practice. AMA Press, Chicago

Guyatt GH, Hayward RS, Richardson WS, Green I, Wilson MC, Sinclair J, Cook D, Glasziou P, Detsky A, Bass E (2002b) Moving from evidence to action. In: Guyatt GH, Rennie D (eds) Users' guide to the medical literature: A manual for evidence-based clinical practice. AMA Press, Chicago

Guyatt GH, Devereaux P, Montori V, Schünemann H, Bhandari M (2004a) Putting the patient first: In our practice, and in our use of language. Evidence Based Medicine 9:6–7

Guyatt GH, Schünemann H, Cook D, Jaeschke R, Pauker S (2004b) Applying the grades of recommendation for antithrombotic and thrombolytic agents. Chest (in press)

Harbour R, Miller J (2001) A new system for grading recommendations in evidence based guidelines. BMJ 323:334–336

Harris R, Helfand M, Woolf SH, Lohr KN, Mulrow CD, Teutsch SM, Atkins D, for the Methods Work Group, Third U.S. Preventive Services Task Force (2001) Current methods of the U.S. Preventive Services Task Force: a review of the process. Am J Prev Med 20(3S):21–35

Haynes RB, Devereaux PJ, Guyatt GH (2002) Clinical expertise in the era of evidence-based medicine and patient choice. ACP J Club 136: A11

Hernandez JL, Riancho JA, Matorras P, Gonzalez-Macias J (2003) Clinical evaluation for cancer in patients with involuntary weight loss without specific symptoms. Am J Med 114(8):631–637

Hill SA, Devereaux PJ, Griffith L, Opie J, McQueen MJ, Panju A, Stanton E, Guyatt GH (2003) Can Troponin I measurement predict short term serious cardiac outcomes in patients presenting to the emergency department with possible acute coronary syndrome. Can J Emerg Med (in press)

Holmes-Rovner M, Llewellyn-Thomas H, Entwistle V, Coulter A, O'Connor A, Rovner DR (2001) Patient choice modules for summaries of clinical effectiveness: a proposal. BMJ 322(7287):664–667

http://www.guidelines.gov/ Accessed March 14, 2004

Hunt S, McKenna S, McEwen J, Backett E, Williams J, Papp E (1980) A quantitative approach to perceived health status: a validation study. J Epidemiol Community Health 34:281–286

Jaeschke R, Singer J, Guyatt GH (1991) Using quality-of-life measures to elucidate mechanism of action. CMAJ 144:35–39

Ladenheim ML, Kotler TS, Pollock BH, Berman DS, Diamond GA (1987) Incremental prognostic power of clinical history, exercise electrocardiography and myocardial perfusion scintigraphy in suspected coronary artery disease. Am J Cardiol 59(4):270–277

Laupacis A, Sackett D, Roberts RS (1988) An assessment of clinically useful measures of the consequences of treatment. N Engl J Med 318:1728–1733

Laupacis A, Wong C, Churchill D (1991) The use of generic and specific quality-of-life measures in hemodialysis patients treated with erythropoietin. Control Clin Trials 12:168S-179S

Ledley RS, Lusted LB (1959) Reasoning foundations of medical diagnosis: symbolic logic, probability, and value theory aid our understanding of how physicians reason. Science 130:9–21

Levine MN, Gafni A, Markham B, MacFarlane D (1992) A bedside decision instrument to elicit a patient's preference concerning adjuvant chemotherapy for breast cancer.[comment]. Ann Intern Med 117(1):53–58

Liang M, Larson M, Cullen K, Schwartz J (1985) Comparative measurement efficiency and sensitivity of five health status instruments for arthritis research. Arthritis Rheum 28:542–547

Lubsen J, Kirwan B (2002) Combined endpoints: can we use them? Stat Med 21:2959–2970

MacKenzie M, Charlson M (1986) Standards for the use of ordinal scales in clinical trials. BMJ 292:40–43

Mahler D, Rosiello R, Harver A, Lentine T, McGovern J, Daubenspeck J (1987) Comparison of clinical dyspnea ratings and psychophysical measurements of respiratory sensation in obstructive airway disease. Am Rev Respir Dis 135:1229–1233

McGinn TG, Guyatt GH, Wyer PC, Naylor CD, Stiell IG (2003) Clinical prediction rules. In: Guyatt GH, Rennie D (eds) Users' guides to the medical literature: A manual for evidence-based clinical practice. AMA Press, Chicago

McKibbon A, Hunt D, Richardson SW, Hayward R, Wilson M, Jaeschke R, Haynes RB, Wyer P, Craig J, Guyatt GH (2002) Finding the evidence. In: Guyatt GH, Rennie D (eds) Users' guides to the medical literature: A manual for evidence-based clinical practice. AMA Press, Chicago

Meier MA, Al-Badr WH, Cooper JV, Kline-Rogers EM, Smith DE, Eagle KA, Mehta RH (2002) The new definition of myocardial infarction: diagnostic and prognostic implications in patients with acute coronary syndromes. Arch Intern Med 162(14):1585–1589

Moher D, Pham B, Jones A, Cook DJ, Jadad AR, Moher M, Tugwell P, Klassen TP (1998) Does quality of reports of randomised trials affect estimates of intervention efficacy reported in meta-analyses? Lancet 352(9128):609–613

National-Guideline-Clearing-House (2004) (http://www.guideline.gov/) Accessed March 14, 2004

CNEP (2001) Executive summary of the third report of the National Cholesterol Education Program (NCEP) Expert Panel on detection, evaluation, and treatment of high blood cholesterol in adults (Adult Treatment Panel III). JAMA 285(19):2486–2497

O'Connor A (2001) Using patient decision aids to promote evidence-based decision making. ACP J Club 135(1):A11–A12

O'Connor AM, Legare F, Stacey D (2003) Risk communication in practice: the contribution of decision aids. BMJ 327:736–740

O'Connor AM, Stacey D, Entwistle V, Llewellyn-Thomas H, Rovner D, Holmes-Rovner M, Tait V, Tetroe J, Fiset V, Barry M, Jones J (2004) Decision aids for people facing health treatment or screening decisions. Cochrane Database of Systematic Reviews 1

Olsson G, Lubsen J, VanEs G, Rehnqvist N (1986) Quality-of-life after myocardial infarction: effect of long term metoprolol on mortality and morbidity. BMJ 292:1491–1493

Osoba D, Aaronson N, Till J (1991) A practical guide for selecting quality-of-life measures in clinical trials and practice. In: Osoba D (ed) Effect of cancer on quality-of-life. CRC Press, Boston

Ott C, Sivarajan E, Newton K, Almes MJ, Bruce RA, Bergner M, Gilson BS (1983) A controlled randomized study of early cardiac rehabilitation: the sickness impact profile as an assessment tool. Heart Lung 12:162–170

Oxman A, Guyatt GH (1993) The science of reviewing research. Ann NY Acad Sci 703:125–133:discussion 133–134

Oxman A, Guyatt GH, Cook D, Montori V (2002) Summarizing the evidence. In: Guyatt GH, Rennie D (eds) Users' guide to the medical literature: A manual for evidence-based clinical practice. AMA Press, Chicago

Oxman AD, Sackett DL, Guyatt GH (1993) Users' guides to the medical literature. I. How to get started. The Evidence-Based Medicine Working Group. JAMA 270(17):2093–2095

Parkerson G, Gehlback S, Wagner E, Sherman A, Clapp N, Muhlbaier L (1981) The Duke-UNC Health Profile: an adult health status instrument for primary care. Med Care 19:806–828

Paul J (1938) Clinical epidemiology. J Clin Invest 17:539–541

Petitti D (1994) Meta-analysis, decision analysis and cost-effectiveness analysis. Oxford University Press, Oxford

PIOPED-Investigators (1990) Value of ventilation/perfusion scan in acute pulmonary embolism. Results of the Prospective Investigation of Pulmonary Embolism (PIOPED). JAMA 263:2753–2759

Protheroe J, Fahey T, Montgomery AA, Peters TJ (2000) The impact of patients' preferences on the treatment of atrial fibrillation: observational study of patient based decision analysis. BMJ 320(7246):1380–1384

Richardson WS (2002) Five uneasy pieces about pre-test probability. J Gen Intern Med 17(11):882–883

Richardson WS, Wilson MC, Nishikawa J, Hayward RS (1995) The well-built clinical question: a key to evidence-based decisions. ACP J Club 123(3):A12-A13

Richardson WS, Wilson MC, Williams JW, Jr., Moyer VA, Naylor CD (2003) Clinical Manifestation of Disease. In: Guyatt GH, Rennie D (eds) Users' guide to the medical literature: A manual for evidence-based clinical practice. AMA Press, Chicago

Sackett D (1969) Clinical epidemiology. Am J Epidemiol 89:125–128

Sackett D (1986) Rules of evidence and clinical recommendations on the use of antithrombotic agents. Arch Int Med 146:464–465

Sackett D (2002) Clinical Epidemiology: what, who, and whither. J Clin Epidemiol 55:1161–1166

Sackett D, Winkelstein W (1967) The relationship between cigarette usage and aortic atherosclerosis. Am J Epidemiol 86:264–270

Sackett D, Chambers L, MacPherson A, Goldsmith C, McAuley R (1977) The development and application of indices of health: general methods and a summary of results. Am J Public Health 67:423–428

Sackett D, Haynes RB, Guyatt GH, Tugwell P (1991) Clinical epidemiology: a basic science for clinical medicine. Little, Brown, Boston, pp 5–17

Sackett D, Straus S, Richardson W, Rosenberg W, Haynes RB (2000) Evidence-based medicine. Churchill Livingston, Toronto, p 166

Schünemann HJ, Best D, Vist G, Oxman AD, for The GRADE Working Group (2003) Letters, numbers, symbols and words: how to communicate grades of evidence and recommendations. CMAJ 169(7):677–680

Schünemann H, Munger H, Brower S, O'Donnell M, Crowther M, Cook D, Guyatt GH (2004) Developing evidence-based guidelines for the ACCP Conference on Antithrombotic and Thrombolytic Therapy. Chest in press

Shekelle PG, Woolf SH, Eccles M, Grimshaw J (1999) Clinical guidelines: developing guidelines. BMJ 318(7183):593–596

Smith D, Baker G, Davies G, Dewey M, Chadwick. D (1993) Outcomes of add-on treatment with Lamotrigine in partial epilepsy. Epilepsia 34:312–322

Smith R, Cokkinides V, Eyre H (2003) American Cancer Society guidelines for the early detection of cancer, 2003. CA Cancer J Clin 53:27–43

Soteriades ES, Evans JC, Larson MG, Chen MH, Chen L, Benjamin EJ, Levy D (2002) Incidence and Prognosis of Syncope. N Engl J Med 347(12):878–885

Sox HC, Blatt MA, Higgins MC, Marton KL (1988) Medical decision making. Butterworths, Boston

Stewart M (1995) Effective physician-patient communication and health outcomes: a review. CMAJ 152:1423–1433

Stiggelbout A, Kiebert G (1997) A role for the sick role. Patient preferences regarding information and participation in clinical decision-making. CMAJ 157:383–389

Strull W, Lo B, Charles G (1984) Do patients want to participate in medical decision making? JAMA 252:2990–2994

Symons MJ, Moore DT (2002) Hazard rate ratio and prospective epidemiological studies. J Clin Epidemiol 55(9):893–899

Szabo E, Moody H, Hamilton T, Ang C, Kovithavongs C, Kjellstrand C (1997) Choice of treatment improves quality of life. A study on patients undergoing dialysis. Arch Intern Med 157:1352–1356

Tandon P, Stander H, Jr. RS (1989) Analysis of quality of life data from a randomized, placebo controlled heart-failure trial. J Clin Epidemiol 42:955–962

Tarlov A, Ware J, Greenfield S, Nelson E, Perrin E, Zubkoff M (1989) The medical outcomes study. JAMA 262:925–930

The CAPRICORN Investigators (2001) Effects of carvedilol on outcome after myocardial infarction in patients with left ventricular dysfunction: the CAPRICORN randomised trial. Lancet 357:1385–1390

Thomson R, Parkin D, Eccles M, Sudlow M, Robinson A (2000) Decision analysis and guidelines for anticoagulant therapy to prevent stroke in patients with atrial fibrillation. Lancet 355:956–962

Torrance G (1986) Measurement of health state utilities for economic appraisal. J Health Econ:1–30

Tugwell P, Bombardier C, Buchanan W, Goldsmith C, Grace E, Bennett K, Williams J, Egger M, Alarcon GS, Guttadauria M (1990) Methotrexate in Rheumatoid Arthritis. Impact on quality of life assessed by traditional standard-item and individualized patient preference health status questionnaires. Arch Intern Med 150:59–62

USPSTF (2002) Screening for prostate cancer: recommendations and rationale. Ann Intern Med 137:915–916

van Walraven C, Hart R, Singer D (2002) Oral anticoagulants vs aspirin in nonvalvular atrial fibrillation: an individual patient meta-analysis. JAMA 288:2441–2448

Ware J, Kozinski M, Bayliss M, McHorney CA, Rogers WH, Raczak A (1995) Comparison of methods for the scoring and statistical analysis of SF-36 health profile and summary measures: Summary of results of the Medical Outcomes Study. Med Care 33:AS264-AS279

Ware J, Sherbourne C (1992) The MOS 36-item short-form health survey (SF-36). Med Care 30:473–483

Weil J, Colin-Jones D, Langman M, Lawson D. Logan R, Murphy M, Rawlins M, Vessey M, Wainright P (1995) rophylactic aspirin and risk of peptic ulcer bleeding. BMJ 310:827–830

Whelan T, Sawka C, Levine M, Gafni A, Reyno L, Willan A, Julian J, Dent S, Abu-Zahra H, Chouinard E, Tozer R, Pritchard K, Bodendorfer I (2003) Helping patients make informed choices: a randomized trial of a decision aid for adjuvant chemotherapy in lymph node-negative breast cancer.[comment]. J Nat Cancer Inst 95(8):581–587

Wiebe S, Guyatt GH, Weaver B, Matijevic S, Sidwell C (2003) Comparative responsiveness of generic and specific quality-of-life instruments. J Clin Epidemiol 56(1):52–60

Weiss N (1996) Clinical epidemiology: the study of the outcome of illness, 2nd edn. Oxford University Press, Oxford

Woolf SH (1994) An organized analytic framework for practice guideline development: using the analytic logic as a guide for reviewing evidence, developing recommendations, and explaining the rationale. In: McCormick KA, Moore S, Siegel RA (eds) Methodology perspectives. US Department of Health and Human Services, Agency for Health Care Policy and Research, Washington, DC

Woolf SH, Grol R, Hutchinson A, Eccles M, Grimshaw J (1999) Clinical guidelines: potential benefits, limitations, and harms of clinical guidelines. BMJ 318(7182):527–530

Pharmacoepidemiology

III.9

Edeltraut Garbe, Samy Suissa

Introduction

In the last two decades we have witnessed a tremendous progress in the medical sciences that has led to the development of a great number of new powerful pharmaceuticals. These new medicines enable us to provide much better medical care, but occasionally they will cause harm and give rise to serious adverse reactions that were unexpected from preclinical studies or premarketing clinical trials. Against this background, pharmacoepidemiology has developed as a scientific discipline at the interface between clinical pharmacology and clinical epidemiology (cf. Chap. III.8 of this handbook). Pharmacoepidemiology can be defined as the application of epidemiologic knowledge, methods, and reasoning to the study of the effects and uses of drugs in human populations (Porta-Serra and Hartzema 1997). The application of epidemiological methods – i.e. the use of nonexperimental observational techniques – , the epidemiological perspective with an emphasis on investigations in large unselected populations and long-term studies, the public health approach and the philosophy of epidemiology are all extended to the scope of clinical pharmacology, i.e. the study of the effects of pharmaceuticals in humans.

Pharmacoepidemiology investigates both beneficial and adverse drug effects. Its focus and the one that receives the greatest attention is the assessment of the risk of uncommon, at times latent, and often unexpected adverse reactions that present for the first time after a drug has been marketed. The greatest challenge of pharmacoepidemiology is then to quantify the risk of a drug accurately, relative to one or several alternatives.

The study of adverse drug effects poses a number of methodological difficulties that must be addressed by pharmacoepidemiological research designs: first, drug exposure is not a stable phenomenon. Drug prescription habits may change due to the development of new pharmaceuticals, better knowledge on already available medications or other reasons. Second, drug exposure can be sensitive to a great number of factors that may also be related to the outcome of interest, such as the indication for prescribing, potential contraindications for drug use, the natural course of the disease or disease severity and compliance. Third, the risk of an adverse drug reaction (ADR) is often not constant, but it may change over time which may have important implications for the design and interpretation of pharmacoepidemiology studies.

In this chapter, we will first discuss limitations of premarketing clinical trials; we will then describe the characteristics of spontaneous reporting systems which have been implemented by regulatory agencies and the pharmaceutical industry for postmarketing surveillance. Another issue will be the use of multipurpose cohorts and large administrative healthcare databases for drug effect studies, which have found widespread application in pharmacoepidemiology. We will further discuss several methodological aspects that are unique to pharmacoepidemiological research: as e.g. the phenomenon of "depletion of susceptibles" which is a form of selection bias; or "confounding by indication" which is also referred to as "confounding by disease severity" or "channelling bias". We will present the use of propensity scores, as a tool to reduce confounding particularly in studies of intended drug effects, and will discuss newer approaches of studying drug effects, such as the case-crossover and case-time-control designs. Characteristics of drug utilization studies and their units of measurement will be discussed.

Limitations of Premarketing Clinical Trials 9.2

Prior to marketing, new drugs are subjected to preclinical animal studies followed by three phases of clinical trials in humans. These phases are divisions of convenience in what is a continuous process of acquiring knowledge on the effects of a new drug in humans. In *phase I studies* humans are exposed to a new drug for the first time. These studies are often conducted in small numbers of healthy volunteers and are intended to explore the tolerability, pharmacokinetic and pharmacodynamic properties of a new drug in humans. In *phase II studies* the optimal dose range of the new drug is investigated and its efficacy and safety are explored in the intended patient population. These studies usually include several hundreds of patients. *Phase III studies* are aimed to prove the efficacy and safety of the new drug under strictly controlled experimental conditions in a larger patient population. They are mostly conducted as randomised controlled clinical trials (RCT) and often include several thousand patients altogether. In spite of the size of phase III studies, these studies have still limited ability to identify rare ADRs, since this would require an even larger number of study participants.

Table 9.1 displays sample size calculations for prospective studies. It shows the number of patients needed to detect a relative risk of a given magnitude in relation to the incidence of the event in the reference group. We can see that for the detection of very rare ADRs with sufficient statistical power, prohibitively large sample sizes in premarketing clinical studies would be needed. It is thus inherent in the drug development process – taking into account the already high cost for development of new pharmaceuticals – that serious rare ADRs will usually only be detected after drug marketing when the drug has been used in large patient populations.

An investigation by the Food and Drug Administration (FDA) into the withdrawal of five pharmaceuticals from the US market between 1997 and 1998 illustrates this point (Friedman et al. 1999). All five drugs were removed from the US market because of the discovery of unexpected serious adverse drug reactions (ADR) in the postmarketing period. The FDA investigated whether this unexpectedly high number of drug removals in only a 12-month-period was related to the expedited drug review and approval process that had been implemented. They calculated the number of patients exposed in the clinical trials before marketing and the approximate number of patients exposed before drug withdrawal (Table 9.2). The figures demonstrate that usually huge numbers of patients need to be exposed before sufficient knowledge on a rare ADR has been accumulated. For example, serious hepatotoxic effects of bromfenac occurred in approximately 1 in 20,000 patients who took the drug for longer than 10 days (Friedman et al. 1999).

Table 9.1. Sample sizes for detection of a given drug risk in a RCT or cohort study (size per study arm)

Relative risk	Incidence of outcome in the control group			
	1/50,000	1/10,000	1/5000	1/1000
2.0	1,177,295	235,430	117,697	23,511
2.5	610,446	122,072	61,025	12,187
3	392,427	78,472	39,228	7832
5	147,157	29,424	14,707	2934
7.5	78,946	15,783	7888	1572
10	53,288	10,652	5323	1059

Calculations are based upon a two-sided significance level α of 0.05, a power of 80% ($\beta = 0.2$), and one control subject per exposed subject

Table 9.2. Drug removals from the US Market between 1997 and 1998. Number of patients exposed to withdrawn drugs in clinical trials compared to actual use after marketing

Removed drug	Number of patients exposed before marketing[1]	Approximate exposure prior to withdrawals
Terfenadine	5000	7,500,000
Fenfluramine	340	6,900,000
Dexfenfluramine	1200	2,300,000
Mibefradil	3400	600,000
Bromfenac	2400	2,500,000

[1] number of patients included in the US premarketing studies

To reliably detect this toxic effect, some 100,000 patients would need to be included in the premarketing clinical studies.

In addition, premarketing clinical studies differ from routine clinical care for a number of other reasons:

1. These studies mostly include a selected study population, defined by strict inclusion and exclusion criteria, which is often not fully representative of subsequent users of the drug. It is well known that premarketing studies tend to under-represent the elderly, patients with comorbid conditions, pregnant women and children. Patients in premarketing trials may even be considered a selected group of patients just because they are willing or able to participate.

2. Premarketing clinical trials are performed at selected sites which are typically better equipped than routine care facilities. They are conducted by specialists in their field and all participating persons have been specially informed and trained. Surveillance of patients is almost by definition more intensive than in routine clinical treatment, if only one considers the frequency and spectrum of laboratory tests or the assessment of therapeutic and unwanted effects.

3. Treatment regimens in premarketing clinical trials are largely fixed and allow almost no individual treatment variations. In contrast, adjustments are constantly made in routine care, depending on the progress of therapy and on the interaction between doctor and patient.

4. Premarketing clinical trials are usually of short duration. This renders it impossible to detect ADRs that only develop after a long induction period or after cumulative drug intake.

For all these reasons, crucial answers to questions of drug safety cannot be provided even by the most valid and complex phase III study.

Characteristics of Spontaneous Reporting Systems 9.3

Description 9.3.1

In the early 1960s, systems evolved in most Western countries that collected spontaneous reports on ADRs from doctors. Establishment of these spontaneous reporting systems was largely a consequence of the "thalidomide disaster", in which children exposed to the hypnotic thalidomide *in utero* were born with phocomelia, a congenital deformity of the limbs resulting from prenatal interference of the drug with the development of the fetal limbs (Wiholm et al. 2000). Worldwide, several thousand cases of limb malformations in newborns observed in the 1950s and 1960s were attributed to the use of thalidomide during pregnancy (Lenz 1987). Based on this experience, spontaneous reporting systems were set up to monitor drug safety in the postmarketing period. In these systems, physicians – in some countries also pharmacists, other health care professionals or patients – report the suspicion of an ADR to the country's drug regulatory agency or to the pharmaceutical company that is marketing the drug. Drug regulatory agencies exchange the ADR reports with the concerned pharmaceutical companies and vice versa. The reports are locally assessed, the reported adverse event terms are coded using a standardized international terminology as e.g. MedDRA (the Medical Dictionary for Regulatory Activities) and are entered in a computerized database. More than 60 countries also forward their ADR reports to the World Health Organization (WHO) Collaborating Centre for International Drug Monitoring in Uppsala (Bate et al. 2002). Through membership in the WHO Programme, one country can know whether similar ADR reports are being made elsewhere.

An ADR report usually contains the patient's demographic information including age and gender; the patient's weight and height; adverse event (AE) information including date and outcome of the event, description of the event, evidence and existing medical history; information of suspect and concomitant medicine(s), including drug name, dose, application and indication for use; whether the event abated after drug use was stopped ("dechallenge"); and whether the event reappeared after the drug was reintroduced ("rechallenge"); and the reporter's name and address.

Each report is assessed for its causality with drug intake by trained reviewers. Causality assessment is usually based on a set of criteria which includes the time interval between drug administration and the onset of the ADR; the course of the reaction when the drug was stopped; the results of re-administration of the drug; the existence of other causes that could also account for the observed reaction such as patient comorbidity or concomitant drug treatment; the pattern of the adverse effect; and the existence of reliable and specific laboratory test results. Causality assessment is not based on the single case report, but will also take into account other available information on the drug(s). In France, causality assessment criteria have been built into an algorithm (the "official method of causality assessment") that is used throughout the country (Benichou 1994). The French method distinguishes "intrinsic imputability" which takes into account only the single case report information from "extrinsic imputability" which is based on all published data on all drugs. Overall, causality assessment from individual case reports is a complex task and often associated with a high degree of uncertainty, since confounding by concomitant drug therapy or the underlying disease can frequently not be ruled out. Rare exceptions are a positive rechallenge to the drug (which is mostly accidental and involuntary, since this is rarely without risks) or positive results of specific laboratory tests such as the detection of drug-dependent antibodies.

Spontaneous reporting systems have several important advantages. They are relatively inexpensive to operate with respect to staff and basic technical equipment. They have the potential to cover the whole patient population and are not restricted to either hospitalised patients or outpatients. Surveillance starts as soon as a drug is marketed and monitoring of drug safety continues throughout the whole postmarketing life cycle of a drug. The suspicion of an ADR is, in theory, based on the experience of all treating physicians and pharmacists. Spontaneous ADR reporting systems can provide an alert to very rare, but nevertheless potentially important drug toxicity. Spontaneous reporting systems have identified many new, i.e. previously unrecognised drug hazards as e.g. clozapine-induced granulocytopenia, captopril-induced cough and amiodarone-induced hepatotoxicity. Further examples can be found in the article by Rawlins et al. (1989).

9.3.2 Limitations

Many of the successes of spontaneous reporting systems have been in the recognition of ADRs occurring shortly after starting therapy. Spontaneous reporting schemes are much less effective in identifying reactions with a long induction period. An example is the oculomucocutaneous syndrome associated with exposure to practolol which was undetected by the yellow card spontaneous reporting scheme in the UK (Venning 1983). For the same reason, spontaneous reporting schemes are not well suited to identify drug-induced cancerogenicity.

ADR reports often do not provide sufficient information to confirm that a drug caused an event. For example, the ADR report may not give enough details on comorbidity or other medications to rule out other possible causes for the event in a remote expert assessment. It may be impossible to exclude confounding by indication, i.e. that the cause for the reported adverse event is rather related to the indication for the drug than to the drug itself. As an example, depression has been reported with the anti-acne medication roaccutane (Wysowski et al. 2001). Depression could, however, also be related to psychological disturbances over severe acne in sensitive teenagers rather than to roaccutane itself.

Recognition of an ADR depends on the level of diagnostic suspicion of the treating physician and may be related to the nature of the adverse event. Some ADRs are more likely to be diagnosed and reported than others because of their known association with drug therapy. For example, acute agranulocytosis is attributable to drug treatment in about 60–70% of cases (Kaufman et al. 1996). It may therefore be more likely to be attributed to drug therapy than a disorder as e.g. acute myocardial infarction that is usually not related to drug treatment (Faich 1986).

Spontaneous reporting systems suffer from serious underreporting of ADRs and various biases that affect reporting. Even in the UK, a country with a relatively high reporting rate in relation to its population size, rarely more than 10% of serious ADRs are notified to the regulatory agency (Rawlins et al. 1989). In France, a recent comparison of ADR reports with data about drug-induced hospitalizations in three pharmacoepidemiology field studies indicates that only 5% of ADRs leading to hospitalisations are actually reported in the spontaneous reporting system (Begaud et al. 2002). Lack of knowledge how to report an ADR and misconceptions about the type of ADR that should be reported are important reasons contributing to underreporting (Eland et al. 1999). On the other hand, it has to be taken into account that spontaneous reporting and published case reports may also lead to numerous false alarms.

Medical or mass media attention can stimulate reporting in a distorted manner and give rise to differential reporting in a dramatic way (Griffin 1986). An example of such "media bias" is that of central nervous side effects following treatment with the benzodiazepine triazolam. After van der Kroef published a case series of these ADR in 1979 (van der Kroef 1979), these side effects received extensive media coverage on Dutch television. As a consequence, the Netherlands received 999 ADR reports related to triazolam in 1979 out of a total of 1912 annual reports in 1979 overall (Griffin 1986). Reporting can also be affected by the market share of the drug; the quality of the manufacturer's surveillance system; reporting regulations and the length of time a drug is on the market (Griffin 1986; Lindquist and Edwards 1993). It has been shown that reporting rates do not remain stable over time, but usually peak during the first or second year after a drug has been introduced into the market and then progressively decline over the following years (Haramburu et al. 1992, 1997).

9.3.3   Statistical Approaches: Reporting Rates and Proportional Reporting Ratio

An ideal early warning system should not only recognize new hazards but also provide an estimate of their incidence. Spontaneous reporting systems may provide alerts of drug hazards, but they cannot be used to calculate incidence rates of adverse events related to a specific drug. Calculation of an incidence rate requires accurate numerator and denominator information, both of which are not available from the spontaneous reporting systems. First, the extent of underreporting for an individual drug is very difficult to assess and may even differ between drugs of the same pharmacological class. Second, the population exposed to the drug (i.e. the population at risk) is unknown and cannot be determined from drug sales data, since the duration of drug use, the dose regimen and compliance in individual patients are unknown.

Instead of the calculation of incidence rates, reporting rates (number of AE reports per market share) based on sales data are sometimes computed as an alternative approach (Pierfitte et al. 2000; Moore et al. 2003). Calculation of reporting rates is based on the assumption that the magnitude of under-reporting is reasonably similar for similar drugs that share the same indication, country and period of marketing (Pierfitte et al. 1999). The comparison of ADR reporting rates should therefore be restricted to drugs of the same category used for the same indication. Factors that may bias the comparison of reporting rates include differences in the length of time the drugs are on the market; differences in exposure populations; secular reporting trends; reporting variations; diagnosis and prescription variation; and the publicity of an ADR. Statistical corrections for year of marketing, secular trends of all-drug-all-adverse event reporting, and drug usage have been proposed (Tsong 1995). These adjustments do not, however, cover all possible sources of bias. In particular do they not erase concerns about differences in the magnitude of under-reporting for different drugs. Interpretation of reporting rates should therefore be conducted with an understanding of their limitations. Differences in reporting rates do not establish differences in incidence rates. They may, however, provide alerts of drug hazards to be investigated by more rigorous pharmacoepidemiological study designs.

The proportional reporting ratio (PRR) has been proposed as another statistical approach for signal generation (Evans et al. 2001). Signals of drug hazards are usually not based on one single ADR report, but on a series of similar suspected reports. The ADR databases maintained by the regulatory authorities and the WHO contain a large number of reports suitable for aggregation, as e.g. 2.5 million reports in the WHO database (Bate et al. 2002), over 2 million reports in the Adverse Event Reporting System (AERS) database maintained by the FDA (Szarfman et al. 2002), and over 350,000 reports in the Adverse Drug Reactions On-line Information Tracking (ADROIT) database of the UK regulatory agency (Evans et al. 2001). The PRR involves calculation of the proportions of specified reactions or groups of reactions for drugs of interest where the comparator is all other drugs in the database. The PRR is the quotient of $a/(a + c)$ divided by $b/(b + d)$ derived from the reported frequencies of all drug-event pairs in the database arranged in a two-by-two table (Table 9.3).

Table 9.3. Calculation of the proportional reporting ratio (PRR) (a, b, c, d are absolute frequencies of the according combination)

	Drug of interest	All other drugs in the database
Event of interest	a	b
All other events	c	d

The PRR behaves in a similar fashion as the relative risk, i.e. the higher the PRR, the greater the strength of the signal. Statistical association is tested using a chi-squared test on 1 degree of freedom for the null hypothesis of independence. Signals can then be identified based on the PRR, the value of the chi-squared test, and the absolute number of reports. In a proof-of-concept study, Evans et al. (2001) defined a signal as a PRR value of at least 2, a value of chi-squared test of at least 4 and a minimum of 3 cases. Using these criteria on the UK ADROIT data base for 15 newly marketed drugs, they identified 481 potential signals, 339 (70%) of which were recognised ADR, 62 (13%) were considered to be related to the underlying disease and 80 (17%) were signals requiring further evaluation. Statistical approaches such as calculation of PRRs are not a substitute for a detailed ADR review, but they may aid in the decision on which series of cases should be investigated next. Similarly, as already mentioned for reporting rates, the PRR may be affected by differential ADR reporting related to notoriety, surveillance and market size effects. A PRR above 1 may therefore just indicate a higher reporting of a possible reaction under a drug, but not necessarily a differential occurrence (Moore et al. 2003). Recently, some modified statistical approaches to ADR data have been proposed for signal generation (Bate et al. 1998; Szarfman et al. 2002). These more complex statistical approaches are, like the PRR, based on a comparison of observed versus expected frequencies of adverse events under a particular drug, but they differ in the way they relate all drug-event combinations in the database to each other and in the use of Bayesian versus frequentist statistical models.

Sources of Data in Pharmacoepidemiological Research   9.4

A great number of pharmacoepidemiology studies are being conducted as field studies, with data being collected for the specific hypothesis under study. These studies are sometimes conducted in an international setting to increase the number of cases and to provide more timely results (Spitzer et al. 1996; Abenhaim et al. 1996; Anonymous 1995b, 1986). Increasingly, already existing data sources are being used for pharmacoepidemiological research. Existing data sources include multipurpose cohort studies or large health databases. Studies utilizing such data can be conducted more quickly and are less expensive than field studies, since the data have already been collected.

9.4.1   Multipurpose Cohorts

Multipurpose cohorts are designed to investigate many different research hypotheses. Their study population usually consists of a subset of a defined population that has not been assembled by a specific exposure, but by other factors. For example, in the US Nurses' Health Studies, study participants were defined by age, female gender and profession (Nurses' Health Study I: 121,700 female nurses aged 30 to 55 years at baseline in 1976; Nurses' Health Study II: 116,671 female nurses aged 25 to 42 years at baseline in 1989). If a multipurpose cohort is used to investigate an association between a specific drug exposure and a disease, its cohort members will usually have sufficient variability in their exposure status for the drug to be investigated: they may currently be exposed or non-exposed, they may be exposed to different doses of the drug, they may have been exposed in the past or they may be exposed in the future. If, in addition, disease occurrence and relevant confounder information has been ascertained, the multipurpose cohort data may be used to investigate a specific pharmacoepidemiological hypothesis. The US Nurses' Health Studies have been extensively used for pharmacoepidemiology research questions. Examples include the association between nonsteroidal anti-inflammatory drugs and risk of Parkinson's disease (Chen et al. 2003), use of estrogens and progestins and risk of breast cancer in postmenopausal women (Colditz et al. 1995), postmenopausal estrogen and progestin use and risk of cardiovascular disease (Grodstein et al. 1996), oral contraceptives and the risk of multiple sclerosis (Hernan et al. 2000), aspirin, other nonsteroidal drugs and risk of ovarian cancer (Fairfield et al. 2002), calcium intake and risk of colon cancer (Wu et al. 2002) and many more associations (Grodstein et al. 1998; Hee and Grodstein 2003; Hernandez-Avila et al. 1990; Weintraub et al. 2002). Other multipurpose cohorts that have been less frequently used for pharmacoepidemiological research include the Health Professionals Follow-up Study (Giovannucci et al. 1994; Chen et al. 2003; Wu et al. 2002); the National Health and Nutrition Examination Survey I (NHANES) epidemiologic follow-up study (Lando et al. 1999; Funkhouser and Sharp 1995); the Framingham cohort study (Worzala et al. 2001; Abascal et al. 1998; Kiel et al. 1987; Felson et al. 1991); and the Rotterdam Study (Schoofs et al. 2003; Beiderbeck-Noll et al. 2003; Feenstra et al. 2002).

9.4.2   Record Linkage Studies

Large health databases have emerged as another important data source for pharmacoepidemiology research. In the United States and Canada, administrative health databases have been set up for the administration of reimbursement payments to health care providers in nationally funded health care systems or managed care organizations. In the United Kingdom, Scotland and some other countries, large health databases consist of data entered by general practitioners (GP) into their practice computers.

Administrative Databases in the US and Canada

These databases usually consist of patient-level information from two or more separate files which can be linked via a unique patient identifier contained in each file. The unique patient identifier often consists of the social security number of the patient which is "scrambled" to ensure patient confidentiality. Information contained in the different files usually consists of demographic patient information; information on drug dispensations from pharmacies; information on hospitalisations; and information on ambulatory physician visits (Fig. 9.1). Through record linkage, person-based longitudinal files can be created for particular research questions. In some databases, record linkage is possible with cancer registries or birth malformation registries to investigate hypotheses of drug carcinogenicity or teratogenicity. Researchers usually have to submit a study protocol for review by an ethics committee and they only receive subsets of the files which are extracted to investigate the particular research hypothesis. Fees are charged for the time needed to extract the necessary data from the entire database. All statistical analyses are done on the anonymized data.

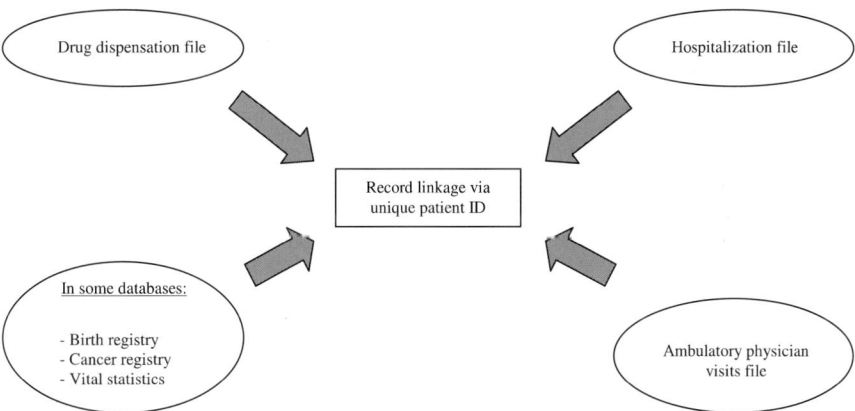

Figure 9.1. Record linkage in administrative health databases

A considerable number of administrative databases in the US and Canada are now available for pharmacoepidemiology research. A brief overview of some of these databases is given in Table 9.4. More detailed information on these databases can be found in the textbook "Pharmacoepidemiology" by Strom (2000).

Saskatchewan's Health Databases have been used extensively for pharmacoepidemiological studies. These databases will be used to illustrate which information may be expected in an administrative healthcare database (Table 9.5, adapted

Table 9.4. Examples of administrative health databases in the US and Canada

Database	Characteristics	Eligible population	Drug dispensations since
Saskatchewan's Health Databases, Saskatchewan, Canada	Provincial health plan	1 million	1975
RAMQ database, Quebec, Canada	Provincial health plan for the elderly	750,000	
Group Health Cooperative, Washington, US	HMO	460,000	1977
Kaiser Permanente, Northern California, US	HMO	2.8 million	1994 (from all pharmacies)
Kaiser Permanente Northwest Division, US	HMO	430,000	1986
Harvard Pilgrim Health Care, New England, US	HMO	1.1 million	
Tennessee Medicaid database, US	Health insurance for recipients of social welfare	1.4 million	1977
New Jersey Medicaid Database	Health insurance for recipients of social welfare	700,000	1980

HMO = Health Maintenance Organizations

from http://www.health.gov.sk.ca/mc_dp_phb_infodoc.pdf). Health Databases in Saskatchewan are based on the universal health insurance programme in this Canadian Province. Differently from the Medicaid program, there is no eligibility distinction based on socio-economic status. Record linkage is possible with the province's cancer registry. Medical records in hospitals are accessible upon approval from individual district health boards and affiliated facilities. Physician records may also be accessed for specific studies. A wide range of conditions has been validated by hospital chart review, including rheumatoid arthritis (Tennis et al. 1993), hip fractures (Ray et al. 1989), gastrointestinal bleeding (Raiford et al. 1996), asthma-related conditions (Spitzer et al. 1992) and others.

Physician-based Databases

The General Practice Research Database (GPRD) is a large physician-based computerized database of anonymized longitudinal patient records from hundreds of general practices in the UK, containing more than 35 million patient years of data. Currently, information is collected on approximately 3 million patients, equivalent to approximately 5% of the UK population. The database was created in June

Table 9.5. Information contained in different files of Health Databases in Saskatchewan

Population registry	Prescription drug database	Hospital separation[1] database	Physician services database
• Name	*Patient information*	*Patient information*	*Patient information*
• HSN[2]	• HSN[2]	• HSN[2]	• HSN[2]
• Sex	• Sex	• Sex	• Age
• Marital status	• Year of birth	• Month and year	• Sex
• Date of birth	• Designation of special	of birth	• Location of
• Date of death	status[3]	*Diagnostic and*	residence
(if applicable)	*Drug information*	*treatment information*	• Indicator for
• Mailing address	• Pharmacologic-	• Up to 3 discharge	registered Indian
• Location code	therapeutic	diagnoses (4-digit	status
• If recipient of	classification	ICD-9)	*Physician information*
Saskatchewan	• Drug identification	• Up to 3 procedures	• Physician specialty
welfare plan	number	(4-digit CCP[4])	• Referring physician
• Dates of	• Active ingredient	• Accident code (ICD-9	• Clinic
coverage	number of drug	external cause code)	• Age
initiation and	• Generic and brand	• Other	• Sex
termination	names	• Admission date	• Place and year
	• Strength and dosage	• Discharge date	of graduation
	forms	• Level of care codes	• Practice type[5]
	• Manufacturer of drug	• Length of stay	*Diagnostic and*
	• Date dispensed	• Admission and	*service information*
	• Quantity dispensed	separation types	• Date of service
	• "No substitution"	• Case mix group	• Type of service
	indicator, if applicable	• Resource intensity	• Primary diagnosis
	Prescriber information	weight	(3-digit ICD-9 code)
	• Prescriber identification	• Attending physician	• Location of service
	number	• Attending surgeon	(e.g., office,
	Dispensing pharmacy	(if applicable)	inpatient,
	information	• Hospital identification	outpatient, home,
	• Pharmacy identification	number	other)
	number		• Billing information
	Cost information		(amount paid, date
	• Unit cost of drug		of payment)
	materials		
	• Dispensing fee		
	• Markup		
	• Consumer share		
	of total cost		
	• Drug plan share		
	of total cost		
	• Total cost		

[1] separation defined as discharge, transfer, or death of an inpatient
[2] health services number [3] e.g. welfare recipient, palliative care registrant, long-term care home resident
[4] CCP: Canadian Classification of Diagnostic, Therapeutic, and Surgical Procedures
[5] solo, association, rural, urban

1987 as the Value Added Medical Products (VAMP) research databank. VAMP provided practice computers and general practice software to general practitioners (GPs) and, in return, GPs consented to undertake data quality training and to contribute anonymized data to a central database for subsequent use in public health research. During the 1990s, VAMP research databank underwent several organisational and management changes. The database was renamed General Practice Research Database (GPRD) in 1994 when it was donated to the UK Department of Health. In 1999, management responsibility for the database was transferred to the UK Medicines Control Agency which became part of the newly created Medicines and Healthcare Products Regulatory Agency (MHRA). The database has been used extensively for pharmacoepidemiology and clinical epidemiology research. A bibliography of studies using GPRD data can be found on the webpage of the GPRD under www.gprd.com.

The database includes the following information: Demographics, including age and gender of patient (information on race is not collected); medical diagnosis, including comments; all prescriptions; events leading to withdrawal of a drug or treatment; referrals to hospitals; treatment outcomes, including hospital discharge reports where patients are referred to hospital for treatment; and miscellaneous patient information e.g. smoking status, height, weight, immunisations, and for a growing number of patients also lab results. Validation studies of the GPRD have shown that the recording of medical data into GPs' computers is almost complete (Garcia Rodriguez and Perez 1998).

Besides the GPRD, other physician-based databases are the MediPlus databases from IMS Health. The MediPlus databases are available in different countries and, like the GPRD, contain anonymized longitudinal patient records. Depending on the particularities of the respective health care system, different data are available for research. A description of the German IMS Disease Analyzer-MediPlus database can be found in an article by Dietlein and Schroder-Bernhardi (2002). The IMS databases have not been used extensively for pharmacoepidemiology research. Studies which examine data validity and comprehensiveness are mostly lacking. The German IMS Disease Analyzer-MediPlus database does not contain patient hospitalisation data. It also lacks diagnostic or treatment information from all physician specialists, since it is usually based on one panel of doctors only, e.g. on a panel of GPs and internists, or gynecologists, or urologists etc. The database derived from the panel of gynecologists would therefore not include information on ambulatory physician contacts in GPs' or internists' offices and vice versa. The German IMS Disease Analyzer-Mediplus database has been used for several drug utilization studies, e.g. on the dosing of cava-cava extracts (Dietlein and Schroder-Bernhardi 2003); whether hospitals influence the prescribing behavior of general practitioners (Schroder-Bernhardi and Dietlein 2002); or how doctors treat Helicobacter pylori infections (Perez et al. 2002) etc. In the UK, the MediPlus database contains similar patient information as the GPRD database.

9.4.3   Advantages and Limitations

Large health databases offer several important advantages:

1. They are usually large, with patient numbers ranging from several hundred thousand to well over several millions. This makes it possible to study rare adverse events of pharmaceuticals in large populations.

2. Medication information is usually more accurate than self-recorded exposure information. Drug histories obtained from patients have limited reliability particularly for drugs that are used only intermittently and not on a regular basis (Kelly et al. 1990). Database information probably represents the most accurate information on drug utilization that can be obtained in elderly patients (Tamblyn et al. 1995). In drug dispensation databases, fairly accurate information can be obtained on drug intake that occurred a long time ago. Exposure information is available also for patients who are deceased or too ill to answer questions, without having to rely on proxy information. There is no potential for recall or interviewer bias which is always of concern with primary data collection.

3. Because the data are collected in an ongoing manner as a by-product of health care delivery, epidemiological studies can be undertaken in reasonable time and at relatively low cost. The study variables are already available in computerized form and need not be obtained in time-consuming and expensive processes of data collection.

4. Some databases provide population-based data which cover the entire population of a geographical region and are thus fully representative of the population. Database studies do not require an informed patient consent and are therefore less prone to selection bias which may be a consequence of a low response rate in the study population.

Use of computerized databases for pharmacoepidemiology research is, however, not undisputed (Shapiro 1989) and there are a number of important limitations. A major concern is related to the validity of the diagnostic information contained in the database. In administrative health databases, diseases are primarily coded for billing and not for research purposes. There is no incentive for the health care provider to use specific codes as e.g. "duodenal ulcer with bleeding" instead of "upper gastrointestinal bleeding otherwise not specified". Diseases are often coded according to the International Classification of Diseases (ICD-9 or ICD-10 coding schemes) and many different ICD-codes may be compatible with the same disease process. A combination of several diagnostic codes into a single "broader" code may therefore be necessary (Garbe et al. 1997, 1998a). Strom and Carson (1990) have described this problem by stating that researchers using diagnostic codes in a computerized database must be "lumpers" rather than "splitters".

The validity of diagnostic coding also depends on the ability of a diagnostic code to rather selectively represent the condition in question and therefore varies with the condition. Strom conducted a validation study of ICD-9 coding of Stevens-Johnson Syndrome in the COMPASS Medicaid database in the US (Strom et al. 1991). Records of 3.8 million patients in five US states were searched for ICD9-CM code 695.1 which codes for Stevens-Johnson syndrome, but also for several other, less serious conditions. In an expert medical record review, only 14.8% of patients with ICD9-CM code 695.1 whose medical records could be reviewed were judged to have Stevens-Johnson syndrome. Thus, studies of Stevens-Johnson-Syndrome in databases with ICD9-coding cannot be conducted without additional validation of the diagnosis. Whenever possible, validity of disease coding should be quantified for each condition studied.

Validation studies usually use the paper medical or pharmacy record as the "gold standard". Access to patient charts for validation purposes is often obtained via the scrambled social security (patient identification) number. All personal-identifying information is removed before copies of the charts are made available. The validation study by Strom also illustrates another problem: Only 51% of the medical records that were sought for in the study could actually be obtained (Strom et al. 1991). The authors state several reasons why they did not obtain access to the medical records: refusal of hospitals (30%); transcription errors (27%); translation of ID-number not possible (17%), no location of medical record possible (22%); other reasons (4%).

Administrative databases usually contain information on large numbers of patients, however, the amount of information per patient is limited:

1. Information about disease severity is mostly lacking and it may not be possible to exclude confounding by disease severity. In some instances, it is possible to construct an index of disease severity based on the patient's pharmacotherapy (Spitzer et al. 1992).
2. Relevant other confounder information for the association under study may not be contained in the database, creating a potential for bias. For example, most administrative databases do not contain information on smoking or alcohol use (Friedman et al. 2000) or age at menopause and reproductive history in women.
3. Administrative databases usually do not contain data on laboratory values or clinical measurements, although, in some databases, linkage with laboratory files has now become possible.
4. If relevant confounder information is missing and additional data collection required, it will make a study considerably more expensive and time-consuming, thereby diminishing some of the advantages connected with database research. It has to be decided on a case-by-case basis whether the information contained in a database is sufficient for the investigation of an association of interest and how much time and cost would be incurred if additional data have to be collected.

Although the medication information in databases is one of their major strengths, it also has some limitations: Information on drugs bought over-the-counter (OTC) and not prescribed by a physician is not available in the database; the patient's compliance with the prescription is unknown; in-hospital medication is usually not contained in the database; the prescribed daily dose is not documented in most databases and the average daily dose has to be calculated instead based on the duration of drug use and the quantity of drug prescribed; the prescription file does not contain the indication for drug prescribing, however, in many instances, this information may be deduced from diagnostic coding in the ambulatory physician file; medication data will be truncated, if the database does not exist long enough or the database only includes elderly subjects. Truncation will limit the study of cumulative drug toxicity. Confounding by previous drug use may be avoided if a prior period of follow-up in the database is defined and the risk is only investigated in new users of the drug (Garbe et al. 1998b); many of the newest and/or most expensive drugs may not be available for study, if they are not included on the drug formulary.

Other important issues include whether the population contained in a database is representative of the source population and stable over time. For example, Saskatchewan Health Databases, which cover the population of the whole province of Saskatchewan, consist of a representative and fairly stable database population (Downey et al. 2003). In contrast, Medicaid Databases in the US are not representative of the US population, since they only include social welfare recipients and thereby over-represent children, females and non-whites in comparison with the total US population (Strom and Carson 1990). The skewedness of Medicaid Databases may not compromise the internal validity of a pharmacoepidemiology study conducted with these databases, but it may be a serious threat to its external validity, particularly when the data are being used for drug utilization research. In Medicaid Databases, turnover of the database population is high due to changing eligibility for Medicaid. Over a five-year time period, only 35% of Michigan and 38% of Tennessee Medicaid enrollees were still in the system, with loss of eligibility being greatest in children and young adults (Ray and Griffin 1989). High patient turnover may also make it difficult to locate patient files for validation studies as has been reported in the study by Strom (Strom et al. 1991). Data from health maintenance databases are also not fully representative of the US population. Members of these organizations tend to be less frequently black or poor and have higher educational achievements. Turnover in membership at HMOs is usually less than in Medicaid databases (Saunders et al. 2000; Friedman et al. 2000).

Methodological Approaches for Pharmacoepidemiology Studies 9.5

The strategies employed to verify hypotheses on drug risks or benefits are similar to those used in other fields of epidemiology. The case-control design is the design of choice for the investigation of rare drug risks, particularly if multiple countries are necessary to attain sufficient power, while the cohort approach is preferably used to assess the risk of more frequent events or if more than one outcome has to be considered simultaneously. The special nature of drug exposure and the availability of existing databases in pharmacoepidemiology have given rise to specific challenges and preferred solutions to estimate risk and benefit.

9.5.1   ## Case-Control Studies

Field studies that employ a case-control design (cf. Chap. I.6 of this handbook) are
not common in the evaluation of the risks and benefits of prescribed drugs. Drugs
available over-the-counter without prescription are not recorded systematically in
computerized databases can therefore not be studied with linked databases. Thus
studies of drugs such as analgesics, vitamin supplements, anorexiants etc, can only
be studied by directly obtaining exposure information from subjects. With this
design, cases with the outcome under study are identified from a given population,
usually in hospitals or specialised clinics since they mostly involve serious outcomes. The approach to select the controls varies across studies. The International
Agranulocytosis and Aplastic Anemia Study (IAAAS) that evaluated the effect
of different analgesics on the risks of agranulocytosis and aplastic anemia used
hospital-based controls (Anonymous 1986). The International Primary Pulmonary
Hypertension Study (IPPHS) of the risk of primary pulmonary hypertension associated with anorexiant agents used patients treated by the same physician as the
source of controls (Abenhaim et al. 1996). The Yale Hemorrhagic Stroke Study assessing the risk of diet and cough/cold remedies containing phenypropalonamine
used population-based controls identified by random-digit dialling (Viscoli et al.
2001) (see also Chap. I.10 of this handbook). Finally, the Transnational study on
oral contraceptive risks used both hospital and population-based controls (Spitzer
et al. 1996). Such field studies that collect information from patients, physicians
or medical charts are the exception because of the resources, expense and time
required to complete the study.

Case-control studies using existing health databases are much more common.
Besides the usual concerns with case-control studies in general, some are specific
to studies conducted from databases. For example, the General Practice Research
Database (GPRD) was used to evaluate the impact of inhaled corticosteroids on the
risk of hip fracture (Hubbard et al. 2002). The entire GPRD was used to identify
16,341 cases of hip fracture and a random sample of 29,889 subjects selected as
controls. This design is attractive because of its efficiency in using only a sample of
subjects to estimate an effect for an entire population. Such an approach, however,
can be deceiving for specific diseases such as asthma because of the illusion of
large sample sizes. Indeed, all cases of hip fracture selected within a population
such as the GPRD suggests a very large sample size for the study, along with
the very large number of controls. However, in assessing the effect of inhaled
corticosteroids, a drug pertinent exclusively to the population of asthma or chronic
obstructive pulmonary disease (COPD) patients, a large proportion of the cases
and the controls are in fact irrelevant to the question at hand. Thus, for example,
for the GPRD case-control study of hip fracture risk, only 878 of the 16,341cases
and 1335 of the 29,889 controls were subjects with asthma or COPD (Hubbard
et al. 2002). With its 16,341 cases and 29,889 controls, the study appears at first
more powerful than the Quebec study, based on 3326 cases of hip fracture and
66,237 controls selected from the asthma/COPD population (Suissa et al. 2004).
In fact, the inference on the effect of inhaled corticosteroids is actually based on

many fewer subjects than believed. This point is particularly relevant for studies that find no significantly increased risk since, despite appearances, conclusions are based on fewer numbers of cases and controls with respiratory disease and thus lower power than expected. Furthermore, the estimate of effect may be biased if the outcome of interest, in this instance fractures, is also associated with the disease itself (asthma or COPD) and not only with the medications used to treat these conditions. In this case, the bias due to the association with the disease can only be eliminated by restricting the analyses to the population of patients who have the disease (Suissa et al. 2004).

Another issue in such database case-control studies is the manner by which controls are selected and particularly the index date for controls. In the GPRD study of the impact of inhaled corticosteroids on the risk of hip fracture, controls were matched to cases on age, sex, general practice and date of entry into the database (Hubbard et al. 2002). While the index date from which exposure was assessed was the fracture date for the cases, the index date for the controls was the same date as the matched case. To allocate such a date, one must be assured that the control is at risk on that date. Indeed, there could be control subjects with the same age, sex, general practice and date of entry, but who are dead or not in the practice at the time of the matched case's fracture. These will be necessarily currently "unexposed", which could bias upward the rate ratio.

Cohort Studies   9.5.2

Observational database studies that use a cohort design (cf. Chap. I.5 of this handbook) differ primarily with respect to their definition of cohort entry or time zero. The Saskatchewan asthma cohorts have defined asthma as well as its onset, by the dispensing of medications used to treat the condition, without the use of diagnostic codes from physicians (Blais et al. 1998b; Suissa et al. 2002). Patients were considered to have asthma as of the first time they received three prescriptions for an asthma medication, including bronchodilators, inhaled steroids and other asthma drugs, on at least two different dates within a one-year period. The date of the third prescription defined the onset and diagnosis of asthma and patients were then followed from that point on for the occurrence of asthma outcomes. Such a definition is not entirely accurate for two reasons: subjects with asthma may be hospitalized at their initial presentation and medications for asthma are used for other conditions such as COPD. In an attempt to exclude patients with COPD, age criteria were used, including only patients to the age of 44, and also excluding oral corticosteroids as one of the defining drugs for asthma.

Alternatively, cohort entry may be defined by calendar time. For example, a cohort formed from a health maintenance organization in eastern Massachusetts defined cohort entry as October 1, 1991 (Donahue et al. 1997; Adams et al. 2002). This cohort of 16,941 asthma patients was followed from this date or registration in the insurance plan to September 30th 1994. Such calendar time based definitions of cohort entry will inherently define cohorts with patients who have varying durations of disease at time zero (cohort entry). Such a "prevalent" cohort, to be distinguished from an "incident" cohort defined by patients with new onset of asthma, can be subject to serious biases when evaluating the association between drug use and asthma outcomes. Indeed, if the risk of the asthma outcome and of being dispensed the drug under study are both associated with the duration of asthma, such prevalent cohorts will produce biased estimates of this association unless the duration of the condition can somehow be adjusted for. A source of selection bias for such prevalent cohorts is that the treatment itself may change because of prior events that are not included in the period of observation. For example, if a patient was hospitalized for asthma in the past and, as a result, was prescribed inhaled corticosteroids, such a patient may be at increased risk of a further hospitalization and of being dispensed inhaled corticosteroids subsequently. For such studies to be valid, information on the history of asthma prior to cohort entry, which includes the duration of the disease and prior outcomes such as asthma hospitalizations as well as prior drug exposures, are required for purpose of adjustment or for testing for effect-modification. A frequent problem with computerized database studies is that these historical data on the duration and history of the disease before cohort entry are rarely available.

The third type of cohort defines cohort entry by a specific clinical event, such as hospitalization, emergency room visit or a physician visit. Here again, these cohorts can be incident or prevalent if these cohort defining events are either the first one ever or rather the first to occur after a certain date. An example of this approach is a study from the Saskatchewan databases of asthma patients, with entry defined by the first time they received three prescriptions for an asthma medication within a one-year period, after a two-year span with no asthma medications. The study cohort consisted of all subjects hospitalized for asthma for the first time after cohort entry and followed until readmission. The use of inhaled corticosteroids subsequent to the first hospitalization was evaluated with respect to the rate of readmission (Blais et al. 1998a). A similar cohort definition was used with the Ontario database, although this cohort was based on elderly COPD patients and the COPD hospitalisation defining cohort entry was not necessarily the first one to occur in their disease (Sin and Tu 2001a).

9.5.3 Nested Case-Control Studies

The complexity in data analysis is greater in the field of database studies because of the technical challenges presented by their large size. Indeed, the asthma cohort formed from the health maintenance organization in eastern Massachusetts included 742 asthma hospitalisations occurring during the three year follow-up period (Donahue et al. 1997). With over 16,000 patients in the cohort, an analysis based on the Cox proportional hazards model with time-dependent exposure (cf. Chap. II.4 of this handbook) would require 742 risk sets (all patients in the cohort on the day of hospitalization) each containing approximately 16,000 observations with information on exposure and confounding factors measured at the point in time when the case occurred. Such an analysis would therefore require to generate close to 12 million observations (742 × 16,000), each with dozens of variables. Another example is the cohort study that included over 22,000 elderly patients hospitalised for COPD in Ontario, Canada, of whom around 8000 either died or were re-admitted for COPD (Sin and Tu 2001a). A proper time-dependent analysis could include up to 140 million observations, creating a serious technical challenge in statistical computing. As a result of this complexity, the temptation to analyse these cohorts with exposures that are assumed not to change over time is attractive but, as described below, can cause severe immortal time bias (see Sect. 9.6.1).

Rather than analyzing such cohort studies with proper but complex time-dependent techniques, methods based on sampling can produce practically the same results at greater efficiency. The nested case-control design (cf. Chap. I.7 of this handbook), nested within the cohort, is precisely such an approach (Suissa 2000; Essebag et al. 2003). It is based on using data on all the cases with the study outcome that occur during cohort follow-up. These represent the case-series. A random sample of person-moments, namely time points during the subjects' follow-up, is then selected from all person-moments in the cohort to provide the control group for the nested case-control approach. For the cases, the index date, on which the timing of the exposure to the drug of interest is based, is simply the time at which the outcome occurred. For controls, the index date is the random person-moment(s) selected for that subject during follow-up, or the same point in time of the corresponding case (Suissa 2000). Because of the highly variable nature of drug exposure over time, it is important that person-moments are selected properly from all person-moments of follow-up for all members of the cohort. Thus, a subject may be selected more than once at different moments of their follow-up, and particularly person-moments preceding the index date of a case are valid control person-moments. For practical reasons and to conform to the Cox proportional hazards model, person-moments are usually selected from the risk set of each case. This approach involves identifying, for each case, all subjects who are at risk of the event at the time that the case occurred (the risk set) and controls are selected from this risk set (incidence density sampling, cf. Chaps. I.6 and I.7 of this handbook). Part of the simplicity of this approach is that all subjects in a risk set are allocated the same index date as the set-defining case.

The advantage of this approach is the direct relationship between the Cox proportional hazard model with time-dependent exposure and the conditional logistic regression analysis (cf. Chap. II.3 of this handbook) that is used to analyse such nested case-control data. Thus, instead of using exposure data on all members of the risk set, as the Cox model would require, data on only a few subjects (usually 4 or 10 controls per case) are sufficient to provide a very efficient estimator of the rate ratio. Such ease of data analysis with the large size databases that are used in pharmacoepidemiology is crucial. As an example, with the asthma cohort study of Donahue, if 10 controls per case were used for each of the 742 cases, the analysis would be based on 7420 observations instead of the 12 million observations necessary with the Cox model analysis.

In studying the effectiveness of drug treatment, one of the major problems is confounding by indication. The nested case-control approach becomes more useful, as it allows cases and controls to be matched on several measures of disease severity. Thus, the effect of a drug can be isolated, independently of the effects of the severity markers. Such a matched nested case-control study was used to evaluate the effectiveness of inhaled corticosteroids on asthma death (Suissa et al. 2000a). In that study, cases were identified from a cohort of over 30,000 asthma patients, from which 66 died of asthma. The Cox analysis would have required almost 2 million observations to be processed. For each case, however, the only members of the risk sets that were identified as controls were those with the same disease severity characteristics as the case, namely: prior hospitalization for asthma, oral corticosteroid use, number of canisters of beta-agonists, use of theophylline and nebulized beta-agonists. Thus, cases and controls were similar on all these severity markers, expect with respect to inhaled corticosteroids. As a result, the effect of inhaled corticosteroids could be assessed independently of these potential confounding factors.

9.5.4   Case-Crossover Design

Pharmacoepidemiology is frequently faced with the assessment of the risk of rare acute adverse events resulting from transient drug effects. Although the case-control approach can be used, the acuteness of the adverse event and the length of the drug's effect, as well as difficulties in determining the timing of drug exposure, induce uncertainty about the proper selection of controls. Moreover, confounding by indication may often be a problematic issue in such a design. In this situation, within-subject approaches have been proposed, including the case-crossover design and its extension the case-time-control design which was devised to counter time trend biases. The principle is that, when studying transient drug effects and acute outcome events, the best representatives of the source population that produced the cases are the cases themselves (cf. Chap. I.7 of this handbook).

To carry out a case-crossover study, three critical points must be considered. First, the study must necessarily be dealing with an acute adverse event which is alleged to be the result of a transient drug effect. Thus, drugs with regular patterns of use which vary only minimally between and within individuals are not easily amenable to this design. Nor are latent adverse events which only occur long after exposure. Second, since a transient effect is under study, the effect period (or time window of effect) must be precisely determined. An incorrect specification of this time window can have important repercussions on the risk estimate. Third, one must obtain reliable data on the usual pattern of drug exposure for each case, over a sufficiently long period of time.

The case-crossover study is simply a crossover study in the cases only. The subjects alternate at varying frequencies between exposure and non-exposure to the drug of interest, until the adverse event occurs, which happens for all subjects in the study, since all are cases by definition. With respect to the timing of the adverse event, each case is investigated to determine whether exposure occurred within the predetermined effect period. In the VACCIMUS study of hepatitis B vaccination and the risk of a multiple sclerosis relapse, spontaneous reports indicated that such an effect could occur within two months of the vaccination (Confavreux et al. 2001). Thus, the case-crossover design used as the risk-period the 2-month period prior to the onset of the relapse and any vaccination in this period to determine exposure status. To obtain control exposure, data on the average drug use pattern are necessary to determine the typical probability of exposure to the time window of effect. This is done by obtaining data for a sufficiently stable period of time prior to time of the event occurrence and its exposure period. For the VACCIMUS study, there were four control periods consisting of the four 2-month periods prior to the 2-month risk period. The estimation of the odds ratio is based on any appropriate technique for matched data (4 controls per case), such as conditional logistic regression.

This design has been used in pharmacoepidemiology (Fagot et al. 2001; Neutel et al. 2002; Etienney et al. 2003; Ki et al. 2003; Confavreux et al. 2001; Barbone et al. 1998; Sturkenboom et al. 1995).

Case-Time-Control Designs

9.5.5

One of the limitations of the case-crossover design, particularly in the context of drug exposures, is that the exposure pattern may have changed over time, and particularly between the control and risk periods. For example, a rapid increase in vaccination rates over time during the span of the case ascertainment for the VACCIMUS study, particularly if this span had been short, would have biased the estimate of the odds ratio. Indeed, this estimate would also include the effect of the natural time trend in exposure. If control subjects are available, the case-time-control design can be used to separate the time effect from the drug effect (Suissa 1995). In simple terms, the time effect is estimated from the case-crossover odds ratio of exposure among the control subjects. The net effect of exposure on event occurrence is then computed by dividing the combined time and drug effect estimated from the case-crossover odds ratio of exposure among the case subjects by the time effect (cf. Chap. I.7 of this handbook).

The approach is illustrated with data from the Saskatchewan Asthma Epidemiologic Project, a study conducted to investigate the risks associated with the use of inhaled β-agonists in the treatment of asthma. Using databases from Saskatchewan, Canada, a cohort of 12,301 asthmatics was followed during 1980–87. All 129 cases of fatal or near-fatal asthma and 655 controls were selected. The amount of β-agonist used in the year prior to the index date, namely high (more than 12 canisters per year) compared with low (12 or less canisters), was found to be associated to the adverse event. Of the 129 cases, 93 (72%) were high users of β-agonists, compared with 241 (37%) of the 655 controls. The resulting crude odds ratio for high β-agonist use is 4.4 (95% confidence interval (CI): 2.9–6.7). Adjustment for all available markers of severity, such as oral corticosteroids and prior asthma hospitalizations as confounding factors, lowers the odds-ratio to 3.1 (95% CI: 1.8–5.4), the "best" estimate one can derive from these case-control data using conventional tools.

The use of inhaled β-agonists, however, is known to increase with asthma severity which also increases the risk of fatal or near-fatal asthma. It is therefore not possible to separate the effects of the drug to the risk from that of disease severity, so that a within-subject design may be preferable. To apply the case-time-control design, exposure to β-agonists was obtained for the one-year current-period and the one-year reference-period. Among the 129 cases, 29 were currently high users of β-agonists and were low users in the reference period, while 9 cases were currently low users of β-agonists and were high users previously. The case-crossover estimate of the odds ratio is thus 29/9 (OR 3.2; 95% CI:1.5–6.8). However, the high use of β-agonists may have increased naturally over time, so that the control subjects were used to estimate this effect. Among the 655 controls, 65 were currently high users of β-agonists and were low users in the reference period, while 25 were currently low users of β-agonists and were high users previously, for an odds ratio of the time trend of 65/25 (OR 2.6; 95% CI:1.6–4.1) . The case-time-control odds ratio, using these discordant pair frequencies for a paired-matched analysis, is given by $(29/9)/(65/25) = 1.2$ (95% CI: 0.5–3.0). This estimate, which excludes the effect of unmeasured confounding by disease severity, indicates a minimal risk for these drugs.

The case-time-control approach provides a useful complement to the case-crossover design when the probability of drug exposure is not stable over time, particularly between the control and risk periods (Donnan and Wang 2001; Hernandez-Diaz et al. 2003). However, its validity is subject to several assumptions, including the homogeneity of the odds-ratio across subjects (Greenland 1996; Suissa 1998).

9.6 Some Methodological Challenges

9.6.1 Immortal Time Bias in Cohort Studies

A challenge of cohort studies is in their data analysis. Since drug therapy, the exposure of interest, often changes over time, data analysis must take this variability into account. However, such variability in exposure over time is not simple to incorporate in the analysis. Due to the complexity of such analyses, several of the studies mentioned above employed a time-fixed definition of exposure, by invoking the principle of intention-to-treat analysis. This principle, borrowed from randomised controlled trials, is based on the premise that subjects are exposed to the drug under study immediately at the start of follow-up. This information is unknown in database studies.

To emulate randomized controlled studies in the context of cohort studies, some authors have looked forward after cohort entry for the first prescription of the drug under study. In this way, a subject who was dispensed a prescription for such drug was considered exposed and a subject who did not was considered unexposed. Different time periods of exposure assessment were used. For instance, in the context of COPD, a prescription for inhaled corticosteroids during the period of 90 days after cohort entry was used to define exposure (Sin and Tu 2001b). In other studies, periods of one year and three years were used to consider subjects exposed to inhaled corticosteroids in assessing their impact on mortality (Sin and Tu 2001a; Sin and Man 2002). This approach, however, leads to immortal time bias, a major source of distortion in the rate ratio estimate (Suissa 2003).

Immortal time bias arises from the introduction of immortal time in defining exposure by looking forward after cohort entry. Indeed, if exposed subjects were classified as such because they were observed to have been dispensed their first prescription for an inhaled corticosteroid 80 days after cohort entry, they necessarily had to be alive on day 80. Therefore, this 80-day period is immortal. While some exposed subjects will have very short immortal time periods (a day or two), others can have very long immortal periods. On the other hand, unexposed subjects do not have any immortal time, and in particular the subjects who die soon after cohort entry, with too little time to receive the drug under study. Therefore, the exposed subjects will have a major survival advantage over their unexposed counterparts because they are guaranteed to survive at least until their drug was dispensed.

This generation of immortal time in exposed subjects, but not in the unexposed subjects, causes an underestimation of the rate of the outcome among the exposed subjects. This underestimation results from the fact that the outcome rate in the exposed is actually composed of two rates. The first is the true rate, based on the person-time cumulated after the date of drug dispensing that defines exposure (post-Rx), while the second is that based on the person-time cumulated from cohort entry until the date of drug dispensing that defines exposure (pre-Rx). The first rate will therefore be computed by dividing all outcome events in that group by the first rate person-time, while the second rate will by definition divide zero events by the second rate person-time. For example, the rate in the exposed

$$\text{rate} = \text{deaths/total person-years}$$

consists in fact of two rates:

$$\text{rate pre-Rx} = 0/\text{person-years pre-Rx}$$

and

$$\text{rate post-RX} = \text{deaths/person-years post-Rx} .$$

The zero component of the rate will necessarily bring down the exposed rate. Since there is no such phenomenon in the unexposed group, the computation of the rate ratio will systematically produce a value lower than the true value because of the underestimation of the exposed rate. In particular, if the drug under study is altogether unrelated to the outcome, so that the true rate ratio is 1, this approach will produce rate ratios lower than 1, thus creating an appearance of effectiveness for the drug.

The immortal time in exposed subjects also causes an overestimation of the rate of the outcome among the unexposed subjects. This is because the zero component of the rate in the exposed group should in fact be classified in the unexposed group. Indeed, subjects are in fact unexposed to the drug under study between cohort entry until the date of drug dispensing that defines exposure. They only start to be exposed after the drug is dispensed. Thus, the zero rate should in fact be combined with the unexposed rate.

Immortal time bias is thus the result of simplistic yet improper exposure definitions and analyses that cause serious misclassification of exposure and outcome events. This situation is created by using an emulation of the randomised controlled trial to simplify the analysis of complex time-varying drug exposure data. However, such studies do not lend themselves to such simple paradigms. Instead, time-dependent methods for analysing risks, such as the Cox proportional hazard models with time-dependent exposures or nested case-control designs, must be used to account for complex changes in drug exposure and confounders over time (Suissa 2003, 2004; Samet 2003).

9.6.2   Confounding by Indication

The indication for which a medication is given may act as a confounder in observational studies, particularly when assessing the effectiveness of a drug (Slone et al. 1979; Horwitz and Feinstein 1981; Strom et al. 1983). Such confounding by indication will be present if the indication for the prescription of the medication under study is also a determinant of the outcome of interest. Generally, a drug is more likely to be prescribed to a patient with more severe disease who, in turn, is more likely to incur an adverse outcome of the disease. Thus, patients prescribed the drug under study will have higher rates of outcome than the subjects not prescribed the drug. Such an appearance of lack of effectiveness could simply be a reflection of the effect of indication, in this case disease severity.

Confounding by indication is often difficult to control, primarily because the precise reason for prescribing is rarely measured. This may preclude the study of drug effectiveness with observational designs (Miettinen 1983). Yet, a clinical trial to answer this question would require the follow-up of thousands of patients over a long time, which may simply be unfeasible. Observational studies become the tool of choice as long as validity of the study is not compromised by intractable confounding by indication (Miettinen 1983). If such an observational study produces lower rates of outcome for the drug under study, one may conclude that these medications are effective. On the other hand, if users of the drug are found to be at equal or increased risk of the outcome relative to nonusers, it would not be possible to conclude on the absence of a protective effect of these medications.

This problem of confounding by indication is compounded with the use of computerized databases, because of their lack of information on important confounders (Shapiro 1989). The absence of information on drug indication precludes the control of confounding by adjustment in the analysis. Thus, control for confounding by indication must be tackled at the design level. One approach is to restrict the study to a group of patients homogeneous with respect to disease severity. For example, in a study of the effectiveness of inhaled corticosteroids in asthma, Blais et al. (1998a) identified a point in time at which users and nonusers of inhaled corticosteroids would have a similar level of asthma severity. The study was thus restricted to patients who had just been hospitalized for asthma, with the discharge date taken as time zero, which would greatly reduce heterogeneity in disease severity. The rate of a readmission for asthma was then assessed according to the use of inhaled corticosteroids after this initial hospitalization.

Another approach is to compare two medications prescribed for the same indication (Strom et al. 1983, 1984). In this case, relative effectiveness as opposed to absolute effectiveness will be evaluated. An example of this approach was also used in a study of the effectiveness of early use of inhaled corticosteroids in asthma. Blais et al. (1998b) identified a cohort of newly treated asthma patients and compared regular users of inhaled corticosteroids with regular users of either anti-allergic agents or theophylline and matched for the duration of asthma at the initiation of therapy.

Depletion of Susceptibles 9.6.3

In general, the risk of an ADR associated with drug use does not remain constant over time, and can change in different ways from the start of its use. The risk may increase with cumulative drug exposure (e.g. the risk of cardiomyopathy associated with cumulative anthracycline exposure or the risk of cataract associated with continued glucocorticoid use), but it may also decrease after an initial period of sharp increased risk. Therefore, in using a case-control study that evaluates the effect of current use of a drug, past history of use of a drug or a class of drugs must be accounted for as it may modify the risk of an ADR associated with current use of the drug.

A decreasing risk after an initial period of increased risk is probably more important than cumulative drug toxicity and may, at the population level, lead to a phenomenon which has been described as "depletion of susceptibles": patients who remain on the drug are those who can tolerate it while those who are susceptible to adverse drug reactions will stop the drug and thereby select themselves out of the exposed cohort (Moride and Abenhaim 1994). Such a pattern has been demonstrated for the gastrointestinal toxicity of nonsteroidal antiinflammatory drugs (NSAIDS). It has been shown that the risk of upper gastrointestinal bleeding (UGIB) was highest after the third NSAID prescription and thereafter decreasing (Carson et al. 1987). Moride and Abenhaim (1994) empirically showed a depletion of susceptibles effect in a hospital-based case-control study of NSAIDS and the risk of UGIB. They investigated the risk of UGIB associated with recent NSAID use stratified by past or no past NSAID use. The risk of UGIB was significantly greater for those patients who used NSAIDS for the first time in 3 years (OR = 22.7) than for those who had used these drugs before (OR = 3.0) (Yola and Lucien 1994).

The enormous importance of accounting for changes in drug risk over time in the design and/or analysis of pharmacoepidemiology studies was highlighted in the debate about the risk of venous thromboembolism (VTE) associated with second or third generation oral contraceptives (OC). Several pharmacoepidemiology studies published in 1995/1996 reported an increased risk of VTE among users of newer OC preparations compared with those of older OC preparations (Bloemenkamp et al. 1995; Anonymous 1995a; Spitzer et al. 1996; Jick et al. 1995). Additional analyses suggested that the magnitude of the risk estimates for individual OC were closely linked with the time of market introduction of the respective OC, with increasing risk for the newer preparations (Lewis et al. 1996). Since a larger proportion of users of older OC preparations were long-term users compared with those using newer OC, a depletion of susceptibles effect was postulated to be active within these studies. It was hypothesized that individuals with good tolerance were preferentially long term users of older OC preparations, whereas groups with shorter duration of use might be more frequently using the newer OC preparations and thereby constitute a different subpopulation.

The phenomenon of depletion of susceptibles can lead, if not accounted for properly, to a comparison of OC medications with different years of entry into the market and result in an overestimation of the risk associated with the most recently introduced medications. To properly account for depletion of susceptibles, the approach to statistical analysis must take account of the duration and patterns of OC use, and of course have the available data to do so. In this example, the pattern and duration of OC use are not confounders, but effect modifiers of the risk of VTE associated with recent OC use. OC pattern and duration can therefore not be simply "adjusted for" in the statistical analysis, but a stratified analysis has to be conducted which compares the risk of VTE for the different OC preparations for the different durations and patterns of use. When the analysis was restricted to the same pattern of OC use, distinguishing between first time users, repeaters and switchers, the risk of VTE as a function of the duration of oral contraceptive use was essentially the same for second and third generation pills relative to never users (Suissa et al. 1997, 2000b) .

9.6.4   Use of Propensity Scores in Pharmacoepidemiology

In a randomized trial, randomization of study subjects to different treatment regimens aims to assure the absence of systematic differences between the patients in terms of measured and unmeasured confounders. In observational studies, direct comparisons of the outcomes of treated and untreated patients may be misleading because of systematic differences between those patients who have and have not received treatment. The propensity score has been proposed as a method of adjusting for covariate imbalances in an observational study and has recently been proposed also for pharmacoepidemiology research (Perkins et al. 2000; Wang and Donnan 2001; Wang et al. 2001). The propensity score

$\pi(X) = Prob(\text{exposed}|X)$ is defined as the conditional probability of receiving a particular treatment (i.e. being exposed) given the set of observed covariates X. The propensity score thus represents a summary of the covariates X that are associated with treatment allocation in the form of a single variable.

The propensity score approach is a two-stage approach. At the first stage, the propensity score is estimated for each study subject based on the values of the observed covariates. The most commonly used approach is to obtain the propensity score estimates in a logistic regression model, where treatment allocation is used as the dependent (response) variable and observed potential confounders X are used as explanatory variables: $\log(\pi(X)/(1 - \pi(X))) = X\beta$, where the regression coefficients β are fitted by maximum likelihood.

Having obtained the estimated propensity score, it can be used by a number of approaches at the second stage: study subjects may be matched or stratified based on their propensity scores or the propensity scores may be adjusted for in a regression model (Wang and Donnan 2001).

Many published applications use stratification by the propensity score. A common approach is to stratify by quintiles of the distribution of the estimated propensity scores and to test the balance of each confounder between the treatment groups in each stratum (Wang and Donnan 2001). Having patients with similar propensity scores in each stratum, it may be assumed that the covariate distributions in the two treatment groups are equally similar within each stratum, so that the treatment assignment within the strata can be functionally regarded as random. If unbalanced confounders are still found, the propensity score model may be re-estimated with modifications until balance is achieved.

Stratification by the propensity score cannot control confounder effects within a single stratum. The somewhat arbitrary choice of five strata can be viewed as a compromise between reduction of bias and robustness of the results: an increasing number of strata will reduce the bias in the stratification estimate, but it will at the same time decrease the robustness of the results when the sample size of the smaller arm in a stratum becomes too small. Control of bias through use of propensity scores is based on the following assumptions:

- All subjects must have some non-zero probability of receiving each treatment (referred to as the "strongly ignorable assumption"). This ensures independence of treatment assignment and response variable within propensity score strata.
- Treatment assignment depends solely on the observed covariates, i.e. *all* confounders are included in the propensity score model.

If *all* confounders were not ascertained or confounder measurement was associated with bias, the use of propensity scores will not eliminate bias. In fact, the study will be subject to the same bias as an observational study that did not measure all confounders and could only incompletely adjust for known confounders. The use of propensity scores may, however, help to detect incomparability between treatment groups (i.e. lack of overlap in covariate values) that may remain undetected in a standard regression model. It also provides an additional tool to assess the performance of the traditional regression model (Wang and Donnan 2001). Propensity scores have more often been used in cohort studies of drug effectiveness (Seeger et al. 2003; Mojtabai and Zivin 2003; Schroder et al. 2003; Young-Xu et al. 2003), but they have also been applied to studies of drug safety (MacDonald et al. 2003). Nevertheless, the use of propensity scores may be a particular challenge in the common situation in pharmacoepidemiology of time-dependent exposures and covariates. Moreover, with the very large sizes of databases used in pharmacoepidemiology, the need to reduce the number of covariates to a single score is not crucial and thus, the advantage of propensity scores compared to including the confounders directly in the model of data analysis becomes less evident.

9.7   Drug Utilization Studies

Drug utilization studies are an important tool in improving rational drug use and providing data for cost/benefit considerations. Drug utilization has been defined as the "prescribing, dispensing, administering, and ingesting of drugs." (Serradell et al. 1991). This definition implies that several steps are involved in drug utilization and that, consequently, in each of these steps problems in drug use can arise. The World Health Organization defines drug utilization in a broader sense as the "marketing, distribution, prescription and use of drugs in a society, with special emphasis on the resulting medical, social and economic consequences" (World Health Organization 1977), thereby including also the effects of drug use on the population. Apart from examining drug use, goals of drug utilization studies include the identification of problems of drug utilization with respect to their importance, causes and consequences; the establishment of a scientific basis for decisions on problem solving and the assessment of the effects of actions taken. Some examples for studies that illustrate these goals are the following: What is the prevalence, pattern and risk factors of use for benzodiazepines in Italy? What is the quality of NSAID prescribing in Croatia and Sweden (Vlahovic-Palcevski et al. 2002)? Are labelled contraindications to the use of cisapride adhered to (Weatherby et al. 2001)? What is the impact of safety alerts on the prescribing of a drug (de la Porte et al. 2002; Weatherby et al. 2001)? After a drug has been withdrawn from the market, in which way does drug utilization of related drugs change (Glessner and Heller 2002)? What are characteristics of physicians and practices that make early use of new prescription drugs (Tamblyn et al. 2003)?

Drug utilization studies can be qualitative and quantitative. *Quantitative* drug utilization studies are conducted for a number of purposes: to ascertain the quantities of drugs consumed in a specific period and in a specific geographical area; to investigate the development of drug utilization over time; to compare and contrast the use of a drug between different geographical areas; to identify possible over- or underutilization of drugs; to determine trends in drug use according to population demographics; to estimate the prevalence of illness based on the consumption of drugs utilised in its treatment and to compare the prevalence of an illness in different areas.

The main aim of *qualitative* drug utilization studies is to determine the appropriateness of drug prescribing. They require the *a priori* establishment of quality indicators against which drug utilization is compared. National or international expert panels are sometimes used to help defining quality indicators in a consensus process (McLeod et al. 1997). Quality indicators may be based on the following parameters: the medical necessity for drug treatment; adherence to labelling with respect to labelled indications, contraindications or interactions; duration and dose of treatment; use of fixed drug combinations when only one of its components would be justified; availability of treatment alternatives which are more effective or less hazardous; availability of an equivalent less costly drug on the market; etc. In North America, these studies are known as drug utilization review (DUR) studies. DUR studies are aimed at detecting and quantifying problems of drug prescribing. They should be distinguished from DUR programs which are interventions in the form of an authorized, structured and ongoing system to improve the quality of drug prescribing (Lee and Bergman 2000). In contrast to DUR studies which provide only minimal feedback to the involved prescribers and are not interventional by their design, DUR programs include efforts to correct inappropriate patterns of drug use, and include a mechanism for measuring the effectiveness of corrective actions taken to normalize undesirable patterns of drug use (Hennessy and Strom 2000).

For quantitative and qualitative studies, it would be ideal to have a count of the number of patients who either ingest a drug of interest during a certain time frame or who use a drug inappropriately in relation to all patients who received the drug during a given time frame. The available data are often only approximations of the number of patients and may be based on cost or unit cost, weight, number of prescriptions written or dispensed and number of tablets, capsules, doses etc sold (Lee and Bergman 2000). Drug cost data have a number of limitations, since the price of a drug is not the same within and across countries. Drug pricing may be affected by different drug distribution channels, the quantities of drugs purchased, exchange rate fluctuations, different import duties and regulatory policies that affect pricing (Serradell et al. 1991). Studies based on the overall weight of a drug sold are similarly limited, since tablet sizes vary which makes it difficult to translate weight even into the number of tablets sold (Lee and Bergman 2000). The number of prescriptions written or dispensed for a particular drug product is a measure that is frequently used in drug utilization studies. However, the number of prescriptions for different patients in a given time interval varies and also the supply of drugs prescribed. To estimate the number of patients, one must divide by the average number of prescriptions per patient. The number of tablets, capsules etc. sold is often used in conjunction with the defined daily dose (DDD) measurement unit for drug use.

The DDD is the assumed average maintenance dose per day for a drug used for its main indication in adults. Use of the DDD underlies two basic assumptions: that patients are compliant and that the doses used for the major indication are the average maintenance doses (Serradell et al. 1991). The DDD dosing levels are assigned per ATC 5th level by the WHO Collaborating Centre for Drug Statistics Methodology in Norway based on recommendations in the medical literature. The DDD provides a fixed unit of measurement independent of the price and formulation of a drug. It can be used to examine changes in drug consumption over time and permits international comparisons. The DDD is a technical unit of measurement and does not necessarily reflect the recommended or prescribed daily dose (PDD). Doses for individual patients and patient groups will often differ from the DDD based on individual patient characteristics such as age, weight, and pharmacokinetic considerations. DDDs may be used to obtain crude estimates of the number of persons exposed to a particular drug or class of drugs and are sometimes used as denominator data for crude estimation of ADR rates (Kromann-Andersen and Pedersen 1988; Leone et al. 2003). This use of the DDD methodology is rather limited in drugs with more than one indication, particularly when the drug dose differs for each indication. It is also limited, when the duration of drug treatment varies greatly between patients. The DDD does not take into account pediatric use of a drug. DDDs are not established for topical preparations, sera, vaccines, antineoplastic agents, allergen extracts, general and local anesthetics and contrast media.

The Defined Daily Dose (DDD) is usually used in conjunction with the Anatomical Therapeutic Chemical (ATC) coding system. Coding for the ATC system at the WHO Collaborating Centre for Drug Statistics Methodology in Norway is based on requests from users including manufacturers, regulatory agencies and researchers. In the ATC system, drugs are classified in groups at five hierarchical levels. The drugs are divided into fourteen main groups (1st level), with one pharmacological/therapeutic subgroup (2nd level). The 3rd and 4th levels are pharmacological/therapeutic and chemical subgroups and the 5th level is the chemical substance. Table 9.6 illustrates the structure of the ATC coding system using metformin as an example. In the ATC system all plain metformin preparations are thus given the code A10B A02.

Table 9.6. The structure of the ATC coding system for metformin

A	Alimentary tract and metabolism (1st level, anatomical main group)
A10	Drugs used in diabetes (2nd level, therapeutic subgroup)
A10B	Oral blood glucose lowering drugs (3rd level, pharmacological subgroup)
A10B A	Biguanides (4th level, chemical subgroup)
A10B A02	Metformin (5th level, chemical substance)

Coverage of the ATC system is not comprehensive: complementary and traditional medicinal products are generally not included in the ATC system; ATC codes for fixed combination drugs are assigned only to a limited extent; some drugs may not be included in the system since no request for coding has been received by the WHO Collaborating Centre; a medicinal product that is used for two or more equally important indications, will usually be given only one code based on its main indication which is decided from the available literature. On the other hand, a medicinal product can have more than one ATC code if it is available in two or more strengths or formulations with clearly different therapeutic uses.

Use of computerized databases has greatly facilitated drug utilization research. Databases can be distinguished into those which include both drug and diagnostic data (examples have been given in Sect. 9.4) and into those which include only drug data (e.g. Denmark's Odense Pharmacoepidemiologic Database, Denmark's Pharmacoepidemiologic Prescription Database of the County of North Jutland, Spain's Drug Data Bank, Sweden's County of Jämtland Project, etc.). Some more databases used in drug utilization research and a description of these databases can be found in references (Lee and Bergman 2000; Serradell et al. 1991).

Interpretation of drug utilization data needs appropriate care. Observed geographic or time differences in drug utilization may be caused by many factors different from prescribing behaviour as e.g. differences in the age and sex distribution, different patterns of morbidity, change in diagnostic criteria, differences in the access to healthcare etc. If used appropriately, drug utilization research provides a powerful scientific tool to identify factors that influence drug prescribing and to develop strategies to modify prescribing behaviour. Further research is needed to determine which characteristics of inappropriate prescribing are susceptible to modification and what are the most efficient intervention strategies.

Conclusions 9.8

Pharmacoepidemiology is still a relatively young scientific discipline. Over the last 20–30 years there has been enormous progress in the improvement of its methods and development of new approaches to studies of drug safety and effectiveness. Pharmacoepidemiology has taken advantage of the rapidly expanding methods in epidemiology and has developed sophisticated methods to cope with problems that are specific to the field. New statistical approaches have been developed for signal generation based on data from the spontaneous reporting systems. Large computerized health databases are now widely used for research into beneficial and harmful drug effects, their use being facilitated by the development of more and more powerful computer technologies. With the experience gained through the use of these data and a careful understanding of the underlying health care system in which the data were generated, computerized databases provide a highly useful data source for pharmacoepidemiology studies. There has been a progressive refinement of case-control and cohort studies and efficient sampling strategies within a cohort are now often employed. The case-crossover and case-time-control designs are being used for the study of acute transient drug effects to eliminate control selection bias and confounding by indication or other factors. Propensity scores are increasingly used as a method to minimize confounding in the study of intended drug effects. Other new methodologies are likely to become of more importance in pharmacoepidemiology over the coming years as e.g. neural networks, sensitivity analysis, etc. Drug utilization review programs are now required in all US hospitals and have been implemented voluntarily in many other health care programs which will lead to further refinement of drug utilization research. A great challenge ahead is linkage of pharmacoepidemiology studies with the latest techniques of genetics, biochemistry, immunology and molecular biology. It is of particular interest to understand why individuals respond differently to drug therapy, both in terms of beneficial and adverse effects. Investigation of the genetic make-up of study patients on a population level will be greatly facilitated through the enormous progress in pharmacogenomics and molecular biology. New study designs may emerge as a consequence of these developments. It remains to be explored to which extent database studies may be used to include moleculargenetic or immunologic investigations.

References

Abascal VM, Larson MG, Evans JC, Blohm AT, Poli K, Levy D (1998) Calcium antagonists and mortality risk in men and women with hypertension in the Framingham Heart Study. Arch Intern Med 158:1882–1886

Abenhaim L, Moride Y, Brenot F, Rich S, Benichou J, Kurz X, Higenbottam T, Oakley C, Wouters E, Aubier M, Simonneau G, Begaud B (1996) Appetite-suppressant drugs and the risk of primary pulmonary hypertension. International Primary Pulmonary Hypertension Study Group. N Engl J Med 335:609–616

Adams RJ, Fuhlbrigge AL, Finkelstein JA, Weiss ST (2002) Intranasal steroids and the risk of emergency department visits for asthma. J Allergy Clin Immunol 109:636–642

Anonymous (1986) Risks of agranulocytosis and aplastic anemia. A first report of their relation to drug use with special reference to analgesics. The International Agranulocytosis and Aplastic Anemia Study. JAMA 256:1749–1757

Anonymous (1995a) Effect of different progestagens in low oestrogen oral contraceptives on venous thromboembolic disease. World Health Organization Collaborative Study of Cardiovascular Disease and Steroid Hormone Contraception. Lancet 346:1582–1588

Anonymous (1995b) Venous thromboembolic disease and combined oral contraceptives: results of international multicentre case-control study. World Health Organization Collaborative Study of Cardiovascular Disease and Steroid Hormone Contraception. Lancet 346:1575–1582

Barbone F, McMahon AD, Davey PG, Morris AD, Reid IC, McDevitt DG, MacDonald TM (1998) Association of road-traffic accidents with benzodiazepine use. The Lancet 352:1331–1336

Bate A, Lindquist M, Edwards IR, Olsson S, Orre R, Lansner A, De Freitas RM (1998) A Bayesian neural network method for adverse drug reaction signal generation. Eur J Clin Pharmacol 54:315–321

Bate A, Lindquist M, Orre R, Edwards IR, Meyboom RH (2002) Data-mining analyses of pharmacovigilance signals in relation to relevant comparison drugs. Eur J Clin Pharmacol 58:483–490

Begaud B, Martin K, Haramburu F, Moore N (2002) Rates of spontaneous reporting of adverse drug reactions in France. JAMA 288:1588

Beiderbeck-Noll AB, Sturkenboom MC, van der Linden PD, Herings RM, Hofman A, Coebergh JW, Leufkens HG, Stricker BH (2003) Verapamil is associated with an increased risk of cancer in the elderly: the Rotterdam study. Eur J Cancer 39:98–105

Benichou C (1994) Imputability of unexpected or toxic drug reactions. The official French method of causality assessment. In: Benichou C (ed) Adverse drug reactions. A practical guide to diagnosis and management. Wiley, Chichester, pp 271–275

Blais L, Ernst P, Boivin JF, Suissa S (1998a) Inhaled corticosteroids and the prevention of readmission to hospital for asthma. Am J Respir Crit Care Med 158:126–132

Blais L, Suissa S, Boivin JF, Ernst P (1998b) First treatment with inhaled corticosteroids and the prevention of admissions to hospital for asthma [see comments]. Thorax 53:1025–1029

Bloemenkamp KW, Rosendaal FR, Helmerhorst FM, Buller HR, Vandenbroucke JP (1995) Enhancement by factor V Leiden mutation of risk of deep-vein thrombosis associated with oral contraceptives containing a third-generation progestagen. Lancet 346:1593–1596

Carson JL, Strom BL, Soper KA, West SL, Morse ML (1987) The association of nonsteroidal anti-inflammatory drugs with upper gastrointestinal tract bleeding. Arch Intern Med 147:85–88

Chen H, Zhang SM, Hernan MA, Schwarzschild MA, Willett WC, Colditz GA, Speizer FE, Ascherio A (2003) Nonsteroidal anti-inflammatory drugs and the risk of Parkinson disease. Arch Neurol 60:1059–1064

Colditz GA, Hankinson SE, Hunter DJ, Willett WC, Manson JE, Stampfer MJ, Hennekens C, Rosner B, Speizer FE (1995) The use of estrogens and progestins and the risk of breast cancer in postmenopausal women. N Engl J Med 332:1589–1593

Confavreux C, Suissa S, Saddier P, Bourdes V, Vukusic S (2001) Vaccinations and the risk of relapse in multiple sclerosis. Vaccines in Multiple Sclerosis Study Group. N Engl J Med 344:319–326

de la Porte M, Reith D, Tilyard M (2002) Impact of safety alerts upon prescribing of cisapride to children in New Zealand. N Z Med J 115:U24

Dietlein G, Schroder-Bernhardi D (2002) Use of the mediplus patient database in healthcare research. Int J Clin Pharmacol Ther 40:130–133

Dietlein G, Schroder-Bernhardi D (2003) Doctors' prescription behaviour regarding dosage recommendations for preparations of kava extracts. Pharmacoepidemiol Drug Saf 12:417–421

Donahue JG, Weiss ST, Livingston JM, Goetsch MA, Greineder DK, Platt R (1997) Inhaled steroids and the risk of hospitalization for asthma. JAMA 277:887–891

Donnan PT, Wang J (2001) The case-crossover and case-time-control designs in pharmacoepidemiology. Pharmacoepidemiol Drug Saf 10:259–262

Downey W, Beck P, McNutt M, Stang M, Osei W, Nichol J (2003) Health databases in Saskatchewan. In: Strom BL (ed) 3rd edition, Pharmacoepidemiology. John Wiley & Sons, Chichester, pp 325–345

Eland IA, Belton KJ, van Grootheest AC, Meiners AP, Rawlins MD, Stricker BH (1999) Attitudinal survey of voluntary reporting of adverse drug reactions. Br J Clin Pharmacol 48:623–627

Essebag V, Genest J, Jr., Suissa S, Pilote L (2003) The nested case-control study in cardiology. Am Heart J 146:581–590

Etienney I, Beaugerie L, Viboud C, Flahault A (2003) Non-steroidal anti-inflammatory drugs as a risk factor for acute diarrhoea: a case crossover study. Gut 52:260–263

Evans SJ, Waller PC, Davis S (2001) Use of proportional reporting ratios (PRRs) for signal generation from spontaneous adverse drug reaction reports. Pharmacoepidemiol Drug Saf 10:483–486

Fagot JP, Mockenhaupt M, Bouwes-Bavinck JN, Naldi L, Viboud C, Roujeau JC (2001) Nevirapine and the risk of Stevens-Johnson syndrome or toxic epidermal necrolysis. AIDS 15:1843–1848

Faich GA (1986) Adverse-drug-reaction monitoring. N Engl J Med 314:1589–1592

Fairfield KM, Hunter DJ, Fuchs CS, Colditz GA, Hankinson SE (2002) Aspirin, other NSAIDs, and ovarian cancer risk (United States). Cancer Causes Control 13:535–542

Feenstra J, Heerdink ER, Grobbee DE, Stricker BH (2002) Association of non-steroidal anti-inflammatory drugs with first occurrence of heart failure and with relapsing heart failure: the Rotterdam Study. Arch Intern Med 162:265–270

Felson DT, Sloutskis D, Anderson JJ, Anthony JM, Kiel DP (1991) Thiazide diuretics and the risk of hip fracture. Results from the Framingham Study. JAMA 265:370–373

Friedman MA, Woodcock J, Lumpkin MM, Shuren JE, Hass AE, Thompson LJ (1999) The safety of newly approved medicines: do recent market removals mean there is a problem? JAMA 281:1728–1734

Friedman DE, Habel LA, Boles M, McFarland BH (2000) Kaiser Permanente Medical Care Program: Division of Research, Northern California, and Center for Health Research, Northwest Division. In: Strom BL (ed) Pharmacoepidemiology. Wiley & Sons, Chichester, pp 263–283

Funkhouser EM, Sharp GB (1995) Aspirin and reduced risk of esophageal carcinoma. Cancer 76:1116–1119

Garbe E, LeLorier J, Boivin JF, Suissa S (1997) Inhaled and nasal glucocorticoids and the risks of ocular hypertension or open-angle glaucoma. JAMA 277:722–727

Garbe E, Boivin JF, LeLorier J, Suissa S (1998a) Selection of controls in database case-control studies: glucocorticoids and the risk of glaucoma. J Clin Epidemiol 51:129–135

Garbe E, Suissa S, LeLorier J (1998b) Association of inhaled corticosteroid use with cataract extraction in elderly patients. JAMA 280:539–543

Garcia Rodriguez LA, Perez GS (1998) Use of the UK General Practice Research Database for pharmacoepidemiology. Br J Clin Pharmacol 45:419–425

Giovannucci E, Rimm EB, Stampfer MJ, Colditz GA, Ascherio A, Willett WC (1994) Aspirin use and the risk for colorectal cancer and adenoma in male health professionals. Ann Intern Med 121:241–246

Glessner MR, Heller DA (2002) Changes in related drug class utilization after market withdrawal of cisapride. Am J Manag Care 8:243–250

Greenland S (1996) Confounding and exposure trends in case-crossover and case-time-control design. Epidemiology 7:231–239

Griffin JP (1986) Survey of the spontaneous adverse drug reaction reporting schemes in fifteen countries. Br J Clin Pharmacol 22:83S–100S

Grodstein F, Stampfer MJ, Manson JE, Colditz GA, Willett WC, Rosner B, Speizer FE, Hennekens CH (1996) Postmenopausal estrogen and progestin use and the risk of cardiovascular disease. N Engl J Med 335:453–461

Grodstein F, Martinez ME, Platz EA, Giovannucci E, Colditz GA, Kautzky M, Fuchs C, Stampfer MJ (1998) Postmenopausal hormone use and risk for colorectal cancer and adenoma. Ann Intern Med 128:705–712

Haramburu F, Tubert-Bitter P, Begaud B (1992) Trends in spontaneous reporting. Post Marketing Surveillance 6:129–134

Haramburu F, Begaud B, Moride Y (1997) Temporal trends in spontaneous reporting of unlabelled adverse drug reactions. Br J Clin Pharmacol 44:299–301

Hee KJ, Grodstein F (2003) Regular use of nonsteroidal anti-inflammatory drugs and cognitive function in aging women. Neurology 60:1591–1597

Hennessy S, Strom BL (2000) Nonsedating antihistamines should be preferred over sedating antihistamines in patients who drive. Ann Intern Med 132:405–407

Hernan MA, Hohol MJ, Olek MJ, Spiegelman D, Ascherio A (2000) Oral contraceptives and the incidence of multiple sclerosis. Neurology 55:848–854

Hernandez-Avila M, Liang MH, Willett WC, Stampfer MJ, Colditz GA, Rosner B, Chang RW, Hennekens CH, Speizer FE (1990) Exogenous sex hormones and the risk of rheumatoid arthritis. Arthritis Rheum 33:947–953

Hernandez-Diaz S, Hernan MA, Meyer K, Werler MM, Mitchell AA (2003) Case-Crossover and Case-Time-Control Designs in Birth Defects Epidemiology. Am J Epidemiol 158:385–391

Horwitz RI, Feinstein AR (1981) Improved observational method for studying therapeutic efficacy. Suggestive evidence that lidocaine prophylaxis prevents death in acute myocardial infarction. JAMA 246:2455–2459

Hubbard RB, Smith CJ, Smeeth L, Harrison TW, Tattersfield AE (2002) Inhaled corticosteroids and hip fracture: a population-based case-control study. Am J Respir Crit Care Med 166:1563–1566

Jick H, Jick SS, Gurewich V, Myers MW, Vasilakis C (1995) Risk of idiopathic cardiovascular death and nonfatal venous thromboembolism in women using oral contraceptives with differing progestagen components. Lancet 346:1589–1593

Kaufman DW, Kelly JP, Jurgelon JM, Anderson T, Issaragrisil S, Wiholm BE, Young NS, Leaverton P, Levy M, Shapiro S (1996) Drugs in the aetiology of agranulocytosis and aplastic anaemia. Eur J Haematol Suppl 60:23–30

Kelly JP, Rosenberg L, Kaufman DW, Shapiro S (1990) Reliability of personal interview data in a hospital-based case-control study. Am J Epidemiol 131:79–90

Ki M, Park T, Yi SG, Oh JK, Choi B (2003) Risk analysis of aseptic meningitis after measles-mumps-rubella vaccination in Korean children by using a case-crossover design. Am J Epidemiol 157:158–165

Kiel DP, Felson DT, Anderson JJ, Wilson PW, Moskowitz MA (1987) Hip fracture and the use of estrogens in postmenopausal women. The Framingham Study. N Engl J Med 317:1169–1174

Kromann-Andersen H, Pedersen A (1988) Reported adverse reactions to and consumption of nonsteroidal anti-inflammatory drugs in Denmark over a 17-year period. Dan Med Bull 35:187–192

Lando JF, Heck KE, Brett KM (1999) Hormone replacement therapy and breast cancer risk in a nationality representative cohort. Am J Prev Med 17:176–180

Lee D, Bergman U (2000) Studies of drug utilization. In: Strom BL (ed) Pharmacoepidemiology. John Wiley & Sons, Chichester, pp 463–481

Lenz W (1987) The Thalidomide hypothesis: How it was found and tested. In: Kewitz H, Roots I, Voigt K (eds) Epidemiological Concepts in Clinical Pharmacology. Springer Verlag, Heidelberg, pp 3–10

Leone R, Venegoni M, Motola D, Moretti U, Piazzetta V, Cocci A, Resi D, Mozzo F, Velo G, Burzilleri L, Montanaro N, Conforti A (2003) Adverse drug reactions related to the use of fluoroquinolone antimicrobials: an analysis of spontaneous reports and fluoroquinolone consumption data from three italian regions. Drug Saf 26:109–120

Lewis MA, Heinemann LA, MacRae KD, Bruppacher R, Spitzer WO (1996) The increased risk of venous thromboembolism and the use of third generation progestagens: role of bias in observational research. The Transnational Research Group on Oral Contraceptives and the Health of Young Women. Contraception 54:5–13

Lindquist M, Edwards IR (1993) Adverse drug reaction reporting in Europe: some problems of comparisons. International Journal of Risk & Safety in Medicine 4:35–46

MacDonald TM, Morant SV, Goldstein JL, Burke TA, Pettitt D (2003) Channelling bias and the incidence of gastrointestinal haemorrhage in users of meloxicam, coxibs, and older, non-specific non-steroidal anti-inflammatory drugs. Gut 52:1265–1270

McLeod PJ, Huang AR, Tamblyn RM, Gayton DC (1997) Defining inappropriate practices in prescribing for elderly people: a national consensus panel. CMAJ 156:385–391

Miettinen OS (1983) The need for randomization in the study of intended effects. Statist Med 2:267–271

Mojtabai R, Zivin JG (2003) Effectiveness and cost-effectiveness of four treatment modalities for substance disorders: a propensity score analysis. Health Serv Res 38:233–259

Moore N, Hall G, Sturkenboom M, Mann R, Lagnaoui R, Begaud B (2003) Biases affecting the proportional reporting ratio (PPR) in spontaneous reports pharmacovigilance databases: the example of sertindole. Pharmacoepidemiol Drug Saf 12:271–281

Moride Y, Abenhaim L (1994) Evidence of the depletion of susceptibles effect in non-experimental pharmacoepidemiologic research. J Clin Epidemiol 47:731–737

Neutel CI, Perry S, Maxwell C (2002) Medication use and risk of falls. Pharmacoepidemiol Drug Saf 11:97–104

Perez E, Schroder-Bernhardi D, Dietlein G (2002) Treatment behavior of doctors regarding Helicobacter pylori infections. Int J Clin Pharmacol Ther 40:126–129

Perkins SM, Wanzhu T, Underhill MG, Zhou XH, Murray MD (2000) The use of propensity scores in pharmacoepidemiologic research. Pharmacoepidemiol Drug Saf 9:93–101

Pierfitte C, Begaud B, Lagnaoui R, Moore ND (1999) Is reporting rate a good predictor of risks associated with drugs? Br J Clin Pharmacol 47:329–331

Pierfitte C, Royer RJ, Moore N, Begaud B (2000) The link between sunshine and phototoxicity of sparfloxacin. Br J Clin Pharmacol 49:609–612

Porta-Serra M, Hartzema AG (1997) The contribution of epidemiology to the study of drug effects. In: Hartzema AG, Porta-Serra M, Tilson HH (eds) Pharmacoepidemiology. The fundamentals. Harvey Whitney, Cincinnati

Raiford DS, Perez GS, Garcia Rodriguez LA (1996) Positive predictive value of ICD-9 codes in the identification of cases of complicated peptic ulcer disease in the Saskatchewan hospital automated database. Epidemiology 7:101–104

Rawlins MD, Breckenridge AM, Wood SM (1989) National adverse drug reaction reporting – a silver jubilee. Adverse Drug Reaction Bulletin 138:516–519

Ray WA, Griffin MR (1989) Use of Medicaid data for pharmacoepidemiology. Am J Epidemiol 129:837–849

Ray WA, Griffin MR, Downey W, Melton LJ, III (1989) Long-term use of thiazide diuretics and risk of hip fracture. Lancet 1:687–690

Samet JM (2003) Measuring the effectiveness of inhaled corticosteroids for COPD is not easy! Am J Respir Crit Care Med 168:1–2

Saskatchwewan Health (2004) (http://www.health.gov.sk.ca/mc_dp_phb_infodoc.pdf) Accessed June 03, 2004

Saunders KW, Davis RL, Stergachis A (2000) Group Health Cooperative of Puget Sound. In: Strom BL (ed) Pharmacoepidemiology. John Wiley& Sons, Chichester, pp 247–262

Schoofs MW, van der KM, Hofman A, de Laet CE, Herings RM, Stijnen T, Pols HA, Stricker BH (2003) Thiazide diuretics and the risk for hip fracture. Ann Intern Med 139:476–482

Schroder D, Weiser M, Klein P (2003) Efficacy of a homeopathic Crataegus preparation compared with usual therapy for mild (NYHA II) cardiac insufficiency: results of an observational cohort study. Eur J Heart Fail 5:319–326

Schroder-Bernhardi D, Dietlein G (2002) Lipid-lowering therapy: do hospitals influence the prescribing behavior of general practitioners? Int J Clin Pharmacol Ther 40:317–321

Seeger JD, Walker AM, Williams PL, Saperia GM, Sacks FM (2003) A propensity score-matched cohort study of the effect of statins, mainly fluvastatin, on the occurrence of acute myocardial infarction. Am J Cardiol 92:1447–1451

Serradell J, Bjornson DC, Hartzema AG (1991) Drug utilization studies: Sources and methods. In: Hartzema AG, Porta MS, Tilson HM (eds) Pharmacoepidemiology: An Introduction. Harvey Whitney Books, Cincinnati Ohio, pp 101–119

Shapiro S (1989) The role of automated record linkage in the postmarketing surveillance of drug safety: a critique. Clin Pharmacol Ther 46:371–386

Sin DD, Man SF (2002) Low-dose inhaled corticosteroid therapy and risk of emergency department visits for asthma. Arch Intern Med 162:1591–1595

Sin DD, Tu JV (2001a) Inhaled corticosteroid therapy reduces the risk of rehospitalization and all-cause mortality in elderly asthmatics. European Respiratory Journal 17:380–385

Sin DD, Tu JV (2001b) Inhaled corticosteroids and the risk of mortality and readmission in elderly patients with chronic obstructive pulmonary disease. Am J Respir Crit Care Med 164:580–584

Slone D, Shapiro S, Miettinen OS, Finkle WD, Stolley PD (1979) Drug evaluation after marketing. Ann Intern Med 90:257–261

Spitzer WO, Suissa S, Ernst P, Horwitz RI, Habbick B, Cockcroft D, Boivin JF, McNutt M, Buist AS, Rebuck AS (1992) The use of beta-agonists and the risk of death and near death from asthma. N Engl J Med 326:501–506

Spitzer WO, Lewis MA, Heinemann LA, Thorogood M, MacRae KD (1996) Third generation oral contraceptives and risk of venous thromboembolic disorders: an international case-control study. Transnational Research Group on Oral Contraceptives and the Health of Young Women. BMJ 312:83–88

Strom BL (ed) (2000) Pharmacoepidemiology. John Wiley & Sons, Chichester

Strom BL, Carson JL (1990) Use of automated databases for pharmacoepidemiology research. Epidemiol Rev 12:87–107

Strom BL, Miettinen OS, Melmon KL (1983) Postmarketing studies of drug efficacy: when must they be randomized? Clinical Pharmacology & Therapeutics 34:1–7

Strom BL, Miettinen OS, Melmon KL (1984) Post-marketing studies of drug efficacy: how? Am J Med 77:703–708

Strom BL, Carson JL, Halpern AC, Schinnar R, Snyder ES, Stolley PD, Shaw M, Tilson HH, Joseph M, Dai WS (1991) Using a claims database to investigate drug-induced Stevens-Johnson syndrome. Stat Med 10:565–576

Sturkenboom MC, Middelbeek A, de Jong van den Berg LT, van den Berg PB, Stricker BH, Wesseling H (1995) Vulvo-vaginal candidiasis associated with acitretin. J Clin Epidemiol 48:991–997

Suissa S (1995) The case-time-control design. Epidemiology 6:248–253

Suissa S (1998) The case-time-control design: further assumptions and conditions [comment]. Epidemiology 9:441–445

Suissa S (2000) Novel approaches to pharmacoepidemiology study design and statistical analysis. In: Strom BL (ed) Pharmacoepidemiology. John Wiley & Sons, Chichester, pp 785–805

Suissa S (2003) Effectiveness of inhaled corticosteroids in COPD: immortal time bias in observational studies. Am J Respir Crit Care Med 168:49–53

Suissa S (2004) Inhaled steroids and mortality in COPD: bias from unaccounted immortal time. European Respiratory Journal 23:391–395

Suissa S, Blais L, Spitzer WO, Cusson J, Lewis M, Heinemann L (1997) First-time use of newer oral contraceptives and the risk of venous thromboembolism. Contraception 56:141–146

Suissa S, Ernst P, Benayoun B, Baltzan M, Cai B (2000a) Low-dose inhaled corticosteroids and the prevention of death from asthma. N Engl J Med 343:332–336

Suissa S, Spitzer WO, Rainville B, Cusson J, Lewis M, Heinemann L (2000b) Recurrent use of newer oral contraceptives and the risk of venous thromboembolism. Hum Reprod 15:817–821

Suissa S, Ernst P, Kezouh A (2002) Regular use of inhaled corticosteroids and the long term prevention of hospitalisation for asthma. Thorax 57:880–884

Suissa S, Baltzan M, Kremer R, Ernst P (2004) Inhaled and nasal corticosteroid use and the risk of fracture. Am J Respir Crit Care Med 169:83–88

Szarfman A, Machado SG, O'Neill RT (2002) Use of screening algorithms and computer systems to efficiently signal higher-than-expected combinations of drugs and events in the US FDA's spontaneous reports database. Drug Saf 25:381–392

Tamblyn R, Lavoie G, Petrella L, Monette J (1995) The use of prescription claims databases in pharmacoepidemiological research: the accuracy and comprehensiveness of the prescription claims database in Quebec. J Clin Epidemiol 48:999–1009

Tamblyn R, McLeod P, Hanley JA, Girard N, Hurley J (2003) Physician and practice characteristics associated with the early utilization of new prescription drugs. Med Care 41:895–908

Tennis P, Bombardier C, Malcolm E, Downey W (1993) Validity of rheumatoid arthritis diagnoses listed in the Saskatchewan Hospital Separations Database. J Clin Epidemiol 46:675–683

Tsong Y (1995) Comparing reporting rates of adverse events between drugs with adjustment for year of marketing and secular trends in total reporting. J Biopharm Stat 5:95–114

van der Kroef KC (1979) Reactions to triazolam. Lancet 2:526

Venning GR (1983) Identification of adverse reactions to new drugs. III: Alerting processes and early warning systems. BMJ 286:458–460

Viscoli CM, Brass LM, Kernan WN, Sarrel PM, Suissa S, Horwitz RI (2001) A clinical trial of estrogen-replacement therapy after ischemic stroke. N Engl J Med 345:1243–1249

Vlahovic-Palcevski V, Wettermark B, Bergman U (2002) Quality of non-steroidal anti-inflammatory drug prescribing in Croatia (Rijeka) and Sweden (Stockholm). Eur J Clin Pharmacol 58:209–214

Wang J, Donnan PT (2001) Propensity score methods in drug safety studies: practice, strengths and limitations. Pharmacoepidemiol Drug Saf 10:341–344

Wang J, Donnan PT, Steinke D, MacDonald TM (2001) The multiple propensity score for analysis of dose-response relationships in drug safety studies. Pharmacoepidemiol Drug Saf 10:105–111

Weatherby LB, Walker AM, Fife D, Vervaet P, Klausner MA (2001) Contraindicated medications dispensed with cisapride: temporal trends in relation to the sending of 'Dear Doctor' letters. Pharmacoepidemiol Drug Saf 10:211–218

Weintraub JM, Taylor A, Jacques P, Willett WC, Rosner B, Colditz GA, Chylack LT, Hankinson SE (2002) Postmenopausal hormone use and lens opacities. Ophthalmic Epidemiol 9:179–190

Wiholm B, Olsson S, Moore N, Waller P (2000) Spontaneous reporting systems outside the US. In: Strom BL (ed) Pharmacoepidemiology. John Wiley & Sons, Chichester, pp 175–192

World Health Organization (1977) The selection of essential drugs. Report of a WHO expert committee. Ser. no. 615. World Health Organization, Geneva

Worzala K, Hiller R, Sperduto RD, Mutalik K, Murabito JM, Moskowitz M, D'Agostino RB, Wilson PW (2001) Postmenopausal estrogen use, type of menopause, and lens opacities: the Framingham studies. Arch Intern Med 161:1448–1454

Wu K, Willett WC, Fuchs CS, Colditz GA, Giovannucci EL (2002) Calcium intake and risk of colon cancer in women and men. J Natl Cancer Inst 94:437–446

Wysowski DK, Pitts M, Beitz J (2001) An analysis of reports of depression and suicide in patients treated with isotretinoin. J Am Acad Dermatol 45:515–519

Young-Xu Y, Chan KA, Liao JK, Ravid S, Blatt CM (2003) Long-term statin use and psychological well-being. J Am Coll Cardiol 42:690–697

Screening

III.10

Anthony B. Miller

10.1   Introduction

10.1.1   General Principles of Screening

Screening, sometimes termed secondary prevention, is one of the major components of disease control, the others comprising primary prevention, diagnosis, treatment, rehabilitation after treatment or disability and palliative care. Ideally, the control of a disease should be achievable, either by preventing the disease from occurring or, if it does occur, by curing those who develop it by appropriate treatment. Complete success from prevention would make treatment obsolete. Complete success from treatment, however, would not make prevention obsolete, as there are costs and undesirable sequelae from the disease and treatment that patients and society would like to avoid if at all possible, especially from diseases such as cancer, diabetes and hypertension. At present, neither is completely successful for most diseases; they will continue to complement each other for a number of conditions, while screening can be regarded as complementary to one or both of the other approaches.

Because of the deep-rooted belief among physicians that "early diagnosis" of disease is beneficial, many regard screening as bound to be effective. However, for a number of reasons discussed below this is not necessarily so, as shown by the failure of screening for lung cancer using sputum cytology or chest X-rays to reduce mortality from the disease, for example (Prorok et al. 1984). It is the purpose of this chapter to attempt to define some of the fundamental issues that are relevant to the consideration of screening in disease control. The approach taken will be from the epidemiology, or public health viewpoint, rather from the clinical standpoint.

Although it is often assumed that screening tests must involve some sort of technological procedure, such as an X-ray or laboratory test, screening can involve simple clinical examinations, such as assessment of blood pressure, or a clinical breast examination. However, it is the advent of expensive technologically-based screening tests in the last few decades which has focused attention on the need for critical evaluation of screening and the importance of soundly based screening programmes.

10.1.2   Definition

Screening was defined by the United States Commission on Chronic Illness (1957) as: "the presumptive identification of unrecognised disease or defect by the application of tests, examinations or other procedures that can be applied rapidly." A screening test is not intended to be diagnostic. Rather a positive finding will have to be confirmed by special diagnostic procedures.

By definition, screening is offered to those who do not suspect that they may have a disease. This is subtly different from being asymptomatic. Symptoms may be revealed by careful questioning related to the organ of interest, not regarded by the individual attending for screening as being related to a possible disease. Further, in a public health programme, open to all comers, it may not be possible to determine that all subjects who enrol are truly asymptomatic. Indeed, many may enrol because they have a suspicion that they have the disease of interest, in the hope that their suspicion will not be confirmed. Thus although it is usual to make the assumption that participants in screening programmes are asymptomatic, this is not a necessary nor an absolute prerequisite for participation in public health based screening programmes.

General Principles Governing the Introduction of Screening

10.2

The principles that should govern the introduction of screening programmes were first enunciated by Wilson and Junger (1968) and refined since (e.g. by Miller 1978, 1996; Cuckle and Wald 1984). These will now be considered.

1. *The disease should be an important health problem.* In practical terms this means that the disease prevalence should be high and the disease should be the cause of substantial mortality and/or morbidity. However, it is important to recognise that the life expectancy of a screened population may be changed little even if the programme is successful. In most technically advanced countries, for example, even if all cancer were to be eradicated, the effect of other competing causes of death is such that life expectancy would be increased only by about 2 1/2 years. The benefits of cholesterol screening to prevent heart disease are measured, at the population level, in days. It is not possible to provide a precise estimate for the level of burden necessary to mount a screening programme. The level of morbidity and mortality considered to be important will depend on a combination of factors such as the age distribution of the population affected, or the severity of the illness. There may be certain circumstances when the major benefit from screening follows, not from reduction in mortality, but from reduction of morbidity consequent upon the diagnosis of the disease in a more treatable phase in its natural history. This could mean that the extent of treatment required and the possibility that treatment may be debilitating or mutilating would be much less. Such advantages may be difficult to quantify; however, as they may be considerable in psychological terms to individuals, and to communities in the lowering in the requirements for extensive rehabilitation services, they should not be overlooked.

2. *The disease should have a detectable preclinical phase (DPCP).* It is important to recognise that this principle is not "The natural history of the disease should include a phase with a detectable precursor". For example for many cancers, including breast and prostate cancer, the DPCP is largely asymptomatic invasive cancer (Fig. 10.1). For cervix cancer, on the other hand, the DPCP probably includes the whole range from dysplasia (CIN 1 or LSIL) through to occult inva-

sive cancer (Fig. 10.2). An alternative name given to the DPCP is sojourn time, meant to indicate the period during which a detectable lesion "sojourns" in the organ. In screening for cardiovascular disease with cholesterol or hypertension, physiological markers of risk are being identified rather than detectable precursors. Nevertheless, such a marker can be considered as synonymous to a preclinical phase.

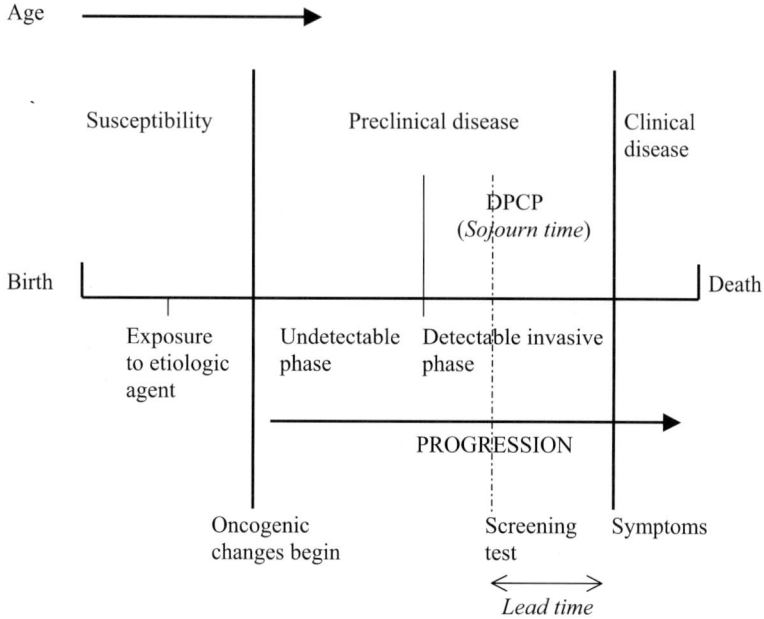

DPCP = detectable preclinical phase

Figure 10.1. The natural history of a cancer when the detectable preclinical phase is asymptomatic invasive disease

3. *The natural history of the condition should be known.* Ideally such a requirement implies that it is known at what stage in the disease process progression, disability and/or death can no longer be prevented. If such information was available and the stage that the development of the disease had reached in individuals was determinable, it would be possible to decide precisely when a screening test should be applied in order to achieve maximum benefit and minimal overutilisation of resources. In a disease such as cervix cancer, it is now recognized that the majority of the preclinical abnormalities detected by the cytology test are not destined to progress, and that the majority will regress, as depicted in Fig. 10.2 (Boyes et al. 1982; Holowaty et al. 1999). This makes it imperative that screening is planned to ensure that gross overtreatment of the majority does not occur. The same requirement may be even more necessary for the test for the primary etiologic agent of the disease, the test for evidence of infection with high risk types of the human papillomavirus

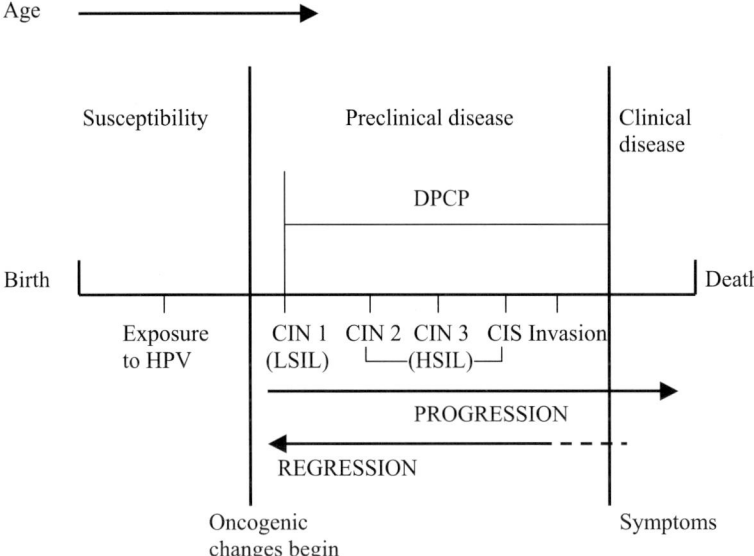

DPCP = detectable preclinical phase
HPV = human papilloma virus
HSIL = high-grade squamous intraepithelial lesion
LSIL = low-grade squamous intraepithelial lesion
CIN = cervical intraepithelial neoplasia

Figure 10.2. The natural history of cancer of the cervix

(Miller 2004). Such conclusions have substantial implications with regard to the optimum frequency of screening examinations. Designing a programme directed to those lesions that, in the absence of screening will progress and more rapidly escape curability, if they can be identified, will be the appropriate approach. Designing a programme which maximises the detection of all cases, the majority with a good prognosis but which in the absence of screening may be unlikely to progress, will waste resources. Such knowledge can be applied to the population in planning screening programmes, but unfortunately it seems unlikely that knowledge will be accumulated to make it possible to determine the natural history of disease in individuals within the population sufficiently precisely. It is recognised that the rate of progression of clinically detected disease from the point of diagnosis to cure or to death varies substantially in different individuals. The distribution of rates of progression of preclinically detectable disease that might be identified by screening is likely to be equally wide. Thus, although an objective for research on screening has to be to determine the extent of the distribution of the sojourn times of the DPCP, in considering the introduction of screening programmes and the scheduling of tests within programmes it is necessary to balance benefits with costs. This means that the schedule will have to be determined that will enable the detection of the maximal number of still curable cases compatible with the longest interval between tests, principles which unfortunately are often anathema to clinicians.

4. *The disease should be treatable, and there should be a recognized treatment for lesions identified following screening.* This principle can be elaborated as follows:

    There should be evidence of the effectiveness of treatment of lesions discovered as a result of screening in reducing disease incidence and/or mortality and the level of improvement expected should be stated,

    and secondly,

    There should be a reasonable expectation that recommendations for the appropriate management of the lesions discovered from a screening programme will be complied with both by the individual with the lesion and by the physician responsible for his (or her) health care.

    Screening programmes should only be set up when there are adequate facilities for treating lesions discovered as a result of screening and functioning referral systems for securing such treatment. There is obviously no point in establishing a screening programme and identifying lesions that should be treated if the facilities, or the infrastructure, are not available for referral, confirmation of diagnosis, and treatment. In general this is not a problem for technically advanced countries, but it can be for developing countries. Unfortunately problems allied to these have occurred. Thus on occasions it has not been certain whether or not lesions identified as a result of screening should be regarded as true disease precursors. When lesions are first identified in a screening programme, information may not be available as to their appropriate treatment, and special studies may be required. Otherwise, errors in terms of observation rather than treatment on the one hand or too extensive treatment on the other are possible. In prostate cancer screening, for example, if too radical treatment is applied in the elderly to the latent or good prognosis prostate cancers that may be identified in a screening programme, the morbidity in terms of incontinence and impotence, and even the mortality from treatment, could offset any benefit from the earlier detection of lesions with truly malignant potential (Chodak and Schoenberg 1989; Miller 1991; Krahn et al. 1994).

    A different sort of difficulty could arise when, as a result of screening, lesions are diagnosed earlier in their natural history, but in spite of this, death is still inevitable. For example, if the available screening methods will not succeed in diagnosing disease before it is outside the range of current therapy, then screening to detect such disease is not worthwhile. The early studies of screening for lung cancer suggested this was not a condition amenable to screening, probably for this reason (Prorok et al. 1984). Recently, evidence has accrued from uncontrolled studies that low dose helical (spiral) computerised tomography of the lung is capable of detecting approximately four times as many small stage 1 lung cancers as chest X-rays, and that these appear likely to have a good prognosis (e.g. Henschke et al. 1999). However, these are peripheral cancers, and are largely adenocarcinomas or related cancers, so that the technique may not be capable of detecting early either the majority of squamous cell or of small cell cancers, and thus may be selectively detecting only those cancers with a good prognosis. If, after spiral CT scanning, the majority of the lung cancers with a poor prognosis continue to occur at about the same time in their natural history as at the present, there could be little overall effect upon lung cancer mortality in the spiral CT screened group. Yet considerable costs will be incurred in treating the peripheral lesions not destined to progress. It is for this reason that large scale trials of this approach are now being initiated in the United States and Europe.

5. *The screening test to be used should be acceptable and safe.*

   In general this implies a non invasive test with high validity. Other criteria of a good screening test include ease of use and relatively low cost. These principles and approaches to assessing validity will now be discussed.

The Validity of a Screening Test   10.2.1

Two measures suffice to describe the validity of screening tests: sensitivity and specificity.

Sensitivity is defined as the ability of a test to detect all those with the disease in the screened population. This is expressed as the proportion of those with the disease in whom a screening test gives a positive result.

Specificity is defined as the ability of a test to correctly identify those free of the disease in the screened population. This is expressed as the proportion of people free of the disease in whom the screening test gives a negative result.

These two terms may be further expressed in terms of test results as follows: sensitivity is calculated as the true positives divided by the sum of the true positives and false negatives and may be expressed as a proportion or a percentage; specificity is calculated as the true negatives divided by the sum of the true negatives and the false positives and may be expressed as a proportion or a percentage (Fig. 10.3). In practice, difficulties with these measures arise over defining a positive result from the test as well as distinguishing the true positives from the false positives among those who test positive, and the true negatives from the false negatives among those who test negative. A relatively imperfect test of a quantitative, continuously distributed measurement can be artificially given a very high sensitivity by setting the boundary between negative and positive to incorporate a high proportion of those who are eventually found to have the disease in the positive category, but at a substantial cost in terms of low specificity. Conversely the same test can be made to appear highly specific, but will then become insensitive, if the boundary between positive and negative is shifted in the opposite direction.

If the test result is expressed in a quantitative form so that the boundaries between what is defined as positive and negative can be varied at will, it is possible to plot a receiver operating characteristic (ROC) curve (Swets 1979). What is plotted is the sensitivity in the vertical axis and 1-specificity (the false positive rate) in the horizontal axis (Fig. 10.4). The point on the curve that is chosen as optimal is often

| | Disease status | |
Test result	Present	Absent
Positive	True positive (TP)	False positive (FP)
Negative	False negative (FN)	True negative (TN)

Then:

$$\text{Sensitivity} = \frac{\text{TP}}{\text{TP} + \text{FN}} \times 100\%$$

$$\text{Specificity} = \frac{\text{TN}}{\text{TN} + \text{FP}} \times 100\%$$

$$\text{Predictive value positive} = \frac{\text{TP}}{\text{TP} + \text{FP}} \times 100\%$$

$$\text{Predictive value negative} = \frac{\text{TN}}{\text{TN} + \text{FN}} \times 100\%$$

Figure 10.3. The relationship between Sensitivity, Specificity, and Predictive Value Positive and Negative

that further from the 45° diagonal, labelled "Chance" in Fig. 10.4, as this represents a test with no better sensitivity or specificity than could be expected by chance. In Fig. 10.4, this point is between 70% and 80% sensitivity, the corresponding 1-specificity being 25%, i.e. a specificity of 75%. This is about the level expected with cervical cytology, and represents rather a poor test. We would hope that even at greater sensitivity, the specificity would be at least 90%, to avoid too many health care costs investigating the false positives. ROC curves are most easily derived for blood tests, but have also been applied to mammography, by varying the extent to which different mammographic abnormalities were regarded as an indication of suspicion of malignancy (Goin and Haberman 1982). Such curves cannot be applied to a test with a dichotomous outcome if the boundaries defining positive and negative are invariant. Further they imply a similar weight to sensitivity and specificity, which as discussed below may not be ideal.

The position of the boundaries that are set between what is regarded as disease and non-(or benign) disease can also considerably influence the numerical values placed on sensitivity and specificity. This arises because of uncertainty as to what truly constitutes an abnormality in the context of a screening programme. In order to come to such a decision it is essential that the conditions identified as a result of screening should have a known natural history. However, as has already been pointed out, such knowledge may not be available at the initiation of a screening programme and may only be obtained as a result of careful study of findings from screening programmes.

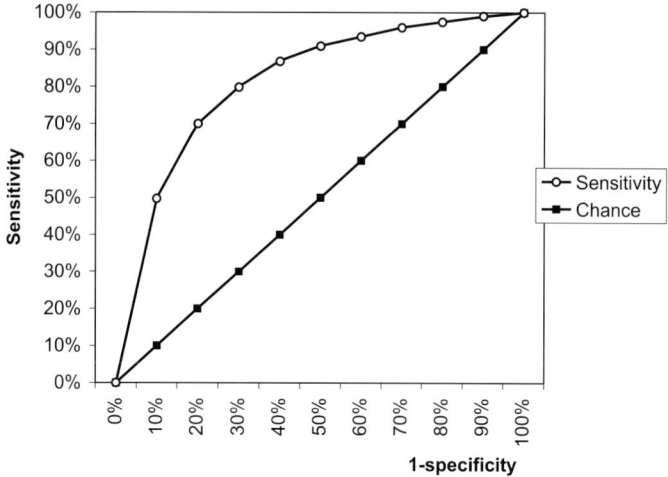

Figure 10.4. Example of an ROC curve

Nevertheless, the definition as to what constitutes disease is crucial in order to determine sensitivity and specificity. Most people have a clear idea as to what they regard as disease in terms of that which surfaces in standard medical practice. By definition, screening is conducted on asymptomatic individuals, so that many conditions that are identified through screening are likely to be at an early stage and may not have the generally recognised clinical characteristics of relatively advanced disease. This difficulty should theoretically be overcome by having clearly defined definitions of disease. However, for cancer, diagnosis is usually made on histology, and histology only imperfectly characterises behaviour, especially for lesions within the DPCP. For cancer one hope for the future is that some of the markers for prognosis currently being evaluated such as markers of oncogene expression or other markers of DNA change may serve to identify those precancerous or in situ components of the DPCP that are likely to progress.

A common error in evaluating potential screening tests is to determine the sensitivity by utilizing the experience of the test in relation to people who have clinical disease. A test that may appear to be highly sensitive under these circumstances may later be found to be much less sensitive when its ability to detect the DPCP is evaluated. A similar error is substituting an intermediate marker as the gold standard for calculating sensitivity and specificity. For example, the test characteristics for a thyroid assay may be compared to a more accurate assay, rather than the presence of the condition in the individual tested. In the screening context, therefore, sensitivity and specificity may vary according to whether they are estimated for early disease or preclinical lesions, and sensitivity for both should be determined in active screening programmes. To do so for specificity is very much easier than for sensitivity. This is because the diagnostic process put in train by a positive screening test generally fairly rapidly identifies those who have the disease and thus distinguishes the true from the false positives. As under most circumstances the proportion of those who have the disease in relation to the total population screened is low, a very good approximation to specificity is obtained by calculating the proportion of all those who tested negative of the sum of the test negatives and false positives. Including the unidentified false negatives in the numerator and denominator of this expression will in practice introduce little error.

Sensitivity, is however a difficult measure to determine initially in a screening programme. The reason for this is that the false negatives are not immediately apparent, as there is no justification to retest all the test negatives just to identify a few false negatives. Only by following the total population who screened negative is it eventually possible to identify those who had the disease at the time the test was administered but were not so identified at the time of screening. This is facilitated if test materials are retained, for example cervical smears or mammograms originally classed negative can be reassessed for those who are found to have disease at the next scheduled screen, or who develop disease during the interval between screens. Such reassessments should preferably be made blind to avoid bias. Such an approach was used in the assessment of the sensitivity of the "reader error" for cervical cancer screening (Boyes et al. 1982) and in the assessment of the sensitivity of mammography in a trial of breast cancer screening (Baines et al. 1988).

When test materials cannot be retained, however, such as in the assessment of the sensitivity of physical examination as a screening test for breast cancer, and for what we have called the "taker error and the biological component" of false negatives in cervical cytology, i.e. disease that was indeed present but was not incorporated in the smear or for some reason did not exfoliate (Boyes et al. 1982), a direct identification of false negatives will not be possible. A usual approach is to assume that disease occurring within a certain period are false negatives, an approach we used in estimating the sensitivity of physical examination of the breasts (Baines et al. 1989). However a possibly more satisfactory approach is to assess the expected detection rate of disease on screening after repeated screens, assuming that most of the false negatives had by then been identified, and to regard the excess disease above this level at the second screen as a measure of the false negatives at the first screen. As a result of such an approach it was determined that the taker and biological component of false negatives was approximately equal to the directly measured reader error, so that the level of sensitivity for cervical cytology approximated to 78% (Miller 1981).

It is generally accepted that:
- The sensitivity and specificity of the screening test to be used should have been evaluated and their expected values stated,
- There should be an acceptable programme of quality control to ensure that the stated levels of sensitivity and specificity are attained and maintained.

Quality control involves issues that concern not only the validity of the screening test but also its safety. There is, for example, the need to ensure that radiation exposure does not drift upwards in a mammography screening programme. Quality control encumbers the training of those who will actually administer and read screening tests, their supervision and the introduction of procedures to check actively on the extent to which those positive or negative are misclassified.

Quality may suffer because of overwork and boredom. One of the reasons why a recommendation was made to change the frequency of examination for most women in cervical cytology screening programmes in Canada was to avoid repetitive rescreening of normal women, with the flooding of laboratories with unnecessary and unrewarding work (Task Force 1976). The Task Force described the mechanisms for ensuring appropriate quality control. It is relevant that these requirements had to be re-emphasized more than a decade later (Miller et al. 1991b).

That such issues are not simple was underlined by consideration of observer variation in mammography reading (Boyd et al. 1982). Relevant to all screening programmes is not only the accuracy with which abnormalities are identified, but if identified, the extent to which appropriate recommendations are made on their management. Our experience suggested that including a category of "probably benign" in a screening mammography report increases the extent of observer variation. Readers differ substantially in the extent they use this category, the extent to which they recommend special observation of individuals placed in this category, and the extent to which they recommend biopsy. Dual reading helps to increase specificity, without much, if any, loss of sensitivity. This permits the simplification of recommendations into two groups, "suspicious of malignancy" and "satisfactory (normal)" examination, and results in far greater consistency. Further, it is compatible with the appropriate separation of findings from screening tests into the probably abnormal (test positive) and probably normal (test negative) dichotomy. The probably abnormal group is subjected to diagnostic tests in the normal way. This approach to use of screening mammography was accepted with difficulty in North America, due to an initial tendency for most radiologists to regard mammography as a diagnostic rather than a screening test. This resulted in greater use of biopsy as a diagnostic test in North America than that reported from Europe (McLelland and Pisano 1992), where more use was made of diagnostic mammography subsequent to screening mammography (often called by European radiologists "complete" mammography) with a consequent reduction in biopsies and a much lower benign to malignant ratio.

Most commentators in the past, when considering the relative weight to be placed on sensitivity and specificity, tended to encourage high sensitivity at the cost of relatively low specificity, as it was felt important to attempt to avoid missing individuals who truly had disease. One vigorous exponent of this view for breast cancer screening was Moskowitz, who coined the term "aggressive screening", as only by such an approach did he feel that the "minimal" breast cancers with an excellent prognosis would be identified (Moskowitz et al. 1976). However, there continues to be little evidence that such cancers are really responsible for the mortality reduction following breast cancer screening. Rather, there is much evidence that the early diagnosis of more advanced disease results in the benefit (Miller 1987, 1994; Miller et al. 2000b, 2002). A disadvantage of aggressive screening was a high benign to malignant ratio, and low specificity of the screen. Although the objective of screening is to identify disease in the DPCP before it gets to the stage of escaping from curability, if a test is made so sensitive that it picks up lesions that would never have progressed in that individuals lifetime, there will be substantial additional costs for diagnosis and treatment (this is one consequence of the "overdiagnosis" bias, which is more fully discussed in relation to survival of cases following screen detection in a later section of this chapter). There is no point in identifying through screening disease which would never have presented clinically, and little point (other than less radical therapy) in identifying early disease that would have been cured anyway if it had presented clinically. Similarly, identifying disease that results in death, even following screen identification and subsequent treatment, only results in greater observation time and no benefit to the screenee. It is only disease that results in death in the absence of screening, but which is cured following treatment after screen detection, from which the real benefit of a screening programme derives. Hence, if high "sensitivity" is largely based on finding more good prognosis disease, but results in lowering specificity, the programme will incur much greater costs without corresponding benefit.

The process measure, as distinct from a measure of validity, that most clearly expresses this difficulty is the predictive value of a positive screen. This is defined as the proportion of those who test positive who truly have the disease (Fig. 10.3). This measure is influenced not only by the sensitivity and specificity of the test, especially the latter, but by the prevalence of disease in the population, whereas sensitivity and specificity are invariant with regard to disease prevalence. If tests are administered under circumstances that incur a low predictive value positive, then not only may costs be high in terms of correctly identifying those who are falsely positive, but also the potential hazard may be high, as an individual classified as positive falsely derives no benefit and potentially a substantial risk from the associated diagnostic procedures. A test with a low positive predictive value rapidly enters into disrepute.

To complete discussion of process measures, the predictive value negative should be defined. This is the proportion of those who test negative who are truly free of the disease. This measure, like sensitivity, is dependent on identifying the false negatives, and therefore is rarely determined while being of little operational value. In practice, however, it is usually high.

As Day (1985) has pointed out, because of the difficulty in identifying false negatives, and because of the overdiagnosis bias, the usual approach to defining sensitivity is not ideal, nor particularly biologically meaningful. He suggested an alternative measure of sensitivity which can be derived if the expected incidence of disease in the absence of screening can be determined, ideally from the control group in a randomised trial, but sometimes in population based programmes from historical data or data from comparable unscreened populations.

The method basically computes the extent a programme is successful in reducing the expected incidence of disease in the absence of screening. The lower the proportion of expected incidence occurring after screening the greater the sensitivity.

The Acceptability of the Test

One of the desirable attributes of a good screening test is that it should be acceptable to the population to which screening is offered and acceptable to those who will administer the test. In general, cervical cytology screening programmes have found acceptance with women and their physicians. Although those who tend to be at highest risk of the disease do not comply as well as those with lower risk, this is not strictly related to acceptability of the test, but rather the fact that such individuals tend to have so many pressing health and social problems, that taking action to reduce an uncertain risk in the future does not have priority with them. Nevertheless, this results in lower effectiveness of programmes than would be the case if all women were to be included. This lack of acceptance is largely related to lower socio-economic status, accompanied by high parity, and often multiple sexual partners.

Breast cancer screening has encountered different problems over acceptability, though this varies substantially in different countries, ranging from the 90% acceptance with screening invitations in the Swedish Two-County trial (Tabar et al. 1985) to the difficulties with both physician and women compliance in the early stages of mammography utilization for breast screening in the United States (Howard 1987). In Europe, a median uptake of 74% has been reported for mammography offered in the population (European Society for Mastology 1993). Perhaps fortunately, those who tend to comply with invitations to attend breast screening programmes tend to be those at higher risk. An exception relates to the misperception of many older women that they are not at risk for the disease, whereas the older they become the greater is their risk.

Another example is screening for colorectal cancer, because of the inevitable distaste of individuals for a procedure that involves manipulation of faeces. In a number of pilot programmes, therefore, the return rates for hemoccult slides have been low, though they have been better in well organised studies (Chamberlain and Miller 1988), and achieved approximately 75% in the Minnesota Colon Cancer Screening Trial (Mandel et al. 1999).

A screening test, therefore, has to be acceptable to the population in its widest sense. The test should be simple and as far as possible easily administered. It should involve procedures that are not unacceptable, and its use should not have unpleasant or potentially hazardous implications. There are also economic advantages in a test being administered or read by allied health professionals, such as use of technologists in screening cervical cytology slides (Anderson 1985), or the use of nurses to perform breast examinations (Bassett 1985; Miller et al. 1991a).

The Ethics of Screening

In general medical practice the special nature of the relationship between a patient and his physician has dictated the need to build up a core of ethical principles that govern this relationship. Further, it is generally accepted that additional issues arise when a patient becomes the subject of a research investigation that is superimposed upon his or her search for and receipt of appropriate medical care. It was not initially appreciated, however, that screening opened up a completely new spectrum of issues, possibly requiring more restrictive boundaries of ethical behaviour than those applied in usual medical care. For example, when a patient goes to see a physician for relief of a symptom or treatment of an established condition, the physician is required to exercise his or her skills only to the extent that knowledge is currently available, while doing what is possible with available expertise and appropriate assistance to help the patient. Treatment may be offered without any implied guarantee that it is necessarily efficacious or will do more than just temporarily relieve the symptoms of which the patient complains. Thus the physician promises to do his or her best for the patient; there is no implied promise that the patient will be cured.

In screening, however, those who are approached to participate are not patients and most of them do not become patients. The screener believes that as a result of screening the health of the community will be better. He or she does not necessarily intend to imply that the condition of every individual will be better. However, screening is often promoted as if it implies a benefit to everyone who is screened. In fact, in some circumstances individuals included in a screening programme may be placed at a disadvantage, as discussed above. Furthermore, the harm from a screening test is not only related to the risk of being false positive or negative. Those that are screened may also incur psychological consequences, sometimes merely from being labelled as being at risk of disease. At the very least, therefore, those planning to introduce a screening programme should be in a position to guarantee overall benefit to the community and a minimum of risk that certain individuals may be disadvantaged by the programme. It was the inability to guarantee overall benefit and lack of disadvantage for those screened that led to the proscription of mammography in women under the age of 50 in the Breast Cancer Detection Demonstration Projects in the United States (Beahrs et al. 1979).

A second ethical issue, which is directed more to the obligations for appropriate care in the community than towards individuals, concerns how limited resources are equitably distributed across the whole community to obtain maximum benefit. Under certain circumstances the offer of screening could diminish the total level of health in a community. This may be a particular problem for developing countries by diverting resources intended for routine health care into screening. Thus, resources diverted to a screening project, which might be regarded as prestigious, especially if involving high technology, could lower the resources available for other more pressing but also more mundane health problems. Although several screening programmes have been proposed for developing countries, there is a particular need for caution and care in order to ensure that they do not overbalance the health care system in the area in which they are introduced.

A final ethical dilemma for screening programmes is how to implement informed consent. Information about risks and benefits of tests and treatments are expected to be provided in usual clinical practice. For screening, providing information about the test alone is not sufficient. Information about the consequences of the test, the diagnostic assessment process and the diseases to be detected and their treatments should also be presented, if a truly informed decision is to be made. Presenting such a large amount of information is obviously difficult, particularly in a primary care setting where several screening tests may be done at the same time. Furthermore, presenting such information becomes even more cumbersome when the evidence base for a screening test is limited, such as is the case with prostate screening with the prostate specific antigen (PSA) test.

Those in charge of screening programmes, therefore, carry an ethical responsibility as least as great as that for medical practice in that approaches to participate are made to ostensibly healthy people. Indeed, the burden of proof for efficacy of the procedures and the necessity to avoid harm are greater than may be required for diagnostic or therapeutic procedures carried out when a patient presents with symptoms to a physician. In screening the physician or public health worker initiates the process and he or she bears the onus of responsibility to be certain that benefit will follow.

The Population to be Included in Screening Programmes

10.4

For a screening programme to be successful, the population to be included should be one in which it is known that the disease has a high prevalence. This will not only encourage a high predictive value for a positive test; it will tend to promote higher quality of performance and assessment of results of screening tests, and will result in lower costs per case detected. Thus in all screening programmes it is desirable to attempt to include only those who are at risk of the disease and to concentrate particularly on those who are at high risk of the disease. This approach was recognized by the Canadian Task Force on Cervical Cytology Screening Programs (Task Force 1976) who carefully defined those whom it believed were at such low risk for the disease that they need not be included in cervical cytology screening programmes, thus defining the remaining "at risk" population on whom major efforts should be concentrated to bring them into screening. In the case of cardiovascular disease, family history and factors such as smoking have been used by some to define populations to be screened.

For other diseases, however, the known risk factors, apart from age, may not suffice to adequately distinguish between those who should be considered for inclusion in screening programmes compared to those who should not. For breast screening, for example, although some discrimination using risk factors has been achieved (Schechter et al. 1986) this has not been sufficient to justify selection on this basis alone. However, age is an important predictor of risk, and for breast cancer in technically advanced countries, all women in the appropriate age group can be regarded as at high risk. Thus for breast cancer currently, it seems unlikely that any programme could justify routine screening of women under the age of 40, while several trials only found a delayed effect of screening women in this age group, and our trial in Canada, the only so far specifically designed to evaluate breast screening at these ages, could not find evidence that screening women age 40–49 with mammography is effective (Miller et al. 2002). As a result, the organised programmes in most European countries and in Canada do not attempt to recruit women under the age of 50 into screening.

One possible approach to concentrating on the relevant segment of the population for screening might be to administer a pre-screening test, especially for a marker for a factor necessary in the causation of the disease. The test for Human Papilloma Virus infection could be used as a pre-screen for cancer of the cervix (Miller et al. 2000a) though a difficulty here is the high proportion of infections that are self-limiting without the development of high grade cervical intraepithelial neoplasia. This means that the test is too non-specific if used among women under the age of 35. However, in older women if found to be negative to a test for oncogenic HPV strains, they can be deemed at low risk for the disease and screened far less frequently than women who are HPV positive.

The development of genetic susceptibility testing opens up the possibility in the future of pre-screening for a range of diseases. Unfortunately the tests that indicate high risks so far only identify individuals in the population responsible for a low proportion of disease. It seems possible that it will be necessary to screen for a combination of genetic polymorphisms each responsible for relatively low relative risks in the population, but with high attributable risk, in order to adequately discriminate at risk from low risk individuals. This will increase the complexity, and costs, of the process considerably.

Nevertheless, in programmes that attempt to select for screening on the basis of risk factors, there will almost invariably be cases occurring in the unscreened group. A consequence of such programmes, however, will be reduced numbers of false positives (in absolute terms) which with the increased prevalence of the disease will result in a higher positive predictive value of the screen. Hakama (1984) coined the terms programme sensitivity and programme specificity which help in understanding the effects of screening concentrating on high risk subjects. The more a programme concentrates on "high risk" groups, the lower the programme sensitivity, as more and more cases will occur in unscreened people. Conversely, however, the programme specificity will increase because of the increase in healthy people unscreened with a reduction in the costs of screening. However, because the reduction in programme sensitivity will result in a reduction in the overall effectiveness of the programme, the overall result of such an approach could be unacceptable.

One other approach to using risk factors is to help determine the optimal periodicity of re-screening. Those judged at high risk could be screened more frequently, as in the example of HPV tests for cervix screening given above. Once again, however, much of the necessary research is incomplete, and we do not know how appropriate such an approach may be. It will probably be necessary to calculate the marginal cost effectiveness of extending screening from high to low risk groups (i.e. the additional cost for such an extension of screening related to the increase in effectiveness of the screening) in order to make the necessary policy decisions.

Diagnosis and Treatment of the Discovered Lesions

10.5

As a screening test is not diagnostic, inevitably the success of the programme will ultimately depend upon the extent those identified as having a positive test accept the procedures offered to them for further evaluation, and the effectiveness of the therapy offered.

A number of difficulties may arise. For example, in the initial phases of many breast cancer screening programmes, it was necessary to demonstrate to the general community of medical practitioners that the abnormalities identified were indeed of importance and that they required care and expertise to biopsy. Indeed in the absence of skills in diagnosis and management, there can be unnecessary biopsy (potentially reducible by the use of diagnostic mammography and fine needle aspiration biopsies) as well as failure to excise the lesion when biopsy is performed. This is part of the spectrum of problems that arise over the fact that lesions may be identified in screening programmes whose biologic features, natural history and other characteristics may be in doubt. The screening participants may require special education programs so that they understand the diagnostic process to reduce as far as possible one of the major adverse consequences of screening, the anxiety accompanying the identification of an abnormality, as well as ensuring that they comply with the recommendations for management. There may even be major disagreements over the histological interpretation of the excised lesions, with uncertainties over the borderline between benign and malignant. Thus the public and the professionals at all levels in a screening programme may require education and/or retraining dependant on their responsibilities. One mechanism to reduce difficulties in the professional area that should be encouraged is the provision of special diagnostic and treatment centres where the necessary expertise in diagnosis and management can be concentrated and where the necessary facilities are available (Miller and Tschechovski 1987). Such diagnosis centres could be regionally based, serving a number of screening centres.

10.6   Evaluation of the Efficacy of Screening

A number of issues have to be noted when evaluating the efficacy of screening. Almost invariably individuals with disease identified as a result of screening will have a longer survival time than those diagnosed in the normal way. Four biases associated with screening explain this (see Box 1). The first is "lead time", defined as the interval between the time of detection by screening and the time at which the disease would have been diagnosed in the absence of screening (depicted in Fig. 10.1). In other words, it is the period by which screening advances the diagnosis of the disease. For example, if as a result of screening, the average point of diagnosis is advanced by one year, then inevitably cases diagnosed by screening will survive one year longer even if there is no long term benefit. It is important to recognise that the lead time for different cases will vary, depending in part on the timing of the screening test in relation to the duration of the DPCP in that case, as well as the rapidity of progression of the DPCP in that individual. Thus there will be a distribution of lead times (Morrison 1985). The lead time for fatal cases will be fairly short, but in one study some fatal cases have been identified as having a lead time of one or more years following mammography screening (Miller et al. 1992).

> **Box 1. The biases associated with survival**
>
> *Lead time:* the period by which screening advances the diagnosis of the disease.
>
> *Length bias:* less rapidly progressive cases are likely to be detected by screening.
>
> *Selection bias:* volunteers for screening are likely to have a better outcome from their disease than those who decline screening.
>
> *Overdiagnosis bias:* lesions identified by screening which would not have progressed to clinical disease in the absence of screening.

The determination of lead time is complex, but models have been developed that do so providing there are control data that permit comparison of screen detection with that expected (Walter and Day 1983).

Differential lead time can be an important factor in comparing the outcome among cases detected by different screening modalities, making it almost impos-

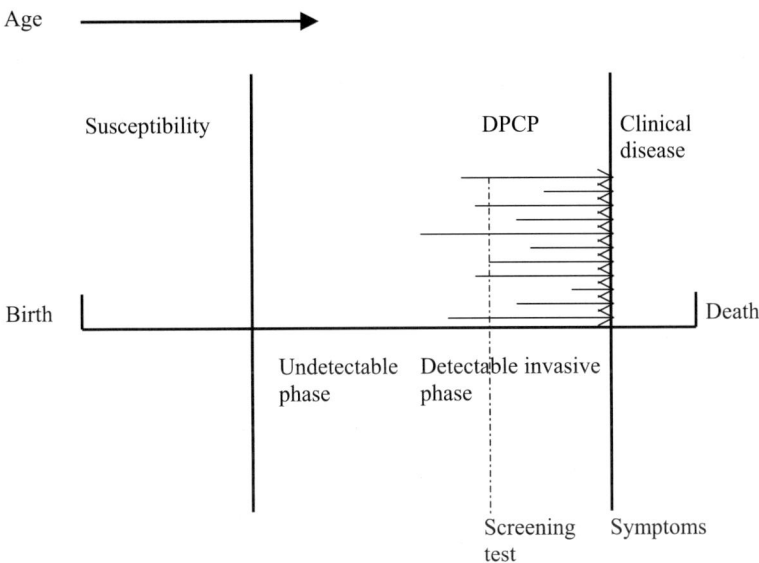

DPCP = detectable preclinical phase

Figure 10.5. The impact of a screening test when the detectable preclinical phase varies in duration – length bias

sible to make a comparison based on survival, unless it is possible to estimate and correct for differential lead time (Walter and Stitt 1987).

The second bias that accounts for improved survival of screen detected cases is "length-biased sampling", or more simply, length bias. This relates to the fact that individuals who have rapidly progressive disease will tend to develop symptoms that cause them to consult physicians directly. Thus only less rapidly progressive cases are likely to remain to be detected by screening. Yet the former have a poorer and the latter a better prognosis, hence the improved survival of screen-detected cases, over and above lead time. An attempt to depict this bias is shown in Fig. 10.5. It is obvious that if the screening test were to be administered just before clinical symptoms occur, nearly all cases would be detected, but by them, some of them would probably have a poorer prognosis. So it is important to try and detect cases earlier in the DPCP, but if one is successful, many of the rapidly progressive cases will be missed. What is more, what is depicted is just at one point in time, rapidly progressive cases that were present at the time the slowly progressive cases become detectable, would have presented with symptoms before the screening test was administered. This bias is most obvious at the initiation of a screening programme, at the first or prevalent screen. However, length-bias will also affect the type of cases detected at rescreening, with the more rapidly progressive cancers diagnosed in the intervals between screens. Hence in evaluating the total impact of programmes, the interval cases must be identified and taken into consideration as well as the screen-detected cases.

The third bias which can artifactually improve survival is selection bias. Those who enter screening programmes are volunteers, and almost invariably more health conscious than those who decline to enter. This means that they are likely, even in the absence of screening, to have a better outcome from their disease than the overall rates in the general population.

The fourth bias is overdiagnosis bias. Simply it means that some lesions identified and counted as disease would not have progressed to present clinically in those individuals during their lifetimes in the absence of screening. It is, in practice, an extreme example of length bias. It is difficult to obtain absolute confirmation of the existence of this bias, though it seems likely that it is at least in part an explanation for the substantial excess of cancers detected by PSA screening for prostate cancer, and it has also been strongly suspected for breast cancer (Miller et al. 2000b, 2002).

The only design that effectively eliminates the effect of all these biases is the randomised controlled trial (Prorok et al. 1984), but only if mortality from the disease (i.e. deaths related to the person-years of observation) is used as the endpoint, rather than survival. Survival could be used in a randomised controlled screening trial only under special circumstances. These are that there is good evidence because of the equivalence in cumulative numbers of cases during the relevant period of observation that there is no overdiagnosis bias; and providing that the start of the period of observation of the cases is taken as the date of randomisation, as that will eliminate differential lead time. This is the approach that will be used in a study of breast self examination in Russia, where it will not be possible to follow all entrants to determine their alive and dead status at the end of the trial (Semiglazov et al. 1993). Length bias and selection bias are not issues, the latter having been equally distributed by the randomisation, and the former by having started at the same point in time, and by including all cases that occur during follow-up in the evaluation.

Outside a randomised trial, if the screening test detects a precursor, reduction in incidence of the clinically detected disease can be expected and evaluated. This effect has been well demonstrated in the Nordic countries in relation to screening for cancer of the cervix (Hakama 1982). It is also anticipated from endoscopy screening for colorectal cancer, with the detection and removal of adenomas. If the screening test does not detect a precursor, or even if it does but the main yield is invasive cancer, then incidence can be expected to increase initially following the introduction of screening, and remain elevated while screening continues, though there may be some reduction towards the baseline after continued screening, if the application of the test results in most at risk subjects being included, and the subsequent screening tests are largely used for rescreening. This seems to have happened with the major rise and then fall, but not to the original levels, of prostate cancer incidence following the opportunistic introduction of the PSA test in North America. Under such circumstances, when further reduction in incidence can not be anticipated, and improvement in survival can not be relied upon because of the biases already discussed, the only valid outcome for assessment of results of a screening programme is mortality from the disease in the total population offered screening in comparison with the mortality that would be expected in the same population if screening had not been offered.

As already emphasized the design of choice for evaluation of changes in mortality is the randomised controlled trial. This can either be an efficacy trial, or an effectiveness trial. Efficacy trials are based on randomisation of the screening test, which answers the biologically relevant question as to whether mortality is reduced in those screened. An effectiveness trial is based on the randomisation of invitations to attend for screening, and more nearly replicates the circumstances that may eventually pertain in practice in a population. Both those who accept the invitation as well as those who refuse will have to be included in the assessment of outcome. Thus it tests the impact of introducing screening in a population. Some trials of this type involve randomisation by cluster. However, cluster randomisation can lead to difficulties in determining whether the trial results are valid, especially if it cannot be confirmed that the randomised groups were balanced, or if there is evidence that they were not. Such problems led to difficulties in determining the validity of some cluster randomised trials of breast screening (IARC 2002).

If for some reason randomisation is believed inappropriate, a second-best method is the quasi-experimental study in which screening is offered in some areas, and unscreened areas as comparable as possible are used for comparison purposes. However, this design is not a cheap and easy way out but demands the same methodological accuracy as required for randomised trials. Further, in view of the substantially larger populations that may have to be studied than in randomised trials, it may prove to be more expensive than the preferred design. Critically, difficulties in analysis may ensue if the baseline mortality in the comparison areas differ (UK Trial of Early Detection of Breast Cancer Group 1988).

Nevertheless, ethical issues may preclude the utilization of randomised trials, particularly for programmes that were introduced before the necessity of utilising trials as far as possible for evaluation was appreciated. This has been the case for screening for cancer of the cervix for example. One approach under these circumstances is to compare the mortality in defined populations before and after the introduction of screening programmes, preferably with data available on the trends in acceptance of screening so that changes in mortality can be correlated with the mortality trends. Such a correlation study will be strengthened if other data that could be related to changes in the outcome variable are entered into a multivariate analysis (Miller et al. 1976).

A case-control study of screening is another approach that can be used to evaluate programmes that were introduced sufficiently long before the study that an effect can be expected to have occurred. Case-control studies depend on comparing the screen histories of the cases with the histories of comparable controls drawn from the population from which the cases arose. Individuals with early stage disease if sampled would be eligible as a control, providing the date of diagnosis was not earlier than that of the case, as diagnosis of disease truncates the screening history. However, a bias would arise if advanced disease is compared only with early stage disease, as the latter is likely to be screen detected, though this is just a function of the screening process, not its efficacy (Weiss 1983). Cases have to reflect the end points used to evaluate screening, i.e. those that would be expected to be reduced by screening. Thus, cases are often deaths from the disease or advanced disease as a surrogate for deaths, or if a precursor of the disease is detected through screening, incident cases in the population. If incident cases are screen detected, the controls should be drawn from those screened in the same programme; if the cases are not screen-detected, the controls should be population based (Sasco et al. 1986).

One difficulty with case-control studies of screening is that they may be affected by selection bias as the health conscious may select themselves for screening. This may be difficult to correct in the analysis, though such a correction should be attempted if the relevant data on risk factors for the disease (confounders) are available. This was possible in a case-control study of breast self-examination nested within the Canadian National Breast Screening Study, in which data on risk factors for breast cancer were collected from all on enrolment (Harvey et al. 1997). Such a bias may not be a problem, however, in other circumstances, if it can be demonstrated that the incidence of cancer in those who declined the invitation to the screening programme is similar to that expected in an unscreened population.

However, even if data are available on risk factors for disease, adjusting for them may not result in avoiding the effect of selection bias. For breast cancer, for example, experience in studies in Sweden and the UK, where case-control studies were performed within trials, show that although those who refused invitations for screening had similar breast cancer incidence to the unscreened controls in the trial, their breast cancer mortality experience was worse than that of those controls. This meant that the estimate of the effect of screening in such case-control studies was greater than could have been expected in the total population (Miller et al. 1990; Moss 1991).

In addition to assessing effectiveness of screening, case-control studies may also be of use to assess other aspects of screening programmes. For example, a method has been proposed for estimation of the natural history of preclinical disease from screening data based on case-control methodology (Brookmeyer et al. 1986).

The cohort study design may also provide an estimate of the effect of screening, an approach in which the mortality from the cancer of interest in an individually identified and followed screened group (the cohort) is compared to the mortality experience in a control population, often derived from the general population. This approach has been used to evaluate the mortality experience in the US Breast Cancer Detection Demonstration Project (Morrison et al. 1988) and in a cohort of women in Finland included in a breast self examination programme (Gastrin et al. 1994). In these studies it has to be recognised that those recruited into a screening programme are initially free of the disease of interest so that it is not appropriate to apply population mortality rates for the disease to the person-years experience of the study cohort. Rather, as is required in estimating the sample size required for a controlled trial of screening, it is first necessary to determine the expected incidence of the cases of interest, then apply to that expectation the expected case-fatality rate from the disease to derive the expectation for the deaths (Moss et al.

1987). In practice, a cohort study of screening suffers from the same problem of selection bias as for case-control studies, so the results have to be interpreted with caution.

Indirect indicators of effectiveness are often desired in evaluating screening programmes, especially one that would predict subsequent mortality. Compliance with screening, and rate of screen-detection, as well as the ratio of prevalence and incidence can be indicators of potentially effective screens (Day et al. 1989). The cumulative prevalence (not the percentage distribution) of advanced disease is one such measure (Prorok et al. 1984). For example, reduction in advanced disease predicted subsequent breast cancer mortality reduction in a trial of mammography screening versus no screening in Sweden (Tabar et al. 1989). However, case detection frequency, numbers of small tumours, and stage shift in percentages of the total should not be used as indicators of effectiveness as they potentially reflect all four screening biases.

In evaluating whether screening programmes are effective in a population, different methods have generally to be used. They are considered in the section on Surveillance, later in this chapter.

Organised Screening Programmes

There are a number of features of effective screening programmes that are largely related to good organization. Indeed there is good evidence, at least for cancer of the cervix, that unorganised or opportunistic screening programmes, which depend on the willingness of individuals to volunteer for screening, and the extent to which their physicians offer screening, often to low risk women, are far less successful (Hakama et al. 1985).

Hakama et al. (1985) defined certain essential elements of organised programmes. These are:

— the target population has been identified;
— the individual women are identifiable;
— measures are available to guarantee high coverage and attendance such as a personal letter of invitation;
— there are adequate field facilities for performing the screening tests;
— there is an organised quality control programme on performing and reading the tests;
— adequate facilities exist for diagnosis and for appropriate treatment of confirmed abnormalities;
— there is a carefully designed and agreed referral system, an agreed link between the participant, the screening centre and the clinical facility for diagnosis of an abnormal screening test, for management of any abnormalities found and for providing information about normal screening tests;
— evaluation and monitoring of the total programme is organised in terms of incidence and mortality rates among those attending, among those not attending,

at the level of the total target population. Quality control of the epidemiological data should be established.

Although these elements are present in many European cancer screening programmes, especially in the Nordic countries, and contribute greatly to their success, several elements are missing from programmes elsewhere, especially those largely based on the private medical care system in North America. In Canada, there are opportunities for introducing some of them, such as the first three, and these were recommended by the two Canadian Task Forces on cervical cancer screening (Task Force 1976, 1982). Unfortunately, only three of the provincial health care authorities (Ontario, Manitoba and British Columbia (the latter having accepted from the beginning the need for centralised laboratory services)) have taken the initiative to establish such programmes. All provinces in Canada that introduced breast screening programmes, however, accepted from the outset the necessity for them to be organised, (Workshop Group 1989), thus attempting to replicate the organisation of breast cancer screening in some of the Nordic countries, the Netherlands and in the United Kingdom.

There has been some debate as to whether organised as distinct from opportunistic screening is most efficacious in reducing the incidence of cancer of the cervix. Nieminen et al. (1999) produced evidence that in Finland, the organised programme is far more effective than opportunistic screening.

10.8   Health Related Quality of Life and Screening

An important evaluation measure for screening is the extent overall quality of life is improved or impaired by screening compared to usual care. Decision making for health care policy is only possible if information is available on quality of life as well as health costs of screened and unscreened participants as well as mortality reduction from screening. For example, it requires an "optimistic" estimate of screening effectiveness to derive an overall benefit from screening for prostate cancer (Krahn et al. 1994). Issues concerning health related quality of life (HRQL) may well vary with different cultural value systems, and different health care systems.

Because of lead time, HRQL events will tend to occur earlier in life than similar events associated with usual care. Given that the adverse quality of life associated with false positive screening tests, and those associated with treatment will tend to occur relatively early, it could be easy to convince oneself (as it has convinced some commentators for prostate cancer screening already) that the HRQL issues are overwhelming and that screening should not be conducted. It will require prolonged follow up, probably more than 10 years, for the detriments associated with advanced disease late in life that may be prevented from occurring in the screened group to appear in the non-screened group (Miller et al. 2001).

If the outcome of screening were to be a major benefit in terms of mortality reduction, the issues related to HRQL would be overwhelmed. It is only if the outcome is a moderate to small mortality reduction that these issues become critical, and paradoxically then it would be necessary for them to have been measured with as much precision as was possible during screening, as, particularly for HRQL, the decrements could not be measured retrospectively with precision. For this reason, in screening trials where adverse HRQL can be anticipated, it is important for such events to be identified and quantified.

Economics of Screening   10.9

Space does not permit a detailed evaluation of the various principles that have to be considered in assessing the economics of screening. In brief, it is necessary to determine the costs of the test and the subsequent diagnostic tests. Also should be included are the costs associated with any hazard of the test as well as the costs of overtreatment. Balancing these costs may be reduced costs of therapy of the primary condition, reduced costs associated with less expenditure on the treatment of advanced disease, and the economic value of the additional years of life gained. This can become quite complex when the value of treatment of disease in years of life gained, transfers such as pensions, and economic productivity are considered. The latter is often disputed, if not regarded with some distaste, so that often what is computed is the cost per year of life saved. Critical may be the marginal costs of additional tests in relation to the benefit, especially when considerations of the frequency of re-screening arise.

Part of the difficulty in economic assessment is that costs are often incurred early, while benefits flow later, so that for proper comparisons of such costs they have to be discounted to the present day. Additional complexity ensues if attempts are made to assess quality of life in economic terms, while the calculations rarely attempt an economic assessment of the fact that if a death is prevented by screening, the relevant individual will inevitably die of some other condition, and that death could be more costly.

It is likely that economic assessments will increasingly guide policy decisions in the future, so it behoves those interested in evaluation of screening to collect the necessary data. Although some economic assessments have suggested that cost-effective programmes are achievable, for example programmes of breast cancer screening using single-view mammography in Sweden (Jonsson et al. 1988), others have suggested that programmes may not be cost-effective, for example breast cancer screening programmes for younger women in the US (Eddy et al. 1988). Economic analysis is particularly important for making decisions *within* screening programmes, for example around screening intervals or method of follow-up. Economic analyses have also facilitated the planning of national breast screening programmes (IARC 2002).

10.10   **Genetic Susceptibility Testing**

The completion of mapping of the human genome holds great promise for disease control. This presages the advent of genetic susceptibility testing. However, the availability of a range of markers for disease susceptibility will lead to increasing controversies about the use of screening tests. While the general principles of screening outlined above will still apply, they will need to be modified. Genetic screening will identify individuals at risk of disease, rather than those with precursors or early stage disease. Although this could lead to focussed application of screening tests on those at higher risk, ideally, primary prevention strategies will be available. Nevertheless, for many conditions, the preventive strategies will be the application of other screening tests implying that diagnostic assessment and treatment strategies will still be required.

10.11   **Surveillance**

Surveillance of a programme is performed to assess its performance, to ensure that it is being as effective as possible. This requires adopting the principles of programme evaluation.

Programme evaluation is "the systematic assessment of the operation and/or outcomes of a programme or policy compared to a set of explicit or implicit standards, as a means of contributing to the improvement of the programme or policy" (Weiss 1998). Continuous evaluation of processes and outcomes of a screening programme is an essential tool for assessing its organisational progress and enhancing its effectiveness.

Monitoring is the process of ongoing evaluation to determine whether a programme is achieving its intermediate objectives. Monitoring uses "process measures", that are designed to indicate whether the programme is on course to achieve its objectives. Of themselves these process measures are not indicators of the success of the programme. Rather they indicate whether or not the programme is on the route to ultimate success, as unless they are achieved, the programme is unlikely to be successful. These process measures cover a number of different aspects of the programme. If the targets, as outlined below, are not met, it should be obvious which aspects of the programme require urgent attention by the programme managers to rectify the situation. Monitoring should be an ongoing activity, carried out as an integral part of the programme, by the programme's own staff.

Evaluation is a process whereby the success of the programme in reaching the targets set for the intermediate outcome, and outcome measures is carefully reviewed and analysed. When carried out during the early phases of the programme it will indicate whether the programme is likely to be successful. When carried out at certain defined time points after the initiation of the programme, it will indicate whether the programme has been successful, and whether in the light of the degree of that success, it should be continued. Evaluation is an intermittent activity. It can be carried out by the programme staff, but it can also be performed by an external consultant to the programme, providing the information system is fully functional and successful in obtaining the data required.

Surveillance and evaluation are essential for all programmes, to ensure that the resources used achieve the benefit expected. Process measures such as the numbers of screens performed, the numbers of positive tests reported, the number (and proportion) of those screened referred for diagnosis and therapy, the numbers of cases of disease diagnosed and the numbers of precursor and benign lesions detected, should be derivable providing the data are collected from the screening centres and the treating institutions and collated. Such data must be analysed by age to confirm that those in the target age group are being screened, and receive appropriate subsequent management. However, such data cannot evaluate the effectiveness in terms of the likely prevention of occurrence of disease or of deaths from the disease, unless the data can be related to that derived from the total population on an ongoing basis, which requires linkage to a pre-existing disease register or vital statistics system, or to a register of cases of the relevant disease established for this purpose.

Depending on the endpoint that should be affected by screening, e.g. deaths from the cancer of interest for cancer screening programmes, the simplest form of surveillance and evaluation that will provide measures of the effectiveness of the programme in the population is to be able to demonstrate a change in the slope of the trend in mortality from the disease in the population. More detailed evaluation requires the identification of all who develop the disease and die from it in the target population and documentation of their screening history. Such documentation could be done by comparing incident cases of disease in the target population with a register of those from the same population who have been screened. This will permit an estimate of the risk in those who have been screened and in those who failed to attend screening and the combined effect can then be compared with the prescreening period. Where such registers have not been established, a screening history should be obtained from subjects with the disease, though this may not be reliable as many are unable to recall whether a screening test has been taken in the past. Efficient surveillance requires a system of linked records. A population register (or available substitute) allows periodic call-back for rescreening at appropriate intervals. The screening programme register, when linked with a disease register, permits the active surveillance of those detected with abnormalities, to ensure recall for diagnosis and therapy. Evaluation of the programme can then be performed with regard to assessment of:

— Management of those screened with positive tests
— Disease diagnosed between the screening interval
— Groups missed in the target population.

10.12   Responsibility for Screening

Responsibility for the efficient management of screening in a country (or region) should preferably be placed on a designated official within a relevant organization. If disease control has been designated to a special agency in a country, this official should have an appointment within that agency. Alternatively, it would be appropriate to designate an official within the Ministry of Health.

In general, it is not appropriate for the Director of the department or laboratory performing the tests to be given responsibility for the overall direction of the whole programme. This is because the responsibilities for direction of the programme are far wider than reading the screening test, but cover aspects from the identification of the target group, through their recruitment, screening, management of abnormalities found to evaluation of the impact of the programme.

The Director should recognise that successful screening programmes:

— Are organised as public-health disease control programmes, and not simply as services for providing clinical investigation,
— Target the age groups at greatest and most immediate risk, concentrating on those who have never had a test,
— Use population registers,
— Have someone in charge who is named, has a telephone number, and can be held to account.

The skills necessary to encompass the responsibility for running a successful programme include epidemiology, public health and management.

10.13   Evaluation of the Effectiveness of Screening Programmes

The principles that underlie the evaluation of screening programmes are that they should be compatible with the programme objectives; there should be standardization of nomenclature, procedures and measurements to facilitate evaluation; and that the programmes should facilitate relevant research.

The *general objectives* of screening programmes are:

— to reduce the incidence of the disease (if a disease precursor is detected); and
— to reduce mortality from the disease.

The *specific objectives* to achieve the general objectives are:

— provision of accessible and acceptable screening services;
— the recruitment of eligible subjects, ensuring that those at high risk are screened;
— ensure adherence to recommended screening schedules;
— quality in taking the test and reading it;

- effective communication of results;
- appropriate follow-up if there is an abnormal test;
- provision of efficient and effective treatment services.

The *components* of programme evaluation should be designed to be compatible with these objectives. They should include:
- population-based information systems;
- quality control systems, both internal and external.

In the absence of population-based information systems specific surveys may provide some of the needed information. They could include surveys of awareness of the need for screening in eligible and especially high risk subjects, and of the practice of screening by the target group and the advice rendered by their physicians.

Specially designed epidemiological studies, most economically of the case-control type, can also be used for programme evaluation, but should in general be part of a specific research project and subject to peer review.

The data requirements for efficient programme evaluation include data on the target population, and a register of all screening tests performed, with identification as to first or repeat (these records must be capable of being linked to provide a longitudinal screening history of each screenee. This requires capturing information on all changes of name, and preferably using unique personal identifying numbers).

Other requirements include:
- a separate register of all abnormal tests, with data on follow-up, management and outcome;
- data on all preclinical lesions diagnosed, classified by the recommended terminology;
- data on all cases of the disease diagnosed;
- data on all deaths from the disease;
- information on cost/manpower items, relevant to every aspect of screening.

For evaluation and monitoring purposes, the data in information systems must be maintained in individually identifiable and linkable form, and the system should be so designed that it is accessible for evaluation and monitoring purposes and research, as well as for the requirements of routine functioning of the programme. The information on the target population should be provided by age, geographical area, and if possible the family physician of those eligible for screening. This will permit the identification of those in the population who are not being screened, who are likely to include those at highest risk, for whom special efforts will be needed to bring them into the programme. Such linkages will enable the success of the measures taken to recruit eligible subjects to be determined.

The *criteria* for success or failure of screening programmes relate to the objectives of the programme. These include:
- increase in awareness of the need for screening in the at risk population;
- increase in participation rates for screening;

- reach members of the target group who have never been screened;
- improve the performance of test centres or laboratories;
- reduce the utilisation of unnecessary medical procedures;
- reduce the incidence of and mortality from the disease.

Thus evaluation should include not only outcome measures, most importantly incidence and mortality from the disease, but also process measures, so that if a programme is not effective the corrective actions needed can be taken.

There has to be some designated authority who will accept responsibility for programme evaluation, assess the success in achieving the programme objectives and ensure corrective action is taken as necessary. Although this may vary by programme and country, the primary responsibility should usually be assumed by government, though government may seek the assistance of non-government organizations in reaching the objectives. It would be desirable for government to appoint a broadly-based advisory committee, with expert members drawn from a variety of disciplines. Acting on the advice of this committee, government may be able to delegate to various organizations responsible for different programme components the responsibility for any corrective action necessary.

Information Systems
10.14 **for Screening Programmes**

A population-based information system is the basic building block of organised screening programmes. Such information systems must be capable of supporting a diversity of goals and objectives (see below) including individual information retrieval and sophisticated aggregate and comparative data analyses.

The range of goals and objectives to which information systems can contribute attest to their importance in assisting screening programmes to achieve positive health outcomes. Information systems for screening programmes should be designed to:
a) identify the target population;
b) identify individuals in the target population;
c) permit the individuals in the target population to be sent letters to:
   1. remind her/him to attend for screening once she reaches the recommended age;
   2. remind her/him to reattend for screening at the recommended intervals;
   3. remind her/him to attend the local diagnosis centre if an abnormality is discovered on self-examination or physician examination;

d) monitor that action has been taken following the discovery of an abnormality;
e) provide long-term follow-up for patients who have received treatment following the diagnosis of disease;

f) permit linkage of individual screens at the individual level;
g) permit evaluation and monitoring of the total system.

Development of information systems will be facilitated by the introduction of permanent individual health care identifiers. However, establishment of data bases to support screening programmes need not be dependent upon unique individual identifiers and should not be delayed where such identifiers are not yet in use.

Goals and Objectives of Information Systems 10.14.1

The *goals* of an information system are:
— to facilitate enrolling the at risk population;
   For a screening programme it is essential that the data base incorporate data on the entire target population.
— to maintain information;
   Information on the screening history of each screenee must be maintained on the data base; in addition, information must be organised and the data elements defined to facilitate analysis and planning.
— to provide the means for follow-up;
   The information system must support communication with individuals concerning test results, the need for screening, rescreening or medical follow-up.
— to support evaluation of quality assurance;
   Design of the information system must incorporate the capacity for qualitative assessment of the programme as a whole.
— to track utilisation of screening by the target population;
   A critical measure of the value of the programme's information system will be its utility to follow patterns of use to determine levels of utilization.
— to monitor compliance.
   Compliance with recommended screening and appropriate follow-up must be monitored by the information system to assist in evaluating the success of the overall programme.

The information system developed to support the screening programme must be designed to meet the following *objectives (action list)*:
— to locate the unscreened and underscreened;
— to provide data to aid programmes to reach special targeted groups such as the elderly;
— to record detected abnormalities;
— to assist in follow-up and treatment;
— to assist in follow-up communications to the target population;
— to support a schedule of testing;
— to evaluate compliance;
— to define high risk groups;
— to facilitate evaluation and planning;
— to determine the cost-effectiveness of the screening programme.

10.14.2   Information System Design

Information system design should not be regarded as simply a technical exercise involving systems experts but must incorporate the views and data requirements of all groups involved in the programme. In other words, wide-ranging consultation and participatory planning is essential. Design of information systems requires collaboration between many disciplines, the clinicians concerned with administering and interpreting screening tests, and the specialists in computer systems that can ensure that the data required to monitor and evaluate a screening programme are collected, coded, collated, and made available for analysis. This process is often very difficult in developing countries. A proposal for a cervical screening information system for developing countries has been published (Marrett et al. 2002).

Without appropriate interaction on system design, opportunities may be overlooked to structure systems in ways which can serve ongoing programme needs. For example, data concerning screening facilities (location, hours, wheelchair accessibility) might be identified as necessary by consumer advocates.

Participatory systems planning and development should include all stakeholders in the success of a screening programme. The process of developing an information system should be sensitive to the needs of diverse interest groups. Among the groups which should be included are:

— consumers – including representatives of health groups, and all minority groups (ethnic minorities, the disabled);
— professional colleges and associations;
— the relevant non-governmental organisation and the Non-Communicable Disease (NCD) control committee;
— government including representation from public health units, health agencies, health promotion agencies;
— the research communities – including epidemiologists and academic researchers in health care and public policy.

10.14.3   Policy Issues and Data Use

Policy makers should understand the need for the information system. In brief the system is justified because it enables the programme to be run on a daily basis, permits its performance to be assessed and enables any necessary improvements to be made; while the system can be used for evaluation and other scientific purposes, i.e. in research. The uses to which data are put are of just as much concern as is the design of the systems from which information is derived. A central concern of custodians of health care data bases is the question of access to information and the protection of individual privacy. Extensive consultation is necessary to ensure that personal privacy is protected, and that appropriate protocols are developed for the use of linked and aggregated data. In addition, other policy issues will arise that will require similar consultation and review.

Components of Information Systems

Information systems developed in support of health programmes usually contain a number of common elements and frequently include: the target population file, a registration file, data linkage capabilities (e.g. for linkage to disease registries, vital statistics systems), and mechanisms for monitoring and evaluation. Despite the likelihood of a substantial commonality of data elements when similar programmes are developed in different jurisdictions, opportunities to improve programme evaluation and delivery may be lost if efforts are not made to coordinate data definitions and standards.

To obtain maximum benefit from the introduction of a screening programme, it is important that common definition of data elements be achieved, through appropriate consultation.

Conclusion on Information Systems

As part of the process of consultation needed to set up information systems for screening, a range of information management issues will have to be addressed. It is anticipated that the consultative policy and planning process advocated will provide the mechanism for addressing them.

Implementation of well-designed and monitored information systems can enhance the benefits of an organised nation-wide screening programme. They can help to ensure quality control by linking testing and treatment with outcomes, increase efficiency, identify under-screening of some risk groups (e.g. the elderly), support programme evaluation, and help in answering research questions. These and other results can be fed back to yield further programme improvement.

Conclusions

There are a number of fundamental issues that have to be resolved when considering disease control by screening. The general principles that govern the introduction of screening programmes include:
— the disease should be an important health problem;
— the disease should have a detectable preclinical phase;
— the natural history of the lesions identified by screening should be known;
— there should be an effective treatment for such lesions; and
— the screening test should be acceptable and safe.

The other issues range from ethics to economics. Critical issues include the population to be included in screening programmes and whether or not it is possible to introduce an organised screening programme. It cannot necessarily be assumed that a screening programme will benefit the population to which it is applied. Not only do ethics demand that only programmes with proven effectiveness be widely disseminated, it is also necessary to ensure that the programme is continually monitored to confirm that effectiveness is maintained. Further, the benefits derived from the programme must be clearly shown to exceed the costs, both in terms of ill health induced by the test and accompanying procedures, and in economic terms. This requires that all programmes are evaluated to ensure that they do meet their objectives.

In spite of these caveats, screening carries the potential for a fairly rapid and important impact on mortality from the disease, often exceeding what can currently be anticipated from other approaches to disease control. Hence the continuing interest in and expectation from existing, and potential programmes.

References

Anderson GH (1985) Cervical cytology. In: Miller AB (ed) Screening for Cancer. Orlando, Academic Press Inc, pp 87–103

Baines CJ, McFarlane DV, Miller AB (1988) Sensitivity and specificity for first screen mammography in 15 NBSS centres. J Can Assoc Rad 39:273–276

Baines CJ, Miller AB, Bassett AA (1989) Physical Examination; evaluation of its role as a single screening modality in the Canadian National Breast Screening Study. Cancer 63:160–166

Bassett AA (1985) Physical examination of the breast and breast self-examination. In: Miller AB (ed) Screening for Cancer. Academic Press Inc, Orlando, pp 271–291

Beahrs OH, Shapiro S, Smart C (1979) Report of the working group to review the National Cancer Institute, American Cancer Society Breast Cancer Detection Demonstration Projects. J Natl Cancer Inst 62:640–709

Boyd NF, Wolfson C, Moskowitz M, Carlile T, Petitclerc M, Ferri HA, Fishell E, Gregoire A, Kiernan M, Longley JD, Simor IS, Miller AB (1982) Observer variation in the interpretation of Xeromammograms. J. Natl Cancer Inst 68:357–363

Boyes DA, Morrison B, Knox EG, Draper GJ, Miller AB (1982) A cohort study of cervical cancer in British Columbia. Clin Invest Med 5:1–29

Brookmeyer R, Day NE , Moss S (1986) Case-control studies for estimation of the natural history of preclinical disease from screening data. Stat Med 5:127–138

Chamberlain J, Miller AB (eds) (1988) Screening for gastrointestinal cancer. Hans Huber, Toronto

Chodak GW, Schoenberg HW (1989) Progress and problems in screening for carcinoma of the prostate. World J Surg 13:60–64

Commission on Chronic Illness (1957) Chronic Illness in the United States: Prevention of Chronic Illness. Harvard University Press, Cambridge

Cuckle HS, Wald NJ (1984) Principles of screening. In. Wald, NY (ed) Antenatal and neonatal screening. Oxford University Press, Oxford

Day NE (1985) Estimating the sensitivity of a screening test. J Epid Comm Hlth 39:364–366

Day NE, Williams DRR, Khaw KT (1989) Breast cancer screening programmes: the development of a monitoring and evaluation system. Br J Cancer 59:954–958

Eddy DM, Hasselblad V, McGivney W, Hendee W (1988) The value of mammography screening in women under age 50 years. JAMA 259:1512–1519

European Society for Mastology (1993) Report of the European Society for Mastology Breast Cancer Screening Evaluation Committee. Consensus conference on breast cancer screening. European Society for Mastology

Gastrin G, Miller AB, To T, Aronson KJ, Wall C, Hakama M, Louhivuori K, Pukkala E (1994) Incidence and mortality from breast cancer in the Mama program for breast screening in Finland, 1973–1986. Cancer 73:2168–2174

Goin JE, Haberman JD (1982) Comments on the logistic function in ROC analysis: Applications to breast cancer detection. Meth Inform Med 21:26–30

Hakama M (1982) Trends in the incidence of cervical cancer in the Nordic countries. In: Magnus K (ed) Trends in cancer incidence. Hemisphere Publ, Washington, pp 279–292

Hakama M (1984) Selective screening by risk groups. In: Prorok PC, Miller AB (eds) Screening for cancer. UICC Technical Report Series, vol 78. International Union Against Cancer, Geneva, pp 71–79

Hakama M, Chamberlain J, Day NE, Miller AB, Prorok PC (1985) Evaluation of screening programmes for gynaecological cancer. Br J Cancer 52:669–673

Harvey BJ, Miller AB, Baines CJ, Corey PN (1997) Effect of breast self-examination techniques on the risk of death from breast cancer. Can Med Assoc J 157:1205–1212

Henschke CI, McCaulay DI, Yankelevitz DF, Naidich DP, McGuinness G, Miettinen OS, Libby DM, Pasmantier MW, Koizumi J, Altorki NK, Smith JP (1999) Early lung cancer action project: overall design and findings from baseline screening. Lancet 354:99–105

Holowaty P, Miller AB, Rohan T, To T (1999) The natural history of dysplasia of the uterine cervix. J Natl Cancer Inst 91:252–258

Howard J (1987) Using mammography for cancer control: an unrealized potential. Cancer 37:33–48

IARC (2002) Breast cancer screening. IARC Handbooks on Cancer Prevention, vol 8. International Agency for Research on Cancer, Lyon

Jonsson E, Hakansson S, Tabar L (1988) Cost of mammography screening for breast cancer: Experiences from Sweden. In: Day NE, Miller AB (eds) Screening for breast cancer. Hans Huber, Toronto, pp 113–115

Krahn MD, Mahoney JE, Eckman MH, Trachtenberg J, Pauker SG, Detsky AS (1994) Screening for prostate cancer: a decision analytic view. JAMA 272:781–786

Mandel JS, Church TR, Ederer F, Bond, JH (1999) Colorectal cancer mortality: effectiveness of biennial screening for fecal occult blood. J Natl Cancer Inst 91:434–437

Marrett LD, Robles S, Ashbury FD, Green B, Goel V, Luciani, S (2002) A proposal for cervical screening information systems in developing countries. Int J Cancer 102:293–299

McLelland R, Pisano ED (1992) The politics of mammography. Radiol Clin North Am 30:235–241

Miller AB (ed) (1978) Screening in cancer. A report of the UICC International Workshop in Toronto. UICC Technical Report Series, vol 40. International Union Against Cancer, Geneva

Miller AB (1981) An evaluation of population screening for cervical cancer. In: Koss LG, Coleman DV (eds) Advances in clinical cytology. Butterworths, London, pp 64–94

Miller AB (1987) Early detection of breast cancer. In: Harris JR, Henderson IC, Hellman S, Kinne DW (eds) Breast diseases. Lippincott, Philadelphia, pp 122–134

Miller AB (1991) Issues in screening for prostate cancer. In: Miller AB, Chamberlain J, Day NE, Hakama M, Prorok PC (eds) Cancer screening. Cambridge University Press, Cambridge, pp 289–293

Miller AB (1994) Screening for cancer: Is it time for a paradigm shift? Annals of the Royal College of Physicians and Surgeons of Canada 27:353–355

Miller AB (1996) Fundamental issues in screening for cancer. In: Schottenfeld D, Fraumeni JF Jr. (eds) Cancer epidemiology and prevention, 2nd edn. New York, Oxford University Press, Oxford, pp 1433–1452

Miller AB (2004) Natural history of cervical cancer. In: Rohan TE, Shah K (eds) Cervical cancer, from etiology to prevention. Kluwer Academic Publishers, Dordecht, pp 61–78

Miller AB, Tsechkovski M (1987) Imaging technologies in breast cancer control: Summary report of a world health organization meeting. AJR 148:1093–1094

Miller AB, Lindsay J, Hill GB (1976) Mortality from cancer of the uterus in Canada and its relationship to screening for cancer of the cervix. Int J Cancer 17: 602–612

Miller AB, Chamberlain J, Day NE, Hakama M, Prorok PC (1990) Report on a workshop of the UICC project on evaluation of screening for cancer. Int J Cancer 46:761–769

Miller AB, Baines CJ, Turnbull C (1991a) The role of the nurse-examiner in the National Breast Screening Study. Can J Publ Hlth 82:162–167

Miller AB, Anderson G, Brisson J, Laidlaw J, Le Pitre N, Malcolmson P, Mirwaldt P, Stuart G, Sullivan W (1991b) Report of a national workshop on screening for cancer of the cervix. Can Med Ass J 145:1301–1325

Miller AB, Baines CJ, To T, Wall C (1992) Canadian national breast screening study: 2. Breast cancer detection and death rates among women age 50–59 years. Can Med Assoc J 147:1477–1488

Miller AB, Nazeer S, Fonn S, Brandup-Lukanow A, Rehman R, Cronje H, Sankaranarayanan R, Koroltchouk V, Syrjanen K, Singer A, Onsrud M (2000a) Report on consensus conference on cervical cancer screening and management. Int J Cancer 86:440-7

Miller AB, To T, Baines CJ, Wall C (2000b) Canadian National Breast Screening Study-2: 13-year results of a randomized trial in women age 50–59 years. J Natl Cancer Inst 92:1490–1499

Miller AB, Madalinska JB, Church T, Crawford D, Essink-Bot, ML, Goel V, de Koning HJ, Maatanem L, Pentikainen T (2001) Review: Health-related quality of life and cost-effectiveness studies in the European randomised study of screening for prostate cancer and the U.S. Prostate, Lung, Colon and Ovary trial. Eur J Cancer 37:2154–2160

Miller AB, To T, Baines CJ, Wall C (2002) The Canadian National Breast Screening Study-1: Breast cancer mortality after 11 to 16 years of follow-up. A randomized screening trial of mammography in women age 40 to 49 years. Ann Intern Med 137:305–312

Morrison AS (1985) Screening in chronic disease. Oxford University Press, Oxford, pp 48–63

Morrison AS, Brisson J, Khalid N (1988) Breast cancer incidence and mortality in the breast cancer detection demonstration project. J Natl Cancer Inst 80:1540–1547

Moskowitz M, Pemmaraju S, Fidler JA, Sutorius DJ, Russell P, Scheinok P, Holle J (1976) On the diagnosis of minimal breast cancer in a screenee population. Cancer 37:2543–2552

Moss SM (1991) Case-control studies of screening. Int J Epidemiol 20:1–6

Moss S, Draper GJ, Hardcastle JD, Chamberlain J (1987) Calculation of sample size in trials of screening for early diagnosis of disease. Int J Epidemiol 16:104–110

Nieminen P, Kallio M, Anttila A, Hakama M (1999) Organised vs. spontaneous Pap-smear screening for cervical cancer: a case-control study. Int J Cancer 83:55–58

Prorok PC, Chamberlain J, Day NE, Hakama M, Miller AB (1984) UICC workshop on the evaluation of screening programmes for cancer. Int J Cancer 34:1–4

Sasco AJ, Day NE, Walter SD (1986) Case-control studies for the evaluation of screening. J Chron Dis 39:399–405

Schechter MT, Miller AB, Baines CJ, Howe GR (1986) Selection of women at high risk of breast cancer for initial screening. J Chron Dis 39:253–260

Semiglazov VF, Sagaidak VN, Moiseyenko VM, Mikhailov EA (1993) Study of the role of breast self-examination in the reduction of mortality from breast cancer. Eur J Cancer 29A:2039–2046

Swets JA (1979) ROC analysis applied to the evaluation of medical imaging technologies. Invest Radiol 14:109–121

Tabar L, Fagerberg CJG, Gad A, Baldetorp L, Holmberg LH, Gröntoft O, Ljungquist U, Lundström B, Månson JC, Eklund G, Day NE (1985) Reduction in mortality from breast cancer after mass screening with mammography: Randomized trial from the breast cancer screening working group of the Swedish National Board of Health and Welfare. Lancet i:829–832

Tabar L, Fagerberg G, Duffy SW, Day NE (1989) The Swedish two county trial of mammographic screening for breast cancer: recent results and calculation of benefit. J Epid Comm Hlth 43:107–114

Task Force (1976) Cervical cancer screening programs. The Walton Report. Can Med Ass J 114:1003–1033

Task Force (1982) Cervical cancer screening programs: Summary of the 1982 Canadian task force report. Can Med Ass J 127:581–589

UK Trial of Early Detection of Breast Cancer Group (1988) First results on mortality reduction in the UK Trial of Early Detection of Breast Cancer. Lancet ii: 411–416

Walter SD, Day NE (1983) Estimation of the duration of a pre-clinical disease state using screening data. Am J Epidemiol 118:865–886

Walter SD, Stitt LW (1987) Evaluating the survival of cancer cases detected by screening. Stat Med 6:885–900

Weiss CH (1998) Evaluation. Prentice Hall, Englewood Cliffs NJ

Weiss NS (1983) Control definition in case-control studies of the efficacy of screening and diagnostic testing. Am J Epidemiol 116:457–460

Wilson JMG, Junger G (1968) Principles and practice of screening for disease. World health Organization, Geneva

Workshop Group (1989) Reducing deaths from breast cancer in Canada. Can Med Ass J 141:199–201

Community-based Health Promotion

John W. Farquhar, Stephen P. Fortmann

Introduction

This chapter describes theories and methods underlying successful *comprehensive community-based health promotion*, and provides four examples. These studies represent well the field of *experimental* epidemiology, involving defined populations and often done following insights derived from *observational* epidemiology. Three of these were designed to reduce risk factors for cardiovascular disease (CVD), and relied heavily on locally available channels of mass communication in addition to community organizing and other education methods, relatively low-cost approaches with the potential to reach and change lifestyle behaviors of entire populations, in contrast to traditional individual or group counseling. One example, studying alcohol-involved trauma, used only community organizing to promote adherence to existing laws, rather than public education for behavior change. By community organizing we mean the process of enlisting community leaders in support of project goals, and also in insuring their continued support. The Stanford Prevention Research Center (SPRC), beginning in 1972, pioneered development of the intervention methods of comprehensive community-based CVD prevention and other methods of health promotion and chronic disease prevention. SPRC was connected to all four examples, either as initiator (for two studies) or collaborator (for two studies). This review also describes the theoretical background, methods of intervention, the past history of such studies, the cultural basis for barriers to change and lessons learned for the future.

A community-based program is defined as one organized locally, and promoted through the community's institutions and communication channels. The traditional definition of a "community" is used in this review (a residential area with legally defined geographic boundaries, where a *local* governmental system regulates many aspects of schools, businesses, transportation, law enforcement, and recreational activities). A community is ordinarily last in a nation's regulatory chain, where education must ultimately occur, although for rural areas (in the United States) the county becomes the governing agent for education.

This chapter will address the following issues:

(1) The advantages are presented for community-wide interventions rather than for more limited locales, such as clinics, hospitals, work sites, or schools.
(2) The theories underlying successful community-based projects are described, including:
   a. community organizing theory, and its relationship to community self-development and diffusion of innovation theories, and
   b. the health communication-behavior change theory, and its relationship to social cognitive theory, social marketing, and to other determinants of successful use of mass media for health promotion.
(3) The methods needed for success are presented, including:
   a. message design through formative research;
   b. process analysis for comprehension of causes for change; and
   c. the role of community activism, advocacy, laws and regulations.

(4) The history of three recent decades of comprehensive community-based health promotion for cardiovascular disease prevention is described.
(5) The cultural basis for barriers to success is outlined.
(6) Lastly, a *Master Plan* for achieving success in this type of health promotion is presented.

Advantages of a Total Community Approach 11.2

Health promotion in schools, work sites, and clinics has a long history of individual success, but synergistic interactive effects can occur when they are imbedded in a *total community* campaign that adds inherently cost-effective mass media and environmental change (Schooler et al. 1997). Evidence for synergism was given by Rogers (1983), who found that diffusion of innovations within a community accelerates when adoption of the innovation reaches about 20% of the population – thus only comprehensive total community education programs have the capacity to achieve such effects. Lifestyles, such as tobacco use, dietary habits and exercise patterns, so strongly influenced by custom and by the media in developed countries, cannot be countered through simple means. Community-wide approaches fit the public health model because the usual medical model can neither prevent most chronic disease nor reach the entire population in need. By the "medical model" we mean the aspects of a nation's health care system, focused on the individual, that rely primarily on clinic outpatient and hospital services provided by physicians. The community provides influence through *locally produced* electronic and print mass media and through work sites, recreation sites, libraries, schools, medical, hospital and pharmacy settings, and social gatherings of many sorts. It offers opportunities for health-promoting regulations, such as providing opportunities for physical activity for all, school fitness classes, healthful school lunches, alcohol sales limits, and preventing tobacco product marketing to children.

Studies at the SPRC have shown that only *multiple and persistent* influences produce meaningful changes in the dietary, exercise, or tobacco-use behavior of adults, adolescents, and children. For adolescents, always resistant to health behavior change, the following influenced success: parents and teachers whose personal habits allow them to be supportive role models; amount and quality of school-based education on tobacco, fitness, and nutrition; peer influence; and amount, duration and quality of community-wide health education. Also, certain personal characteristics were influential – for example, the presence before the education's onset of *self-efficacy* toward one's behavior-change abilities (Fortmann et al. 1995).

11.3   Underlying Theories

Community-based health education carried out by SPRC and by some analogous projects have been guided by two major theories (community organizing and health communication-behavior change), with success dependent upon a judicious blending of the two (Flora et al. 1989; Farquhar et al. 1991).

11.3.1   Community Organizing Theory

Community organizing theory describes methods of identifying the health problem (and resources needed or available), mobilizing the community's opinion leaders and organizations, gaining populace support, forming coalitions, launching and maintaining education programs, achieving regulatory changes, and *empowering communities* to reach and maintain their goals. Community organizing for health requires continued attention similar to the accepted role of political leaders – to assess periodically the needs of both governmental and nongovernmental organizations, and, in the case of health promotion, to aid in planning and coordinating health promotion campaigns. Community organizing as defined here has analogies to "community self-development" as described by Green and Kreuter (1991) and it also relies on elements of diffusion theory (Rogers 1983) – which has shown how innovations are adopted through natural social networks, aided by a community's opinion leaders. Rogers' account of "failure of water-boiling in a Peruvian village" provided an excellent example of the need to identify and work with a community's opinion leaders as a prerequisite for the success of a health innovation initiated solely by self-appointed "experts" who are not seen as trustworthy by the community's residents.

11.3.2   The Health Communication-Behavior Change Theory

The health communication-behavior change theory provides the basis for designing, sequencing and distributing messages for the total population and its subgroups based on their health needs, cultural attributes, social networks, media habits, attitudes, motivation, knowledge and self-management skills. It describes theories underlying educational *content*, such as social cognitive theory (Bandura 1986), which is primarily based on an individual's capacity for self-directed change. Bandura's research confirms that "learning by doing" is more effective than "learning from observing" (modeling a behavior), and both are more effective than an "information-only" approach that changes knowledge alone. These principles are contained in his *social cognitive theory*, which posits that guided practice in a new behavior can lead to increased self-efficacy and to greater behavior change (Bandura 1986). Thus, "knowledge-only" campaigns have been found less effective than those that apply Bandura's recommendations.

The health communication-behavior change theory also incorporates methods of reaching the total population using principles described as "social marketing"

(Kotler 1975; Lefebvre and Flora 1988). These marketing principles described first by Kotler as "product, price and promotion" lead to insuring the relevance of the "product" (health messages), and to the low material and psychological cost of attending to the health message. Additionally, successful social marketing occurs only when the health messages are promoted and distributed efficiently to a large proportion of the populace.

Another behavior change method included within the communication-behavior change theory is the method of teaching counter-arguing skills, as described by Roberts and Maccoby (1973). This method, also called "inoculation", can be presented either through the media or face-to-face, and teaches the learner how to best argue against a deleterious message, such as an advertisement promoting cigarette use. This "inoculation" method was found to be very effective in prevention of adolescent substance abuse when used in a manner that can be incorporated into comprehensive community-based health promotion (Robinson et al. 1987).

Lastly, Carwright's (1949) pioneering work on mass persuasion principles is also quite germaine to the health communication-behavior change theory. He described the need to change not only a person's knowledge and motivation, but that changes in "action structure" were also needed. These principles, when combined with Bandura's methods for self-management skills training and with certain elements of Rogers' diffusion theory, leads to a logical sequence of steps recommended for both the delivery and behavioral objectives, as derived from the health communication-behavior change theory (Table 11.1).

Table 11.1. The health communication-behavior change components (adapted from Farquhar et al. 1991)

Communication inputs	Communication functions (for the sender)	Behavior objectives (for the receiver)
Face-to-face messages	Determine receiver's needs	Become aware
Mediated messages	Gain attention (set the agenda)	Increase knowledge
Community events	Provide information	Increase motivation and interest
Environmental cues	Provide incentives	Take action, assess outcomes
	Provide training	Maintain action, practice self-management skills
	Provide cues to action, including environmental change	Become an opinion leader (exert peer group influence)

Methods

11.4

Initial Steps

11.4.1

Problem Identification. The initiating agency, group or person can emanate either from within or outside of the community. The first task is to identify the problem.

Local (community) interventions should ideally coexist with and interact with national programs and must be linked to scientific support from the national or international level, which has indicated that both CVD prevention (WHO 1986) and alcohol sales control (Holder and Wallack 1986) are problems requiring *local* action. Other than the initial steps of problem identification and formation of a coalition, most of the methods to be described are relevant only to the three CVD prevention examples described in this chapter. However, any chronic disease that requires widespread education designed to change "lifestyle" behaviors (such as exercise, diet and cigarette use) will require analogous methods.

Coalition Formation.   Key political and opinion leaders as well as relevant organizations must form a coalition. This coalition must create a resource inventory, obtain populace support, and plan the intervention. Relevant organizations are listed below under Sect. 11.4.3 and include the following: the County Medical Society, municipal hospital community affairs departments, city parks and recreation departments and voluntary health agencies (i.e. the local branches of national heart, lung, cancer and diabetes organizations, as well as the Red Cross). Any organization that will act as a conduit (or "channel") for the distribution of mediated instruction or classes must also be represented (i.e. television and radio stations, local newspapers, schools, churches, libraries, pharmacies, clinics and physicians and dentists offices). As the coalition grows in size, a "steering committee" made up of about 6 members needs to be formed to carry out more detailed planning, including formation of expert groups in education and evaluation and "task forces" assigned to particular topics (Flora et al. 1989; Farquhar et al. 1991).

11.4.2   Planning

Formative Evaluation.   As the term "formative" indicates, these activities form (create) the education effort and can be divided into categories of audience needs analysis, message design, pre-testing of education programs and evaluation of education programs. The needs analysis, message design and pre-testing phases are part of the social marketing aspect of health communication-behavior change theory. Also, the evaluation of education programs, although properly labeled as "formative" is also often termed "process" evaluation since it determines the contributions to success of different components of each education program (Farquhar et al. 1991). Process analysis is also done at the completion of the total program as part of "summative evaluation", although the distinction between formative and summative is sometimes quite arbitrary, depending on the intent of the evaluator (Farquhar et al. 1991).

11.4.3   Implementation

Need for a Comprehensive Approach.   Interventions must go beyond attempting to change knowledge, the usual goal of an educational system, by providing training in behavior-change *skills*. They must also go well beyond the individual, enlisting multiple community organizations in campaigns for change and seeking changes in the social environment and in regulations that promote access to the facilities and resources needed for healthful practices. Multiple communication channels (such as radio, television, newspapers, mass-distributed print products, schools and the internet) are needed to reach different subgroups, recognizing differing media usages, knowledge, and desire for change. A comprehensive intervention should involve schools, work sites, senior citizens' centers, voluntary health agencies (such as the local branches of any national organization that deals with cardiovascular disease, diabetes and cancer), churches, and facilities for sport, recreation, and health. These organizations and others can serve as education conduits, with the community's electronic and print mass media organizations assisting in message design, content and delivery. The Internet provides a new channel, whose community education role is now becoming better defined (Baker et al. 2003). Interactive computer learning, now becoming common in classrooms, can be designed for large groups – an emerging variant of mass media.

Comprehensiveness requires variety. For example, in tobacco control programs of SPRC's community campaigns, local medical clinics, dental offices, pharmacies, and libraries distributed a low-cost skills-training Quit Kit; a local smoking cessation class was shown on television; many newspaper articles and columns appeared; a local business supported costs of a smoking cessation contest; and all newspapers and electronic media "cross-advertised" activities designed for mass audiences (Altman et al. 1987). Formative evaluation must be continued throughout the entire implementation period of any planned intervention campaign. Success requires a well designed mix and sequence of programs delivered through varied channels. This integration, with goals set in advance and goal changes based on early results, is analogous to a commercial marketing campaign, hence the term "social marketing". The distinction from commercial marketing is that social marketing uses marketing methods for social betterment without a commercial or profit-making intent. As described above, social marketing is the explanatory term for the needs analysis, message design and pre-testing phases of formative evaluation. These phases require message tailoring to fit any subgroup's needs and preferences, respecting cultural differences, learning styles, and preferred learning sites. A message sequence should increase awareness, then, increase knowledge, and last, increase motivation and provide training in the skills needed for adoption and maintenance of a new behavior (Bandura 1986). Electronic media can carry out the first two parts of this sequence and stimulate use of the more information-dense print media of newspapers and booklets, which are inherently more effective in *skills training* than are electronic media (Flora et al. 1997).

Message Characteristics.   Messages must be clear, focused, and salient. Salience requires broad reaching media, arousing interest and awareness – topics must break through passive indifference engendered by the information overload of many societies and become "on the public agenda". Given the large advertising budgets of today's mass media, health agencies' messages must be of sufficient production quality to compete for the public's attention. The competition for the public's attention is great indeed since the average adult in the United States is exposed annually to 35,000 television advertisements, equaling 292 hours of exposure (Fortmann et al. 1995). Formative evaluation must continue during a campaign and alter message content in accordance to the state of readiness of the population. Thus, early in a campaign, messages should increase knowledge and awareness, followed by those that increase motivation and provide skills training – with resultant behavior change (Schooler et al. 1997).

11.4.4   The Amount of Intervention Needed

The amount of intervention (the "dose" of intervention) needed depends on many factors: lesser amounts are needed in smaller communities, at earlier stages in a country's adoption of a "health innovation", and when the advocated behavior change is reasonably simple (such as mammography, hypertension screening and immunization campaigns). Clearly, more complex changes are needed in individuals and in society's norms to alter eating or exercise patterns or to control tobacco use. Complexity in respect to nutrition arises from many sources, including long-standing cultural beliefs and practices; entrenched methods in agriculture, food production, and retailing; advertising of "unhealthful" foods; and the advent of widespread fast-food chains that are dominated by commercial interests unresponsive to local demands and needs. Few projects have measured intervention dose, except in very general terms that do not allow accurate estimates of the amount of exposure. One excellent method records the total number and duration of messages distributed over a defined time period, albeit with a defect due to lack of message quality measures (Farquhar et al. 1990). This method's use increased evaluation costs (which comprised almost two-thirds of total expenses) in the Stanford Five-City Project (FCP – see below). This expense may explain why others have not used it nearly to the same degree of completeness. However, it is clear that public health education would be served if more campaigns were analyzed this thoroughly. The following describes this method's use in the Stanford Five-City Project (see Sect. 11.5.3). The number of adults aged 18–74 were known in the communities receiving the education programs, and they were used for the analysis. The number and duration of messages from TV/radio, newspaper, other print messages and face-to-face messages (largely classes) were enumerated each year for five years. The number of messages from newspaper, other print and face-to-face encounters were obtained from the education group's records. The TV broadcast hours were obtained from the Neilsen (A.C. Neilsen Co, Chicago IL) monitoring system, which records the proportion of households viewing a particular TV station for all hours for each major community area in the United States. Radio hours were obtained from the local radio station survey data. Calculations are then made for the number of messages for each education channel and their duration for the average adult in the community (Flora et al. 1989; Farquhar et al. 1990).

Evaluation

Comprehensive community-based campaigns aiming for widespread behavior change in the community's population need the following types of evaluation: (1) Formative evaluation to plan and test messages (as described in Sect. 11.4.2); (2) Summative evaluation to determine the effects of the campaign at different levels (the individual, in organizations, and in community's social or physical environment); and (3) Process evaluation to study the effects of each individual educational activity. Formative evaluation determines the likelihood that a message, class or group activity will reach the intended audience. Process evaluation examines the success or failure of a program component, and also allows insight into why it succeeded (or failed). As mentioned in Sect. 11.4.2, process analysis may be classified under either "formative" or "summative", depending on timing and purpose. (Flora et al. 1989; Farquhar et al. 1991). Summative evaluation methods are generally more rigorous than formative evaluation methods, and, in the case of chronic disease prevention interventions, often will entail measures of physiological states (such as blood pressure), as well as attitudes, knowledge or behavior (such as cigarette use) (Farquhar et al. 1977, 1990). The unit of analysis is commonly the individual, although both the Stanford Three Community Study (Williams et al. 1981) and the Five-City Project (Farquhar et al. 1990) also analyzed risk factor change by the more conservative method, with the community as the unit of analysis.

Additional Methods Needed

Successful community-based health promotion requires effective leaders, community activists with the courage and charisma to advocate health innovations. Advocacy campaigns derived from international, national, state, or provincial sources can provide a local activist leader with the popular support to fight entrenched bureaucrats who defend the status quo. Tobacco control in Australia and the United States provide examples. National and state advocacy groups with access to mass media created a strong mass movement for change, allowing advocates to enlist popular support for local tobacco control measures. In both California and Australia's State of Victoria this popular support led to statewide increases in tobacco taxes, with some retained for education against tobacco, a measure that had been resisted by state legislators who had long been influenced by tobacco lobbyists – an example of community activism moving up the "ladder" of bureaucracy to a higher political level (Victorian Health Promotion Foundation 1994; Pierce et al. 1994; Catalonia Declaration 1996).

Changes in policies, laws and regulations (PLR) are needed for success, especially for long-term success. Local PLR can affect alcohol and tobacco sales, and create environments that improve nutrition and enhance physical activity. However, national, state, or provincial actions can magnify local PLR and education efforts on topics such as tobacco taxation, automobile seat-belt laws, food and drug safety, school nutrition, school physical activity policies, and (in the United

States) laws on firearms. As described above, widespread popular attitude changes in numerous communities can also affect the political process at the state, province or federal level.

11.5   History of Comprehensive Community Health Promotion

The history of the past three decades described in this chapter is restricted largely to 13 formal research projects designed to affect cardiovascular disease (CVD) risk factors. They involved entire populations of at least one *education* community, compared to at least one *control* community. Three of the four examples to follow are drawn from these 13 projects. Dissemination worldwide into practical applications of community organizing and mass communication technologies, derived in part from these research projects, occurred throughout these three decades.

11.5.1   The First Two Examples: the First Decade

The first and second example, the Stanford Three-Community Study (TCS), in three small agricultural marketing towns in California (total population 45,000), and the North Karelia Study (NKS), in two adjoining predominately rural Finnish counties (North Karelia population about 180,000), each began in 1972.

TCS, the first Stanford project, was carried out from 1972–1975 in both English and Spanish, comparing effects of mass media alone in one community and mass media plus 10-session risk reduction classes for some high-risk adults in a second, with a third as a control (Farquhar et al. 1977; Schooler et al. 1997). Groups exposed to varied education amounts showed a dose-response change in smoking, blood pressure, and blood cholesterol, with a proportionately larger effect in the Spanish-speaking residents than in the Anglo majority. This minority population outcome required intervention resources in Spanish to be proportionately larger than those provided in English to the Anglo majority. A composite CVD risk reduction of about 23% and 30% occurred in the mass media/only and mass media/plus classroom conditions, respectively. The risk score (a probability) was derived from each adult's "before-after" risk levels (age, gender, systolic blood pressure, blood total cholesterol level, cigarette use and relative weight). These risk parameters were entered into a multiple logistic regression model to predict the 12-year future probability of a coronary heart disease event (myocardial infarction, sudden death or angina pectoris). The scoring system was based on coronary events experienced by adults in the long-term prospective Framingham Heart Study (Truett et al. 1967). Thus, a relatively modest amount of mass media (about 30 television and radio "spots", weekly newspaper columns on heart health, and four separate mass mailings of booklets) was sufficient to change the population's body weight, cholesterol and blood pressure levels, and smoking prevalence.

The education followed the principles outlined in Sect. 11.3 for the community organizing and health communication-behavior change theories. As an example of community organizing, close cooperative relationships were created with two influential opinion leaders (a local Anglo physician, and the Hispanic program director of the local Spanish language radio station). As an example of the social marketing aspect of the health communication-behavior change theory, message design for the smoking cessation print materials were different in the English and Spanish languages, as dictated by formative evaluation. Both the eight session classes held for a high-risk subset of the population and the print products mailed to households incorporated some of Bandura's self-management principles, such as building awareness, making a clear commitment (i.e. a written "contract") and adopting gradual, stepwise changes in behavior designed to increase confidence in one's ability to achieve the desired behavior change.

NKS evaluated two matched, rural Finnish counties that contained many villages with farming and lumbering as the main occupations. North Karelia (about 180,000 population) received an education campaign that began in 1972, continuing to the present. After ten years, CVD risk factor changes comparable to the TCS occurred, and significant net reductions in CVD events occurred (Puska et al. 1985; Schooler et al. 1997). This study was marked by extensive community organizing, resulting in strong partnerships with residents and their organizations. The NKS influence on its country's policies was unparalleled among the CVD projects, providing its most important lesson – that a well done project led by respected scientists can move an entire country. As examples, Finland's food and agricultural industries made large changes: Fertilizers were supplemented with selenium (a substance low in Finland's soil that is needed for health), milk pricing was changed (based on protein instead of fat content), programs were created to replace dairy farms with berry farms, a new canola industry replaced jobs lost in dairying, and increased production of low-saturated fat foods occurred (Puska et al. 1985; Puska 1995; Catalonia Declaration 1996).

In 1972 population-wide nutrition change and smoking cessation interventions were an innovation internationally, which may partly explain the success of these two pioneering programs (TCS and NKS).

Early International Diffusion, 1977–1983   11.5.2

Studies similar to the TCS were done in Italy (The Martignacco Project, 1977–1983, one treatment, mass media and screening, one control – CHD risk fell in men only); Australia (The North Coast Project, 1978–1980, similar to TCS, one mass media, one mass media plus classes – effects on smoking, greater in the mass media "plus" community); Switzerland (two treatment, two control pairs, German and French speaking, mass media, classes, environment changes – effects on smoking, blood pressure and obesity); and South Africa (similar to TCS, one mass media, one mass media plus classes plus community events – decreased CHD risk, blood pressure, smoking; both treatments were equivalent). All four studies, reviewed in Schooler et al. (1997), reported significant risk factor changes, adding evidence for the effectiveness of the TCS model, namely that a predominately community-wide mass media campaign is effective, but that supplemental face-to-face instruction usually adds some extra effects (Farquhar et al. 1991). It is noteworthy that all of these studies were done in rather small communities (population sizes of about 12,000 to 15,000 residents), thus these effects may be more difficult to achieve in larger and more complex communities.

The Second and Third Decades:
11.5.3   Projects Begun in the 1980s and 1990s

The third example is the Stanford Five-City Project (FCP) (USA). Its intervention phase from 1980–1986 extended TCS methods to larger populations (total population of about 360,000) with multifactor CVD prevention directed at two northern California cities. There were three control cities (Farquhar et al. 1990). It differed from TCS in the larger size of the communities, in greater use of community organizing and in greater collaboration with the communities' health, media, and education organizations in planning and implementing programs. It was similar in generous use of mass media, both print and electronic. The *number* of messages received by the average adult over 5 years of education was as follows: television and radio 67%, newspaper 28%, other print (such as booklets and "tip" sheets) 4% and face-to-face 1%. Duration of exposure over 5 years was as follows: television and radio 35%, newspaper 18%, other print 41% and face-to-face 5%. It was unique in measuring total dose of education (about 5 hours/year and about 100 episodes of exposure/year to all forms of media and classroom education) (Flora et al. 1989; Farquhar et al. 1990). This means that an "average adult" who has followed the whole program on mass media and in classrooms would have experienced 100 single episodes (including TV, radio, newspaper or other print, workshop training, or community sponsored exercise sessions) which add up to 5 hours duration in total in each year.

FCP's initial year of television messages (defined as "high reach/low involvement") stimulated the public's use of print media, which supplied more effective training than from television in the skills needed for smoking cessation, healthful food purchasing or preparation, learning appropriate exercise habits or ways to lose or control body weight (Flora et al. 1997). However, television can be quite effective in skills training. For example, the FCP presented an 8 week "live" TV broadcast of a local smoking cessation class, which contained considerable modeling of the smoking cessation skills being learned by the class attendees (such as behavioral problem solving, self monitoring, tapering, goal setting, deep muscle relaxation and group social support) (Altman et al. 1987). Results were comparable to the TCS (about a 15% fall in Framingham composite risk of CVD) (Truett et al. 1967), with a major impact on blood pressure (4–5%) and smoking (13%) (Farquhar et al. 1990). Health bureaucracies, usually timid, should gain courage from the FCP's "David and Goliath" demonstration that only 3 hours/year of high quality television health education can counteract the public's exposure to about

100 hours/year of television advertising devoted to unhealthy nutrition. The exposure of the US population is estimated as 292 hours of TV advertisement based on the Neilsen monitoring system (cf. Sect. 11.4.4). Michael Jacobson of the Center for Science in the Public Interest estimated that about one third of these are for "unhealthy" nutrition (personal communication). Almost all TV nutrition advertising is "unhealthy" since the food industry is so inclined. For example, after the nutritionists and preventive medicine scientists succeeded, through education, in decreasing egg and butter intake, the counterattack began to bring the US population back to their previous unhealthy consumption. Although all preceding CVD studies showed effects in small towns and/or rural districts, FCP showed benefit in *cities* (with populations as high as 100,000). Also, these effects occurred despite the advent (at least in the state of California) in the 1980s of dual working families and increasing public use of fast food, factors that made achieving nutrition-behavior change more difficult.

FCP's modest resources and greater effects, as compared to similar projects, support the benefits of the mass media presentation components of the health communication-behavior change theory, including its adaptation of the skills training aspects of Bandura's social cognitive theory. Perhaps the most practical lesson to policymakers is that adult residents saved 30 times more money from their decreased cigarette purchases ($120/adult/year) than the cost of the campaign ($4/adult/year) – savings retained by the individuals of the community, not counting savings in long-term health costs and short-term decrease in absenteeism from the individual's employment. Lastly, the communities expanded the health promotion activities of the county's Department of Health and adopted FCP's technologies, later applying them to seat-belt promotion and violence and adolescent pregnancy prevention.

Other successful CVD projects, both large and small, occurred in these decades in the United States, Sweden, Denmark, Canada, Germany, the Czech Republic, and China. Also, World Health Organization-sponsored projects began in about 23 other countries (Schooler et al. 1997) and have expanded beyond that since 1997. In all instances, they borrowed heavily from the experiences of the three exemplars and in many instances received training from either the Stanford or the North Karelia groups. In some of these projects, changes seen were less than was the case in the Stanford and North Karelia projects. Although it is difficult to know the reasons for a relative lack of success (for example, the magnitude of the interventions was incompletely described), in some instances the cause appeared to be related to inadequate use of mass media.

Community Projects in Other Health Topics   11.5.4

Interventions on alcohol, mammography, tobacco control, immunization, motor vehicle injuries and HIV/AIDS are prominent examples of other community-based projects done in developed countries, but with fewer well-controlled studies than in CVD. Also, many community studies have been done in developing countries, where effective recruiting methods and effective mass media use (often using radio messages) have been reported, but a review of these is beyond the scope of this chapter. One well-controlled U.S. study, Preventing Alcohol Trauma (PAT)[1], is the fourth example. This five-year study of three U.S. communities showed a 10% decrease in alcohol-related traffic injuries and a 50% decrease in adolescent alcohol use (Holder et al. 1997). The traffic injuries were analyzed for three years prior to the study, and were compared to police and hospital records for the five year study duration. The alcohol use data were compiled from various records, prior to and during the study. These records included: (1) arrest records of adolescents under the age of 18 for drinking while driving, and, (2) sales records from retail liquor stores and bars or taverns, using under-age adolescents as attempted purchasers (to test the system). Coalition building and organizational behavior change among the police, alcohol sales outlets, and alcohol servers (such as bar tenders and restaurant personnel) were the main interventions. The public responded to a fear, instilled through publicity, of the penalties of greater enforcement of existing laws on underage alcohol purchases or drinking and driving. Therefore, in contrast to the three CVD exemplars, PAT showed that *major* public education is not needed for large public behavior changes. PAT estimated a cost saving of $2.88 for every dollar invested, a number close to that found in many work-site health promotion studies, where the "return on investment" was $3 to $6 for each dollar invested, measured in two to five years of the program (Aldana 2001). The cost savings came from decreased medical costs secondary to the reduced rate of alcohol-related automobile injuries. PAT found their communities had the required infrastructure for the campaigns, requiring only training provided by one indigenous community coordinator, a part-time clerk, an imaginative plan, and the will to proceed.

TCS, the first, and PAT, the fourth example, are opposites: TCS had a maximum of mass media education and a minimum of organizing, whereas PAT had the opposite. Thus, either model works, but to change complex behaviors, community educators must use sophisticated behavior-change methods, such as those of the health communication-behavior change theory described above. If fear of arrest for breaking existing laws on alcohol use suffices to change personal drinking-and driving-habits, then the education process is simpler.

11.6   Past Experience Leads to a "Master Plan"

A five-step approach emerges from these studies:
(a) Define the problem. Does the community need a health promotion campaign? A decision can be made from national or local survey data.
(b) Organize the community, creating a campaign that includes education, continued organizing, training of community organizations, empowerment of the public and the community's organizations, and future maintenance of programs developed during an initial phase of about two years.

---

[1] The Stanford Prevention Research Center collaborated with the investigators of this study.

(c) Implement an intervention, delivering 3–5 hours of education exposure per year for two years, using in year one, about 70% television/radio to arouse interest and provide knowledge, about 15% from more specific and instructive print media (emphasizing newspapers, if available) and 15% from community events and programs (such as health fairs, contests, and classes). In the second year, decrease TV/radio to about 40% and increase print to 30% and community events and programs to 30%.

(d) Evaluate the intervention, using the process and summative methods described above. Insure that adequate tracking of exposure to the intervention (the independent variable) is done, with calculations of both the amount and type of intervention.

(e) Institutionalize programs. The community becomes a demonstration project, with its "empowered" organizations functioning as health promotion resource centers for a wider region.

(f) Use the new community resources and its residents' potential power to advocate for local, regional, and national governmental regulations and laws that will increase local intervention effects and extend them beyond the community.

Any individual or organization that wishes to engage in community-based health education should gain courage from the words of the now deceased anthropologist, Margaret Mead, as quoted in the closing passage of the Catalonia Declaration (1996, p 75), "Never doubt the capacity of a few dedicated individuals to change the world, in fact, it is the only way it ever has."

The Cultural Basis for Barriers to Success   11.7

A *healthy city* has been defined by the absence of crime, crowding, and poverty and by the presence of educated residents and enlightened (and trained) organizations. Together these lead to a community empowered to solve its social problems (i.e., to increase its social capital) (Travers 1997).

Considering barriers, MacIntyre (2000) found Glasgow's environmental factors to be major barriers to healthful exercise behavior. Certain macroeconomic factors inherent in *globalization*, such as capital flight and increased wealth and income gaps, have been described as barriers to planned change (Cahill 1983; Bezruchka 2000). All such barriers threaten *community stability*, inhibiting greatly the success of health promotion attempts. However, wise compensatory resource allocation can overcome many barriers, as was shown in the Hispanic minority of the TCS. Therefore, the challenge for the future is: Responsibility for success in community-based health interventions lies with the interventionist, not with the community's residents! Secondly, it is clear that successful community-based health promotion requires attention to the cultural, environmental and social determinants of health that underlie the modern epidemics of chronic disease. Colditz (2001) reminds us of Rudolph LK Virchow's words, to paraphrase, that: "The history of epidemics is therefore the history of disturbances of human culture." Certainly the increasing worldwide prevalence of obesity, the spread of tobacco use and the urban barriers to physical activity fit Virchow's definition of "disturbances of human culture". As Colditz points out, many scientific endeavors put false hope in the search for new risk factors, rather than in applying the now well-established means and economic benefits of reducing the culturally determined risk factors for chronic disease. For example, Aldana (2001) cites evidence for cost savings of from 3 to 6 times the cost of health promotion for life-style change in large worksites. Despite this and other extensive evidence for the benefits of primary prevention (The Victoria Declaration 1992; The Catalonia Declaration 1996), many countries, including the U.S., spend less than 5% of total health care expenditures on prevention activities of all kinds (including immunizations, mammography and health promotion) (Medical News and Perspective 1994; World Health Report 1997). Although the reasons for the *unreasonable* diversion of a nation's resources from disease prevention to disease treatment are many, it certainly includes pressure exerted by the pharmaceutical and medical device industries. Also, the tobacco industry is still a prosperous growth industry worldwide, especially in middle and low income countries (The Osaka Declaration 2001). Therefore, from a political economy perspective, success in chronic disease prevention requires vigorous governmental policy changes (i.e., on taxation, advertising, promotion of tobacco use to minors, etc.), not only more economic resources (The Osaka Declaration 2001).

11.8   Conclusions

Three decades of the "total community" health promotion approach in developed countries strongly support the feasibility, at relatively low cost, of achieving transfer of public education technologies to a community's infrastructure (public health, media, schools, etc.), resulting in significant changes in health habits of populations. Although most studies derive from small communities, recent successes in Tianjin (China), a city of 400,000 (two exemplars examined populations of > 100,000), suggest that the model also works in large populations (Schooler et al. 1997). Organizing and educating communities requires *advocacy, activism, coalition building*, and *leadership*; success is enhanced by *regulatory change*. Theory matters: When the population gains self-efficacy through education, the result – *community efficacy* – enhances capacity to change institutional policy and practice, thus maintaining community change.

Science cannot serve society if its evidence for educational benefit is ignored. This is not a new concept. As written over 2000 years ago in the Chinese *Book of Lessons*, "If a virtuous and learned scholar aims to influence the people as a whole, one must first educate the people".

References

Aldana S (2001) Financial impact of health promotion programs: a comprehensive review of the literature. Am J Health Promotion 15:296–320

Altman DG, Flora JA, Fortmann SP, Farquhar JW (1987) The cost-effectiveness of three smoking cessation programs. Am J Public Health 77:162–165

Bandura A (1986) Social foundations of thought and action: A social cognitive theory. Prentice-Hall, Englewood Cliffs, NJ

Baker L, Wagner TH, Singer S, Bundorf MK (2003) Use of the internet and e-mail for health care information: Results from a national survey. JAMA 289:2400–2406

Bezruchka S (2000) Is globalization dangerous to our health? Western J of Medicine 172:332–334

Cahill J (1983) Structural characteristics of the macroeconomy and mental health: Implications for primary prevention research. Am J Community Psychology 11:553–571

Cartwright D (1949) Some principles of mass persuasion. Hum Relations 2:253–267

The Catalonia Declaration: Investing in Heart Health (1996) Declaration of the Advisory Board, Second International Heart Health Conference 1995. Department of Health and Social Security of the Autonomous Government of Catalonia, Barcelona, Spain

The Chinese Classics: The Great Learning, one of four books written 2000 years ago

Colditz GA (2001) Cancer culture: Epidemics, human behavior, and the dubious search for new risk factors. Am J Public Health 91:357–359

Farquhar JW, Maccoby N, Wood P, Alexander JK, Breitrose H, Brown BW, Haskell WL, McAlister AL, Meyer AJ, Nash JD, Stern MP (1977) Community education for cardiovascular health. Lancet 1:1192–1195

Farquhar JW, Fortmann S P, Flora JA, Taylor CB, Haskell WL, Williams PT, Maccoby N, Wood PD (1990) The Stanford Five-City Project: Effects of community-wide education on cardiovascular disease risk factors. JAMA 264:359–365

Farquhar JW, Fortmann SP, Flora JA, Maccoby N (1991) Methods of communication to influence behaviour. In: Holland WW, Detels R, Knox G (eds) Oxford textbook of public health, 2d edn, vol. 2. Oxford University Press, Oxford

Flora JA, Maccoby N, Farquhar JW (1989) Communication campaigns to prevent cardiovascular disease: The Stanford studies. In: Rice R, Atkin C (eds) Public communication campaigns. Sage, Beverly Hills, CA, pp 233–252

Flora JA, Saphir MN, Schooler C, Rimal RN (1997) Toward a framework for intervention channels: Reach, involvement and impact. Ann Epidemiol S7: S104–S112

Fortmann SP, Flora JA, Winkleby MA, Schooler C, Taylor CB, Farquhar JW (1995) Community intervention trials: Reflections on the Stanford Five-City Project. Am J Epidemiol 142(6):576–586

Green LW, Kreuter MW (1991) Health promotion planning: an educational and environmental approach, 2nd edn. Mayfield Publishing, Mountain View (CA)

Holder HD, Wallack L (1986) Contemporary perspectives for prevention of alcohol problems: An empirically-derived model. J Public Health Policy 7:324–330

Holder HD, Salz RF, Grube JW, Treno AJ, Reynolds RI, Voas RB, Gruenewald PJ (1997) Summing up: Lessons from a comprehensive community prevention trial. Addiction 92 (S2):S293–S301

Kotler P (1975) Marketing for nonprofit organizations. Prentice Hall, Englewood Cliffs, New Jersey

Lefebvre RC, Flora JA (1988) Social marketing and public health interventions. Health Educ Q 15:299–315

MacIntyre S (2000) The social patterning of exercise behaviours: The role of personal and local resources. British J of Sports Medicine 34:6

Medical News and Perspective (1994) New disease prevent effort goes by the book. JAMA 13: 993–994

Pierce JP, Evans N, Farkas NJ (1994) Tobacco use in California. An evaluation of the Tobacco Control Program 1989–1993. La Jolla (California), University of California, San Diego

Puska P, Nissinen A, Tuomilehto J, Salonen JT, Koskela K, McAlister A, Kottke TE, Maccoby N, Farquhar JW (1985) The community-based strategy to prevent coronary heart disease: Conclusions from the ten years of the North Karelia Project. Ann Review of Public Health 6:147–193

Puska P (1995) Experience with major subprogrammes and examples of innovative interventions. In: Puska P, Nissinen A, Vartianinen E (eds) The North Karelia Project. Helsinki University Printing House, Helsinki, pp 159–167

Robinson TN, Killen JD, Taylor CB, Telch MJ, Bryson SW, Saylor KE, Maron DJ, Maccoby N, Farquhar JW (1987) Perspectives on adolescent substance abuse: A defined population study. JAMA 258:2027–2076

Roberts DF, Maccoby N (1973) Information processing and persuasion: counter-arguing behavior. In: Kline F, Clarke P (eds) Sage Communication Research Annuals, vol II. Sage Publications, Beverly Hills, CA

Rogers E (1983) Diffusion of innovations. Free Press, New York

Schooler C, Farquhar JW, Fortmann SP, Flora JA (1997) Synthesis of findings and issues from community prevention trials. Ann Epidemiol S7: S54–S68

The Osaka Declaration, health, economics and political action: stemming the global tide of cardiovascular disease (2001) Declaration of the policy board. The Fourth International Heart Health Conference, Osaka

Travers KD (1997) Reducing inequities through participatory research and community empowerment. Health Education and Behavior 24:344–356

Truett J, Cornfield J and Kannel E (1967) Multivariate analysis of the risk of coronary heart disease in Framingham. J Chronic Disease 20:511–524

Victoria Declaration on Heart Health (1992) Declaration of the Advisory Board, First International Heart Health Conference. Health and Welfare Canada, Victoria (Canada)

Victorian Health Promotion Foundation (1994) Annual report, 1994. VicHealth, Victoria (Australia)

Williams PT, Fortmann SP, Farquhar JW, Varady A, Mellen S (1981) A comparison of statistical methods for evaluating risk factor changes in community-based studies: An example from the Stanford Three Community Study. J Chron Disease 34:565–571

World Health Organization (1986) Report of a WHO Expert Committee. Community prevention and control of cardiovascular disease. Technical Report Series No. 732. World Health Organization, Geneva

World Health Report (1997) Conquering suffering, enriching humanity. World Health Organization, Geneva

Part IV
Research Areas in Epidemiology

Infectious Disease Epidemiology

Susanne Straif-Bourgeois, Raoult Ratard

Introduction

The following chapter intends to give the reader an overview of the current field of applied infectious disease epidemiology. Prevention of disease by breaking the chain of transmission has traditionally been the main purpose of infectious disease epidemiology. While this goal remains the same, the picture of infectious diseases is changing. New pathogens are identified and already known disease agents are changing their behavior. The world population is aging; more people develop underlying disease conditions and are therefore more susceptible to certain infectious diseases or have long term sequelae after being infected.

Infectious diseases are not restricted to certain geographic areas anymore because of the increasing numbers of world travelers and a worldwide food distribution. The fear of a bioterrorist attack adds a new dimension in infectious disease epidemiology, and health departments enhance their surveillance systems for early detection of suspicious disease clusters and for agents used as weapons of mass destruction.

Improvements in laboratory techniques and mapping tools help to expand the knowledge of transmission of disease agents and enhanced surveillance techniques are feasible as a result of software progress and reporting of diseases via secure internet sites.

Surveillance and outbreak investigations remain the major responsibilities in public health departments. Epidemiologic methods and principles are still the basis for these tasks but surveillance techniques and outbreak investigation are changing and adapting to improvements and the expanded knowledge.

Conducting surveys is a useful way to gather information on diseases where surveillance data or other data sources are not available, especially when dealing with emerging or re-emerging pathogens. Program evaluation is an important tool to systematically evaluate the effectiveness of intervention or prevention programs for infectious diseases.

The Global Burden of Infectious Diseases

Infectious diseases are a major cause of human suffering in terms of both morbidity and mortality. In 1995, out of an estimated total of 52 million deaths, 17 million were due to infectious diseases (WHO 2000a,b). The most common cause of infectious disease deaths were pneumonia (5 million), diarrhea (3 million) followed by tuberculosis, malaria, AIDS and hepatitis B. Not surprisingly, there is a large imbalance in diseases between developing and industrialized countries (see Table 1.1).

Morbidity due to infectious diseases is very common in spite of the progress accomplished in recent decades. Even in industrialized countries, the prevalence of infection is very high for some infectious agents. Serologic surveys found that by young adulthood the prevalence of antibodies was 80% against herpes simplex virus type 1, 15–20% against type 2, 95% against human herpes virus, 33%

Table 1.1. Proportion of principal causes of deaths

	Developing countries	Industrialized countries
Infectious diseases	43%	1%
Cardiovascular diseases	24%	46%
Cancer	10%	21%
Respiratory diseases	10%	8%

Source: WHO, World Health Report 2000

against *Hepatitis A*, 2% against *Hepatitis C*, 5–8% against *Hepatitis B*, and 50% against *Chlamydia pneumoniae* (American Academy of Pediatrics 2003; Mandell et al. 2000). Annually, approximately 267,000,000 episodes of diarrhea leading to 612,000 hospitalizations and 3000 deaths occur among adults in the United States (Mounts et al. 1999). The Center for Disease Control and Prevention (CDC) estimates that each year 76 million people in the US get sick, more than 300,000 are hospitalized and 5000 die as a result of foodborne illnesses (CDC 2004). Every year influenza circulates widely, infecting from 10% to 40% of the world population.

1.1.2   The Importance of Infectious Disease Epidemiology for Prevention

It is often said that epidemiology is the basic science of preventive medicine. To prevent diseases it is important to understand the causative agents, risk factors and circumstances that lead to a specific disease. This is even more important for infectious disease prevention, since simple interventions may break the chain of transmission. Preventing cardiovascular diseases or cancer is much more difficult because it usually requires multiple long term interventions requiring lifestyle changes and behavior modification, which are difficult to achieve.

In 1900, the American Commission of Yellow Fever, headed by Walter Reed, was sent to Cuba. The commission showed that the infective agent was transmitted by the mosquito *Aedes aegypti*. This information was used by the then Surgeon General of the US Army William Gorgas, to clean up the 200 year old focus of yellow fever in Havana by using mosquito proofing or oiling of the larval habitat, dusting houses with pyrethrum powder and isolating suspects under a mosquito net. This rapidly reduced the number of cases in Havana from 310 in 1900 to 18 in 1902 (Goodwin 1996).

A complete understanding of the causative agent and transmission is always useful but not absolutely necessary. The most famous example is that of John Snow who was able to link cholera transmission to water contamination during the London cholera epidemic of 1854 by comparing the deaths from those households served by the Southwark & Vauxhall Company versus those served by another water company. John Snow further confirmed his hypothesis by the experiment of removing the Broad street pump handle (Wills 1996a).

The Changing Picture
of Infectious Disease Epidemiology

Over the past three decades, more than 40 new pathogens have been identified, some of them with global importance: *Bartonella henselae, Borrelia burgdorferi, Campylobacter, Cryptosporidium, Cyclospora, Ebola virus, Escherichia coli* 0157:H7, *Ehrlichia, Hantaan virus, Helicobacter, Hendra virus, Hepatitis C* and *E, HIV, HTLV-I & II, Human herpesvirus 6* and *8, Human metapneumovirus, Legionella,* new variant Creutzfeldt-Jakob disease agent, *Nipah virus, Parvovirus B19, Rotavirus,* severe acute respiratory syndrome (SARS) etc..

While there are specific causative agents for infectious diseases, these agents may undergo some changes over time. The last major outbreak of pneumonic plague in the world occurred in Manchuria in 1921. This scourge, which had decimated humans for centuries, is no longer a major threat. The plague bacillus cannot survive long outside its animal host (humans, rodents, fleas) because it lost the ability to complete the Krebs cycle on its own. While it can only survive in its hosts, the plague bacillus also destroys its hosts rapidly. As long as susceptible hosts were abundant, plague did prosper. When environmental conditions became less favorable (lesser opportunities to sustain the host to host cycles), less virulent strains had a selective advantage (Wills 1996b).

Changes in Etiologic Agent

The influenza virus is the best example of an agent able to undergo changes leading to renewed ability to infect populations that had been already infected and immune. The influenza virus is a single stranded RNA virus with a lipophilic envelope. Two important glycoproteins from the envelope are the hemagglutinin (HA) and neuraminidase (NA). The HA protein is able to agglutinate red blood cells (hence its name). This protein is important as it is a major antigen for eliciting neutralizing antibodies. *Antigenic drift* is a minor change in surface antigens that result from point mutations in a gene segment. Antigenic drift may result in epidemics, since incomplete protection remains from past exposures to similar viruses. *Antigenic shift* is a major change in one or both surface antigens (H and/or N) that occurs at varying intervals. Antigenic shifts are probably due to genetic recombination (an exchange of a gene segment) between influenza A viruses, usually those that affect humans and birds. An antigenic shift may result in a worldwide pandemic if the virus can be efficiently transmitted from person to person.

Changes in Populations at Risk

In the past three decades throughout the world, there has been a shift towards an increase in the population of individuals at high risk for infectious diseases.

In industrialized nations, the increase in longevity leads to higher proportion of the elderly population who are more prone to acquiring infectious diseases and developing life threatening complications. For example, a West Nile Virus (WNV) infection is usually asymptomatic or causes a mild illness (West Nile fever); rarely does it cause a severe neuro-invasive disease. In the 2002 epidemic of West Nile in Louisiana, the incidence of neuro-invasive disease increased progressively from 0.3 per 100,000 in the 0 to 14 age group to 9 per 100,000 in the 60 to 75 year old age group and jumped to 32 per 100,000 in the age group 75 and older. Mortality rates showed the same pattern, a gradual increase to 0.7 per 100,000 in the 60 to 75 age group with a sudden jump to 11 per 100,000 for the oldest age group of 75 and older.

Improvement in health care in industrialized nations has caused an increase in the number of immune-deficient individuals, be it cancer survivors, transplant patients or people on immuno-suppressive drugs for long term auto-immune diseases. Some of the conditions that may increase susceptibility to infectious diseases are: cancers, particularly patients on chemo or radiotherapy, leukemia, lymphoma, Hodgkin's disease, immune suppression (HIV infection), long term steroid use, liver disease, hemochromatosis, diabetes, alcoholism, chronic kidney disease and dialysis patients. For example persons with liver disease are 80 times more likely to develop *Vibrio vulnificus* infections than are persons without liver disease. Some of these infections may be severe, leading to death.

In developing countries a major shift in population susceptibility is associated with the high prevalence of immune deficiencies due to HIV infections and AIDS. In Botswana which has a high prevalence of HIV (sentinel surveillance revealed HIV seroprevalence rates of 36% among women presenting for routine antenatal care), tuberculosis rates increased from 202 per 100,000 in 1989 to 537 per 100,000 in 1999 (Lockman et al. 2001) while before the HIV/AIDS epidemics, rates above 100 were very rare.

Changes in lifestyles have increased opportunities for the transmission of infectious disease agents in populations previously at low risk. Intravascular drug injections have increased the transmission of agents present in blood and body fluids (e.g. HIV, hepatitis B and C). Consumption of raw fish, shell fish and ethnic food expanded the area of distribution of some parasitic diseases. Air travel allows people to be infected in a country and be half-way around the globe before becoming contagious.

By the same token, insects and other vectors have become opportunistic global travelers. *Aedes albopictus*, the Asian Tiger mosquito, was thus imported in 1985 to Houston, Texas inside Japanese tires. Subsequently, it has invaded 22 US states.

Changes in Knowledge About Transmission of Disease Agents

With the advent of nucleic acid tests, it has become possible to detect the presence of infectious disease agents in the air and environmental surfaces. For example, the use of air samplers and polymerase chain reaction analysis has shown that *Bordetella pertussis* DNA can be found in the air surrounding patients with *B. pertussis* infection, providing further evidence of airborne spread (Aintablian et al. 1998) and thus leading to re-evaluate the precautions to be taken. However the presence of nucleic acids in an environmental medium does not automatically mean that transmission will occur. Further studies are necessary to determine the significance of such findings.

Bioterrorism Adds a New Dimension

Infectious disease agents, when used in bioterrorism events, have often been re-engineered to have different physical properties and are used in quantities not usually experienced in natural events. There is little experience and knowledge about the human body's response to large doses of an infectious agent inhaled in aerosol particles that are able to be inhaled deep into lung alveolae. During the 2001 anthrax letter event, there was considerable discussion about incubation period, recommended duration of prophylaxis, and minimum infectious dose. This lack of knowledge base has led to confusion in recommendations being made.

New Approaches in Infectious Disease Epidemiology

1.2

Although the basics of infectious disease epidemiology have not changed and the discipline remains strongly anchored on some basic principles, technological developments such as improved laboratory methods and enhanced use of informatics (such as advanced mapping tools, web based reporting systems and statistical analytical software) have greatly expanded the field of infectious disease epidemiology.

Improved Laboratory Methods

1.2.1

Molecular techniques are being used more and more as a means to analyze epidemiological relationships between microorganisms. Hence the term molecular epidemiology refers to epidemiologic research studies made at the molecular level.

The main microbial techniques used, target plasmids and chromosomes. More specifically, plasmid fingerprinting and plasmid restriction endonuclease (REA) digestion, chromosomal analysis including pulse field gel electrophoresis (PFGE), restriction fragment length polymorphism (RFLP), multi-locus sequence type (MLST) and spa typing to name a few of these techniques. Polymerase chain reaction (PCR) is used to amplify the quantity of genomic material present in the specimen. Real-time PCR detection of infectious agents is now possible in a few hours. These techniques are becoming more widely used, even in public health laboratories for routine investigations.

It is beyond the scope of this text to describe these methods in more detail.

Applications of molecular epidemiology methods have completely changed the knowledge about infectious disease transmission for many microorganisms.

The main application is within outbreak investigations. Being able to characterize the nucleic acid of the microorganisms permits an understanding of how the different cases relate to each other.

Molecular epidemiology methods have clarified the controversy about the origin of tuberculosis cases: is it an endogenous (reactivation) or exogenous (re-infection) origin? Endogenous origin postulates that *Mycobacterium tuberculosis* can remain alive in the human host for a lifetime and can start multiplying and producing lesions. On the other hand exogenous origin theory postulates that reinfection plays a role in the development of tuberculosis. The immunity provided by the initial infection is not strong enough to prevent another exposure to *Mycobacterium tuberculosis* and a new infection leads to disease. In countries with low tuberculosis transmission, for example the Netherlands, most strains have unique RFLP fingerprints. Each infection is unique and there are hardly any clusters of infections resulting from a common source. Most cases are the result of reactivation. This is in contrast with areas of high endemicity where long chains of transmission can be identified with few RFLP fingerprinting patterns (Alland et al. 1994). In some areas, up to 50% of tuberculosis cases are the result of reinfection.

Numerous new immunoassays have been developed. They depend on an antigen-antibody reaction, either using a test antibody to detect an antigen in the patient's specimen or using a test antigen to detect an antibody in the patient's specimen.

An indicator system is used to show that the reaction has taken place and to quantify the amount of patient antigen or antibody. The indicator can be a radioactive molecule (radioimmunoassay [RIA]), a fluorescent molecule (fluorescent immunoassay [FIA]), a molecule with an attached enzyme that catalyzes a color reaction (enzyme-linked immunoassay [ELISA or EIA]), or a particle coated with antigen or antibody that produces an agglutination (latex particle agglutination [LA]).

The reaction can be a simple antigen/antibody reaction or a "sandwich" immunoassay where the antigen is "captured" and a second "read out" antibody attaches to the captured antigen. The antibody used may be polyclonal (i.e. a mixture of immunoglobulin molecules secreted against a specific antigen, each recognizing a different epitope) or monoclonal (i.e. immunoglobulin molecules of single-epitope specificity that are secreted by a clone of B cells). It may be directed against an antigen on an epitope (i.e. a particular site within a macromolecule to which a specific antibody binds).

1.2.2   Mapping as an Epidemiological Tool

Plotting diseases on a map is one of the very basic methods epidemiologists do routinely. As early as 1854 John Snow, suspecting water as a cause of cholera, plotted the cases of cholera in the districts of Golden Square, St. James and Berwick, in London. The cases seemed to be centered around the Broad Street pump and less dense around other pumps. The map supplemented by other observations led to the experiment of removing the handle on the Broad Street pump and subsequent confirmation of his hypothesis (Snow 1936).

Geographical information systems (GIS) have been a very useful tool in infectious disease research. GIS are software programs allowing for integration of a data bank with spatial information. The mapping component includes physical layout of the land, towns, buildings, roads, administrative boundaries, zip codes etc. Data may be linked to specific locations in the physical maps or to specific aggregates. A GIS system includes tools for spatial analysis. Climate, vegetation and other data may be obtained through remote sensing and combined with epidemiologic data to predict vector occurrence.

However, these tools should be used with caution. They can be useful to generate hypotheses and identify possible associations between risk of disease and environmental exposures. Because of potential bias, mapping should never be considered as more than an initial step in the investigation of an association. "The bright color palettes tend to silence a statistical conscience about fortuitous differences in the raw data" (Boelaert et al. 1998). For statistical methods in geographical epidemiology see Chap. II.8 of this handbook.

Computer Reporting and Software Progress 1.2.3

Web based reporting, use of computer programs and developments of sophisticated reporting and analytical software have revolutionized epidemiologic data collection and analysis. These tools have provided the ability to collect large amounts of data and handle large databases. However this has not been without risks. It remains crucial to understand the intricacies of data collected to avoid misinterpretation. For example, one should be aware that diseases and syndromes are initially coded by a person who may not be very software proficient, using shortcuts and otherwise could enter data of poor quality.

What Are the Questions to Be Answered? 1.3

Too often one sees epidemiologists and statisticians preparing questionnaires, carrying out surveys, gathering surveillance information, processing data and producing reports, tables, charts and graphs in a routine fashion. Epidemiology describes the distribution of health outcomes and determinants for a purpose. It is important to question the goals and objectives of all epidemiologic activities and tailor these activities to meet these objectives.

The description of disease patterns includes analysis of demographic, geographical, social, seasonal and other risk factors.

Age groups to be used differ depending on the disease e.g. diseases affecting young children should have numerous age groups among children; sexually transmitted diseases require detailed age groups in late adolescence and early adulthood. Younger age groups may be lumped together for diseases affecting mainly the elderly. Gender categorization, while important for sexually transmitted diseases and other diseases with a large gender gap (such as tuberculosis), may not be important for numerous other diseases.

Geographical distribution is important to describe diseases linked to environmental conditions but may not be so useful for other diseases.

1.4   Surveillance Issues

Surveillance, both active and passive, is the systematic collection of data pertaining to the occurrence of specific diseases, the analysis and interpretation of these data, and the dissemination of consolidated and processed information to contributors to the program and other interested persons (CDC 2001b).

1.4.1   Passive Surveillance

In a *passive surveillance system* the surveillance agency has devised and put a system in place. After the placement, the recipient waits for the provider of care to report.

Passive case detection has been used for mortality and morbidity data for decades. It is almost universal. Most countries have an epidemiology section in the health department that is charged with centralizing the data in a national disease surveillance system collecting mortality and morbidity data.

In theory, a passive surveillance system provides a thorough coverage through space and time and gives a thorough representation of the situation. Practically, compliance with reporting is often irregular and incomplete. In fact, the main flaws in passive case detection are incomplete reporting and inconsistencies in case definitions.

The main advantages are the low cost of such a program and the sustained collection of data over decades. The purpose is to produce routine descriptive data on communicable diseases, generate hypotheses and prompt more elaborate epidemiologic studies designed to evaluate prevention activities.

Some conditions must be met to maximize compliance with reporting:

1. Make reporting easy: Provide easy to consult lists of reportable diseases, provide pre-stamped cards for reporting, provide telephone or fax reporting facilities.
2. Do not require extensive information: Name, age, sex, residence, diagnosis. Some diseases may include data on exposure, symptoms, method of diagnosis etc.
3. Maintain confidentiality and assure reporters that confidentiality will be respected.
4. Convince reporters that reporting is essential: provide feedback; show how the data are used for better prevention.

Confidentiality of data is essential, particularly for those reporting health care providers who are subject to very strict confidentiality laws. Any suspicion of failure of maintaining secure data would rapidly ruin a passive surveillance program.

1.4.2   Active Surveillance

In an *active surveillance system,* the recipient will actually take some action to identify the cases.

   In an active surveillance program, the public health agency organizes a system by searching for cases or maintaining a periodic contact with providers. Regular contacting boosts the compliance of the providers. Providers are health agencies but also as in passive case detection, there may be day care centers, schools, long term care facilities, summer camps, resorts, and even public involvement. The agency takes the step to contact the health providers (all of them or a carefully selected sample) and requests reports from them at regular intervals. Thus no reports are missing.

   Active surveillance has several advantages:
— It allows the collection of more information. A provider sees that the recipient agency is more committed to surveillance and is therefore more willing to invest more time her/himself.
— It allows direct communication and opportunities to clarify definitions or any other problems that may have arisen.

Active surveillance provides much better, more uniform data than passive case detection but active case detection is much more expensive (see Tables 1.2 and 1.3).

Table 1.2. Reports per 100 physicians of cases of hepatitis, salmonellosis, measles, and rubella by active and passive reporting, Monroe County (NY), 1980–1981

Disease	Active	Passive	Ratio
Hepatitis	78	27	2.9
Measles	11	8	1.4
Rubella	7	3	2.3
Salmonellosis	44	9	4.9
Total	140	48	2.9

Table 1.3. Comparison of Health Department estimated costs for active and passive surveillance systems, Vermont 1981

	Type of surveillance system	
	Active ($)	Passive ($)
Paper	114	80
Mailing	185	48
Telephone	1947	175
Personnel		
Secretary	3000	2000
Public health nurses	14,025	0
State laboratory	700	500
Post exposure prophylaxis	10,890	8250
Total	30,861	11,053

Active Surveillance Through Active Case Detection

Active surveillance systems are usually designed when a passive system is deemed insufficient to accomplish the goals of disease monitoring. This type of surveillance is reserved for special programs, usually when it is important to identify every single case of a disease. Active surveillance is implemented in the final phases of an eradication program: smallpox eradication, poliomyelitis eradication, Guinea worm eradication and malaria eradication in some countries. Active surveillance is also the best approach in epidemic or outbreak investigations to elicit all cases.

In the smallpox eradication program, survey agents visited providers, asking about suspected cases and actually investigating each suspected case. In polio eradication programs, all cases of acute flaccid paralysis are investigated.

In malaria eradication programs and some malaria control programs, malaria control agents go from house to house asking who has fever or had fever recently (in the past week or month for example). A blood smear is collected from those with fever.

1.4.3   Case Register

A case register is a complete list of all the cases of a particular disease in a definite area over a certain time period. Registers are used to collect data on infections over long periods of time. Registers should be population based, detailed and complete. A register will show an unduplicated count of cases. They are especially useful for long term diseases, diseases that may relapse or recur and diseases for which the same cases will consult several providers and therefore would be reported on more than one occasion.

Case registers contain identifiers, locating information, disease, treatment, outcome and follow-up information as well as contact management information. They are an excellent source of information for epidemiologic studies. In disease control, case registers are indispensable tools for follow up of chronic infections disease such as tuberculosis and leprosy.

The contents and quality of a case register determine its usefulness. It should contain

— Patient identifiers with names (all names), age, sex, place and date of birth, complete address with directions on how to reach the patient,
— Name and address of a "stable" relative that knows the patient's whereabouts,
— Diagnosis information with disease classification, brief clinical description (short categories are better than detailed descriptions),
— Degree of infectiousness (bacteriological, serological results),
— Circumstances of detection,
— Initial treatment and response with specific dose, notes on compliance, side effects, clinical response,
— Follow-up information with clinical response, treatment regimen, compliance, side effects,
— Locating information; for some diseases contact information is also useful.

Updating a register is a difficult task. It requires cooperation from numerous persons. Care must be taken to maintain the quality of data. It is important to only request pertinent information for program evaluation or information that would remind users to collect data or to perform an exam. For example, if compliance is often a neglected issue, include a question on compliance. Further details concerning the use of registries in general are given in Chap. I.4 of this handbook.

Sentinel Disease Surveillance   1.4.4

For sentinel disease surveillance, only a sample of health providers is used. The sample is selected according to the objectives of the surveillance program. Providers most likely to serve the population affected by the infection are selected, for example child health clinics and pediatricians should be selected for surveillance of childhood diseases. A sentinel system allows cost reduction and is combined with active surveillance.

A typical surveillance program for influenza infections includes a selected numbers of general practitioners who are called every week to obtain the number of cases presented to them. This program may include the collection of samples for viral cultures or other diagnostic techniques. Such a level of surveillance would be impossible to maintain on the national level.

Evaluation of a Surveillance System   1.4.5

Surveillance systems are evaluated on the following considerations (CDC 2001b):
- Usefulness: Some surveillance systems are routine programs that collect data and publish results; however it appears that they have no useful purpose – no conclusions are reached, no recommendations are made. A successful surveillance system would provide information used for preventive purposes.
- Sensitivity or the ability to identify every single case of disease is particularly important for outbreak investigations and eradication programs.
- Predictive value positive (PVP) is the proportion of reported cases that actually have the health-related event under surveillance. Low PVP values mean that non-cases might be investigated, outbreaks may be exaggerated or pseudo outbreaks may even be investigated. Misclassification of cases may corrupt the etiologic investigations and lead to erroneous conclusions. Unnecessary interventions and undue concern in the population under surveillance may result.
- Representativeness ensures that the occurrence and distribution of cases accurately represent the real situation in the population.
- Simplicity is essential to gain acceptance, particularly when relying on outside sources for reporting.
- Flexibility is necessary to adapt to changes in epidemiologic patterns, laboratory methodology, operating conditions, funding or reporting sources.
- Data quality is evaluated by the data completeness (blank or unknown variable values) and validity of data recorded (cf. Chap. I.13 of this handbook).

- Acceptability is shown in the participation of providers in the system.
- Timeliness is more important in surveillance of epidemics.
- Stability refers to the reliability (i.e., the ability to collect, manage and provide data properly without failure) and availability (the ability to be operational when it is needed) of the public health surveillance system.

1.4.6   # Elements of a Surveillance System

The major elements of a surveillance system as summarized by WHO are: Mortality registration, morbidity reporting, epidemic reporting, laboratory investigations, individual case investigations, epidemic field investigations, surveys, animal reservoir and vector distribution studies, biologics and drug utilization, knowledge of the population and the environment. Traditional surveillance methods rely on counting deaths and cases of diseases. However, these data represent only a small part of the global picture of infectious disease problems.

Mortality Registration

Mortality registration was one of the first elements of surveillance implemented. The earliest quantitative data available on infectious disease is about mortality. The evolution of tuberculosis in the US for example, can only be traced through its mortality. Mortality data are influenced by the occurrence of disease but also by the availability and efficacy of treatment. Thus mortality cannot always be used to evaluate the trend of disease occurrence.

Morbidity Reporting

Reporting of infectious diseases is one of the most common requirements around the world. A list of notifiable diseases is established on a national or regional level. The numbers of conditions vary; it ranges usually from 40 to 60 conditions. In general, a law requires that health facility staff, particularly physicians and laboratories, report these conditions with guaranteed confidentiality. It is also useful to have other non-health related entities report suspected communicable diseases such as day care centers, schools, restaurants, long term care facilities, summer camps and resorts. Regulations on mandatory reporting are often difficult to enforce. Voluntary compliance by the institution's personnel is necessary. Reporting may be done in writing, by phone or electronically in the most advanced system. Since most infectious diseases are confirmed by a laboratory test, reporting by the laboratory may be more reliable. The advantage of laboratory reporting is the ability to computerize the reporting system. Computer programs may be set up to automatically report a defined set of tests and results.

For some infectious diseases, only clinical diagnoses are made. These syndromes may be the consequences of a large number of different microorganisms for which laboratory confirmation is impractical.

When public or physician attention is directed at a specific disease, reporting may be biased. When there is an epidemic or when the press focuses on a particular disease, patients are more prone to look for medical care and physicians are more likely to report. Reporting rates were evaluated in several studies. In the US, studies show report rates of 10% for viral hepatitis, *Hemophilus influenzae* 32%, meningococcal meningitis 50% and shigellosis 62%.

Morbidity Case Definition

It is important to have a standardized set of definitions available to providers. Without standardized definitions, a surveillance system may be counting different entities from one provider to another. The variability may be such that the epidemiologic information obtained is meaningless.

Most case definitions in infectious disease epidemiology are based on *laboratory tests*, however some clinical syndromes such as toxic shock syndrome do not have confirmatory laboratory tests. Most case definitions include a brief *clinical description* useful to differentiate active disease from colonization or asymptomatic infection. Some diseases are diagnosed based on epidemiologic data. As a result many case definitions for childhood vaccine preventable diseases and foodborne diseases include epidemiologic criteria (e.g., exposure to probable or confirmed cases of disease or to a point source of infection). In some instances, the anatomic site of infection may be important; for example, respiratory diphtheria is notifiable, whereas cutaneous diphtheria is not (CDC 1997).

Cases are classified as a confirmed case, a probable or a suspected case. An epidemiologically linked case is a case in which 1) the patient has had contact with one or more persons who either have/had the disease or have been exposed to a point source of infection (including confirmed cases) and 2) transmission of the agent by the usual modes is plausible. A case may be considered epidemiologically linked to a laboratory-confirmed case if at least one case in the chain of transmission is laboratory confirmed. Probable cases have specified laboratory results that are consistent with the diagnosis yet do not meet the criteria for laboratory confirmation. Suspected cases are usually cases missing some important information in order to be classified as a probable or confirmed case.

Case definitions are not diagnoses. The usefulness of public health surveillance data depends on its uniformity, simplicity and timeliness. Case definitions establish uniform criteria for disease reporting and should not be used as the sole criteria for establishing clinical diagnoses, determining the standard of care necessary for a particular patient, setting guidelines for quality assurance, or providing standards for reimbursement. Use of additional clinical, epidemiological and laboratory data may enable a physician to diagnose a disease even though the formal surveillance case definition may not be met.

Which Stage of Disease Should Be Collected?
The Morbidity Iceberg

Surveillance programs collect data on the overt cases diagnosed by the health care system. However these cases may not be the most important links in the chain of transmission. Cases reported are only the tip of the iceberg. They may not at all be representative of the true endemicity of an infectious disease.

There is a continuous process leading to an infectious disease: exposed, colonized, incubating, sick, clinical form, convalescing, cured. Even among those who have overt disease there are several disease stages that may not be included in a surveillance system:

— some have symptoms but do not seek medical attention
— some do get medical attention but do not get diagnosed or get misdiagnosed
— some get diagnosed but do not get reported

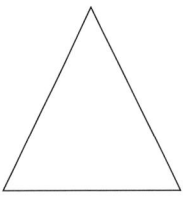

Cases reported
Cases diagnosed but not reported
Cases who seek medical attention but were not diagnosed
Cases who were symptomatic but did not seek medical attention
Cases who were not symptomatic

Infectious disease cases play different roles in the epidemiology of an infectious disease; some individuals are the indicators (most symptomatic), some are the reservoir of microorganisms (usually asymptomatic, not very sick), some are amplifiers (responsible for most of the transmission), some are the victims (those who develop severe long term complications). Depending on the specific disease and the purpose of the surveillance program, different disease stages should be reported. For example

— In a program to prevent rabies in humans exposure to a suspect rabid animal (usually a bite) needs to be reported. At the stage where the case is a suspect, prevention will no longer be effective.
— For bioterrorism events, reporting of suspects is of paramount importance to minimize consequences. Waiting for confirmation causes too long of a delay. In the time necessary to confirm cases, opportunities to prevent co-infections may be lost and secondary cases may already be incubating, depending on the transmissibility of the disease.
— Surveillance for West Nile viral infections best rests on the reporting of neuro-invasive disease. Case reports of neuro invasive diseases are a better indicator than West Nile infection or West Nile fever cases that are often benign, go undiagnosed and are reported haphazardly.
— For Gonorrhea, young males are the indicators because of the intensity of symptoms. Young females are the main reservoir because of the high proportion of asymptomatic infections. Females of reproductive age are the victims because of pelvic invasive disease (PID) and sterility.
— A surveillance program for hepatitis B that only would include symptomatic cases of hepatitis B could be misleading. A country with high transmission of hepatitis B from mother to children would have a large proportion of infected newborn becoming asymptomatic carriers and a major source of infection during their lifetime. Typically in countries with poor reporting of symptomatic hepatitis, the reporting of acute cases of hepatitis B would be extremely low in

spite of high endemicity which would result in high rates of chronic hepatitis and hepatic carcinoma.

Individual Cases or Aggregate Data?

Most morbidity reporting collects data about individual cases. Reporting of individual cases includes demographic and risk factor data which are analyzed for descriptive epidemiology and for implementation of preventive actions. For example, any investigation leading to contact identification and prophylaxis requires a start from individual cases.

However, identification of individuals may be unnecessary and aggregate data sufficient for some specific epidemiologic purposes. Monitoring an influenza epidemic for example, can be done with aggregate data. Obtaining individual case information would be impractical since it would be too time consuming to collect detailed demographics on such a large number of cases. Aggregate data from sentinel sites consists of a number of influenza-like illnesses by age group and the total number of consultants or the total number of 'participants' to be used as denominators. Such data is useful to identify trends and determine the extent of the epidemic and geographic distribution.

Collection of aggregate data of the proportion of school children by age group and sex is a useful predictive tool to identify urinary schistosomiasis endemic areas (Lengeler et al. 2002) without having to collect data on individual school children.

Investigations of Cases, Outbreaks, Epidemics and Surveys

Epidemics of severe diseases are almost always reported. This is not the case for epidemics of milder diseases such as rashes or diarrheal diseases. Many countries do not want to report an outbreak of disease that would cast a negative light on the countries. For example, many countries that are tourism dependent do not report cholera or plague cases. Some countries did not report AIDS cases for a long time.

Case investigations are usually not undertaken for individual cases unless the disease is of major importance such as hemorrhagic fever, polio, rabies, yellow fever, any disease that has been eradicated and any disease that is usually not endemic in the area.

Outbreaks or changes in the distribution pattern of infectious diseases should be investigated and these investigations should be compiled in a comprehensive system to detect trends. While the total number of infectious diseases may remain the same, changes may occur in the distribution of cases from sporadic to focal outbreaks. For example the distribution of WNV cases in Louisiana shifted from mostly focal outbreaks the first year the West Nile Virus arrived in the state in 2002, to mostly sporadic cases the following year in 2003 (see Fig. 1.1).

Surveys are a very commonly used tool in public health, particularly in developing countries where routine surveillance is often inadequate (cf. Chap. IV.6 of this handbook). Survey data needs to be part of a comprehensive surveillance database. One will acquire a better picture from one or a series of well constructed surveys than from poorly collected surveillance data. Surveys are used in control

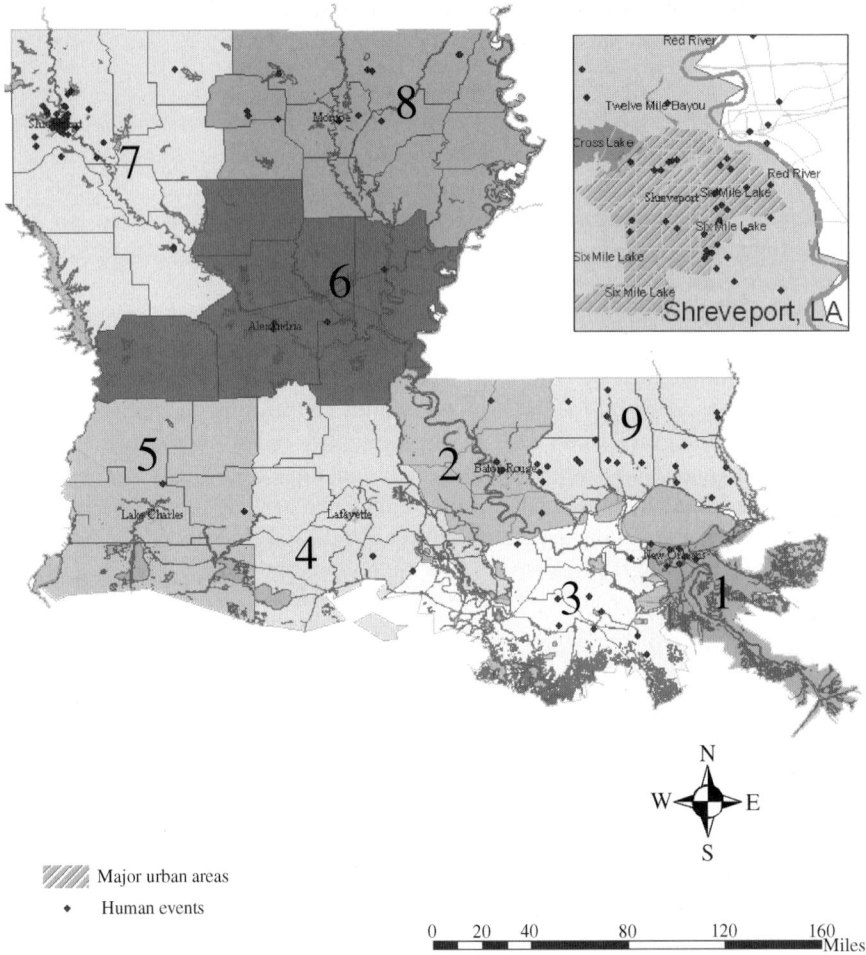

Figure 1.1. Human West Nile Virus Cases Louisiana 2003

programs designed to control major endemic diseases: spleen and parasite surveys for malaria, parasite in urine and stools for schistosomiasis, clinical surveys for leprosy or guinea-worm disease and skin test surveys for tuberculosis.

Surveillance of Microbial Strains
Surveillance of microbial strains is designed to monitor, through active laboratory based surveillance, the bacterial and viral strains isolated. Examples of these systems are:

— In the US, the *PulseNet program* is a network of public health laboratories that performs DNA fingerprinting of bacteria causing foodborne illnesses (Swaminathan et al. 2001). Molecular sub-typing methods must be standardized to allow comparisons of strains and the building of a meaningful data bank.

The method used in PulseNet is pulse field gel electrophoresis. The use of standardized subtyping methods has allowed isolates to be compared from different parts of the country, enabling recognition of nationwide outbreaks attributable to a common source of infection, particularly those in which cases are geographically separated.

— The US National Antimicrobial Resistance Monitoring System (NARMS) for enteric bacteria is a collaboration between CDC, participating state and local health departments and the US Food and Drug Administration (FDA) to monitor antimicrobial resistance among foodborne enteric bacteria isolated from humans. NARMS data are also used to provide platforms for additional studies including field investigations and molecular characterization of resistance determinants and to guide efforts to mitigate antimicrobial resistance (CDC 2003).

— Monitoring of antimicrobial resistance is routinely done by requiring laboratories to either submit all, or a sample of their bacterial isolates.

Surveillance of Animal Diseases

Surveillance for zoonotic diseases should start at the animal level, thus providing early warning for impending increases of diseases in the animal population.

— Rabies surveillance aims at identifying the main species of animals infected in an area, the incidence of disease in the wild animals and the prevalence of infection in the asymptomatic reservoir (bats). This information will guide preventive decisions made when human exposures do occur.

— Malaria control entomologic activities must be guided by surveillance of *Anopheles* population, biting activities, *Plasmodium* infection to biting acivities and *Plasmodium* infection rates in the *Anopheles* population.

— Surveillance for dead birds, infection rates in wild birds, infection in sentinel chickens and horse encephalitis are all part of West Nile encephalitis surveillance. These methods provide an early warning system for human infections.

— The worldwide surveillance for influenza is the best example of the usefulness of monitoring animals prior to spread of infection in the human population. Influenza surveillance programs aim to rapidly obtain new circulating strains to make timely recommendations about the composition of the next vaccine. The worldwide surveillance priority is given to the establishment of regular surveillance and investigation of outbreaks of influenza in the most densely populated cities in key locations, particularly in tropical or other regions where urban markets provide opportunities for contacts between humans and live animals (Snacken et al. 1999).

Rationale of Selecting Diseases for Surveillance Purposes

The rationale for selecting infectious diseases and an appropriate surveillance method is based on the goal of the preventive program. Table 1.4 shows a few examples of different surveillance methods based on the disease and the objectives of the surveillance.

Table 1.4. Examples of different surveillance methods based on the disease and the objectives of the surveillance system

Disease	Objectives	Surveillance method
Anthrax	Limit bioterrorism event	Active or passive syndromic surveillance
Antibiotic resistance	Description	Active laboratory reporting of antibiograms
Aseptic meningitis	Sentinel event for West Nile Identification of outbreak	Passive surveillance by health care providers
Gonorrhea	Description of epidemic Treatment of cases	Passive case detection by health care practitioners Systematic screening of young females (Family planning, pre-natal, student health services etc.)
Hepatitis B	Description of endemicity	Survey of representative groups
Hepatitis B	Prevention of perinatal transmission	Screening of pregnant women
Influenza	Quantify epidemic	Sentinel surveillance with aggregate data from physicians' offices, emergency departments, nursing homes and schools
Poliomyelitis	Identification of residual cases before complete eradication	Active surveillance of acute flaccid paralysis
Rabies	Prevent human cases	Passive reporting of exposure to potentially rabid animals
Staphylococcus aureus Methicillin resistant (MRSA)	Provide information for management of suspected staphylococcal infections	Active laboratory surveillance of aggregate data on proportion of staphylococci resistant to Methicillin
Staphylococcus aureus Vancomycin resistant (VRSA)	Identification of an emerging infection	Laboratory submission of specimens
Tuberculosis	Description of endemicity Case management	Case register
West Nile	Early warning for public and mosquito control	Passive reporting of dead birds by the public, passive reporting of encephalitic horses, sentinel chicken serology, survey of wildlife by serologic methods
West Nile	Description of epidemic	Passive and active case finding of neuro-invasive disease

1.5   Outbreak Investigations

Outbreaks of acute infectious diseases are common and investigations of these outbreaks are an important task for public health professionals, especially epidemiologists. In 2001, a total of 1238 foodborne outbreaks with 25,035 cases involved were reported in the US (CDC 2004) with Norovirus being the most common confirmed etiologic agent associated with these outbreaks (see Table 1.5).

Table 1.5. Confirmed etiologic agents of foodborne outbreaks in the US in 2001

Etiology	Number of Outbreaks
Bacillus cereus	5
Brucella spp.	1
Campylobacter spp.	16
Clostridium botulinum	3
Clostridium perfringens	30
Enterohemorrhagic Escherichia coli	4
Enterohemorrhagic Escherichia coli O157:H7	16
Enterotoxigenic Escherichia coli	2
Listeria monocytogenes	1
Salmonella spp.	112
Shigella spp.	15
Staphylococcus aureus	23
Vibrio spp.	4
Yersinia enterocolitica	3
Total Bacteria	235
Ciguatera	23
Histamin	10
Other Chemical	1
Scrombroid	18
Total Chemical	52
Cyclospora cayetanensis	2
Giardia lamblia	1
Trichinella spp	2
Total Parasitic	5
Hepatitis A	6
Norovirus	150
Total Viral	156

Source: CDC Foodborne Outbreak Response and Surveillance Unit, 2004

Outbreaks or epidemics are defined as the number of disease cases above what is normally expected in the area for a given time period. Depending on the disease, it is not always known if the case numbers are really higher than expected and some outbreak investigations can reveal that the reported case numbers did not actually increase.

The nature of a disease outbreak depends on a variety of circumstances, most importantly the suspected etiologic agent involved, the disease severity or case fatality rate, population groups affected, media pressure, political inference and investigative progress. There are certain common steps for outbreak investigations as shown in Table 1.6. However, the chronology and priorities assigned to each phase of the investigation have to be decided individually, based on the circumstances of the suspected outbreak and information available at the time.

Table 1.6. Common steps in outbreak investigations

1.	"Outbreak" detected based on initial report or analysis of surveillance data
2.	Collect basic numbers and biologic specimens
3.	Investigate or not?
4.	Think prevention first
5.	Get information on the disease or condition
6.	Sometimes numbers do not count
7.	Is the increase real or artificial?
8.	Verify the diagnosis
9.	Prepare a case definition
10.	Put the information in a database
11.	Find additional cases
12.	Basic descriptive epidemiology (time, place and person)
13.	Hypothesis testing and measures of association
14.	Final report and communications

For example, in 2002, 21 outbreaks of acute gastroenteritis on cruise ships with travel destinations outside the US were reported to the CDC (CDC 2002). In only five of these outbreaks about 1400 persons, with an average 280 cases per cruise, had symptoms of viral acute gastroenteritis. Norovirus outbreaks begin usually as a food or water borne disease but often continue because of the easy person to person transmission in a closed environment and low infectious dose (100 viral particles can be infectious) (CDC 2001a).

1.5.1 Basic Steps in Outbreak Investigations

1. The initial report can originate from very different sources. Examples are:
    — A physician is calling the local or state health department about an increase of number of patients seen and diagnosed with a specific disease,
    — A high number of patients with similar signs and symptoms are showing up in the emergency room,
    — A school principal or daycare owner is reporting a high number of absent students,
    — A nursing home health care professional is seeing a lot of residents with gastrointestinal illnesses,
    — A person is complaining to the health department that she/he got sick after eating at a certain restaurant.

Another way to detect an increase of cases is if the surveillance system of reportable infectious diseases reveals an unusually high number of people with the same diagnosis over a certain time period at different health care facilities.

Outbreaks of benign diseases like self-limited diarrhea are often not detected because people are not seeking medical attention and therefore medical services are not aware of them. Furthermore, early stages of a disease outbreak are often undetected because single cases are diagnosed sporadically. It is not until a certain threshold is passed, that it becomes clear that these cases are related to each other through a common exposure or secondary transmission. Depending on the infectious disease agent, there can be a sharp or a gradual increase of number of cases. It is sometimes difficult to differentiate between sporadic cases and the early phase of an outbreak. In the 2001 St. Louis Encephalitis (SLE) outbreak in Louisiana, the number of SLE cases increased from 9 to 18 between week one and two and then the numbers gradually decreased over the next 9 weeks to a total of 63 cases (Jones et al. 2002).

2. After the initial report is received, it is important to collect and document basic information: Contact information of persons affected, a good and thorough event description, names and diagnosis of hospitalized persons (and depending on the presumptive diagnosis their underlying conditions and travel history), laboratory test results and other useful information to get a complete picture and to confirm the initial story of the suspected outbreak. It also might be necessary to collect more biological specimens such as food items and stool samples for further laboratory testing.

3. Based on the collected information the decision to investigate must be made. It may not be worthwhile to start an investigation if there are only a few people who fully recovered after a couple of episodes of a self-limited, benign diarrhea. Other reasons not to investigate might be that this type of outbreak occurs regularly every summer or that it is only an increase in number of reported cases which are not related to each other.

On the other hand, however, there should be no time delay in starting an investigation if there is an opportunity to prevent more cases or the potential to identify a system failure which can be caused, for example, by poor food preparation in a restaurant or poor infection control practices in a hospital or to prevent future outbreaks by acquiring more knowledge of the epidemiology of the agent involved. Additional reasons to investigate include the interest of the media, politicians and the public in the disease cluster and the pressure to provide media updates on a regularly basis. Another fact to consider is that outbreak investigations are good training opportunities for newly hired epidemiologists.

Sometimes lack of data and lack of sufficient background information make it difficult to decide early on if there is an outbreak or not. The best approach then is to assume that it is an outbreak until proven otherwise.

4. Prevention of more cases is the most important goal in outbreak investigations and therefore a rapid evaluation of the situation is necessary. If there are precautionary measures to be recommended to minimize the impact of the outbreak and the spread to more persons, they should be implemented

before a thorough investigation is completed. Most likely control measures implemented by public health professionals in foodborne outbreaks are:
  — Recall or destruction of contaminated food items,
  — Restriction of infected food handlers from food preparation,
  — Correction of any deficiency in food preparation or conservation.

5.   After taking immediate control measures, the next step is to know more about the epidemiology of the suspected agent. The most popular books for public health professionals include the "Red Book" (American Academy of Pediatrics 2003), the "Control of Communicable Diseases Manual" from the American Public Health Association (APHA 2000) or other infectious disease epidemiology books as well as the CDC website (www.cdc.gov). If the disease of interest is a reportable disease or a disease where surveillance data are available, baseline incidence rates can be calculated. Then a comparison is made to determine if the reported numbers constitute a real increase or not. Furthermore, the seasonal and geographical distribution of the disease is important as well as the knowledge of risk factors. Many infectious diseases show a seasonal pattern such as Rotavirus or *Neisseria meningitides*. For example in suspected outbreaks where cases are associated with raw oyster consumption, the investigator should know that in the US Gulf states *Vibrio* cases increase in the summer months because the water conditions are optimal for the growth of the bacteria in water and in seafood. This kind of information will help to determine if the case numbers show a true increase and if it seems likely to be a real outbreak.

6.   For certain diseases, numbers are not important. Depending on the severity of the disease, its transmissibility and its natural occurrence, certain diseases should raise a red flag for every health care professional and even a single case should warrant a thorough public health investigation. For example a single confirmed case of a rabid dog in a city (potential dog to dog transmission within a highly populated area), a case of dengue hemorrhagic fever or a presumptive case of smallpox would immediately trigger an outbreak investigation.

7.   Sometimes an increase of case numbers is artificial and not due to a real outbreak. In order to differentiate between an artificial and a natural increase in numbers, the following changes have to be taken into consideration:
  — Alterations in the surveillance system,
  — A new physician who is interested in the disease and therefore more likely to diagnose or report the disease,
  — A new health officer strengthening the importance of reporting,
  — New procedures in reporting (from paper to web based reporting),
  — Enhanced awareness or publicity of a certain disease that might lead to increased laboratory testing,
  — New diagnostic tests,
  — A new laboratory,
  — An increase in susceptible population such as a new summer camp.

8. It is important to be sure that reported cases of a disease actually have the correct diagnosis and are not misdiagnosed. Is there assurance that all the cases have the same diagnosis? Is the diagnosis verified and were other differential diagnoses excluded? In order to be correct, epidemiologists have to know the basis for the diagnosis. Are laboratory samples sufficient? If not, what kind of specimens should be collected to ascertain the diagnosis? What are the clinical signs and symptoms of the patient?

    In an outbreak of restaurant associated botulism in Canada only the 26th case was correctly diagnosed. The slow progression of symptoms and misdiagnosis of the dispersed cases made it very difficult to link these cases and identify the source of the outbreak (CDC 1985, 1987).

9. The purpose of a case definition is to standardize the identification and counting of the number of cases. The case definition is a standard set of criteria and is not a clinical diagnosis. In most outbreaks the case definition has components of person, place and time, such as the following: Persons with symptoms of X and Y after eating at the restaurant Z between Date1 and Date2. The case definition should be broad enough to get most of the true cases but not too narrow so that true cases will not be misclassified as controls. A good method is to analyze the data, identify the frequency of symptoms and include symptoms that are more reliable than others. For example, diarrhea and vomiting are more specific than nausea and headache in the case definition of a food related illness.

10. What kind of information is necessary to be collected? It is sufficient to have a simple database with basic demographic information such as name, age, sex and information for contacting the patient. More often, date of reporting and date of onset of symptoms are also important. Depending on the outbreak and the potential exposure or transmission of the agent involved further variables such as school, grade of student or occupation in adults might be interesting and valuable.

11. During an outbreak investigation it is important to identify additional cases that may not have been known or were not reported. There are several approaches:
    - Interview known cases and ask them if they know of any other friends or family members with the same signs or symptoms,
    - Obtain a mailing list of frequent customers in an event where a restaurant is involved,
    - Set up an active surveillance with physicians or emergency departments,
    - Call laboratories and ask for reports of suspected and confirmed cases.

Another possibility is to review surveillance databases or to establish enhanced surveillance for prospective cases. Occasionally it might be worthwhile to include the media for finding additional cases through press releases. However the utility of that technique depends on the outbreak and the etiologic agent; the investigator should always do a benefit risk analysis before involving the media.

12. After finding additional cases, entering them in the database and organizing them, the investigator should try to get a better understanding of the situation by performing some basic descriptive epidemiology techniques such as sorting the data by time, place and person. For a better visualization of the data, an epidemic or "epi" curve should be graphed. The curve shows the number of cases by date or time of onset of symptoms. This helps to understand the nature and dynamic of the outbreak as well as to get a better understanding of the incubation period if the time of exposure is known. It also helps to determine whether the outbreak had a single exposure and no secondary transmission (single peak) or if there is a continuous source and ongoing transmission. Figures 1.2 and 1.3 show "epi" curves of two different outbreaks: a foodborne outbreak in a school in Louisiana, and the number of WNV human cases in Louisiana in the 2002 outbreak, respectively.

Sometimes it is useful to plot the cases on a map to get a better idea of the nature and the source of an outbreak. Mapping may be useful to track the spread by water (see John Snow's cholera map) or by air or even a person to person transmission. If a contaminated food item was the culprit, food distribution routes with new cases identified may be helpful. Maps, however, should be taken with caution and carefully interpreted. For example, WNV cases are normally mapped by residency but do not take into account that people might have been exposed or bitten by an infective mosquito far away from where they live. For outbreak investigations, spot maps are usually more useful than rate maps or maps of aggregate data.

Depending on the outbreak it might be useful to characterize the outbreak by persons' demographics such as age, sex, address and occupation or health status. Are the cases at increased susceptibility or at high risk of infection?

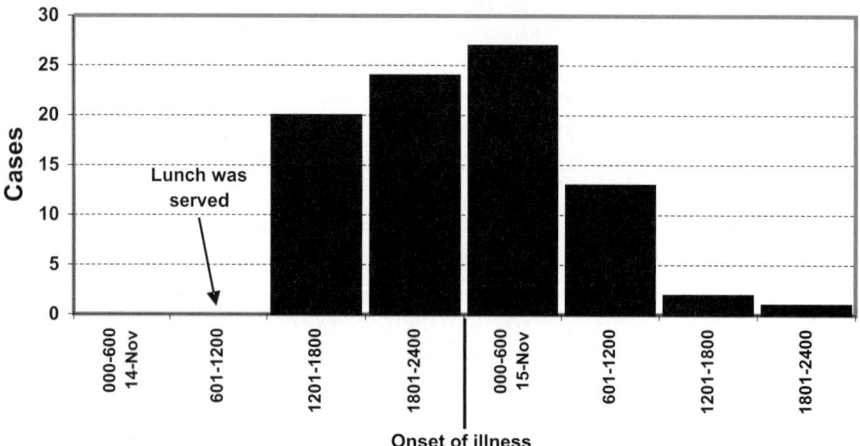

Figure 1.2. Gastroenteritis outbreak in a school in Louisiana, 2001

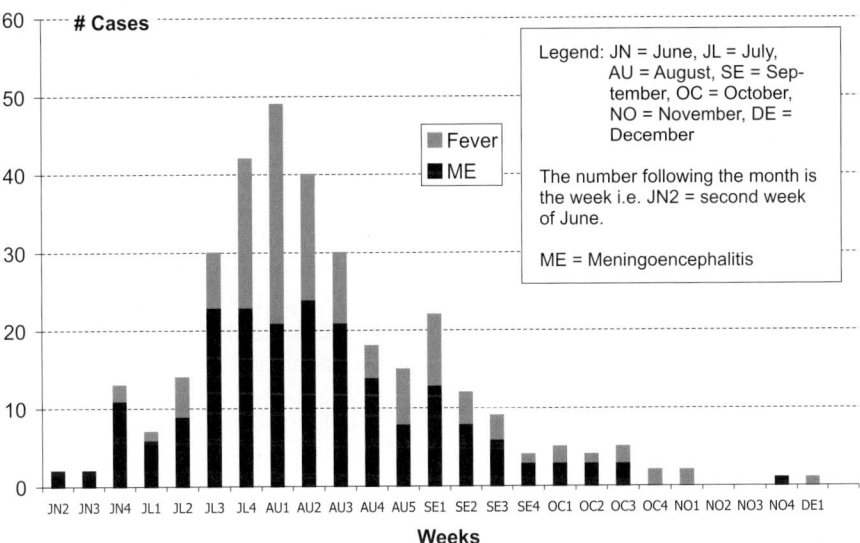

Figure 1.3. Human West Nile Virus cases, Louisiana 2002

These kinds of variables might give the investigator a good idea if the exposure is not yet known. For typical foodborne outbreaks however, demographic information is not very useful because the attack rates will be independent of age and sex. More details on methods used in descriptive epidemiology are given in Chap. I.3 of this handbook.

13. Based on the results of basic descriptive epidemiology and the preliminary investigation, some hypotheses should be formulated in order to identify the cause of the outbreak. A hypothesis will be most likely formulated such as "those who attended the luncheon and ate the chicken salad are at greater risk than those who attended and did not eat the chicken salad". It is always easier to find something after knowing what to look for and therefore a hypothesis should be used as a tool. However, the epidemiologist should be flexible enough to change the hypothesis if the data do not support it. If data clues are leading in another direction, the hypothesis should be reformulated such as "those who attended the luncheon and ate the baked chicken are at greater risk than those who attended and did not eat the baked chicken".

To verify or deny hypotheses, measures of risk association such as the relative risk (RR) or the odds ratio (OR) have to be calculated (as described in Chaps. I.2, I.5, and I.6 of this handbook). The CDC has developed the software program 'EpiInfo' which is easy to use in outbreak investigations, and, even more importantly, free of charge. It can be downloaded from the CDC website (http://www.cdc.gov/epiinfo/). Measures of association, however, should be carefully interpreted; even a highly significant measure of association can not give enough evidence of the real culprit or the contaminated food item. The measure of association is only as good and valid as the data. Most people have recall problems when asked what they ate, when they ate and when their symptoms started. Even more biases or misclassifications of cases and controls can hide an association. A more confident answer comes usually from the laboratory samples from both human samples and food items served at time of exposure. Agents isolated from both food and human samples that are identified as the same subtype, in addition to data results supporting the laboratory findings, are the best evidence beyond reasonable doubt.

14. As the last step in an outbreak investigation, the epidemiologist writes a final report on the outbreak and communicates the results and recommendations to the public health agency and facilities involved. In the US, public health departments also report foodborne outbreaks electronically to CDC via a secure web based reporting system, the Electronic Foodborne Outbreak Reporting System (EFORS).

1.5.2   Types of Outbreaks

The "Traditional" Foodborne Outbreak

The "traditional" foodborne outbreak is usually a small local event such as family picnic, wedding reception, or other social event and occurs often in a local restaurant or school cafeteria. This type of outbreak is highly local with a high attack rate in the group exposed to the source. Because it is immediately apparent to those in the local group such as the group of friends who ate at the restaurant or the students' parents, public health authorities are normally notified early in the outbreak while most of the cases are still symptomatic. Epidemiologists can start early on with their investigation and therefore have a much better chance to collect food eaten and stool samples of cases with gastroenteritis for testing and also to detect the etiologic agent in both of them.

In a 2001 school outbreak in Louisiana, eighty-seven persons (sixty-seven students and twenty faculty members) experienced abdominal cramps after eating at the school's annual "Turkey Day" the day before. Stool specimens and the turkey with the gravy were both positive for *Clostridium perfringens* with the same pulse field gel electrophoresis (PFGE) pattern (Merlos 2002). The inspection of the school cafeteria revealed several food handling violations such as storing, cooling and reheating of the food items served. Other than illnesses among food handlers, these types of improper food handling or storage are the most common causes of foodborne outbreaks.

New Types of Outbreaks

A different type of outbreak is emerging as the world is getting smaller. In other words persons and food can travel more easily and faster from continent to continent and so do infectious diseases with them. Foodborne outbreaks related to imported contaminated food items are normally widespread, involving many states and countries and therefore are frequently identified. In 1996, a large outbreak of *Cyclospora cayetanensis* occurred in 10 US states and Ontario, Canada and was linked to contaminated raspberries imported from South America. Several hundred laboratory confirmed cases were reported, most of them in immunocompetent persons (CDC 1996).

A very useful molecular tool to identify same isolates from different geographic areas is sub-typing enteric bacteria with PFGE. In the US, the PulseNet database allows state health department to compare their isolates with other states and therefore increase the recognition of nationwide outbreaks linked to the same food item (Swaminathan et al. 2001).

In a different scenario, a widely distributed food item with low-level contamination might result in an increase of cases within a large geographic area and therefore might be not get detected on a local level. This kind of outbreak might only be detected by chance if the number of cases increased in one location and the local health department alerts other states to be on the lookout for a certain isolate.

Another type of outbreak is the introduction of a new pathogen into a new geographic area as it happened in 1991 when *Vibrio cholerae* was inadvertently introduced in the waters off the Gulf Coast of the United States. In the U.S., however, most cases are usually traced back to people who traveled to areas with a high cholera risk or to people who ate food imported from cholera-risk countries and only sporadic *Vibrio cholerae* cases are associated with the consumption of raw or undercooked shellfish from the Gulf of Mexico (CDC 1999b).

Food can not only be contaminated by the end of the food handling process i.e. by infected food handlers but also can be contaminated by any event earlier in the chain of food production. In 1996, an ice cream outbreak of *Salmonella enteritidis* in a national brand of ice cream resulted in 250,000 illnesses. The outbreak was detected by routine surveillance because of a dramatic increase of *Salmonella enteritidis* in South Minnesota. The cause of the outbreak was a basic failure on an industrial scale to separate raw products from cooked products. The ice cream premix was pasteurized and then transported to the ice cream factory in tanker trucks which had been used to haul raw eggs. This resulted in the contamination of the ice cream and subsequent salmonella cases (Hennessey et al. 1996).

Surveys   1.6

Surveys are useful to provide information for which there is no data source or no reliable data source. Surveys are time consuming and are often seen as a last choice to obtain information. However, too often unreliable information is used because it is easily available. For example, any assessment of the *Legionella* problem using passive case detection will be unreliable due to under-diagnosis and under-reporting. Most cases of legionellosis are treated empirically as community acquired pneumonias and are never formally diagnosed.

In developing countries, surveys are often necessary to evaluate health problems since data collected routinely (disease surveillance, hospital records, case registers) are often incomplete and of poor quality. In industrialized nations, although many sources of data are available, there are some circumstances where surveys may be necessary.

Prior to carrying out surveys involving human subjects, special procedures need to be followed. In industrialized countries, a human subject investigation review board has to evaluate the project's value and ethics. In developing countries, however, such boards may not be formalized but it is important to obtain permission from medical, national and local political authorities before proceeding.

1.6.1   Survey Methods

Surveys of human subjects are carried out by mail, telephone, personal interviews, and behavioral observations. In infectious diseases, the collection of biological specimens in humans (i.e. blood for serologic surveys) or the collection of environmental samples (food, water, environmental surfaces) is very common. Personal interviews and specimen collection require face to face interaction with the individual surveyed. These are carried out in offices or by house to house surveys.

Non-respondents are an important problem for infectious disease surveys. Those with an infection may be absent from school, may not answer the door or may be unwilling to donate blood for a serologic survey, thus introducing a systematic bias into the survey results.

Since surveys are expensive, they cannot be easily repeated. All field procedures, questionnaires, biological sample collection methods and laboratory tests should be tested prior to launching the survey itself. Feasibility, acceptability and reliability can be tested in a small scale pilot study. More details on survey methods are to be found in Chap. I.10 of this handbook.

1.6.2   Sampling

Since surveys are labor intensive, they are rarely carried out on an entire population but rather on a sample. To do a correct sampling, it is necessary to have a sampling base (data elements for the entire population) from which to draw the sample. Examples of sampling bases are population census, telephone directory (for the phone subscriber population), school roster or a school list. In developing countries such lists are not often available and may have to be prepared before sampling can start. More information on sampling designs can be found in Chap. IV.5 of this handbook.

1.6.3   Community Surveys (House to House Surveys)

Most community surveys are carried out in developing countries because reliable data sources are rare. The sampling base often ends up to the physical layout of the population. A trip and geographical reconnaissance of the area are necessary.

The most common types of surveys undertaken in developing countries are done at the village level; they are based on maps and a census of the village.

In small communities, it is important to obtain the participation of the population. Villagers are often wary of government officials counting people and going from door to door. To avoid misinterpretations and rumors, influential people in the community should be told about the survey. Their agreement is indispensable and their help is needed to explain the objectives of the survey and particularly its potential benefits. Increasing the knowledge about disease, disease prevention and advancing science are abstract notions that are usually poorly understood or valued by villagers who are, in general, very practical people. If a more immediate benefit can be built into the survey, there will be an increase in cooperation of the population. Incentives such as offering to diagnose and treat an infection or drugs for the treatment of common ailments such as headaches or malaria enhance the acceptance of the survey.

In practically all societies the household is a primary economic and social unit. It can be defined as the smallest social unit of people who have the same residency and maintain a collective organization. The usual method for collecting data is to visit each household and collect samples or administer a questionnaire.

Medical staff may feel left out or even threatened whenever a medical intervention (such as a survey) is done in their area. A common concern is that people will go to their medical care provider and ask questions about the survey or about specimen collection and results. It is therefore important to involve and inform local medical providers as much as practical.

A rare example of a house to house survey in an industrialized nation was carried out in Slidell, Louisiana for the primary purpose of determining the prevalence of West Nile infection in a southern US focus. Since the goal was to obtain a random sample of serum from humans living in the focus, the only method was a survey of this type. A cluster sampling design was used to obtain a representative number of households. The area was not stratified because of its homogeneity. Census blocks were grouped so that each cluster contained a minimum of 50 households. The probability of including an individual cluster was determined by the proportion of houses selected in that cluster and the number of persons participating given the number of adults in the household. A quota sampling technique was used, with a goal of enlisting 10 participating households in each cluster.

Inclusion criteria included age (at least 12 years of age) and length of residence (at least 2 years). The household would be included only if an adult household resident was present. A standardized questionnaire was used to interview each participant. Information was collected on demographics, any recent febrile illness, knowledge, attitudes, and behaviors to prevent WNV infection and potential exposures to mosquitoes. A serum sample for WNV antibody testing was drawn. In addition, a second questionnaire regarding selected household characteristics and peridomestic mosquito reduction measures was completed. Informed consent was obtained from each participant, and all participants were advised that they could receive notification of their blood test results if they wished. Institutional Review Board approvals were obtained.

Logistics for specimen collection, preservation and transportation to the laboratory were arranged. Interpretation of serologic tests and necessary follow up were determined prior to the survey and incorporated in the methods submitted to the ethics committee.

Sampling weights, consisting of components for block selection, household-within-block selection, and individual-within-household participation, were used to estimate population parameters and 95% confidence intervals (CI). Statistical tests were performed incorporating these weights and the stratified cluster sampling design.

In this survey, 578 households were surveyed (a 54% response rate), including 1226 participants. There were 23 IgM seropositive persons, for a weighted seroprevalence of 1.8% (with a 95% confidence interval of 0.9%–2.7%) (Vicari et al. 2003).

1.7   Program Evaluation

Program evaluation is a systematic way to determine if prevention or intervention programs for the infectious disease of interest are effective and to see how they can be improved. It is beyond the scope of this chapter to explain program evaluation in detail however there is abundant information available i.e. the CDC's Framework for Program Evaluation in Public Health (CDC 1999a) as well as text books on program evaluation (Fink 1993).

Most importantly, evaluators have to understand the program such as the epidemiology of the disease of interest, the program's target population and their risk factors, program activities and resources. They have to identify the main objectives of the control actions and determine the most important steps. Indicators define the program attributes and translate general concepts into measurable variables. Data are then collected and analyzed so that conclusions and recommendations for the program are evidence based.

Evaluating an infectious disease control program requires a clear understanding of the microorganism, its mode of transmission, the susceptible population and the risk factors. The following example of evaluation of tuberculosis control shows the need to clearly understand the priorities.

Most of tuberculosis transmission comes from active pulmonary tuberculosis cases who have positive sputum smear (confirmed as tuberculosis *Mycobacteria* on culture). To a lesser extent, smear negative culture positive pulmonary cases are also transmitting the infection. Therefore priority must be given to find sputum positive pulmonary cases. The incidence of smear positive tuberculosis cases is the most important incidence indicator. Incidences of active pulmonary cases and of all active cases (pulmonary and extra-pulmonary) are also calculated but are of lesser interest. The following proportions are used to detect anomalies in case finding or case ascertainment:

— all tuberculosis cases who are pulmonary versus extra-pulmonary,
— smear positive, culture positive, pulmonary cases versus smear negative, culture positive, pulmonary cases,
— culture positive, pulmonary cases versus culture negative, pulmonary cases.

Poor laboratory techniques or low interest in obtaining sputa for smears or cultures may result in underestimating bacteriological confirmed cases. Excessive diagnosis of tuberculosis with reliance on chest X-rays on the other hand may overestimate unconfirmed tuberculosis cases.

Once identified, tuberculosis cases are placed under treatment. Treatment of infectious cases is an important preventive measure. Treatment efficacy is evaluated by sputum conversion (both on smear and culture) of the active pulmonary cases. After 2 months of an effective regimen, 85% of active pulmonary cases should have converted their sputum from positive to negative. Therefore the rate of sputum conversion at 2 months becomes an important indicator of program effectiveness. This indicator must be calculated for those who are smear positive and with a lesser importance for the other active pulmonary cases.

To ensure adequate treatment and prevent the development of acquired resistance, tuberculosis cases are placed under directly observed therapy (DOT). This measure is quite labor intensive. Priority must therefore be given to those at highest risk of relapse. These are the smear positive culture proven active pulmonary cases. DOT on extra-pulmonary cases is much less important from a public health standpoint.

The same considerations apply to contact investigation and preventive treatment in countries that can afford a tuberculosis contact program. A recently infected contact is at the highest risk of developing tuberculosis the first year after infection; hence the best preventive return is to identify contacts of infectious cases. Those contacts are likely to have been recently infected. Systematic screening of large population groups would also identify infected individuals but most would be 'old' infections at lower risk of developing disease. Individuals infected with tuberculosis and HIV are at extremely high risk of developing active tuberculosis. Therefore the tuberculosis control program should focus on the population at high risk of HIV infection.

Often, program evaluation is performed by epidemiologists who have not taken the time to understand the dynamics of a disease in the community. Rates or proportions are calculated, no priorities are established and precious resources are wasted on activities with little preventive value. For example, attempting to treat all tuberculosis cases, whether pulmonary or not with DOT, investigating all contacts regardless of the bacteriologic status of the index case, would be wasteful.

1.8 Conclusions

Today the world is smaller than ever before, international travel and a worldwide food market make us all potentially vulnerable to infectious diseases no matter where we live.

New pathogens are emerging such as the SARS or spreading through new territories such as WNV. WNV introduced in the US in 1999, became endemic in the US over the next years. Hospital-associated and community-associated Methicillin Resistant Staphylococcus Aureus (MRSA) and resistant tuberculosis cases and outbreaks are on the rise. Public health professionals are concerned that a novel recombinant strain of influenza will cause a new pandemic.

But not only the world and the etiologic agents are changing, the world population is changing as well. In industrialized countries, the life expectancy is increasing and the elderly are more likely to acquire a chronic disease, cancer or diabetes in their lifetime. Because of underlying conditions or the treatment of these diseases, older populations also have an increased susceptibility for infectious diseases and are more likely to develop life-threatening complications.

Knowledge in the field of infectious disease epidemiology is expanding. While basic epidemiological methods and principles still apply today, improved laboratory diagnoses and techniques help to confirm cases faster, see how cases are related to each other and therefore can support the prevention of spread of the specific disease. Better computers can improve the data analysis and internet allows access to in depth disease specific information. Computer connectivity improves disease reporting for surveillance purposes and the epidemiologist can implement faster preventive measures if necessary and is also able to identify disease clusters and outbreaks on a timelier basis.

The global threat of bioterrorism adds a new dimension. The intentional release of anthrax spores, and the infection and death of persons who contracted the disease created a scare of contaminated letters in the US population.

With all these changes, there is renewed emphasis on infectious disease epidemiology and makes it a challenging field to work in.

References

Aintablian N, Walpita P, Sawyer MH (1998) Detection of Bordetella pertussis and respiratory syncytial virus in air samples from hospital rooms. Infect Control Hosp Epidemiol 19:918-923

Alland D, Kalkut GE, Moss AR, McAdam RA, Hahn JA, Bosworth W, Drucker E, Bloom BR (1994) Transmission of tuberculosis in New York City. An analysis by DNA fingerprinting and conventional epidemiologic methods. NEJM 330(24):1710–1716

American Academy of Pediatrics (AAP) (2003) In: Pickering LK (ed) Red Book: 2003. Report of the Committee on Infectious Diseases, 26th edn. AAP, Elk Grove Village, IL

American Public Health Association (2000) In: Chin J (ed) Control of communicable diseases manual, 17th edn. United Book Press Inc, Baltimore, MD

Boelaert M, Arbyn M, Van der Stuyft P (1998) Geographical Information System (GIS), gimmick or tool for health district management? Trop Med Int Health 3:163–165

CDC (1985) Update: International outbreak of restaurant-associated botulism – Vancouver, British Columbia, Canada. MMWR 34(41):643

CDC (1987) Epidemiologic notes and reports restaurant associated botulism from mushrooms bottled in-house – Vancouver, British Columbia, Canada. MMWR 36(7):103

CDC (1996) Outbreaks of Cyclospora cayetanensis infection – United States, 1996. MMWR 45(25):549–551

CDC (1997) Case definitions for infectious conditions under public health surveillance. MMWR 46(10):1–55

CDC (1999a) Framework for program evaluation in Public Health. MMWR 48(11):1–40

CDC (1999b) Summary of infections reported to *Vibrio* surveillance system (http://www.cdc.gov/ncidod/dbmd/diseaseinfo/files/VibCSTE99web.pdf) Accessed May 25, 2004

CDC (2001a) "Norowalk-like viruses": Public health consequences and outbreak management. MMWR 50 (9):1–17

CDC (2001b) Updated guidelines for evaluating public health surveillance systems: Recommendations from the Guidelines Working Group. MMWR 50(13): 1–35

CDC (2002) Outbreaks of gastroenteritis associated with noroviruses on cruise ships – United States, 2002. MMWR 51(49):1112–1115

CDC (2003) National antimicrobial resistance monitoring system for enteric bacteria (NARMS): 2001 Annual Report. U.S. Department of Health and Human Services, Atlanta, Georgia

CDC (2004) Diagnosis and management of foodborne illnesses: A primer for Physicians and other health care professionals. MMWR 53(4):1–33

EpiInfo (http://www.cdc.gov/epiinfo/) Accessed May 25, 2004

Fink A (1993) Evaluation fundamentals: Guiding health programs, research and policy. Sage, Newbury Park, CA

Goodwin LG, Gordon Smith CE (1996) Yellow fever. In: Cox CR (ed) The Wellcome Trust illustrated history of tropical diseases. Wellcome Trust, London, p 147

Hennessy TW, Hedberg CW, Slutsker L, White KE, Besser-Wiek JM, Moen ME, Feldman J, Coleman WW, Edmonson LM, MacDonald KL, Osterholm MT (1996) A national outbreak of salmonella enteritidis Infections from ice cream. NEJM 334(20): 1281–1286

Jones SC, Morris J, Hill G, Alderman M, Ratard RC (2002) St. Louis encephalitis outbreak in Louisiana in 2001. J La State Med Soc 154:303–306

Lengeler C, Makwala J, Ngimbi D, Utzinger J (2000) Simple school questionnaires can map both Schistosoma mansoni and Schistosoma haematobium in the Democratic Republic of Congo. Acta Trop 74(1):77–87

Lockman S, Sheppard JD, Braden CR (2001) Molecular and conventional epidemiology of Mycobacterium tuberculosis in Botswana: A population-based prospective study of 301 pulmonary tuberculosis patients. J Clin Microbiol 39 (3):1042–1047

Mandell GL, Bennett JE, Dolin R (eds) (2000) Mandell, Douglas, and Bennett's principles and practice of infectious diseases, 5th edn. Churchill Livingstone, Philadelphia

McMahon B, Pugh TF (1970) Epidemiology, principles and methods. Little, Brown and Company, Boston, p 149

Merlos II (2002) An uninvited guest at "Turkey Day" Louisiana morbidity report 13(1): 1–2 (http://www.oph.dhh.state.la.us/infectiousdisease/docs/Lmr/janfeb02.pdf) Accessed May 25, 2004

Mounts AW, Holman RC, Clarke MJ, Bresee JS, Glass RI (1999) Trends in hospitalizations associated with gastroenteritis among adults in the United States, 1979–1995. Epidemiol Infect 123:1–8

Snacken R, Kendal AP, Haaheim LR, Wood JM (1999) The next influenza pandemic: Lessons from Hong Kong, 1997. Emer Inf Dis 5 (2):195–203

Snow J (1936) On the mode of communication of cholera. In: Snow on cholera. A reprint of two papers by John Snow. The Commonwealth Fund, New York, pp 1–175

Swaminathan B, Barrett TJ, Hunter SB, Tauxe RV, and the CDC PulseNet Task Force (2001) PulseNet: The Molecular Subtyping Network for Foodborne Bacterial Disease Surveillance, United States. Emer Inf Dis 7 (3):382–389

Vicari SA, Zielinski-Gutierrez E, Montgomery S, Chow C, O'Leary D, Grayson K, Biggerstaff B, Martin D, Ratard R, Campbell C, Bunning M (2003) Household-based seroepidemiologic survey of West Nile Virus infection-Slidell, Louisiana, 2002. Late-breaker report presented at the CDC "Annual Epidemic Intelligence Service Conference" held in Atlanta, GA, on April 4, 2003

WHO (2000a) World health report 2000 (http://www.who.int/whr2001/2001/archives/index.htm) Accessed May 25, 2004

WHO (2000b) World health report 2000. Statistical annex. (http://www.who.int/whr2001/2001/archives/2000/en/pdf/StatisticalAnnex.pdf) Accessed May 25, 2004

Wills C (1996a) Cholera, the Black one. In: Yellow fever black goddess, the co-evolution of people and plagues. Addison-Wesley Publishers, Reading, MA, p 115

Wills C (1996b) Four tales from the new decameron. In: Yellow fever black goddess, the coevolution of people and plagues. Addison-Wesley Publishers, Reading, MA, p 84

Cardiovascular Diseases

IV.2

Darwin R. Labarthe

2.1

Introduction

Coronary heart disease (CHD) and stroke are the first and second leading causes of death and are major contributors to disability worldwide (Murray and Lopez 1996). Accordingly, they represent the foremost cardiovascular disease (CVD) challenges of our time. They are prominent in public health and clinical importance and have been under extensive epidemiologic investigation over the past half-century. As a result, with parallel clinical and laboratory research, understanding of the causes of and means to prevent CHD and stroke have become well established, and their present and immediate future global impact is becoming recognized (Labarthe 1998).

This chapter begins with a discussion of the scope and basic concepts of CVD epidemiology. As the focus of the chapter, the atherosclerotic and hypertensive diseases are defined, several aspects of their epidemiology are highlighted, and applications of the main types of epidemiologic methods in CVD are briefly illustrated. Against this backdrop, the sections that follow address four broad questions, with illustrative examples from classic studies in the field: How can we describe the occurrence of CVD from a population perspective? What factors account for differences in CVD incidence and mortality among populations and for differences in risk among individuals within a given population? What do we understand to be the causes of these differences, and what preventive strategies follow from this understanding? And, what are the foremost issues for the immediate future in CVD epidemiology?

2.2   Scope and Basic Concepts

2.2.1   Atherosclerotic and Hypertensive Diseases

CHD and stroke are the main consequences of atherosclerosis and hypertension. Also termed ischemic heart disease, CHD is a manifestation of reduced blood supply – and hence reduced oxygen supply – via the coronary arteries to the myocardium (muscle of the heart). Sudden loss of oxygen supply may result in injury or death to the muscle cells, constituting a myocardial infarction (heart attack). Disturbance of normal rhythmic contraction of the heart may occur, and this arrhythmia often causes sudden death unless effective emergency aid is administered promptly. A less severe – but also ominous, perhaps equally painful, and recurring – condition is unstable angina, which represents transient impairment of blood flow. The typical culprit lesion in the artery wall common to these varied circumstances is the atherosclerotic plaque, which may itself grow gradually over years to narrow or occlude the artery or may suddenly rupture and trigger the rapid formation of an occlusive thrombus (blood clot) within the artery. Survival from an acute coronary event may be accompanied by disability from residual cardiac impairment and entails a high risk of recurrent events or progressive heart failure.

Stroke results from injury to the brain in a manner sometimes analogous to myocardial infarction: interruption of the arterial blood supply by a thrombotic occlusion. But other mechanisms may also cause stroke, chiefly occlusion by lodging of an embolus (a blood clot that has arisen, for example, in a damaged heart and carried through the circulation to the brain) or by hemorrhage (when a blood vessel within the brain ruptures). Regardless of the mechanism, interruption of blood flow may produce injury and death of brain cells. The event may be rapidly fatal or may be followed by survival, with a high risk of recurrence and often with significant disability. The main underlying condition leading to thrombosis is atherosclerosis, whereas hemorrhage is especially attributable to hypertension.

Chronic heart failure may develop as a consequence of either CHD or hypertension, greatly increases the risk of stroke, and causes disability due to impaired circulatory function. It may also result from several other cardiac disorders, but in populations where CHD is a frequent condition, heart failure as a late consequence of CHD has become increasingly common, especially among older adults.

These five interrelated conditions – atherosclerosis, hypertension, CHD, stroke, and heart failure – comprise the greater part of 'cardiovascular diseases', or 'CVD', as used throughout this chapter. Other important cardiovascular conditions, such as atherosclerotic peripheral arterial disease, aortic aneurysm, cardiomyopathies, rheumatic heart disease, Chagas' disease, congenital heart disease, deep vein thrombosis, and pulmonary embolism, while important vascular conditions, are beyond the scope of this review.

Cardiovascular Diseases in Epidemiologic Perspective 2.2.2

Measures of CVD in the population are fundamental to epidemiologic investigation and understanding. Terms such as mortality, incidence, or prevalence introduced e.g. in Chaps. I.1, I.2 and I.3 of this handbook have their particular use and importance in CVD epidemiology. *CVD mortality* can be studied insofar as deaths are registered and classified in accordance with reliable and standardized procedures and the current census of the underlying population is known. Such data have been collected for several decades in many countries but have yet to be recorded at all in many others. The most informative data are those presented for specific age and sex groups within a population, and for other subgroups as appropriate. Adherence to practices for the *International Statistical Classification of Diseases and Related Health Problems, Tenth Revision* (World Health Organization (WHO) 1992) is now required for national death registration systems. For epidemiologic research, case validation can be conducted through well-standardized procedures such as those of the WHO MONICA Project (WHO MONICA Project Principal Investigators 1988). Case validation is especially important for unobserved and out-of-hospital deaths in which CHD or stroke is suspected but documentation regarding diagnostic criteria is unavoidably incomplete.

The CVD burden of a population may be estimated, and comparisons among populations made, by surveys to determine the proportion of the population affected, or *CVD prevalence*. Prevalence of CVD is influenced by both the rate at which new cases occur and the duration of their survival in the population. Sampling methods and selective factors in survey participation, such as disease-related disability, must be taken into account in evaluating findings. Standard cardiovascular survey methods have been published since the 1960s (Blackburn et al. 1960; Rose and Blackburn 1968) and updated subsequently. The prevalence of CVD and related conditions such as high blood pressure, high blood cholesterol concentration, and smoking history can be assessed with reasonable efficiency, although a low CHD or stroke prevalence in some populations may make this approach impractical.

The frequency with which newly detected cases of CVD occur in a population, or *CVD incidence*, is measured by long-term (several years) follow-up among persons found at the baseline survey to be disease free and for whom first events can be ascertained by periodic re-examination, surveillance of hospitalizations or deaths, or a combination of these approaches. Issues in evaluation of findings relate especially to chances for missed or misdiagnosed cases, and losses to follow-up. Detection of new cases also allows assessment of the proportion of events leading to death in the short term (*case-fatality*; usually within 28 days of symptom onset) and *long-term survival* (for any specified period beyond 28 days post-event).

Other concepts basic to CVD epidemiology relate to the progression from cardiovascular health to disease and the corresponding array of intervention strategies and approaches that apply across this continuum. These concepts provide a framework for public health action to prevent heart disease and stroke (Fig. 2.1). They are addressed briefly here as background for the more detailed discussions of the sections that follow.

The lower panel of Fig. 2.1 represents as "the present reality" a well-established series of connections characterizing the progression from unfavorable social and environmental conditions, through the adverse behavioral patterns that they foster, to the emergence of the major CVD risk factors. Not shown are the typical long-term development of subclinical (undetected) disease and the immediate precipitating factors that link the major risk factors to the first event – whether heart attack, stroke, or episode of heart failure. Sudden death may rapidly end the course, or survival may extend it, often with significant disability and high risk of recurrent CVD events. Paralleling this progression is the dimension of the life course of CVD, from possible maternal and fetal influences where earliest environmental factors may operate; to childhood and adolescence where behavioral patterns often become established and risk factors begin to emerge; and on to early, middle, and late adulthood with the acute events and their consequences. The counter to this present reality is a vision of the future (upper panel), in which the opposite of each of these states has been achieved.

The means of change toward this vision are the intervention approaches identified in the center panel of Fig. 2.1. Each approach has potential application from its first point of intervention throughout the further progression of CVD. For example, policy and environmental change can be applied to health care settings, work sites, and schools as well as to society at large (Association of State and Territorial Directors of Health Promotion and Public Health Education 2001). Risk factor detection and control applies not only before any clinical events but also,

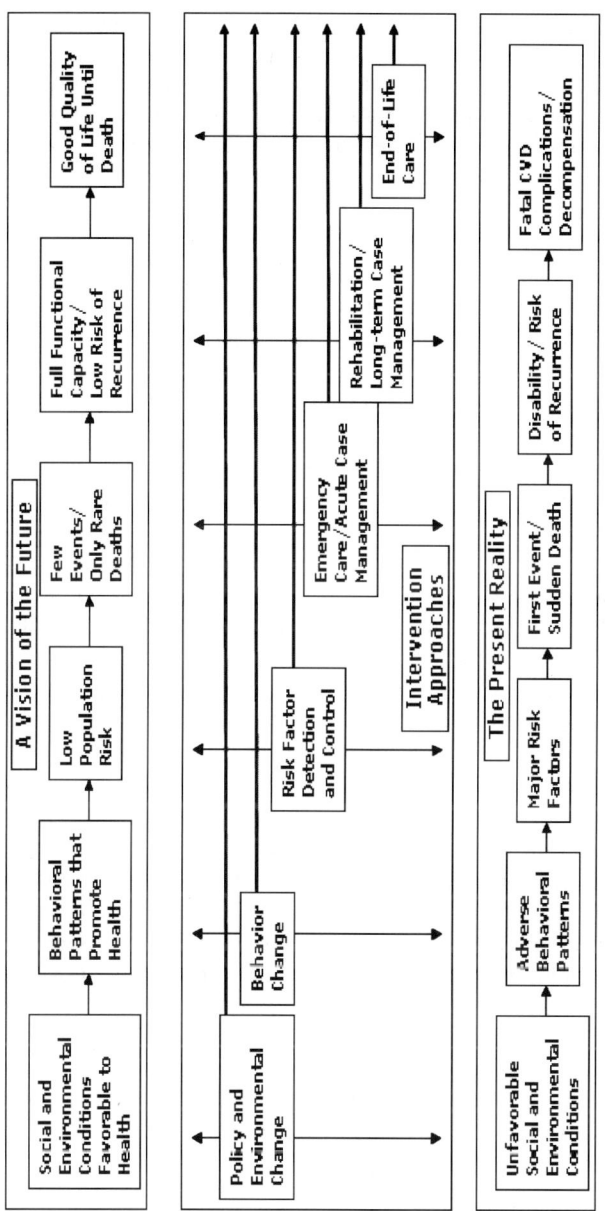

Figure 2.1. Action framework for a comprehensive public health strategy to prevent heart disease and stroke (adapted from US Department of Health and Human Services (2003))

for persons who survive, to lifelong care to prevent recurrent CVD events. These and the more familiar concepts of secondary, primary, and primordial prevention and of high-risk and population-wide strategies are discussed further below.

2.2.3   **Epidemiologic Methods in Cardiovascular Diseases**

CVD exemplifies the chronic or non-communicable diseases (NCDs), whose public health importance and epidemiologic investigation gained increasing attention
in the mid-twentieth century. Population-based studies were conducted in many
places throughout the world, stimulating development and widespread application of standardized research methods. The now-commonplace epidemiologic
approaches to studying chronic diseases were devised or greatly refined in subsequent decades, very often as a means of investigating CVD. The knowledge
summarized here represents the cumulative results of this research and illustrates
the approaches whose principles and methods are presented in Part I of this handbook (see Chaps. I.5–I.8):

- *Analysis of vital statistics*, specifically comparison of death rates (mortality)
  from cardiovascular causes, was an early strategy in CVD epidemiology and
  continues to be of value in demonstrating differences between population
  groups or trends over time in national or other geopolitical areas. A classic
  example was the work of Gordon (1957) in recognizing that men of Japanese
  ancestry living in Japan, Hawaii, and California experienced strikingly different patterns of mortality from CHD and stroke (CHD being low in Japan,
  intermediate in Hawaii, and high in California, and the opposite gradient for
  stroke). A major strength of this approach is ready availability of vital data over
  decades or longer for many countries and their subdivisions. Serious limitations include the lack of data especially for low- and middle-income countries
  and the need to take into account changes in classification of causes of death
  over time and variable data quality.
- *Population surveys* (cross-sectional surveys, conducted in principle at a point
  in time and typically in a defined geographic area) in their simplest design provide essential background information about the proportion of a population
  affected by a particular disease (disease prevalence) and related factors. But
  such surveys can extend to multiple-population comparisons or be repeated
  periodically, thereby addressing population differences or secular trends, including testing of hypotheses about predicted findings. In this way, for example,
  the INTERSALT Study demonstrated an association between the slope of increasing blood pressure with age and urinary electrolyte excretion in adults
  among 52 study centers in 32 countries (INTERSALT Co-operative Research
  Group 1986); rapid change was shown in blood pressure among Luo tribesmen
  migrating from rural to urban Kenya (Poulter et al. 1990); favorable trends
  were seen in the distribution of systolic blood pressure over 40 years in the
  U.S. population (Goff et al. 2001); and comparison of the prevalence of hypertension in six European countries, Canada, and the United States revealed
  a previously unrecognized higher prevalence in Europe (Wolf-Maier et al. 2003).
  Strengths of the population survey include versatility of design, e.g. permitting geographic or temporal comparisons, and fundamental simplicity and
  relative expediency of execution. Limitations include the cross-sectional property that necessarily restricts observation to prevalent cases and constrains

collection of historical data on exposures that may have preceded onset of disease.

— *Cohort studies* to determine the rate of occurrence of new cases among persons free of disease at first (baseline) observation (measuring disease incidence in relation to baseline characteristics of interest) were initiated in the 1950s to yield early insights into causes of CHD and stroke. Three leading examples of cohort studies conducted within a single population or for comparison of multiple populations to assess risk factors for cardiovascular events are the Framingham Study, with nearly 50 years of multigenerational observation of CVD in one U.S. community (Dawber et al. 1951); the Whitehall Study of British civil servants, which also provided long-term follow-up and insight to individual risks (Rose and Shipley 1986); and the Seven Countries Study of factors accounting for differences in CHD rates between European, Japanese, and North American populations (Keys 1980). Cohort studies are unique among observational designs in permitting direct assessment of disease incidence in relation to baseline or interim risk characteristics (relative risk). They require large populations, long-term follow-up, or both to generate sufficient person-years of experience to afford reliable estimates of incidence and risk and are correspondingly demanding of resources and skill.

— The *case-control study* is used to identify already affected persons (the case group) and assess characteristics of interest among them, with comparable assessment among a suitable non-affected group (the control group) to judge whether exposures among cases may be linked in a meaningful way with the presence of disease. In recent years, for example, the case-control approach has been applied in a large-scale multinational collaborative study of the association between the presence of stroke and other vascular conditions among women by their history of oral contraceptive use (WHO Collaborative Study of Cardiovascular Disease and Steroid Hormone Contraception 1996). This approach is widely used to study conditions of relatively low incidence, a situation in which demands of cohort studies noted above are difficult to satisfy. The fundamental issue in design, conduct and interpretation of case-control studies is evaluation of possible bias or confounding in the comparison of cases and controls.

— *Combinations of approaches* have also been used to monitor CHD and stroke in populations, as illustrated by the especially comprehensive WHO MONICA (Monitoring Trends and Determinants in Cardiovascular Disease) Project (WHO MONICA Project Principal Investigators 1988; Tunstall-Pedoe 2003). In this major collaboration among 38 populations in 21 countries, repeated cross-sectional surveys were used to assess trends in risk factors and treatment of cases, continuous community-wide and hospital-based surveillance identified new and recurring cases and case-fatality, and death rates based on validated cause of death in accordance with the MONICA Project surveillance protocol were used to evaluate the corresponding vital statistics systems. In some centers, cohort designs were incorporated as well. Composite study designs combine both advantages and limitations of each approach that is included.

— The many "clues to causation" generated from the kinds of studies described above (collectively the "observational study" approaches) have ultimately led to a very large body of experimental research, such as the intervention trials also addressed in Chap. I.8 of this handbook. In CVD epidemiology, this research has ranged from *clinical trials* among selected individuals to evaluate the efficacy of treatments among patients (*secondary prevention trials*) or of measures to reduce risk of first events (*primary prevention trials*), to long-term *community-based trials* and *demonstration projects* to test the effectiveness of interventions for the population at large (cf. Chap. III.11 of this handbook). One example of early clinical trials that stimulated subsequent population-based trials and strongly influenced policy and practice is the U.S. Veterans Administration Trial of the Treatment of Hypertension (Freis 1990). Community trials and demonstrations are well illustrated by the North Karelia Project (Puska et al. 1998) and by examples in the United States and elsewhere (Blackburn 1992; Labarthe 1998).

The Major Atherosclerotic and Hypertensive Diseases: an Epidemiologic Description

2.3

2.3.1   Overview

A half-century of CVD epidemiology, developing and applying the methods highlighted above, has provided a comprehensive understanding of the natural history of these conditions (see, e.g. Marmot and Elliott 1992; Labarthe 1998). Several broad features of this extensive body of work can be described.

— CVD is pervasive throughout the world. In the mid-twentieth century CVD, and especially CHD, came to be regarded as a public health problem of the Western industrialized nations. Before the end of the century, CVD (principally expressed as CHD or stroke) was recognized as a public health problem of global importance and a significant deterrent to social and economic development in low- and middle-income countries.

— Change in population burdens of CVD, as reflected in the crude, late measure of cause-specific mortality, can occur rapidly and with abrupt and unpredicted change in direction or may be sustained over several decades and result in a twofold or greater change in rates. Such rapid change is unequivocal evidence of powerful environmental factors whose influence is highly variable over time and place. In addition, migration of population subgroups has demonstrated change in CVD rates such that rates for migrants come to resemble those of the new population setting in contrast to rates for the non-migrating members of the source population. Such observations suggest that environmental factors are potentially subject to interventions to establish or maintain social and environmental conditions protective against CVD.

— Epidemiologic investigation of the pathology of atherosclerosis strongly supports the view of early-life onset and life long progression of this vascular disorder, which underlies CHD and many strokes. Studies of military casualties dying of non-CVD causes have shown that unrecognized coronary atherosclerosis may be extensive even in early adulthood. Thus true prevention of atherosclerosis and its complications requires effective intervention as early as childhood and adolescence.

— National vital statistics systems that provide reliable data on cause-specific mortality are sometimes adequate for gauging the population burden of CVD, but these data are incomplete or lacking for many countries. Additional information is needed to fully characterize a population's CVD profile, and efforts to compile such data on a worldwide basis have revealed serious shortcomings even in high-income countries, such as the United States, where data on disease incidence are typically lacking except in specific localities with special epidemiologic studies. Characterizing the global burden thus faces serious obstacles.

— Notwithstanding these limitations, serious efforts to project the global burden of CVD and other major causes of death and disability, and the potential impact of selected interventions against these conditions, have provided a view of the world's health two decades hence. The results indicate that CHD and stroke have been the first and second leading causes of death worldwide since 1990 and would remain so through 2020, barring greatly intensified public health efforts in prevention.

Classic studies in the field of CVD epidemiology are reviewed below to illustrate a twentieth-century historical perspective, studies of pathology, the present global burden, and projections for the decades ahead.

Illustrations
2.3.2

Historical Perspective
Studying long-term CVD mortality trends in one or more countries can provide valuable epidemiologic insight. A leading example of this approach is the work of Omran (1971), who studied mortality from multiple causes in the United States and elsewhere from 1900 through 1970. On the basis of these observations, he presented the concept of "epidemiologic transition" to describe the relative shift in frequency between infectious and circulatory diseases as causes of death (Table 2.1). According to this concept, the proportion of deaths from circulatory disease can be expected to increase from only 5–10 percent to 35–55 percent of deaths as a society progresses from the "age of pestilence and famine" to the "age of degenerative and man-made diseases." Following Omran, two further phases of transition were

added by others. The first was a declining proportional circulatory mortality in an "age of delayed degenerative diseases," explained by improvement in risk factors due to education and resulting behavioral changes (Olshansky and Ault 1986). These contributions are combined in the representation of the concept in Table 2.1 (Pearson et al. 1993). Next was a second wave of rising proportional mortality attributable to disruption of supports for CVD prevention and health promotion due to social and political upheavals (not shown in Table 2.1) (Yusuf et al. 2001).

Table 2.1. The epidemiologic transition (from Pearson et al. (1993))

Phase of Epidemiologic Transition	Deaths from Circulatory Disease (%)	Circulatory Problems	Risk Factors
Age of pestilence and famine	~ 5–10	Rheumatic heart disease; infectious and deficiency-induced cardiomyopathies	Uncontrolled infection; deficiency conditions
Age of receding pandemics	10–35	As above, plus hypertensive heart disease and hemorrhagic stroke	High-salt diet leading to hypertension; increased smoking
Age of degenerative and man-made diseases	35–55	All forms of stroke; ischemic heart disease	Atherosclerosis from fatty diets; sedentary lifestyle; smoking
Age of delayed degenerative diseases	Probably under 50	Stroke and ischemic heart disease[a]	Education and behavioral changes leading to lower levels of risk factors

[a] At older ages. Represents a smaller proportion of deaths

In its simplest form, the concept of epidemiologic transition is useful in calling attention to the massive shifts in causes of death that can accompany social and economic change. Yet these shifts do not necessarily represent replacement of one burden with another but may result in the "double burden" of continued occurrence of infectious diseases with superimposed NCDs, of which circulatory conditions are a major part. Further, the shifts resulting from the latter conditions may change direction as underlying social conditions change. The question is the extent to which the rise in frequency of CHD and stroke can be slowed or reversed to reduce, to the greatest possible degree, the burden they pose for countries throughout the world, especially the low- and middle-income countries which can least afford this burden.

In general, it has been considered that Western industrial nations have undergone such a transition within the twentieth century, whereas developing countries have yet to do so. The concept of epidemiologic transition implies that

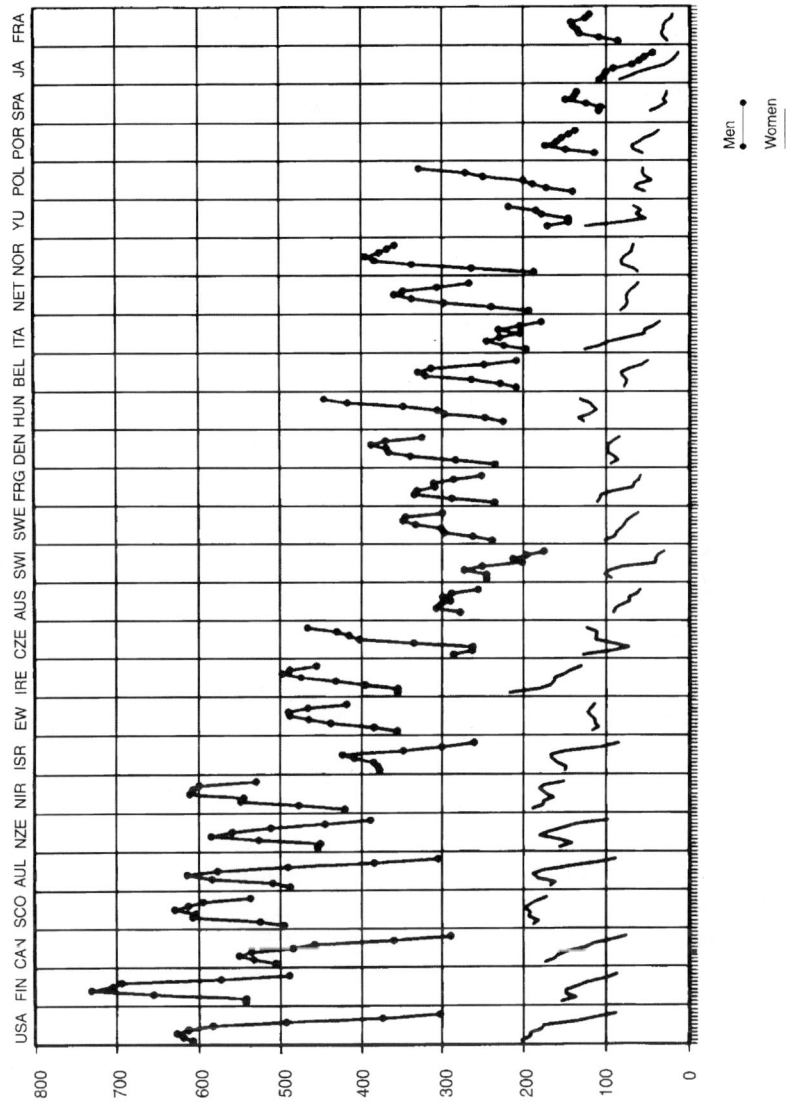

Figure 2.2. Coronary heart disease mortality in 27 countries, 1950–1987 (from Thom et al. (1992))

circulatory conditions therefore are less important in developing than industrialized countries. But 1985 estimates of death rates from ischemic heart disease and stroke by geopolitical or economic regions of the world, presented by the World Bank, point to a different interpretation (Pearson et al. 1993). *Proportional mortality* from circulatory conditions remained low (20 percent or less) in non-

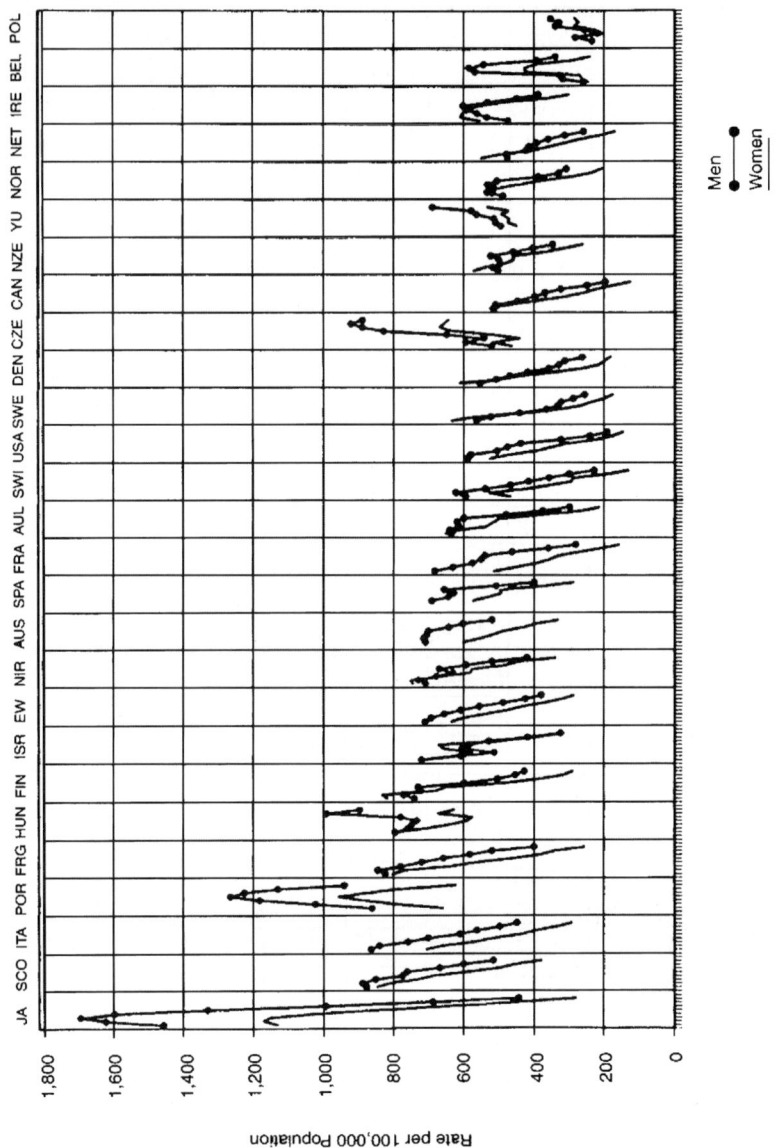

Figure 2.3. Stroke mortality in 27 countries, 1950–1987 (from Thom et al. (1992))

industrialized regions of the world, but estimated *absolute death rates* for these
conditions were nearly as high (or for stroke, even higher than) in all but the
industrial non-market economies. Thus among most regions of the world CVDs
present a similar burden that is masked by attention to proportional mortality
alone.

Analysis of national secular trends in cardiovascular mortality over the latter half of the twentieth century demonstrates several important aspects of the epidemiology of CHD and stroke over this period (Thom et al. 1992). The data illustrated in Fig. 2.2 represent CHD mortality among persons aged 45–64 years in 27 countries for consecutive time periods from 1950–54 to 1984–87[1]. These countries were included because they had reported reliable annual mortality data to the WHO over the entire 38 years.

This figure shows a universal excess in rates for men relative to those for women; a wide range of rates among countries – as much as 6-fold; marked changes in rates within countries over successive 5-year intervals; and generally similar trends for women and men in the same country. These observations indicate strong time-dependent and regionally or nationally distinct environmental influences that commonly, though not invariably, affected women and men in similar ways. Because population genetics do not change so rapidly, such changes are attributable to environmental factors.

An analogous figure for stroke (Fig. 2.3) shows notable epidemiologic differences from CHD. Here the age range is 65–74 years, because the rates of stroke death are lower and generally less reliably estimated at earlier ages. The following features are most striking: the same 27 countries appear in quite different order (for example, Japan is first, in contrast to its position next to last for CHD); rates for men and women were generally similar within each country; and overall rates and trends were quite homogeneous among countries with few exceptions (JA, POR, HUN, CZE, YU, POL). Stroke does not closely match CHD epidemiologically. It does, however, share the aspect of marked change in mortality in a rather short historical period that indicates strong environmental influences, here operating in a generally similar way between sexes and among countries.

Epidemiologic Studies of Pathology

Epidemiologic study of atherosclerosis has included a substantial body of work by pathologists that is well represented by two studies, the International Atherosclerosis Project and the Pathobiological Determinants of Atherosclerosis in Youth (PDAY) Study. The International Atherosclerosis Project was essentially a cross-sectional multinational survey of coronary and aortic atherosclerosis (Tejada et al. 1968). Sections of coronary arteries and aortas were obtained from more than 23,000 autopsies for non-CVD deaths at ages 10–69 years in 14 countries, including Latin America as well as the United States and South Africa. Wide variation among the populations was found in the average extent of coronary atherosclerosis at any given age, and this measure and the CHD mortality rates corresponded

---

[1] USA, United States; FIN, Finland; CAN, Canada; SCO, Scotland; AUL, Australia; NZE, New Zealand; NIR, Northern Ireland; ISR, Israel; EW, England and Wales; IRE, Ireland; CZE, Czechoslovakia; AUS, Austria; SWI, Switzerland; SWE, Sweden; FRG, Federal Republic of Germany; DEN, Denmark; HUN, Hungary; BEL, Belgium; ITA, Italy; NET, Netherlands; NOR, Norway; YU, Yugoslavia; POL, Poland; POR, Portugal; SPA, Spain; JA, Japan; FRA, France. Each point represents the sex-specific average annual mortality for one period. Countries are arrayed in descending order of mortality for men in the first interval.

closely within the respective countries. Where the extent of coronary atherosclerosis was greatest, males had more extensive lesions than females did, but little difference by sex was evident in populations were coronary involvement was least. No sex differences in the extent of aortic disease were observed.

A strong age gradient in degree of atherosclerosis at death was also observed in six of the countries studied: from a range of 0–25 percent of intimal surface involvement with fibrous plaques at age 20, the percentage approximately doubled by age 30 in each population and continued to increase, although less steeply, to later ages at death. These findings confirmed marked population differences in the extent of coronary atherosclerosis, especially at early ages. They also supported earlier observations indicating that onset of atherosclerosis was common before age 20 and that males exhibited more extensive coronary atherosclerosis than females did.

The PDAY Study conducted standardized postmortem examinations of coronary and aortic specimens among black or white decedents aged 15–34 years from non-CVD causes at eight centers in the United States (Pathobiological Determinants of Atherosclerosis in Youth (PDAY) Research Group 1990). Beyond pathology alone, this study introduced assessment of CVD risk factors based on blood samples and other materials obtained at death. This study demonstrated that the extent and severity of atherosclerosis at these early ages was strongly related to adverse blood lipid profiles and to smoking (as assessed by serum thiocyanate concentration). Earlier, the Bogalusa Heart Study had begun conducting postmortem studies of atherosclerosis in participants in their school-based surveys who died years later from non-CVD causes (Berenson et al. 1992). Risk factor measurements in school, including blood lipids, blood pressure, smoking and obesity, were associated with the extent and severity of coronary atherosclerosis at death. The findings from these two studies established a critical link between risk factors and pathology at ages well before clinical CVD typically appears. This link is important for strategies of CVD prevention and strengthened evidence for the progressive development of atherosclerosis in early life, as conceptualized decades earlier by Holman and colleagues (Holman et al. 1958).

Present Burden

The present burden of CVD can be described in considerable detail in many countries, although limitations of data in even some of the most economically advanced countries, including the United States, remain to be overcome. The World Heart Federation (WHF) has assessed the global situation in a recent report, *Impending Global Pandemic of Cardiovascular Diseases: Challenges and Opportunities for the Prevention and Control of Cardiovascular Diseases in Developing Countries and Economies in Transition* (Chockalingam and Balaguer-Vintró 1999) (see also www.worldheart.org). This report addressed the need for international cooperation, the role of the WHF, the profile and magnitude of the global CVD burden, current activities and resources, and strategies for global action. It compiled results of surveys from member WHF countries concerning existing policies, programs, and guidelines for CVD prevention, resource requirements and funding sources, human resources, and cardiology infrastructure and practices. Several indicators of the CVD burden as of 1990 are provided in Table 2.2.

Table 2.2. Proportionate contributions to selected CVD conditions by geopolitical region (adapted from Chockalingam and Balaguer-Vintró (1999))

	Geopolitical Region		
	Established Market Economies	Economies in Transition[a]	Developing Countries
CVD mortality (%)	22.0	15.0	63.0
Coronary mortality (%)	30.3	21.7	48.0
Cerebrovascular mortality (%)	17.0	14.3	68.7
CVD-related disability life years lost (%)	14.9	11.5	73.6

[a] Chiefly the countries of the former USSR and others in Eastern Europe

The World Health Report 2002: Reducing Risks, Promoting Healthy Life (World Health Organization 2002) provides a further development of such estimates for the year 2001 (see also www.who.int) (Table 2.3). This table presents estimated numbers of deaths and numbers of disability-adjusted life years (DALYs) lost[2], by cause, overall and for each of the six WHO Regions (AFR = Africa, AMR = the Americas, EMR = Eastern Mediterranean, EUR = Europe, SEAR = South-East Asia, and WPR = Western Pacific). Although each region is subclassified by mortality pattern in the source tables, data are summarized here for entire WHO Regions, for ischemic heart disease and cerebrovascular disease.

Table 2.3. Estimated numbers of deaths and numbers of DALYs lost due to ischemic heart disease and cerebrovascular disease by WHO Region, 2001 (from World Health Organization (2002))

Measure of burden	WHO Region						
	AFR	AMR	EMR	EUR	SEAR	WPR	Total
Deaths ($\times$1000)							
Ischemic heart disease	333	967	523	2423	1972	963	7181
Cerebrovascular disease	307	454	218	1480	1070	1926	5455
DALYs lost ($\times$1000)							
Ischemic heart disease	3258	6506	5353	16,000	20,236	7373	58,726
Cerebrovascular disease	3318	4057	2364	10,443	9952	15,736	45,870

Of all deaths worldwide, 22.3 percent were estimated to be due to these two conditions, as were 7.1 percent of all DALYs lost. Each region contributes substantial numbers to these measures of the CVD burden, without including rheumatic, hypertensive, or inflammatory heart disease. Relative contributions to ischemic

---

[2] 1 DALY lost = 1 full year of healthy life expectancy lost, 2 years lived with 50% disability, etc.

heart disease and stroke vary strikingly among regions, being about equal in Africa, with clear predominance of cerebrovascular disease in the Western Pacific and of ischemic heart disease in all other regions. The relative frequencies of these two conditions as contributors to the CVD burden are about equivalent for both deaths and DALYs lost. Beyond these estimates of current burden, the WHO report provides an extensive analysis of the major risks to health, strategies to reduce these risks, how to strengthen risk prevention policies, and how to take action to prevent risks.

Projections

While communicable disease epidemiologists commonly use mathematical models to project the course of epidemics, such efforts have only rarely been described in connection with NCDs. However, through a joint undertaking of WHO, the World Bank, and the Harvard University School of Public Health, the Global Burden of Disease Study was conducted to estimate incidence, prevalence, mortality, and disability related to more than 100 diseases and causes of injury as of the year 1990 and to project the global disease burden to the year 2020 (Murray and Lopez 1996). The Global Burden of Disease Study identified ischemic heart disease and stroke as leading causes of death and disability worldwide in both 1990 and 2020. Among the many findings of importance in the CVD projections are the following, for change in total CVD death rates from 1990 to 2020: world, +16.2%; established market economies, +1.8%; economies in transition, +19.4%; and developing countries, +28.2%.

These forecasts remain the best available data from which to anticipate the near-term course of CVD in the world population. They suggest that even in the established market economies the death rates will increase. The impact in the two other major geopolitical regions will be substantially greater unless measures can be taken to reverse these projected trends.

2.4 Risk Factors and Determinants

2.4.1 Overview

Many factors contribute to development of CVD. They may be as remote as conditions of fetal development or as immediate as precipitators of plaque rupture in a coronary artery. They may be as distal in their influences as community-level poverty and lack of education or as proximate as an individual's blood concentration of low density lipoprotein (LDL)-cholesterol. "Risk factors", "determinants", and other related terms are commonly used interchangeably. Here, "determinants" is generally used for the whole array of these influences, including social determinants (such as income or relative poverty, education, and housing quality) and risk factors (such as personal, behavioral, metabolic, physiologic characteristics). All influences can be viewed as either population based or individual based. For example, the social determinants (which are population characteristics) affect individuals, and the risk factors (which are individual traits) have their corresponding distributions and trends in populations. The major established risk factors for CVD are highlighted briefly here; details of their epidemiology are addressed elsewhere (Stamler 1992; Labarthe 1998).

In broad terms, these many factors are considered to relate to the progressive development of CVD as represented in Fig. 2.1, bottom row. That is, social and environmental conditions such as level of literacy contribute importantly to health-related behavior, in part through establishing the range of societal or individual choices available; behavioral patterns such as dietary habits reflect in part policies affecting food production, distribution, and pricing and produce specific risk factors such as adverse blood lipid profile or high blood pressure; and major risk factors (discussed below) account for the greater part of population differences in CVD rates as well as individual differences in risks within a population. These factors in combination influence the probability of surviving a first acute event, experiencing and surviving recurrences, and ultimately dying from CVD. Several aspects of the determinants of CVD can be summarized as follows (Labarthe 1998):

— Age, sex, race or ethnicity, and heredity intersect with all other determinants. The risks of atherosclerotic and hypertensive diseases are strongly related to age and often differ by sex and by race or ethnicity. Heredity, whether considered in terms of family history (which reflects sharing of both genes and environment among related persons) or individual genetic traits, is also related in some respects to CVD risk.

— Age, sex, race or ethnicity, and heredity are often considered as unmodifiable risk factors in that they are fixed characteristics of individuals. In contrast, modifiable risk factors are behavioral, metabolic, or physiologic characteristics that can in principle be changed through intervention. It is important to consider the extent to which the risks attributed to the unmodifiable factors may actually reflect variation in modifiable risk factors associated with these traits.

— Dietary imbalance can be considered in three senses – unfavorable macronutrient composition of the diet, excessive sodium intake relative to physiologic requirements, and excessive energy intake relative to energy expenditure. It represents in each of these forms a fundamental behavioral pattern in the progressive development of CVD. Its critical role has been established by decades of epidemiologic, clinical and laboratory research that has addressed numerous aspects of diet (for example, types and amounts of animal fats – especially saturated fats –, relative to fruits, vegetables, and legumes, and the amount of salt and total energy intake).

— Physical inactivity, as a concomitant of the typical social and economic characteristics of contemporary industrial societies, contributes to CVD risk through the failure of matching energy expenditure with energy intake and potentially through numerous biological mechanisms related to cardiac metabolism and physiology. As a consequence of reduced physical work for personal locomotion and physical exertion in most occupations, research attention turned to leisure-time physical activity. But leisure time has increasingly become devoted to sedentary pursuits (such as watching television), so that average population levels of physical activity have become very low in many countries.

— Both the dietary imbalance and physical inactivity common to contemporary industrial societies represent vast changes from human evolutionary norms and earlier post-agricultural nutritional patterns that can be inferred from an-thropological research and other sources (WHO Study Group 1990; Blackburn 1983; President's Council on Physical Fitness and Sports 1996). From this per-spective, there is considerable room for progression toward more natural and health-promoting dietary habits, with due regard to modern understanding of human nutritional requirements for optimum growth and function.

— Dietary imbalance contributes directly to the development of adverse blood lipid profiles (high concentration of low-density lipoprotein [LDL-] cholesterol is the most essential factor in atherogenesis) and to high blood pressure. Along with physical inactivity, dietary imbalance produces overweight or obesity, which contributes further to these risk factors and to impaired glucose tolerance and diabetes. The major metabolic and physiologic risk factors for CVD are thus dependent on these two adverse behavioral patterns, and extensive evidence from trials demonstrates that these risk factors can be prevented or controlled by appropriate interventions.

— Smoking of tobacco has long been recognized as an established major risk factor for CVD and for other common chronic diseases. Targeting of youth and the populations of developing countries by tobacco marketers has been a mounting concern of national and international health organizations. The projected excess mortality attributable to smoking throughout the world in the coming decades contributed to the adoption of the Framework Convention for Tobacco Control, a landmark international treaty that supports governments combating the tobacco epidemic (WHO 2003).

— Both adverse psychosocial patterns at the level of the individual and broad societal conditions or social determinants of health have been studied with great interest in relation to CVD. These aspects are implicit in Fig. 2.1 where, in "the present reality", they are reflected in the adverse social and environmental conditions and resulting adverse behavioral patterns that contribute to devel-opment of the major CVD risk factors. Alternatively, "a vision of the future" in the figure contemplates social and environmental conditions favorable to health and behavioral patterns that promote health, with consequently reduced risk and rates and severity of CVD events in the population (US Department of Health and Human Services 2003). These determinants of health are addressed in some detail under social epidemiology in Chap. III.1 in this handbook.

2.4.2   Illustrations

Important contributions of epidemiologic research to understanding CVD deter-minants include both studies of between-population differences in rates of disease and studies of between-individual differences in risk within selected populations. Classic studies of both types are illustrated below.

Population Differences

The role of nutrition in causing atherosclerosis and hypertension – and therefore CHD, stroke, and related conditions – has been a dominant theme throughout the past half-century of epidemiologic investigation. The profound influence of nutrition on population differences in CHD occurrence has been central to this field and was demonstrated most effectively by Keys and colleagues through their decades-long Seven Countries Study (Keys 1980). As a backdrop to this work, Keys highlighted anecdotal evidence from China and Indonesia suggesting that adoption of a Western-style dietary pattern, in contrast to traditional ones, accompanied the development of atherosclerosis, which was otherwise rare or absent from these populations (Keys 1983). Keys also reviewed the observations of Malmros and others on marked short-term fluctuations in mortality attributable to atherosclerosis associated with changes in food supply in Northern Europe during and immediately after the Second World War (Malmros 1950). These changes appeared to be closely synchronous and supported the idea that dietary composition, especially with respect to animal fats, was an essential underlying factor in determining population rates of CHD.

Changes in many conditions of life affect the health of populations, both within the Western world and in the developing world as urbanization, industrialization, and globalization take place. Changes in dietary patterns, transition to an increasingly sedentary lifestyle, and multinational marketing of tobacco products are only a few of these changes, important in the present context for their direct relevance to risk of CVD (Labarthe 1998). The extensive evidence for a necessary role of dietary composition that is disproportionately high in saturated fats includes a large body of animal laboratory, pathological, and clinical research that cannot be reviewed here but is summarized and documented elsewhere (e.g., Stamler 1992; Committee on Diet and Health 1989).

Building further on his prior work on the postulated link between diet, blood cholesterol concentration, and atherosclerosis, Keys undertook development of his monumental Seven Countries Study (Keys 1980). The organization and implementation of this unique and seminal program are presented in detail by Blackburn and others who provide exceptional accounts of this formative work in CVD epidemiology (Blackburn 1995; Kromhout et al. 1993). This program was designed to test the hypothesis that population differences in CHD incidence were largely determined by differences in dietary saturated fat intake, with blood cholesterol concentration as the principal intermediate factor.

Men aged 40–59 years were examined in 16 cohorts in the seven countries they represented (12,763 men in all). Baseline examinations took advantage of standardized methods whose development was in part stimulated by the requirements for this study. To assess dietary intake, repeated weighed diet samples were obtained for men in 12 of the 16 cohorts, and questionnaire methods were used in the remaining 4. Baseline examinations began in four cohorts in 1958 and were completed in 1964. Follow-up was accomplished by re-examination at 10 years in 14 of the cohorts. A major report of findings, based on this 10-year follow-up, addressed each of the main exposure variables and CHD outcomes (Keys 1980). Many additional reports, including 25-year and still later follow-ups, have provided further evidence on the central hypothesis and other questions.

The 25-year findings relating intake of saturated fatty acids (as a percentage of calories or energy intake per day, or "En%") – to CHD mortality in the 16 cohorts is illustrated in Fig. 2.4 (Kromhout et al. 1995). Intake of saturated fatty acids varied from less than 5% to nearly 25% of calories, and 25-year CHD mortality ranged from less than 5% to nearly 30% percent; the correlation coefficient *r* was 0.88. Clearly lowest in both saturated fat intake and CHD mortality were Tanushimaru (T) and Ushibuka (U), Japan; Corfu (G) and Crete (K), Greece; and Dalmatia (D), former Yugoslavia. Intermediate cohorts were those in Rome railroad workers (R), Montegiorgio (M), and Crevalcore (C), Italy; and Velika Krsna (V), Zrenjanin (Z), Slavonia (S), and Belgrade (B) in former Yugoslavia. Highest in intake and mortality were East (E) and West (W) Finland; Zutphen (N), the Netherlands; and U.S. railroad workers (A).

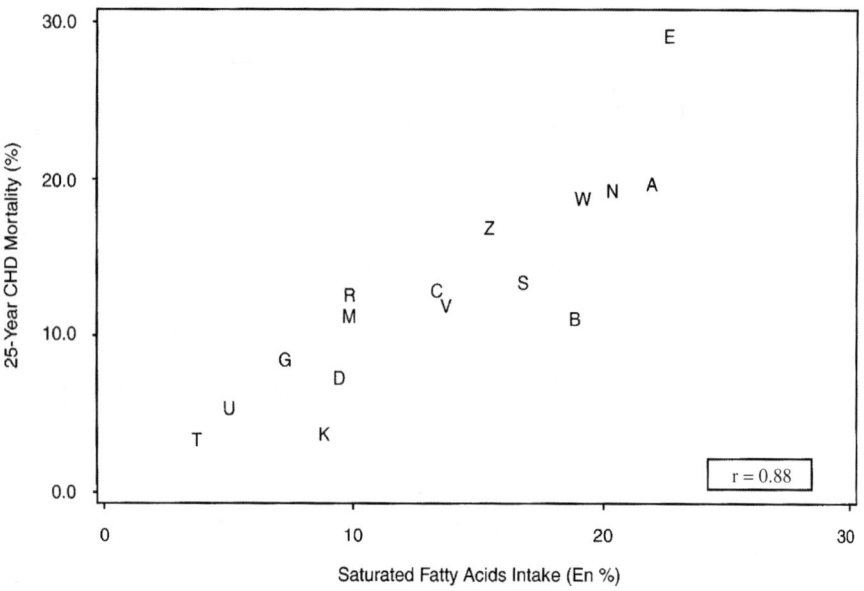

Figure 2.4. Association between average intake of total saturated fatty acids and 25-year coronary heart disease mortality, Seven Countries Study (*r* = 0.88, correlation coefficient; see text for key to alphabetic characters) (from Kromhout et al. (1995))

Similarly based on the 25-year mortality follow-up, the relationship between serum total cholesterol concentration and CHD mortality was present for the cohorts within groups defined by geographic area (Verschuren et al. 1995). Within each of six geographic areas, the multiple cohorts were pooled where applicable

(Fig. 2.5). Cholesterol distributions overlapped between Northern Europe and the United States, between the Mediterranean and inland Southern Europe, and between Serbia and Japan. In all areas except Japan, where cholesterol concentration was only rarely greater than 200 mg/dl, an upward gradient of mortality was evident in relation to cholesterol concentration. But within each of these three pairs of areas having similar ranges of cholesterol concentration, the first-mentioned had somewhat greater mortality. Overall, a three- to four-fold range of mortality was found at any given level of cholesterol concentration. In general, the higher the range of values in the cholesterol distribution, the steeper was the mortality gradient. These observations support the role of serum total cholesterol in explaining population differences in CHD mortality. They also indicate that, at any given cholesterol level in a population, additional factors are needed to explain the observed mortality.

From the 10-year report, two other factors were clearly related to population differences in CHD mortality (Keys 1980). Median systolic blood pressure ranged from approximately 128 to 146 mmHg, and mortality varied from 0 to nearly 70 per 1000 men in 10 years (Fig. 2.6). The regression analysis supported the investigators' prediction that systolic blood pressure would be an important influence on differences in coronary mortality between populations.

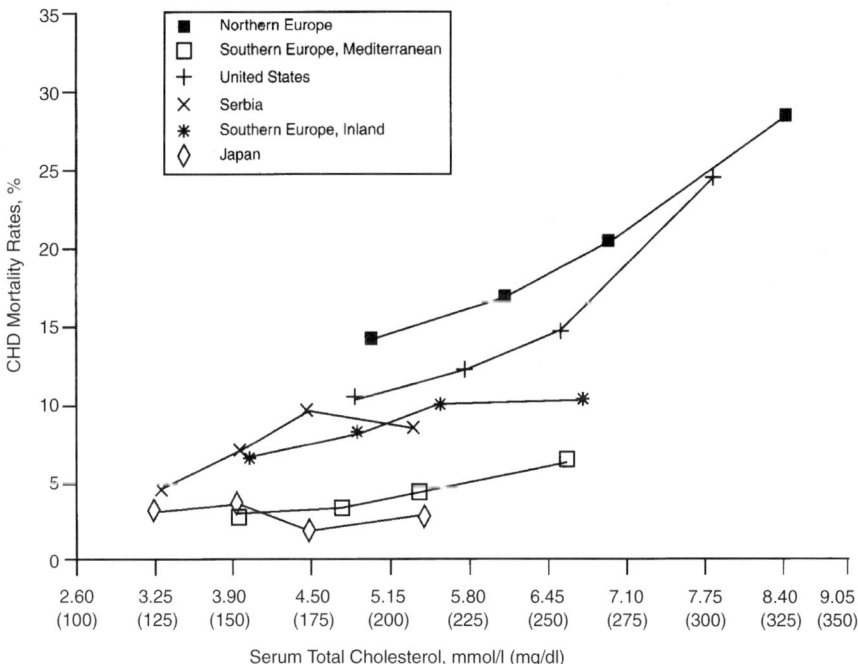

Figure 2.5. Twenty-five year coronary death and quartiles of serum cholesterol concentration, adjusted for age, cigarette smoking, and systolic blood pressure, Seven Countries Study (from Verschuren et al. (1995))

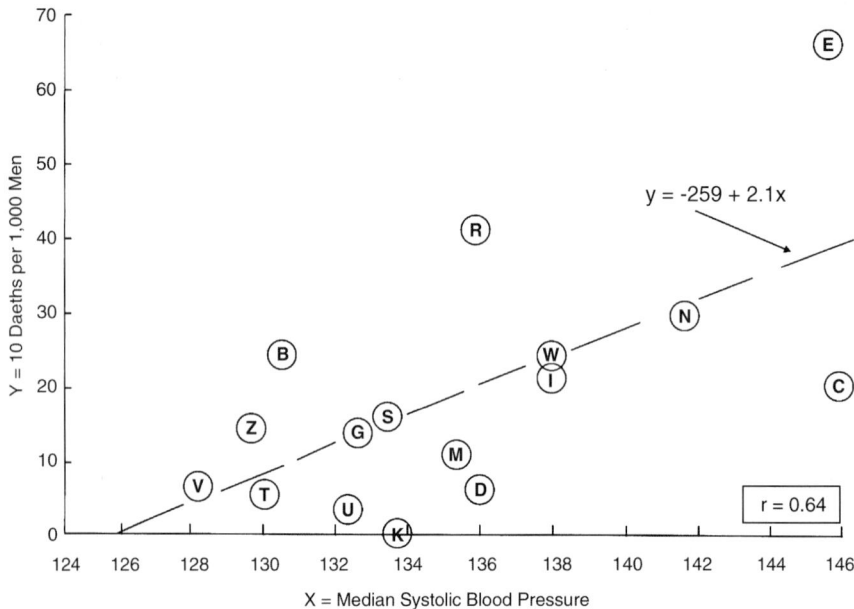

Figure 2.6. Ten-year mortality in relation to median levels of systolic blood pressure, Seven Countries Study ($r = 0.64$, correlation coefficient; $y = -259 + 2.1x$, regression equation for mortality on systolic blood pressure; see text following Fig. 2.4 for key to alphabetic characters) (from Keys (1980))

"Cigarette habit" (smoking) was examined in a manner analogous to that for cholesterol concentration, after grouping cohorts by three geographic areas (Fig. 2.7). Smoking appeared related to mortality differences both within and among these designated regions. That is (as for the other factors), event rates differed both among cohorts within a region, by level of smoking, and among regions at any given level of smoking. Smoking was quantitatively related to event rates in every region and was most strongly related in the region with the highest rates, Northern Europe.

In addition to the landmark Seven Countries Study, two other studies on population differences in CVD rates added especially to this research. First was the Ni-Hon-San Study (NI-Nippon, HON-Honolulu, SAN-San Francisco), a comparison of men of Japanese ancestry among three population settings: migrants to the mainland United States living in the San Francisco Bay Area, migrants to Honolulu, Hawaii, and non-migrants still living in Hiroshima, Japan (Worth et al. 1975; Kagan and Yano 1996). Stimulated by the differences in CHD and stroke mortality among these three groups that were reported by Gordon (1957), the Ni-Hon-San Study sought to determine whether these differences were reflected in variation in disease prevalence in the three areas and could be accounted for by differences in risk factors.

The most extensive comparisons were made on the basis of long-term follow-up of the Hawaii cohort (through the Honolulu Heart Program) and the Japan

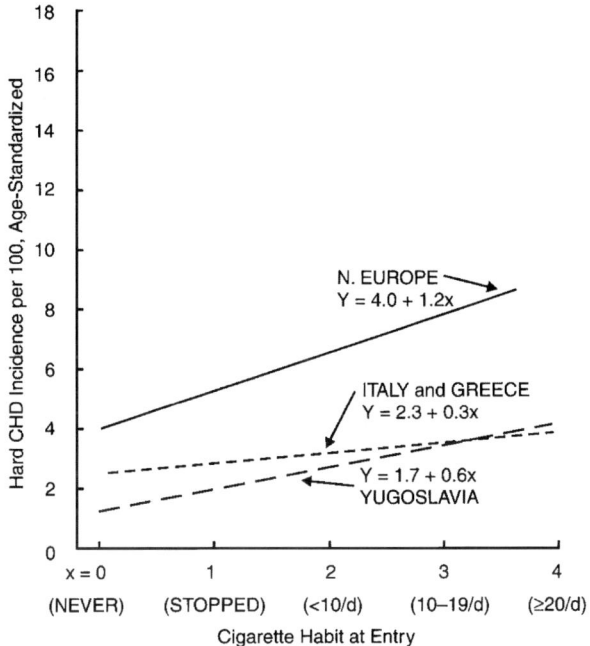

Figure 2.7. Ten-year incidence of "hard" coronary heart disease by smoking class, Seven Countries Study (regression lines and their corresponding equations are given for each of three regions based on combined cohorts within the respective geographic areas) (from Keys (1980))

cohort (through the Radiation Effects Research Foundation). In general, predicted differences among the three populations in relative frequency of CHD (lowest in Japan and higher in Hawaii and California) and stroke (highest in Japan and lower in Hawaii and California) were confirmed. Risk factor differences partly explained these differences. Among the most important findings of the Ni-Hon-San Study was confirmation that these three groups differed in CVD occurrence in association with the broad environmental changes attendant on migration – differences not attributable to change in population genetics.

The second further example is that of the WHO MONICA Project (World Health Organization MONICA Project 1988; Tunstall-Pedoe 2003). This extensive study was undertaken in 38 geographically defined populations in 21 countries. Study areas were predominantly in Europe but also included Australia, New Zealand, China, and the United States. The study aim was to investigate the separate associations between 10-year trends in survival and in coronary event rates to changes in CHD mortality and the contributions to these associations from changes in risk factors and coronary care from the mid-1980s to the mid-1990s. Through development and implementation of detailed protocols for all aspects of data collection, centralized data management, and quality control procedures, the study aim was accomplished and the main results were reported in 1999 and 2000.

First, decreases in both incidence and case fatality contributed to observed declines in CHD mortality. The contribution of decreased incidence was twice that of decreased case fatality (Tunstall-Pedoe et al. 1999). Second, the relationship of trends in population-level risk factors to corresponding CHD event rates appeared weaker than anticipated, possibly because of difficulties of measurement and analytic issues, including the appropriate time lag to be used between trends in risk factors and events (Kuulasmaa et al. 2000). Were this study the only basis for identifying major CVD risk factors, it would have failed in this respect; but in view of the limitations of the design for such a purpose (recalling the combined limitations of a composite study design discussed above) these results do not lead to a conclusion that other, unmeasured factors must be invoked to explain the disease event trends. Third, changes in both acute and post-event coronary care contributed strongly to decreased rates of coronary end-points (Tunstall-Pedoe et al. 2000).

Taken together, these three observations indicate that measurable changes in CHD incidence, case fatality, and mortality can occur within a decade in widely diverse populations; the most readily demonstrable impact on decreasing event rates is treatment of cases; and risk factor improvements, while associated with benefit in these populations, were more difficult to evaluate partly because of inherent limitations of the study. Reduced mortality was dependent foremost on reduced incidence of events. Also deserving mention are the further contributions of the WHO MONICA Project to development of current standardized methods for population-base surveillance for CHD and stroke events, risk factors, and treatment and in training local teams for the needed work.

Individual Differences

In contrast to between-population differences, addressing differences in CVD risk at the individual level required long-term studies in which large numbers of individual study participants could be examined at a common starting point in time and observed over several years to determine whether and when each person might develop detectable CVD. Which baseline characteristics were predictive of CVD events could then be assessed through appropriate statistical analysis. Among the earliest and best-known examples of this type of epidemiologic approach is the Framingham Study, whose purpose and design were reported more than 50 years ago (Dawber et al. 1951). That report is instructive about the limited knowledge at the time for planning the study design with respect to sample size, follow-up time, and many other aspects. The impact of the study belies its restriction to one small community in the northeastern United States, with only 5200 participants drawn both from a probability sample of residents and additional volunteers. Nonetheless, the intensive biennial examination schedule, long-term continuity of follow-up and investigator involvement, and incorporation of new design components over its decades-long history have made this a uniquely rich source of data on individual risks of CVD events.

A landmark report of the Framingham Study, based on the first 6 years of follow-up, identified serum cholesterol concentration, blood pressure, and electrocardiographic evidence of left ventricular hypertrophy as predictors of CHD development, as assessed through records of death or hospitalization or changes in electrocardiographic findings at biennial follow-up examinations (Kannel et al. 1961). It was in this report that the Framingham Study investigators introduced the term "risk factor" to describe such predictive characteristics.

Concurrent U.S. studies in CVD epidemiology included several community- or work-site-based cohort studies with designs and methods similar to those of the Framingham Study. These similarities allowed combining the studies in order to estimate more precisely, based on much larger numbers of events, the relationships between selected baseline characteristics and incident CHD events. Thus the U.S. National Cooperative Pooling Project was conceived, combining into a single data set the experience of five studies (Albany Civil Servants, Chicago Gas Company, Chicago Western Electric Company, Framingham, and Tecumseh, Michigan) (Pooling Project Research Group 1978). Altogether 8422 men aged 40–64 years and free of CHD at entry were followed for an average of 8.6 years, providing 72,011 person-years of observation and 658 first major coronary events. New statistical methods, the multivariate regression analysis of Truett et al. (1967), were devised to examine multiple baseline characteristics in relation to outcomes. This analysis demonstrated the joint predictive relationship of serum cholesterol concentration, diastolic blood pressure, and cigarette smoking to incidence of CHD and, in the conclusions of the 1978 report, established that these were unequivocal causal factors. According to the derived multivariate model, the highest risk quintile group experienced more than a six-fold risk relative to that of the lowest-risk quintile group.

Concurrent community- or work-site-based population studies were undertaken in the United States, the United Kingdom, Europe, and Japan (where the primary interest was in stroke). Often these studies laid the foundation for long-term follow-up, even to the present, by re-examination of surviving participants or through death notification or other indirect procedures. Some cohorts of the Seven Countries Study continue to be followed today.

This review of risk factors and determinants is of course not exhaustive of all factors that could be discussed. Also to be noted are glucose intolerance, insulin resistance and diabetes, obesity, alcohol consumption, antioxidants, hemostatic factors, hyperhomocysteinemia, vascular and endothelial factors, genetic factors, and others. Sex, race/ethnicity, income and education are further dimensions of variation in CVD experience (Labarthe 1998). This review has emphasized those factors that have the longest history of investigation, most extensive body of supporting evidence, and most immediate applicability for prevention, to which we turn in the section that follows.

2.5   **Causation and Prevention**

2.5.1   Overview

Together with countless other studies, observational epidemiologic research has identified a plethora of factors possibly associated with the development of CVD. Some of the findings were first identified decades ago and were replicated in multiple subsequent studies, and others were only recently reported or were isolated findings. The former are generally regarded as 'established' (or sometimes 'traditional') and the latter as 'emerging' risk factors. As early as 1981, it was reported that 246 CVD risk factors had been described in the literature, each meeting the criterion of a reported p-value of < 0.05 in at least one study (Hopkins and Williams 1981). With all the research conducted since then, including many epidemiologic studies addressing pathogenetic mechanisms and elements of physiologic or metabolic regulatory systems, the number of qualifying factors has surely increased several-fold. Which of these are causal factors, and which offer practical means of prevention?

Several points may be useful in thinking about these questions before considering examples of causal models in CVD epidemiology or concepts of CVD prevention (see also Chap. III.11 of this handbook) and the role of trials:

— Identifying causes on the basis of associations found in observational epidemiologic studies generally rests on the outcome of what might be termed a 'differential diagnosis of causation': (1) critical assessment identifies flaws, bias, or confounding that may underlie a spurious association (cf. Chaps. I.9 and I.13 of this handbook); (2) statistical assessment addresses the potential role of random variation that may produce a chance association; and (3) consideration of several properties of the evidence (for example, greater strength of association, consistency of the finding across multiple studies, and specificity, among other considerations) may increase confidence that an association is causal. Application of these considerations is illustrated by the Pooling Project report with respect to serum cholesterol concentration, diastolic blood pressure, and smoking (Pooling Project Research Group 1978).

— Such differential diagnosis of causation is not always applied, however, and how many of the 246 factors listed by Hopkins and Williams might have passed this more stringent procedure, then or now, is unknown. Even the first reported use of the term "risk factor" noted that evidence was insufficient to conclude that the associations described were causal and that further study was needed (Kannel et al. 1961). Thus it would be inappropriate to interpret references to "risk factors" throughout the literature of CVD epidemiology as necessarily meaning "causal factors" in the strict sense suggested above.

— Experimental evidence is sometimes regarded as indispensable in establishing a causal role for a risk factor, but recent experience with hormonal replacement therapy (found protective against CHD in women in observational studies but ineffective or harmful in prevention trials) heightens caution in this regard.

The contribution of experimental studies of intervention in humans to understanding causation is indirect, however, because rather than introducing exposure to a suspected causal factor, such experiments test interventions to remove or reduce that exposure. Further, because exposure has been present for some time and its reduction or removal requires a new exposure (that of the intervention), the outcome is not necessarily equivalent to absence of the exposure of interest in the first place.

Illustrations

Variations on Causal Models

Beyond differences in procedures for reaching conclusions about causation, differences in concepts or models of causation must also be recognized. These can be appreciated, and causation of CVD can be better understood, by considering several contrasts: One cause, or many? One outcome, or many? Immediate causes, or "fundamental causes"? All causes, or only a few? Causes of cases, or causes of incidence? Each of these contrasts can be illustrated briefly as follows:

One Cause or Many?   Conditions such as CHD and stroke are generally accepted to be consequences of multiple factors acting in concert ("multifactorial causation"). Admitting multiple risk factors, however, may deny credibility to any one of them (McCormick and Skrbanek 1988; Stehbens 1992). This view stems from the ancient concept of one "necessary and sufficient cause" as the whole explanation of a phenomenon. This concept was generally abandoned for the chronic diseases during the 1950s and 1960s in the effort to explain the consistently incomplete conjunction of any one exposure and disease. That is, exposure and disease overlap when they are causally related, but neither does every case result from the same exposure nor does exposure uniformly produce the same disease. Models of CVD causation have advanced by taking into account the multivariate setting, in which single causal factors operating together tend to multiply risk above that attributable to the sum of effects of the individual factors. As a result, multivariate risk scores have been calculated for use both as the outcome variable in intervention studies and as a tool for assessing risk of a future CVD event as a basis for deciding whether treatment is warranted (Farquhar et al. 1990; De Backer et al. 2003). Currently the multifactorial view strongly prevails.

One Outcome or Many?   A theme of CVD epidemiology in its early years, rediscovered only recently, was that increased susceptibility resulting from any social factor should be expected to be non-specific in its disease expression. Therefore factors increasing the risk of CHD should be studied as factors in illness generally and not for CHD alone. In this view, causes could have quite varied outcomes, so that a causal model specific to one disease outcome must be inherently incomplete and therefore subject to misinterpretation or misunderstanding. Echoing this theme, Stallones (1980) argued that models of causation that converge on a single disease outcome should be superseded by considering "the interdependence of a number of diseases, characteristics of individuals, and environmental and social variables as elements in a constellation which is n-dimensional" (p 76). The tendency to focus on single diseases, even specific ones within the array of CVD, tends to predominate in current epidemiological thinking. However, wider appreciation of the "n-dimensional" constellation of elements in a causal framework may follow from the recent resurgence of concepts of "social determinants of health" and "population health".

Immediate Causes or "Fundamental Causes"?   Here the argument is that a focus on immediate or proximal causes of disease, and interventions to mitigate their effects, is inherently flawed. For example, high blood pressure may be causally associated with rates and risks of stroke, but to concentrate public health efforts on detection and control of high blood pressure is to miss the greater public health need. This need is to address population characteristics such as poverty, illiteracy, unemployment, and other social ills that would diminish health and well-being by countless other mechanisms, even if high blood pressure were completely removed as a public health problem. The differential diagnosis of causation includes specificity of an association as one consideration, in the sense that an association which uniquely links a particular exposure with a particular disease may more reasonably be thought causal than one in which both the exposure and the disease are related to multiple other conditions. The "fundamental causes" are in principle non-specific and partly for that reason fail to satisfy narrower, more immediate, and disease-specific concepts of "cause".

All Causes or Only a Few?   The all-inclusive view of CVD causes recognizes that innumerable factors influence risk, some in adverse and others in protective ways. This view finds excitement in the "emerging risk factors" whose novelty and interest reinforce confidence in the advances of science and the sense of being at the leading edge. In this view, CVD epidemiology may be at the threshold of an era of unprecedented discovery with the advent of population genomics. One causal model for CHD portrays, in one tier, simply "genes"; an indefinitely large array of individual genes is linked through multiple connections from the first to the second tier, a "network of intermediate traits" (hemostasis, lipid metabolism, carbohydrate metabolism, and blood pressure regulation); and these four traits converge to act on the third tier, the "probability of CHD", which is represented graphically as a surface that represents age and environment (Sing et al. 1992). The biological complexity depicted by this scheme represents a rich body of knowledge whose growth is almost inevitable as science advances at all three levels and the connections between them are continually elaborated. And this represents only the convergence of factors on one outcome, not the "n-dimensional array" conceived by Stallones (1980).

The "only a few" point of view focuses on only those factors regarded as useful for widespread intervention to arrest and reverse the CVD epidemic around the world. Those few factors, variously termed the major or established or traditional risk factors, consistently include blood lipids, blood pressure, and smoking. Stamler (1992) identifies four factors: "... 'rich' diet, diet-related above-optimal levels of serum total cholesterol (TC) and blood pressure (BP), and cigarette smoking". He explains (p 36):

> All four of these risk factors are designated *established* because substantial amounts of data from many disciplines have demonstrated their significant role in the aetiology of epidemic CHD. They are designated *major* for three reasons: their high prevalence in populations, particularly in Western industrialized countries, their strong impact on coronary risk, and their preventability and reversibility, primarily by safe improvements in population life-styles, from early childhood on. (Age and male gender are known risk factors, but are not amenable to influence and hence are not designated major; diabetes is a known risk factor, but of lower prevalence than cigarette smoking and elevated TC and BP in most populations, and hence is not designated major.) … 'Rich' diet is pivotal among these four – the primary and essential cause of the coronary epidemic.

These two views, all versus few, are commonly seen as conflicting. From the "all" point of view, the "few" perspective ignores evidence for many new and emerging factors and fails to see the potential of genetic epidemiology, for example, to provide invaluable and perhaps radically new insights about causation and prevention of CVD. On the other hand, from the "few" perspective, preoccupation with these factors is a significant and unwelcome distraction from the needed focus on applying knowledge of the major risk factors and research to make that application as effective as possible for prevention. Perhaps from the perspective of "fundamental causes" this polarity of views is irrelevant, as the main issues are the broadest social determinants of health and quality of life, of which CVD is only one aspect.

A resolution of these seemingly conflicting views is found in the point made by Stallones (1980), who suggested that models of causation depend for their value on their utility, and that utility depends in turn on the purpose for which a model is used. If the dual purposes of intellectual pursuit and public health practice are accepted as complementary in CVD epidemiology and prevention, the views of "all" and "few" can both be embraced. "Epidemiology and public health have the luxury as well as the necessity of entertaining both views of causation in pursuit of the complementary purposes of advancing knowledge and serving the health of the public" (Labarthe 1998, p 463).

Causes of Cases or Causes of Incidence? This last contrast addresses a distinction between two kinds of causal questions posed by Rose (1985) (p 33):

> The first seeks the causes of cases, and the second seeks the causes of incidence. "Why do some individuals have hypertension?" is a quite different question from "Why do some populations have much hypertension, whilst in others it is rare?" The questions require different kinds of study, and they have different answers.

The distinction emphasizes that what appear to be causal factors (from studies of individual risks within populations) may instead be only markers of susceptibility to true causal factors to which exposure is very common throughout the population, and that detection of true causal factors requires comparison of populations with different incidence rates to identify the determinants of those differences. As with each of the preceding contrasts, this distinction relates closely to concepts of prevention and has direct implications for thinking about individual and population-wide levels of intervention.

Concepts of CVD Prevention and the Role of Trials

As the foundation of epidemiologic knowledge about CVD expanded, recommended approaches to CVD prevention evolved correspondingly. For example, under the aegis of the former WHO Cardiovascular Disease Unit, expert meetings were convened on many occasions from the 1960s through the mid-1990s to address CHD prevention, primary prevention of hypertension, prevention in childhood and youth of adult CVD, and other topics. Official recommendations and intervention guidelines have been developed by such national organizations as the American Heart Association and American College of Cardiology, and the U.S. National Heart, Lung, and Blood Institute and at a regional level by such joint efforts as those of the European Society of Cardiology, the European Atherosclerosis Society, and the European Society of Hypertension.

Concepts of prevention reflected in these many recommendations and guidelines often embrace two broad approaches articulated in the early 1980s by Rose (1981) – the individual (or high-risk) approach and the population-wide approach. The first approach addresses reduction of risk for cardiovascular events among persons with already manifest CVD or risk factors, and the second addresses risk factor reduction across the whole population. These two approaches are complementary. "The 'high-risk' strategy of prevention is an interim expedient, needed in order to protect susceptible individuals, but only for so long as the underlying causes of incidence remain unknown or uncontrollable; if causes can be removed, susceptibility ceases to matter" (Rose 1981, p 38).

The high-risk approach has been considerably refined so as to identify, on the basis of multiple factors (such as sex, current smoking, age, systolic blood pressure, and total cholesterol concentration) persons whose combined risk characteristics predict a specified probability of a major cardiovascular event within the ensuing 10 years (De Backer et al. 2003). Based on such scoring, policy decisions are made regarding which intervention will be recommended and perhaps financed for which risk levels. The population-wide approach has evolved to include not only interventions to shift unfavorable distributions of the major risk factors across the whole population, but also prevention of adverse levels and distributions of these risk factors in the first place, wherever this might be possible. This latter concept of "primordial prevention" contemplates prevention of risk factor epidemics themselves as an essential approach to CVD prevention, especially in developing countries (Strasser 1978).

The high-risk approach to risk reduction as conceived by Rose (1981) would today encompass both secondary prevention (applied to individuals already manifesting CHD or stroke) and primary prevention (applied to individuals at high risk but without manifest CVD). The population-wide approach to risk reduction would consist of that part of primary prevention applied to the population as a whole; it may be complemented by prevention of risk factors in the first place (primordial prevention). In relation to the intervention approaches represented in Fig. 2.1, the high-risk approach extends from risk factor detection and control through end-of-life care, all at the individual level. The population-wide approach extends, in turn, from policy and environmental change through behavior change, at the population level. For completeness, "health promotion" can be regarded generally as coextensive with the population-wide approach, in contrast to the high-risk approach to individuals.

Epidemiologic evidence for causation of CVD has come primarily from observational studies and has sometimes been supported indirectly by experimental studies in which exposure to suspected factors has been reduced by intervention. The balance of evidence for causation is heavily weighted toward observational studies. How is evidence for CVD prevention obtained? Evidence from observational studies may be considered sufficient to establish causation, but different requirements are often, perhaps typically, applied to prevention – primarily experimental evidence of the efficacy and safety of a proposed intervention.

This question thus calls attention to the role of trials or, more broadly, intervention studies. These studies encompass a wide variety of study questions and designs and include clinical trials of secondary or primary prevention, population-based trials of primary prevention or health promotion, and community demonstrations of intervention that may include combinations of health promotion, primary prevention, and secondary prevention. It is beyond the scope of this review to detail the evidence for prevention; such commentaries are available elsewhere (Blackburn 1992; Labarthe 1998). For a general discussion we also refer to Chap. III.11 of this handbook. It is useful, however, to summarize briefly the general types of intervention studies on which CVD prevention is based:

— The great preponderance of experimental studies in CVD prevention have been *clinical trials in secondary prevention*. These are designed to test the efficacy and safety of individual-level interventions to prevent recurrent CVD events or related outcomes among survivors of first events or persons otherwise known to have pre-existing CVD. The typical multicenter organization of such trials, the recruitment and enrollment of hundreds or thousands of participants, and the multi-year periods of follow-up combine to make these studies epidemiologic in scale, even though they may be altogether clinically based and not referable to any definable population beyond the participating institutions.

— *Primary prevention trials* are designed to test the efficacy and safety of individual-level interventions, but the participants are initially free of known CVD. The outcome is usually the first qualifying CVD event, be it an acute coronary event, stroke, or other defined outcome, depending on the question under study. For example, in studies of primary prevention of high blood pressure, progression of blood pressure levels may be the outcome of interest. Study participants may be identified in clinical settings or drawn from defined communities, as volunteers or through systematic sampling, such as from work sites or geographic residential areas. Eligible participants must be apparently well, so only interventions relatively free of known adverse effects or other impediments to long-term adherence to study treatment guidelines are good candidates for evaluation. Because participants' average risk of CVD outcomes is relatively lower in primary than in secondary prevention trials, thousands of participants and follow-up periods of several years are typically needed to observe a sufficient number of outcomes for satisfactory analysis.

— *Community trials* in CVD prevention are used to study intervention in whole populations defined by geographical area of residence, place of work, or otherwise. If insufficient numbers of study units such as schools or factories are involved to permit true random allocation, as is usually the case, the term "quasi-experimental study" is sometimes used. Systematic comparison among similar communities with and without intervention is still implied, even if the number of intervention and comparison units is small. Fatal or non-fatal CVD events could be the primary end point in such trials, but these studies are often designed to address risk factor or behavioral outcomes instead. The choice of interventions shares the same considerations as described for primary prevention trials.

— A *community demonstration* of intervention represents a distinct shade of meaning from "community trials" in that intervention may be implemented in a single community, with or without a control community for comparison. Community demonstrations may combine multiple intervention strategies into a secondary and primary prevention program to influence individuals' practices as well as community-wide aspects whose target is the population as a whole. Evaluating the impact of such an intervention may be based on CVD events, but practical constraints often arise. Evaluation may therefore be limited to the procedures by which the intervention was delivered and such proximate outcomes as changes in behavior or risk factor levels.

Analogous to the question of causation in epidemiologic studies is the question of whether a given intervention actually produces the intended outcome. The most convincing evidence comes from well-designed and properly conducted randomized trials; however, population-wide public health interventions may only rarely be amenable to evaluation through trials of this kind. This circumstance leads to the seeming dilemma of holding population-wide interventions to a standard of evidence that can rarely, if ever, be attained in practice and therefore giving rise to the perception that population-wide interventions are only rarely, if ever, scientifically justified. However, the essence of the question for a proposed public health intervention is whether it is better supported by all the relevant scientific evidence than is the status quo, as represented by current conditions or policies. If so, intervention would be appropriate if other due considerations were met, and rigorous evaluation of the intervention's effect once implemented could provide further evidence as to its benefit, cost-effectiveness, and long-term feasibility.

Among a great many potential examples of intervention studies, one with broad implications for prevention policy is especially convenient for illustration. The North Karelia Project provides a classic example; detailed published accounts of its organization, design, implementation, and evaluation are provided elsewhere (Vartiainen et al. 1994; Puska et al. 1998; Puska 2002).

As shown in Fig. 2.2, Finnish men experienced exceptionally high CHD mortality that had increased sharply in the 1950s. Since 1959, studies in East and West Finland as part of the Seven Countries Study had documented the problem in some detail and confirmed the highest CHD rates to be in Eastern Finland. Concern about this led to implementation in 1972 of a multifaceted community-based prevention project in which North Karelia (population 210,000) and Kuopio (population 250,000), both in Eastern Finland, would be intervention and control communities, respectively. Among the many components of the project were programs targeting high blood cholesterol concentration, high blood pressure, and smoking. Extensive community involvement and engagement with health services were major aspects of these programs. Risk factor distributions and other characteristics in both communities were assessed by sample surveys among adults aged 30–59 years in 1972 and every five years until 1992, and mortality was monitored from 1969 through 1992.

Twenty-year changes in risk factors for women included reductions in cholesterol concentration by 18% and in diastolic blood pressure by 13%, while smoking increased from 11 to 25%. Corresponding changes for men were reductions of 13% and 9%, and a decrease in smoking from 53 to 37%. Changes in dietary habits and physical activity underlying the change in risk factor distributions have also been described.

Changes in CHD mortality were predicted from the actual risk factor distributions observed in the serial cross-sectional surveys. These results are displayed in Fig. 2.8 for women and Fig. 2.9 for men. The predicted mortality effects of change in each risk factor separately and together are shown in each figure, as well as the observed decrease in mortality (by 68% for women and 55% for men) which closely paralleled but actually exceeded the cumulative predicted changes.

What was the contribution of intervention to these changes? Changes in risk factors were greater in the intervention area, North Karelia, than in the control area, Kuopio, only in the first five years; thereafter they were similar. Change in mortality was not limited to the study areas: overall, in the whole of Finland, CHD mortality declined by 50% from 1970 to 1992 and stroke mortality declined markedly. Interpretation of the effect of intervention in North Karelia is conditioned by the study design (comparison of two selected communities and not a randomized trial in a large number of communities), but the investigators addressed these issues and supported the conclusion that the mortality decline was a direct consequence of

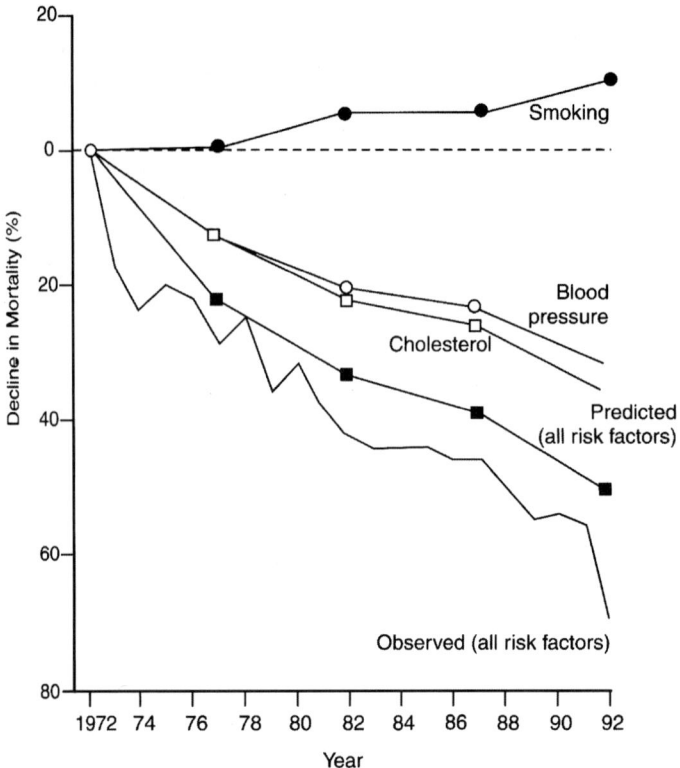

Figure 2.8. Observed and predicted decline in mortality from ischemic heart disease in women aged 35–64 in Finland (from Vartiainen et al. (1994))

the risk factor changes (Vartianinen et al. 1994; Puska et al. 1998). That the project began to influence policy nationwide after its first five years probably accounts for the broader evidence of risk factor and mortality change in Finland as a whole that has continued to the present and makes it difficult to isolate the intervention effects to North Karelia alone. It was recognized that improvements in treatment of coronary events could also have contributed, a factor that would be evaluated further with Finland's participation in the WHO MONICA Project.

From the perspective advanced by Rose (1981), the Finnish experience supports the view that the major determinants of incidence have been identified, and population-wide efforts to modify these determinants have made it possible to prevent the mass occurrence of CVD in whole populations. At the broadest level of community change and population-wide intervention, coupled with health care system interventions to improve services for risk factor detection and control, the North Karelia Project is a powerful demonstration of the potential for an integrated, coordinated, and sustained public health effort to affect the major cardiovascular conditions of our time, CHD and stroke.

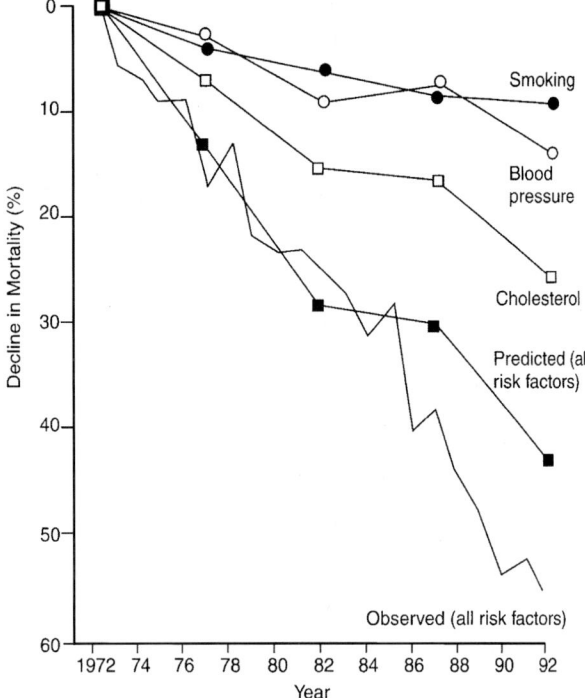

Figure 2.9. Observed and predicted decline in mortality from ischemic heart disease in men aged 35–64 in Finland (from Vartiainen et al. (1994))

Conclusions

Several of the topics introduced in this chapter in a historical context can be revisited from a current perspective and with a view to the future.

Childhood and Adolescence/Maternal and Fetal Influences. Atherosclerosis begins in childhood and youth and the major risk factors – high cholesterol concentration, high blood pressure and smoking – contribute beginning from adolescence or earlier (Berenson 1986; Mahoney et al. 1991). Yet this knowledge has failed to stimulate the needed programs on a sufficient scale to avert development of risk factors and subclinical disease in the whole population. Guidelines to address CVD risk factors in early life have been published repeatedly, but few large-scale programs have been mounted to assess the impact of the recommended interventions. The need for such programs to advance policy development in CVD prevention seems clear, and research in this area – beginning with implementation and evaluation of currently available approaches – is a high priority. The question of how important maternal and fetal influences are on development of CVD, from risk factors levels in childhood to overt CVD in adults, continues to be debated (Barker 1992, 1998). In view of the potential impact on health generally as well as CVD in particular, resolving this question by conducting trials of optimum nutritional and other supportive maternal care, coupled with postnatal nutrition to evaluate benefits on metabolic and physiologic mechanisms involved in later risk factor development, is important.

Genomics/Population Genetics.   The current level of investment in research on genomics and CVD is partly based on expectations of findings that will revolutionize CVD prevention and treatment. It is important to appreciate the contemplated results of this research and to anticipate the need for epidemiologic assessment of its findings as they pertain to public health applications. At the same time, balance among CVD research priorities is needed. Real progress in applying what is already known about means of CVD prevention will require a major increase in support for prevention research, including especially systematic evaluation of programs implemented in other countries today on a scale proportionate to the North Karelia Project in the 1970s.

Research Capacity.   The need for applied research in CVD epidemiology far exceeds current capacity. This is due in part to the persistence of CVD as leading cause of death throughout the world and forecasts for its continuation in this position at least through the next two decades. Training and engagement in substantial epidemiologic research projects and programs, as well as ongoing and expanding activities in monitoring and surveillance, are essential for building this capacity. A model program for such training is illustrated by the International Ten-Day Teaching Seminars on Epidemiology and Prevention of Cardiovascular Diseases, a program now in its 37th year and sponsored principally by the WHF (Labarthe et al. 1998). Other international training programs (such as that conducted in developing countries under the auspices of the Department of Social and Preventive Medicine, University of Lausanne) offer additional models, all of which should be replicated many times over to reach much-increased numbers of health professionals. It is of course also necessary to develop funded research to provide settings where trained epidemiologists and others in CVD prevention can do the needed work, extend their skills, and provide mentorship and training to others.

Organizational Arrangements.   The role of supporting organizations and agencies in CVD epidemiology and prevention has been critical in the past and may be even more so in the immediate future. WHO, WHF, the World Bank, the Global Forum for Health Research, and other agencies with global reach are essential partners for the kind of network cited by WHO Director-General Brundtland in her proposed global strategy for NCD prevention and control (WHO 1999). National organizations in many countries are also important. In the United States, for example, the National Center for Chronic Disease Prevention and Health Promotion of the Centers for Disease Control and Prevention, Department of Health and Human Services, is committed to global health efforts. This interest is an integral part of *A Public Health Action Plan to Prevent Heart Disease and Stroke* (US Department of Health and Human Services 2003), which provides for regional and global partnerships in cardiovascular health in pursuit of common aims and in the expectation of mutual gain from sharing information and experience.

Developing Countries. The so-called "impending epidemic" of CVD in developing countries is already present and well-established, resulting in many countries in a "double burden" in the presence of the continuing health problems of an earlier era. The world has been slow to awaken to this reality, although for two decades or more WHO and, more recently the World Bank and other organizations, have been calling attention to the need for action. The economies in transition must be included in this call if the adverse trends in mortality in these countries are to be addressed. Efforts of the Global Forum for Health Research and its Initiative for Cardiovascular Health Research in Developing Countries require support if these activities will achieve their goals and contribute in meeting the global challenge of CVD.

Global Strategies. CVD shares with other "non-communicable diseases" the paradoxical aspect of being strongly influenced from communication of culture, lifestyles and behavior that contribute to the development of risk as a population-wide phenomenon. Global concern about tobacco control and success in adoption by the World Health Assembly of the Framework Convention on Tobacco Control in April 2003 illustrated recognition of this circumstance (WHO 2003). Through a series of conferences and published declarations, the International Heart Health Society has been a consistent advocate for global efforts to prevent CVD and to promote cardiovascular health (WHF et al. 2004). WHO has convened expert groups who have recommended that all countries develop policies and programs for CVD prevention and has proposed a global strategy for NCD prevention and control, including the launching of integrated efforts to address tobacco use, unhealthy diet, and physical inactivity (WHO Expert Committee 1990; WHO 1999). The call by WHO to strengthen a global network for NCD prevention and control as a major part of the global strategy gives national and multinational organizations and agencies a clear opportunity to collaborate. Understanding the global forces that influence the course of the CVD epidemic, monitoring their impact, and learning how to put their influence to work in the interest of cardiovascular health are pressing needs.

Societal Change. CVD epidemiology over the past half-century has established understanding of the causes of epidemic CHD and stroke as well as strategies to prevent these diseases. The challenge that lies immediately ahead is to apply this knowledge effectively to the benefit of the world's population. Societal change is needed to achieve the goals of longer, healthier life free of significant disability due to CVD and other major chronic conditions, and free of disparities in the occurrence of these conditions within and among countries. Societal change will occur regardless whether epidemiology and public health are considered, as change is a continuing – albeit sometimes fitful and unpredictable – process with its own powerful impetus from many sources. But change that is best will be informed and influenced by knowledge of consequences for CVD, and for health generally. Positive change can be accomplished best to the extent that epidemiologists and others who hold that knowledge contribute to the direction of this change.

References

Association of State and Territorial Directors of Health Promotion and Public Health Education (2001) Policy and environmental change: new directions for public health (executive summary). US Centers for Disease Control and Prevention, Atlanta

Barker DJP (ed) (1992) Fetal and infant origins of adult disease. BMJ Books, London

Barker DJP (1998) Mothers, babies and health in later life. Second edition. Churchill Livingston, Edinburgh

Berenson GS (1986) Causation of cardiovascular risk factors in children: perspectives on cardiovascular risk in early life. Raven, New York

Berenson GS, Wattigney WA, Tracy RE, Newman WP III, Srinivasan SR, Webber LS, Dalferes ER Jr, Strong JP (1992) Atherosclerosis of the aorta and coronary arteries and cardiovascular risk factors in persons ages 6 to 30 years and studied at necropsy (the Bogalusa Heart Study). Am J Cardiol 70:851–858

Blackburn H (1983) Physical activity and coronary heart disease: a brief update and population view (Part I). J Card Rehabil 3:101–111

Blackburn H (1992) Community programs in coronary heart disease prevention and health promotion: changing community behaviour. In: Marmot M, Elliott P (eds) Coronary heart disease epidemiology: from aetiology to public health. Oxford University Press, Oxford, UK, pp 495–514

Blackburn H (1995) On the trail of heart attacks in seven countries. The Country Press, Middleborough

Blackburn H, Keys A, Simonson E, Rautaharju P, Punsar S (1960) The electrocardiogram in population studies: a classification system. Circulation 21:1160–1175

Chockalingam A, Balaguer-Vintró I (eds) (1999) Impending global pandemic of cardiovascular diseases: challenges and opportunities for the prevention and control of cardiovascular diseases in developing countries and economies in transition. Prous Science, Barcelona

Committee on Diet and Health, Food and Nutrition Board, Commission on Life Sciences, National Research Council. Diet and Health (1989) Implications for Reducing Chronic Disease Risk. National Academy Press, Washington, DC

Dawber TR, Meadors GF, Moore FE Jr (1951) Epidemiological approaches to heart disease: the Framingham Study. Am J Public Health 41:279–286

De Backer G, Ambrosioni E, Borch-Johnsen K, Brotons C, Cifkova R, Dallongeville J, Ebrahim S, Faergeman O, Graham I, Mancia G, Cats VM, Orth-Gomér K, Perk J, Pyörälä K, Rodicio JL, Sans S, Sansoy V, Sechtem U, Siolber S, Thomsen T, Wood D (2003) Executive summary: European guidelines on cardiovascular disease prevention in clinical practice. Third Joint Task Force of European and Other Societies on Cardiovascular Disease Prevention in Clinical Practice. Eur Heart J 24:1601–1610

Farquhar JW, Fortmann SP, Flora JA, Taylor B, Haskell WL, Williams PT, Maccoby N, Wood PD (1990) Effects of community wide education on cardiovascular disease risk factors: the Stanford Five-City Project. JAMA 264:359–365

Freis ED (1990) Reminiscences of the Veterans Administration Trial of the Treatment of Hypertension. Hypertension 16:472–475

Goff DG, Howard G, Russell GB, Labarthe DR (2001) Birth cohort evidence of population influences on blood pressure in the United States, 1887–1994. Ann Epidemiol 11:271–279

Gordon T (1957) Mortality experience among the Japanese in the United States, Hawaii, and Japan. Public Health Rep 72:543–553

Holman RL, McGill HC, Strong JP, Geer JC (1958) The natural history of atherosclerosis. Am J Pathol 34:209–235

Hopkins PN, Williams RR (1981) A survey of 246 suggested coronary risk factors. Atherosclerosis 40:1–52

INTERSALT Study Co-operative Research Group (1986) An international co-operative study on the relation of blood pressure of electrolyte excretion in populations. I: Design and methods. Hypertension 4:781–787

Kagan A, Yano K (1996) Ni-Hon-San Study. In: Kagan A (ed) The Honolulu Heart Program: an epidemiological study of coronary heart disease and stroke. Harwood Academic, Amsterdam, pp 21–32

Kannel WB, Dawber TR, Kagan A, Revotskie N, Stokes J III (1961) Factors of risk in the development of coronary heart disease – six-year follow-up experience: the Framingham Study. Ann Intern Med 55:33–50

Keys A (1980) Seven Countries: a multivariate analysis of death and coronary heart disease. Harvard University Press, Cambridge, MA

Keys A (1983) From Naples to Seven Countries – a sentimental journey. Prog Biochem Pharmacol 19:1–30

Kromhout D, Menotti A, Blackburn H (1993) The Seven Countries Study: a scientific adventure in cardiovascular disease epidemiology. Brouwer Offset bv, Utrecht

Kromhout D, Menotti A, Bloemberg B, Aravanis C, Blackburn H, Buzina R, Dontas AS, Fidanza F, Giampaoli S, Jansen A, Karvonen M, Katan M, Nissinen A, Nedeljkovic S, Pekkanen J, Pekkarinen M, Punsar S, Räsänen L, Simic B, Toshima H (1995) Dietary saturated and trans fatty acids and cholesterol and 25-year mortality from coronary heart disease: the Seven Countries Study. Prev Med 24:308–315

Kuulasmaa K, Tunstall-Pedoe H, Dobson A, Fortmann S, Sans S, Tolonen H, Evans A, Ferrario M, Tuomilehto J for the WHO MONICA Project (2000) Estimation of contribution of changes in classic risk factors to trends in coronary-event rates across the WHO MONICA Project populations. Lancet 355:675–687

Labarthe DR (1998) Epidemiology and prevention of cardiovascular diseases: a global challenge. Aspen, Gaithersburg, MD

Labarthe DR, Khaw K-T, Thelle D, Poulter N (1998) The Ten Day International Teaching Seminars on Cardiovascular Epidemiology and Preventions: a 30-year perspective. CVD Prev 1:156–163

Mahoney LT, Lauer RM, Lee J, Clarke WR (1991) Factors affecting tracking of coronary heart disease risk factors in children: the Muscatine Study. Ann N Y Acad Sci 623:120–132

Malmros H (1950) The relation of nutrition – a statistical study on the effect of war-time on atherosclerosis, cardiosclerosis, tuberculosis and diabetes. Acta Med Scand (Suppl) 246:137–153

Marmot M, Elliott P (eds) (1992) Coronary heart disease epidemiology: from aetiology to public health. Oxford University Press, Oxford, UK

McCormick J, Skrbanek P (1988) Coronary heart disease is not preventable by population interventions. Lancet 2:839–841

Murray CJL, Lopez AD (eds) (1996) The global burden of disease: a comprehensive assessment of mortality and disability from diseases, injuries, and risk factors in 1990 and projected to 2020. Harvard School of Public Health, Boston

Olshansky SJ, Ault AB (1986) The fourth stage of the epidemiologic transition: the age of delayed degenerative diseases. Milbank Q 64:355–391

Omran AR (1971) The epidemiological transition: a theory of the epidemiology of population change. Milbank Q 49:509–538

Pathobiological Determinants of Atherosclerosis in Youth (PDAY) Research Group (1990) Relationship of atherosclerosis in young men to serum lipoprotein cholesterol concentrations and smoking. JAMA 264:3018–3024

Pearson TA, Jamison DT, Trejo-Gutierrez J (1993) Cardiovascular disease. In: Jamison DT, Mosley WH, Measham AR, Bobadilla JL (eds) Disease control priorities in developing countries. Oxford University Press, Oxford pp 577–594

Pooling Project Research Group (1978) Relationship of blood pressure, serum cholesterol, smoking habit, relative weight and ECG abnormalities to incidence of major coronary events: final report of the Pooling Project. J Chronic Dis 31:201–306

Poulter NR, Khaw KT, Hopwood BEC, Mugambi M, Peart WS, Rose G, Sever PS (1990) The Kenyan Luo Migration Study: observations on the initiation of a rise in blood pressure. BMJ 300:967–972

President's Council on Physical Fitness and Sports (1996) Physical activity and health: a report of the Surgeon General. National Center for Chronic Disease Prevention and Health Promotion, Centers for Disease Control and Prevention, US Dept of Health and Human Services, Atlanta

Puska P (2002) Successful prevention of non-communicable diseases: 25-year experiences with North Karelia Project in Finland. Public Health Med 4: 5–7

Puska P, Tuomilehto J, Nissinen A, Vartiainen E (eds) (1998) The North Karelia Project: 20 year results and experiences. National Public Health Institute, KTL, Helsinki

Rose G (1981) Strategy of prevention: lessons from cardiovascular disease. BM J 282:1847–1851

Rose G (1985) Sick individuals and sick populations. Int J Epidemiology 14:32–38

Rose GA, Blackburn H (1968) Cardiovascular survey methods. World Health Organization, Geneva

Rose G, Shipley M (1986) Plasma cholesterol concentration and death from coronary heart disease: 10 year results of the Whitehall Study. BMJ 293:306–307

Sing CF, Haviland MB, Templeton AR, Zerba KE, Reilly SL (1992) Biological complexity and strategies for finding DNA variations responsible for inter-individual variation in risk of a common chronic disease, coronary artery disease. Ann Med 24:539–547

Stallones RA (1980) To advance epidemiology. Annu Rev Public Health 1:69–82

Stamler J (1992) Established major risk factors. In: Marmot M, Elliott P (eds) Coronary heart disease epidemiology: from aetiology to public health. Oxford University Press, Oxford, UK, pp 35–66

Stehbens WE (1992) Causality in medical science with particular reference to heart disease and atherosclerosis. Perspect Biol Med 36:97–119

Strasser T (1978) Reflections on cardiovascular diseases. Interdisciplinary Sci Rev 3:225–230

Tejada C, Strong JP, Montenegro MR, Restrepo C, Solberg LA (1968) Distribution of coronary and aortic atherosclerosis by geographic location, race, and sex. Lab Invest 18:509–526

Thom TJ, Epstein FH, Feldman JJ, Leaverton PE, Wolz M (1992) Total mortality and mortality from heart disease, cancer and stroke from 1950 to 1987 in 27 countries: highlights of trends and their interrelationships among causes of death. NIH Publication 92-3088. National Heart, Lung and Blood Institute, National Institutes of Health, Public Health Service, US Dept of Health and Human Services, Bethesda, MD

Truett J, Cornfield J, Kannel E (1967) Multivariate analysis of the risk of coronary heart disease in Framingham. J Chronic Disease 20:511–524

Tunstall-Pedoe H (ed) (2003) MONICA monograph and multimedia source book. World Health Organization, Geneva

Tunstall-Pedoe H, Kuulasmaa K, Mähönen M, Tolonen H, Ruokokoski E, Amouyel P for the WHO MONICA Project (monitoring trends and deter-minants in cardiovascular disease) (1999) Contribution of trends in survival and coronary-event rates to changes in coronary heart disease mortality: 10-year results from 37 WHO MONICA Project populations. Lancet 353:1547–1557

Tunstall-Pedoe H, Vanuzzo D, Hobbs M, Mähönen M, Cepaitis Z, Kuiulasmaa K, Keil U, for the WHO MONICA Project (2000) Estimation of contribution of changes in coronary care to improving survival, event rates, and coronary heart disease mortality across the WHO MONICA Project populations. Lancet 355:688–700

US Department of Health and Human Services (2003) A public health action plan to prevent heart disease and stroke. Centers for Disease Control and Prevention, US Dept of Health and Human Services, Atlanta

Vartiainen E, Puska P, Pekkanen J, Tuomilehto J, Jousilahti P (1994) Changes in risk factors explain changes in mortality from ischemic heart disease in Finland. BMJ 309:23–27

Verschuren WMM, Jacobs DR, Bloemberg BPM, Kromhout D, Menotti A, Aravanis C, Blackburn H, Buzina R, Dontas AS, Fidanza F, Karvonen MJ, Nedeljković S, Nissinen A, Toshima H (1995) Serum total cholesterol and long-term coronary heart disease mortality in different cultures: twenty-five year follow-up of the Seven Countries Study. JAMA 274:131–136

Wolf-Maier K, Cooper RS, Banegas JR, Giampoli S, Hense H-W, Joffres M, Kastarinen M, Poulter N, Primatesta P, Rodríguez-Artalejo F, Stegmayr B, Thamm M, Tuomilehto J, Vanuzzi D, Vescio F (2003) Hypertension prevalence and blood pressure levels in 6 European countries, Canada, and the United States. JAMA 289:2363–2369

World Health Organization (1992) International statistical classification of diseases and related health problems: tenth revision. World Health Organization, Geneva

World Health Organization (1999) Report by the Director-General: global strategy for the prevention and control of noncommunicable diseases. World Health Organization, Geneva

World Health Organization (2002) The world health report 2002: reducing risks, promoting healthy life. World Health Organization, Geneva (www.who.int). Accessed May 05, 2004

World Health Organization (2003) WHO framework convention on tobacco control. World Health Organization, Geneva

World Health Organization Collaborative Study of Cardiovascular Disease and Steroid Hormone Contraception (1996) Haemorrhagic stroke, overall stroke risk, and combined oral contraceptives: results of an international, multicenter, case-control study. Lancet 348:505–510

World Health Organization Expert Committee (1990) Prevention in childhood and youth of adult cardiovascular diseases: time for action. WHO Technical Report Series 792. World Health Organization, Geneva

World Health Organization MONICA Project Principal Investigators (1988) The World Health Organization MONICA Project (monitoring trends and determinants in cardiovascular disease): a major international collaboration. J Clin Epidemiol 41:105–114

World Health Organization Study Group (1990) Diet, nutrition, and the prevention of chronic diseases. WHO Technical Report Series 797. World Health Organization, Geneva

World Heart Federation (www.worldheart.org). Accessed 05 May, 2004

World Heart Federation, Centers for Disease Control and Prevention, International Heart Health Society (2004) International action on cardiovascular disease: a platform for success. World Heart Federation, Geneva (in press)

Worth RM, Kato H, Rhoads GG, Kagan A, Syme SL (1975) Epidemiologic studies of coronary heart disease and stroke in Japanese men living in Japan, Hawaii and California: mortality. Am J Epidemiol 102:481–490

Yusuf S, Reddy S, Óunpuu S, Anand S (2001) Global burden of cardiovascular diseases. Part I: general considerations, the epidemiologic transition, risk factors, and the impact of urbanization. Circulation 104:2746–2753

Cancer Epidemiology

Paolo Boffetta

IV.3

Introduction

Cancer encompasses a family of several hundreds of diseases which are distinguished in humans by site, morphology, clinical behaviour and response to therapy. Whether considered from a biological, a clinical or a public health point of view, it is the malignant and invasive nature of many of these diseases that is of dominant importance.

Although the words 'cancer' and 'carcinoma' refer to malignant tumours arising from epithelial tissues, they are often used to include all malignant neoplasms. These are characterized by progressive and variable growth of tissue with structural and functional changes with respect to the normal tissue. In many cases, the alterations can be so important that it becomes difficult to identify the tissue of origin.

Knowledge about the causes of and the possible preventive strategies for malignant neoplasms has greatly advanced during the last century. This was largely due to the findings from cancer epidemiology. In parallel to the identification of the causes of cancer, primary preventive strategies have been developed. Secondary preventive approaches have also been proposed and, in some cases, they have been shown to be effective. A careful consideration of the achievements of cancer research, however, suggests that the advancements in knowledge about the causes of cancer have not been followed by an equally important reduction in the burden of cancer. Part of this paradox is explained by the long latency occurring between exposure to carcinogens and development of the clinical disease. Changes in exposure to risk factors are therefore not followed immediately by changes in disease occurrence. The main reason for the gap between knowledge and public health action, however, rests with the cultural, societal and economic aspects of exposure to most carcinogens.

Scope and Approaches in Cancer Epidemiology

Cancer epidemiology investigates the distribution and determinants of the incidence, mortality and prevalence of cancer in human populations (Adami and Trichopoulos 2002). Many approaches have been used in cancer epidemiology which can be classified according to different dimensions, as shown in Table 3.1. Although most studies in cancer epidemiology are observational in nature, intervention (experimental) studies are conducted to evaluate the efficacy of prevention strategies, such as screening programmes and chemoprevention trials (clinical trials are usually considered to be outside the scope of cancer epidemiology). Observational studies are traditionally classified in descriptive, analytical (or etiological) and ecological studies (for a detailed description of the different types of epidemiological studies see Chaps. I.3–I.8 of this handbook).

Table 3.1. Approaches used in cancer epidemiology

Dimension	Approaches	Examples
Nature of observation	Experimental	Chemoprevention trial
	Observational	Cohort study
Purpose of investigation	Description	Time-trend analysis
	Etiological research	Case-control study
	Evaluation	Community trial of screening modalities
Unit of observation	Grouped data	Ecological study of environmental exposure
	Individual data	Case-control study with questionnaire data
Sampling strategy*	Census-based	Cohort study
	Sample-based	Case-control study
Source of information on exposure	Routine collection	Record-linkage study
	Ad-hoc collection	Questionnaire-based study

* In studies based on individual data

Descriptive cancer epidemiology is a particularly flourishing branch of the discipline, thanks to the availability of high-quality population-based cancer registries in many areas of the world and to the possibility to use mortality data to estimate the incidence of highly lethal cancers. As an illustration, Fig. 3.1 shows the estimated incidence of cancer among women in all countries of the world: these estimates are derived mainly from data from cancer registries and mortality statistics. Although subject to various sources of error, such estimates are more precise than those available for any other chronic disease. An additional useful distinction of etiological studies concerns the nature of the information on exposure: while some studies use data routinely collected for other purposes, such as census records and hospital files, in other circumstances ad-hoc information on exposure is collected following a variety of approaches, including record abstraction, questionnaires, pedigree reconstruction, environmental monitoring and measurement of biological markers.

Given the importance of cancer in developed countries and the efforts to prevent it, cancer epidemiology has acquired a recognized status in medicine and has developed into a separate profession. For this reason, and thanks to the availability of high-quality data on the outcomes of interest, it has played an important role in the development of modern epidemiology. The criteria for causal inference in observational research (with the corollary of methodological studies on bias, confounding and statistical power) have been largely shaped following the discovery of the important role of tobacco smoking as a human carcinogen (Doll 1998); modern statistical approaches such as multivariable logistic and Poisson regressions have originally been proposed for use in cancer studies (Breslow and

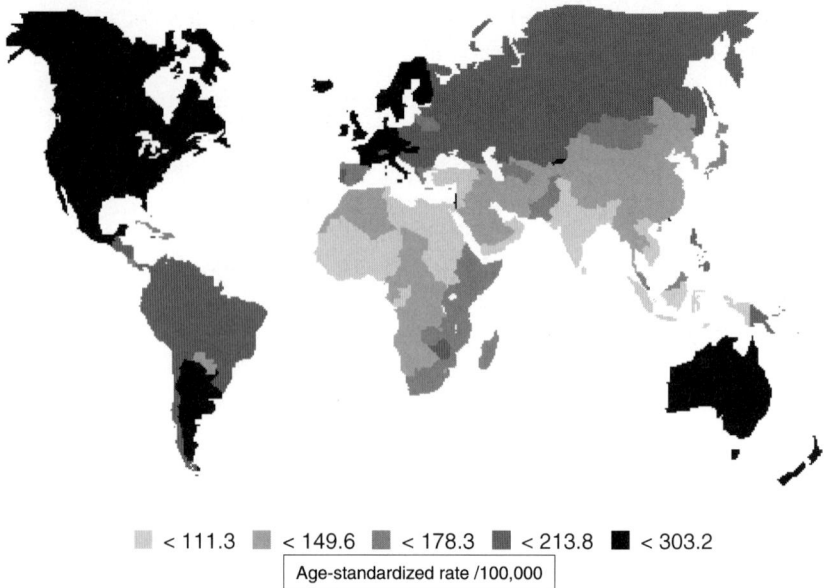

Figure 3.1. Estimated incidence rate of cancer in women, by country (year 2000). From (Ferlay et al. 2001)

Day 1980, 1987; see also Chap. II.3 of this handbook); molecular epidemiology has developed as a discipline bridging different areas of cancer research (Perera 2000; see also Chap. III.6 of this handbook); and methodological advances in genetic epidemiology have stemmed from familial studies of cancer (Thomas 2000; see also Chap. III.7 of this handbook).

3.3 The Global Burden of Cancer

The number of new cases of cancer that occurred worldwide in 2000 has been estimated at about 10 million (Table 3.2) (Ferlay et al. 2001), including 5.3 million in men and 4.7 million in women. About 4.7 million cases occurred in developed countries (North America, Japan, Europe including Russia, Australia and New Zealand) and 5.3 million in developing countries. Among men, lung, stomach, colorectal, prostate and liver cancers are the most common malignant neoplasms (Fig. 3.2), while breast, cervical, colorectal, lung and ovarian cancers are the most common neoplasms among women (Fig. 3.3).

Such global statistics are of limited interest, given the complexity of the factors affecting the risk of each neoplasm and the reader is referred to specialized publications for a more detailed review (Ferlay et al. 2001; Parkin et al. 1997). Some general trends can however be identified:

— A decrease in stomach cancer incidence in most countries;

Table 3.2. Estimated number of new cases of cancer (incidence) and of cancer deaths (mortality) in 2000, by gender and geographical area (Ferlay et al. 2001)

	Men	Women	Total
Incidence:			
Developed countries	2,503,700	2,176,000	4,679,700
Developing countries	2,814,100	2,561,700	5,375,800
Total	5,317,800	4,737,700	10,055,500
Mortality:			
Developed countries	1,488,200	1,157,600	2,645,800
Developing countries	2,034,200	1,528,700	3,562,900
Total	3,522,400	2,686,300	6,208,700

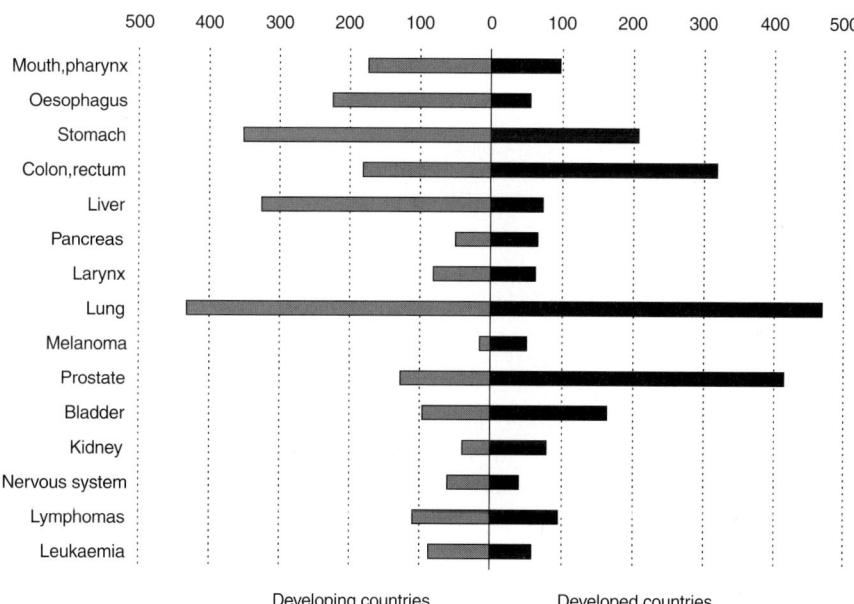

Figure 3.2. Estimated number of new cancer cases ($\times 1000$) in men, (year 2000). From Ferlay et al. (2001)

— a plateau or decrease in the incidence of lung cancer and, to some extent, other tobacco-related cancers among men from developed countries, and a corresponding increase among men in developing countries and women in developed countries;

— a very modest improvement in survival, in particular for highly lethal cancers.

The number of deaths from cancer was estimated at about 6.2 million in 2000 (Table 3.2) (Ferlay et al. 2001). No global estimates of survival from cancer are

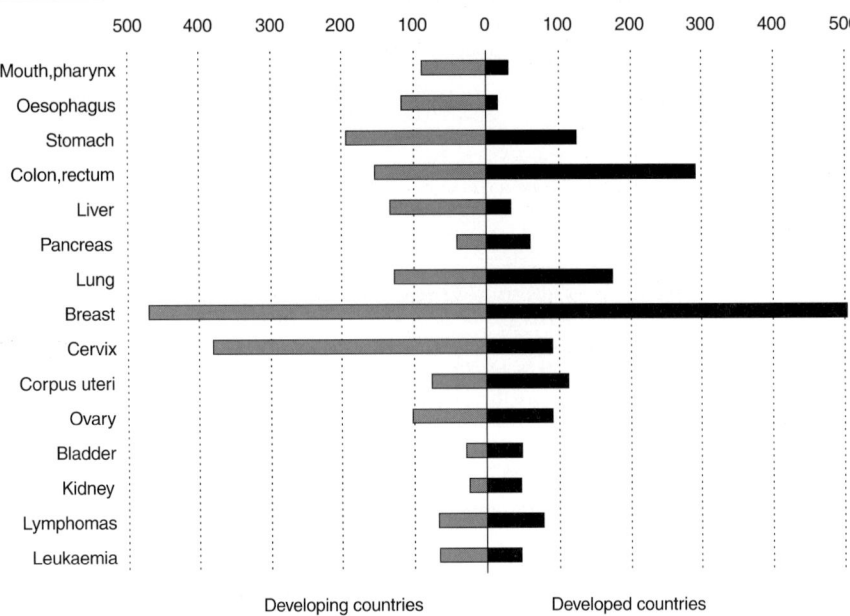

Figure 3.3. Estimated number of new cancer cases ($\times 1000$) in women, (year 2000). From Ferlay et al. (2001)

available: data from selected registries suggest wide disparities between developed and developing countries for neoplasms with effective but expensive treatment, such as leukaemia, while the gap is narrow for neoplasms without an effective therapy, such as lung cancer (Berrino et al. 1999; Kosary et al. 1995; Sankaranarayanan et al. 1998) (Fig. 3.4). The overall five-year survival of cases diagnosed during 1985–1989 in European Union countries was 41% (Berrino et al. 1999).

3.4 Causes and Prevention of Human Cancer

In the following sections, the current knowledge about the risk factors and the strategies for primary and secondary prevention of cancer is summarized. For more details, the reader is referred to systematic reviews (Adami et al. 2002; Boffetta et al. 2002; Peto 2001).

Table 3.3 shows the results of reviews of the contribution of known causes of cancer in developed countries (Doll and Peto 1981; HCCP 1996; Peto 2001). Such estimates are subject to assumptions and uncertainties and should be interpreted as approximations. However, it is worth noting that the estimate of the relative importance of the major causes of cancer is fairly consistent. No systematic estimate has been proposed for developing countries, where the contribution of infectious agents is likely to be very important.

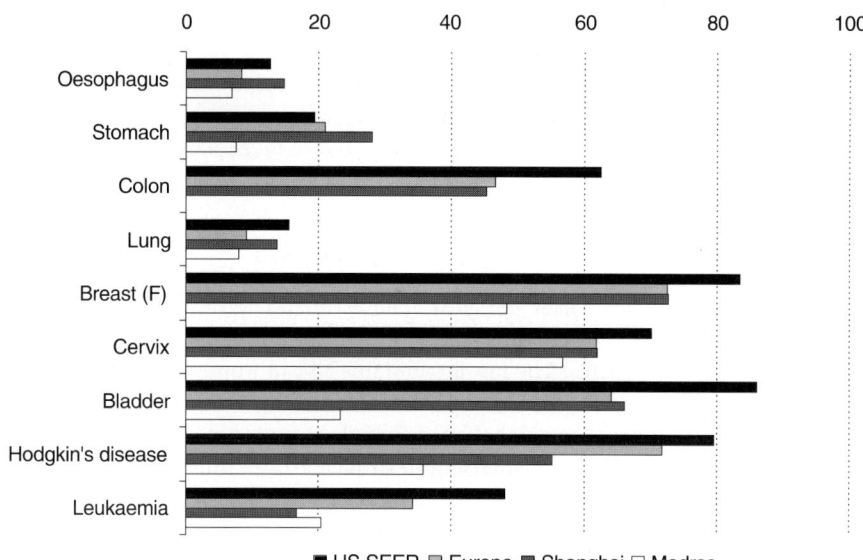

Figure 3.4. Five-year relative survival from cancer in selected populations. From Berrino et al. (1999) and Sankaranarayanan et al. (1998)

Table 3.3. Quantifications of contribution of major causes to human cancer burden (attributable fractions in percent)

Cause	Peto 2001*		HCCP 1996	Doll and Peto 1981
	Smokers	Non-smokers		
Tobacco	60	0	30	30
Dietary factors	4–12?	10–30?	30	35
Obesity	4	10	30	N/A**
Sedentary life	0.4	1	5	N/A
Biological agents	2	5	5	10?
Occupation	0.4	1	5	4
Alcohol	0.4	1	3	3
Environmental factors	0.4	1	2	2
UV/ionizing radiation	0.4	1	2	3***
Reproductive factors	N/A	N/A	3	7
Medical factors	N/A	N/A	1	1
Food additives	N/A	N/A	1	< 1
Perinatal factors	N/A	N/A	5	N/A
Socio-economic factors	N/A	N/A	3	N/A
Genetic factors	N/A	N/A	5	N/A

* Avoidable causes
** Not available *** Geophysical factors

3.4.1   Tobacco Smoking

Tobacco smoking is the main single cause of human cancer worldwide. It is a cause of cancers of the oral cavity, pharynx, oesophagus, stomach, liver, pancreas, nasal cavity, larynx, lung, cervix, kidney and bladder, and of myeloid leukaemia (IARC 2004). It is commonly considered that tobacco smoking causes up to one third of human cancers (Table 3.3); a detailed review of the number of cancers attributable to tobacco smoking in 1985, which was based on very strict criteria for attribution of cases, resulted in the estimate of at least 15% (Parkin et al. 1994), corresponding to about 1.5 million new cases per year. The estimates were 25% in men and 4% in women and, in both genders, they were 16% in developed countries and 10% in developing countries. The low attributable risk in women (and, to a lesser extent, in developing countries) is due to the low consumption of tobacco in past decades: the recent upward trend that has taken place among women and in many developing countries will obviously result in a much greater number of cancers in the future.

The risk of tobacco-related cancers among smokers relative to non-smokers depends on the different characteristics of the habit; in Table 3.4 are reported

Table 3.4. Relative risk of ever smoking and proportion of cancer attributable to tobacco smoking

Cancer	Relative risk for ever smoking*	Attributable risk**	
		Men	Women
Oral cavity, pharynx	2–3	41%	11%
Oesophagus	2–5 (squamous cell carcinoma) < 2 (adenocarcinoma)	45%	11%
Stomach	1.5	13%***	7%***
Liver	2	N/A****	N/A
Pancreas	2–4	27%	11%
Nasal cavity and sinuses	2 (squamous cell carcinoma)	N/A	N/A
Larynx	10–15	67%	28%
Lung	10–15 (small cell and squamous cell carcinoma) 3–5 (adenocarcinoma)	85%	46%
Cervix	2	N/A	N/A
Kidney	2 (renal cell carcinoma) 3 (cancer of the renal pelvis)	38%	4%
Bladder	3	37%	14%
Leukaemia	1.2 (myeloid)	N/A	N/A

* Derived from IARC (2004) and Kuper et al. (2002)
** Derived from Parkin et al. (1994) unless stated otherwise
*** Derived from Tredaniel et al. (1997) **** Not available

relative risks found for ever-smokers in Europe and North America. In different populations, risk estimates have been produced for increasing levels of duration and amount of tobacco smoking: in general, a separate effect has been shown for both dimensions of smoking, with a stronger role of the former (IARC 2004). The effect of duration of smoking on the risk of smoking-related cancers, and of lung cancer in particular, is so strong that it is difficult to determine whether there is an independent contribution of other factors, such as age and age at starting smoking. Smoking of filtered cigarettes and cigarettes with reduced tar content results in a lower risk of lung and other cancers than smoking of cigarettes without filter and with high tar content, although by no means the former products should be seen as 'risk-free' (IARC 2004). Smoking of black tobacco cigarettes entails a higher risk of most smoking-related cancers than smoking of blond tobacco cigarettes (IARC 2004). A carcinogenic effect of cigar and pipe smoking has been demonstrated for cancers of the oral cavity, pharynx, larynx, lung and bladder (IARC 2004). Similarly, smoking of local tobacco products, such as papirossi in Russia, bidis in India and yaa muan in Thailand, entails an increased risk of cancer of the lung and other organs.

A benefit of quitting tobacco smoking in adulthood has been shown for most cancers causally associated with the habit (Table 3.5). This result emphasizes the need to devise anti-smoking strategies that address avoidance of the habit among the young as well as reduction of smoking and quitting among adults. There is strong evidence of a protective effect of quitting smoking at any age (Peto et al. 2000). The decline in tobacco consumption that has taken place during the last 20 years among men in North America and several European countries, and which has resulted in decreased incidence of and mortality from lung cancer, has resulted primarily from the increase in the number of smokers quitting at middle age.

With the identification of tobacco as a carcinogen for the lung, the causal nature of an association between a chronic disease and a risk factor was for the first time established beyond doubt, representing an important contribution to the development of epidemiology. The association was replicated in various populations, using different approaches, namely cohort and case-control studies. This discovery was facilitated by several aspects of tobacco smoking: firstly, it is a potent carcinogen, containing – at high concentrations – several agents

Table 3.5. Effect of quitting tobacco smoking on risk of selected cancers (Kuper et al. 2002)

Cancer	Effect of quitting
Oral cavity, pharynx	Long-term quitters have risk close to that of never-smokers
Oesophagus	Risk decreases, but significant increase persists
Pancreas	Up to 50% risk reduction in long-term quitters
Larynx	Long-term quitters have risk close to that of never-smokers
Lung	Sharp decline in risk, some excess risk persists
Kidney	Up to 25% risk reduction in long-term quitters
Bladder	Up to 60% risk reduction in long-term quitters

acting on different stages of the carcinogenic process; secondly, a sizable group in most populations is composed of heavy smokers, exposing themselves to high doses; and thirdly, exposure is easier to quantify compared to most other agents, since smokers can report with a good degree of precision their present and past consumption.

3.4.2   Use of Smokeless Tobacco Products

There is conclusive epidemiological evidence that use of smokeless tobacco products is associated with an increased risk of head and neck cancer (IARC 1985). Chewing of tobacco-containing products is particularly prevalent in southern Asia, where it represents a major cause of cancer of the oral cavity, pharynx, oesophagus and larynx, either alone or in combination with smoking.

3.4.3   Dietary Factors

Despite considerable research efforts in cancer epidemiology, the exact role of dietary factors in causing human cancer remains largely obscure. The World Cancer Research Fund (WCRF 1997) has published a systematic review of the evidence of an association between intake of foods, food groups and nutrients and different cancers. Their evaluations are summarized in Table 3.6 and, with one exception, are valid today. The evidence of a protective role of vegetable and, to a lesser degree, fruit intake has been evaluated as convincing for a number of important human tumours. However, a formal IARC evaluation which has taken place in March 2003 concluded that there is no definite evidence for a cancer protective effect of high intake of fruits and vegetables, although such an effect is probable for cancer of the esophagus, stomach, colon/rectum and lung (IARC 2003). For the remaining dietary factors, few evaluations of convincing or probable associations have been made by WCRF, and in most cases the conclusion was a possible increase or decrease in risk. This is namely the case for high intake of total and saturated fat, and of micronutrients such as carotenoids, vitamin E and selenium. In addition, the International Agency for Research on Cancer (IARC) has concluded that there is evidence suggesting lack of cancer-preventive activity for preformed vitamin A (IARC 1998a) and for β-carotene when used at high doses (IARC 1998b). In recent years the evidence has grown for a carcinogenic role of excess caloric intake, disregarding the source of calories, resulting in overweight and obesity (see Sect. 3.4.4).

The mechanisms of dietary-related carcinogenesis are not well understood. Dietary factors are likely to play a role in most if not all steps of the process, including genotoxicity, interference in the metabolism of other carcinogens, methylation of cancer genes, alteration of DNA repair and apoptotic mechanisms, alteration of DNA and cell replication, and cell proliferation (for a review see WCRF 1997). In particular, it is plausible that fresh fruits and vegetables act at least in part via control of endogenously formed radical oxygen species. In addition, insulin and insulin-like Growth Factor-I (IGF-I), which are produced as a result of caloric intake, stimulate anabolic processes resulting in inhibition of apoptosis, and cell proliferation (see Sect. 3.4.4).

Several suspected dietary carcinogens have been widely studied in cancer epidemiology. Grilled and barbecued meat and fish contain carcinogenic polycyclic aromatic hydrocarbons and heterocyclic amines: high intake of these foods has been suggested to increase the risk of stomach and colorectal cancer. Similarly, high intake of cured and processed meat is a probable cause of digestive tract cancer: nitrosamines might be among the relevant carcinogens. High intake of salt probably increases the risk of stomach cancer (WCRF 1997). Intake of Chinese-style salted fish increases the risk of cancer of the nasopharynx (IARC 1993) and consumption of other types of salted fish might represent a risk factor in South-East Asia and the Arctic. Other preserved foods used as weaning food in different areas of China have also been associated to nasopharyngeal cancer: chung choi (a salted root), salted shrimp paste, salted eggs and preserved fruits. The high rates of this tumour in Northern Africa might be due to consumption of dried mutton, touklia (a spiced mixture of peppers) or harissa (a hot sauce).

In several areas of Asia and Africa, high incidence of liver cancer is due to food contamination by mycotoxins, including aflatoxins (Stuver and Trichopoulos 2002). A role of another group of mycotoxins – fumonisins – in oesophageal cancer risk is suspected (IARC 2002a). The application of exposure biomarkers to the study of aflatoxin-related liver cancer represented a major success of molecular cancer epidemiology and has allowed to elucidate the role of this important group of carcinogens (Ross et al. 1992). In Japan, eating bracken fern has been associated with an elevated oesophageal cancer risk (Alonso-Amelot and Avendano 2002). In Central Europe, a chronic renal disease called Balkan Endemic Nephropathy has been described, which is associated with an increased risk of kidney cancer and is likely to be due to ochratoxin contamination of foodstuff (IARC 1993).

Intake of large amounts (more than one litre per day) of hot maté, a herbal tea, is a risk factor for oesophageal cancer in Southern Brazil, Uruguay and Northern Argentina (Castellsague et al. 2000). It is unclear, however, whether the effect is due to components of maté or to the high temperature: studies from other regions suggest that intake of hot beverages (e.g., hot tea in Iran, Singapore and Japan, hot coffee in Puerto Rico, and hot drinks or soups in Hong Kong) increases the risk of oesophagitis and oesophageal cancer, although the evidence is less consistent than in the case of maté (Nyren and Adami 2002a).

The investigation of dietary carcinogens presents major challenges because of the difficulties to assess precisely the relevant carcinogenic (or preventive) factors. In most populations, diet varies greatly during the life of an individual, because of changes in personal choices and in societal aspects (availability of different food items, modification of eating patterns, etc.). Furthermore, many nutritional factors are strongly correlated, making it difficult to disentangle the effect of each factor, and variability in exposure within relatively homogeneous

Table 3.6. Assessment of associations between dietary factors and human cancer (WCRF 1997)

Factor (high intake)	Oral cavity and pharynx	Oesophagus	Stomach	Colon and rectum	Liver	Pancreas	Lung	Breast	Cervix	Endometrium	Ovary	Prostate	Kidney	Bladder
Starch			[-]	[+]										
Fibres			{-}	[-]		[-]		[-]						
Sugar				[+]		{+}								
Total fat				[+]			[+]	[+]		{+}	{+}	[+]		{+}
Saturated fat				[+]			[+]	[+]		[+]	{+}	[+]		
Cholesterol						[+]	[+]	(=)		{+}				
Animal protein								{+}						
Carotenoids		[-]	[-]	[-]			(-)	[-]	[-]					{-}
Vitamin C	[-]	[-]	(-)	{-}		[-]	[-]	{-}	[-]	{-}	{-}			{-}
Retinol			[=]	{-}			[=]	[=]	[=]			[=]		{-}
Vitamin E			[=]	{-}			[-]	[-]	[-]					
Folate				{-}					[=]					
Selenium			{-}	[=]	{-}		[-]							
Iron				{+}	{+}									
Vitamin D				{-}										
Calcium				[=]										
Allium compounds			[-]											

table to be continued

Table 3.6. (continued)

Factor (high intake)	Oral cavity and pharynx	Oeso-phagus	Sto-mach	Colon and rectum	Liver	Pan-creas	Lung	Breast	Cervix	Endo-metrium	Ovary	Pros-tate	Kidney	Bladder
Cereals				{–}										
Whole grain cereals			[–]											
Refined cereals		[+]												
Vegetables	[–]	–	–	–	[–]	(–)	–	(–)	[–]	[–]	[–]	[–]	[–]	(–)
Fruits	[–]	–	–			(–)	–	(–)	[–]	[–]	[–]			(–)
Meat				(+)		[+]		[+]				[+]	[+]	
Eggs				[+]		[+]					{+}		[=]	[=]
Fish				[=]		{+}		{–}			{–}			
Milk & dairy products												[+]	[+]	
Coffee	[+]		(+)	{–}		(=)		=				[=]	(=)	[+]
Maté	[+]	[+]												
Black tea			(=)					[=]					(=)	(=)
Green tea			[–]											

Direction of the effect: + increased risk; – decreased risk; = no relationship
Strength of the evidence: no brackets: convincing evidence of an association
    round brackets: probable association
    squared brackets: possible association
    curly brackets: insufficient evidence to fully assess the association

populations might not be large enough to allow the detection of carcinogenic effects. Dietary retrospective exposure assessment is complicated by recall bias and unavailability of valid biomarkers, making the case-control approach particularly unsuitable. Even the evidence derived from prospective (e.g., cohort) studies, however, is far from being unequivocal: as an example, the fairly established notion that high intake of fat, mainly of saturated fat from animal foods, might be a risk factor for breast cancer was recently challenged by the results of prospective studies based on detailed dietary assessment (Holmes et al. 1999). The equivocal evidence, however, might depend on a different effect of fat intake on the risk of premenopausal and postmenopausal breast cancer (Cho et al. 2003). For a general discussion of nutritional epidemiology see Chap. III.4 of this handbook.

3.4.4   Overweight and Obesity

Overweight, defined as body mass index (BMI) over 25 kg/m^2, increases the risk of colon, breast (post-menopausal), endometrial and kidney cancer and of adenocarcinoma of the oesophagus (IARC 2002b). The risk of these cancers is linearly related to severity of overweight and obesity, where obesity is defined as BMI over 30 kg/m^2; adult weight gain is a strong and consistent predictor of risk. In the case of colon cancer, body fat distribution expressed as waist to hip circumference ratio, might have an effect independent from that of body mass. It is likely that obesity exerts a carcinogenic effect via alteration of endogenous hormone metabolism, involving in particular insulin resistance and chronic hyperinsulinaemia, modulation of adrenal cortical hormones, and increased bioavailability of estrogens. Other possible mechanisms include interference with carcinogen metabolism, accumulation of reactive oxygen species and alteration of mechanisms regulating cell proliferation, resulting in enhanced proliferation and reduced apoptosis, as well as induction of angiogenesis in tissues other than the fat. The magnitude of the excess risk is not very high (for most cancers the relative risk ranges between 1.1 and 1.5 for overweight and between 1.3 and 2 for obesity), however, the attributable risk in industrialized countries is large because of the high prevalence of overweight people: estimates for Europe suggest that about 6% of all cancers in women and 3% in men are attributable to overweight and obesity (Table 3.7).

3.4.5   Physical Activity

Regular sustained workplace or recreational physical activity (e.g., at least 30 minutes/day) decrease the risk of colon and breast cancer; a protective effect is also likely for endometrial and prostate cancer (IARC 2002b). The magnitude of risk reduction for colon and breast cancer is in the order of 40%, and a dose-response relationship has been shown for both neoplasms. Up to 13% of cases of colon cancer in the USA can be attributed to physical inactivity (Slattery 1997). Although

Table 3.7. Cancer risk attributable to overweight and obesity in European Union countries (Bergström et al. 2001)

Cancer	Relative risk		Attributable fraction (%)		Attributable
	Overweight	Obesity	Women	Men	cases
Breast	1.12	1.25	8.5	–	12,870
Colon	1.15	1.33	10.7	11.1	21,610
Endometrium	1.59	2.52	39.2	–	14,230
Prostate*	1.06	1.12	–	4.4	4990
Kidney	1.36	1.84	24.5	25.5	10,380
Gallbladder*	1.34	1.78	23.7	24.8	6460
Total	–	–	6.4	3.4	70,540

* Evidence of a causal role of overweight considered less than conclusive by IARC (2002b)

regular physical activity contributes to weight control, the epidemiological evidence suggests that two factors also act independently. The mechanisms through which physical activity contributes to cancer prevention are not fully understood, but they may include enhancement of immune function, interference with sex steroids, and insulin and IGF-I pathways (IARC 2002b).

Alcohol Drinking   3.4.6

There is convincing epidemiological evidence that the consumption of alcoholic beverages increases the risk of cancers of the oral cavity and pharynx, oesophagus, and larynx. The risks tend to increase with the amount of ethanol drunk, in the absence of any clearly defined threshold below which no effect is evident; an interaction has been shown between alcohol drinking and tobacco smoking (Fig. 3.5). The evidence of differences in carcinogenicity among alcoholic beverages is inconclusive. Alcohol might act as co-carcinogen, enhancing the effect of tobacco and dietary carcinogens; in addition, a direct carcinogenic effect of acetaldehyde, the main metabolite of ethanol cannot be excluded. An increased risk has also been reported for colorectal cancer and liver cancer, although the effect on the latter might be mediated by development of liver cirrhosis. Breast cancer risk is also increased among drinkers (CGHFBC 2002a): although weak (relative risk in the order of 1.07 for each 10 g/day increase in alcohol intake), the association is of importance because of the apparent lack of a threshold, the large number of women drinking large amounts of alcohol, and the high incidence of the disease.

The carcinogenic effect of alcohol should be considered in the light of other health effects, notably the increased mortality from chronic digestive diseases and accidents and the reduced mortality from cardiovascular diseases among moderate drinkers (Vogel 2002). In middle-aged and old people, the benefit on cardiovascular disease is likely to offset the increased cancer risk, up to a level of approximately 20 g/day among men and 10 g/day among women.

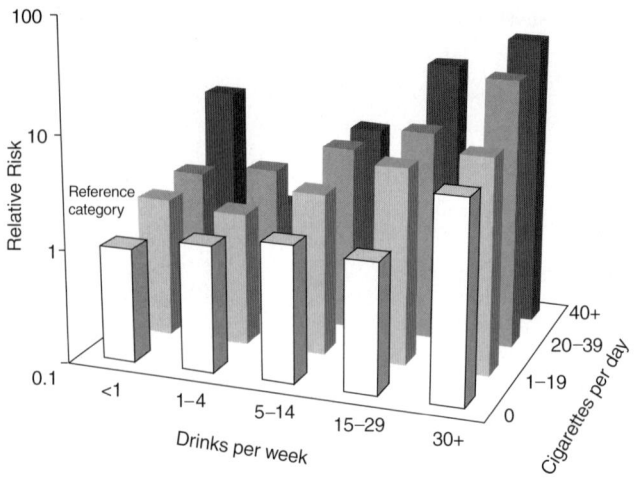

Figure 3.5. Risk of oral cancer, tobacco smoking and alcohol drinking. From Blot et al. (1988)

3.4.7   ## Infectious Agents

There is growing epidemiological evidence that chronic infection with some viruses, bacteria and parasites represents a major cause of human cancer, in particular in developing countries. A number of infectious agents have been evaluated within the IARC Monograph Programme (Table 3.8), and the evidence of a causal association has been classified as sufficient for several of them. Human Papilloma virus (HPV) is detected in almost all cases of cervical cancer: several oncogenic HPV types have been identified, with HPV 16 and 18 being the most prevalent ones (Munoz et al. 2003). Chronic infection with Hepatitis B virus (HBV) or Hepatitis C virus (HCV) is a major cause of liver cancer worldwide; an interaction has been shown between HBV infection and other causes of liver cancer such as aflatoxin exposure. Additional carcinogenic viruses include Epstein-Barr virus, a major cause of Hodgkin's disease and of some types of non-Hodgkin lymphoma, Human Herpes virus 8 (HHV8), which causes Kaposi sarcoma, Human Immunodeficiency virus I, which causes various types of non-Hodgkin lymphoma, and Human T-cell leukaemia/lymphoma virus I. In addition, childhood leukaemia is likely linked to one or more viruses that have not yet been identified.

Infection with Helicobacter pylori is associated with an approximately six-fold increased risk of non-cardia gastric cancer, after controlling for other risk factors of the disease (Nyren and Adami 2002a). Unplanned control of Helicobacter infection via widespread antibiotic use and improved living conditions is likely to be an important component of the decline in stomach cancer incidence, which occurred in many countries during recent decades. Infestation with several parasites has been linked with occurrence of human cancer in tropical countries: the evidence is particularly strong for Schistosoma haematobium, causing bladder

Table 3.8. Assessment of associations between infections and human cancer (IARC 1994a,b, 1995, 1996a, 1997a)

	Evidence*	Target organs**
Viruses:		
Hepatitis B virus	S	Liver
Hepatitis C virus	S	Liver, (lymphoma)
Hepatitis D virus	I	Liver
Human papilloma virus types 16, 18	S	Cervix, anus, penis, (oral cavity)
Human papilloma virus types 31, 33	L***	(Cervix)
Human papilloma virus, other types	I***	
Human immunodeficiency virus 1	S	Kaposi's sarcoma, non-Hodgkin's lymphoma
Human immunodeficiency virus 2	I	
Human T-cell lymphotrophic virus I	S	Adult T-cell leukaemia/lymphoma
Human T-cell lymphotrophic virus II	I	
Epstein-Barr virus	S	Burkitt's lymphoma, Hodgkin's disease, nasopharynx
Human herpes virus 8	L***	(Kaposi's sarcoma)
Bacterium:		
Helicobacter pylori	S	Stomach cancer, gastric lymphoma
Parasites:		
Schistosoma haematobium	S	Bladder
Schistosoma japonicum	L	(Liver, stomach)
Schistosoma mansoni	I	
Opistorchis viverrini	S	Liver
Opistorchis felineus	I	
Clonorchis sinensis	L	Liver

* I, inadequate; L, limited; S, sufficient
** Established target organs without brackets; suspected target organs in brackets
*** The evidence of a causal role of these agents has become stronger since the IARC evaluation

cancer in North Africa and the Middle East, and Chlonorchis siniensis, causing cholangiocarcinoma in South East Asia (IARC 1994a,b).

Global estimates of the number of cases of cancer attributable to biological agents suggest that at least 16% of all neoplasms worldwide are due to infection (Table 3.9) (Pisani et al. 1997). HBV- and HCV-related liver cancer, HPV-related cervical cancer and Helicobacter-related stomach cancer each account for approximately 30% of the total. Because of the high prevalence of most carcinogenic agents in developing countries, the estimate of the attributable risk is higher in this part of the world.

More than for other causes of cancer, a carcinogenic role of infectious agents is strongly suggested by extreme variability in cancer risk observed among populations in descriptive epidemiological studies. Thus, an infectious agent had

Table 3.9. Cancer risk attributable to infectious agents (Pisani et al. 1997)

Cancer	Agent	Developing countries AF%	Developing countries N cases	Developed countries AF%	Developed countries N cases
Liver	HBV, HCV	91	352,644*	51	46,762
Stomach	H. pylori	54	299,636	60	205,292
Cervix	HPV	91	335,946	82	80,420
Female genital	HPV	91	20,816	82	10,219
Lymphoma**	HIV, EBV	33	57,987	27	32,316
Leukaemia	HTLV-I	1.4	2200	0.5	500
Bladder	S. haematobium	7.7	10,249	0	0
Total		21	1,079,443	9.1	375,509

AF attributable fraction
* Including 808 cases of cholangiocarcinoma attributable to infestation with 0. viverrini
** Including Kaposi sarcoma (no cases attributed to HHV8)

been suspected for a long time for a number of human neoplasms (e.g., Kaposi sarcoma), before sensitive and specific assays became available for the identification of the responsible agent. In addition, the investigation of infectious causes of cancer poses special problems of reverse causality: the detection of an agent in a tumour, as compared to the normal tissue of the patients or controls, does not imply an etiological role, since the altered environment resulting from the neoplasm might favour the growth of the micro-organism above detection levels. Cohort studies with repeated samples of the target tissue or surrogate material (typically serum) represent the strongest approach to establish causality.

3.4.8   Occupational Exposures

Twenty-nine occupational agents, groups of agents and mixtures, as well as 12 exposure circumstances, are classified as carcinogenic by IARC (Table 3.10) (IARC 1972–2004). An additional 31 compounds and 3 exposure circumstances are classified as probable carcinogens (Table 3.11). While some (e.g., mustard gas) are mainly of historical interest, exposure is still widespread for important carcinogens such as asbestos, coal tar and other mixtures of polycyclic aromatic hydrocarbons, heavy metals and silica. Although the overall burden of occupational cancer is relatively small, these cancers concentrate among exposed subjects (mainly male blue-collar workers), among whom they may represent a sizeable proportion of total cancers (Boffetta et al. 1995). Furthermore, unlike lifestyle factors, exposure is involuntary and can be, to a large extent, avoided. In fact, reduction of exposure to occupational and environmental carcinogens has taken place in industrialized countries during recent decades and represents one of the successes of cancer epidemiology.

The epidemiological approach to study occupational causes of cancer was traditionally based on the historical cohort design. Groups of workers were identified

Table 3.10. Occupational agents, classified by the IARC Monographs programme as carcinogenic to humans

Agents, mixture, circumstance	Main industry, use
Agents, groups of agents:	
4-Aminobiphenyl	Pigment
Arsenic and arsenic compounds	Glass, metal, pesticide
Asbestos	Insulation, filter, textile
Benzene	Chemical, solvent
Benzidine	Pigment
Beryllium and beryllium compounds	Aerospace
Bis(chloromethyl)ether and chloromethyl methyl ether*	Chemical intermediate
Cadmium and cadmium compounds	Dye/pigment
Chromium[VI] compounds	Metal plating, dye/pigment
Dioxin	Chemical
Ethylene oxide	Sterilant
Mustard gas*	War gas
2-Naphthylamine	Pigment
Nickel compounds	Metallurgy, alloy, catalyst
Plutonium-239 and its decay products	Nuclear industry
Radium-226 and its decay products*	Luminizing industry
Radium-228 and its decay products*	Luminizing industry
Radon-222 and its decay products	Mining
Silica, crystalline	Stone cutting, mining, glass
Solar radiation	Agriculture
Talc containing asbestiform fibres	Paper, paints
Vinyl chloride	Plastics
X- and γ-radiation	Medical
Mixtures:	
Coal-tar pitches	Construction, electrode
Coal-tars	Fuel, construction, chemical
Mineral oils, untreated	Metal
Shale-oils	Fuel
Soots	Pigment
Wood dust	Wood
Exposure circumstances:	
Aluminium production	
Auramine, manufacture of*	Pigment
Boot and shoe manufacture and repair	
Coal gasification	
Coke production	

* Agent mainly of historical interest

table to be continued

Table 3.10. (continued)

Agents, mixture, circumstance	Main industry, use
Furniture and cabinet making	
Haematite mining (underground) with exposure to radon	
Iron and steel founding	
Magenta, manufacture of*	Pigment
Painter (occupational exposure as a)	
Rubber industry	
Strong inorganic-acid mists containing sulphuric acid	Metallurgy

* Agent mainly of historical interest

via company or union records, and their cancer mortality or incidence was compared with that of a reference population, most commonly that of the country or the region, leading to the estimate of indirectly standardized mortality (or incidence) ratios. In recent decades, alternative approaches gained popularity, including: (1) community-based case-control studies, leading to the simultaneous estimate of the risk from exposure to a large number of agents (see for example the multi-site study conducted in Montreal by Siemiatycki (1995)); and (2) comparisons within subgroups of cohort members, based on reconstructed (often model-based) estimates of exposure to one or more agents of interest. Occupational cancer research has also been a field of successful application of biomarkers of exposure, as in the case of the identification of ethylene oxide as a human carcinogen following the detection of protein adducts in exposed workers and in animals showing an increased incidence of neoplasms (IARC 1994c).

The main reasons for the success of the application of epidemiology to the field of occupational cancer are the possibility to identify clearly defined groups of exposed individuals and the availability of historical measures of exposure. For more details on occupational epidemiology see Chap. III.2 of this handbook.

3.4.9 Environmental Agents

Exposure to many occupational carcinogens listed in Tables 3.10 and 3.11 also occurs in the general environment; for two additional agents, the naturally-occurring fibre erionite and short-lived radioiodine isotopes, the main source of exposure is the general environment. Overall, the available evidence suggests, in most populations, a small role of purely environmental sources of exposure to carcinogens (air, water, soil pollution): global estimates are in the order of 1% or less of total cancers. This is in contrast with public perception, which often identifies environmental pollution as a major cause of human cancer. It should be stressed, however, that in selected areas (e.g., residence near asbestos processing plants or in areas with drinking water contaminated by arsenic) environmental exposure to carcinogens may represent an important cancer hazard (Armstrong and Boffetta 1998).

Table 3.11. Occupational agents, classified by the IARC Monographs programme as probably carcinogenic to humans

Agents, mixture, circumstance	Main industry, use
Agents, groups of agents:	
Acrylamide	Chemical, construction
Benz[a]anthracene	Combustion fumes
Benzidine-based dyes	Paper, leather, textile dyes
Benzo[a]pyrene	Combustion fumes
1,3-Butadiene	Plastics, rubber
Captafol	Fungicide
α-Chlorinated toluenes	Chemical intermediate
4-Chloro-ortho-toluidine	Dye/pigment manufacture, textiles
Dibenz[a,h]anthracene	Combustion fumes
Diethyl sulfate	Chemical intermediate
Dimethylcarbamoyl chloride	Chemical intermediate
Dimethyl sulfate	Chemical intermediate
Epichlorohydrin	Plastics/resins monomer
Ethylene dibromide	Chemical intermediate, fumigant
Formaldehyde	Plastics, textiles, laboratory agent
Glycidol	Chemical intermediate
4,4′-Methylene bis(2-chloroaniline) (MOCA)*	Rubber manufacture
N-Nitrosodimethylamine*	Chemical intermediate
Styrene-7,8-oxide	Plastics, chemical intermediate
Tetrachloroethylene	Solvent, dry cleaning
ortho-Toluidine	Dyestuff, rubber
Trichloroethylene	Solvent, dry cleaning, metal
1,2,3-Trichloropropane	Solvent, chemical intermediate
Tris(2,3-dibromopropyl)phosphate	Plastics, textiles, flame retardant
Vinyl bromide	Plastics, textiles, monomer
Vinyl fluoride	Chemical intermediate
Mixtures:	
Creosotes	Wood preservation
Diesel engine exhaust	Transport
Non-arsenical insecticides (spraying and application)	Agriculture
Polychlorinated biphenyls	Electrical components
Exposure circumstances:	
Art glass, glass container and pressed ware (manufacturing of)	
Hairdresser and barber	
Petroleum refining	

* Agent mainly of historical interest

The search for environmental causes of cancer has been particularly elusive to the epidemiological approach. The main reason for such relative lack of success lies in several biases affecting the assessment of exposure to most environmental carcinogens and leading to false negative results: low-level exposure is often widespread and the range of dose is limited; exposure levels vary with time and most available measurements refer to the present or recent past; individuals are unable to validly and precisely reconstruct their past exposure. For more details on these problems please refer to Chap. III.3 of this handbook.

3.4.10   Reproductive Factors

The epidemiological evidence of a carcinogenic effect of reproductive factors is strongest for breast cancer: early age at menarche, low parity, late age at first pregnancy and late age at menopause are all associated with an increased risk, while spontaneous and induced abortions are not (Hankinson and Hunter 2002). In addition, breastfeeding protects from breast cancer. A large pooled analysis resulted in an estimated 4.3% (95% confidence interval (CI) 2.9–5.8) decrease in risk for every 12 months of breastfeeding, in addition to a decrease of 7.0% (95% CI 5.0–9.0) for each birth (CGHFBC 2002b). The same reproductive factors seem to exert an effect on endometrial cancer risk similar to that played on breast cancer, while the evidence of an effect on other cancers is inadequate, although there is limited evidence that nulliparity increases the risk of ovarian cancer. No detailed estimates are available on the contribution of reproductive factors to the global burden of cancer. Some authors have, however, proposed figures in the order of 3% (HCCP 1996). An extensive discussion of methodological problems in reproductive epidemiology can be found in Chap. III.5 of this handbook.

3.4.11   Other Lifestyle Factors

A number of other lifestyle factors have been shown or suggested in epidemiological studies to cause cancer in humans. Poor oral hygiene and ill-fitting dentures are likely to represent additional risk factors for oral cancer. The use of mouthwash with high alcohol content has also been associated with oral cancer (Mucci and Adami 2002). Herbs of the *Aristolochia* genus, used in traditional Chinese medicine as anti-rheumatics and diuretics and included in weight-loss regimens, cause a rapidly progressive renal disease called Chinese Herb Nephropathy, as well as cancer of the urinary tract (IARC 2002a).

3.4.12   Hormones

Increased levels of endogenous estrogens are associated with an increased risk of breast and endometrial cancers, and a similar effect is likely to be played by endogenous androgens (Hankinson and Hunter 2002; Persson and Adami 2002). The role of other hormones, such as progesterone and prolactin, in these cancers is not clearly known, nor is the role of endogenous androgens in prostate cancer.

There is growing evidence that growth hormones, in particular IGF-I, have a strong effect on the risk of breast, colon, prostate and possibly other cancers (Furstenberg and Senn 2002), and that chronic hyperinsulinaemia is a cause of cancers of the colon, pancreas, breast and endometrium (Kaaks et al. 2002).

There is a large body of epidemiological studies on cancer risk following exposure to exogenous hormones. Current and recent (up to 10 years) use of oral contraceptives entails a small increase in breast cancer risk, but no excess risk is apparent 10 or more years after cessation of use (CGHFBC 1996). Long-term use of oral contraceptives is associated with an increased risk of liver cancer, while the risk of endometrial and ovarian cancer is decreased following oral contraceptive use (IARC 1999a).

Post-menopausal hormonal therapy increases the risk of breast and endometrial cancer (CGHFBC 1997; IARC 1999a). In the case of breast cancer, the effect is stronger for combined estrogen-progestagen combinations than for other types of hormonal therapy (Beral et al. 2003). The evidence for other organs is inconclusive.

Tamoxifen is widely used for treatment of breast cancer: beyond its therapeutic effects, it decreases the risk of contralateral breast cancer but it increases the risk of endometrial cancer (IARC 1996b).

Perinatal Factors

3.4.13

Excess energy intake early in life is possibly associated with breast and colon cancer (IARC 2002b). The role of attained height, growth factors, and other factors such as insulin resistance or sensitivity in this association is unclear. In addition, high birth weight is possibly linked with an increased risk of breast cancer. Perinatal factors have been proposed to cause up to 5% of human cancers, but this estimate is subject to uncertainty. The implications of these findings for preventive strategies will be clarified by a more detailed understanding of the underlying carcinogenic mechanisms (HCCP 1996).

Ionizing and Non-ionizing Radiation

3.4.14

The available epidemiological studies of populations exposed to ionizing radiation following military actions, accidents, occupational exposure and medical treatments represent a very comprehensive database, which has been used beyond the assessment of radiation carcinogenicity, notably to elaborate models of carcinogenesis in humans and of quantitative risk assessment (Moolgavkar et al. 1999). Ionizing radiation causes acute lymphoblastic leukaemia, acute myeloid leukaemia, chronic myeloid leukaemia and breast, lung and thyroid cancers (IARC 2000). Bone, rectal and brain cancers may develop following prolonged therapeutic exposure. There is evidence of a linear dose-response relationship between radiation dose and cancer risk. However, levels at which people are commonly exposed to man-made radiation in most countries carry little risk and the main exposure comes from natural radiation, including indoor radon (IARC 2000). The estimates of the global contribution of ionizing radiation to human cancer range from 1% to 3% (Table 3.3).

The study of cancer risk following exposure to ionizing radiation represented one of the main paradigms of chronic disease epidemiology. In most exposure circumstances, doses – including those in the past – are known with great precision. In addition, they are characterized by different intensity and dose rates, allowing the separate investigation of different components of the carcinogenic effect.

Solar (ultraviolet) radiation is carcinogenic to the skin and the lip, and it might increase the risk of other neoplasms such as non-Hodgkin lymphoma (IARC 1992). Over 90% of skin neoplasms are attributable to sunlight; however, because of the low fatality of non-melanocytic skin cancer, solar radiation is responsible for only 1% to 2% of total cancer deaths (Table 3.3). Epidemiological studies have contributed to elucidate the contribution of dose rate and time of exposure in ultraviolet-related carcinogenesis. The evidence of a carcinogenic effect of other types of non-ionizing radiation, in particular electric and magnetic fields, is inconclusive (IARC 2002c).

3.4.15   Medical Procedures and Drugs

In addition to post-menopausal hormonal therapy, oral contraceptives and tamoxifen, other drugs may cause cancer. Many cancer chemotherapy drugs are active on the DNA, in order to block the replication of cancer cells. This, however, might result in damage to normal cells, including cancer transformation. The main neoplasm associated with chemotherapy treatment is leukaemia, although the risk of solid tumours is also increased (Boffetta and Kaldor 1994). A second group of carcinogenic drugs includes immunosuppressive agents, which have been studied in particular in transplanted patients (Kinlen 1996). Non-Hodgkin lymphoma is the main neoplasm caused by these drugs. Phenacetin-containing analgesics increase the risk of cancer of the renal pelvis (Lindblad and Adami 2002).

There is strong evidence from observational studies that aspirin reduces the risk of colorectal cancer (IARC 1997b), an effect probably shared by other non-steroidal anti-inflammatory drugs.

No precise estimates are available for the global contribution of drug use to human cancer. It is unlikely, however, that drugs represent more than 1% in developed countries (Table 3.3). Furthermore, the benefits of such therapies are usually much greater than the potential cancer risk.

Use of ionizing radiation for diagnostic purposes is likely to carry a small risk of cancer, which has been demonstrated only for childhood leukaemia following intrauterine exposure (IARC 2000). Radiotherapy increases the risk of cancer in the irradiated organs. There is no clear evidence of an increased cancer risk following other medical procedures, including surgical implants (IARC 1999b).

The epidemiological investigation of the carcinogenicity of drugs and medical procedures shares several characteristics of occupational cancer research: well-defined groups of exposed individuals and valid records of exposure, often in the form of prescription or hospital discharge databases, in addition to the strong potency of several medical agents. These factors explain the relatively large number of drugs identified as human carcinogens.

Medical Conditions 3.4.16

Changes in immunological function are likely to play an important role in human cancer, but epidemiological studies have been largely unable to identify specific factors determining an increased or a decreased risk. Both severe immunosuppression and immunostimulation are associated with an elevated risk of cancer (Kinlen 1996). On the one hand, individuals infected with the Human Immuno-deficiency Virus (HIV) and patients undergoing immunosuppressive treatments, such as transplant recipients, are at increased risk of lymphoma and skin cancer (Kinlen 1996). On the other hand, patients suffering from systemic autoimmune diseases are also at increased risk of lymphoma and possibly other neoplasms (Kinlen 1996). The significance of less severe disturbances of the immunological competence is poorly known.

Several chronic inflammatory conditions represent a risk factor for cancer: the epidemiological evidence is particularly strong in the case of colorectal cancer following inflammatory bowel disease and of lymphoma following chronic infectious diseases such as tuberculosis, malaria and herpes zoster (Melbye and Trichopoulos 2002; Potter and Hunter 2002).

Recent epidemiological studies have clearly shown that gastro-oesophageal reflux is an important cause of adenocarcinoma of the lower oesophagus, a neoplasm whose incidence is increasing in developed countries (Nyren and Adami 2002b).

Genetic Factors 3.4.17

The notion that genetic susceptibility plays an important role in human cancer is well-established, and early studies have demonstrated an increased risk of several types of cancer in individuals with a familial history of the same or related cancers. Several familial conditions entailing a very high risk of cancer have been identified, such as the Li-Fraumeni syndrome and familial polyposis of the colon (Haiman and Hunter 2002). It is only recently that, thanks to the development of molecular tools in human genetics, specific high-risk cancer genes have been identified. Inherited mutations of such high-penetrance cancer genes increase dramatically the risk of some neoplasms (Table 3.12). However, these are rare conditions in most populations and the number of cases globally attributable to them is rather small.

A familial aggregation has been shown for most types of cancers, in non-carriers of known high-penetrance genes. This is notably the case for cancers of the breast, colon, prostate and lung. The relative risk is in the order of 2 to 4, and is higher for cases diagnosed at young age. Although some of the aggregation can be explained by shared risk factors among family members, it is plausible

Table 3.12. High penetrance cancer predisposition genes (Haiman and Hunter 2002)

Gene	Syndrome	Main targets
RET	Multiple endocrine neoplasia 2	Medullary thyroid carcinoma, pheochromocytoma, parathyroid adenoma
MET	Familial papillary renal cancer syndrome	Papillary renal cancer
APC	Familial adenomatous polyposis	Colorectal cancer
VHL	von Hippel-Lindau syndrome	Clear-cell renal carcinoma, hemangioblastoma, retinal angioma, pheochromocytoma
WT1	Wilms' tumour syndrome	Bilateral Wilms' tumour
RB1	Hereditary retinoblastoma	Retinoblastoma
NF1	Neurofibromatosis 1	Neurofibroma, neurofibrosarcoma, optic glioma
NF2	Neurofibromatosis 2	Vestibular schwannoma, meningioma
p53	Li-Fraumeni syndrome	Sarcoma, leukaemia, breast, brain, lung, pancreas and skin cancers, others
p16/DCK4	Hereditary melanoma syndrome	Melanoma
PTCH	Nevoid basal cell carcinoma syndrome	Basal cell carcinoma
MEN1	Multiple endocrine syndrome 1	Tumours of parathyroids, gastrointestinal endocrine tissues and anterior pituitary
BRCA1	Hereditary breast-ovarian cancer syndrome	Breast, ovary, prostate and colon cancer
BRCA2	Hereditary breast-ovarian cancer syndrome	Breast (also male) and ovary cancer
PTEN	Cowden syndrome	Hamartoma, breast and thyroid cancer
hMSH2, hMLH1, hPMS1, hPMS2	Hereditary nonpolyposis colon	Colon, endometrium, ovary, stomach cancers, others
ATM	Ataxia-telangiectasia	Leukaemia, lymphoma, breast cancer
XP(A-G)	Xeroderma pigmentosum	Skin cancer
BLM	Bloom syndrome	Leukaemia, lymphoma, most cancers
FAC, FAA	Fancomi anaemia	Acute myeloid leukaemia, others
WRN	Werner syndrome	Sarcoma, melanoma, thyroid carcinoma

that a true genetic component exists for most human cancers. This takes the form of an increased susceptibility to exogenous carcinogens. The knowledge of low-penetrance genes responsible for such susceptibility is still very limited, although research has currently focused on genes encoding for metabolic enzymes, DNA repair, cell cycle control and hormone receptors (Haiman and Hunter 2002). Current estimates of the global contribution of genetic factors to human cancer are in the range of 5% to 10%, of which less than 1% is attributable to high-penetrance genes.

The investigation of high- and medium-penetrance genetic cancer risk factors relies mostly on specific methodological approaches whose discussion goes beyond the scope of this chapter (please refer to Chap. III.7 of this handbook for more details). In the case of low-penetrance genes, however, association studies have been successful in identifying genetic susceptibility factors. Given the lack of dependence of genetic markers of time and disease development, the case-control approach is particularly suitable for this type of investigation.

Screening for Cancer   3.5

Screening is considered to be an effective approach to reduce cancer mortality, because human neoplasms go through several pre-neoplastic stages before they become biologically relevant and clinically detectable. For most cancers, this process takes years or even decades. The possibility to detect preclinical lesions with the potential to develop to a full cancer is highly appealing and is an area of very active research. The slow evolution of cancer, however, is a strong argument to avoid intervention on lesions that do not have the potential to develop to a full cancer during the lifespan of the individual, in order to avoid undue medical procedures such as surgery or chemotherapy. Furthermore, any screening technique has to be carefully evaluated in terms of efficacy to reduce mortality, compliance and costs. Carefully conducted trials with mortality as main outcome are needed to demonstrate the effectiveness of screening. In practice, however, the available evidence is often restricted to observational data.

Oral inspection aimed at identifying pre-neoplastic lesions might be an effective approach for secondary prevention of oral cancer. The inspection can be performed by medically certified professionals, but also, in particular in high-risk areas in developing countries such as India, by specifically trained health workers. Large-scale preventive trials are on-going, which should provide evidence in favour or against this approach (Sankaranarayanan et al. 2000).

Surveillance via flexible sigmoidoscopy, involving removal of adenomas, is a recommended measure for secondary prevention of colorectal cancer. An additional approach consists of the detection of occult blood in the faeces. The method suffers from low specificity and, to a lesser extent, low sensitivity, in particular in the ability to detect adenomas. However, trials have shown a reduced mortality from colorectal cancer after annual tests, although this is achieved at a high cost due to an elevated number of false positive cases. Current recommendations for individuals aged 50 and over include either annual faecal occult blood testing or flexible sigmoidoscopy every five years (Cuzick 1999).

The most suitable approach for secondary prevention of breast cancer is mammography. The effectiveness of screening by mammography in women older than 50 years has been demonstrated, and programmes have been established in various countries (IARC 2002d). The effectiveness of mammography in women younger than 50 is not demonstrated. The benefit of other screening approaches, such as physical examination and self-examination, is not known (Moss 1999).

Cytological examination of exfoliated cervical cells (the Papanicolaou smear test) is effective in identifying precursor lesions, resulting in a decrease in incidence of and mortality from invasive cervical cancer. The benefit is in the order of a two- to four-fold decreased incidence. There is no conclusive evidence, however, regarding the optimal timing of the test (Miller 1999). Cytological smears are not applicable, however, in countries with limited availability of cytologists and pathologists, and alternative approaches for secondary prevention have therefore been proposed, including visual inspection of the cervix with possible enhancement of precursor lesions by acetic acid (Sankaranarayanan et al. 1999). Use of HPV testing as a screening method, either as a first choice for general application or as the triage method of inconclusive cytological diagnoses, is also under trial (Kulasingam et al. 2002).

Secondary prevention has been proposed for prostate cancer, based on digital rectal examination and measurement of prostate-specific antigen. There is no evidence from controlled trials that either procedure decreases the mortality from prostate cancer (Schröder 1999). Despite this lack of evidence, these procedures, in particular the prostate-specific antigen testing, have gained popularity in many countries.

Despite a large body of research since the 1970s, no effective screening method has yet been identified for lung cancer (Black 1999). Spiral computerized tomography scanning has been shown to be able to identify small, subclinical lesions in the lung of high-risk individuals (Henschke et al. 1999), and the effectiveness of this method to reduce mortality is currently under investigation. For a general discussion of the methodological problems of screening see Chap. III.10 of this handbook.

3.6 Conclusions

The application of principles of modern epidemiology to cancer research leads to some methodological considerations of a more general nature. Cancer epidemiology is relatively young, yet it has gained an important status in medicine and is practiced by many professionals around the world. In many respects, cancer epidemiology exemplifies the strengths and the weaknesses of the discipline at large.

On the one hand, cancer epidemiology has the privilege of complete and good-quality disease registries in many populations, covering a broad spectrum of rates and exposures. The network of cancer registries not only provides important clues in terms of etiological and clinical research, for example via the analysis of geographical and temporal differences in incidence, mortality and prevalence of different neoplasms, but also allows in many countries the conduct of large-scale, high-quality (and relatively low-cost) record linkage studies (cf. Chap. I.4 of this handbook). Examples of such studies include the analysis of cancer risk in migrants by region of origin and length of stay in the host country, the linkage between census and cancer registry data to assess risk from employment in specific occupations, the analysis of second primary neoplasms in cancer patients, and the risk of cancer following diagnosis of (or hospitalization for) non-neoplastic conditions.

On several occasions, cancer epidemiology has been the key tool to demonstrate the causal role of important cancer risk factors. The best example is the association between tobacco smoking and lung cancer, which led in the early 1960s to the establishment of criteria for causality in observational research (Doll 1998). Other contributions of epidemiology to the elucidation of important causes of human cancer include the demonstration of the role of HPV in cervical cancer, the role of Helicobacter pylori in stomach cancer, and that of solar radiation exposure in skin cancer, as well as the growing body of evidence for a major role of overweight and obesity in the aetiology of several important neoplasms. These findings have brought important regulatory and public health initiatives as well as lifestyle changes in many countries of the world. For example, Box 1 shows the European Code Against Cancer, which adequately summarizes the current evidence for cancer prevention: these recommendations are mainly based on evidence accumulated via epidemiological studies.

These epidemiological 'discoveries' share two important characteristics: they involve potent carcinogens, and methods are available to reduce misclassification of exposure to the risk factor of interest and to major possible confounders. It has therefore been possible to consistently demonstrate an association in different human populations. It should be noted that it is not necessary for the prevalence of exposure to be high (although this obviously has an impact on the population attributable risk): examples are the many occupational exposures and medical treatments for which conclusive evidence of carcinogenicity has been established on the basis of epidemiological studies conducted in small populations of individuals with well-characterized high exposure.

On the other hand, when these conditions are not met, the evidence accumulated from epidemiological studies is typically inconsistent and difficult to interpret (Taubes 1995). The history of cancer epidemiology presents many examples of premature conclusions, which have not been confirmed by subsequent investigations and have damaged the reputation of the discipline. Misclassification of the relevant exposure (cf. Chap. I.11 of this handbook), uncontrolled confounding (cf. Chaps. I.1 and I.9) and inadequate statistical power (cf. Chap. II.1) are the most common limitations encountered in cancer epidemiology. Two solutions have been proposed to overcome these problems. First, epidemiological studies

Box 1. European Code Against Cancer (Boyle et al. 2003)

Many aspects of general health can be improved, and many cancer deaths prevented, if we adopt healthier lifestyles:

1. Do not smoke; if you smoke, stop doing so. If you fail to stop, do not smoke in the presence of non-smokers.
2. Avoid obesity.
3. Undertake some brisk, physical activity every day.
4. Increase your daily intake and variety of vegetables and fruits: eat at least five servings daily. Limit your intake of foods containing fats from animal sources.
5. If you drink alcohol, whether beer, wine or spirits, moderate your consumption to two drinks per day if you are a man or one drink per day if you are a woman.
6. Care must be taken to avoid excessive sun exposure. It is specifically important to protect children and adolescents. For individuals who have a tendency to burn in the sun active protective measures must be taken throughout life.
7. Apply strictly regulations aimed at preventing any exposure to known cancer-causing substances. Follow all health and safety instructions on substances which may cause cancer. Follow advice of National Radiation Protection Offices.

There are public health programmes that could prevent cancers developing or increase the probability that a cancer may be cured:

8. Women from 25 years of age should participate in cervical screening. This should be within programmes with quality control procedures in compliance with *European Guidelines for Quality Assurance in Cervical Screening*.
9. Women from 50 years of age should participate in breast screening. This should be within programmes with quality control procedures in compliance with *European Guidelines for Quality Assurance in Mammography Screening*.
10. Men and women from 50 years of age should participate in colorectal screening. This should be within programmes with built-in quality assurance procedures.
11. Participate in vaccination programmes against hepatitis B virus infection.

should be very large in size. This is achieved either by conducting multicentre studies including thousands of cases of cancer (see for example the analysis of pure cigar and pipe smokers in a study based on 5621 cases of lung cancer and 7255 controls (Boffetta et al. 1999)) or by performing pooled and meta-analyses of independent investigations (see the pooled analyses of risk factors for breast can-

Table 3.13. Examples of important contributions of molecular epidemiology

Class of biomarkers	Agent, exposure	Reference
Dose marker	Aflatoxin	Ross et al. 1992
Viral infection	HPV	Munoz et al. 1992
Adducts	Ethylene oxide	Schulte et al. 1992
Acquired p53 mutations	Tobacco	Hernandez-Boussard and Hainaut 1998
Chromosomal aberrations	Individual susceptibility	Hagmar et al. 1998
Metabolic polymorphisms	NAT2*	Marcus et al. 2000

* N-acetyltransferase 2

cer including more than 50,000 cases (CGHFBC 1996, 1997, 2002a,b)). Second, the use of biological markers of exposure and early effect has been proposed to reduce exposure misclassification, increase the prevalence of the relevant outcomes, and shed light on the mechanism of action of the carcinogen under study (Boffetta and Trichopoulos 2002). In a few cases, biomarker-based studies have led to important advances in cancer epidemiology (Table 3.13). Assessment of exposure to aflatoxins, enhanced sensitivity and specificity of assessment of past viral infection, detection of protein and DNA adducts in workers exposed to reactive chemicals such as ethylene oxide, are among the examples in which molecular epidemiology has greatly contributed to the understanding of human cancer (cf. Chap. III.6). In many other cases, however, initial, promising results have not been confirmed by subsequent, usually methodologically sounder, investigations. They include in particular the search for susceptibility to environmental carcinogens by looking at polymorphism for metabolic enzymes (Vineis et al. 1999). If biomarkers offer new opportunities to overcome some of the limitations of epidemiology, their added value over traditional approaches should be systematically assessed. Biomarkers should be validated; consideration of sources of bias and confounding in molecular epidemiology studies should be no less stringent than in other types of epidemiological studies. Similarly, other aspects of the study (e.g., determination of required sample size, statistical analysis, reporting and interpretation of results) should be approached with the same rigour used in other areas of cancer epidemiology.

References

Adami H-O, Trichopoulos D (2002) Concepts in cancer epidemiology and etiology. In: Adami H-O, Hunter D, Trichopoulos D (eds) Textbook of cancer epidemiology. Oxford University Press, Oxford, pp 87–112

Adami H-O, Hunter D, Trichopoulos D (eds) (2002) Textbook of cancer epidemiology. Oxford University Press, Oxford

Alonso-Amelot ME, Avendano M (2002) Human carcinogenesis and bracken fern: a review of the evidence. Curr Med Chem 9:675–686

Armstrong BK, Boffetta P (1998) Environmental cancer. In: Boffetta P (ed) Cancer chapter, Encyclopaedia of occupational health and safety, vol I, 4th edn. International Labour Office, Geneva, pp 2.8–2.14

Beral V, Million Women Study Collaborators (2003) Breast cancer and hormone-replacement therapy in the Million Women Study. Lancet 362:419–427

Bergström A, Pisani P, Tenet V, Wolk A, Adami H-O (2001) Overweight as an avoidable cause of cancer in Europe. Int J Cancer 91:421–430

Berrino F, Capocaccia R, Estève J, Gatta G, Hakulinen T, Micheli A, Sant M, Verdecchia A (eds) (1999) Survival of cancer patients in Europe: the EUROCARE-2 study. IARC Scientific Publications No 151. International Agency for Research on Cancer, Lyon

Black WC (1999) Lung cancer. In: Kramer BS, Gohagan JK, Prorok PC (eds) Cancer screening: theory and practice. Marcel Dekker, New York, pp 327–377

Blot WJ, McLaughlin JK, Winn DM, Austin DF, Greenberg RS, Preston-Martin S, Bernstein L, Schoenberg JB, Stermhagen A, Fraumeni JF Jr (1988) Smoking and drinking in relation to oral and pharyngeal cancer. Cancer Res 48: 3282–3287

Boffetta P, Kaldor JM (1994) Secondary malignancies following cancer chemotherapy. Acta Oncol 33:591–598

Boffetta P, Trichopoulos D (2002) Biomarkers in cancer epidemiology. In: Adami H-O, Hunter D, Trichopoulos D (eds) Textbook of cancer epidemiology. Oxford University Press, Oxford, pp 73–86

Boffetta P, Kogevinas M, Simonato L, Wilbourn J, Saracci R (1995) Current perspectives on occupational cancer risks. Int J Occup Environ Health 1:315–325

Boffetta P, Pershagen G, Jöckel K-H, Forastiere F, Gaborieau V, Heinrich J, Jahn I, Kreuzer M, Merletti F, Nyberg F, Rösch F, Simonato L (1999) Cigar and pipe smoking and lung cancer risk: a multicenter study from Europe. J Natl Cancer Inst 91:697–701

Boffetta P, Brennan P, Saracci R (2002) Neoplasms. In: Detels R, McEwen J, Beaglehole R, Tanaka H (eds) Oxford textbook of public health, vol 3, The practice of public health, 4th edn. Oxford University Press, Oxford, pp 1155–1192

Boyle P, Autier P, Bartelink H, Baselga J, Boffetta P, Burn J, Burns HJ, Christensen L, Denis L, Dicato M, et al. (2003) European Code Against Cancer and scientific justification: third version. Ann Oncol 14:973–1005

Breslow NE, Day NE (1980) Statistical methods in cancer research, vol I, The analysis of case-control studies. IARC Scientific Publications No 32. International Agency for Research on Cancer, Lyon

Breslow NE, Day NE (1987) Statistical methods in cancer research, vol II, The design and analysis of cohort studies. IARC Scientific Publications No 82. International Agency for Research on Cancer, Lyon

Castellsague X, Munoz N, De Stefani E, Victora CG, Castelletto R, Rolon PA (2000) Influence of mate drinking, hot beverages and diet on esophageal cancer risk in South America. Int J Cancer 88:658–664

CGHFBC (Collaborative Group on Hormonal Factors in Breast Cancer) (1996) Breast cancer and hormonal contraceptives: collaborative reanalysis of individual data on 53,297 women with breast cancer and 100,239 women without breast cancer from 54 epidemiological studies. Lancet 347:1713–1727

CGHFBC (Collaborative Group on Hormonal Factors in Breast Cancer) (1997) Breast cancer and hormone replacement therapy: collaborative reanalysis of data from 51 epidemiological studies of 52,705 women with breast cancer and 108,411 women without breast cancer. Lancet 350:1047–1059

CGHFBC (Collaborative Group on Hormonal Factors in Breast Cancer) (2002a) Alcohol, tobacco and breast cancer – collaborative reanalysis of individual data from 53 epidemiological studies, including 58,515 women with breast cancer and 95,067 women without the disease. Br J Cancer 87:1234–1245

CGHFBC (Collaborative Group on Hormonal Factors in Breast Cancer) (2002b) Breast cancer and breast feeding: collaborative reanalysis of individual data from 47 epidemiological studies in 30 countries, including 50,302 women with breast cancer and 96,973 women without the disease. Lancet 360:187–195

Cho E, Spiegelman D, Hunter DJ, Chen WY, Stampfer MJ, Colditz GA, Willett WC (2003) Premenopausal fat intake and risk of breast cancer. J Natl Cancer Inst 95:1079–1085

Cuzick J (1999) Colorectal cancer. In: Kramer BS, Gohagan JK, Prorok PC (eds) Cancer screening: theory and practice. Marcel Dekker, New York, pp 219–265

Doll R (1998) Uncovering the effects of smoking: historical perspective. Stat Methods Med Res 7:87–117

Doll R, Peto R (1981) The causes of cancer. Oxford University Press, Oxford

Ferlay J, Bray F, Pisani P, Parkin DM (2001) Globocan 2000: cancer incidence, mortality and prevalence worldwide. IARC CancerBases No 5. International Agency for Research on Cancer, Lyon

Furstenberg G, Senn HJ (2002) Insulin-like growth factors and cancer. Lancet Oncol 3:298–302

Hagmar L, Bonassi S, Stromberg U, Brogger A, Knudsen LE, Norppa H, Reuterwall C (1998) Chromosomal aberrations in lymphocytes predict human cancer: a report from the European Study Group on Cytogenetic Biomarkers and Health (ESCH). Cancer Res 58:4117–4121

Haiman C, Hunter D (2002) Genetic epidemiology of cancer. In: Adami H-O, Hunter D, Trichopoulos D (eds) Textbook of cancer epidemiology. Oxford University Press, Oxford, pp 54–72

Hankinson S, Hunter D (2002) Breast cancer. In: Adami H-O, Hunter D, Trichopoulos D (eds) Textbook of cancer epidemiology. Oxford University Press, Oxford, pp 301–339

HCCP (Harvard Center for Cancer Prevention) (1996) Harvard report on cancer prevention, vol 1, Causes of human cancer. Cancer Causes Control 7, S3–S58

Henschke CI, McCauley DI, Yankelevitz DF, Naidich DP, McGuinness G, Miettinen OS, Libby DM, Pasmantier MW, Koizumi J, Altorki NK, Smith JP (1999) Early Lung Cancer Action Project: overall design and findings from baseline screening. Lancet 354:99–105

Hernandez-Boussard TM, Hainaut P (1998) A specific spectrum of p53 mutations in lung cancer from smokers: review of mutations compiled in the IARC p53 database. Environ Health Perspect 106:385–391

Holmes MD, Hunter DJ, Colditz GA, Stampfer MJ, Hankinson SE, Speizer FE, Rosner B, Willett WC (1999) Association of dietary intake of fat and fatty acids with risk of breast cancer. JAMA 281:914–920

IARC (1972–2003) IARC Monographs on the Evaluation of Carcinogenic Risks to Humans, vols 1–83. International Agency for Research on Cancer, Lyon

IARC (1985) Tobacco habits other than smoking; betel-quid and areca-nut chewing; and some related nitrosamines. IARC Monographs on the Evaluation of the Carcinogenic Risk of Chemicals to Humans, vol 37. International Agency for Research on Cancer, Lyon

IARC (1992) Solar and Ultraviolet Radiation. IARC Monographs on the Evaluation of Carcinogenic Risks to Humans, vol 55. International Agency for Research on Cancer, Lyon

IARC (1993) Some naturally occurring substances: food items and constituents, heterocyclic aromatic amines and mycotoxins. IARC Monographs on the Evaluation of Carcinogenic Risks to Humans, vol 56. International Agency for Research on Cancer, Lyon

IARC (1994a) Hepatitis viruses. IARC Monographs on the Evaluation of Carcinogenic Risks to Humans, vol 59. International Agency for Research on Cancer, Lyon

IARC (1994b) Schistosomes, liver flukes and helicobacter pylori. IARC Monographs on the Evaluation of Carcinogenic Risks to Humans, vol 61. International Agency for Research on Cancer, Lyon

IARC (1994c) Ethylene oxide. In: Some industrial chemicals. IARC Monographs on the Evaluation of Carcinogenic Risks to Humans, vol 60. International Agency for Research on Cancer, Lyon, pp 73–159

IARC (1995) Human papillomaviruses. IARC Monographs on the Evaluation of Carcinogenic Risks to Humans, vol 64. International Agency for Research on Cancer, Lyon

IARC (1996a) Human immunodeficiency viruses and human T-cell lymphotropic viruses. IARC Monographs on the Evaluation of Carcinogenic Risks to Humans, vol 67. International Agency for Research on Cancer, Lyon

IARC (1996b) Some pharmaceutical drugs. IARC Monographs on the Evaluation of Carcinogenic Risks to Humans, vol 66. International Agency for Research on Cancer, Lyon

IARC (1997a) Epstein-Barr virus and Kaposi's sarcoma herpesvirus/human herpesvirus 8. IARC Monographs on the Evaluation of Carcinogenic Risks to Humans, vol 70. International Agency for Research on Cancer, Lyon

IARC (1997b) Non-steroidal anti-inflammatory drugs. IARC Handbooks of Cancer Prevention, vol 3. International Agency for Research on Cancer, Lyon

IARC (1998a) Vitamin A. IARC Handbooks of Cancer Prevention, vol 3. International Agency for Research on Cancer, Lyon

IARC (1998b) Carotenoids. IARC Handbooks of Cancer Prevention, vol 2. International Agency for Research on Cancer, Lyon

IARC (1999a) Hormonal contraception and post-menopausal hormonal therapy. IARC Monographs on the Evaluation of Carcinogenic Risks to Humans, vol 72. International Agency for Research on Cancer, Lyon

IARC (1999b) Surgical implants and other foreign bodies. IARC Monographs on the Evaluation of Carcinogenic Risks to Humans, vol 74. International Agency for Research on Cancer, Lyon

IARC (2000) Ionizing radiation, Part 1, X- and gamma (γ)-radiation and neutrons. IARC Monographs on the Evaluation of Carcinogenic Risks to Humans, vol 75. International Agency for Research on Cancer, Lyon

IARC (2002a) Some traditional herbal medicine, some mycotoxins, naphthalene and styrene. IARC Monographs on the Evaluation of Carcinogenic Risks to Humans, vol 82. International Agency for Research on Cancer, Lyon

IARC (2002b) Weight control and physical activity. IARC Handbooks of Cancer Prevention, vol 6. International Agency for Research on Cancer, Lyon

IARC (2002c) Non-ionizing radiation, Part I, Static and extremely low frequency (ELF) electric and magnetic fields. IARC Monographs on the Evaluation of Carcinogenic Risks to Humans, vol 80. International Agency for Research on Cancer, Lyon

IARC (2002d) Breast cancer screening. IARC Handbooks of Cancer Prevention, vol 7. International Agency for Research on Cancer, Lyon

IARC (2003) Fruit and vegetables. IARC Handbooks of Cancer Prevention, vol 8. International Agency for Research on Cancer, Lyon

IARC (2004) Tobacco smoking and involuntary tobacco smoke. IARC Monographs on the Evaluation of the Carcinogenic Risk of Chemicals to Humans, vol 83. International Agency for Research on Cancer, Lyon (in press)

Kaaks R, Lukanova A, Kurzer MS (2002) Obesity, endogenous hormones, and endometrial cancer risk: a synthetic review. Cancer Epidemiol Biomarkers Prev 11:1531–1543

Kinlen LJ (1996) Immunologic factors, including AIDS. In: Schottenfeld D, Fraumeni JF Jr (eds) Cancer epidemiology and prevention, 2nd edn. Oxford University Press, New York, pp 532–545

Kosary CL, Ries LAG, Miller BA, Hankey BF, Harras A, Edwards BK eds (1995) SEER cancer statistics review, 1973–1992: tables and graphs. NIH Publication No 96–2789. National Cancer Institute, Bethesda, MD

Kulasingam SL, Hughes JP, Kiviat NB, Mao C, Weiss NS, Kuypers JM, Koutsky LA (2002) Evaluation of human papillomavirus testing in primary screening for cervical abnormalities: comparison of sensitivity, specificity, and frequency of referral. JAMA 288:1749–1757

Kuper H, Boffetta P, Adami H-O (2002) Tobacco use and cancer causation: association by tumour type. J Internal Med 252:206–224

Lindblad P, Adami H-O (2002) Kidney cancer. In: Adami H-O, Hunter D, Trichopoulos D (eds) Textbook of cancer epidemiology. Oxford University Press, Oxford, pp 467–485

Marcus PM, Vineis P, Rothman N (2000) NAT2 slow acetylation and bladder cancer risk: a meta-analysis of 22 case-control studies conducted in the general population. Pharmacogenetics 10:115–122

Melbye M, Trichopoulos D (2002) Non-Hodgkin's lymphoma. In: Adami H-O, Hunter D, Trichopoulos D (eds) Textbook of cancer epidemiology. Oxford University Press, Oxford, pp 535–555

Miller AB (1999) Cervix cancer. In: Kramer BS, Gohagan JK, Prorok PC (eds) Cancer screening: theory and practice. Marcel Dekker, New York, pp 195–217

Moolgavkar S, Krewski D, Schwarz M (1999) Mechanisms of carcinogenesis and biologically based models for estimation and prediction of risk. In: Moolgavkar S, Krewski D, Zeise L, Cardis E, Møller H (eds) Quantitative estimation and prediction of human cancer risks. IARC Scientific Publications No 131. International Agency for Research on Cancer, Lyon, pp 179–237

Moss SM (1999) Breast cancer. In: Kramer BS, Gohagan JK, Prorok PC (eds) Cancer screening: theory and practice. Marcel Dekker, New York, pp 143–170

Mucci L, Adami H-O (2002) Oral and pharyngeal cancer. In: Adami H-O, Hunter D, Trichopoulos D (eds) Textbook of cancer epidemiology. Oxford University Press, Oxford, pp 115–136

Munoz N, Bosch FX, de Sanjose S, Tafur L, Izarzugaza I, Gili M, Viladiu P, Navarro C, Martos C, Ascunce N, et al. (1992) The causal link between human papillomavirus and invasive cervical cancer: a population-based case-control study in Colombia and Spain. Int J Cancer 52:743–749

Munoz N, Bosch FX, de Sanjose S, Herrero R, Castellsague X, Shah KV, Snijders PJ, Meijer CJ (2003) Epidemiologic classification of human papillomavirus types associated with cervical cancer. N Engl J Med 348:518–527

Nyren O, Adami H-O (2002a) Stomach cancer. In: Adami H-O, Hunter D, Trichopoulos D (eds) Textbook of cancer epidemiology. Oxford University Press, Oxford, pp 162–187

Nyren O, Adami H-O (2002b) Esophageal cancer. In: Adami H-O, Hunter D, Trichopoulos D (eds) Textbook of cancer epidemiology. Oxford University Press, Oxford, pp 137–161

Parkin DM, Pisani P, Lopez AD, Masuyer E (1994) At least one in seven cases of cancer is caused by smoking: global estimates for 1985. Int J Cancer 59:494–504

Parkin DM, Whelan SL, Ferlay J, Raymond L, Young J eds (1997) Cancer incidence in five continents, vol VII. IARC Scientific Publications No 143. International Agency for Research on Cancer, Lyon

Perera FP (2000) Molecular epidemiology: on the path to prevention? J Natl Cancer Inst 92:602–612

Persson I, Adami H-O (2002) Endometrial cancer. In: Adami H-O, Hunter D, Trichopoulos D (eds) Textbook of cancer epidemiology. Oxford University Press, Oxford, pp 359–377

Peto J (2001) Cancer epidemiology in the last century and the next decade. Nature 411:390–395

Peto R, Darby S, Deo H, Silcocks P, Whitley E, Doll R (2000) Smoking, smoking cessation, and lung cancer in the UK since 1950: combination of national statistics with two case-control studies. BMJ 321:323–329

Pisani P, Parkin DM, Munoz N, Ferlay J (1997) Cancer and infection: estimates of the attributable fraction in 1990. Cancer Epidemiol Biomarkers Prev 6: 387–400

Potter JD, Hunter D (2002) Colorectal cancer. In: Adami H-O, Hunter D, Trichopoulos D (eds) Textbook of cancer epidemiology. Oxford University Press, Oxford, pp 188–211

Ross RK, Yuan JM, Yu MC, Wogan GN, Qian GS, Tu JT, Groopman JD, Gao YT, Henderson BE (1992) Urinary aflatoxin biomarkers and risk of hepatocellular carcinoma. Lancet 339:943–946

Sankaranarayanan R, Black RJ, Parkin DM eds (1998) Cancer survival in developing countries. IARC Scientific Publications No 145. International Agency for Research on Cancer, Lyon

Sankaranarayanan R, Shyamalakumary B, Wesley R, Sreedevi Amma N, Parkin DM, Nair MK (1999) Visual inspection with acetic acid in the early detection of cervical cancer and precursors. Int J Cancer 80:161–163

Sankaranarayanan R, Mathew B, Jacob BJ, Thomas G, Somanathan T, Pisani P, Pandey M, Ramadas K, Najeeb K, Abraham E (2000) Early findings from a community-based, cluster-randomized, controlled oral cancer screening trial in Kerala, India. Cancer 88:664–673

Schröder FH (1999) Prostate cancer. In: Kramer BS, Gohagan JK, Prorok PC (eds) Cancer screening: theory and practice. Marcel Dekker, New York, pp 461–514

Schulte PA, Boeniger M, Walker JT, Schober SE, Pereira MA, Gulati DK, Wojciechowski JP, Garza A, Froelich R, Strauss G et al. (1992) Biologic markers in hospital workers exposed to low levels of ethylene oxide. Mutat Res 278: 237–251

Siemiatycki J (1995) Future etiologic research in occupational cancer. Environ Health Perspect 103 (Suppl 8):209–215

Slattery ML, Potter J, Caan B, Edwards S, Coates A, Ma KN, Berry TD (1997) Energy balance and colon cancer - beyond physical activity. Cancer Res 57: 75–80

Stuver S, Trichopoulos D (2002) Cancer of the liver and biliary tract. In: Adami H-O, Hunter D, Trichopoulos D (eds) Textbook of cancer epidemiology. Oxford University Press, Oxford, pp 212–232

Taubes G (1995) Epidemiology faces its limits. Science 269:164–169

Thomas DC (2000) Genetic epidemiology with a capital "E". Genet Epidemiol 19:289–300

Tredaniel J, Boffetta P, Buiatti E, Saracci R, Hirsch A (1997) Tobacco smoking and gastric cancer: review and meta-analysis. Int J Cancer 72: 565–573

Vineis P, d'Errico A, Malats N, Boffetta P (1999) Overall evaluation and research perspectives. In: Vineis P, Malats N, Lang M, d'Errico A, Caporaso N, Cuzick J, Boffetta P (eds) Metabolic polymorphisms and susceptibility to cancer. IARC Scientific Publications No 148. International Agency for Research on Cancer, Lyon

Vogel RA (2002) Alcohol, heart disease, and mortality: a review. Rev Cardiovasc Med 3:7–13

WCRF(1997)Food,nutritionandthepreventionofcancer:aglobalperspective.World CancerResearchFund&AmericanInstituteforCancerResearch,Washington,DC

Musculoskeletal Disorders

IV.4

Hilkka Riihimäki

4.1 Introduction

Musculoskeletal disorders are a significant public health problem in industrialised countries. They are one of the leading causes of short- and long-term disability and cause high costs due to loss of productivity, burden on health care services and social security systems. It has been estimated that the cost of back pain only is 1–2% of the gross national product. About 10% is due to direct health care costs and 90% due to indirect costs (Norlund and Waddell 2000). In this chapter the focus is in morbidity and aetiology of musculoskeletal disorders. The social consequences, such as disability are not discussed, because disability-related issues depend on the societal context, such as cultural factors and social security regulations, to the extent that cross-national comparisons cannot be made. Firstly, an overview is given of the occurrence and risk factors of the most common musculoskeletal disorders, back and neck disorders, osteoarthritis, upper limb disorders, and osteoporosis. Secondly, some methodological problems in epidemiological research, characteristic for musculoskeletal disorders, are discussed including general study design, and assessment of both health outcome and exposure.

4.2 Occurrence and Risk Factors

4.2.1 Back Disorders

Dorsopathies or back disorders are classified in the International Classification of Diseases 10 (ICD-10) (World Health Organisation, WHO, 1992) into deforming dorsopathies (kyphosis and lordosis, scoliosis, spinal osteochondrosis and others), spondylopathies (ankylosing spondylitis, other inflammatory spondyloses, spondylosis, others), and other dorsopathies (intervertebral disc disorders, other dorsopathies not classified elsewhere, and dorsalgia with several subcategories). This classification is not very useful from the point of view of epidemiological research. For acute back pain it has been estimated that for 70% of the cases a specific diagnosis cannot be determined, i.e. most of the cases fall into the category dorsalgia in the ICD-10. A large proportion of the societal burden due to back disorders is attributable to non-specific back pain. An underlying mechanism in back pain is disc degeneration, but the relationship between low back pain and disc degeneration continues to be controversial.

Occurrence

The prevalence estimates of low back pain (LBP) vary widely from one study to another depending on the population characteristics and assessment methods. In a systematic literature review (Walker 2000), the point prevalence in the general population varied from 12–33%, one-year prevalence from 22–65% (Table 4.1), and life-time prevalence from 30–84% in studies with acceptable quality. The crude prevalence of LBP increases with increasing age reaching its peak around 55–64 years and declining after that towards older age groups (Deyo and Tsui-Wu 1987; Heliövaara et al. 1993). In a national sample of the U.S. population aged 25 years or more the lifetime prevalence of low back pain on most days for at least two weeks was 14%, the lifetime prevalence of sciatica was 2%, and also 2% of the subjects had been told that they had a ruptured disc in the low back (Deyo and Tsui-Wu 1987). In very few studies clinically verified low back syndromes have been studied. One example is the Mini-Finland Health Survey, in which a representative sample of 3322 Finnish men and 3895 women aged 30 years or more were examined. The point prevalence of clinically verified low back pain syndrome was 17.5% in men and 16.3% in women (age-adjusted estimates). For sciatica or herniated disc the estimates were 5.1 and 3.7%, respectively (Heliövaara et al. 1991, 1993).

Table 4.1. One-year prevalence of low back pain in community-based good-quality studies (data from Walker 2000)

Author	Country	Sample size	Age (years)	Prevalence (%)
Harreby et al. (1996)	Denmark	481	38	60/65*
Rafnsson et al. (1989)	Iceland	672	16–65	55
Leboeuf-Yde et al. (1996)	Denmark	1370	30–50	54
Biering-Sorensen (1982)	Denmark	928	30, 40, 50, 60	45
Hillman et al. (1996)	England	3184	25–64	39
Mason (1994)	England	6000	16+	37
Walsh et al. (1992)	England	2667	20–59	36
Lau et al. (1995)	Hong Kong	652	18+	22

* men/women

Very little data are available on the incidence of low back disorders. Biering-Sorensen (1982) reported 6% one-year cumulative incidence in a Danish community sample aged 20, 30, 40 and 50 years and Hillman et al. (1996) observed 4.7% annual incidence in an English community sample aged 25–64 years. In an occupational cohort the three-year cumulative incidence of LBP was 26.6% (Hoogendoorn et al. 2000a). Most prospective studies among adults have not shown marked influence of age on the incidence of LPB.

An increasing interest in low back disorders among children and adolescents has emerged. A large study of Danish twins, representative of the population aged 12–41 years, showed that the prevalence of LBP increases sharply from 12–20 years of age (Leboeuf-Yde and Kyvik 1998). In different countries the prevalence of back pain varies from 1 to 8% among the 11-year-olds, from 1 to 14% among the 13-year-olds, and from 2 to 22% among the 15-year-olds. The prevalence is little higher among girls than boys (Waddell and Waddell 2000). There is an increasing trend from lower to upper social classes.

Time trends in the prevalence of low back pain have been reported in Finland from 1978 to 1992, based on questionnaires sent annually to a random sample of 5000 Finns 15–64 years of age (Leino et al. 1994). On average, the one year prevalence of back disease verified or treated by a doctor was about 15%, and there was no significant change over time. Likewise, the one-month prevalence of back pain was about 36% in women and 34% in men, again without any significant time trend. These results support the view that there have been no major changes in the occurrence of back pain during the past 20 years.

The prevalence rates of radiographically detectable degenerative changes of the lumbar spine in a community sample over 34 years of age were described by Lawrence in 1969. The prevalence of disc degeneration (grades 1–4) was 51% in men aged 35–44, increasing to 91% at 65 or older. In women the prevalence rates were 40% and 78%, respectively. The corresponding rates for more severe disc degeneration (grades 3 and 4) were 5% and 38% in men and 3% and 24% in women. The most probable explanation for the gender difference is men's higher exposure to physical load; the prevalence was highest in men in physically strenuous occupations. A more sensitive method of detection, magnetic resonance imaging (MRI), has revealed high prevalence of disc degeneration even in symptom-free subjects, 6% in women 20 years of age or younger and 79% in those 60 years or older (Powel et al. 1986).

The relationship between degenerative changes in the lumbar spine and low back pain is controversial. Van Tulder et al. (1997) found in their systematic review that radiographically detected degeneration of the lumbar spine was associated with non-specific LBP with odds ratios ranging from 1.2 to 3.3. No association was found between spinal deformities (spondylolysis and -olisthesis, spina bifida, transitional vertebra, etc.) and low back pain. A recent MRI study of 115 monozygotic male twin pairs found that disc height and annular tears were associated with low back pain, but the within pair differences of these findings accounted for only 6–12% of the total variance of LBP when genetic and other familial influences were controlled for (Videman et al. 2003).

Risk Factors

Several comprehensive reviews on risk factors of low back disorders have been published. In Table 4.2 the evidence of risk factors of back pain is given based on the review by Hoogendoorn et al. (1999). There is strong evidence that manual materials handling, frequent bending and twisting of the trunk and whole-body vibration at work are risk factors of back pain. Moderate evidence exists for heavy physical work in general, but there is no evidence for sitting, walking or standing. Other reviews have reported similar results with some deviations in the grading of the evidence level. The National Research Council (NRC) (2001) reported estimates of attributable fractions (AF among the exposed) for the physical work-related risk factors. The AF ranged from 11 to 66% for manual materials handling, from 19 to 57% for frequent bending and twisting, and from 18 to 80% for whole-body vibration. Recently published case-control and cohort studies (Norman et al. 1998; Hoogendoorn et al. 2000a; Vingård et al. 2000) have provided further support for

Table 4.2. Physical risk factors of back and neck pain. Level of evidence according to two systematised reviews

	Back pain Hoogendoorn et al. (1999)	Neck pain Ariëns et al. (2000)
Work-related		
Manual materials handling/lifting/ forceful movements	strong	
Bending and twisting/ awkward posture	strong	some
Heavy physical work	moderate	
Standing or walking	no evidence	
Sitting	no evidence	some
Whole body vibration	strong	
Neck postures		inconclusive
Arm force and posture		inconclusive
Hand-arm vibration		inconclusive
Workplace design factors		inconclusive
Leisure time		
Sports activities/exercise	no evidence	inconclusive
Golf, cycling, athletic training	no evidence	
Total physical activity	no evidence	
Car driving	no evidence	inconclusive

manual materials handling and bending and twisting of the trunk to be risk factors of back pain.

Current knowledge on the physical risk factors of LBP is mainly qualitative and little is known about quantitative exposure-response relationships. The prospective study by Hoogendoorn et al. (2000a) indicated that trunk flexion more than 60 degrees for more than 5% of the working time, trunk rotation more than 30 degrees for more than 10% of the working time, and lifts of more than 25 kg more than 15 times per working day increase the risk of LBP by 30–60%. The accumulated evidence suggests that reduction of occupational physical load carries potential for the prevention of LBP, but data are sparse to define safety levels for exposure. Also little evidence exists of the effectiveness of workplace interventions affecting physical work load.

Much research has addressed the role of work-related psychosocial factors in back pain. According to a review by Hoogendoorn et al. (2000b) the evidence is strong for low social support and low job satisfaction, but the evidence is insufficient for other psychosocial factors (Table 4.3). The National Research Council

Table 4.3. Psychosocial risk factors of low back and neck pain. Level of evidence according to two systematised reviews

	Back pain Hoogendoorn et al. (2000b)	Neck pain Ariëns et al. (2001c)
Work-related		
Work pace, high quantititavie demands	insufficient	some
High qualitative demands[a]	insufficient	
Poor job content[b]	insufficient	
Low job control[c] or low decision latitude[d]	insufficient	some
Low social support	strong	some
Low job satisfaction	strong	some
High or low skill discretion		some
High job strain		inconclusive
Low job security		inconclusive
Conflicts		inconclusive
Lack of break opportunities		inconclusive
Private life	insufficient	
Low social support		inconclusive
Conflicts		inconclusive

[a] conflicting demands, interruption, intense concentration for long periods
[b] monotonous; few possibilities to learn new things, to develop knowledge and skills
[c] autonomy, influence
[d] poor content and control

reported AF estimates ranging from 28 to 48% for low social support and from 17 to 69% for low job satisfaction.

Some studies have shown that leisure time physical activities, such as total physical activity, exercise, sports, or athletics training increase the risk of back pain, but recent systematised reviews did not find the evidence to be convincing (Table 4.2). Likewise, the evidence of a possible protective effect of physical activity is sparse. People who contract a low back disorder may either increase or decrease physical activity, which makes it difficult to study their relationship. Also for the psychosocial factors in private life the evidence is insufficient (Tables 4.2 and 4.3). According to a review by Nachemson and Vingård (2000), there is some evidence for smoking as a risk factor of low back pain, but not of sciatica. They also found some evidence that tall men have an increased risk of sciatica, but moderate obesity was not found to be a risk factor. The epidemiologic evidence of individial risk factors is, however, contradictory; Burdorf and Sorock (1997) did not find convincing evidence for any of these factors in occupational studies.

Low back disorders are complex and the aetiology is multifactorial: there is an interplay between mechanical load, psychosocial factors and also individual host factors. From the point of view of primary prevention, the evidence base seems sufficient for workplace interventions targeted to both physical load on the back as well as on psychosocial work environment and work organisation. Leisure time physical exercise and sports may have a deleterious effect on the back due to injuries but on the other hand, they may also have a protective effect by improving physical fitness. Although good physical fitness is generally considered to protect the back, epidemiologic literature does not provide strong support for this view. For overweight and smoking the case is not very strong either. Anyway, public health programs aiming at improved health behaviour with sufficient physical exercise, avoidance of overweight or weight reduction and quitting smoking may be beneficial for the health of the back.

Neck Disorders   4.2.2

In the ICD-10, neck disorders are classified as subcategories of back disorders or dorsopathies identifiable at the 3 to 4 digit level of the classification. The situation is analogous to that for back disorders: in the majority of the cases a specific diagnosis cannot be set but most of them fall into the category of non-specific neck pain (cervicalgia, "tension neck", etc.). Accordingly, in most epidemiological studies the health outcome has been neck pain.

Occurrence

Neck pain is nearly equally common as back pain. In Table 4.4 prevalence rates are given in the general population of different countries. The rates vary from one study to another due to different age distributions and definitions of neck pain in the surveys. The lifetime prevalence is about 70%, 12-month prevalence varies between 26 and 40%, and point prevalence between 13 and 25%. In specific occupational groups, 12-month prevalence rates as high as 76% have been reported (Ariëns et al. 2001c). The prevalence of neck pain is a little higher in women than in men. The prevalence increases with increasing age until the age of 65, but after that there is a decline (Mäkelä et al. 1991). Little data are available on the incidence rates of neck pain. Among Dutch workers in various industrial and service branches, who had been free of neck pain for at least 12 months, the three-year cumulative incidence of neck pain was 14% (Ariëns et al. 2001a). The highest 12-month prevalences have been observed among secretaries and typists (31%), tailors (28%), loaders, un-loaders and packers (24%), bricklayers and carpenters (23%), and administrative workers (23%) (Blatter and Bongers 1999). In general, neck pain is less disabling and leads less frequently to sick leave or disability pension than back pain.

Risk Factors

Very few cohort or case-control studies have been done on risk factors of neck pain and therefore, the evidence is sparse (Tables 4.2 and 4.3). Several reviews with concordant results have been recently published. According to a review by Ariëns et al. (2000), some evidence exists only for bending and twisting, and sitting at work, but for all other work- and leisure-time-related physical factors the evidence is inconclusive. A prospective cohort study by Ariëns et al. (2001a) added to the

Table 4.4. Prevalence of neck pain in the general population (data from Nachemson et al. (2000))

Authors	Country	Age	Lifetime prevalence	12-month prevalence	Point prevalence
Coté et al. (1998)	Canada	20–69	67		22
van der Donk et al. (1991)	Netherlands	20–65			13
Palmer et al. (2001)	Great Britain	16–65		34	20
Mäkelä et al. (1991)	Finland	30+	71		men 15* women 13*
Westerling and Jonsson (1980)	Sweden	18–65		men 16 women 20	
Hasvold and Johnsen (1993)	Norway	20–56			men 15 women 25
Bovim et al. (1994)	Norway	18–67		men 29 women 40	

* chronic neck pain syndrome

evidence that neck flexion (more than 20 degrees more than 70% of work time) and prolonged sitting (more than 90% of work time) increase the risk of neck pain. Another prospective study among workers in repetitive monotonous jobs with one-year follow-up found a relative risk (RR) of 1.8 for high repetitiveness, 2.0 for high force and 2.3 for the combination of high repetitiveness and high force (Andersen et al. 2002). In a prospective industrial cohort study on neck pain radiating to the upper limb, female gender, high body mass index, smoking, work with hand above shoulder level, mental stress and other musculoskeletal pains were associated with an increased risk (Viikari-Juntura et al. 2001).

The evidence of psychosocial factors as risk factors of neck pain is presented in Table 4.3 according to Ariëns et al. (2001c). Some evidence exists for high quantitative job demands, low social support, low job control, high or low skill discretion and for low job satisfaction. The prospective cohort study by Ariëns et al. (2001b) provided further evidence for high quantitative job demands (RR 2.1), low co-worker support (RR 2.4), and low decision authority (RR 1.6). Andersen et al. (2002) found in their prospective study a RR of 1.8 for female gender, and 1.6 for low pressure pain threshold (Andersen et al. 2002).

Less epidemiologic studies have been conducted on neck than back disorders, but it seems that they share similar multi-factorial aetiology, in which both physical load and psychosocial factors have a role. Even though the evidence base for neck disorders is weaker, it suggests that workplace interventions aiming at reduction of harmful physical load on the neck region and improving psychosocial aspects of work carry potential for the prevention of neck disorders.

4.2.3   Osteoarthritis

Osteoarthritis (OA) is a degenerative process in the joints, in which loss of cartilage is seen as joint space narrowing on radiography. Bony changes include sclerosis in the subchondral bone, osteophyte formation, and bone cysts. Clinical signs of osteoarthritis include pain and restricted range of motion in the joint. In particular, osteoarthritis of the two large weight bearing joints, the hip and knee, is common in elderly people and it causes pain, limits daily activities, and worsens many people's quality of life.

Occurrence

The prevalence estimates of hip OA vary considerably (Table 4.5). In 55–64-year-olds the prevalence varied from 7 to 19% in men and from 3 to 12% in women in radiographic studies. In the Mini-Finland Health Survey osteoarthritis was defined based on symptoms and clinical findings (Heliövaara et al. 1993). The age-specific prevalence rates accorded with those based on radiographic examination in a Dutch population sample (van Saase et al. 1989). The prevalence increased with increasing age.

The prevalence of knee OA also increases with age. It is much more common in women than in men (Table 4.5). In various studies knee OA was detected radiographically in 5–28% of men and in 8–40% of women of age 55 to 64 years. In the Framingham Study repeated radiographs were taken in 1983–1985 (baseline) and 1992–1993 (Felson et al. 1997). The mean age of the subjects without radiographically detectable knee OA at baseline was 70.5 years. During the follow-up 11.1% of the men and 18.1% of the women developed moderate or severe knee OA.

The prevalence of OA of the hand joints increases with increasing age and it is more common in women than in men (Table 4.6). It occurs most frequently in the proximal interphalangeal joints. In the Framingham study the prevalence of symptomatic hand OA (symptoms and radiological findings) was 26.2% in women and 13.4% in men aged at least 71 years (Zhang et al. 2002).

Risk Factors

Mechanical load seems to be important in the inception and development of OA. Systemic factors, such as obesity, bone density, nutrients, oestrogen use, and genetics influence the process (Sowers 2001; Felson et al. 2000). Furthermore, local factors play a role. Extrinsic local factors include physical activity and injury and the intrinsic factors include alignment (varus, valgus), muscle strength (quadriceps), joint laxity, and proprioception (Sharma 2001).

Lievense et al. (2001) and Vingård (2001c) have reviewed the evidence concerning the influence of work on hip OA. Moderate evidence was detected for a positive association between previous heavy physical workload and hip OA, moderate to strong evidence for farming for 10 years or more, or lifting heavy weights ($\geq$ 25 kg). There is also evidence for a positive association between knee OA and heavy physical work, and squatting and kneeling at work (Maetzel et al. 1997; Vingård 2001d). Several studies have indicated that occupational factors such as repetitive work with hands increase also the risk of hand OA (Hadler et al. 1978; Lehto et al. 1990; Felson et al. 2000).

Lievense et al. (2002) found in their systematic review moderate evidence for a positive association between obesity and hip OA, with an odds ratio of ap-

Table 4.5. Prevalence of hip and knee osteoarthritis in general population (%)

Age	Mini-Finland Health Survey[a]		Northern England (Leigh)[b]		The Netherlands (Zoetermeer)[c]		HANES-I[d]	
	Men	Women	Men	Women	Men	Women		
Hip	(n = 3322)	(n = 3895)	(n = 173)	(n = 207)	(n = 1359)	(n = 1598)	Both sexes (n = 2358)	
30–44	0.3	0.7						
45–54	1.9	2.8			2.5	2.3		
55–64	6.6	7.9	18.6	12.0	7.8	3.1	2.3	
65–74	11.9	11.7			8.5	12.5	3.9	
75–	16.4	21.2			10.5	19.1		
Total (age-adjusted)	4.6	5.5						
			Men	Women	Men	Women	Men	Women
Knee			(n = 550)	(n = 566)	(n = 1359)	(n = 1598)	(n = 2498)	(n = 2765)
30|35–44	0.3	1.6	5.5	4.0			1.2	1.2
45–54	4.0	9.7	8.2	13.1	9.3	14.2	2.2	3.6
55–64	9.0	24.2	28.1	40.0	16.8	18.6	5.1	7.5
65–74	12.8	33.0	26.4	49.1	20.9	36.1	9.0	20.3
75–	15.7	38.4			22.1	45.9		
Total (age-adjusted)	5.5	14.5						

[a] Heliövaara et al. (1993), symptom history and clinical examination; [b] Lawrence et al. (1966); [c] van Saase et al. (1989) (right hip and knee); [d] Anderson and Felson (1988)

Table 4.6. Prevalence of hand osteoarthritis (Kellgren grade ≥ 2) by age in two populations

Joint	Men					Women				
	30–44	45–54	55–64	65–74	75+	30–44	45–54	55–64	65–74	75+
Distal interphalangeal										
Finland[a]	0.4–2.3	3.7–10.9	11.4–26.7	21.3–36.4	24.0–51.0	0.2–1.2	5.7–11.8	24.2–40.0	40.3–62.1	48.2–68.9
Zoetermeer[b]	4.2	18.7	44.3	54.3	59.3	4.6	30.5	61.5	75.5	73.1
Proximal interphalangeal										
Finland	0–0.6	0–1.3	2.3–6.5	5.1–11.1	12.5–22.9	0–0.4	0.8–2.1	5.5–9.5	15.1–27.1	21.8–36.3
Zeotermeer	0.8	4.1	12.1	18.9	27.9	0.9	6.3	24.6	32.7	45.9
Metacarpophalangeal										
Finland	0–1.5	0–3.5	0.6–11.7	1.6–21.0	1.0–30.2	0–0.4	0.2–2.2	0–6.1	3.2–15.1	2.6–20.7
Zoetermeer	6.1	12.9	34.2	44.8	43.0	5.2	18.5	36.6	55.4	60.3
Carpometacarpal										
Finland	0.4	1.3–1.6	4.3–7.7	7.5–9.9	17.7–18.6	0.2	3.1–3.7	8.7–12.5	20.1–24.5	27.5–31.6
Zoetermeer	1.9	7.7	17.8	20.4	37.2	2.6	13.3	29.0	43.9	54.6

[a] Haara et al. (2003) Range of joint-specific prevalence rates. General Finnish population
[b] van Saase et al. (1989) Overall prevalence rate. General population of Zoetermeer, The Netherlands

proximately 2. The associations were stronger in studies in which the diagnosis was based on both radiological criteria and clinical symptoms. For knee osteoarthritis obesity is a well-established risk factor (Felson et al. 2000; Riihimäki and Viikari-Juntura 2000). Obesity is more strongly related with bilateral OA in the knee than in the hip (Stürmer et al. 2000). Overweight is associated also with hand OA which indicates that the influence may be due to systemic effects.

In a large prospective study with 25-year follow-up, high levels of physical activity increased the risk of hip OA (self-report of OA diagnosed by a doctor) among men younger that 50 years but not among women or older men (Cheng et al. 2000). In a cross-sectional study with retrospective history of recreational physical activity as teenager, at age 30, and at age 50, it was found that among elderly women the risk of moderate to severe radiographic hip OA was modestly increased in those who had had highest physical activity as a teenager (odds ratio, OR, 1.7), at age 50 (OR 1.4), and weight bearing activities at age 30 (OR 1.4) (Lane et al. 1999). For symptomatic hip OA the respective ORs were a little higher (2.0–1.6). The authors concluded that recreational physical activities before menopause may increase the risk of radiographic and symptomatic hip OA. Physical exercise has beneficial effect on bone density, but on the other hand, there is evidence that high bone density is associated with an increased risk of osteoarthritis.

Hip injuries have been linked to hip OA in several cross-sectional and case-control studies but prospective cohort studies are rare (Riihimäki and Viikari-Juntura 2000). Gelber et al. (2000) followed 1321 former medical students, initially 22 years of age, for a median duration of 36 years. Hip and knee injury at cohort entry or during the follow-up increased the risk of OA in the corresponding joint.

Several studies are available on genetic influences on knee OA. Twin and family studies have shown a large familial and genetic component of OA heritability ranging from 39–65% (Felson et al. 2000; Loughlin 2001). One twin pair study has suggested that genetic influence may be stronger in females than males (Kaprio et al. 1996). Association studies of candidate genes suggest that genes for type II collagen (COL2A1) and the vitamin D receptor gene (VDR) may encode for OA susceptibility (Loughlin 2001). Uitterlinden et al. (2000) reported from a population-based study that COL2A1 gene and vitamin D receptor gene are involved in radiographic knee OA, but in separate features. The COL2A1 gene was associated with a two-fold increased risk of joint space narrowing and the VDR gene was associated with osteophytes. Carriers of COL2A1 4B allele did not show an increased risk of radiographic knee OA, the risk was 1.8-fold among carriers of VDR 1 allele and 2.7-fold among carriers of the combination, as compared with non-carriers. The involvement of these two genes in the aetiology of clinically relevant OA remains, however, to be established.

Based of the epidemiological evidence, weight control, avoidance of excessive physical load, and prevention of joint injuries should be the targets in preventive programs of OA. Moderate-level physical activity and exercise may have a protective effect.

Upper Limb Disorders 4.2.4

Upper limb disorders rank high among compensated occupational diseases or injuries and they are also one of the leading causes of sick leaves. Over the years, many "umbrella" concepts have been used for these disorders, such as occupational overuse syndrome, repetitive strain injury, and cumulative trauma disorder, indicating work-related aetiology. Several specific disorders can be diagnosed: rotator cuff syndrome, epicondylitis, neural impingement syndromes (cubital tunnel syndrome, radial tunnel syndrome, carpal tunnel syndrome, Guyon canal syndrome) and tenosynovitis or peritendinitis of the wrist-forearm region – including de Quervain's disease. Yet a great proportion of the problem manifests only as non-specific symptoms. In this section only the most common syndromes are discussed.

Occurrence

Little data are available on the occurrence of hand-wrist tendon syndromes (tendinitis, tenosynovitis, peritendinitis) in the general population. In occupational studies the point prevalence has varied from 0 to 13.5% in the non-exposed reference groups and from 0.9 to 56% in the exposed groups (Bernard 1997). Leclerc et al. (2001) studied wrist tendinitis in jobs with repetitive work (assembly line work, work in clothing, shoe and food industry, packaging, and supermarket cashiering). The prevalence of proved or suspected wrist tendinitis was 11.2%, 19.1% among men and 7.9% among women. The three-year cumulative incidence was 5.7%. Age did not influence the prevalence or incidence (Table 4.7). In Finland Kurppa et al. (1991) obtained the incidence rates ranging from less than 1 to 25/100 workers/year depending on gender and hand strain at work.

The prevalence of epicondylitis in the Swedish general population was estimated 1–3%, but it reached 10% in 40–45-year old women (Allander 1974). In the study by Leclerc et al. (2001) the prevalence of lateral epicondylitis was 12.2%, 9.6% among men and 13.3% among women. The three-year cumulative incidence was 12.2%. Both the prevalence and incidence increased with increasing age (Table 4.7).

For carpal tunnel syndrome the prevalence estimates in the general population range from 0.5% in the U.S.A. (Tanaka et al. 2001) to 9% in women and 1% in men in The Netherlands (de Krom et al. 1992). Among French workers in repetitive work the prevalence was 21.9% (Leclerc et al. 2001, Table 4.7). Nordstrom et al. (1998) reported the incidence rate of 3.5/1000 person-years in a US general population (selected zip code areas in Wisconsin) and Leclerc et al. (2001) found three-year cumulative incidence of 12.2% in the French workers in hand-strenuous jobs. The incidence increased with increasing age in the U.S. general population but not among the French workers. In the former study the incidence rate varied by occupation from 1.5 cases per 1000 person-years among sales workers to 9.9 cases per 1000 person-years among handlers and labourers.

Risk Factors

All the upper limb disorders discussed above have been associated with repetitive movements of the hand, use of hand force, non-neutral wrist postures and hand-

Table 4.7. Prevalence and three-year incidence of upper limb disorders (proven or possible) by age in workers exposed to repetitive work (Leclerc et al. 2001)

Age (years)	Wrist tendinitis	Lateral epicondylitis	Carpal tunnel syndrome
Prevelence (%)			
≤ 29	17.9	4.3	13.7
30–39	11.1	8.4	23.1
40–49	6.9	17.2	25.1
≥ 50	13.2	26.4	22.6
Total	11.2	12.2	21.9
	NS	$P = 0.01$	NS
Three-year incidence (%)			
≤ 29	6.2	4.5	11.9
30–39	7.5	11.2	15.6
40–49	3.2	17.9	10.5
≥ 50	6.5	15.4	4.9
Total	5.7	12.2	12.2
	NS	$P = 0.01$	NS

arm vibration. The evidence of repetition and combination of these risk factors is strong for carpal tunnel syndrome but limited for the other risk factors. For epicondylitis and wrist-hand tendon disorders the evidence is moderate to limited for all these risk factors and their combinations (Vingård 2001a,b; Bernard 1997). In the National Research Council's review (2001) the AF estimates ranged from 44 (vibration) to 93% (repetition + force). The role of psychosocial factors is controversial (NRC 2001). Carpal tunnel syndrome has been related to hormonal factors in older women, obesity and previous history of other musculoskeletal complaints.

Criteria for the upper limb disorders are not standardised and varying criteria have been used in different studies, which contributes partly to the obtained differences in the occurrence estimates. The occurrence rates are rather high particularly among workers in hand strenuous jobs which indicates that preventive action is needed. The gradient across occupational groups seems to be most prominent for carpal tunnel syndrome.

4.2.5   Osteoporosis

Osteoporosis has been defined as a systemic skeletal disorder characterised by low bone mass and microarchitectural deterioration of bone tissue, with a consequent increase in bone fragility and susceptibility to fracture (Anonymous 1993). Osteoporosis is often identified by the occurrence of characteristic low trauma fractures (fragility fractures), the most serious of which are fractures of the hip and vertebrae. One of the strongest risk factors of fractures is low bone mineral density (BMD). High-precision methods to identify BMD are dual energy X-ray absorptiometry (DEXA) and quantitative computed tomography. DEXA is widely accepted as the reference method (Pafumi et al. 2002), but its use in large-scale population studies is restricted by the availability of the equipment. For screening purposes quantitative ultrasonometry (QUS) of the calcaneal bone can be used.

The World Health Organisation (1994) has recommended four categories to classify osteoporosis: *normal*: BMD not more than 1 standard deviation (SD) below the mean of young adults; *osteopenia*: BMD between 1 and 2.5 SD below the mean of young adults; *osteoporosis*: BMD more than 2.5 SD below the mean of young adults; *severe osteoporosis*: BMD more than 2.5 SD below the mean of young adults and one or more fragility fractures. The criteria are useful in population-based surveys but less useful in assessing individual risks (Jordan and Cooper 2002).

Occurrence

In Table 4.8 the prevalence of osteoporosis is presented by age for men and women 50 years or older in a sample of the general population, Rochester, Minnesota. A clear increase with increasing age is seen, but it is less steep for the lumbar spine than for other sites. This may be due to age-related artifacts that mask bone loss from the vertebral body (Melton 2003). The total prevalence of osteoporosis in the lumbar spine, wrist, and all sites combined was higher in women as compared to men, but the genders had similar prevalences for the hip. In some other studies, in which the same absolute bone density cut-off level for men and women has been used, lower prevalence rates have been obtained for men (Melton 2003).

Risk Factors

Bone mass is generally lower in Caucasians and Asians than among other races, but the underlying factors explaining the difference are largely unknown (Melton 2003). The Study of Osteoporotic Fractures Research Group found higher age, mother's fracture history, current smoking, gastric surgery, and lifetime caffeine intake to be risk factors of low BMD among elderly white women. Higher weight and height, oestrogen use, muscle strength, thiazide use, dietary calcium intake, noninsulin-dependent diabetes and recent or past physical activity proved to be protective of bone loss. These determinants, however, explained only 20–34% of the variance in bone density at various sites (Orwoll et al. 1996). Twin studies have confirmed genetic influence on bone mass and some candidate genes involved have been identified (Walker-Bone et al. 2002). Also early developmental factors such as tall maternal height and low rate of childhood growth seem to have an influence (Cooper et al. 2001).

With the expected demographic shift towards older age groups in the industrialised countries the number of affected people, women in particular, will increase substantially. Prevention of osteoporosis is an important public health issue. Optimising maternal nutrition and fetal growth, improving calcium intake and general nutrition in growing children, and increasing the level of physical exercise through-

Table 4.8. Prevalence of osteoporosis among an age-stratified sample of residents of Rochester, Minnesota. World Health Organisation criteria (2.5 SD or more below sex-specific young normal mean). (Adapted from Melton 2003)

Age (years)	n	Hip (%)	Lumbar spine (%)	Wrist (%)	Hip or spine or wrist (%)
Postmenopausal women					
50–59	50	4.0	2.0	6.0	8.0
60–69	50	10.0	8.0	28.0	30.0
70–79	51	19.6	17.6	56.9	56.9
> 80	50	40.0	4.0	78.0	82.0
Total	201	13.6[a]	7.7[a]	32.9[a]	34.7[a]
Men					
50–59	49	12.2	2.0	4.1	12.2
60–69	50	16.0	0	4.0	18.0
70–79	51	15.7	2.0	11.8	21.6
> 80	50	26.0	2.0	30.0	40.0
Total	200	15.8[a]	1.4[a]	8.8[a]	19.4[a]

[a] Prevalence per 100, age-adjusted to the 1990 U.S. white population ≥ 50 years old

out the population have been suggested to be included in the preventive strategies (Walker-Bone et al. 2002).

Methodological Problems in Epidemiological Research

4.3

4.3.1   Aspects of Study Design

Most epidemiologic studies have used a cross-sectional study design. These studies serve well administrative purposes providing descriptive information of the magnitude of the problem in different populations, but they are not good for etiological considerations due to well-known inherent biases (cf. Chap. I.3 of this handbook). A wide range of potential determinants have been explored in cross-sectional settings, but to advance the knowledge of risk factors of musculoskeletal disorders more rigorous study designs are required in the future.

Case-control studies of musculoskeletal disorders are rare because of the difficulties in case definition and catchment (cf. Chap. I.6 of this handbook). The majority of people with musculoskeletal problems is treated in primary health care. Generally accepted diagnostic criteria are not available and the use of diagnostic labels varies remarkably among practitioners. In some studies cases have been identified from health care providers (e.g. Vingård et al. 2000) or from registers (e.g. Heliövaara et al. 1987). In such studies one needs to be aware of potential bias in etiological considerations due to differential proneness across exposure groups to file a claim or seek care or to get treatment. This bias can be minimized by restricting the cases to only severe cases, which will be treated in a similar way irrespective of e.g. social class or demands on physical performance (e.g. Manninen et al. 2002).

Another question to consider in case-control studies is the validity and relevance of exposure assessment (cf. Chap. I.11 of this handbook). Often the only feasible option for data collection is to use retrospective questionnaires or interviews providing data susceptible to recall error. This error can be differential between the cases and referents. Due attention should be paid to the relevant time windows for exposure assessment in reference to the inception of the disease of interest and induction period. In very few studies this matter has been considered, but some examples can be found (Vingård et al. 1991a). In cases where the inception and induction periods are not known, assumptions can be made and tested. For studying the triggering factors of musculoskeletal disorders a case-crossover design may be the approach of choice (cf. Chap. I.7 of this handbook). This approach is appropriate, for instance, for sudden-onset overexertion injuries. Even though the degenerative process of the spine, chronic in nature, may be the underlying cause for back and neck disorders, these disorders characteristically manifest as painful episodes. Little is known of the possible triggering causes of such spells.

During the past ten years an increasing number of cohort studies on musculoskeletal disorders have been published (cf. Chap. I.5 of this handbook). The exposures of interest and other determinants have been measured at baseline and used as predictors of new-onset musculoskeletal pain or incident cases of musculoskeletal disorders. According to the general principles of etiological cohort studies, persons already afflicted by the index disorder should be excluded. This simple principle turns out to be quite difficult to follow for disorders with a chronic underlying process, such as disc or cartilage degeneration, which manifest as intermittent pain episodes. The date of inception for such disorders is not easy to define and operational definitions, preferably based on assumed or known pathomechanisms, should be employed. For example, for osteoarthritis a natural proxy is the time of the first occurrence of "arthritic" pain in the afflicted joint.

In prospective cohort studies health outcome can be assessed using repeated surveys including symptom questionnaires or interviews, imaging or functional performance tests, or clinical tests allowing exact diagnostics, if appropriate. When available, register data are useful particularly in large scale epidemiological studies (e.g. Heliövaara et al. 1987) (cf. Chap. I.4 of this handbook).

Health Outcome Assessment

4.3.2

Questionnaire Surveys

The occurrence of pain has been the most common outcome measure in epidemiologic studies on musculoskeletal disorders. The occurrence parameter has been one-, three-, or 12-month, or lifetime period prevalence or cumulative incidence in follow-up studies. One of the major drawbacks of symptom data is its non-specificity; pain due to minor sprains may not be differentiated from more chronic and severe conditions although this would be important in both etiologic and prognostic studies. Pain perception is person-dependent and it can be modified by several factors such as prior experience, culture, coping mechanisms, etc. Pain experience may also depend on physical activity at work and leisure, because physical activity provokes musculoskeletal pain. This can lead to spurious associations in studies on physical risk factors.

No generally agreed symptoms questionnaires are available. One of the most commonly employed forms is the Nordic questionnaire (Kuorinka et al. 1987). Lack of consensus in defining such fundamental concepts as new onset cases, acute, recurrent and chronic cases and an episode hampers the development of epidemiologic research focussing on pain and other symptoms. A scoring system for pain intensity proposed by von Korff et al. (1990) is gaining acceptance among research scientists in the field.

Better characterization of the temporal aspects of musculoskeletal disorders is needed. Von Korff (1994) proposed definitions for transient, recurrent, chronic, acute, first-onset and flare-up back pain. Nachemson (2000) proposed time limits to define *acute* (0 to 3 weeks' duration of pain or disability), *subacute* (4 to 12 weeks' duration of pain or disability) and *chronic back or neck pain* (more than 12 weeks' duration of pain or disability) and *recurrent problems* (patients seeking help after at least 1 month of not seeking care or not being on sick leave after at least 1 month of working). These definitions serve mainly prognostic epidemiology. De Vet et al. (2002) made a proposal to define episodes of low back pain. Croft and Raspe (1995) have written an overview of the classification of back pain.

Table 4.9 summarizes the characteristic of pain and indicates the most commonly used measuring methods (for references see the original article).

Clinical Tests

Clinical examination, laboratory tests and functional performance tests usually do not provide very useful information for the case definition of back and neck disorders. For the back a comprehensive review of the repeatability of different function measurements concluded that recommendations for tests to be used in epidemiological studies can not be made (Essendrop et al. 2002). For upper limb disorders a criteria document has been published proposing diagnostic criteria based on symptoms and clinical findings (Sluiter et al. 2001). For osteoarthritis, clinical examination has been used for classification, e.g., the American College of Rheumatology has presented criteria (www.rheumatology.org/publications/classification).

Imaging

Radiological site-specific definition of osteoarhtritis is recognised as the method of choice in epidemiologic studies of osteoarthritis (Hart and Spector 1995, 2000). Exposure to radiation is a matter of concern especially when taking radiographs of

Table 4.9. Characteristics of back pain and their measurement (adapted from Croft and Raspe 1995)

Characteristic		Measurements
Back pain	Location	Pain drawing
	Intensity	Visual Analogue Scale
		Numerical rating
		Verbal rating
	Quality	McGill Short Form
	Temporality	Duration of current episode
		Number of days of back pain in defined
		period (6 or 12 months)
Bodily symptoms	Other pains	Pain drawing
	Other complaints	Area checklist
		MSPQ*
		Symptom-Checklist 90R
Psychological features	Emotions	General Health Questionnaire
		Zung Depression Index
		Hospital Anxiety Depression Scale
	Cognitions	Pain-related control scale
		Fear Avoidance Beliefs
	Behaviour	Inappropriate symptoms
	Psychiatric disorders	DSM-III[#]
Signs	Systemic	Fever, ESR, weight loss
	Local back	Tender points
	Local other	SLR[§]: active, passive to reproduce leg pain
		Femoral stretch
		Schober's test
		Lateral flexion
		Inappropriate signs

* MSPQ = Modified Somatic Perceptions Questionnaire
[#] DSM III = Diagnostic and Statistical Manual of the American Psychiatric Association (American Psychiatric Association 1980).
[§] SLR = Straight leg raise

the hip, pelvic or lumbar spine area. Kellgren and Lawrence presented already in 1957 (Kellgren and Lawrence 1957; Kellgren 1963) classification criteria, which have been widely used. In this system osteoarthritis is classified using grades from 0 to 4. The grading is based on a presumption of sequential appearance of osteophytes, loss of joint space, subchondral sclerosis, and cyst formation, but it relies heavily on the presence of osteophytes. Criticism has been presented against this classification and there is growing consensus that semi-quantitative grading of osteophytes and joint space narrowing, using validated atlases, should be separately recorded. Based on these data also aggregate measures can be constructed (Hart and Spector 1995, 2000).

For the imaging of the spine, magnetic resonance imaging (MRI) has provided a sensitive method to study the degenerative process of the spinal tissues, the intervertebral disc, in particular. No known adverse health effects are involved, but high costs and availability of the equipment limit the use of MRI in large-scale epidemiologic studies. No generally agreed classification criteria exist, but for disc degeneration a system based on the morphology of the disc (inhomogeneity of disc structure, clarity of the distinction between the annulus and nucleus, and collapse of the disc space) has been proposed (Pfirrmann et al. 2001). Instead of using aggregate grading systems combining different features of disc degeneration, it seems advisable to record different features (morphology, signal intensity, bulging) separately in epidemiologic studies.

Bone Mineral Density Measurements

Bone mineral density (BMD) can be measured with high-precision using dual-energy X-ray absorptiometry (DEXA). It is based on the attenuation of X-rays passing through the bone. With this technique it is possible to detect bone mass reduction that carries increased risk of fracture. DEXA is widely accepted as the reference method to diagnose osteoporosis and fracture risk (Pafumi et al. 2002). The use of DEXA in large epidemiological studies is limited by the availability of the equipment that is usually located in specialized centres. Another method, quantitative ultrasonometry (QUS) of the calcaneal bone, has several advantages. The equipment is cheaper, it is transportable and the execution of the measurement is rapid. However, QUS is more suitable to assess bone density in younger (up to 55 years) than old people (Pafumi et al. 2002).

Registers

Register data of occupational injuries, users of social security benefits such as sick leave and disability pension, or of users of health care services (hospital discharge registers, registers from health care providers) can be used for descriptive epidemiology to find gradients across different population groups (e.g. Leino-Arjas et al. 2002; Vingård et al. 1991b). Register-based case assessment of musculoskeletal disorders in etiological studies carries a potential for bias due to differential proneness across population groups to file a workers compensation claim, seek or get treatment, to go on sick leave or pension. Another weakness is non-uniform use of diagnostic labels among medical doctors. In some countries a national register of arthroplasties is being kept making it easy to identify severe cases of osteoarthritis (Manninen et al. 2002).

4.3.3   Exposure Assessment

Assessment of exposure to mechanical load is a challenging task in epidemiologic studies. For many other risk factors, such as anthropometric measures and life-style factors standardized and validated methods are available. Also for psychosocial factors validated questionnaires are available, as an example the Job Content Questionnaire to assess psychosocial job characteristics (Karasek et al. 1998).

Exposure to physical or mechanical load as a risk factor is conceptually problematic. Everybody is "exposed" to materials handling, awkward postures, repetitive movements and most also to vibration, the known risk factors of musculoskeletal disorders. Sedentary life-style is becoming more common and has raised concern of too low "exposure" levels to mechanical load leading to deterioration of people's physical condition. A crucial question is, at what level mechanical load starts having adverse effects on musculoskeletal system.

Mechanical exposure involves exertion, motion and posture. Each of these can be characterized by level (amplitude), frequency (repetitiveness) and duration. Dynamic movement characteristics, velocity and acceleration, may also be important. Furthermore, for different musculoskeletal disorders the relative importance of peak and cumulative exposures varies. This makes mechanical exposure very complex to assess and for the planning of the assessment strategy one should have prior knowledge or hypotheses of the pathomechanisms of the disorders. Using biomechanical modelling, the internal exposure can be estimated and even a common metrics has been proposed for the assessment of physical workload (Wells et al. 1997)

In epidemiologic studies mechanical exposure can be assessed using self-reports, observation methods or direct measurement. Winkel and Mathiassen (1994) have described the feasibility of different assessment methods. Capacity, versatility, and generality decrease whereas exactness and cost increase from self-reports to observations to direct measurements. With modern sophisticated measuring technology it is possible to get accurate measures for current exposure to various dimensions of physical load at work. Direct measurements may not be feasible for large studies and the accuracy of measurements is of value only if current exposure is relevant with regard to study objective. Also, if current exposure can be considered as a proxy of past exposure direct measurements are warranted. However, often this may not be the case, and other means of past exposure assessment, such as interview or expert assessment based on occupational history, must be utilized. Several validation studies of self-assessment of physical exposures have shown that the accuracy is not always very good but for some exposures such data are usable in epidemiologic studies. As an example, Mortimer et al. (1999) studied the validity of self-reported duration of work postures in a population based study. The validation was done against observations and technical measurements. They concluded that time spent in sitting, standing or walking with hands above shoulder level and standing or walking with hands below knuckle level may be accurate enough to be used in epidemiological studies. Likewise, Viikari-Juntura et al. (1996) studied the validity of self-reported physical work load by questionnaire and logbook against task analysis and observations among industrial workers. They found the validity to be acceptable for frequency of manual handling, duration of trunk flexion, neck rotation, hands above shoulder level, and squatting and kneeling. The duration of some postures was overestimated in the questionnaires and less so in the logbooks.

Different techniques to assess posture, including observational methods, videotaping and computer-aided observational methods, direct measurements, as well as self-reports, have been reviewed and discussed by Li and Buckle (1999). Precision, cost and feasibility of different techniques to assess postural load, mechanical load, psychophysical load, and physiological load in epidemiologic studies has been compared by Burdorf et al. (1997). Also van deer Beek and Frings-Dreesen

(1998) have reviewed mechanical exposure assessment methods and strategies in epidemiologic studies. Direct measurements, such as electromyography, can be used for more accurate assessment. Methods for data reduction have been developed, such as exposure variation analysis (EVA, Mathiassen and Winkel 1991) or its modification, clustered EVA (Anton et al. 2003).

4.4   Conclusions

In epidemiology of musculoskeletal disorders steady progress has been made during the past decades. Even though longitudinal and case-control studies are still sparse, their number is increasing. Systematized reviews have collected the available evidence of the risk factors of musculoskeletal disorders. Major risk factors have been identified qualitatively but little is known of exposure-effect relationships. More studies with rigorous study designs are needed with valid methods to assess both exposures and health outcomes.

The lack of knowledge on exposure-effect relationships makes it difficult to plan preventative programs and agree on standards and guidelines to reduce the risk of musculoskeletal disorders. The knowledge base is, however, sufficient to plan interventions aiming at prevention. In workplace interventions a good starting point is to reduce exposure to highest loads. Reviews of intervention studies have revealed that high-quality studies are rare and all the reviews conclude that randomized controlled studies are needed to provide convincing evidence of the effectiveness of the interventions.

For low back and neck pain it has been shown that both physical load and psychosocial factors play a role. When subjective perception of non-specific pain is the health outcome, the question remains, how much physical load acts as a symptom provoking or aggravating factor and how much it is a causal factor for back morbidity. Likewise it can be questioned to what extent psychosocial factors modify the pain perception of the subjects. This question is relevant, because in experimental studies it has been shown that pain perception of individuals varies very much when exposed to a standardized pain-inducing stimulus. For the future development of epidemiology of back and neck disorders it is important that effort is put to identifying more specific and also clinically relevant entities of low back and neck disorders. For upper limb disorders better diagnostic criteria are available but the specific diagnoses cover only a part of all upper limb complaints. It is equally important to develop exposure assessment methods that are valid and feasible also for large-scale population-based studies.

Recent studies have revealed that the prevalence of low back and neck disorders starts to increase already in the adolescence. There also seems to be an association between the development of disc degeneration and low back pain among the young (Salminen et al. 1999). These results suggest that follow-up studies of young cohorts are needed to learn more about the temporal relationships between low back and neck pain and the degenerative process of the intervertebral disc. Another question of interest is the inception and natural course of low back and neck disorders from the adolescence through adulthood to older age.

Genetic epidemiology is emerging also in the field of musculoskeletal disorders. Twin studies have provided information of the familial and genetic influences on musculoskeletal disorders of the back and joints, in particular. Some candidate genes have been identified, but much remains to be done in unraveling the genes involved and their influences. A future challenge is to learn about the interactions between genetic susceptibility and environmental factors.

References

Allander E (1974) Prevalence, incidence, and remission rates of some common rheumatic diseases and syndromes. Scand J Rheumatol 3:145–153

American College of Rheumatology. Classification criteria for rheumatic diseases (www.rheumatology.org/publications/classification). Accessed April 08, 2004

Anderson JJ, Felson DT (1988) Factors associated with osteoarthritis of the knee in the first national health and nutrition examination survey (HANES I). Evidence for an association with overweight, race, and physical demands of work. Am J Epidemiol 128:179–189

Andersen JH, Kaergaard A, Frost P, Thomsen JF, Bonde JP, Fallentin N, Borg V, Mikkelsen S (2002) Physical, psychosocial, and individual risk factors for neck/shoulder pain with pressure tenderness in the muscles among workers performing monotonous repetitive work. Spine 27:660–667

Anonymous (1993) Consensus development conference: Diagnosis, prophylaxis and treatment of osteoporosis. Am J Med 94:646–650

Anton D, Cook TM, Rosecrance JC, Merlino LA (2003) Method for quantitatively assessing physical risk factors during variable noncyclic work. Scand J Work Environ Health 29:354–362

Ariëns GAM, van Mechelen W, Bongers PM, Bouter LM, van der Wal G (2000) Physical risk factors for neck pain. Scand J Work Environ Health 26:7–19

Ariëns GAM, Bongers PM, Douwes M, Miedema M, Hoogendoorn WE, van der Wal G, Bouter LM, van Mechelen W (2001a) Are neck flexion, neck rotation, and sitting at work risk factors for neck pain? Results from a prospective cohort study. Occup Environ Med 58:200–207

Ariëns GAM, Bongers PM, Hoogendoorn WE, Houtman IL, van der Wal G, van Mechelen W (2001b) High quantitative job demands and low coworker support as risk factors for neck pain: Results of a prospective cohort study. Spine 26:1896–1901

Ariëns GAM, van Mechelen W, Bongers PM, Bouter LM, van der Wal G (2001c) Psychosocial risk factors for neck pain: A systematic review. Am J Ind Med 39:180–193

Bernard BP (ed) (1997) Musculoskeletal disorders and workplace factors. A critical review of epidemiologic evidence for work-related musculoskeletal disorders of the neck, upper exptremity, and low back. U.S. Department of Health and Human Services CDC (NIOSH), DHHS (NIOSH) Publication No. 97–141, Cincinnati

Biering-Sorensen F (1982) Low back trouble in a general population of 30-, 40-, 50-, and 60-years-old men and women. Study design, representativeness and basic results. Dan Med Bull 29:289–299

Blatter BM, Bongers PM (1999) Work related neck and upper limb symptoms (RSI): High risk occupations and risk factors in the Dutch working population. TNO-report 4070117/r9800293. TNO Work and Employment, Hoofddorp

Bovim G, Schrader H, Sand T (1994) Neck pain in the general population. Spine 19:1307–1309

Burdorf A, Rossignol M, Fathallah FA, Snook SH, Herrick RF (1997) Challenges in assessing risk factors in epidemiologic studies on back disorders. Am J Ind Med 32:142–152

Burdorf A, Sorock G (1997) Positive and negative evidence of risk factors for back disorders, Scand J Work Environ Health 23:243–256

Cheng Y, Macera CA, Davis DR, Ainsworth BE, Troped PJ, Blair SN (2000) Physical activity and self-reported, physician diagnosed osteoarthritis: Is physical activity a risk factor? J Clin Epidemiol 53:315–322

Cooper C, Eriksson JG, Forsen T, Osmond C, Tuomilehto J, Barker DJ (2001) Maternal height, childhood growth and risk of hip fractures in later life. Osteoporosis Int 12:623–629

Coté P, Cassidy JD, Carroll L (1998) The Saskatchewan health and back pain survey: The prevalence of neck pain and related disability in Saskatchewan adults. Spine 23:1689–1698

Croft P, Raspe H (1995) Back pain. Baillière's Clin Rheumatol 9:565–583

de Krom MCTFM, Knipschild PG, Kester ADM, Thijs CT, Boekkooi PF, Spaans F (1992) Carpal tunnel syndrome: Prevalence in the general population. J Clin Epidemiol 45:373–376

de Vet HCW, Heymans MW, Dunn KM, Pope DP, van der Beek AJ, Macfarlane GJ, Bouter LM, Croft PR (2002) Episodes of low back pain. A proposal for uniform definitions to be used in research. Spine 27:2409–2416

Deyo RA, Tsui-Wu Y-J (1987) Descriptive epidemiology of low-back pain and its related medical care in the United States. Spine 12:264–268

Essendrop M, Maul I, Läubli T, Riihimäki H, Schibye B (2002) Measures of low back function: A review of reproducibility studies. Clin Biomechanics 17:235–249

Felson DT, Zhang Y, Hannan MT, Naimark A, Weissman B, Aliabadi P, Levy D (1997) Risk factors for incident radiographic knee osteoarthritis in the elderly. Arthritis Rheum 40:728–733

Felson DT, Lawrence RC, Dieppe PA, Hirsch R, Helmick CG, Jordan JM, Kington RS, Lane NE, Nevitt MC, Zhang Y, Sowers M, McAlindon T, Spector TD, Poole AR, Yanovski SZ, Ateshian G, Sharma L, Buckwalter JA, Brandt KD, Fries JF (2000) Osteoarthritis: New insights. Part 1: The disease and its risk factors. Ann Intern Med 133:635–646

Gelber AC, Hochberg MC, Mead LA, Wang NY, Wigley FM, Klag M (2000) Joint injury in young adults and risk for subsequent knee and hip osteoarthritis. Ann Intern Med 133:321–328

Haara M, Manninen P, Kröger H, Arokoski JPA, Kärkkäinen A, Knekt P, Aromaa A, Heliövaara M (2003) Osteoarthritis of finger joints in Finns aged 30 or over: Prevalence, determinants, and association with mortality. Ann Rheum Dis 62:151–158

Hadler NM, Gillings DB, Imbus HR, Levitin PM, Makuc D, Utsinger PD, Yount WJ, Slusser D, Moskowitz N (1978) Hand structure and function in an industrial setting. Arthritis Rheum 21:210–220

Hart DJ, Spector TD (1995) The classification and assessment of osteoarthritis. Bailliéres Clin Rheumatol 9:407–432

Hart DJ, Spector TD (2000) Definition and epidemiology of osteoarthritis of the hand: A review. Osteoarthritis Cartilage 8(Suppl A):S2–S7

Harreby M, Kjer J, Hesselsoe G, Neergaard K (1996) Epidemiological aspects and risk factors for low back pain in 38-year-old men and women: A 25-year prospective cohort study of 640 school children. Eur Spine J 5:312–318

Hasvold T, Johnsen R (1993) Headache and neck or shoulder pain: Frequent and disabling complaints in the general population. Scand J Health Care 11:219–224

Heliövaara M, Knekt P, Aromaa A (1987) Incidence and risk factors of herniated lumbar intervertebral disc or sciatica leading to hospitalization. J Cron Dis 40:251–258

Heliövaara M, Mäkelä M, Knekt P, Impivaara O, Aromaa A (1991) Determinants of sciatica and low-back pain. Spine 16:608–614

Heliövaara M, Mäkelä M, Sievers K (1993) Tuki- ja liikuntaelinten sairaudet Suomessa. [Musculoskeletal diseases in Finland]. Publication of the Social Insurance Institution AL:35, Helsinki

Hillman M, Wright A, Rajaratnam G, Tennant A, Chamberlain MA (1996) Prevalence of low back pain in the community: Implications for service provision in Bradford, UK. J Epidemiol Community Health 50:347–352

Hoogendoorn WE, van Poppel MNM, Bongers PM, Koes BW, Bouter LM (1999) Physical load during work and leisure time as risk factors for back pain. Scand J Work Environ Health 25:387–403

Hoogendoorn WE, Bongers PM, de Vet HCW, Douwes M, Koes BW, Miedema MC, Ariëns GAM, Bouter LM (2000a) Flexion and rotation of the trunk and lifting at work are risk factors for low back pain: Results of a prospective cohort study. Spine 25:3087–3092

Hoogendoorn WE, van Poppel MNM, Bongers PM, Koes BW, Bouter LM (2000b) Systematic review of psychosocial factors at work and private life as risk factors for back pain. Spine 25:2114–2125

Jordan KM, Cooper C (2002) Epidemiology of osteoporosis. Best Pract Res Clin Rheumatol 16:795–806

Kaprio J, Kujala U, Peltonen L, Koskenvuo M (1996) Genetic liability to osteoarthritis may be greater in women than men. Br Med J 313:232

Karasek R, Brisson C, Kawakami N, Houtman I, Bongers P, Amick B (1998) The job content questionnaire (JCQ): An instrument for internationally comparative assessment of psychosocial job characteristics. J Occup Health Psychol 3:322–355

Kellgren JH (1963) The epidemiology of chronic rheumatism. Atlas of standard radiographs, vol 2. Blackwell Scientific, Oxford

Kellgren JH, Lawrence JS (1957) Radiological assessment of osteoarthritis. Ann Rheum Dis 16:494–501

Kuorinka I, Jonsson B, Kilbom Å, Vinterberg H, Biering-Sorensen F, Andersson G, Jorgensen K (1987) Standardised Nordic questionnaire for the analysis of musculoskeletal symptoms. Appl Ergon 18:233–237

Kurppa K, Viikari–Juntura E, Kuosma E, Huuskonen M, Kivi P (1991) Incidence of tenosynovitis or peritendinitis and epicondylitis in a meat–processing factory. Scand J Work Environ Health 17:32–37

Lane NE, Hochberg MC, Pressman A, Scott JC, Nevitt MC (1999) Recreational physical activity and the risk of osteoarthritis of the hip in elderly women. J Rheumatol 26:849–854

Lau EMC, Egger P, Coggon D, Cooper C, Valenti L, O'Connell D (1995) Low back pain in Hong Kong: Prevalence and characteristics compares with Britain. J Epidemiol Community Health 49:492–494

Lawrence JS (1969) Disc degeneration. Its frequency and relationship to symptoms. Ann Rheum Dis 28:121–138

Lawrence JS, Bremner JM, Bier F (1966) Osteo-arthrosis. Prevalence in the population and relationship between symptoms and X-ray changes. Ann Rheum Dis 25:1–23

Leboeuf-Yde C, Klougart N, Lauritzen T (1996) How common is low back pain in the Nordic population? Data from a recent study on a middle-aged general Danish population and four surveys previously conducted in the Nordic countries. Spine 21:1518–1525

Leboeuf-Yde C, Kyvik KO (1998) At what age does low back pain become common problem? A study of 29,424 individuals aged 12–41 years. Spine 23:228–234

Leclerc A, Landre MF, Chastang JF, Niedhammer I, Roquelaure Y, Study Group on Repetitive Work (2001) Upper limb disorders in repetitive work. Scand J Work Environ Health 27:268–278

Lehto TU, Rönnemaa TE, Aalto TV, Helenius HYM (1990) Roentgenological arthrosis of the hand in dentists with reference to manual function. Community Dent Oral Epidemiol 18:37–41

Leino P, Berg M-A, Puska P (1994) Is back pain increasing? Results from national surveys in Finland during 1978/9–1992. Scand J Rheumatol 23:269–276

Leino-Arjas P, Kaila-Kangas L, Notkola V, Keskimäki I, Mutanen P (2002) Inpatient hospital care for back disorders in relation to industry and occupation in Finland. Scand J Work Environ Health 28:304–313

Li G, Buckle P (1999) Current techniques for assessing physical exposure to work-related musculoskeletal risks, with emphasis on posture-based methods. Ergonomics 42:674–695

Lievense A, Bierma-Zeinstra S, Verhagen A, Verhaar J, Koes B (2001) Influence of work on the development of osteoarthritis of the hip: A systematic review. J Rheumatol 28:2520–2528

Lievense AM, Bierma-Zeinstra SM, Verhagen AP, van Baar ME, Verhaar JA, Koes BW (2002) Influence of obesity on the development of osteoarthritis of the hip: A systematic review. Rheumatology (Oxford) 41:1155–1162

Loughlin J (2001) Genetic epidemiology of primary osteoarthritis. Curr Opin Rheumatol 13:111–116

Maetzel A, Mäkelä M, Hawker G, Bombardier C (1997) Osteoarthirtis of the hip and knee and mechanical occupational exposure – a systematic overview of the evidence. J Rheumatol 24:1599–1607

Manninen P, Heliövaara M, Riihimäki H, Suomalainen O (2002) Physical work-load and risk of severe knee osteoarthritis. Scand J Work Environ Health 28: 25–31

Mason V (ed) (1994) The prevalence of back pain in Great Britain. A report on OPCS Omnibus Survey Data produced on behalf of the Department of Health. Her Majesty's Stationery Office, London, p 3

Mathiassen SE, Winkel J (1991) Quantifying variation in physical load using exposure-vs-time data. Ergonomics 34:1455–1468

Melton LJ III (2003) Epidemiology worldwide. Endocrinol Metab Clin N Am 32:1–13

Mortimer M, Hjelm EW, Wiktorin C, Pernold G, Kilbom Å, Vingård E (1999) Valid-ity of self-reported duration of work postures obtained by interview. MUSIC-Norrtälje Study Group. Appl Ergon 30:477–486

Mäkelä M, Heliövaara M, Sievers K, Impivaara O, Knekt P, Aromaa A (1991) Preva-lence, determinants and consequences of chronic neck pain in Finland. Am J Epidemiol 134:1356–1367

Nachemson AL (2000) Introduction. In: Nachemson AL, Jonsson E (eds) Neck and back pain. The scientific evidence of causes, diagnosis, and treatment. Lippincott Williams & Wilkins, Philadelphia, pp 1–12

Nachemson AL, Vingård E (2000) Influences of individual factors and smoking on neck and low back pain. In: Nachemson AL, Jonsson E (eds) Neck and back pain. The scientific evidence of causes, diagnosis, and treatment. Lippincott Williams & Wilkins. Philadelphia, pp 79–96

Nachemson AL, Waddell G, Norlund AI (2000) Epidemiology of neck and low back pain. In: Nachemson AL, Jonsson E (eds) Neck and back pain. The scientific evidence of causes, diagnosis, and treatment. Lippincott Williams & Wilkins, Philadelphia, pp 165–187

National Research Council and the Institute of Medicine (2001) Musculoskeletal disorders and the workplace: Low back and upper extremities. Panel on Muscu-loskeletal Disorders and the Workplace. Commission on Behavioral and Social Sciences and Education. National Academy Press, Washington, DC

Nordstrom DL, DeStefano F, Vierkant RA, Layde PM (1998) Incidence of di-agnosed carpal tunnel syndrome in a general population. Epidemiology 9: 342–345

Norlund AI, Waddell G (2000) Cost of back pain in some OECD countries. In: Nachemson AL, Jonsson E (eds) Neck and back pain. The scientific evidence of causes, diagnosis, and treatment. Lippincott Williams & Wilkins. Philadelphia, pp 421–425

Norman R, Wells R, Neumann P, Frank J, Shannon H, Kerr M (1998) A comparison of peak vs cumulative physical work exposure as risk factors and the reporting of low back pain in the automotive industry. Clin Biomech (Bristol, Avon) 13:561–573

Orwoll ES, Bauer DC, Vogt TM, Fox KM (1996) Axial bone mass in older women: Study of Osteoporotic Fractures Research Group. Ann Intern Med 124:187–196

Pafumi C, Chiarenza M, Zizza G, Roccasalva L, Ciotta L, Farina M, Pernicone G, Russo A, Maggi I, Bandiera S, Giardina P, Cavallaro A, Cianci A (2002) Role of DEXA and ultrasonometry in the evaluation of osteoporotic risk in post-menopausal women. Maturitas 42:113–117

Palmer KT, Walker-Bone K, Griffin MJ, Syddall H, Pannett B, Coggon D, Cooper C (2001) Prevalence and occupational associations of neck pain in the British population. Scand J Work Environ Health 27:49–56

Powell MC, Wilson M, Szypryt P, Symonds EM, Worthington BS (1986) Prevalence of lumbar disc degeneration observed by magnetic resonance in symptomless women. Lancet i:1366–1367

Pfirrmann CWA, Metzdorf A, Zanetti M, Hodler J, Boos N (2001) Magnetic Resonance classification of lumbar intervertebral disc degeneration. Spine 26:1873–1878

Rafnsson V, Steingrimsdottir OA, Olafsson MH, Sveinsdottir T (1989) Muskulose-letala besvär bland islänningar. Nord Med 104:104–107 (in Swedish)

Riihimäki H, Viikari-Juntura E (2000) Back and limb disorders. In: McDonald C (ed) Epidemiology of work-related diseases, 2nd edn. BMJ Publishing Group, Bristol, pp 233–265

Salminen JJ, Erkintalo MO, Pentti J, Oksanen A, Kormano MJ (1999) Recurrent low back pain and early disc degeneration in the young. Spine 24:1316–1321

Sharma L (2001) Local factors in osteoarthritis. Curr Opin Rheumatol 13:441–446

Sluiter JK, Rest KM, Frings-Dresen MHW (2001) Criteria document for evaluating the work-relatedness of upper extremity musculoskeletal disorders. Scand J Work Environ Health 27:Suppl 1

Sowers M (2001) Epidemiology of risk factors for osteoarthritis: Systemic factors. Curr Opin Rheumatol 13:447–451

Stürmer T, Gunther KP, Brenner H (2000) Obesity, overweight and patterns of osteoarthritis: The Ulm Osteoarthritis Study. J Clin Epidemiol 53:307–313

Tanaka S, Petersen M, Cameron L (2001) Prevalence and risk factors of tendini-tis and related disorders of the distal upper extremity among U.S. workers: Comparison to carpal tunnel syndrome. Am J Ind Med 39:328–335

Uitterlinden AG, Burger H, van Duijn CM, Huang Q, Hofman A, Birkenhager JC, van Leeuwen JP, Pols HA (2000) Adjacent genes, for COL2A1 and the vitamin D receptor, are associated with separate features of radiographic osteoarthritis of the knee. Arthritis Rheum 43:1456–1464 van der Beek AJ, Frings-Dresen MHW (1998) Assessment of mechanical exposure in ergonomic epidemiology. Occup Environ Med 55:291–299

van der Donk J, Schouten JSAG, Passchier J, van Romunde LK, Valkenburg HA (1991) The associations of neck pain with radiological abnormalities of the cervical spine and personality traits in a general population. J Rheumatol 18:1884–1889

van Tulder MW, Assendelft WJJ, Koes BW, Bouter LM (1997) Spinal radiographic findings and nonspecific low back pain. A systematic review of observational studies. Spine 22:427–434

van Saase JLCM, van Romunde LKJ, Vandenbroucke JP, Valkenburg HA (1989) Epidemiology of osteoarthritis: Zoetermeer Survey. Comparison of radiological osteoarthirtis in a Dutch population with that in 10 other populations. Ann Rheum Dis 48:271–80

Videman T, Battié MC, Gibbons LE, Maravilla K, Manninen H, Kaprio J (2003) Associations between back pain history and lumbar MRI findings. Spine 28:582–588

Viikari-Juntura E, Rauas S, Martikainen R, Kuosma E, Riihimäki H, Takala E-P, Saarenmaa K (1996) Validity of self-reported physical work load in epidemiologic studies on musculoskeletal disorders. Scand J Work Environ Health 22:251–259

Viikari-Juntura E, Martikainen R, Luukkonen R, Mutanen P, Takala E-P, Riihimäki H (2001) Longitudinal study on work related and individual risk factors affecting radiating neck pain. Occup Environ Med 58:345–352

Vingård E (2001a) Epicondylitis and work (in Swedish with English summary) In: Hansson T, Westerholm P (eds) Arbete och besvär i rörelseorganen. En vetenskaplig värdering av frågor om samband. National Institute of Working Life, Stockholm. Arbete och Hälsa 12:161–171

Vingård E (2001b) Carpal tunnel syndrome (in Swedish with English summary) In: Hansson T, Westerholm P (eds) Arbete och besvär i rörelseorganen. En vetenskaplig värdering av frågor om samband. National Institute of Working Life, Stockholm. Arbete och Hälsa 12:173–183

Vingård E (2001c) Hip osteoarthrosis and work (in Swedish with English summary) In: Hansson T, Westerholm P (eds) Arbete och besvär i rörelseorganen. En vetenskaplig värdering av frågor om samband. National Institute of Working Life, Stockholm. Arbete och Hälsa 12:185–194

Vingård E (2001d) Knee osteoarthrosis and work (in Swedish with English summary) In: Hansson T, Westerholm P (eds) Arbete och besvär i rörelseorganen. En vetenskaplig värdering av frågor om samband. National Institute of Working Life, Stockholm. Arbete och Hälsa 12:195–203

Vingård E, Alfredsson L, Fellenius E, Goldie I, Hogstedt C, Köster M (1991a) Coxarthrosis and physical work load. Scand J Work Environ Health 17:104–109

Vingård E, Alfredsson L, Goldie I, Hogstedt C (1991b) Occupation and osteoarthrosis of the hip and knee: A register-based cohort study. Int J Epidemiol 20:1025–1031

Vingård E, Alfredsson L, Hagberg M, Kilbom A, Theorell T, Waldenstrom M, Hjelm EW, Wiktorin C, Hogstedt C, MUSIC-Norrtalje Study Group (2000) To what extent do current and past physical and psychosocial occupational factors explain care-seeking for low back pain in a working population? Results from the Musculoskeletal Intervention Center-Norrtalje Study. Spine 25:493–500

von Korff M, Dworkin SF, Le Resche L (1990) Graded chronic pain status: An epidemiologic evaluation. Pain 40:270–291

von Korff M (1994) Studying the natural history of back pain. Spine 19(suppl):2041–2046

Waddell G, Waddell H (2000) A review of social influences on neck and back pain and disability. In: Nachemson AL, Jonsson E (eds) Neck and back pain. The scientific evidence of causes, diagnosis, and treatment. Lippincott Williams & Wilkins, Philadelphia, pp 13–55

Walker BF (2000) The prevalence of low back pain: A systematic review of the literature from 1966 to 1998. J Spin Disorders 13:205–217

Walker-Bone K, Walter G, Cooper C (2002) Recent developments in the epidemiology of osteoporosis. Curr Opin Rheumatol 14:411–415

Walsh K, Cruddas M, Coggon D (1992) Low back pain in eight areas in Britain. J Epidemiol Community Health 46:227–230

Wells R, Norman R, Neumann P, Andrews D, Frank J, Shannon H (1997) Assessment of physical workload in epidemiologic studies: Common measurement metrics for exposure assessment. Ergonomics 40:51–61

Westerling D, Jonsson BG (1980) Pain from the neck-shoulder region and sick leave. Scand J Soc MEd 8:131–136

Winkel J, Mathiassen SE (1994) Assessment of physical load in epidemiologic studies: Concepts, issues, and operational considerations. Ergonomics 37:979–988

World Health Organisation (WHO) (1992) International statistical classification of diseases and related health problems, 1989 revision. WHO, Geneva

World Health Organisation (WHO) (1994) Assessment of fracture risk and its application to screening for postmenopausal women. WHO Technical Report Series 843. WHO, Geneva 6

Zhang Y, Niu J, Kelly-Hayes M, Chaisson CE, Alibadi P, Felson DT (2002) Prevalence of symptomatic hand osteoarthritis and its impact on functional status among the elderly: The Framingham Study. Am J Epidemiol 156:1021–1027

Health Services Research

Thomas Schäfer, Christian A. Gericke, Reinhard Busse

Introduction

After a brief introduction into the general field of health services research, a large section deals with the specific issues arising when epidemiological or statistical methods are used to study health services. This is followed by sections describing the main fields of investigation which are usually thought of as pertaining to the wider realm of health services research. These are studies of demand, need, utilisation and access to health services which have the interface between the patient and health services in common. The next section describes the importance of financial resources, structure, and organisation for the delivery of effective and efficient health care. This is followed by a description of the processes and outcomes of health care, including concepts such as effectiveness and appropriateness of care and their use, e.g. in physician profiling or in hospital rankings. In the section on outcomes, special emphasis is put on health status measurement and the evaluation of health systems in international comparisons. Important health economic concepts, such as cost-effectiveness and efficiency, are covered in various sections. The chapter concludes with describing common pitfalls and caveats in interpreting health services research.

Health Services Research Defined

Health services research (HSR) attempts to answer questions about the best medical treatment or preventive course of action, the quality of care provided by a hospital or a physician, the efficient delivery of services to all populations, and their costs. The Institute of Medicine (1994) defines HSR as "A multi-disciplinary field of inquiry, both basic and applied, that examines access to, and the use, costs, quality, delivery, organisation, financing, and outcomes of health care services to produce new knowledge about the structure, processes, and effects of health services for individuals and populations". The three basic dimensions of care studied are: (1) the process of deciding what care to provide, (2) the process of providing care in the best possible manner, and (3) the outcomes that result from care. Many HSR projects study aspects of care that span all three dimensions under the rubric "quality of care" (Brook and Lohr 1985). As Scott and Campbell (2002) pointed out, this frequently used but rarely defined phrase encompasses notions of effectiveness, efficiency, safety, access, and consumer satisfaction and is thus not a very precise title for scientific investigation. HSR challenges the dominant biomedical model in which disease occurs, leading to illness, which is then treated (Black 1997). In contrast to the clinical view focussing on individual patients, it adopts a population perspective and considers other determinants of the use of health care (Black 1997), such as socioeconomic status, local availability or acceptability of health services. HSR thus often challenges medical claims about the value of specific interventions.

HSR cannot be defined as a methodological discipline. It draws upon and uses multiple methodologies and is multidisciplinary in nature. The majority of quantitative research in the field is done using epidemiological methods and epidemiologists increasingly work in this field of research.

This multidisciplinary approach is seen by many authors as characteristic of this field of investigation, which is reflected in Last's definition of HSR as "The integration of epidemiologic, sociologic, economic, and other analytic sciences in the study of health services. HSR is usually concerned with relationships between need, demand, supply, use, and outcome of health services. The aim is evaluation, particularly in terms of structure, process, output, and outcome" (Last 2001).

The ultimate goal of HSR however is to provide unbiased, scientific evidence to influence health services policy at all levels so as to improve the health of the public (Black 1997).

5.1.2   The Input–Output Model of Health Care

Different models have been proposed for the study of health services. These include operational models, e.g. the patient-flow model or the social sciences model. The patient-flow model starts with the assumption of a healthy population, where a patient's way through the different health care institutions is followed once a disease manifests itself (Bennett 1978). The social sciences model attempts to consider the main social and political influences, causal relationships, and environmental conditions on the process of service delivery in a health care system. Social experiences, values, priorities, importance of societal resources and structures are the focus of the analysis (Weinermann 1971). A causal or epidemiological model is also possible, which analyses care along known or supposed hypothetical causal biosocial links (de Miguel 1971). The drawback of such a model is its complexity.

For many analyses simpler models are more adequate. We prefer a model adapted from engineering sciences in which some components of the other models have been integrated – the input–output model – which takes structure, processes, outputs and outcomes into account (Schwartz and Busse 2003).

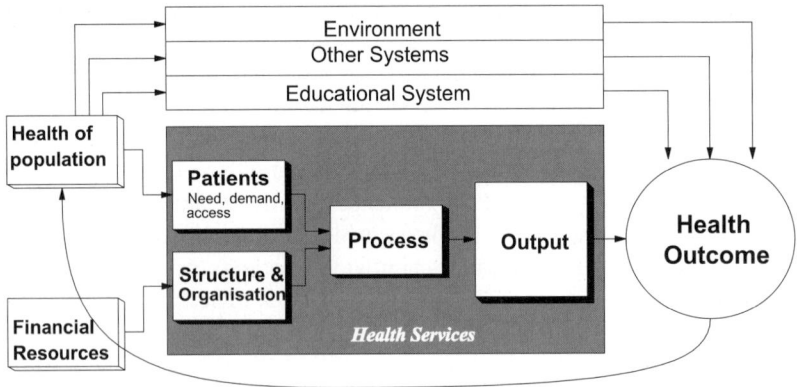

Figure 5.1. The input–output model (Busse and Wismar 2002)

In this model, statistical data can be structured in an easy and transparent manner. Political debates on health services also often follow this structure.

The input of the health care system is divided into (Schwartz and Busse 2003):

— Patient-side input, i.e. the health status of the population as well as its access to care.
— Resource-orientated input, i.e. the input in terms of financial and non-financial resources, such as human resources and infrastructure, as well as organisational structures, responsibilities and interdependencies between actors and organisations.

Throughput forms the centre of the model – encompassing all processes of care in a health care system.

The output of the health care system is divided into two sequential elements (Schwartz and Busse 2003):

— Direct results of the processes, i.e. output measures in the classical sense, also termed intermediary outcomes, e.g. the number of cardiac catheterisations performed.
— Outcomes in terms of changes in health status, which are often only measurable in the long-term, e.g. the mortality avoided by a specific intervention.

Common to all models deployed is the problem of causal inference. Although some problems are also encountered by epidemiological research, like the establishment of precedence in time in case-control studies or in historical cohorts (Hill 1965), these problems are much more important in health services research and thus make the latter more prone to biased or confounded results. The main problem is the complexity of the system with multiple interdependencies which result in the dilemma of "before the intervention is after the intervention". A good example is the evaluation of health care reforms, which often come in a piece-meal fashion, and which are only half-way executed before the next reform measures start. Assigning observed changes in an evaluation study to one particular reform package then becomes difficult and, as with all uncontrolled before-and-after studies, the results of such studies have to be interpreted with great caution (Grimshaw et al. 2001). However, in particular for the evaluation of health reforms such before-and-after studies are often the only possible research method, as conducting controlled studies is often not feasible.

Level of Analysis   5.1.3

A complementary approach to the one described is the analysis of the level at which processes of care take place (Schwartz and Busse 2003):

— The macro level – consisting of the health system as a whole and national health policy.
— The meso level – research focussing on inter-organisational structures and processes, e.g. between health care payers and providers, or the relationships between providers in a specific region.
— The micro level – analysis of individual care services and technologies.

Aday et al. (1998) attempted to match research methods to the level of analysis, illustrated in Table 5.1. In their model, the macro level refers to a population perspective on the determinants of the health of communities as a whole ("health of population" in the model), and the micro level represents a clinical perspective on the factors that contribute to the health of individuals at the system, institution, or patient level (Aday et al. 1998). Their intermediary system level encompasses both the macro and meso level in our model. It refers to the resources (money, people, physical infrastructure, and technology) and the organisational configurations used to transform these resources into health care services either for the country as a whole (macro level) or within a specific region (meso level).

Table 5.1. Levels of analysis in health services research. Adapted from Aday et al. (1998)

Data sources	Level of analysis			
	Population	System	Institution	Patient
Census	×			
Public Health Surveillance Systems	×			
Vital statistics	×			
Surveys				
Population	×			
Organisations		×	×	
Providers		×	×	
Patients		×	×	×
Insurance records/ administrative data				
Enrolment	×	×	×	×
Encounters		×	×	×
Claims		×	×	×
Medical records		×	×	×
Qualitative studies				
Participant observation	×	×	×	×
Case studies		×	×	×
Focus groups	×		×	×
Ethnographic interviews	×			×

5.2 Methodological Considerations

Generally all types of data can be analysed for the purposes of HSR. We find experimental data from randomised controlled trials as well as observational data from case-control or cohort studies, registers or surveys. But many analyses in HSR make use of data from large administrative databases that are abstracted from medical or hospital discharge records, prescriptions and bills of payments for delivered health services.

Study Designs

Randomised Controlled Trials

When alternative approaches to the delivery of health care have to be evaluated, a randomised controlled trial (RCT) is considered the gold standard, i.e. the most rigorous method available. RCTs are performed in order to avoid bias and confounding. It is the effect of randomisation that provides equality of study and control group in all relevant characteristics except the intervention being tested.

Regardless of this advantage one has to keep in mind some critical issues when considering the RCT methodology. First the recruitment of participants (or other experimental units like communities or schools etc.), who meet all eligibility criteria, may be difficult and expensive. Furthermore a randomised assignment of treatments to patients may not be feasible because of ethical reasons (for instance if you want to compare a treatment that is widely believed to be efficacious with "no treatment" or with a placebo). The study population is frequently not representative of the target population. Thus, it is true that a RCT has a high level of "internal" validity, as study group and control group are really comparable, but this tends to be connected with a low level of "external" validity which is an important consideration in HSR as it aims to examine effects under actual conditions and not under trial conditions. The results of a RCT refer solely to efficacy (a treatment is called efficacious if the desired effect is obtained under optimal conditions) but not necessarily to effectiveness (a treatment is called effective if the desired effect is obtained under everyday conditions).

Accordingly, the role of RCTs in HSR is more limited than in other areas of health research, and RCTs have only been carried out in certain areas of HSR. For example the efficacy of cholesterol-lowering treatment in the prevention of coronary heart disease in men with high cholesterol was demonstrated by a multi-centre, randomised, double-blind clinical trial, the *Lipid Research Clinics Coronary Primary Prevention Trial* (Lipid Research Clinics Program 1984). As Kelsey et al. (1998) report, the most expensive research study ever sponsored by the US-National Institutes of Health – the Women's Health Initiative (Buring and Hennekens 1992) – consists of a series of RCTs to test the hypotheses, whether a low-fat dietary pattern protects against breast cancer and colon cancer, whether hormone replacement therapy reduces risk for coronary heart disease, and whether calcium and Vitamin D supplementation protects against hip fractures. Even in the context of evaluating organisational change RCTs had been carried out. The so called *Health Insurance Experiment* (Newhouse 1974) was designed as an RCT to evaluate the effect of different levels of cost sharing in health insurance on utilisation, expenditures and health status (for more details see Sect. 5.3.2). But regardless of such examples the majority of RCTs are designed to evaluate a new (drug) therapy and are performed in clinical settings (randomised *clinical* trials).

Observational Studies

An overwhelming part of HSR is based on observational studies. In a pure epidemiological setting case-control and cohort studies are used to estimate and evaluate the association between a specific exposure and a specific disease. In addition exposure and outcome are frequently mapped into binary variables. In HSR exposures and outcomes have a higher degree of variety than in chronic disease epidemiology.

Typical exposures are:

— Conditions that may lead to inequalities in access to care, e.g. low income status, rural area of residence
— Health states that define certain needs for care, e.g. mental illness
— Medical interventions, e.g. stent implants vs. bypass surgery to prevent heart attacks
— Different health care delivery systems, e.g. Health Maintenance Organisations (HMO) vs. capitated Preferred Provider Organisations (PPO) vs. a traditional indemnity plan with fee for service (FFS) payments,
— Programmes that aim to improve the quality of care, e.g. disease management programmes
— Programmes to contain the costs of care, e.g. drug formularies.

Typical study outcomes are:

— Access to care, e.g. preventive services (e.g. vaccination), therapeutics
— Health status, e.g. incidence of pre-specified (tracer) diagnoses
— Life years gained, i.e. reduction of mortality
— Patient reported outcomes, e.g. health related quality of life
— Quality of care scores, e.g. measures of the Health Plan Employer Data and Information Set (HEDIS)
— Appropriateness of care measures, e.g. an appropriateness evaluation protocol (AEP)
— Cost of care, e.g. increases (additional costs or losses) or decreases (savings).

The general limitations of observational studies are dealt with among others in Chaps. I.5, I.6, I.7, I.9, and I.12 of this handbook. The absence of randomisation gives reason for special concerns, i.e. a special type of selection bias, when the goal of the study is to evaluate interventions. Persons who choose a particular intervention – or are advised by a physician to undergo it – are often on a different level of risk for the outcome of interest compared with persons who are not assigned to or did not choose to use this intervention (Selby 1994). Particularly in the case of an open intervention programme persons who pay attention to their health may be more likely to participate and comply with a recommendation (e.g. to undergo a screening examination) than persons who do not (Kelsey et al. 1998).

Case-Control Studies. The methodology of case-control studies is treated in great detail in Chap. I.6 of this handbook. Because of its obvious merits (a case-control study can be carried out at relatively low cost and comparably quickly) it is used with increasing frequency in HSR, especially in order to asses the adverse effects of drugs and other therapies and to evaluate the efficacy of preventive interventions (Kelsey et al. 1998).

Examples for the application of the case-control approach in HSR are numerous. This includes evaluations of vaccine efficacy and vaccination effectiveness, assessments of medical therapies, of screening programmes for cervical, breast and colon cancers and of a number of programmatic activities in the community (Armenian 1998).

Cohort Studies. Primary data collection for classical epidemiological cohort studies (cf. Chap. I.5 of this handbook) is relatively rare in HSR compared to chronic disease epidemiology. One reason might be that health systems change fast in small scales, i.e. in trends in coding diagnoses, and in large scales as e.g. completely new reimbursement structures like Diagnosis Related Groups (DRGs), so that information from long lasting follow-up studies may often be outdated and not worth the expense.

The majority of cohort studies in HSR is based on administrative data collected for purposes other than research and is focused on the outcomes of a medical treatment or a preventive intervention. The outcomes vary and may include mortality, morbidity, functional status, quality of life, costs, and satisfaction with care. The studies frequently use historical cohorts. For example the investigation of short-term (30-day) and long-term (5-year) mortality in a cohort of members of a large HMO with hip fractures was a historical study that used computer-stored hospital discharge data linked with computer-stored data from death certificates (Petitti and Sidney 1989). A different type of cohort analysis in HSR focuses on the description of changes in symptoms, functional status, or quality of life in patients who undergo a treatment or are the subject of a preventive intervention (Petitti 1998a).

Cross-sectional Studies. If the goal of data analysis is related to health planning or the assessment of needs for services, prevalence rates are often more useful than incidence rates. Cross-sectional studies therefore represent an important tool for health planning and evaluation. In outcome research the common methodological approach of *variance in practice* (e.g. to assess the quality of medical care or the outcome of the health system of a county) is tightly connected to a cross-sectional design, mostly based on administrative data, with organisations (e.g. hospitals), providers (e.g. surgeons), counties, states or even countries as the units of analysis.

Cross-sectional studies are also used to establish research priorities based on consideration of the burden of disease (Kelsey et al. 1998). In a study on the prevalence of chronic gynaecologic conditions among US women of reproductive age, for example, it was found that the most common conditions were menstrual disorders, adnexal conditions, and uterine fibroids. The results stressed the need for more effective treatments for these disorders, and moreover, suggested that more research on their aetiology would be highly desirable (Kjerulff et al. 1996).

Cross-sectional studies are of course less useful to examine hypotheses on causal effects. Mainly because of the lack of knowledge on the temporal sequence of hypothetical causes and potential effects, but also because cross-sectional studies include both, new and old cases. This results in a case group which has more than its fair share of individuals with disease of long duration, because those who die or recover quickly will be underrepresented (Kelsey et al. 1998).

5.2.2 Complex Models for Data Analysis

In several health systems, available claims data are characterised by a longitudinal structure with long strings of repeated measures of health services for individual patients. Such data structures demand appropriate analytical designs. To make full use of them, complex longitudinal data analysis techniques must be applied that can handle time-varying exposures, repeated outcomes and intra-person correlations.

The lack of detailed information on the severity of disease in claims data sometimes is a reason to use case-based study designs as for instance case-crossover studies to allow cases to be their own controls (cf. Chap. I.8 of this handbook).

Another complicating factor is that observations in health care delivery systems are often not independent. For many observational studies, the level of observation is a patient (characterised by a vector of patient attributes). A cluster of patients will be seen by the same physician (characterised by a vector of physician attributes) and will therefore experience similar treatment patterns so that their outcomes cannot be expected to be completely independent. Physicians often practice in groups sharing similar practice styles. These groups may practice in a larger health care delivery system that imposes constraints to treatment choices, e.g. drug formularies or payment by capitation (a lump sum per patient or per enrollee), which will make practice styles of groups within a health plan more similar than groups outside the plan. This clustering of observations on multiple levels has led to the adoption of multi-level regression models as standard tools of HSR.

5.2.3 Data Sources

Primary data collection in a randomised controlled trial, a case-control or a cohort study, is certainly an important, although unusual data source of HSR. Primary data, when used in HSR, are more frequently collected from the general population (or subgroups) by questionnaire. The majority of data that are analysed in HSR stem from large administrative databases, as pointed out before.

Surveys

Survey research is frequent in HSR. For a detailed description of survey methods see Chap. I.10 of this handbook. On the one hand it can be used to provide snapshots of the current state of a health care system. On the other hand survey subjects often become re-interviewed in regular intervals to form a longitudinal data structure or a panel. Further possibilities to classify surveys are given by the

- unit of observation (patients, patient-provider contacts or providers),
- target population (total population or subgroups),
- type of data collected (interview data, data of medical examination or both) and
- access to information (personal interview, mail survey or telephone interview).

A well-known German survey – the *EVaS-Study* (*Study among office-based ambulatory care physicians in the Federal Republic of Germany*, Schwartz and Schach 1989) – was a cross-sectional survey with patient-physician (or patient-office) contacts as units of observation. The concept followed the US-*National Ambulatory Medical Care Survey* (*NAMCS*, Tenney et al. 1974) to some extent. The target population was defined by a number of selected regions in Germany, a fixed study period and the exclusion of a few medical specialties concerning the involved physicians. The data were collected by mail using an induction interview questionnaire, a reporting form and a final questionnaire. The final data record covers data of the patient as well as data provided by the physician's office (including e.g. the diagnosis corresponding to the patient's major reason for encounter, the assessment of the severity of the problem, the services delivered and the duration of the encounter).

The recent *German National Health Interview and Examination Survey* however (carried out from October 1997 to March 1999) targeted the general population aged between 18 and 79 years (Bellach et al. 1998).[1] The units of observation had been residents who were interviewed and medically examined. The data are available for research as a public use file. One of the results of this survey for example concerned the utilisation of medical services available in Germany in statutory sickness fund facilities. About 90% of all Germans had seen their doctor at least once a year. Half of the population had consulted a doctor during the past four weeks and, on average, a medical practitioner was consulted 11 times a year (Bergmann and Kamtsiuris 1999).

Another frequently cited German survey is based on a representative, regionally stratified sample of 0.4% of all prescription forms, which are completed by office-based physicians for members of statutory sickness funds. This survey is supported in cooperation by the federal associations of the office-based physicians, the statutory sickness funds and the free-standing pharmacies. It is carried out each year. The annually published results include an analysis of the sales increase with respect to its components referring to prices, volumes and structural composition (Schwabe and Paffrath 2002).

---

[1] This survey had three predecessors in the years 1984–1986, 1987–1989 and 1990–1991 and will be supplemented by *The German National Health Interview and Examination Survey for Children and Adolescents* that started in May 2003 and is scheduled to run for three years. The target population are children and adolescents aged between 0 and 18 and living in Germany (Kurth et al. 2002).

The US-*Medicare Current Beneficiary Survey (MCBS)* is an example of a survey that is designed as a panel. MCBS began in 1991 as a continuous panel in order to provide a more complete picture of the use of health services, expenditures, and sources of payment for the Medicare population. It is an ongoing computer-assisted personal survey of Medicare beneficiaries residing in the United States and Puerto Rico. Each person is interviewed three times per year over four years (regardless of whether he or she resides in the community or a long-term care facility), following a four-year rotating panel design. The MCBS thus contains four overlapping panels of Medicare beneficiaries. Each year one panel is dropped from the survey and a new one is added. This design produces three calendar years of medical utilisation data for each sample person. The data are collected over a four-year period in which sample persons are interviewed twelve times. The first interview collects baseline information on the beneficiary. The next 11 interviews are used to collect three complete years of utilisation data. Included are medical expenditure data as well as detailed data on health conditions, health status, use of medical care services, charges and payments, access to care, satisfaction with care, health insurance coverage, income, and employment (Adler 1994). The data are used to produce calendar year public use files on access to care, cost and use. The nation wide MCBS data are released – as usual for public use files – only under a data use agreement. In addition, requests for regional or supplementary data must include a study protocol with specific justification for the additional data required, along with an identifiable data use agreement (see http://cms.gov/mcbs).

Another excellent population-based US-panel, created by the (former) Agency for Health Care Policy and Research and the National Center for Health Statistics, is the *Medical Expenditures Panel Survey (MEPS)* which collects data from several sources to provide a complete picture of the health status and health care utilisation of a random sample of citizens (Cohen 1997).

In addition to other sampling methods, computer-assisted telephone interviews have become more frequently used in HSR. This method has comparatively low costs and guarantees an approximate full coverage of the general resident population in developed countries which have high rates of telephone access. Even unlisted households can be covered by means of random digit dialling. The increasing use of cellular phones will probably jeopardise this approach in the future. Data are checked for correctness, completeness and plausibility and stored continuously in the course of the interview. Separate steps for data input and examination are not necessary. Germany started the first *National Telephone Health Survey* in September 2002. About 8000 German speaking residents aged 18 years and older had been questioned on diseases, health-related behaviour and utilisation of the health care system (Ziese et al. 2003). This survey was supplemented by a regional one in Bavaria (Meyer et al. 2002).

Official Statistics

Official mortality and other health or demographic statistics, especially vital statistics (births, marriages, deaths, etc.) have been extensively used in HSR. An early well-known and frequently cited example in the context of equity research is the study on differential mortality in the United States (Kitagawa and Hauser 1973). The comparison of mortality rates and the proportions of money from the national accounts that are spent on health is a popular starting point for health economists in analysing the efficiency of a particular health system. But official statistics – mostly based on law – resemble routine registries and share their limitations (cf. Chap. I.4 of this handbook and Sörensen 2001). The validity of mortality statistics in particular is strongly dependent on the rate of autopsies in a country. In a German survey of institutes of pathology within universities and in community hospitals in the year 2000 a median value of 23.3% and 13.3% of autopsies among hospital deaths was found, respectively. This was considered clearly below the recommended value of 30% (Schwarze and Pawlitschko 2003).

Administrative Databases

Administrative data are abstracted from medical or hospital discharge records, prescriptions and bills of payments. Thus they have several advantages. They are routinely collected data representing the reality of health care delivery. They need no additional time and money to gain access to large patient populations over long periods of time with repeated recordings of most health care encounters of each subject. But the advantage of quick and easy access to large and representative populations is counterbalanced by data that may be incomplete and suffer from voluntary and involuntary miscoding. Although the quality of these data appears to improve over time it has to be kept in mind that the primary reason for creating them was to document medical diagnoses and interventions obtained from medical records and manage the flow of payments for delivered health services obtained from claims data.

Since the advantages, particularly of electronic claims data, are so obvious, researchers try to better understand the consequences of the data limitations and develop analytical methods to adjust for them. See for example the approach of Newhouse and McClellan (1998) used to overcome the typical selection problem they were confronted with in analysing the data of catheterisation of patients with acute myocardial infarction. As data limitations are unique to each administrative database, a very good understanding of how data were generated is crucial for interpreting analytical findings.

Examples of administrative databases in the USA include the national Medicare and Medicaid databases as well as claims files for privately insured patients or members of a particular health facility. Data from the Medicare programme, run by the *Centers for Medicare & Medicaid Services (CMS)*, are confidentiality-protected, longitudinally linked, person-level records that track virtually all elderly US citizens from their 65th birthday onwards until death, through geographical moves and changes in providers.[2] The data sets include the types and amounts of health services used (e.g. hospitalisations, office visits, home health care, surgeries,

---

[2] About 10% of Medicare enrollees are younger, disabled persons, who are tracked from their time of certification.

and diagnostic tests), the medical problems being treated (diagnoses), provider characteristics (site of service and physician training), and charges. Information on long-term care services and outpatient prescription drugs, not covered by CMS, is not included (Diehr et al. 1999).

In Germany, administrative databases which do not find their ways into an official statistic or a survey are scattered across the statutory sickness funds or other agencies of social security. Due to comparably strict data protection rules they are generally case-based and allow no longitudinal analysis of health status or services delivered for one patient. Moreover record linkage is not a common practice in Germany because of data protection issues.

The abundance of information in claims databases in various states is often overwhelming. Many redundant measures are recorded and researchers must identify the underlying variables that represent the concepts they want to evaluate. Since researchers on the other side hate to discard already recorded information, *data reduction techniques* including co-morbidity scores or propensity scores are increasingly applied to condense data while preserving information. For a detailed discussion of pharmacoepidemiological databases we refer to Chap. III.9 of this handbook.

5.2.4   Measurement Error (Misclassification)

In HSR measurement errors (nondifferential and differential as well; cf. Chap. II.5 of this handbook) for all variables of interest are considered to be higher than in a traditional epidemiological setting for several reasons:

— Some data that are collected and stored but are not directly used for reimbursement or other administrative purposes (e.g. job or social status of an enrolled person) are likely to be not up to date.
— Diagnostic information on claims is documented to justify reimbursement; a bill for tests to rule out cancer e.g. may contain a diagnostic code for "cancer" even if the tests were negative.
— The information on clinical conditions in administrative data is in the form of diagnoses coded using the International Classification of Diseases (ICD) which is revised from time to time. Currently ICD-10 (the tenth revision) is in use. Several countries (e.g. the USA) prefer ICD-10-CM, a clinical modification of the ICD. Some diseases such as arthritic or psychiatric disorders are difficult to classify because of lack of clearly defined diagnostic criteria. Less serious or vague conditions have a high probability of inconsistent coding. Regional and temporal variations of coding patterns may additionally reduce the reliability of coded diagnostic information.
— Especially the reliability of ambulatory diagnoses is a major concern. An analysis by the Medicare Payment Advisory Commission – MedPAC (1998) demonstrated the inaccuracy of outpatient diagnosis coding. For the purposes of the study, MedPAC selected beneficiaries whose Medicare Part B claims in 1994 showed a diagnosis of one of 11 serious diseases, then checked for claims for the same diagnosis in 1995. As shown in Table 5.2, the likelihood of a claim in

1995 was only about 50–60% for each of the 11 diagnoses (cf. Newhouse et al. 1999). Part B Medicare covers the costs for medical service by general practitioners, for a small selection of pharmaceuticals, for ambulatory treatments in hospitals and other therapeutic and care services that are not covered by Part A Medicare.

— Moreover, administrative data used to reimburse hospitals or physicians are subject to some problems that are not familiar to epidemiologists, called "up-coding", "coding proliferation" and "gaming". Upcoding of diagnoses to more serious conditions is the process of assigning a diagnosis code or codes to a patient that may maximise the provider's reimbursement (e.g. ischaemia to myocardial infarction) as it has occurred with some DRG payment systems (Dunn et al. 1996). Coding proliferation means the increase in the coding of all related conditions affecting treatment. Both types of distortion are relevant sources of measurement errors in HSR. Gaming is a serious problem that is dealt with in Sect. 5.5.2 because it cannot be subsumed under the term "misclassification" seamlessly.

In summary, the quality of claims data may be adequate for some purposes, but it is important to remember that claims are generated to justify reimbursement rather than to facilitate research.

Table 5.2. Persistence in Diagnostic Coding of Those Identified in 1994

Diagnosis on 1994 Part B Claim	Percent with Part B Claim in 1995
Hypertension	59
Coronary Artery Disease	53
COPD	62
Congestive Heart Failure	61
Stroke	51
Dementia	59
Rheumatoid Arthritis	55
High Cost Diabetes	58
Renal Failure	56
Quadriplegia/Paraplegia	52
Dialysis	59

Source: Medicare Payment Advisory Commission 1998, p 17. Note: Excludes those who died in 1994 or 1995.

Sampling Issues   5.2.5

A considerable part of data analysed in HSR is based on samples from the population of interest (this is called the "target population" or the "population being sampled"). Sampling can help to save time and money. Sampling may also result in an increase of accuracy of measurement, since more effort can be spent on this issue if only a manageable number of units of observation is included. Scientifically sound sampling methods are indispensable tools for designing an efficient sample, and to provide consistent and unbiased projections from complex samples. Scientific sampling means *probability sampling*, i.e. the probabilities of selection must be under control. Non-random samples based on volunteers or on the judgement of the sampler are not covered by this concept and are not recommended for use in HSR.

The sampling procedure is called *simple random sampling* if each of the possible samples of a given size has an equal chance to be selected. It follows that every one of the sampling units in the population has the same chance of being included in the sample. This is occasionally offered as the definition of simple random sampling (e.g. Kelsey et al. 1998) without realising that there are other sampling procedures (e.g. systematic sampling, see below), which also have this property (Sukhatme and Sukhatme 1970). Simple random sampling is simple in theory but less so in practice because one needs a complete list of the population to draw the sample.[3] In many instances it may not be the most efficient method of sampling. Therefore – apart from telephone sampling – it is not much used in practice.

Systematic sampling is a common type of sampling based on selecting every k-th individual from a list or a file after choosing a random number from 1 to k as starting point. It is based on a fixed rule and is not limited to selection from an actual file. Thus, selection of all those born on the (randomly chosen) third day of any month or of everyone whose social security number ends in (the randomly chosen digits) 17, 48 or 76 is similar to systematic sampling procedures yielding approximately 3% samples.[4] Because of these properties systematic sampling is often simpler to administer under field conditions than simple random sampling. But systematic sampling has a severe handicap: differently from other sample designs it is impossible to estimate the variance from one single sample. For an unbiased estimate you need repeated sampling. Several (biased) approximations are used in practice to estimate the variance. One of these consists in treating the systematic sample as if it were a random sample of n units (Sukhatme and Sukhatme 1970).

When the population can be divided into *strata* in such a way that each stratum is more homogenous than the population as a whole, one can reduce the sampling error compared to a simple random error. Examples of variables that are often used for stratification are region, age, gender, race, and socio-economic status. Following a *stratified sampling* design, a separate sample is drawn from each stratum and the results are then appropriately combined in the analysis. If much of the measured total variance is between the strata, but we sample within them, the combined results are completely free of the variability between strata. An additional advantage

---

[3] Random digit dialling in order to sample for computer assisted telephone interviews is considered as a way to handle this problem if no such complete list exists.

[4] Of course, the choice of the sampling scheme has to be relevant to the population being sampled. A population that is not completely covered by social security would be unsuitable for sampling by means of social security number.

of stratified sampling is that one can be sure that members of each stratum are represented in the overall sample. Finally, the strata can be constructed so that those who are least expensive to include or who provide the highest amount of variability, can be sampled with the highest weight, simultaneously reducing cost and increasing precision.

Cluster sampling has contrasting properties compared to stratified sampling. It is a simple random sample applied to groups of population members (*clusters*) that usually leads to a substantial loss of precision. But because of operational improvements of access to the units to be selected one often achieves a heavy decrease of collecting-costs and thereby an increase in precision per unit of cost. Examples of clusters that could be sampled are hospital wards, villages, schools, families etc. If clusters are positively correlated within themselves, i.e. they have a high positive *intraclass-correlation coefficient (ICC)*, indicating more homogeneity than would result from chance alone, cluster sampling variance will be larger than simple random sampling variance. This is a situation frequently observed in real life. Only when the ICC is negative (a rare event in practice) the investigator benefits from cluster sampling both by reduced variance for fixed sample size and by reduced costs. As ICCs are positive in most cases, simple sampling variance can grossly underestimate the true cluster sampling variance. The ratio of the latter to the first-mentioned variance is called the *cluster effect*.

In a *multistage sampling design* stratification and clustering may be combined on several stages of the sampling procedure forming a complex random sample. Stratified sampling for example may be used to ensure that schools are represented in the sample according to different socio-economic areas in a large city, and cluster sampling of classrooms within the selected schools might then be employed for efficiency. The above mentioned EvaS-Study also was designed as a two-stage sample: In the first stage, a stratified sample of office-based physicians was drawn with their specialities defining the strata. In the second stage, a systematic sampling approach was used to sample patient-physician encounters of the selected physicians (Schach 1989).

The analysis of data from a complex sample procedure that includes cluster sampling requires a sound knowledge of sampling theory or statistical advice. There are a series of textbooks on sampling theory (e.g. Hansen et al. 1953; Kish 1965; Stuart 1968; Sukhatme and Sukhatme 1970; Cochran 1968, 1972; Stenger 1986; Levy and Lemeshow 1991) and many handbooks or textbooks on statistics contain at least a chapter on sampling theory (e.g. Kendall and Stuart 1958; Kahn and Sempos 1989; Krishnaiah and Rao 1994; Voß 2003). The use of a special software (e.g. Sudaan), or a special module of one of the common large statistical packages (e.g. SAS, Stata or SPSS) is inevitable. They allow for variance weighting in the statistical procedures to adjust for the specific sampling design. Otherwise, as cluster sampling variance may be many times larger than the variance calculated by assuming a simple random sample (Abraham 1986), and the analysis can result in severely misleading conclusions about the significance of the study findings.

Confounding and Risk Adjustment

For general principles of control for confounding see Chap. I.9 of this handbook. Health services researchers tend to summarise methods to adjust for confounding under the term "risk adjustment". With respect to the large databases analysed, standardisation and multivariate modelling are more frequently used to control for confounding than the traditional approach of stratification.

Any level of comparison can be affected by confounding. This includes the mapping of health care needs, the evaluation of clinical strategies and programmes, studies of the effectiveness of quality improvement initiatives, or the evaluation of cost containment measures. Typical confounders are age, gender, ethnicity, income, smoking, or other risk variables. In outcome studies confounding is a major concern because of differences in severity of illness and co-morbidity.

The most frequent approach to control for confounding in HSR is to include the potential set of confounders as predictors in the regression model (cf. Chap. II.3 of this handbook) to predict the outcome of interest:

— Ordinary least squares (OLS) regression when the outcome has a continuous distribution (ideally a normal distribution) as e.g. the logarithm of costs.
— Poisson (or negative binomial) regression when the outcome is described by counts (as for example the number of hospital admissions in a specified year).
— Binomial (logistic) regression when the outcome variable is binary, indicating e.g. the occurrence of disease or death.

When a large database is used for the analysis, co-morbidity is often taken into account by including a lot of so-called "dummy", i.e. binary 0/1 variables in the regression model that indicate the presence (or absence respectively) of each out of a list of classified co-morbidities. When using samples of small or moderate size this approach may not be possible. In this case a pre-modelled aggregated index of co-morbidity can be included in the analysis (Schneeweiss et al. 2001).

Including a potential confounder variable in the analysis requires its storage in the database. This is crucial whenever "second hand" data are analysed. Especially in a country like Germany where record linkage is not a common practice one cannot expect to have full control over all relevant confounders (ambulatory diagnoses for example are not stored in routine data sets, and even many socio-economic characteristics are available only in survey research).

Omission of one or several confounders usually leads to a violation of the assumptions underlying the estimation procedure in the OLS regression model

$$Y_i = \beta_1 x_{i1} + \beta_1 x_{i2} + \ldots + \beta_k x_{ik} + \varepsilon_i, \quad i = 1, \ldots, n,$$

as the k predictors x_{ij}, $j = 1, \ldots, k$, and the random errors ε_i, $i = 1, \ldots, n$, are no longer uncorrelated where n denotes the number of subjects, Y_i the response variables, and β_j the regression coefficients.

In this situation the introduction of one or more of so-called *instrumental variables* can help to establish a consistent estimation of the interesting effects (i.e. β_j). This has been a well known technique of econometric analysis (IV-technique) for over half a century which is described in almost every econometric textbook (e.g. Greene 2003). But it is very rarely applied to HSR problems because a sound econometrical or statistical background is needed. Instrumental variables should be correlated with the predictor variable as much as possible, and at the same time they should be (at least asymptotically) uncorrelated with the random errors. The skill of the technique consists in finding such variables which are already in the database or could be added to it at a tolerable cost.

An illuminating example of the usefulness of IV-technique is presented by Newhouse and McClellan (1998) who explain the instrumental variable convincingly as a device that achieves a pseudo-randomisation. The authors analysed the effect of catheterisation and associated revascularisation of acute myocardial infarction on mortality in the years following treatment. For IV-estimation of this effect they used the differential distances of the patients' place of residence to the nearest catheterisation, revascularisation, and high-volume hospital as instrumental variables.

Demand, Need, Utilisation, and Access to Health Care

5.3

A main focus of HSR is the assessment of demand, need, utilisation and access to health services, which represent closely related but distinct fields of investigation. In the input–output model they represent the endogenous, risk-related input, which is, among others, determined by population health – representing the exogenous risk-related input in the model.

Demand is a general economic concept, which can be defined as the "quantity of a good buyers wish to buy at a conceivable price" (Begg et al. 1997a). Demand for health and health care is in many respects different from demand for other goods and services. The demand for health care is a derived demand as health care is not sought in itself but as a means to improve one's health or to prevent its deterioration. Health care itself is indeed often rather unpleasant (McPake et al. 2002). Health is not something that can be traded and both health and health care are surrounded by uncertainty. What people want in essence from health care, is to buy access to care in case they need it, i.e. insurance (McPake et al. 2002). Another aspect is that health is both a consumption good and a capital good (McPake et al. 2002). Especially politicians and health care funders often focus on the consumption side and neglect the potential of investing in health as a durable good which is an important prerequisite for economic growth.

The notions of need, utilisation, access, and the relationships between them will be discussed in more detail in the following sections.

Assessing Health Needs

The concept of "need" for health and health care links directly to population health. Initially it appears simple and is often used by politicians in health policy discussions, but quickly becomes complicated and is therefore avoided by many analysts (Kindig 1997). Instead many policy analysts, in particular in the United States, prefer to use the economic demand and supply framework, where it is assumed that if someone "needs" something, he or she will express this desire by purchasing the item that is needed in the marketplaces, and as a consequence, supply will increase (Kindig 1997).

An alternative concept of need as the "capacity to benefit" has been proposed by Williams (1974) and Culyer (1993). Their concept also goes beyond the perspective of an initial baseline level of health, because unhealthy individuals and populations cannot be said to need more health care without regard to their potential for improving their health status (Kindig 1997). Capacity to benefit also rules out health services which might be desired by individuals or providers but which do not make a positive contribution to health adjusted life expectancy (Kindig 1997). It also goes beyond a mere epidemiological description of health needs in terms of ill-health or shortcomings in care in a specified population as it incorporates the notion of effectiveness of the intervention. Some authors use the terms "felt need", "normative need" and "expressed need". The "felt need" reported by patients is often substantially different from the "normative need" as judged by health professionals. "Expressed need" represents the need expressed by action, e.g. visiting a doctor (Wright 2001).

Three main approaches to health needs assessment exist (Wright 2001):

— Epidemiologically-based needs assessment – combining epidemiological approaches, such as specific health status assessments, with assessment of the effectiveness and possibly cost-effectiveness of interventions.
— Comparative needs assessment – comparing levels of service receipt between different populations.
— Corporate needs assessment – canvassing the demands and wishes of professionals, patients, politicians, and other stakeholders.

In practice, comprehensive health needs assessments often combine all three approaches. Practical applications are manifold, such as to highlight areas of unmet need and to provide a clear set of objectives to meet these needs, to decide how to use resources to improve the local population's health, and to influence policy, interagency collaboration, or research and development priority setting (Wright 2001).

A good example for a health needs assessment is a study contrasting the epidemiological need for carotid endarterectomy with actual service provision in an English region (Ferris et al. 1998). The authors estimated the need for a carotid endarterectomy on the basis of demographic and epidemiological data, assuming that the rate of endarterectomies in their region should match the rate of patients with symptomatic carotid disease – the patient group for whom carotid endarterectomy is proven to prevent strokes. Based on estimates of the incidence of transient ischaemic attacks ($77/10^6$ population/year) and minor strokes ($76/10^6$/year) they calculated that the need for endarterectomy was $153/10^6$/year, which contrasted with operation rates of $35/10^6$/year in 1991–92 and $89/10^6$/year in 1995–96. The ratio of use to need was 0.47 (95% confidence interval (CI) from 0.4 to 0.54), which was far from being satisfactory. Furthermore, they noted a disconcerting variation in the use to need ratios between districts, ranging from 0.28 (95% CI: 0.19 to 0.38) to 0.81 (95% CI: 0.62 to 1.06), and lower use to need ratios in elderly and female patients – indicative of inequity in access in relation to need. The epidemiological needs assessment was supplemented with a corporate needs assessment comprising interviews with vascular surgeons and a joint purchaser-provider workshop. These indicated that the low operation rates were primarily due to low rates of referral for diagnostic assessment by general practitioners. The variation between districts partly reflected the concentration of services – districts with a high use to need ratio tended to have one of the main provider sites. This study clearly demonstrates the usefulness of such research in identifying the main levers for improvement of current service provision – in this case raising awareness for the clinical indications for carotid endarterectomy in general practitioners, in particular those located in rural areas without access to a local vascular surgical service.

Assessing Utilisation and Access to Services   5.3.2

Studies assessing the utilisation of services attempt to improve our understanding of who uses health care services and why (Black 1997). In the previous sections it has already become clear that many factors determine whether a patient utilises a health care service, amongst them whether the patient suffers from a condition for which an effective intervention is available, and whether he or she demands that service. Three other common determinants of utilisation have become apparent in the example of the health needs assessment for carotid endarterectomy in England – clinician's judgement, distance from facilities, and gender. If a general practitioner does not consider that referral to a specialist is necessary, it is unlikely that the patient will end up having the procedure nonetheless – resulting in unmet need and underutilisation of health services. Other important factors influencing utilisation and access are patients' knowledge and the cost of services to the patient.

A well recognised example for the influence of gender on utilisation are higher rates of appendectomy in women than in men (Black 1997). After the primary assertion that appendicitis is more frequent in women was not supported by evidence, the more likely explanations were as follows: Appendicitis-like symptoms are more common in women, probably arising from ovarian dysfunction; in some cultures young women prove their independence by undergoing an operation; operation rates are dependent on the availability of services – the more surgical services are available, the higher the gender difference in operation rates (Black 1997).

The influence of clinicians' judgement on health service delivery has been investigated in a series of studies comparing hospital care and related costs between

Boston and New Haven in the United States – two cities with similar demographics where most hospital care is provided by university hospitals (Wennberg et al. 1987, 1989). However, in 1982 expenditures per head for inpatient care in Boston were about twice as high as in New Haven ($889 vs. $451) (Wennberg et al. 1987). The excess utilisation in Boston compared to New Haven totalled $300 million and 739 hospital beds per year. In a subsequent study in 1985, Wennberg and colleagues showed that the variation in operation rates between the two areas did not result in statistically significant differences in mortality between the two cities (Wennberg et al. 1989). The authors concluded that the lower rate of hospital use in New Haven was not associated with a higher overall mortality rate in the populations concerned and consequently that hospital care was overutilised in Boston and not underutilised in New Haven.

The influence of geographical and financial barriers to access is also well documented. Black and colleagues (Black et al. 1995) attempted to identify the reasons for geographical variation in the use of coronary revascularisation in the United Kingdom in a cross-sectional study. They found considerable variation in revascularisation rates between districts, which arose from differences in supply factors, notably the distance to a regional revascularisation centre and the existence of a local cardiologist. The level of coronary heart disease mortality in the population and the lack of use of alternative treatments not only failed to explain the observed variation but was inversely associated with the rate of revascularisation (Black et al. 1995). This inverse relationship between need and provision of care has been observed in many settings and has been termed the "inverse care law" by Julian Tudor-Hart (Tudor-Hart 1971, 2000). It has to be kept in mind that in measuring the utilisation of health care facilities only those patients are counted, who have surmounted barriers to access – be it long distances, fear of an operation, lack of public transport, waiting lists – and are thus biased (Schwartz and Busse 2003). These barriers to access also exist in countries which grant a legal right to health care to every citizen, in particular among socially disadvantaged groups in society. These differences in access to care are even more pronounced in countries without such a right to health care and where direct financial barriers to care exist on top of other barriers to access.

The effect of financial barriers to accessing health services has been studied in many countries at different levels of development. The most famous study is the RAND Health Insurance Study (see also Sect. 5.2.1) on the effect of cost-sharing measures on utilisation (Newhouse 1974; Newhouse et al. 1981; Brook et al. 1983). Between 1974 and 1977, about 2000 non-elderly families were randomly assigned to different insurance plans. Participants were assigned to either pre-paid group practices or to one of 14 fee-for-service insurance plans, which varied in their co-insurance rates and in maximum spending per family and year (Newhouse 1993). The authors found that the more families had to pay out of pocket, the fewer health care services they used. Families on the plan with the highest co-insurance (95%) up to a $1000 limit on annual family expenditure reduced expenditure by 25–30% compared to a plan which was free to the family (Newhouse 1993). Interestingly, the use of all types of services, whether physicians, hospitals, pharmaceuticals, dental, or mental health services fell with cost-sharing to a similar degree, except hospital admissions of children which did not respond to plan (Newhouse 1993). While the reduced utilisation had no negative effect on the health for the average person, health among the "sick poor" – the most disadvantaged 6% of the population – was adversely affected (Newhouse 1993). Especially the poor who began the experiment with elevated blood pressure had their blood pressures lowered more on the free care plan than on the cost-sharing plans, and mortality rates predicted on the presence of major risk factors were 10% lower among those insured on the free plan (Newhouse 1993). Free care at the point of delivery also improved both near and far corrected vision, increased the likelihood that a decayed tooth would be filled, and the prevalence of anaemia among poor children was lower (Newhouse 1993). All observed adverse health effects of cost-sharing hit the poor and less educated disproportionately more.

A number of other factors can limit access to services, in particular gender, age, professional status, race, and religion (Schwartz and Busse 2003). The discrepancy between need in terms of ill-health and capacity to benefit from intervention and utilisation is a commonly used measure of equity.

Financial Resources, Structure, and Organisation of Health Services

5.4

Health care financing can be described from different perspectives:
- The first one looks for the ultimate sources of funding. Here, intermediary sources of financing (government, social security funds, private social insurance and private households above all) have to be tracked back to their origin.
- The second one, commonly used in National Health Accounts, aims at a breakdown of expenditure on health into the complex network of third-party-payments plus the direct payments by households or direct funders (OECD 2000).
- The third one focuses on the allocation of the available resources. Health planning and management of health care among others includes the continuous task of distributing the financial resources, e.g. to distinct segments in the natural history of disease (as reflected in prevention, cure, rehabilitation, and care), to alternative treatments for a specific disease, to different regions, to various groups of providers, or simultaneously with respect to some of these categories.

When comparing the developed countries with respect to financing from the first perspective we can find two marked types of health services systems: systems that are funded by taxes and typically have a National Health Service (NHS) – so-called NHS-type or Beveridge-type systems – and systems that are predominantly financed by contributions of employees and employers (so-called Bismarck-type

Table 5.3. International Classification for Health Accounts (ICHA) – one- and (partly) two-digit level (from OECD 2000)

HP Code	Classification of Health Care Provider (HP) Description
1	Hospitals*
2	Nursing and residential care facilities*
3	Providers of ambulatory health care
31	Offices of physicians
32	Offices of dentists
33	Offices of other health practitioners
34	Out-patient care centers
35	Medical and diagnostic laboratories
36	Providers of home health care services
39	Other providers of ambulatory health care
4	Retail sale and other providers of medical goods
41	Dispensing chemists
42	Retail sale and other suppliers of optical glasses
43	Retail sale and other suppliers of hearing aids
44	Retail sale and other suppliers of other medical appliances
49	All other miscellaneous suppliers of medical goods
5	Provision and administration of public health programmes
6	General health administration and insurance
61	Government administration of health
62	Social security funds
63	Other social insurance
64	Other (private) insurance
69	All other providers of health administration
7	Other industries (rest of the economy)
71	Establishments as providers of occupational health care
72	Private households as providers of home care
79	All other industries as secondary producers of health care
9	Rest of the world

* two digit level omitted

table to be continued

systems). In the real world we find, of course, mixed systems including all the common forms of public and private financing. The UK is generally considered to be the classic example of a NHS-type health service system and the German health system, as established by Bismarck in the late nineteenth century, naturally acts as the model of all Bismarck-type systems.

Health services systems also vary considerably in the overall health insurance coverage rates. In all EU Member States, nearly 100% of the population has coverage of some type of public or private health insurance, whereas in the USA 43.6 million persons (corresponding to 15.2% of the population) had no coverage at all during

Table 5.3. (continued)

HF Code	Classification of Health Care Financing (HF) Description
1	General Government
11	Gen. Gov. excluding social security funds
12	Social security funds
2	Private sector
21	Private social insurance
22	Private insurance (other than social insurance)
23	Private households
24	Non-profit institutions serving households
25	Corporations (other than health insurance)

HC Code	Functional Classification (HC)* Description
	Personal Health Care Services and goods
1	Services of curative care
2	Services of rehabilitative care
3	Services of long-term nursing care
4	Ancillary services to health care
5	Medical goods dispensed to out-patients
	Collective health care services
6	Prevention and public health services
7	Health administration and health insurance
HCR	Health-related functions
1	Capital formation of health care provider institutions
2	Education and training of health personnel
3	Research and development in health
4	Food, hygiene and drinking water control
5	Environmental health
6	Administration and provision of social services in kind to assist living with disease and impairment
7	Administration and provision of health-related cash-benefits

* two digit level omitted

the entire year 2002 (U.S. Census Bureau 2003), which constitutes an important barrier to access as seen above.

International comparisons of health care spending is hampered by a variety of definitions and classifications, used by the national statistical agencies, resembling the different organisational structures of health care delivery (van Mossefeld 2003). To improve comparability of health accounting data Eurostat, the statistical office of the European Union (EU), and the Organisation for Economic Co-operation and

Development (OECD) jointly developed a conceptual basis of rules for the statistical reporting of health accounts together with EU Member States (OECD 2000). This so-called *System of Health Accounts (SHA)* corresponds to the new German health expenditure data system which was developed simultaneously (Brückner 1997; Statistisches Bundesamt 2000a,b). The SHA includes expenditures of private households, is consistent with the System of National Accounts (SNA) methodology (OECD 1993), and covers three dimensions: functions of health care, providers of health care and sources of funding (Table 5.3). Core of the SHA is a newly developed *International Classification for Health Accounts (ICHA)* that is based on a three digit code (in Table 5.3 the three digit level is completely omitted).

The ICHA gives a first impression of the potential variations among health systems in structure and organisation of health care and the share of work between the various providers. One remarkable distinction between health services systems, when looking at the organisation, refers to outpatient care. In many countries patient-physician contacts take place only in offices of general practice. Contacts with medical specialists are limited to hospital visits no matter whether the patient has been admitted to the hospital or not. But there are other countries, among them Germany and France, where outpatient specialised curative care is predominantly provided by office-based specialists.

There are many additional differences in the structure and organisation of health services systems in spite of the fact that in all developed countries patients with a specific health condition receive more or less the same treatment, provided that quality standards are observed. The package of activities in health care seems to be stable over the health systems, while the providers are different. This statement was the starting point of another important study, sponsored by the European Commission, to improve comparability of data on health services in Europe. The project, *Towards Comparable Health Care Data in the European Union (Eucomp)*, among others, produced a refinement of the functional classification of the ICHA in establishing activities of the providers (actors) and introduced an additional dimension of classification, the so-called *Mode of Production* (inpatient care/day care/outpatient care/home care) to sub-categorise both functions and activities in order to allow for the identification of provider differences. The core of the Eucomp-project was to establish a metadata-base[5] on the European health services systems that should provide efficient retrieval modes as well as conceptual clarity (clear definitions, well-determined units, references to broadly recognised classifications), concise insight in data collection and processing, measuring instruments, availability of data, etc. In this metadata-base the total number of actors and their activities in the field of health care for all European countries will be described in all European languages. The ultimate goal of the ongoing Eucomp-project is the establishment of an internet-based information retrieval system, covering the metadata-base as well as glossaries in the national languages together with country profiles of national health care systems as provided by the Euro-

---

[5] A particular example of such a metadata system is provided by the Australian Institute of Health and Welfare (1998).

pean Observatory on Health Systems and Policies (2004) (European Commission 2000).

International studies of health care systems based on comparable data sets, as called for by Eucomp, are rare. One of the outstanding examples is the WHO/International Collaborative Study of Medical Care Utilisation – WHO/ICS-MCU (Kohn and White 1976). The data collection process of this carefully designed and methodically ambitious study included a cross-national multilingual household survey (by personal interviews), and standardised forms relating to health services resources and organisational factors. The study included almost 48,000 respondents representing over 15 million persons in twelve study areas scattered over Europe and America. One of the striking results of the WHO/ICS-MCU study was that study areas with the highest estimates of societal interest in health were also the areas with the lowest totals for per capita health expenditure and for health expenditure as a percentage of national income.

Allocation of Resources   5.4.1

Health related decision makers in government, regional authorities, insurance companies or other institutions are faced with the task of allocating resources. Examples are allocating research funds to different areas of HSR, Medicaid funds to treatments, Medicare funds to HMOs, or global funds to local authorities. Regional allocation is a main concern of all NHS-type health care systems. Risk-adjusted capitation payments to insurers or to providers is a related topic that has been discussed extensively in several non NHS-type countries (e.g. the USA, the Netherlands, and Germany).

There is no unique method for resource allocation analysis. Different levels and variable purposes of resource allocation analysis require different methods:

— For economic evaluation, e.g. of drugs, surgical procedures, other types of clinical interventions or of community intervention programmes, limits on health care resources mandates resource-allocation decisions guided by considerations of cost in relation to expected benefits (Weinstein and Stason 1977).
— The UK-approach of weighted capitation has become the principal method of allocating health care finance to regions (Rice and Smith 1999).
— Risk-adjusted capitation, whereby capitated payments are adjusted to reflect the expected cost of individual enrolees, is commonly based on multivariate regression models to predict health care expenditure (Van de Ven and Newhouse 2000).

While economic evaluation are mostly based on RCTs and observational studies (mainly on effectiveness and costs), risk-adjusted capitated payments and formulas of weighted capitation are generally based on official statistics (e.g. census or mortality statistics) or on large samples from administrative databases. For an example see Sect. 5.4.1.

Economic Evaluation, Especially Cost-Effectiveness Analysis

Economic evaluation can be defined as the comparative analysis of alternative courses of action in terms of both their costs and consequences (Drummond et al. 1997). There are four main types of economic evaluation (see Table 5.4). But in practice most of the health economic evaluations apply the cost-effectiveness methodology. *Cost-benefit analysis* is rarely used in public health and health care settings, because of methodological difficulties to measure the value of human life and low acceptability of its results on the side of health policy decision-makers and health professionals. *Cost-utility analysis (CUA)* is considered by many to be a sub-type of *cost-effectiveness analysis (CEA)* where the effectiveness measure includes societal or individual preferences for the outcomes – a customary effectiveness measure in CUA is the quality-adjusted life year (QALY) (cf. Sect. 5.6.1; Chap. I.3 of this handbook) – compared to natural units as effectiveness measure in CEA, e.g. life years gained or mmHg blood pressure reduction. Most of the important methods and concepts applicable to cost-effectiveness studies are also applicable to cost-utility and cost-minimisation studies. Cost-of-illness studies may be identified as a fifth type of economic study in HSR. Their goal is to estimate the total societal costs of caring for persons with a specific illness compared to persons without this illness, irrespective of any intervention. Such studies are carried out to demonstrate the (relative) burden of illness. They are not full economic evaluations because alternatives are not compared (Drummond et al. 1997).

Table 5.4. Types of Health Economic Evaluations

Type of Analysis	Assumption/Question Addressed
Cost-minimisation	The effectiveness (or outcome) of two or more interventions is the same. Which intervention is the least costly?
Cost-effectiveness	The effectiveness of two or more interventions differs. What is the comparative cost per unit of outcome for the intervention?
Cost-utility	The question is the same as for cost-effectiveness analysis. The outcome is a preference measure that reflects the value patients or society places on the outcome
Cost-benefit	The effectiveness (or outcome) of two or more interventions differs. What is the economic trade-off between interventions when all of the costs and benefits of the intervention and its outcome are measured in monetary terms?

Source: Epstein and Sherwood (1996)

One limitation that is common to all types of economic evaluation arises from the difficulty in obtaining a true estimate of costs, particularly in a health care or public health setting where high proportions of fixed costs and little flexibility in changing the labour pool are typically found (Petitti 1998b).

A common understanding of cost-effectiveness claims that one of three criteria has to be met (Doubilet et al. 1986). First, an intervention is cost-effective when it is less costly and at least as effective as its alternative. Second, an intervention is cost-effective when it is more effective and more costly, but the added benefit is "worth" the added cost. Third, an intervention is cost-effective when it is less effective and less costly, and the added benefit of the alternative is not "worth" the added cost.

Cost-effectiveness is measured as a ratio of cost to effectiveness. Two concepts to calculate this ratio should be distinguished (Detsky and Naglie 1990): An average cost-effectiveness ratio is estimated by dividing the cost of the intervention by a measure of effectiveness. An incremental cost-effectiveness ratio is an estimate of the cost per unit of effectiveness of switching from one intervention to another. In estimating an incremental cost-effectiveness ratio, both the numerator and denominator of the ratio represent differences between alternative interventions (Weinstein and Stason 1977). Often the terms "marginal" and "incremental" are used interchangeably in the literature, although *marginal costs* are strictly speaking the costs of producing one extra unit of output, whereas *incremental costs* usually refer to the difference, in cost or effect, between the two or more programmes being compared in the economic evaluation (Drummond et al. 1997).

Estimating *average cost-effectiveness ratios* can be useful for service planning and for resource allocation decisions between very different health programmes, e.g. an influenza vaccination programme and liver transplantations. However, for resource allocation decisions between interventions for the same disease, e.g. two different antihypertensive drugs, *incremental cost-effectiveness ratios* should be used. The importance of using incremental cost-effectiveness ratios for decision making in some settings, is best illustrated with the example of the sixth Guaiac stool test to screen for colorectal cancer, which had been endorsed by the American Cancer Society, and which has later been shown to have an incremental cost of $47 million per case detected compared to an average cost of $2451 per case detected (Neuhauser and Lewicki 1975).

The unspecified implicit alternative to an intervention is usually doing nothing. But doing nothing has costs and effects that should be taken into account in the analysis (Detsky and Naglie 1990). Furthermore, explicit declaration of "doing nothing" as the alternative intervention helps to frame discussions of the desirability of the intervention (Petitti 1998b).

Costs seem to be a straightforward notion, well understood by everybody. But actually it is a rather complex term that consists of various components: direct costs, indirect costs and intangible costs. Costs that are directly related to an intervention (and to side effects and other consequences) are summed up to the total of *direct costs*. By *indirect costs* health economists understand the monetary value of lost wages and productivity due to morbidity and death of a person affected. *Intangible costs* refer to consequences that are difficult to measure and value, such as the value of improved health or the pain and suffering associated with illness or treatment (Drummond et al. 1997). The rationale of economic evaluation is based on the concept of *opportunity cost*, i.e. the benefits forgone by not deploying resources for the next best alternative use.

As costs are seen differently from different *perspectives* (e.g., perspectives of health insurers, corporations, hospitals, physicians, and patients), it is also important to define a cost perspective in CEA and state it explicitly (Petitti 1998b). A common goal in CEA is the societal perspective, so that the total costs of the intervention to all payers for all persons are included in the analysis.

Costs and benefits, after all, must be discounted before comparing them by calculating the ratio of cost to effectiveness. *Discounting* is the usual procedure in economics used to determine the present value of future money. This analysis gives a greater weight to costs and benefits the earlier they occur. High positive discount rates favour alternatives with costs that occur later or benefits that occur earlier. This clearly favours curative vs. preventive health programmes. In the business world there is no fixed rate of return on investment and the use of a private sector return rate for public sector program cost may not be correct (Sudgen and Williams 1990). Most published CEA in developed countries use discount rates between 3 and 5%. An expert panel commissioned by the US Public Health Service, based on the "shadow price of capital", recommended using a discount rate of 3% for economic evaluation in the public health sector (Gold et al. 1996). Whether benefits should also be discounted, and if so at what rate, is highly controversial.

Estimates of benefits and costs in a CEA may be uncertain because of imprecision in both underlying data and modelling assumptions. Therefore major assumptions should be varied and the net present value and other outcomes computed repeatedly to determine how sensitive outcomes are to changes in the assumptions. This so-called *sensitivity analysis* is typically the last step in a CEA. A sensitivity analysis varying the discount rate from 0% up to 7% should always be done (Gold et al. 1996).

As illustrated by Oregon's Medicaid reform efforts in 1990/91, CEA or other types of economic evaluation cannot be used as sole basis for allocating scarce resources because the question of equity and ethical issues are not addressed by this method. In Oregon, CEA was only one of 13 factors used to prioritise funding of services for the poor (Petitti 1998b).

Since Sir William Petty found out in 1667 that public health expenditures to combat the plague would achieve a benefit-cost ratio of 84 to 1 (Fein 1971), numerous studies of economic evaluation have been carried out, most of them using ratios of cost to effectiveness. The list of interventions that were economically evaluated within the last ten year spans from influenza vaccination of healthy school-aged children (White et al. 1999) to colonoscopy in screening for colorectal cancer (Sonnenberg and Delco 2002), and preoperative autologous blood donation (Etchason et al. 1995) to reducing the population's intake of salt (Selmer et al. 2000).

Weighted Capitation in NHS-Type Health Systems

The central aim of weighted capitation is to distribute a global health budget between geographical areas in accordance with population needs and thus provide equal opportunity of access for equal needs. Currently used formulas of weighted capitation can be described as a modified age standardisation of health care expenditure. The UK Resource Allocation Working Party (RAWP) originally recommended in 1976 that the resources for the hospital and community health services (HCHS) be distributed on the basis of population size, weighted by age and sex, the need for health care and the costs of providing services (Carr-Hill 1989; ACRA 1999). Standardised mortality ratios (SMRs) were used as a proxy measure for relative needs. However, this had been criticised for failing to fully reflect the demand for health care resources related to chronic disease and deprivation.

In 1995 a new weighted capitation formula for HCHS was introduced. This comprises an age index (based on estimates of national resources spent per capita in eight age groups) and an "additional needs" index (additional to that accounted for by demographic variables). The need weighting index takes the form of four indices for acute, psychiatric, non-psychiatric community, and community psychiatric services, which are based on 1991 small-area census socio-economic variables. It is derived from an empirical model that identified its needs indicators as those census-derived health status and socio-economic variables which, having been adjusted for the independent effects of supply, were most closely correlated with the national average pattern of hospitalisation (Carr-Hill et al. 1994).

For all its merits, however, this formula, also called English formula, and the models on which it is empirically based have been criticised. The fundamental criticism relates to the use of utilisation-based models to assess need for health care, which implies that historical patterns of service uptake between different care groups (as revealed by utilisation) are appropriate (Mays 1995).

Against this background, some scientists pleaded for a radically new approach to health resource allocation, one that distributes NHS resources on the basis of direct measures of morbidity rather than indirect proxies such as health service utilisation or deprivation. The Welsh steering group on Allocation (Townsend 2001) for example recommended the use of a morbidity-based budgeting approach. In a recent study of target allocations for the inpatient treatment of coronary heart disease in a sample of 34 primary care trusts in different areas in England, it was shown that a morbidity-based model would result in a significant shift in hospital resources away from deprived areas, towards areas with older demographic profiles and towards rural areas (Asthana et al. 2004). In the discussion of their findings, the authors concluded by calling for greater clarity between the goals of health care equity and health equity.

Risk-adjusted Capitation

When competition is an essential component of a health care system, it is a widespread belief that capitated payments create incentives to contain costs and to compete on quality. But they also create undesirable incentives for risk selection ("cream skimming" or "cherry picking"), i.e. to attract profitable patients (or enrolees) and to avoid unprofitable ones, and to decrease service intensity.

Risk adjustment is an important tool to reduce cream skimming while encouraging desirable cost and quality competition. This method controls for confounding (co-morbidity above all) by calculating the expected health care costs (or some other measure of an outcome) for members of health plans or insurance companies. This control is realised either by stratification (*cell-based approach*) or by multi-variate modelling (*regression approach*). In many developed countries around the world, health care organisations have established some sort of risk adjustment procedure for resource allocation. Examples exist for the following countries: Austria, Brazil, Canada, Chile, Germany, Hong Kong, Israel, the Netherlands, Spain, Switzerland, Taiwan, and the USA. Most of the risk adjustment procedures are based on a regression model to predict future health expenditure. Models differ with respect to the set of included predictors, the procedure of grouping diagnostic information, and the populations used for calibration.

The exclusive reliance on risk-adjusted capitated payments has been criticised, e.g., by Newhouse et al. (1999), who pointed out that the common risk adjusters (predictors of cost) are not likely to reduce risk selection problems to negligible levels. This concern was confirmed by a study of Shen and Ellis (2001) who examined the maximum potential profit that plans could hypothetically gain by using their own private information to select low-cost enrolees when payments are made using one of four commonly-used risk adjustment models. Their findings – based on simulations using a privately-insured sample – suggested that risk selection profits remain substantial (Shen and Ellis 2001).

Against this background it was recommended to move the financing of health services to partial capitation payments. Partial capitation for an individual enrolee combines capitation methods and some reflection of that person's actual use of services, i.e. a fee for service payment. Partial capitation would reduce plans' incentives to select good risks – the intent of risk adjustment – and also reduce the financial incentive to under-serve or stint on care (Newhouse et al. 1999).

The General Form of Regression-based Risk Adjustment Model.   Frequently used are regression models with untransformed costs as the dependent variable, estimated by ordinary least square (OLS). The standard assumptions of that type of statistical model (namely a normal distribution, homoscedasticity, and independent observations) are not satisfied sufficiently by utilisation data, but for predicting of future costs the model has shown to work about as well as more complex models in real situations (Diehr et al. 1999).

Occasionally a two-part model is applied: One equation predicts the probability that a person has any use and a second equation predicts (on a log scale) the level of use for users only. In a two-part model the regression coefficients of the first equation are estimated by logistic regression analysis and those of the second equation by OLS regression. Two-part models tend to meet the assumptions better than one-part models and provide insight into the utilisation process, but they are not recommended when the goal is to predict future costs, because transformations cause complications in this context (Diehr et al. 1999).

The list of possible predictors of a model for risk-adjusted capitation includes age, gender and other demographic or socio-economic variables as well as binary variables to indicate that a person has been assigned to a diagnosis belonging to a special group from a system of diagnostic groups or has received a drug prescription belonging to a special group from a system of drug categories. To incorporate information on morbidity, some models use hospital diagnoses alone, while others use both inpatient and outpatient diagnoses. It has, however, to be noted, that previous utilisation is a strong predictor of future utilisation (for chronically ill patients the costs in one year heavily depend on utilisation in the year before). Thus, as in any regression analysis, it is important not to control for this variable lying on the causal pathway (Diehr et al. 1999).

The estimated regression coefficients ("regression weights") refer to the so-called calibration population. For diagnosis-based models generally this is also the population used to establish the diagnostic classification system, the "grouper". Recalibration of a model without a refinement of the grouper therefore may lead to biased estimation. Generally the models are calibrated prospectively (i.e., the data of the predictor set refers to the previous year, while the cost data refer to the actual year), but in order to evaluate the predictive power current calibration (both types of data refer to the same year) has been performed as well.

The standard summary measure of model performance in prediction is R^2, the percentage of the total variance of the dependent variable that is explained by the model. Usually the values of R^2 in prospectively calibrated models do not exceed 20%. Newhouse et al. (1989) used theoretical and empirical arguments to estimate that the maximum possible R^2 in the context of utilisation data is about 15% for total expenditure (prospectively modelling).

In addition to the grouper and the regression module any risk adjustment methodology finally requires a module that links the estimated costs to the payment system or the resource allocation procedure respectively, i.e. a mechanism that controls the way payments or the allocation of resources are based on the predicted health care expenditure.

Risk Adjustment in the US Setting.   Up to 1999, Medicare paid the HMO's 95% of the *adjusted average per capita cost (AAPCC)*, an estimate of the expected cost of treating Medicare beneficiaries in the fee-for-service sector in each local area. The AAPCC methodology adjusted for differences between the HMO's enrolees and fee-for-service users with respect to age, gender, welfare status, and whether or not they were in a nursing home (Ellis et al. 1996).

Since its implementation in 1985 the AAPCC had prompted concern about its fairness and accuracy and it was shown that only about one percent of total variance of the cost of treatment was explained by this concept (Newhouse 1986; Ash et al. 1989). Against this background the *Health Care Financing Agency (HCFA)* sponsored the development of alternative approaches that include diagnostic information as predictors in the regression-based risk adjustment model, among them the *Diagnostic Cost Groups (DCG)* family and the *Adjusted Clinical Group (ACG)* methodology (Ingber 1998). In the years 2000 to 2003, AAPCC has been stepwise replaced by the *Principal Inpatient Diagnostic Cost Group model (PIP-DCG)* which uses socio-demographic variables and hospital diagnoses to predict next years cost

(Pope et al. 2000). In 2004, a 100 percent comprehensive risk adjustment scheme (using full encounter diagnostic data) should be established (Ingber 2000). In view of the widespread concern about the quality of ambulatory diagnoses, the DCG family was supplemented in 2001 by a model that uses outpatient pharmacy data, grouped into 127 mutually exclusive categories, instead of ambulatory diagnoses (Zhao et al. 2001).

Medicaid supported the development of the *Chronic Illness and Disability Payment System (CPDS)* which groups the Medicaid beneficiaries according to a hierarchical diagnostic classification system (Kronick et al. 1996). CPDS, which was reconstructed and recalibrated later on to predict expenditures also for Medicare beneficiaries, has now been established in several US states (Kronick et al. 2002).

Risk Adjustment in a Bismarck-Type European Setting.   In European countries with a predominating Bismarck-type organisation of health services we find competition among all insurance companies and even among the statutory sickness funds. The main goal of risk-adjustment in these settings is to reduce risk selection by the sickness funds and to establish a fair system of income-related contributions. HSR has played a major role in designing and reforming these systems.

Like in the USA, the starting point of risk-adjustment in Europe has been set by models based on age, gender and other socio-demographic variables. The Netherlands for example started in 1992 with a prospectively used age and gender based model. In 1995 region and disability were included as predictors, and a "high risk pool" was established in addition. Since 2002, dummy variables were added to the model that indicate prescriptions of drugs falling into one out of 13 mutually exclusive categories, the *Pharmacy-based Cost Groups (PCGs)*, each of them closely related to a serious chronic disease (Lamers 1999). From 2004 onwards, the Dutch risk-adjustment methodology will be further supplemented by an inpatient DCG module that uses hospital diagnoses only.

In 1994, Germany introduced a retrospective risk-adjustment procedure among statutory sickness funds which was based on the following variables: age, gender, and two dummy variables indicating invalidity or disability pension and the entitlement for sickness allowance. The procedure was also designed to adjust for different incomes because the beneficiaries pay income-related contributions. The largest share of the risk-adjusted financial transfers between sickness funds (up to 60%) results from differences in per capita income of the beneficiaries. From 2002 on, the German risk-adjustment methodology has been extended. First, a retrospective "high cost pool"[6] was established, and second, a dummy variable was added to the set of risk adjusters indicating that a beneficiary is registered in an accredited disease management programme. In a long term perspective it is planned to introduce a morbidity-based risk adjusted formula and a high risk pool (Buchner and Wasem 2003).

---

[6] The high cost pool consists of insured with high cost in the past year (above a fixed threshold) which are shared by all statutory sickness funds.

Evaluating Effects
of Organisational Characteristics and Change

As health services systems in the developed countries tend to go through one reform after another and are more or less continuously exposed to change, evaluation is a permanent task of HSR. But the preconditions do not favour the establishment of scientifically sound research designs. Experimental designs are extremely rare. The above-cited RAND Health Insurance Study on the effect of cost-sharing measures on utilisation is one of the most famous exceptions. In some circumstances it is even difficult to implement a quasi-experimental design including a control group. Particularly in countries like Germany, where benefits and programmes are uniform but the organisational responsibilities are widely scattered over local authorities and institutions, evaluation research is very complex.

Suggested by the structure of available data, perhaps the most frequently used quasi-experimental design for analysing aggregated annual data in the context of programme evaluation is the time-series experiment. It can be characterised by a periodic measurement process on some group and the introduction of an experimental change X into this time series of measurements O_i. Adapting a diagram by Campbell and Stanley (1966) the time series design can be outlined as follows (whereby the number of observations before or after X, occurring here in year five, may be smaller or larger as in a real problems):

$$O_1, O_2, O_3, O_4, X, O_6, O_7, O_8, O_9 \ .$$

The main problem of (internal) validity inherent in a time series design is revealed by seeking likely alternative explanations of the shift in the time series other than the effect of X. This problem, of course, could be settled to a great extent by establishing a suitable control group (comparison series) that shares all intervening factors except X with the study group.

A natural approach for analysing data from a time series design is *segmented* or *piecemeal regression* (e.g. Neter and Wasserman 1974). This method is appropriate when the considered response variable has a linear trend over the range before X (segment one) followed by another linear trend over the range after X (segment two). The year which divides the segments (year five in the above diagram) is known as the join point (or break point). When the hypothetical change of trend line refers only to the slope and not to the intercepts (that means no discontinuity between the both lines), the regression equation for analysing data from a design as diagrammed above can be specified as follows:

$$E(Y) = \beta_0 + \beta_1 x_1 + \beta_2 x_1 x_2 \ ,$$

where Y is the response variable, x_1 is the year ($x_1 = 1, 2, 3, 4, 6, 7, 8, 9$) and x_2 is a dummy variable indicating that the year is greater than 5. The parameter β_2 measures the difference in slopes between the lines. If the same trend continues from the first segment to the second segment, then $\beta_2 = 0$. The β_j are estimated, and the hypothesis $\beta_2 = 0$ is tested, using standard procedures in regression. It is easy to expand segmented regression to more than two segments and even to allow for discontinuities between segmented regression lines. Autocorrelated errors or heteroskedasticity can be handled by using standard techniques (e.g. Greene 2003).

A good example for applying this type of analysis to evaluate the impact of a programme on the basis of aggregated data is the study of the effect of a regionalised perinatal care programme in North Carolina (established in 1965) on perinatal and postneonatal mortality (Gillings et al. 1981). A similar – but due to autocorrelation more complex – analysis was carried out to evaluate the effects of patient-level payment restrictions for prescription drugs under Medicaid in the years 1981–83. By this analysis, supplemented by survival analysis to measure the rate of admissions to hospital and nursing homes, it could be shown that the decline in the use of drugs after the cap (a limit of three paid prescriptions per month) had been associated with an increase in rates of admission to nursing homes (Soumerai et al. 1987, 1991).

Regardless of these examples there is only limited use of OLS-regression models for evaluation because of several restrictions. First, costs or the logarithm of costs or other continuously distributed responses are only one type of outcome measure used for evaluation. Counts of specific events, e.g. contacts, prescriptions, hospital admissions etc. and binary response variables like death, accident or first occurrence of a specific disease are equally important - in some situations even more important measures. Second, if individual longitudinal data are available, to make full use of the data structure, the model used should be able to handle clustered (correlated) response data, arising from repeated measurements and time-varying covariates. *Generalised linear models* (Nelder and Wedderburn 1972; McCullagh and Nelder 1983) and the related *generalised estimating equations* (GEEs) (Liang and Zeger 1986) form the methodological framework of an advanced approach of statistical modelling for evaluation. Consistent parameter estimates in these models are achieved by maximising likelihood- or quasi-likelihood functions using some sort of Gauss–Newton algorithm. Several of the common packages of statistical software, among them SAS, provide corresponding procedures.

The standard model to analyse count data, for example, is the *Poisson regression model*, which is a non-linear regression model that can be formulated as a generalised linear model. Poisson regression is robust insofar as consistent estimation of the regression coefficients does not require that the dependent variable is Poisson distributed. Only a correct specification of the conditional mean is required (Cameron and Trivedi 1998). But Poisson regression is prone to overdispersion. Therefore the condition that the variance equals the mean has to be relaxed by introducing a dispersion parameter that must be estimated as well. Otherwise testing hypotheses on the regression coefficients could yield misleading rejections of null hypotheses (Cameron and Trivedi 1998).

Poisson regression can also be used to analyse correlated counts from repeated measurements. The within-patients correlation is then estimated in the framework of GEEs, whereas the effects of the covariates can be modelled as a generalised linear model. For example, the introduction of reference pricing for angiotensin-converting-enzyme (ACE) inhibitors for patients of 65 years of age or older in

British Columbia, Canada, in January 1997, was evaluated by using such a type of analysis (Schneeweiss et al. 2002). Several covariates were included in the model, among them age, gender, the household adjusted income and a chronic disease score computed from prescription medications for every quarter and treated as a time-varying covariate. This ambitious study was based on computerised administrative health databases covering a large proportion of the population, including all types of claims, hospital admissions, admissions for long-term care, diagnoses, and the medications, dose, and dispensed quantity of all prescriptions. Even the deaths within the study cohort were included.

A similar analysis has never been done in Germany, though reference-based prices (RBP) for the beneficiaries of the statutory sickness funds were established in 1992/93. For reasons of privacy and data protection, cross-institutional linkage of existing scattered administrative databases on drug utilisation, ambulatory diagnoses and medical services, and hospital data on an individual level need extensive data protection procedures in Germany or even the informed consent by each patient. Thus the effects of RBP can be only evaluated on the basis of aggregated data. But any conclusions on the overall economic and public health impact, if obtained solely on the basis of aggregated data, are distorted because of the introduction of fixed drug budgets and the effects of the reunification of Germany (among other confounders) that both took place in the beginning of the 1990s, more or less simultaneously with RBP (Schneeweiss et al. 1998).

Sometimes one has to balance the advantage of using individual longitudinal data – without having a control group – against the advantage of having a control group at the price of rather limited capacities of analysis based on aggregated data. For example, in a study of the effect of premium rebate to reward low utilisation of services for beneficiaries of one statutory sickness fund in Germany, the effect on expenditure mainly was analysed using a long time series of aggregated data together with a control series. In a second step this analysis was combined with an examination of the effects on non-monetary measures of utilisation based on short time series of beneficiary-related data that were primary collected by the sickness fund in order to support administration of premium rebates (Schäfer and Nolde-Gallasch 1999).

Process of Health Care: Effectiveness, Appropriateness and Quality

5.5

Research on the process of health care considers questions like: Which services are provided in which quantity, by whom, where, and how (Schwartz and Busse 2003)? The production of health care is a complex result of financing arrangements and of demand and supply-side factors. The interaction of these different factors is not well understood. An interest in investigating these questions arouse after substantial and unexplained variation in procedures and hospital admissions was observed between similar hospitals. Some examples for these variations have already been presented in Sect. 5.3.2, e.g. the Boston-New Haven Study (Wennberg et al. 1987, 1989). These studies demonstrated the importance of supply-side factors on utilisation patterns and frequency, if patient-related factors are controlled for, such as age, gender, case mix, and socio-economic status. The supply-side of a region is primarily described by the density of physicians, hospital beds, and the availability of medical technologies. However, most studies do not analyse the effects of these provider or supply-side characteristics on the health status of the populations concerned (Brook and Lohr 1985).

More refined supply-side characteristics determining the use of services comprise provider payment mechanisms, experience and gender of health professionals, organisation and equipment of physicians' practices, size and type of hospital, as well as referral patterns between different providers (Schwartz and Busse 2003). "Self-referral" of patients has been identified as an important determinant of small area variation in the use of medical technologies (Childs and Hunter 1972). Self-referral describes the phenomenon of providing expensive medical technology, e.g. X-ray examinations, for patients in general practitioners', physicians', or orthopaedic surgeons' practices without referring the patient to a radiologist. In comparisons between countries with a comparable standard of health care, the possibility of self-referral for X-ray examinations compared to countries with X-ray examinations exclusively provided by a radiologist increases the overall rate of X-rays by a factor of 4 (Busse 1995). Within a country, differences in examination frequency between doctors with the possibility of self-referral compared to doctors who have to refer patients to a radiologist yield comparable results. In Germany, the rates for X-ray examination for patients with chronic pain was increased by a factor of 2.7, the rates for abdominal ultrasound for patients presenting with gastrointestinal symptoms by a factor of 3.0 in practices with a possibility of self-referral compared to practices who had to refer their patients to other practices (Busse 1995). Of course this observation is linked to the method of physician remuneration. It is a phenomenon which is primarily observed in countries with fee-for-service remuneration such as the United States and Germany. The effects of the structure of financial incentive systems and resulting overutilisation on a system level tend to be underestimated. In Germany, fee-for-service remuneration combined with the possibility of self-referral and the widespread practice of non-radiologists to provide X-ray examinations in their practices resulted in 1655 X-ray examinations being performed per 1000 inhabitants in 1997 (Deutsche Röntgengesellschaft 2002) – about twice the rate observed in other European countries. It is estimated that unnecessary X-ray examinations during the last decades now cause around 2000 incident cases of cancer in the country annually (Berrington de Gonzalez 2004).

The extreme variation in health service provision raises the question whether diagnostic and therapeutic procedures are appropriately used in the process of care. To judge whether a procedure is appropriate, knowledge about the effectiveness of the procedure for certain indications or clinical presentations is required. However, this is not the case for the majority of indication-procedure pairs.

Assessing Effectiveness and Appropriateness of Care   5.5.1

In general, the effectiveness of a health care professional or service is the degree to which the desired outcomes are achieved (Gray 1997). However, the proposition that an intervention is effective implies that there is only one outcome of care and only one objective in the design of that intervention – which is rarely the case (Gray 1997). In addition to a number of beneficial outcomes of care, such as lower mortality and morbidity, the possibility of harmful effects of care has to be considered. Effectiveness research attempts to answer questions, such as "What is the right thing to do?" or "What care confers significant health benefit for a given clinical situation?" (Scott and Campbell 2002).

Another frequently used concept is that of efficacy, which is the impact of an intervention in the best possible circumstances (Gray 1997). These can be achieved in randomised clinical trials (RCTs). However, the reverse conclusion that RCTs always produce efficacy results is not true, as not all RCTs satisfy high quality standards. The distinction between efficacy and effectiveness is important, as the latter represents the impact of an intervention under routine care conditions. The difference between the two concepts in terms of health status outcomes is illustrated in Fig. 5.2 using the example of complications of radical prostatectomy. Data on effectiveness in the example are derived from a meta-analysis of Medicare routine data, efficacy data are taken from a meta-analysis of RCTs.

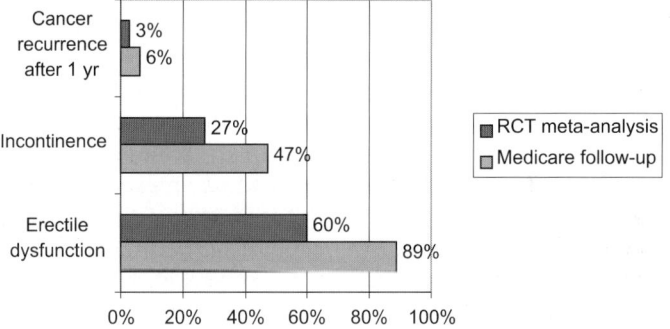

Figure 5.2. Comparison of effectiveness and efficacy using the example of radical prostatectomy (adapted from Fowler et al. 1993)

An important aspect of both efficacy and effectiveness is that they apply to groups of patients. However, the impact of an intervention on the health status of an individual depends to a large extent on individual factors. To answer the question of whether the most appropriate care was provided given the clinical circumstances is the realm of appropriateness research. An intervention can be considered appropriate, if the expected health benefit exceeds the expected negative consequences by a large enough margin to justify performing the procedure rather than other alternatives (Herrin et al. 1997).

Appropriateness research also addresses the questions of overuse, underuse or misuse of interventions (Scott and Campbell 2002). We have already discussed the effect of provider remuneration systems and organisational features of a health system on utilisation rates. Another major determinant of utilisation is clinical judgement. A historical study on clinicians' judgement variation is a study from New York in the 1920s, in which one thousand 11-year-olds had their throats examined (American Child Health Association 1934) cited by Black (1997). In 61% of these children a tonsillectomy was performed. Of the remaining 39% the examining doctor thought half would require a tonsillectomy. The half with healthy tonsils were examined by another doctor, who thought that half of them required surgery. The healthy children were again examined by yet another doctor, who declared that half of them required a tonsillectomy, which means that after four examinations only 65 out of 1000 children would have escaped with their tonsils intact (Black 1997).

During the last 10 years a number of studies using the RAND/UCLA appropriateness method have been performed. This basically consists in collecting an expert opinion on the appropriateness of an intervention using the Delphi technique. The experts are asked to judge a number of possible indications (i.e. case descriptions with clinical information including co-morbidity, age, and sex) on whether a specific intervention was appropriate, inappropriate or even harmful in these cases. In a second step, these judgements are applied to real patient groups in order to determine in how many cases the procedure was appropriate or inappropriate. Most studies using the RAND/UCLA appropriateness method reported appropriate interventions in the range of 50 to 85% of all interventions performed. Non-US expert groups consistently thought that more procedures were inappropriate compared to US expert groups. This has to be kept in mind when interpreting results from appropriateness studies. An example is a review of the appropriateness of coronary angiography, upper gastrointestinal endoscopy and carotid endarterectomy performed on 4564 patients in the USA in 1988. The review which was based on a literature review and on an expert panel consensus concluded that, respectively, only 77%, 76%, and 36% of these procedures had been appropriate (Brook et al. 1990). Inappropriate care is more than a nuisance. It can be harmful to health. For example in a prospective observational study on congestive heart failure admissions, 7% of admissions were found to be the result of improper medical treatment, including fluid overload, procedures, and misuse of drugs. Hospital mortality for this group of patients was 32% compared to 9% in patients without inappropriate treatment (Rich et al. 1996).

5.5.2 Assessing Quality of Care: Clinical Practice Performance

Measures of clinical practice performance continue to be under constant discussion, particularly when they are published routinely, as is the case, for example, for hospitals in the United States and the United Kingdom. There is broad agreement on the dominant paradigm, established by Donabedian (1980), of measuring quality of clinical care in terms of *structure*, *process* and *outcome*, but each category has advantages and disadvantages which must be assessed in relation to the type and the speciality of the service (e.g., inpatient versus outpatient care or surgery versus drug therapy), the condition being treated (e.g., diabetes, hypertension, acute myocardial infarction, or mental disorders), the case-mix of the patients, the role of the comparative information, and a variety of other context variables (Shojania et al. 2001).

The type of assessment of clinical practice performance heavily depends on the perspective on quality. Blumenthal (1996) distinguishes four main perspectives on quality: the health care professional perspective, the perspective of health care plans and organisations, the purchaser perspective, and the patient perspective. Health care professionals tend to emphasise technical excellence and the characteristics of interaction between patient and professional (Donabedian 1988). Health care plans and organisations place greater emphasis on the general health of the enrolled population and on the function of the organisation (Leape 1994). Purchasers, of course, additionally incorporate the price and the effectiveness of the delivery of care. Taking into account the preferences and values of patients leads to a definition of quality that emphasises outcomes such as functional status, morbidity, mortality, or quality of life, and encompasses satisfaction with care (Petitti and Amster 1998).

Indicators of Structural Quality

Structural measures characterise the resources in the health system. They describe the setting in which care occurs and the capacity of that setting to produce quality (Donabedian 1980, Brook et al. 1996). Quality assurance programmes and organisations such as the Joint Commission on the Accreditation of Health Care Organisations (JCAHO) and the National Committee on Quality Assurance (NCQA) in the USA or the associations of statutory health insurance physicians in Germany, rely on structural measures (as listed below) to infer quality and confer accreditation on this basis.

For providers, structural measures include professional characteristics like speciality or board certifications etc. For hospitals, they include ownership, number of beds, teaching status, licensure status, availability of sophisticated technologies, qualification of personnel and other organisational factors for inpatient care (e.g., staff-to-patient ratio, closed intensive care units, dedicated stroke units, or the presence of a clinical information system). One frequently used structural measure of quality is patient volume (Shojania et al. 2001). The growing use of this indicator reflects an extensive literature, which documents superior outcome for hospitals and physicians with higher patient volumes for certain indications and procedures (e.g., Luft et al. 1979; Hannan et al. 1989; Phibbs et al. 1996; Thiemann et al. 1999).

When using structural indicators to measure quality of care, the implicit assumption is that structure affects outcome. This is certainly true for the compliance with minimum standards of structure (e.g., rules for hygiene in operating rooms). But on higher levels of structural quality the link between structure and outcome is less clear (Shojania et al. 2001). For example, specialist care as a quality measure not always results in better outcomes. This is demonstrated by the findings that even cardiologists fail to provide proven therapies to many eligible patients with acute myocardial infarction (Brand et al. 1995). These findings promote the case to measure the processes of health care delivery directly instead.

Indicators of Process Quality

Process indicators permit a glimpse into the inside of the care-delivering units, allowing measurement of the care patients actually receive. They measure the net effect of physicians' clinical decision-making. Clinical choices about the use of surgery, medication or diagnostic tests, admission to a hospital, and length of stay account for a large proportion of the costs of services and of outcomes experienced by the patients. Sometimes generic process measures are used (e.g., number of prescriptions, average length of stay, or day case surgery rate). But mostly they are specific to specialities and certain conditions (e.g., antibiotics within eight hours for patients with community-acquired pneumonia, prophylaxis for venous thromboembolism, or beta-blockers for patients with acute myocardial infarction).

Process measures can be reported for individual physicians, groups of practitioners, for hospitals, hospital units, or hospital trusts, or for the entire system of care. They are favoured by providers to indicate quality because they are directly related to what providers do. Frequently they are derived from evidence-based clinical guidelines and facilitate individual physician quality improvement. If proven diagnostic and therapeutic strategies are monitored, quality problems can be detected long before demonstrable outcome differences occur (Brook et al. 1996).

Even so there are some arguments against process-based measurement of the quality of care. First, process measures are not necessarily good predictors of outcome, and allocating resources to processes which do not affect outcomes may increase cost without producing any improvement in health (Ellwood 1988). Moreover, collecting process data may be a comparatively elaborate procedure. Finally, it may not be possible to achieve consensus on the recommended process for many clinical problems (Petitti and Amster 1998).

Indicators of Outcome Quality and Adjustment for Case-Mix

The quality-relevant health outcomes have been described as the "five Ds" – death, disease, disability, discomfort, and dissatisfaction (Elinson 1987), or, more positively turned, when measuring quality of care, health outcomes could be summarised as survival, states of physiologic, physical and emotional health, and patient satisfaction (Lohr et al. 1988). Broader definitions of outcomes include psychosocial functioning, quality of life, resource utilisation and costs of care (Iezzoni 1994).

The use of outcome measures to assess the quality of clinical performance has been criticised for several reasons. First, even for common conditions, it may take years to detect differences in outcomes between groups of patients (Palmer 1997). Moreover, such differences may not be under the control of providers but reflect, among others, patient factors, variations in admission practices, or chance rather than differences in quality of care (Shojania et al. 2001). Many outcomes (e.g., mortality) are rare and comparisons of quality based on such outcomes often have low statistical power (Brook et al. 1996).

Considerable concern is related to perverse incentives for "upcoding" and "gaming" (McGlynn 1998), whereby gaming means a change of treatment to more expensive forms which are frequently more stressful for the patient and result in a reduced quality of care (e.g. a surgical procedure instead of a drug prescription, an inappropriate hospitalisation or a short hospital admission for a marginal diagnosis).

Incentives for gaming may arise from the criteria used to define target patient populations. For example, restricting inpatient mortality to deaths that literally occur in the hospital allows hospitals to lower their mortality rates simply by discharging patients to die at home or in other institutions (Jencks et al. 1988). Additionally, the incentive for physicians or hospitals to avoid caring for sicker patients remains a substantial concern for outcome-based performance measurement (Hofer et al. 1999). Proliferation of diagnoses related to co-morbidity or coding of diagnoses related to severity of illness (upcoding) were observed after the introduction of the prospective payment system for HMO-enrolled beneficiaries of Medicare (Keeler et al. 1990).

The most important concern of research related to outcome-based quality measures focused on the development of case-mix adjustment models for hospital mortality rates. Case-mix adjustment and risk adjustment are based on similar methods, but they use different data sources: Case-mix indices are based on medical records from hospitals or physicians, while risk adjustment is based on administrative data, e.g. from health insurances. Models that have originally been designed to predict financial rather than clinical outcomes (see Sect. 5.4.1) did not perform sufficiently well in this context. Progress has been made in adopting models to identify the case-mix of a group of patients by focusing on specific subgroups of patients instead of overall hospital mortality and using clinical rather than administrative data (Iezzoni 1994).

Examples for Performance Assessment 5.5.3

Comparison of HMOs Based on a Performance Indicator System

The federal Centers for Medicare and Medicaid Services (CMS), formerly known as the Health Care Financing Administration (HCFA), and the private sector in the USA have supported the development of several performance indicator systems in order to compare the quality of care delivered by HMOs. Perhaps the most popular system, the Health Employer Data and Information Set (HEDIS), was introduced in 1993 and was revised in 1995 and again in 1997. It can be considered as the model for many other performance measurement efforts (Petitti and Amster 1998).

HEDIS was designed by the National Committee for Quality Assurance (NCQA) to evaluate several aspects of health plan performance including clinical quality of care, access to care, satisfaction with care, utilisation of services, and the financial performance of the HMO. The clinical quality-of-care indicators included in HEDIS were chosen to address aspects of the care process for which there was strong evidence in the literature to support the relationship between medical care process and desired outcomes (Petitti and Amster 1998). These included indicators for low birth-weight babies, childhood immunisation status, breast cancer screening, eye exams for people with diabetes, and beta-blocker treatment after heart attack.

Hospital Ranking

In NHS-type countries the assessment of the quality of clinical performance focuses on the health of the general population and the function of the health care system with a special concern on inpatient care. For example, in the United Kingdom, in order to rank hospitals, the publication of clinical indicators in the form of so-called league tables has a long history. As far back as 1983, a set of performance indicators was published covering five areas, one of which was clinical activity. Since then the set of indicators has been revised several times (British Medical Association 2000).

Currently the published UK league tables are compiled by the Dr Foster organisation (separately for England, Wales, Scotland and Northern Ireland). They are based on the Department of Health's Episode Statistics (HES) and data collected through questionnaires. The indicators fall into five broad categories: standardised mortality rates, waiting times and volumes, staff to bed ratios, and – for England only – patient and staff satisfaction and other rating based scales (clean hospital, good food etc.). The mortality rates are standardised for age, sex, length of stay, and type of admission (elective or emergency admission). SMRs are calculated for each of 80 ICD9 three-digit primary diagnoses (accounting for 80 per cent of all in-hospital deaths) cited in the final episode of care. The expected deaths for each hospital[7] (the denominator of the SMRs) are calculated by multiplying the number of hospital admissions in each stratum or cell by the national death rates for that stratum and adding across all strata. Hospitals are classified as high or low with respect to a SMR if their 95% confidence intervals do not include unity. A supplementary indicator based on HES is the diagnosis-specific standardised admission ratio (SAR) for each Primary Care Trust (PCT) area. The SAR is calculated like a SMR where the denominator is built up by the number of admissions expected for the PCT population assuming it had the same admission rate as the national average, taking into account age, sex and the different diagnoses (Dr Foster 2004a,b). The league tables are criticised for several reasons. The first concern refers to an insufficient control for case-mix relating to severity, co-morbidity, deprivation, and the availability of places for people to be discharged to nursing homes or hospices. The second refers to the use of HES, which are based on finished consultant episodes (the NHS's measure of hospital activity), whereas no conversion to hospital spells is provided (HES are not designed to collect detailed clinical data). Third, the primary diagnosis has been questioned, as diagnostic criteria change. Finally the focus on inpatient mortality is considered a shortfall because

---

[7] The SMRs for England are calculated at trust level only.

an increasing proportion of deaths occur outside the hospital (Jacobson et al. 2003).

In the United States an annual index of hospital quality ("America's Best") is published by *U.S. News & World Report*. This hospital ranking methodology was devised in 1993 by the statistics and methodology department of the National Organization for Research (NORC) at the University of Chicago, which carries out the analysis and refines it as needed. The index is designed to be used by patients who are looking for the best hospital to treat their health problems. The 2003 hospital ranking is broken down into 17 specialities. It is based on reputation, mortality and other factors. The reputational scores of a hospital in each of the 17 specialities are based on a survey. 150 randomly selected board-certified physicians were asked to list up to five hospitals they believed to be tops in their speciality, without considering cost or location. The mortality score is adjusted for case-severity. The severity adjustments were derived using the All Patient Refined Diagnosis Related Group (APR-DRG) method designed by 3M Health Information Systems. The APR-DRG adjusts expected deaths for severity of illness by means of principle diagnosis and categories of secondary diagnoses. Most of the data that are summed up to the "other factors" (e.g., data on nursing care and technology availability) came from the 2001 annual survey of hospitals by the American Hospital Association (O'Muircheartaigh et al. 2003).

The ranking of hospitals on behalf of the *U.S. News & World Report* is not the only one published in the United States. The Hospital Association of Southern California (HASC) states that an "incredible proliferation of hospital record cards by all sorts of organizations is bombarding the public and the membership" (Barber 2003). HASC has established a Hospital Quality Committee that, among others, has the task to analyse hospital ranking report cards, including source data, data aggregation, weighting, risk adjustment, sample thresholds and presentation style (Qureshi 2003).

In Germany, there is no published ranking of hospitals except for some studies of limited impact, e.g., of the University of Bayreuth (Institut für Medizinmanagement und Gesundheitswesen 2004), that are connected to credit rating required by the new guidelines of the banks of the Group of Ten countries (Basel Committee on Banking Supervision 2003).

Physician Profiling

The Physician Payment Review Commission of the American Medical Association (AMA) defines physician profiling as "an analytical tool that uses epidemiological methods to compare practice patterns of providers on the dimensions of cost, service use, or quality (process and outcome) of care." Profiles can be developed for an individual physician, a group of physicians, or physicians within a hospital or managed care plan. They can be broken down by geographic area, speciality, type of practice or other characteristics. Profiling can focus on many different types of outcome or resource measures. Those resources may be defined globally (e.g., overall charges/costs for the care of a person or group of persons) or they may represent certain subcategories of services (e.g., laboratory, X-ray, physician services, or pharmaceuticals). Profiling is usually applied to compare resources used by cohorts of patients to get a sense of whether their providers do or do not practice efficiently. Even when profiles are not used to modify payment, they may be used to select or reject providers or to determine appropriate patient caseloads for salaried practitioners (Tucker et al. 2002).

The core element of any profiling methodology is risk adjustment by calculating an SMR-like figure, i.e., a ratio of observed to expected values of the considered measure. The expected value is adjusted with respect to age, sex of the patients and to the diagnostic groups that were assigned by the used grouper. Most of the sellers of common models of diagnosis based risk adjustment (e.g., ACG and DCG) offer the use of their predictive models for profiling.

Profiling may serve as a tool to feed information on care back to the physicians. Also, managed care organisations as a whole have had considerable experience with profiling in order to monitor plan activity. For example, profiling reports, adjusted for case-mix, can be used to distribute bonus or set-aside funds that are marked to recognise how well resource management goals are achieved among managed care providers (Tucker et al. 2002). A review of profiling in practice is given by Sutton (2001).

Concerns about physician profiling encompass the following issues (Zastrow 2001): Although managed care organisations and hospitals overtly justify profiling as a means to improve quality or conduct utilisation review, they may act without any concern for cost-effectiveness. Profiling is thus mainly based on billing/claim data that are considered not only to be limited in nature, but also to be grossly incorrect. Profiling methods are frequently flawed as they do not take into account sample size, and regional or physician speciality variation. The underlying assumption that the "average" standard of care is the best, is questionable. Although profiling saves money, it adds cost back into the system. There has also been controversy surrounding who has access to profile information. For physician groups who profile their own members, feedback to individual physicians is routinely given as an educational measure. However, this is not always the case for health plans (Zastrow 2001). Against the background of these concerns the American Medical Association (AMA) compiled a position paper describing principles to guide the collection, release and use of physician-specific health care data (AMA 2000).

In 1996, the Commonwealth of Massachusetts became one of the first states to implement a comprehensive physician profiling programme available to consumers over the Internet. Many other states have adopted similar systems since. In the beginning of the year 2001, physician profiles were available in 30 states, with legislation pending in eight others (Sutton 2001).

In Germany, profiling of physicians has been based on crude measures. Up to now they have been compared with the average of the regional group of physicians belonging to the same speciality, but a medium-term change to the risk adjusted profiling system, mandated by law, is scheduled.

Outcomes of Health Care

Assessing Output and Outcomes of Care

A frequently cited definition of outcomes was given by Donabedian (1985): "Outcomes are those changes, either favourable or adverse, in the actual or potential health status of persons, groups or communities that can be attributed to prior or concurrent care."

The most conventional method of measuring the health status of populations is by means of vital statistics, including statistics of birth and death. Disease-specific incidence rates, cause-specific mortality rates or other population-based indicators are extensively used to assess the health status of communities, counties, or health systems in general (see Sect. 5.6.3). For example, the Centers for Disease Control (CDC) established a set of 18 population-based health status indicators in 1991 for use at all administrative levels in the United States (Freedman et al. 1991).

Vital statistics may be considered as the key feature of outcomes research to study health care and the effect of intervention on a broad range of outcomes, both humanistic and clinical (Petitti 1998a). As population-based measures of health and methods of adjustment are dealt with in Chaps. I.2 and I.9 of this handbook and in several sections of this chapter, in the following we focus on further approaches to measure health status used in outcomes research, including patient-based outcomes measurement, adjusted life expectancy, and patient satisfaction. A common feature of most of these outcomes measures is that data are collected by questionnaires directly from patients, residents, employees, insured, or HMO-enrolled beneficiaries.

Patient-based Measures of Health Status

Clinicians can make use of a variety of measures which are disease-specific, system or organ-specific, function-specific (such as instruments that examine sleep or sexual function), or problem-specific (such as back pain) to explore the full range of patients' experience. Disease-specific health status measures have been developed for nearly all chronic conditions, including, for example, asthma, cancer sites, cardiovascular diseases, diabetes, rheumatoid arthritis, prostate disease, epilepsy, hypertension, pneumonia, and migraine (Guyatt et al. 1995). But if there is interest to go beyond the specific illness and to compare the impact of treatments on health-related quality of life (HRQL) across diseases or conditions, one will require a more comprehensive assessment. None of the disease-specific, system or organ-specific, function-specific or problem-specific measures are adequate for comparisons across conditions. These comparisons require generic measures designed for administration to people with any underlying health problem (or no problem at all) that cover all relevant areas of HRQL (Guyatt et al. 1995).

Generic health-status questionnaires are usually designed to establish separate scales including physical, mental and social health, as suggested by the well known definition of health by the WHO (1947). There are numerous generic health-status measures – for a review and description see, e.g., Spilker (1995) or McDowell and Newell (1996). Three of these are very popular and have become standard in the health status field: The 36-Item Short Form Questionnaire (SF-36) (Ware and Sherbourne 1992), the Sickness Impact Profile (SIP) (Bergner et al. 1981) and the Quality of Well-Being Scale (QWB) (Kaplan and Anderson 1988). The psychometric properties of these instruments are sufficiently tested and the reliability is considered high (Petitti 1998a).

In particular the SF-36 (a shortened version of a battery of 149 health status questions) is one of the most widely accepted, extensively translated and tested instruments around the world (Tseng et al. 2003). It satisfies rigorous psychometric criteria for validity and internal consistency. Clinical validity was shown by the distinctive profiles generated for each condition, each of which differed from that in the general population in a predictable manner. Furthermore, SF-36 scores were lower in referred patients than in patients not referred and were closely related to general practitioners' perceptions of severity (Garratt et al. 1993).

The SF-36 was designed for use in clinical practice and research, health policy evaluations, and general population surveys. It includes one multi-item scale that assesses eight health concepts:

1. limitations in physical activities because of health problems;
2. limitations in social activities because of physical or emotional problems;
3. limitations in usual role activities because of physical health problems;
4. bodily pain;
5. general mental health (psychological distress and well-being);
6. limitations in usual role activities because of emotional problems;
7. vitality (energy and fatigue); and
8. general health perceptions.

See also the measurement concept in Fig. 5.3 and an excerpt of the questionnaire in Fig. 5.4. The survey was constructed for self-administration by persons 14 years of age and older, and for administration by a trained interviewer in person or by telephone (Ware and Sherbourne 1992).

In the late 1980s a European group of researchers started to develop a generic health-status measure – the European Quality of Life Scale (EQ-5D) – simultaneously in several European languages (EuroQol Group 1990; Brooks 1996). The EuroQol Group consisted originally of a network of international multidisciplinary researchers from Europe, but nowadays includes members from Canada, Japan, New Zealand, Singapore, South Africa and the USA. The EQ-5D self-report questionnaire comprises five dimensions of health (mobility, self-care, usual activities, pain/discomfort anxiety/depression) rated on three levels (no problems, some/moderate problems/extreme problems). A unique EQ-5D health state is defined by combination of these dimensions. EQ-5D is a public domain instrument (http://www.euroqol.org/index.htm).

Items   Scales   <u>Summary Measures</u>

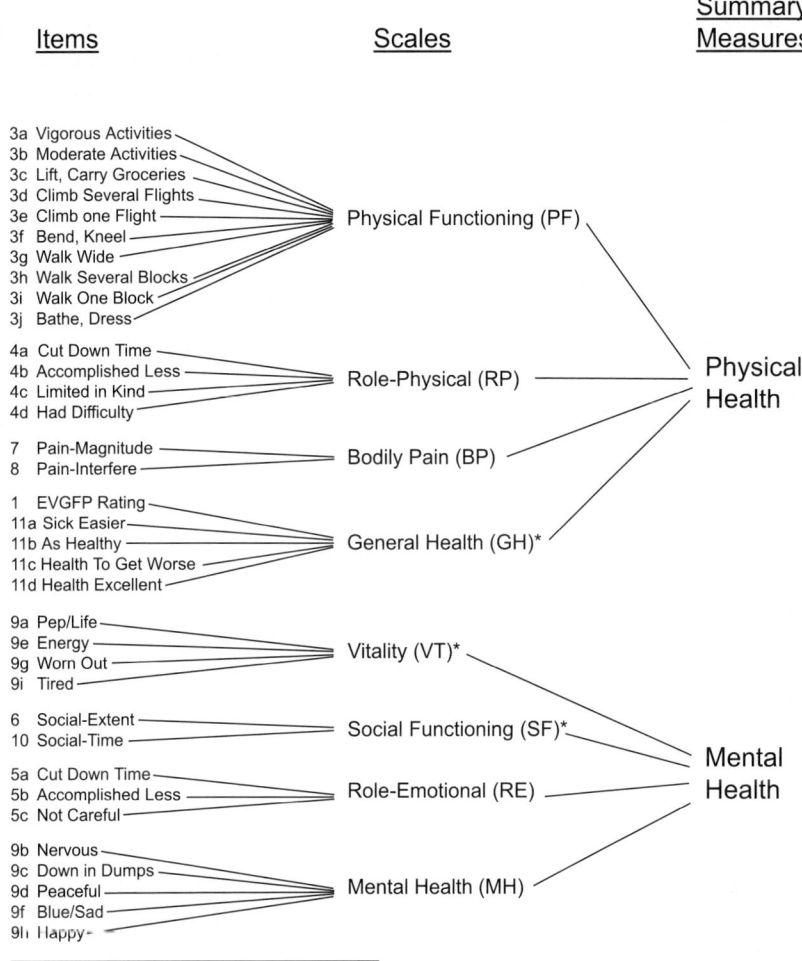

* Significant correlation with other summary measure

Figure 5.3. The SF-36 measurement concept (adapted from SF-36 Psychometric Considerations; http://www.sf-36.org/tools/sf36.shtml)

Adjusted Life Expectancy

Life expectancy, even without any adjustments, is already a rather complex measure. It is defined as the average future lifetime of a person at birth and is calculated from a current life table (the key tool of actuaries for some 200 years). Consider a large group, or "cohort", of persons, who were born on the same day. If an actuary could follow the cohort from birth until death, he or she could record the number of individuals alive at each birthday – age x, say – and the number dying during the following year. The ratio of these is the probability of dying at

9. These questions are about how you feel and how things have been with you during the <u>past 4 weeks</u>. For each question, please give the one answer that comes closest to the way you have been feeling. How much of the time during the <u>past 4 weeks</u>...

	All of the time	Most of the time	A good bit of the time	Some of the time	A little of the time	None of the time
a Did you feel full of pep?	☐1	☐2	☐3	☐4	☐5	☐6
b Have you been very nervous person?	☐1	☐2	☐3	☐4	☐5	☐6
c Have you felt so down in the dumps that nothing could cheer you up?	☐1	☐2	☐3	☐4	☐5	☐6
d Have you felt calm and peacefull?	☐1	☐2	☐3	☐4	☐5	☐6
e Did you have a lot of energy?	☐1	☐2	☐3	☐4	☐5	☐6
f Have you felt downhearted and blue?	☐1	☐2	☐3	☐4	☐5	☐6
g Did you feel worn out?	☐1	☐2	☐3	☐4	☐5	☐6
h Have you been a happy person?	☐1	☐2	☐3	☐4	☐5	☐6
i Did you feel tired?	☐1	☐2	☐3	☐4	☐5	☐6

Figure 5.4. Excerpt from the SF-36 questionnaire: Item 9 (from SF-36 Health Survey Scoring Demonstration; http://www.sf-36.org/demos/SF-36.html)

age x, usually denoted by $q(x)$. It turns out that once the $q(x)$'s are all known, the life table is completely determined. In practice such "cohort life tables" are rarely used, in part because individuals would have to be followed for up to 100 years, and the resulting life table would reflect historical conditions that may no longer have relevance. Instead, one generally works with a period, or current, life table. This summarises the mortality experience of persons of all ages in a short period, typically one year or three years. More precisely, the death probabilities $q(x)$ for every age x are computed for that short period, often using census information gathered at regular intervals (for example, every ten years in the U.S.). These $q(x)$'s are then applied to a hypothetical cohort of 100,000 people over their life span to create a current life table (Strauss and Shavelle 2000).

Several approaches have been developed to adjust life expectancy for aspects of health-related quality of life (Drummond et al. 1997). Most often used are the concepts of quality-adjusted life years (QALY) on the one hand and the concept of disability-adjusted life years (DALY) on the other hand (cf. Chap. I.3 of this handbook).

A quality-adjusted life year is a measure that assigns a (utility) value, often called Q, between 0 and 1 to each health state of a year with 0 representing death and 1 representing perfect health. The Q factors are then multiplied with the time spent in the corresponding health states and these weighted times finally are summed up to achieve the QALY.

Three methods are used alternatively to establish a set of consistent Q values, all derived from consumer choice theory, which describes how consumers decide what to buy on the basis of two fundamental elements: their budget constraints and their preferences. Consumer preferences for different consumables are often represented by the concept of "utility" (Torrance et al. 1972, 1987; Mankiv 1998). The techniques proposed to measure the utility of specific health states on a linear scale were the von Neumann-Morgenstern "standard gamble", the "time trade-off" method, and direct scaling techniques (e.g. category rating). These were claimed to produce equivalent and reliable results, but the time trade-off is easier to administer than each of the other two techniques (O'Connor 1993). The results of a simultaneous test of all three methods were that subjects found the time trade-off task the easiest, the standard gamble slightly more difficult (but probably impossible without some props), and the direct scaling task the most difficult. Only the time trade-off task was considered to be capable of being executed without a well trained interviewer (Torrance 1976; O'Connor 1993). Nevertheless direct scaling methods are commonly used to derive preferences (Petitti 1998a), probably without observing the necessary methodological diligence.

In a standard gamble the rater (i.e. the person to establish the utilities) must choose between two alternatives. One alternative has a certain outcome (that is the health state to be rated) and the other involves a gamble with two possible outcomes: the best health state (usually complete health), which is described as occurring with a probability, p, or an alternative state, the worst state (usually death) which is described as occurring with probability $1 - p$. The probability p is varied until the rater is indifferent to the alternative which is certain and the gamble that may bring the better health state. The time trade-off task also entails a choice between two alternatives, but neither is a gamble. Each is a different health state, but for differing periods of time. The rater is asked to value a choice of being in a less desirable health state for a longer time followed by death compared with being in a more desirable state for shorter period of time followed by death. The time in the less desirable health state then is decreased to the point of indifference. In category rating, raters sort the health states into a specified number of categories, and equal changes in preference between adjacent categories are assumed to exist (Petitti 1998a).

QALYs have been widely criticised on ethical, conceptual, operational and methodological grounds. To begin with the last ones: Prieto and Sacristán (2003) have recently pointed to a considerable problem, which results from the numerical nature of its constituent parts. The appropriateness of the QALY arithmetical operation is compromised by the essence of the utility scale: while life-years are expressed in a ratio scale with a true zero, the utility is an interval scale where 0 is an arbitrary value for death. In order to be able to obtain coherent results, both scales would have to be expressed in the same units of measurement. The different nature of these two factors jeopardises the meaning and interpretation of QALYs. By a simple general linear transformation of the utility scale the authors demonstrate that the results of the multiplication are not invariant, and offer a mathematically solution to these limitations through an alternative calculation of QALYs by means of operations with complex numbers, so that the new QALYs have a real part (length of life) and an imaginary part (utility). The revisited formulation of the QALYs provides a less dramatic adjustment of years of life than that implied by the multiplicative model. The maximum penalization represented by living in a sub-optimal state of health is capped at 30% of the total time lived in that state, in contrast to the case of the multiplicative model, where the penalization can reach 100% (Prieto and Sacristán 2003).

Ethical concerns arise when QALYs are used in cost-effectiveness or cost-utility analysis for evaluation of alternative health policies, treatment programmes, or setting of priorities. A simple ratio cost/QALY is commonly calculated in this type of analysis in order to compare cost-effectiveness of treatments, intervention and programmes etc. But is has been pointed out, among other arguments, that investing in the interventions that have the lowest cost per QALY ignores the principle of equity (Drummond 1987). In addition, QALYs share a problem of life-expectancy as a measure of outcome: they discriminate against the aged and the disabled, because these groups of persons have fewer life years to gain from an intervention (Harris 1987).

The main other type of commonly used summary measure which combines information on mortality and morbidity is the disability-adjusted life year. The DALY is the best known example of a "health gap" summary measure, which quantifies the gap between a population's actual health and a defined goal used to quantify the burden of disease in a country, region, or on the global level (Murray and Lopez 1996). However, DALYs share most of the methodological and ethical difficulties with QALYs, such as utility-weighting and discounting health benefits. The discrimination of elderly people is even more pronounced than with QALYs as an additional age-weighting is performed when constructing DALYs, whereby years lost during the productive phase of life get a higher weight than years lost in childhood or at a more advanced age (Gericke and Busse 2003). Related concepts are Disability Free Life Years (Sullivan 1971) and Healthy Life Expectancy (Robine and Ritchie 1991) which may be based on surveys. DALYs can be calculated exclusively based on life tables from census data and cross-sectional data from official disability statistics (if necessary on a sample base). The so-called Sullivan method to adjust the conventional life table for disability consists of applying disability rates calculated from cross-sectional data to the person-years of the conventional life table. This calculation results into new estimates of the person-years lived in disability, and the complement of the later, the person-years lived free of disability, the DALYs (Guend et al. 2002).

A related measure is disability-adjusted life expectancy (DALE) used by WHO in a controversial report to display the burden of disease by cause, sex and mortality stratum in WHO regions (WHO 2000). The disability rates used in the WHO calculations relied on subjective and expert assessment and not on empirical data, due to data limitations in many nations.

Patient Satisfaction

Interest in measuring satisfaction with healthcare has grown considerably in recent years around the world and there is a large and expanding literature in this field. Patient satisfaction and its measurement are undoubtedly important issues for public policy analysts, healthcare managers, practitioners, and users. Nevertheless measurement of satisfaction often lacks a clear definition. In particular, it is not always well understood by the people who measure it that satisfaction is a relative concept which can be measured only against individuals' expectations, needs or desires (Wüthrich-Schneider 2000; Crow et al. 2003). Despite problems with establishing a tangible definition of "satisfaction" and difficulties with its measurement (among other things those which are predicted by the well-known theory of cognitive dissonance, cf. Festinger 1957) the concept continues to be widely used. However, in many instances when investigators claim to be measuring satisfaction, more general evaluations of healthcare services are being undertaken that tend to result in high levels of satisfaction being recorded (Crow et al. 2003).

Historically patient satisfaction surveys have focused on inpatient health care services but in recent years investigations of patient satisfaction have been carried out in outpatient settings as well. In Germany, for example, a recently developed questionnaire to measure patient satisfaction in generalist and specialist ambulatory medical care comprises 27 single items divided into the four dimensions: "professional competence", "physician-patient interaction", "information", and "organisation of the practice". This concept has been tested in a survey of 3487 patients in 123 physician practices (Gericke et al. 2004). A former international study of patients' priorities with respect to general practice care collected data by postal surveys in UK, Norway, Sweden, Denmark, the Netherlands, Germany, Portugal and Israel. The study results show that patients in different cultures and health care systems have many views in common, particularly concerning doctor-patient communication and accessibility of services (Grol et al. 1999).

Assessing Efficiency of Care   5.6.2

In addition to measuring the output of health care in terms of healthy life gained, efficiency is another important dimension in assessing health services output. Unfortunately, the word efficiency is often used inappropriately to describe productivity, i.e. relating episodes of care or number of procedures to the inputs or costs (Gray 1997). Efficiency refers to the health system's ability to use whatever resources it has to maximum effect (Le Grand 1998). Efficiency has three levels: technical, productive and allocative efficiency. Technical efficiency answers the narrow question of whether the same or a better outcome could be obtained by using less of one type of input (Palmer and Torgerson 1999). It is based on effectiveness. Productive or internal efficiency is achieved when the maximum possible improvement in outcome is obtained from a given level of resource inputs or when costs are minimised to obtain a given level of output (Donaldson and Gerard 1993; Palmer and Torgerson 1999). Prerequisite for productive efficiency is technical efficiency.

Allocative or external efficiency refers to the way resources are divided between alternative uses within the health sector (Barr 1998). It implies productive efficiency (Donaldson and Gerard 1993). The theoretical foundation of allocative efficiency rests on the Pareto criterion: a resource allocation is efficient if it is impossible to move to an alternative allocation which would make some people better off and nobody worse off (Begg et al. 1997b). Among other conceptual difficulties, strict adherence to this principle would preclude changes that would make many people much better off at the expense of a few made slightly worse off (Palmer and Torgerson 1999). Therefore, an operational utilitarian decision rule is often used instead: allocative efficiency is achieved when resource allocation maximises social welfare (Palmer and Torgerson 1999). Cost-effectiveness studies as a tool to put the concept of operational efficiency in health care into practice have already been summarised in Sect. 5.4.1. Cost-benefit studies can address questions of allocative efficiency comparing interventions between different sectors, as output of care is measured in monetary units. As this is politically and ethically difficult to accept for many non-economists, cost-benefit analyses of health interventions are seldom performed.

5.6.3   Assessing the Outcome of Health Systems

In principle the same methods are used to assess the outcome of health systems which are used to assess the outcome of health services within a country. However, problems with data quality, definitions and comparability across different cultures make comparisons between different health systems more difficult than health services research limited to a particular country (Schwartz and Busse 2003). As decision-makers in countries of all levels of development are faced with common problems as they struggle to make appropriate choices to improve the performance of their health systems, the interest of politicians and scientists in comparative health systems research has grown rapidly during the last two decades. A common goal of researchers is to provide policy decision-makers and managers with the best available evidence in order to inform policy decision making. In analogy to evidence-based medicine this movement has been termed evidence-based health policy or evidence-based health care (Gray 1997). However, the evidence-base on how to improve the performance of health systems is still weak (Murray and Evans 2003).

Cross-sectional Comparisons

Two methodological approaches are commonly used in comparative health systems research. A cross-sectional approach comparing a number of parameters at a particular point in time, and a longitudinal approach comparing the development of parameters over a defined time period. To illustrate the advantages and disadvantages of both approaches we will focus here on two examples. The first is a summary of the approach taken by the World Health Organization (WHO) to assess health systems performance on a global scale. In 1998 WHO embarked on a project to assess the health system performance of its member states, culminating in the World Health Report 2000, in which countries' health systems were ranked according to their performance. Health system performance was measured according to the level and distribution of population health, responsiveness, and fairness in financing (World Health Organization 2000; Murray and Evans 2003). Although the provision of comparative data on health system characteristics is recognised as important in improving health care systems, the report has elicited heavy criticism, summarised by Gravelle et al. (2003). These included the purpose of the exercise (Williams 2001), the definition of some of the performance measures (Braveman et al. 2001), the quality of data (McKee 2001; Williams 2001), and mixed messages (Navarro 2000). Gravelle et al. (2003) furthermore demonstrated that the efficiency rankings and estimates of the magnitude of inefficiency in countries were not robust when compared with other, no less reasonable, methodological choices concerning the econometric methods used. The final rankings for a number of EU countries and ranking results concerning patient satisfaction with health systems are illustrated in Table 5.5, and compared to a number of other parameters which are commonly used to measure the input, process, and outcome of a health system.

It can be noted that parameters differ widely between countries at a similar level of national income and development. Some factors show a close correlation, e.g. the health score with patient satisfaction or hospital bed provision with hospital utilisation. On the other hand, satisfaction with the health system does not correlate at all with the overall WHO ranking of the health system performance. This results in contradictory results for countries like Denmark and Finland on the one hand, and Spain on the other (Schwartz and Busse 2003). Table 5.5 illustrates some of the issues surrounding the interpretation of cross-sectional data. Different data sources can vary substantially on the same measure. Such discrepancies – if detected at all – demand a thorough investigation of possible causes. A common cause are differences in the numerator, e.g. differences between licensed and practising doctors or beds in acute care hospitals or in all hospitals. Differences in the denominator are also important. For instance for the measurement of neonatal mortality it makes a difference whether all births on the territory of a country are counted or all births of nationals of that country (Schwartz and Busse 2003).

The most important difficulty with cross-sectional comparisons of health systems from a policy perspective is probably that health output measured in terms of reduced mortality and health systems performance are correlated in a contradictory way. If a country reacts in an appropriate way to high mortality rates and invests in health system infrastructure, mortality would fall as a result assuming effectiveness of the measures taken. This longitudinal result cannot be measured in cross-sectional studies. Therefore cross-sectional comparisons cannot indicate whether a high level of inputs in a particular country has obviated even higher mortality rates and we only see average mortality in this country or whether there truly exists an inefficient input–output relation.

Longitudinal Comparisons

The other approach consists in comparing the development of input, process and output parameters in different health systems in a longitudinal perspective. The

Table 5.5. Selected input, process and outcome parameters for some European countries, around 1997. Data from the OECD Health Dataset 2001, the WHO Health for All database 2003, and the World Health Report 2000 (World Health Organization 2000). Adapted from Schwartz and Busse (2003)

	Financial input: % of GDP (1998)	Structure: Hospital beds/1000 population (1997)	Structure: Doctors/ 1000 population (1997)	Process: Hospital cases/100 pop./year (1996)	Process: Hospital days/ capita (1996)	Process: ambulatory doctor-patient contacts/year (1996)	Outcome: Neonatal mortality/ 1000 (1998)	Outcome: Satisfaction with health system in % [Ranking within EU] (1998)	Outcome: Overall ranking of health system within EU (1999)
Austria	8.0	9.1	2.9	25.1	2.6	6.3	4.9	72.7 [3]	4
Belgium	8.6	7.3	3.7	20.0	2.2	8.0	5.6	62.8 [7]	11
Denmark	8.3	4.6	3.3	19.8	1.4	5.7 (6.6)*	4.7	90.6 [1]	15
Finland	6.9	7.9	3.0	26.9	3.2	4.3	4.1	81.3 [2]	14
France	9.4	8.6	3.0	22.5	2.6	6.5	4.6	65.0 [6]	1
Germany	10.3	9.4	3.4	19.7	2.8	6.5	4.7	57.5 [9]	13
Greece	8.4	5.0	4.1	–	1.2	–	5.7 (6.7)*	15.5 [15]	6
Ireland	6.8	–	2.1	15.1	1.1	–	6.2	57.9 [8]	10
Italy	8.2	5.8	5.8	18.5	1.7	–	5.3	20.1 [13]	2
Luxembourg	6.0	8.1	3.0 (2.4)*	–	2.8	2.9	5.0	66.6 [5]	7
Netherlands	8.7	11.3 (5.3)*	–	11.1	3.6	5.4	5.0	69.8 [4]	8
Portugal	7.7	4.1	3.1	11.4	1.1	3.2	5.9	16.4 [14]	5
Spain	7.0	–	2.9	11.4 (10.0)*	1.1	–	5.7 (4.9)*	43.1 [12]	3
Sweden	7.9	4.0 (5.2)*	3.1	18.1	1.3	2.9	3.5	57.5 [9]	12
United Kingdom	6.8	4.4	1.7	15.0 (23.1)*	1.3	6.1	5.7	57.0 [11]	9

* More than 10 per cent difference between OECD and WHO datasets.

1980s time series analyses on "avoidable mortality" marked the first attempts at international longitudinal comparisons (Bunker et al. 1994; Charlton and Velez 1986). A common measure for comparing health systems in a longitudinal way is life expectancy. In Fig. 5.5, the development of life expectancy at birth is depicted for a number of selected European countries compared to the EU average for the time period 1970 to 2000.

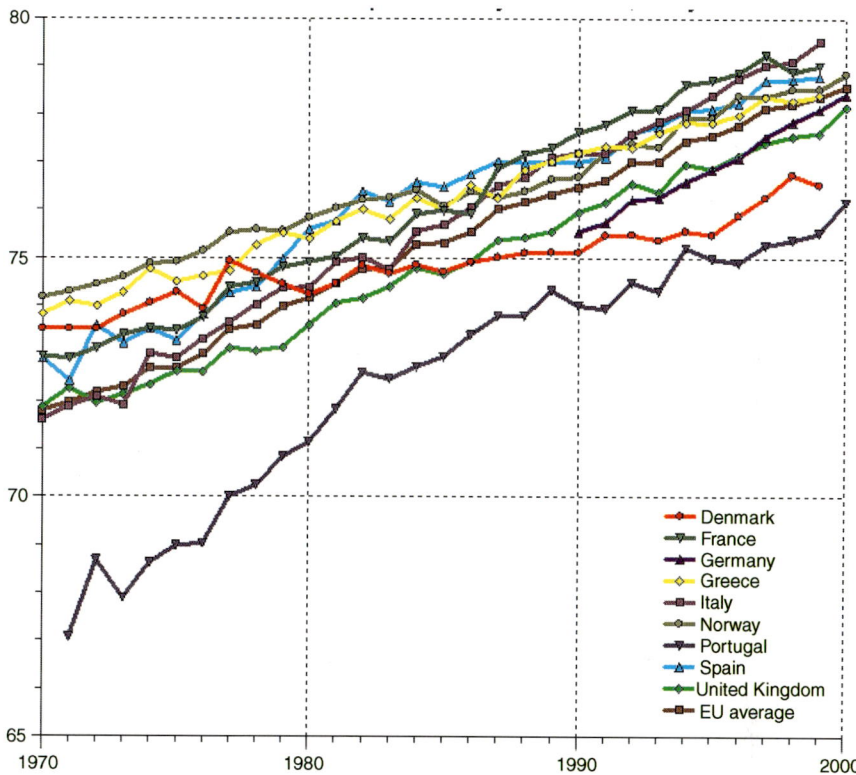

Figure 5.5. Life expectancy at birth in selected member countries of the European Union 1970 to 2000. Calculated with data from WHO Health for All Database 2003

This is often done although it is well known that life expectancy is influenced by many variables outside the scope of the health system, such as the level of socio-economic development. However, in general, mortality (on which the calculation of life expectancy is based) is an output measure which is relatively insensitive to common health services endeavours (Schwartz and Busse 2003):

— The overwhelming part of mortality is not amenable to health services activity ("avoidable mortality") but natural mortality.

— In particular for men a substantial proportion of deaths is due to traffic accidents.

— The commonplace argument that mortality figures do not respond quickly to changes had to be revised after the experience in Russia after the breakdown of the Soviet Union, where life expectancy at birth for males fell by approximately 6 years between 1990 and 1994. On the other hand, life expectancy in the Eastern part of Germany increased substantially in the 1990s.

Relative changes over time are of particular importance for evaluation and policy decision-making. This is illustrated in the development of life expectancy at birth in Denmark and Portugal. Whereas both countries had an average life expectancy at birth of 76 years in the year 2000, Portugal has massively improved on this measure since 1970, up from 67 years. Although life expectancy in Denmark has nominally also increased since 1970, up from 74 years, it has had the smallest relative increase in Western Europe – which is in fact a rather negative development and not an improvement.

5.7   Conclusions

As demonstrated in the examples discussed above, the combination of simple inputs and outputs can be of particular political importance, despite all the methodological difficulties and caveats. The fact, that even if life expectancy were a good indicator of health production in the health care system, the question of why a good result has occurred, i.e. examining structure and process, would not have been answered. There is little consensus on how international comparisons of structures and processes should be performed. How inappropriate simplification of health system comparisons can be misleading is demonstrated by the "state versus free market" debate in Germany. Financing of German hospital care on the basis of per diem payments has been coined as inefficient, as this payment mechanisms creates an incentive for longer hospital stays. Some economists have compared the German system with the US system, where hospital stays are usually shorter, claiming that this was due to payments according to diagnostic-related groups (DRGs). However, they did not consider that at that time only hospital services for 15% of the population covered under the Medicare scheme were remunerated according to DRGs and that hospital costs per case in the USA were about twice as high as in Germany, "despite" the DRGs. Likewise, the expected rise in ambulatory care costs to compensate for early hospital discharge was not considered (Schwartz and Busse 2003). International comparisons of health system outcomes along one-dimensional hypotheses have thus to be treated with great caution, in particular because they are easily misunderstood by policy decision-makers (Schwartz and Busse 2003).

References

Abraham S (1986) Analysis of data from a complex sample: the Health Examination Surveys. Am J Clin Nutr 43:839–843

ACRA (1999) A brief history of resource allocation in the NHS, 1948–98. Advisory Committee on Resource Allocation, Department of Health, London

Aday LA, Begley CE, Lairson DR, Slater CH (1998) Evaluating the healthcare system. Effectiveness, efficiency, and equity. Health Administration Press, Chicago

Adler GS (1994) A profile of the Medicare Current Beneficiary Survey. Health Care Financing Review 15(4):153–163

American Child Health Association (1934) Physical defects: the pathway to correction. ACHA, New York

American Medical Association (AMA) (2000) Board of Trustees Report 31-I-00, American Medical Association, House of Delegates, Chicago

Armenian HK (1998) Case-control methods. In: Amenian HK, Shapiro S (eds) Epidemiology and health services. Oxford University Press, New York, Oxford, pp 135–155

Ash A, Porell F, Gruenberg L Sawitz E, Beiser A (1989) Adjusting Medicare capitation payments using prior hospitalization data. Health Care Financ Rev 10(4):17–29

Asthana S, Gibson A, Moon G, Dicker J, Brigham P (2004) The pursuit of equity in NHS resource allocation: should morbidity replace utilisation as the basis for setting health care capitations? Soc Sci Med 58:539–551

Australian Institute of Health and Welfare (ed) (1998) National health data dictionary, Version 7.0. Australian Institute of Health and Welfare, Canberra

Barber J (2003) Hospital quality reports, May 30 (http://www.hcncc.org/doc/Hospital%20Qual%20Ratings.pdf) Accessed May 28, 2004

Barr N (1998) The economics of the welfare state. Oxford University Press, Oxford

Basel Committee on Banking Supervision (2003) Consultative document – overview of the new Basel capital accord. Bank for international settlements, Basel

Begg D, Fischer S, Dornbusch R (1997a) Demand, supply, and the market. In: Economics. McGraw Hill, London, pp 30–43

Begg D, Fischer S, Dornbusch R (1997b) Introduction to welfare economics. In: Economics. McGraw Hill, London, pp 240–259

Bellach B-M, Knopf H, Thefeld W (1998) Der Bundesgesundheitssurvey 1997/98. Gesundheitswesen 60 (Suppl 2):59–68

Bennett AC (1978) Improving management performance in health care institutions. American Hospital Association, Chicago

Bergmann F, Kamtsiuris F (1999) Inanspruchnahme medizinischer Leistungen. Gesundheitswesen 61 (Spec Issue):138–144

Bergner M, Bobbitt RA, Carter WB Gilson BS (1981) The sickness impact profile: development and final revision of a health status measure. Med Care 19:787–805

Berrington de Gonzales A, Darby S (1994). Risk of cancer from diagnostic X-rays: estimates for the UK and 14 other countries. Lancet 363:345–351

Black N (1997) Health services research: saviour or chimera? Lancet 349:1834–1836

Black N, Langham S, Petticrew M (1995) Coronary revascularisation: why do rates vary geographically in the UK? J Epidemiol Community Health 49:408–412

Blumenthal D (1996) Quality of care: what is it? N Engl J Med 335:891–894

Brand DA, Newcomer LN, Freiburger A, Tian H (1995) Cardiologists' practices compared with practice guidelines: use of beta-blockade after acute myocardial infarction. J Am Coll Cardiol 26:1432–1436

Braveman P, Starfield B, Geiger HJ (2001) World Health Report 2000: how it removes equity from the agenda for public health monitoring and policy. BMJ 323:678–681

British Medical Association (2000) Clinical indicators (League tables) – a discussion paper. British Medical Association, London

Brook RH, Lohr KN (1985) Efficacy, effectiveness, variations, and quality. Boundary-crossing research. Med Care 23:710–722

Brook RH, McGlynn EA, Cleary PD (1996) Quality of health care. Part 2: Measuring quality of care. N Engl J Med 335:966–970

Brook RH, Park RE, Chassin MR, Solomon DH, Keesey J, Kosecoff J (1990) Predicting the appropriate use of carotid endarterectomy, upper gastrointestinal endoscopy, and coronary angiography. N Engl J Med 323:1173–1177

Brook RH, Ware JE, Jr, Rogers WH, Keeler EB, Davies AR, Donald CA, Goldberg GA, Lohr KN, Masthay PC, Newhouse JP (1983) Does free care improve adults' health? Results from a randomized controlled trial. N Engl J Med 309:1426–1434

Brooks R (1996) EuroQol: the current state of play. Health Policy 37:53–72

Brückner G (1997) Developing a new system of health care statistics. A major challenge for all participants? Federal Statistical Office, Wiesbaden

Buchner F, Wasem J (2003) Needs for further improvement: Risk adjustment in the German health insurance system. Health Policy 65:21–35

Bunker JP, Frazier HS, Mosteller F (1994) Improving health: measuring effects of medical care. Milbank Q 72:225–258

Buring JE, Hennekens CH (1992) The women's health study: summary of the study design. J Mycardial Ischemia 4:27–29

Busse R (1995) Radiologie, Gesundheitsstrukturreform und Gesundheitssystemforschung – Stand, Entwicklungen und Herausforderungen. Akt Radiologie 5:127–130

Busse R, Wismar M (2002) Health target programmes and health care services – any link? A conceptual and comparative study (part 1). Health Policy 59:209–221

Cameron AC, Trivedi PK (1998) Regression analysis of count data. Cambridge University Press, Cambridge New York Melbourne

Campell DT, Stanley JC (1966) Experimental and quasi-experimental designs for research. Rand McNally & Co, Chicago

Carr-Hill R (1989) Allocating resources to health care: RAWP (Resources Allocation Working Party) is dead-long live RAWP. Health Policy 13:135

Carr-Hill R, Hardman G, Martin S, Peacock S, Sheldon T, Smith P (1994) A formula for distributing NHS revenues based on small area use of hospital beds. University of York: Centre of Health Economics. Joint Health Surveys Unit, University College London, London

Carr-Hill R, Sheldon T, Smith P, Martin, S, Peacock S, Hardman G (1994) Allocating resources to health authorities:development of method for small area analysis of use of inpatient services. BMJ 309:1046%

Charlton JR, Velez R (1986) Some international comparisons of mortality amenable to medical intervention. BMJ 292:295–301

Childs AW, Hunter ED (1972) Non-medical factors influencing use of diagnostic X-ray by physicians. Med Care 10:323–335

Cochran WG (1968) Sampling techniques. John Wiley, New York

Cohen SB (1997) Sample design of the 1996 Medical Expenditure Panel Survey Household Component. Meps Methodol Rep No 2. AHCPR Pub. No 97–0027, Rockville

Crow R, Gage H, Hampson S, Hart J, Kimber A, Storey L (2002) The measurement of satisfaction with healthcare: implications for practice from a systematic review of the literature. Health Technology Assessment 2002, vol 6, no 32

Culyer A (1993) Health, health expenditures, and equity. In: VanDoorslaer E (ed) Equity in the finance and delivery of health care. Oxford University Press, Oxford

de Miguel JM(1971) A framework for the study of national health systems. Inquiry 12:10–24

Detsky AS, Naglie IG (1990) A clinician's guide to cost-effectiveness analysis. Ann Intern Med 113:147–154

Deutsche Röntgengesellschaft (2002) Pressemitteilung anlässlich des 83. Deutschen Röntgenkongresses vom 8.–11. Mai 2002 in Wiesbaden (http://www.drg.de/data/wichtige_infos/PMRoekon2002.htm) Accessed May 19, 2004

Diehr P, Yanez D, Ash A, Hornbrook M, Lin DY (1999) Methods for analyzing health care utilization and costs. Ann Rev Public Health 20:125–144

Donabedian A (1980) Explorations in quality assessment and monitoring. Health Administration Press, Ann Arbor, MI

Donabedian A (1985) The methods and findings of quality assessment and monitoring. Health Administration Press, Ann Arbor, Ml

Donabedian A (1988) The quality of care: how can it be assessed? JAMA 260:1743–1748

Donaldson C, Gerard K (1993) Economics of health care financing. The visible hand. Macmillan, London

Doubilet P, Weinstein MC, McNeil JB (1986) Use and misuse of the term 'cost-effectiveness' in medicine. N Engl J Med 314:253–256

Dr Foster (ed) (2004a) Hospital guide – methodology. (http://www.drfoster.com/ghg/objectlist.aspx?w=9&p=320) Accessed May 31, 2004

Dr Foster (ed) (2004b) consultant guide – methodology. (http://www.drfoster.com/consultant/methodology.asp) Accessed May 31, 2004

Drummond MF (1987) Ressource allocation decisions in health care. A role for quality of life assessments? J Chron Dis 40:605–616

Drummond MF, O'Brien B, Stoddart GL, Torrance GW (1997) Methods for the economic evaluation of health care programmes, 2nd edn. Oxford University Press, Oxford

Dunn DL, Rosenblatt A, Taira DA, Lattimer E, Bertko J, Stoiber T (1996) A comparative analysis of methods of health risk assessment. Society of Actuaries, Schaumburg, IL

Elinson J (1987) Advances in health assessment discussion panel. J Chronic Dis 40 (Suppl 1):83S–91S

Ellis R, Pope G, Iezzoni L, Ayanian J, Bates D, Burstin H, Ash A (1996) Diagnosis-based risk adjustment for Medicare capitation payments. Health Care Financing Review 17(3):101–128

Ellwood PM (1988) Outcomes management: a technology of patient experience. N Engl J Med 318:1549–1556

Epstein RS, Sherwood LM (1996) From outcomes research to disease management. A guide for the perplexed. Ann Intern Med 124:832–837

Etchason J, Petz L, Keeler E, Calhoun L, Kleinman S, Snider C, Fink A, Brook R (1995) The cost effectiveness of preoperative autologous blood donations. N Engl J Med 332:719–724

European Commission (2000) Eucomp – towards comparable health care data in the European Union. Statist Netherlands, Voorburg/Herlen

European Observatory on Health Systems and Policies (2004) Health care systems in transition – HiTs (http://www.euro.who.int/observatory/Hits/TopPage) Accessed May 28, 2004

EuroQol Group (1990) EuroQol – a new facility for the measurement of health-related quality of life. Health Policy 16:199–208 (http://www.euroqol.org/index.htm) Accessed May 31, 2004

Fein R (1971) On measuring economic benefits of health programs. In: McLachlan G, McKeown T (eds) Medical history and medical care. Oxford University Press, London

Ferris G, Roderick P, Smithies A, George S, Gabbay J, Couper N, Chant A (1998). An epidemiological needs assessment of carotid endarterectomy in an English health region. Is the need being met? BMJ 317:447–451

Festinger L (1957) A theory of cognitive dissonance. Stanford University Press, Stanford, CA

Fowler FJ, Jr, Barry MJ, Lu-Yao G, Roman A, Wasson J, Wennberg JE (1993) Patient-reported complications and follow-up treatment after radical prostatectomy. The national Medicare experience: 1988–1990 (updated June 1993). Urology 42:622–629

Freedman MA in collaboration with the CDC Health Status Indicators Consensus Work Group (1991) Health status indicators for the year 2000. National Center for Health Statistics vol 1, no 1

Garratt AM, Ruta DA, Abdalla MI, Buckingham JK, Russell IT (1993) The SF36 health survey questionnaire: an outcome measure suitable for routine use within the NHS? BMJ 306:1440–1444

Gericke C, Busse R (2003) Gesundheitsökonomische Aspekte der Pharmakothera-
pie älterer Menschen. Arzneimittelforschung Drug Research 53:918–921.

Gericke CA, Schiffhorst G, Busse R, Häussler B (2004) Messung der Patientenzufriedenheit in ambulanter haus- und fachärztlicher Behandlung
mit dem QUALISKOPE-A. Diskussionspapier 2004/10, Technische Universität Berlin, Fakultät Wirtschaft und Management, Berlin (http://www.ww.tu-
berlin.de/diskussionspapiere/2004/dpa10–2004.pdf) Accessed May 31, 2004

Gillings D, Makuc D, Siegel W (1981) Analysis of interrupted time series mortality
trends; an example to evaluate regionalized perinatal care. Am J Public Health
71:38–46

Gold MR, Siegel JE, Rusek KB, Weinstein MC (1996) Cost-effectiveness in health
and medicine. Oxford University Press, New York

Gravelle H, Jacobs R, Jones AM, Street A (2003) Comparing the efficiency of national
health systems: a sensitivity analysis of the WHO approach. Appl Health Econ
Health Policy 2:141–147

Gray JAM (1997) Assessing the outcomes found. In: Evidence-based healthcare.
Churchill Livingstone, New York, pp 103–154

Greene WH (2003) Econometric Analysis, 5th edn. Prentice and Hall, Upper Saddle
River, New Jersey

Grimshaw JM, Wilson B, Campbell M, Eccles M, Ramsay C (2001) Epidemiological
methods. In: Fulop N, Allen P, Clarke A, Black N (eds) Studying the organisation
and delivery of health services. Research methods. Routledge, London, pp 56–72

Grol R, Wensing M, Mainz J, Ferreira P, Hearnshaw H, Hjortdahl P, Olesen F,
Ribacke M, Spenser T, Szecsenyi J (1999) Patients' priorities with respect to
general practice care: an international comparison. Fam Pract 16:4–11

Guend H, Stone-Newsom R, Swallen K, Lasker A, Kindig D (2002) State disability adjusted life expectancy using census disability. University of Wisconsin,
Madison

Guyatt GH, Naylor CD, Juniper E, Heyland DK, Jaeschke R, Cook RD for the Evidence Based Medicine Working Group (1995) How to use articles about health-
related quality of life measurements. Centre for Health Evidence, Edmonton
(http://www.cche.net/usersguides/life.asp) Accessed on May 28, 2004

Hannan EL, O'Donnell JF, Kilburn H, Jr, Bernard HR, Yazici A (1989) Investigation of the relationship between volume and mortality for surgical procedures
performed in New York State hospitals. JAMA 262:503–510

Hansen MH, Hurwitz WN, Madow WG (1953) Sample survey methods and theory,
vol I and vol II. Wiley publication, New York, London

Harris J (1987) QUALYfying the value of life. J Med Ethics 13:117–123

Herrin J, Etchason JA, Kahan JP, Brook RH, Ballard DJ (1997) Effect of panel composition on physician ratings of appropriateness of abdominal aortic aneurysm
surgery: elucidating differences between multispecialty panel results and specialty society recommendations. Health Policy 42:67–81

Hill AB (1965) The environment and disease: Association or causation? Proc R Soc
Med 58:295–300

Hofer TP, Hayward RA, Greenfield S, Wagner EH, Kaplan SH, Manning WG (1999) The unreliability of individual physician "report cards" for assessing the costs and quality of care of a chronic disease. JAMA 281:2098–2105

Iezzoni LI (1994) Risk and outcome. In: Iezzoni LI (ed) Risk adjustment for measuring healthcare outcomes. Health Administration Press, Ann Arbor, Michigan, pp 1–28

Ingber MJ (1998) The current state of risk adjustment technology for capitation. Journal Ambulatory Care Management 21(4):1–28

Ingber MJ (2000) Implementation of risk adjustment for Medicare. Health Care Financing Review 21(3):119–126

Institut für Medizinmanagement und Gesundheitswesen der Universität Bayreuth (2004) Krankenhausrating (http://www.krankenhausrating.de/) Accessed May 28, 2004

Institute of Medicine (1994) Health services research: Opportunities for an expanding field of inquiry – An interim statement. National Academies Press, Washington, DC

Jacobson B, Mindell J, McKee M (2003) Hospital mortality league tables. BMJ 326:777–778

Jencks SF, Williams DK, Kay TL (1988) Assessing hospital-associated deaths from discharge data. The role of length of stay and comorbidities. JAMA 260:2240–2246

Kahn HA, Sempos CT (1989) Statistical methods in epidemiology. Oxford University Press, New York, Oxford

Kaplan RM, Anderson JP (1988) A general health policy model: update and applications. Health Serv Res 23:203–205

Keeler EB, Kahn KL, Draper D, Sherwood MJ, Rubenstein LV, Reinisch EJ, Kosecoff J, Brook (1990) Changes in sickness at admission following the introduction of the prospective payment system. JAMA 264:1962–1968

Kelsey JL, Petitti DB, King AC (1998) Key methodologic concepts and issues. In: Brownson RC, Petitti DB (eds) Applied epidemiology. Oxford University Press, New York, Oxford, pp 35–69

Kendall MG, Stuart A (1958) Advanced theory of statistics, vol 1. Charles Griffin and Co., London

Kindig DA (1997) Different populations, different needs? In: Purchasing population health. Paying for results. The University of Michigan Press, Ann Arbor, pp 133–148

Kish L (1965) Survey sampling. John Wiley and Sons, New York

Kitagawa EM, Hauser PM (1973) Differential mortality in the United States – a study in socioeconomic epidemiology. Harvard University Press, Cambridge

Kjerulff KH, Erickson BA, Langenberg PW (1996) Chronic gynecological conditions reported by U.S. women: finding from the National Health Interview Survey 1984 to 1992. Am J Public Health 86:195–199

Kohn R, White KL (eds) (1976) Health care – an international study. Oxford University Press, Oxford New York Toronto

Krishnaiah PR, Rao CR (eds) (1994) Handbook of statistics 6 – Sampling, 2nd edn. Elsevier Science Publishers, Amsterdam

Kronick R, Dreyfus T, Lee L, Zhou Z (1996) Diagnostic risk adjustment for Medicaid: The disability payment aystem. Health Care Financing Review 17(3): 7–33

Kronick R, Gilmer T, Dreyfus T, Ganiats T (2002) CDPS-Medicare: The chronic illness and disability payment system modified to predict expenditures for Medicare beneficiaries. Final peport to CMS. University of California, San Diego

Kurth B-M, Bermann KE, Dippelhofer A, Hölling A, Kamtsiuris P, Thefeld W (2002) Die Gesundheit von Kindern und Jugendlichen in Deutschland. Bundesgesundheitsblatt-Gesundheitsforschung-Gesundheitsschutz 11:852–858

Lamers LM (1999) Pharmacy costs groups: A risk-adjuster for capitation payments based on the use of prescribed drugs. Medical Care 37(8):824–830

Last JM (2001) A dictionary of epidemiology, 4th edn. Oxford University Press, Oxford

Le Grand J (1998) Financing health care. In: Feachem Z, Hensher M, Rose L (eds) Implementing halth sector reform in Central Asia. World Bank, Washington, DC, pp 75–85

Leape LL (1994) Error in medicine. JAMA 272:1851–1857

Levy PS, Lemesshow S (1991) Sampling of populations: methods and applications. John Wiley, New York

Liang KY, Zeger SL (1986) Longitudinal data analysis using generalized linear models. Biometrika 73:13–22

Lipid Research Clinics Program (1984) The lipid researchs clinics coronary primary prevention trial results I. Reduction in incidence of coronary heart disease. JAMA 251:351–364

Lohr KN, Yordi KD, Their SO (1988) Current issues in quality of care. Health Affairs 7:5–18

Luft HS, Bunker JP, Enthoven AC (1979) Should operations be regionalized? The empirical relation between surgical volume and mortality. N Engl J Med 301:1364–1369

Mankiw NG (1998) Principles of economics Harcourt. Brace & Co, Boston

Mays N (1995) Geographical resource allocation in the English National Health Service, 1974–1994: The tension between normative and empirical approaches. International Journal of Epidemiology 24:96–102

McCullagh P, Nelder JA (1983) Generalized linear models. Chapman and Hall, London, New York

McDowell I, Newell C (1996) Measuring health. A Guide to rating scales and questionnaires, 2nd edn. Oxford University Press, New York, Oxford

McGlynn EA (1998) The outcomes utility index: will outcomes data tell us what we want to know? Int J Qual Health Care 10:485–490

McKee M (2001) Measuring the efficiency of health systems. The world health report sets the agenda, but there's still a long way to go. BMJ 323:295–296

McPake B, Kumaranayake L, Normand C (2002) The demand for health and health services. In: Health economics. An international perspective. Routledge, London, New York, pp 12–19

Medicare Payment Advisory Commission (1998) Report to the Congress: Context for a changing Medicare program. Medicare Payment Advisory Commission, Washington

Meyer N, Fischer R, Weitkunat R, Crispin A, Schotten K, Bellach B-M, Überla K (2002) Evaluation des Gesundheitsmonitorings in Bayern mit computerassistierten Telefoninterviews (CATI) durch den Vergleich mit dem Bundesgesundheitssurvey 1998 des Robert Koch-Instituts. Gesundheitswesen 64:329–335

Murray CJL, Lopez AD (1996) The Global Burden of Disease. A comprehensive assessment of mortality and disability from diseases, injuries, and risk factors in 1990 and projected to 2020. Harvard University Press, Cambridge, MA

Murray JL, Evans DB (2003) Health systems performance assessment: goals, framework and overview. In: Murray JL, Evans DB (eds) Health systems performance assessment: Debates, methods and empiricism. World Health Organization, Geneva, pp 3–20

Navarro V (2000) Assessment of the World Health Report 2000. Lancet 356:1598–1601

Nelder JA, Wedderburn EWM (1972) Generalized linear models. J R Statist Soc A 135:370–384

Neter J, Wasserman W (1974) Applied linear statistical models. Richard D. Irwin Inc., Homewood IL

Neuhauser D, Lewicki AM (1975) What do we gain from the sixth stool guaiac? N Engl J Med 293:226–228

Newhouse JP (1974) A design for a health insurance experiment. Inquiry 11:5–27

Newhouse JP (1986) Rate adjuster for Medicare under capitation. Health Care Financ Rev (Spec No):45–55

Newhouse JP (1993) Free for all? Lessons from the RAND Health Insurance Experiment. Harvard University Press, Cambridge, MA

Newhouse JP, McClellan M (1998) Econometrics in outcomes research: the use of instrumental variables. Ann Rev Public Health 19:17–34

Newhouse JP, Buntin MB, Chapman JD (1999) Risk adjustment and Medicare. The Commonwealth Fund (http://www.cmwf.org/programs/medfutur/newhouse_riskadj_revised_232.asp) Accessed May 28, 2004

Newhouse JP, Manning WG, Keeler EB, Sloss EM (1989) Adjusting capitation rates using objective health measurers and prior utilization. Health Care Financ Rev 10(3):41–54

Newhouse JP, Manning WG, Morris CN, Orr LL, Duan N, Keeler EB, Leibowitz A, Marquis KH, Marquis MS, Phelps CE, Brook RH (1981) Some interim results from a controlled trial of cost sharing in health insurance. N Engl J Med 305:1501–1507

O'Muircheartaigh C, Burke A, Murphy W (2003) The 2003 Index of Hospital Quality. U.S. News & World Report's, Washington DC

O'Connor R (1993) Issues in the measurement of health-related quality of life. Working Paper 30. NHMRC National Centre for Health Program Evaluation Melbourne, Australia

OECD (1993) System of national accounts. OECD, Paris

OECD (2000) A system of health accounts, Version 1.0. OECD, Paris

Palmer RH (1997) Process-based measures of quality: the need for detailed clinical data in large health care databases. Ann Intern Med 127:733–738

Palmer S, Torgerson DJ (1999) Definitions of efficiency. BMJ 318:1136

Petitti DB (1998a) Epidemiological issues in outcomes research. In: Brownson RC, Petitti DB (eds) Applied epidemiology. Oxford University Press, New York, Oxford, pp 249–275

Petitti DB (1998b) Economic evaluation. In: Brownson RC, Petitti DB (eds) Applied epidemiology. Oxford University Press, New York, Oxford, pp 277–298

Petitti DB, Amster A (1998) Measuring the quality of health care. In: Brownson RC, Petitti DB (eds) Applied epidemiology. Oxford University Press, New York, Oxford pp 299–321

Petitti DB, Sidney S (1989) Hip fracture in women: incidence, in-hospital mortality, and five-year survival probabilities in members of prepaid health plan. Clin Orthopaedics 246:150–155

Phibbs CS, Bronstein JM, Buxton E, Phibbs RH (1996) The effects of patient volume and level of care at the hospital of birth on neonatal mortality. JAMA 276:1054–1059

Pope GC, Ellis RP, Ash AS, Liu C-F, Ayanian JZ, Bates DW, Burstin H, Iezzoni LI, Ingber MJ (2000) Principal inpatient diagnostic cost group model for Medicare risk adjustment. Health Care Financ Rev 21(3):93–118

Prieto L, Sacristán JA (2003) Problems and solutions in calculating quality-adjusted life years (QALYs). Health and Quality of Life Outcomes 1:80 (http://www.hqlo.com/content/1/1/80) Accessed May 28, 2004

Qureshi A (2003) Hospital Quality Committee Report – Selecting optimal attributes for public reporting of hospital quality ratings: key points. Briefs Focus, Special supplement for HASC members, May 30: 1–2 (http://www.hasc.org/resources/download.cfm?ID=333) Accessed May 28, 2004

Rice N, Smith P (1999) Approaches to capitation and risk adjustment in health care: an international survey. ACRA paper 09, Department of Health, London

Rich MW, Shah AS, Vinson JM, Freedland KE, Kuru T, Sperry JC (1996) Iatrogenic congestive heart failure in older adults: clinical course and prognosis. J Am Geriatr Soc 44:638–643

Robine JM, Ritchie K (1991) Healthy life expectancy: Evaluation of global indicator of change in population health. BMJ 302:457–460

Schach S (1989) Stichprobenplan. In: Zentralinstitut für die kassenärztliche Versorgung in der Bundesrepublik Deutschland (ed) Die EvaS-Studie. Eine Erhebung über die ambulante medizinische Versorgung in der Bundesrepublik Deutschland. Deutscher Ärzte-Verlag, Köln, pp 237–245

Schäfer T, Nolde-Gallasch A (1999) Modellversuch zur Beitragsrückzahlung bei den AOKs Lindau und Ostholstein – Bericht der wissenschaftlichen Begleitung. Technical report, University of Applied Science Gelsenkirchen, Bocholt (forthcoming, Federal Association of the AOK, Bonn)

Schneeweiss S, Schöffski O, Selke GW (1998) What is Germany's experience on reference based drug pricing and the etiology of adverse health outcomes or substitutions? Health Policy 44:253–260

Schneeweiss S, Seeger J, Maclure M, Wang P, Avorn, J, Glynn RJ (2001) Performance of comorbidity scores to control for confounding in epidemiologic studies using claims data. Am J Epidemiol 154:854–864

Schneeweiss S, Walker AM, Glynn RJ, Maclure M, Dormuth C, Soumerai SB (2002) Outcomes of reference pricing for angiotensin-converting-enzyme inhibitions. N Engl J Med 346:822–829

Schwartz FW, Busse R (2003) Denken in Zusammenhängen: Gesundheitssystemforschung. In: Schwartz FW, Badura B, Busse R, Leidl R, Raspe H, Siegrist J, Walter U (eds) Public Health. Gesundheit und Gesundheitswesen. Urban & Fischer, München, Jena, pp 518–545

Schwartz FW, Schach E (1989) Summary. In: Zentralinstitut für die kassenärztliche Versorgung in der Bundesrepublik Deutschland (ed): Die EvaS-Studie. Eine Erhebung über die ambulante medizinische Versorgung in der Bundesrepublik Deutschland. Deutscher Ärzte-Verlag, Köln, pp 31–42

Schwarze E-W, Pawlitschko J (2003) Autopsie in Deutschland: Derzeitiger Stand, Gründe für den Rückgang der Obduktionszahlen und deren Folgen. Dtsch Arztebl 100:A2802–2808

Scott I, Campbell D (2002) Health services research: what is it and what does it offer? Intern Med J 32:91–99

Selby JV (1994) Case-control evaluations of treatment and program efficiency. Epidemiol Rev 16:90–101

Selmer RM, Kristiansen IS, Haglerød A, Graff-Iversen S, Larsen HK, Meyer HE, Bønaa KH, Thelle DS (2000) Cost and health consequences of reducing the population intake of salt. J Epidemiol Community Health 54:697–702

SF-36 Health Survey Scoring Demonstration (http://www.sf-36.org/demos/SF-36.html) Accessed May 31, 2004

SF-36 Psychometric Considerations (http://www.sf-36.org/tools/sf36.shtml) Accessed May 31, 2004

Shen Y, Ellis RP (2001) How profitable is risk selection? A comparison of four risk adjustment models. http://econ.bu.edu/Ellis/Papers/shen1.pdf

Shojania KG, Showstack J, Wachter RM (2001) Assessing hospital quality: A review for clinicians. Effective Clinical Practice 4:82–90

Sonnenberg A, Delco F (2002) Cost-effectiveness of a Single Colonoscopy in Screening for Colorectal Cancer. Arch Intern Med 162:163–168

Sörensen HT (2001) Routine registries. In: Olsen J, Saracci R, Trichopoulos D (eds) Teaching epidemiology. Oxford University Press, Oxford New York, pp 99–106

Soumerai SB, Avorn J, Ross-Degnan D, Gortmaker S (1987) Payment restrictions for prescription drugs under Medicaid. N Engl J Med 317:550–556

Soumerai SB, Ross-Degnan D, Avorn J, McLaughlin JT, Choodnovskiy I (1991) Effects of Medicaid drug-payment limits on admission to hospitals and nursing homes. N Engl J Med 325:1072–1077

Spilker B (ed) (1995) Quality of life and pharmacoeconomic clinical trials. Lippincott-Raven, Phildelphia, PA

Statistisches Bundesamt (ed) (2000a) Gesundheitsbericht für Deutschland. Metzler-Poeschel, Stuttgart

Statistisches Bundesamt (ed) (2000b) Konzept einer Ausgaben- und Finanzierungsrechnung für die Gesundheitsberichterstattung des Bundes. Metzler-Poeschel, Stuttgart

Stenger H (1986) Stichproben. Physica Verlag, Heidelberg Wien

Strauss DJ, Shavelle RM (2000) University of California life expectancy project (http://www.lifeexpectancy.com/index.shtml) Accessed May 28, 2004

Stuart A (1968) Basic ideas of scientific sampling. Charles Griffin and Co, London

Sudgen R, Williams A (1990) The principles of practical cost-benefit analysis. Oxford University Press, Oxford

Sukhatme PV, Sukhatme BV (1970) Sampling theory of surveys with applications. Asia Publishing House, London

Sullivan DF (1971) A single index of morbidity and mortality. HSMHA Health Reports 86:347–355

Sutton JH (2001) Physician data profiling proliferates. Bulletin of the American College of Surgeons 86:20–24

Tenney JB, White KL, Williamson JW (1974) National Ambulatory Medical Care Survey: Background and methodology. In: National Center for Health Statistics (ed) Vital and Health Statistics Series 2: Data evaluation and methods research No. 61. U.S. Government Printing Office, Washington DC

Thiemann DR, Coresh J, Oetgen WJ, Powe NR (1999) The association between hospital volume and survival after acute myocardial infarction in elderly patients. N Engl J Med 340:1640–1648

Torrance GW (1976) Social preference for health status. SocioEcon Plan Sci 10:129–136

Torrance GW (1987) Utility approach to measuring health-related quality of life. J Chronic Disease 40:593–600

Torrance GW, Thomas WH, Sackett DL (1972) A utility maximisation model for evaluation of health care programs. Health Serv Res 7:118–133

Townsend (2001) NHS resource allocation review: Targeting poor health (vol I). In: Welsh Assembly's National Steering Group on the Allocation of NHS Resources. National Assembly for Wales, Cardiff

Tseng H-M, Lu J-f R, Gandek B (2003) Cultural issues in using the SF-36 Health Survey in Asia: Results from Taiwan. Health and Quality of Life Outcomes 1:72 (http://www.hqlo.com/content/1/1/72) Accessed May 28, 2004

Tucker MA, Weiner JP, Abrams C (2002) Health-based risk adjustment: Application to premium development and profiling. In: Wrightson C (ed) Financial strategy for managed care organizations: Rate setting, risk adjustment, and competitive advantage. Health Administration Press, Chicago, pp 165–225

Tudor-Hart J (1971) The inverse care law. Lancet 1:405–412

Tudor-Hart J (2000) Commentary: three decades of the inverse care law. BMJ 320:18–19

U.S. Census Bureau (2004) Health insurance coverage: 2002 (http://www.census.gov/hhes/hlthins/hlthin02/hlth02asc.html) Accessed May 28, 2004

Van de Ven WPMM (2001) Risk selection on the sickness fund market. The European Journal of Health Economics 2:91–95

Van de Ven WPMM, Ellis RP (2000) Risk adjustment in competitive health plan markets. In: Culyer AJ, Newhouse JP (eds) Handbook of health economics. Vol. 1A. Elsevier/North Holland, New York, pp 755–845

Van Mossfeld CJPM (2003) International comparison of health care expenditure. Statistics Netherlands, Voorburg/Herlen

Voß W (ed) (2003) Taschenbuch der Statistik, 2nd edn. Carl Hanser Verlag, München, Wien

Ware JE, Sherbourne CD (1992) The MOS 36-item short-form health survey (SF-36). I. Conceptual framework and item selection. Med Care 30:473–483

Weinermann JE (1971) Research on comparative health services systems. Med Care 9:272–290

Weinstein MC, Stason WB (1977) Foundations of cost-effectiveness analysis for health and medical practices. New Engl J Med 296:716–721

Wennberg JE, Freeman JL, Culp WJ (1987) Are hospital services rationed in New Haven or over-utilised in Boston? Lancet 1:1185–1189

Wennberg JE, Freeman JL, Shelton RM, Bubolz TA (1989) Hospital use and mortality among Medicare beneficiaries in Boston and New Haven. N Engl J Med 321:1168–1173

White T, Lavoie S, Nettleman, MD (1999) Potential cost savings attributable to influenza vaccination of school-aged children. Pediatrics 103:73e

Williams A (1974) "Need" as a demand concept (with special reference to health). In: Culyer A (ed) Economic policies and social goals. Martin Robertson, London

Williams A (2001) Science or marketing at WHO? A commentary on 'World Health 2000'. Health Econ 10:93–100

World Health Organization (1947) The constitution of the World Health Organization. WHO Chronicle 1:6–24

World Health Organization (2000) World Health Report 2000. Health systems: Improving performance. WHO, Geneva

Wright J (2001) Assessing health needs. In: Pencheon D, Guest C, Melzer D, Muir Gray JA (eds) Oxford handbook of public health practice. Oxford University Press, Oxford, pp 38–46

Wüthrich-Schneider E (2000) Patientenzufriedenheit – wie verstehen? Teil 1. Schweizerische Ärztezeitung 81:1046–1048

Zastrow RJ (2001) Physician practice profiling. Homepage of the Medical College of Wisconsin – Milwaukee School of Engineering joint Masters degree program in Medical Informatics web site for course MI-13203: Health Care Decision Support (http://home.wi.rr.com/zastrow/profiling.htm) Accessed May 28, 2004

Zhao Y, Ellis RP, Ash AS, Calabrese D, Ayanian JZ, Slaughter JP, Weyuker L, Bowen B (2001) Measuring population health risks using inpatient diagnoses and outpatient pharmacy data. Health Services Research 26(6 Part II):180–193

Ziese T, Neuhauser H, Kohler M, Rieck A, Borch S (2003) Flexible Ergänzung der Gesundheitssurveillance in Deutschland: Gesundheitssurveys per Telefon. Gesundheitsberichterstattung des Bundes, Berlin (http://www.rki.de/GBE/) Accessed May 28, 2004

Epidemiology in Developing Countries

IV.6

Klaus Krickeberg (A General),
Anita Kar, Asit Kumar Chakraborty (B The Example India)

Introduction

Modern epidemiology can boast of a precise definition, clearly formulated basic concepts, and well elaborated methods, all of them described elsewhere in this handbook. These are in principle the same in developing and in developed countries. What is different is the *framework*, the choice of *topics* and of *applications* to be treated given local necessities, but also the battery of *tools* adapted to typical tasks and available under local conditions and the type of *difficulties* that epidemiologic work is facing.

This chapter attempts to outline these differences. Still, both developing and developed countries vary enormously also between themselves. Moreover, many countries belong to one of the two categories when applying certain criteria like income but to the other one regarding other aspects like education. We will therefore not adhere throughout to a fixed definition of a developing or a developed country. Nevertheless, many common features exist in each of the two groups of countries regardless how they are defined.

In Sect. A, after a short description of essential features that are specific to health systems in developing countries, we review the main needs of these countries in the realm of epidemiology. The last four sections are devoted to the methods of acquiring and applying epidemiologic knowledge. Of these, global health information systems are a particularly striking specific component of the health structures in developing countries because they practically exist only there. Sample surveys also play a more important role than in developed countries, whereas the opposite is true for more advanced epidemiologic studies.

The context for epidemiological investigations in India has to be placed against the background of some ground realities. India is the second most populous country in the world with a population of over 1 billion in 2001 and an annual birth cohort of approximately 25 million (Census of India 2001). This gigantic population is distributed through diverse geographical terrains and show a wide spectrum of socio-economic development, cultural heterogeneity, and linguistic diversity. The phenomenon of developmental planning including health planning is relatively recent, initiated after Independence, less than sixty years ago. The historic evolution of the health sector has witnessed the development of both public and private health sectors. The latter is poorly regulated, and currently there is no information on the number of active practitioners in the private sector. Adding to this complexity is the fact that India has plural systems of medicine, namely, Indian systems of medicine such as ayurveda, unani, siddha, naturopathy as well as allopathy and homeopathy. These diverse factors enhance the challenge of collecting accurate, reliable and up-to-date morbidity and mortality data.

In Sect. B, we will address two aspects of epidemiology in India. In the first part, we comment on the availability of demographic and health statistics in the country. Data on age specific mortality is available in the country, although reliable information on overall morbidity is unavailable. We illustrate the challenge of establishing and maintaining disease registers, by presenting the intricate organizational structure of the health sector in India that imposes enormous complexity in data management.

In the second part, we use tuberculosis epidemiology as a case study, to illustrate the trajectory between epidemiological investigations and their role in shaping national tuberculosis control strategies. Tuberculosis accounts for the largest cause of infectious morbidity and mortality in the country. Globally, India is ranked first amongst the twenty-two high burden countries listed by the World Health Organization. We discuss the issues of estimating disease incidence and prevalence in the absence of complete and accurate morbidity data. We conclude with the obvious statement that in a resource starved country like India, an accurate, reliable and timely disease reporting system is an urgent requirement to ensure evidence-based rather than ad hoc health policies.

General (by K. Krickeberg)

A

The Framework: Health in Developing Countries

6.1

The specific form of epidemiologic research and applications in a given country is conditioned to a large extent by the way health care is organized and functioning. There we encounter many differences on principle between developed and developing countries. The former are generally richer and can spend more money on health in absolute terms, but usually also in relative terms as measured in relation to national income.

More specifically, the way curative care is organized differs substantially between the two groups. This is especially true for primary health care in the classical sense of health care that begins at the time of the first encounter between a patient and a provider of health service. In developed countries it rests essentially with the general practitioner who is a trained physician, and to a lesser extent with doctors in hospitals and policlinics. In developing countries it is mostly offered by *communal health centres* (CHCs) or comparable health facilities that are mainly staffed with health workers like nurses and midwives who are less trained but sometimes more efficient than physicians. Regarding secondary health care, hospitals in the least developed countries tend to be concentrated in large cities, especially in the capital, to the detriment of the rest of the country.

General hygiene and specific preventive measures in developing countries suffer particularly from the lack of material means and knowledge. Bureaucratic weak administrative structures and lack of management training and experience also have much bearing on Public Health and so do insufficient civil registries and other records, especially demographic ones. It is in this environment that, for instance, the burden of AIDS has been incommensurably heavier than in developed regions of the world.

The main reason next to poverty for which the health system in developing countries has taken such a different path from that of developed ones is founded in their historical evolution and in particular in the role of contributions from outside. These were twofold.

Firstly, health care in colonies was initially built up to a large extent by missionaries and then by the colonial masters, the latter adapting it mainly to their own needs, sometimes to the detriment of indigenous medicine. This building up continued later in the form of bilateral cooperation with developed countries, especially training, and also embraced developing countries that had never been colonies like Thailand or Turkey, often in synergy with national efforts. In general, it emphasized individual health care and often suffered from the concentration of hospitals in urban centres. Again, there were exceptions, some developing countries like Vietnam succeeding in making substantial progress in Public Health, too, and in creating networks of CHCs and small hospitals that covered the entire country.

Secondly, international programmes have been a very important source of contributions from outside. They were mostly designed by WHO but implemented by organizations like UNICEF, international or national non-governmental organizations, and national health authorities or institutes like ministries of health or national hygiene institutes. They are installed and run *vertically*, from their respective top administrations down to the basic providers of health care. They tend to strengthen Public Health and are sometimes curative, sometimes preventive, and sometimes both. They have shaped large sectors of the health system of developing countries. Since they usually involve a lot of epidemiologic work, we will list some of them here. For details, see the relevant publications of WHO.

The first major international programmes after World War II concerned tuberculosis and malaria. Other programmes directed against particular diseases followed, e.g. against smallpox which lead to its eradication, poliomyelitis, goiter, cataract, and finally HIV. There were some programmes of more regional importance like leprosy, schistosomiasis, onchocerciasis (river blindness), meningitis, and arthropod-borne virus diseases, especially yellow fever and dengue fever.

In addition, WHO-programmes of a different type appeared which were not meant to prevent or cure a specific disease but to prevent death caused by certain unspecific manifestations of any of a whole group of acute ailments: CDD and ARI. The core of CDD (Control of Diarrhoeal Diseases) consisted in preventing death from dehydration of children under the age of 5 who suffered from acute diarrhoea. The main method was *oral rehydration* regardless of the cause of the diarrhoea. Hygienic measures to prevent diarrhoeas were included but not the main objective. The philosophy of ARI (Acute Respiratory Infections) was similar, namely to prevent the death of children under 5 who had caught an acute respiratory infection like pneumonia by a non-specific antibiotic standard treatment. Preventive action against the infections themselves was a side issue.

Essential Drugs is a WHO-programme of still a different nature, and so is Reproductive Health, which often boils down to plain family planning.

The most beneficial WHO-programme is probably EPI (Extended Programme on Immunization) by which a high number of cases of severe diseases and deaths have been prevented. Its objective is the systematic vaccination of all children under one or two years of age against measles, poliomyelitis, diphteria, tetanus, and pertussis (whooping cough), plus a dose of BCG that is, however, controversial and no longer generally recommended. Moreover, the programme includes a vaccination of all women in childbearing age against neonatal tetanus. The vaccination of children against hepatitis B was added later.

Many other international programmes of varying importance exist or have existed, above all MCH (Mother and Child Health), but also Nutrition, Vitamin A Deficiency, Rehabilitation of War Victims, etc. All the vertical programmes have unfortunately been very little coordinated with each other. Moreover, EPI was often overly stressed and drew many of the resources of the health system to itself to the detriment of other activities, detracting in particular from the normal routine. The conceptual and operational bases of an integration of the various aspects of primary health care have been expounded long ago (Krickeberg 1989), but it is only recently that a programme "Integrated Management for Childhood Diseases" was launched by WHO.

We are now going to outline the role that epidemiologic work plays and, more importantly, ought to play within this framework.

Epidemiologic Needs of Developing Countries

6.2

In the area of descriptive epidemiology in the classical sense, i.e. *health statistics*, the needs of developing countries are in principle hardly different from those of developed ones: incidence or prevalence of major diseases by sex, age, time, and place of residence plus disease specific mortality, infant mortality, maternal mortality, etc. (cf. Chap. I.3 of this handbook). These statistics are one of the pillars of the *management* of the health system, especially yearly budgeting. They ought to be used also for rational planning and implementing *global health strategies* but this aspect still leaves much to be desired apart from international vertical programmes. They are often presented in official health statistics publications, e.g. health yearbooks that sometimes appear to be their main justification.

The actual differences between the needs for descriptive epidemiology within the two groups of countries result from the different weight that the various categories of disease have or that health authorities attribute to them. Infectious diseases certainly weigh much more in developing countries than in developed ones in spite of their resurgence in the latter (cf. Chap. IV.1 of this handbook). Incidence figures should be available regularly, and classical *epidemic surveillance* is of course of utmost importance.

Health authorities in developing countries often tend to neglect non-infectious ailments like cancer, cardio-vascular diseases, and osteoarthritis, and hence few reliable statistics are available about them. There is reason to believe that their incidence, prevalence, and mortality is in some of these countries of the same order of magnitude as that of the main infectious diseases. Very few indicators are known on *nicotine addiction*, one of the most menacing epidemics in developing countries.

The most *specific* requirements regarding incidence or prevalence usually emanate from the managers of special programmes, mainly international vertical ones, who need them for planning, running, monitoring, and evaluating their programmes.

In the domain of *observational epidemiology*, i.e. the study of risk factors, the needs of developing countries have been less pronounced than in that of health statistics. There has been a tendency to rely on results obtained in developed countries or by teams from there who found interesting study objects in a developing country but often contributed little to furthering the epidemiologic capacities of their hosts.

Moreover, for infectious diseases, the principal risk factor being the infective agent itself, there has been less motivation to investigate contributing factors like genetic, social, and environmental ones. Studies have mainly centred on the pathways of the pathogen and their effect on infections including mathematical modelling. Their practical conclusions regarding e.g. hygiene are more or less known. For concrete illustrations it suffices to think of diarrhoea and AIDS. However, studies of general risk factors of the type mentioned above in view of preventive measures are direly needed in developing countries. For example, in the realm of the programme ARI, what is the effect of smoke in dwellings on acute respiratory diseases? Which factors influence the malaria cycle, and how?

Regarding observational epidemiology of non-infectious diseases, specific to developing countries, there is obviously an urgent need regarding, above all, the investigation of nutritional risk factors and of environmental exposures in large cities, but also of infections, e.g. viral infections as causes of cancer.

The epidemiologic needs described up to here are *global* in the sense that they concern a whole country. They are mainly recognised by health authorities at the top of the hierarchy. In addition, there is what WHO once called "epidemiology at the basis". This is *local* epidemiology which is tied to a smaller geographic or administrative entity, usually a commune. For example, knowing the relative frequencies of the various diseases including traumata which appear at a CHC not only has a practical value for managing the centre but also an educative one; it may be a motivation for the health worker as well. The same holds for other simple activities in local observational epidemiology like linking an incidence to a social factor or a geographic one, e.g. stagnant waters to shigellosis. While nurses often design ingenious charts, maps, and other devices to monitor certain epidemiologic features of their community including rules how to apply them, a general and systematic approach is wanting.

In experimental epidemiology including intervention activities, the needs of developing countries are manifold. They arise in all branches of that area. There is *clinical* epidemiology both in the form of studies in diagnostics and of clinical trials of curative treatments, and there are trials to evaluate preventive actions. All of them play a particular role in vertical programmes. Let us elaborate a bit and look at a few examples.

As said above, diagnostics and curative treatment in developing countries are often very different from what is customary in the developed world. To a large extent they take place in CHCs and are performed by only partly trained health workers under poor material conditions, in particular in the absence of laboratory equipment. Therefore, simplified and *standardized decision rules* for case management have been designed.

For example, diagnoses have usually to be made on the basis of only some clinical symptoms without any laboratory analysis. In regions of Cambodia where malaria is endemic, the symptoms "fever" and "headache" will normally entail the preliminary diagnosis "malaria". Similarly, a differential diagnosis of amoebic and bacterial dysentery (shigellosis) must often be founded on the clinical symptoms "headache", "fever", "blood in the stool", and "mucus in the stool". In both cases, a more reliable diagnosis may take time because a blood or stool analysis can only be done in a laboratory that is far away, or it may not be possible at all. However, it is usually both necessary and common to treat the patient at once, having only a preliminary diagnosis at one's disposal. If one wants to judge the merits or dangers of this strategy, one needs to know the epidemiologic characteristics of the underlying preliminary diagnostic decision rule, i.e. its *sensitivity, specificity*, and *prognostic values*. One may also wish to compare this clinical decision rule with alternatives of the same type in order to select the best one.

The programme CDD is another example. Here, the result of the diagnosis is not expressed in the form of a particular disease but as a degree of dehydration, either 0, I, II, or III, determined as a simple function of a few easily recognizable clinical symptoms. The treatment, too, has a standardized form and depends only on this degree, in particular oral rehydration in case II. Again, the epidemiologic characteristics of the diagnostic rule need to be known in order to evaluate the usefulness of the entire strategy. ARI works analogously.

The preceding discussion of diagnosis applies in a similar way to simple standardized curative treatments that are largely being used in developing countries. Their efficacy ought to be estimated by appropriate clinical trials.

Traditional medicine, too, is an area where the epidemiologic necessities of developing and developed countries obviously differ. In order to bridge the gap between traditional curative treatments and those taught in medical schools at universities and to integrate the useful part of the former into the health system of developing countries, clinical trials including meta-analyses are required. There is in principle no difference between the two curative systems. After all, much of the "Western" pharmacopoeia had its origin in traditional medicinal plants, e.g. quinine and aspirin and, more recently, viagra. Unfortunately, until not long ago, medical herbs and animals that were known for centuries if not millennia have been studied only from a purely pharmacologic and chemical point of view, to extract the "active principle", without raising the question of their actual efficacy. It is only recently that traditional cures of any kind have been subjected to epidemiologic scrutiny, first in India and China, and then in developed countries, too.

Let us conclude this section by looking at epidemiologic needs that arise when taking preventive measures. The principal measures in developing countries are on the one hand person-based *interventions* of the type treated in Chap. I.8 of this handbook, especially *immunizations* in the framework of EPI, and, on the other hand, community-based *health promotion* as described both in Chaps. I.8 and III.11, often connected with vertical programmes. As examples we can quote classical hygiene, treating bednets against anopheles, and urging the community to cooperate in a given programme. Campaigns for healthier nutrition or against smoking are still in their infancy and so are screening programmes along the lines of those presented in Chap. III.10 for developed countries. The problem at hand is to evaluate the effect of such activities.

Regarding *immunizations*, there is a tendency to make do with the results about their efficacy obtained in developed countries. Sometimes, however, the situation may be different. A case in point is the problem of the optimal period for vaccinating against *measles*, the so-called "window". In developed countries, this vaccination can wait until the maternal antibodies still present in the infant's blood can no longer interfere with its immunizing action. In developing countries, however, the infectious potential around a child is often very high from the beginning. The child's maternal antibodies do not protect it sufficiently, hence early vaccination is called for. To overcome this dilemma, WHO decided to advocate the use of a higher-titre vaccine of the "Edmonston-Zagreb" type in spite of the existence of epidemiologic studies which gave rise to the fear that this might lead to a higher overall-mortality among vaccinated female children. This was indeed observed in later studies, and the vaccine had to be withdrawn (Das Gupta et al. 1997; in particular the article Aaby 1997).

The epidemiologic judgment of community-based interventions in developing countries does not in principle differ from those in developed ones. Like the actions themselves, their evaluations are often much more poorly designed and executed, though. Similarly, rigorous person-based intervention trials are largely lacking.

We now turn to the question of how and to which extent the epidemiologic needs of developing countries can be satisfied in theory and practice. We will first describe the most important tool, health information systems, and then, in the remaining three sections, examine the contributions of this tool and of the two other ones, i.e. health surveys and epidemiologic studies.

6.3 Health Information Systems in Developing Countries

A health information system (HIS) links different institutions that are concerned with health between each other. It consists of mechanisms to *collect, transmit, analyze*, and *exploit* information on health in the widest sense. This is mostly done regularly, in a *routine* fashion, but may be supplemented by an ad hoc exchange of information. For example, most hospitals have their own, sometimes computerized, system by which information flows between its various wards and administrative units.

Here, we will be dealing only with HISs which go beyond a single institution, and where information is transmitted between CHCs, policlinics, hospitals, and public health institutions and administrations. For instance, a central disease register as described in Chap. I.4 of this handbook amounts to a HIS where reports from physicians, hospitals, and laboratories are directed to the office where the data are stored and handled.

We are going to restrict our scope further by focussing on much larger HISs that may deal with many sorts of information and link institutions of very different nature. In the extreme case, such a system may be founded on *regular reports* on *all* major events and activities from *all* health institutions of a *whole country* to higher health authorities, culminating in the Ministry of Health. The bulk of information emanates from the basic health institutions that are in direct contact with the population for curative or preventive activities: private practitioners, health centres, policlinics, small hospitals, individual wards of large hospitals, hygiene teams etc.

Developing countries have, as a rule, started very early to build HISs, sometimes rudimentary, sometimes quite elaborate. They were motivated by the need to manage scarce resources efficiently, including traditional budgeting, and to control the functioning of the various components of the health system. Epidemiologic information for planning and implementing health strategies played originally a secondary role apart from simple health statistics based on statistics of treatments, but over the years HISs have become an essential, and often the main source of epidemiologic knowledge.

In spite of the necessity felt by health planners to be equipped with a reliable HIS, the systems actually constructed have almost consistently been suffering from serious deficiencies. In some countries, e.g. in Africa and Central America, they did not reach far enough into the countryside nor did they cover the essential subject matter sufficiently well. In others, on the contrary, especially in socialist countries, they were usually too heavy and bureaucratic, attempting to cover everything and containing many redundant or superfluous elements that impeded their functioning. Neither the former nor the latter were designed following clear ideas and guidelines including a rational logical structure.

In the beginning HISs were installed by the central health authorities, usually the Ministry of Health. They tried to build a more or less centralized HIS under which basic health institutions had to send reports on their general activities routinely following a hierarchical path, e.g. from CHCs to district health administrations, from there to provincial health authorities, and ending up in the Ministry. Unfortunately, given the deficiencies of such systems mentioned above, in some countries other central institutions had to build their own HIS that ran parallel to that of the Ministry. For example, a national hygiene institute would set up a separate reporting system on *infectious diseases* including *epidemic surveillance*. Similar systems were needed by a central tuberculosis or malaria institute. All of this caused a lot of extra work in basic institutions, especially in CHSs.

The worst confusion, however, resulted from the management of international programmes. As said above, managers usually felt the need for a centralized and *vertical* approach, working from the top to the bottom. This involved specific systems for providing the required information in the form of basic demographic, epidemiologic, sociologic, and economic indicators, and of indicators to be updated all the time, for instance on the logistics of drugs or on vaccination coverage. Thus a plethora of information systems emerged for the various programmes. As a rule these manifold HISs were coordinated neither with each other nor with the system of the Ministry and other existing systems. The burden of writing and filing all the required reports rested mainly with the local health workers who were naturally more interested in their purely medical activities. It became frequently unbearable. The situation in Vietnam as described in a recent report (Krickeberg 1999) is a good example though there are great differences between countries.

The question of how to design a *single* information system that could be handled efficiently and at the same time serve all the essential needs of health care, i.e. a so-called *integrated* HIS, has therefore been discussed occasionally. Although some developing countries have in fact set up reasonable HISs, e.g. Cuba, the principles on which such systems should rest have been investigated only recently in a systematic way (Krickeberg 1994, 2003; Lippeveld et al. 2000). The remaining part of this section will be devoted to a short presentation of these principles, starting with the functions of HISs, passing on to the properties which they should have in order to do what we want them to do, and finally looking at their structure. More details can be found in the three references just quoted.

Regarding functions, *budgeting* and all *health management* that go beyond the smallest entities of the health system, require a good HIS. This holds for the general standing health system as well as for special vertical programmes that rely, for instance, on an efficient logistics for drugs or vaccines. *Health insurance* could in principle get from an integrated HIS all the information it needs for planning and running. An important specific application would be to estimate from it the average cost caused by a case of a particular disease. In the context of this handbook, though, we are only dealing with the epidemiologic functions of a HIS, to be described in the following section.

Regarding desirable properties, they are largely dictated by experience. The system should be *integrated*, i.e. cover all health institutions and all kind of numerical information. In particular, the medical and epidemiologic aspects must not be separated from the economic and managerial components. So-called "Health Management Information Systems" usually cover *some* clinical and epidemiologic information but not enough; in most cases, the term is misleading.

The HIS ought to have a *transparent, logical structure*. This is not only indispensable for designing and running the system efficiently, but also constitutes, as again many experiences have shown, a powerful motivation for the health workers who handle it. Moreover, only a well-structured HIS can be computerized although there have been quite a few, always futile, attempts at saving a bad system by using computers.

The system needs to be shaped in view of *well-defined objectives*, and incorporate rules how to analyze and exploit the information obtained in order to reach these objectives.

Given its objectives, it has to be *minimal*, free of superfluous elements and in particular of redundancies, and has to function at minimal cost. This has, in particular, an implication regarding the *flow of information* between institutions: routine reports must be filed only from and to institutions as really needed, and following operational priorities.

The system should be *flexible* so it can be adapted to changes of all kind, in particular to varying epidemiologic situations, but also to alterations of the structure of the health system or of health strategies and medical knowledge and techniques, economic and social changes of the country, and new information technology.

The information obtained must be as *reliable* as one can realistically hope for.

There have to be clearly defined rules indicating what to do about *wrong* or *missing information*, and there have to exist *error-correcting* procedures.

Moving on to the underlying structural and technical principles we have to recall first a few elementary definitions because there is no general agreement about them. As always in statistics when talking about information in a concrete context, we need to specify first a *population* (set) of *units* (elements), e.g. all children under 5 living at a given moment in a given village, or all consultations done during a certain month in a certain health centre. Information has either the form of *data* or of *indicators*. Data are the values of a *variable*, which is a function defined on a population, like the function *age* which assigns, to each of these children, his or her age, or the function *diagnosis* that attributes to every consultation the diagnosis made, properly coded. A *register* is a concrete, explicit representation of the data of one or several variables as described in Chap. I.4 of this handbook, usually on paper or on a computer disk. We will not enter into technical details like sub-registers or linked registers.

An *indicator*, in contrast to data, concerns a population as a whole, but not individual units. It depends on one or several variables defined on the same population. Two examples, concerning our first and second example of a variable, respectively: the mean age of these children, and the number of "diarrhoea" cases recorded. In practice, an indicator is computed from *all* the values of the underlying variables as given in a register. Let us note in passing that WHO has given a completely different definition of an indicator.

Registers are *the* fundamental, and often neglected, components of a HIS. They need to obey the following "golden" rule: in any basic institution, there is *only one register for a given population*, i.e. for a given type of unit. For example, it is compulsory that there exists, in a health centre or a ward of a hospital, only one register of consultations, not a "general" one for the Ministry, and one more for each vertical programme and for other special purposes.

Well-designed registers are in particular the main tool for the local use of the HIS, both clinical and epidemiologic, to be sketched in the following section. Their multiple functions demand a clear definition of the variables involved.

The second function of a register, namely to serve as the basis for the routine reports to be filed, should also follow rigorous structural rules. This applies both to paper-based and computer-based HISs. We note first that most information contained in routine reports is in the form of *indicators*, be they epidemiologic, economic, or others. The transmission of *data* on individual units, e.g. on cases, is indeed rare and mainly restricted to epidemic surveillance and registers of special diseases. For indicators resulting from clinical activities which are the most prominent ones, the structural rule in question looks like this: the clinical act giving rise to the data, the immediate use of these data in the act, the filling in of the relevant register, and the drawing up of the reports based on these data, have to be *integrated conceptually* and *technically*. In particular, the *layout* of the register and that of the reporting forms need to be closely coordinated so as to allow calculating the indicators and writing the report in a single, transparent, and almost automatic operation.

In this way, many indicators of quite a different nature can be easily computed and transmitted to various institutions and according to needs that may change, all based on the *same* registers and on the *same* variables. However, on no account should there exist a register that is not tied operationally to some function within the health system and whose only purpose is to calculate and report indicators.

There have been attempts, e.g. by WHO, at designing HISs by starting with a list of the indicators to be covered in view of the goals of the system. This idea may be tempting at first sight but is in fact naïve. Such lists have always been long and subject to debate, they leave no room for flexibility, and they are at variance with the basic structural principles as outlined above. What we have to fix in the beginning are the *variables* needed; to do this well is crucial. The second step will then be the design of the *registers*.

Reliability of the information is a particularly difficult problem in the context of a developing country. Standard procedures to assure quality as those described in the Chaps. I.10 and I.13 of this handbook can only be applied to a rather limited extent. Motivation of the health worker is a somewhat more efficient measure but gaps and errors will remain. The topic of what to do when confronted with them has many facets. The Chaps. II.5 and II.6 concern errors and missing data in a *single* epidemiologic study. In the realm of HISs, however, we have to handle them *routinely*, e.g. for every monthly report of a district health administration to its superiors. To this end, simple rules and algorithms need to be developed which can function under the specific conditions (Krickeberg 1994, 2003).

Let us now try to elucidate to which extent, and how, HISs can serve the epidemiologic functions enumerated in Sect. 6.2.

Epidemiologic Insights from Health Information Systems

It is a truism that, *potentially*, epidemiologic needs can be satisfied via a HIS to the extent, and only to the extent, that the necessary data or combinations of data are recorded in the system. The practice is a bit different but let us look at the mechanisms anyway.

Existing HISs have usually been built in view of establishing various health statistics and of managing health activities albeit in a rudimentary fashion, e.g. yearly budgeting. In addition, we have sketched the principles for reforming older HISs or building new ones. In any case, we are facing the following questions: What kind of registers are there? Which variables are being recorded and how? How is information extracted from the registers and transmitted to its destinations?

As stated in the preceding section, a register is tied in a natural way to a particular operation that is routinely executed in the health system, above all a clinical one. Thus the main register in a CHC is the register of *consultations*. Next to the date of the consultation and data to identify the patient it features variables like symptoms or syndrome, sometimes a tentative diagnosis, and treatment. Recording of the relevant data serves, in the first place, the clinical act "consultation" itself. Clearly defined variables may indeed help the health worker to decide about his diagnosis and treatment as explained in Sect. 6.2 for CDD and ARI cases.

The main epidemiologic function of the register of consultations is to allow calculating the incidence of symptoms like injury, stomach-ache, diarrhoea or acute respiratory infection, but also of tentative diagnoses that can be regarded as more or less satisfactory surrogates for a correct diagnosis of certain ailments, especially of frequent infectious diseases like measles. This is obviously conditional on the training of the health worker whom the patient is consulting.

As said in the preceding section, these calculations and the filing of the corresponding reports ought to be integrated with the data entry into the registers. The details depend of course on whether the register is on paper or on a computer disk. In any case, the report should display the epidemiologic situation reported also immediately to the health worker himself in a vivid fashion in the spirit of the "epidemiology at the basis". In fact, "local mastership" over information is one of the main roles of a good HIS, in contrast to the old bureaucratic idea that such a system exists mainly to produce indicators for higher-up administrations. This local mastership must not be taken away from the basic health institutions. The often advocated "feedback" is useful but after all a poor substitute for local use of information.

Incidences calculated and reported may sometimes be *corrected* later, i.e. replaced by *estimates* that will generally be closer to the true incidences and should therefore be used in health statistics and for health planning (Krickeberg 1994). A very rough procedure actually in use is the multiplication of every indicator obtained from the records by a constant "correcting factor" that had been estimated beforehand; an interesting application concerns maternal mortality (Ministerio de

Salud Pública y Asistencia Social 2002) where the factor 1.58 is being used. Slightly more elaborate but still elementary estimations could use simple extrapolations or Bayesian methods (Krickeberg 2003).

When well organized, the register of consultations in a CHC can serve the *epidemiologic surveillance* of infectious diseases as well. Moreover, by defining the values of the variable "symptoms" or "syndrome" appropriately so as to identify the consultations that belong to a programme like CDD, ARI, malaria or tuberculosis, a separate register of consultations for these programmes becomes superfluous at the level of the commune without making the general register of consultations any more complicated. The latter will furnish all the incidences required.

The register of consultations of a CHC may also allow some rough but illuminating *experimental epidemiology*. In some CHCs this register contains an additional variable "outcome" which can take the value "cured" or "deceased" among others. Strictly speaking, this variable concerns the larger unit "case" and not a "consultation" but in the absence of a register of cases, it can easily be recorded in a paper-based register of consultations by going back to the first consultation for a case, provided that the outcome becomes known not too late, e.g. for acute diseases. When using computers, recording an outcome which may occur much later, or even deriving a register of cases from that of consultations, is fairly easy. The variables "treatment" and "outcome" now permit both the local health workers and health administrators, in particular those of vertical programmes, to monitor standard treatments. To this end, they can peruse the complete register during a certain period or, usually more efficiently, employ *sampling from records*, i.e. random sampling from the units of a register, an unfortunately fairly neglected method although classical in hospitals of developed countries.

Sampling from records in CHCs also enables health authorities to estimate some of the epidemiologic characteristics of the preliminary clinical diagnoses described in Sect. 6.2. If the true diagnosis will *eventually* be known for most cases as it happens with malaria, it suffices to retrieve this diagnosis for the subjects included in the sample from the relevant records of district or provincial malaria stations, hospitals etc. In the opposite case, e.g. for dysentery, a laboratory-based diagnosis for the sampled subjects needs to be done.

In addition to the register of consultations, CHCs frequently have a register for the programme MCH whose underlying unit is not always well-defined. In principle, it should serve the needs of EPI, too, making an EPI-register superfluous. It can fulfil some epidemiologic functions analogously to the one of consultations.

Some CHCs have also set up a register of all *families* or *households* of the commune which can furnish certain epidemiologic insights, e.g. on infectious diseases or the role of socio-economic factors in health.

Registers in policlinics, hospitals, specialized malaria or tuberculosis stations, and the like concern mainly the units "out-patient consultation", "hospitalization", "discharge", and various "laboratory tests". Rare are the hospitals in developing countries that have a so-called *Central Register* whose unit is a "patient". Most of the more elaborate incidence and prevalence statistics which appear for example in health yearbooks originate from hospitals where diagnoses are on the whole more precise. Many of the health problems handled only in CHCs are lost in this way, though. The old problem of linking records in primary, secondary, and eventually tertiary health care usually does not get sufficient attention.

However, when remaining within the secondary and tertiary health system the issues are not basically different in developing and in developed countries. In particular, the part of the HIS based on consultations and treatments in hospitals may still be quite incomplete. For instance, in Vietnam the cancer incidences reported within that system and published in the Health Yearbook are much lower than the figures obtained from the Central Cancer Registry that has been operating for some time in a few regions (Krickeberg 1999).

Epidemiologic Sample Surveys 6.5

Let us start again with a truism that does not have much weight in practice either: sample surveys should be done and *only* be done if the results are not readily available from registers. For example, in developing countries many cases of measles do not lead to a contact of the patient with the health system, and are therefore registered nowhere, not even with a tentative diagnosis. This is the so-called iceberg problem. In such a situation, to get an idea of measles incidence, sample surveys are required. We will also discuss situations where they are *not* required.

In the present section we will restrict ourselves to sample surveys whose purpose is to estimate indicators that depend on a *single* variable, e.g. the incidence or prevalence of a disease, or mortality. Epidemiologic studies to investigate the *association* between several variables like those between a risk factor and a disease, or between a treatment and the outcome, will be taken up in the last section, although the borderline is not everywhere well-traced. Cross-sectional studies, in particular, usually have outwardly the form of a classical sample survey.

The most frequent *units* of a sample survey, i.e. elements of the "target population", are a person, a family (household), or a community, e.g. a hamlet or a commune, but a unit like a CHC may also occur if one wishes to evaluate the performance of such centres.

It is customary that for every new vertical programme a sample survey is launched in order to estimate the so-called "baseline indicators", and often this survey is repeated later to monitor changes that may reflect the impact of the programme. Such indicators are for instance incidences or prevalences of the relevant diseases; case fatalities; infant, child or maternal mortalities; indicators describing the nutritional status of children; vaccination coverages; or sometimes plain demographic indicators.

Surveys outside of any vertical programme that include an epidemiologic component have mostly been organized in the form of a large international project. An early model was the World Fertility Survey of the International Statistical Institute (Cleland and Scott 1987) that had been conducted between 1974 and 1982 in 42 developing and a few developed countries. Its methods including software were subsequently incorporated into the baseline surveys of some family planning programmes. UNFPA (United Nations Fund for Population Activities) organized demographic health surveys in many countries, often repeatedly, and these were later also conducted by private firms. Household surveys done by the United Nations have been a similar global venture (United Nations 1984).

Unfortunately, in a given developing country, these multitudinous surveys have practically never been coordinated with each other regarding their purpose, choice and definition of variables and indicators, methodology, and availability of the results. Therefore they cannot be compared with each other and exploited only with difficulty or not at all. Often, they duplicate existing knowledge, or the results are buried in the files of the relevant programme office, or both. By contrast, the World Fertility Survey is an early model of good quality and availability of its results, usually published locally.

Moreover, the definition of variables and indicators employed by most sample surveys is usually not compatible with that of existing HISs. The fundamental question to which extent an information system could have furnished the same result is rarely asked. For example, in a country like Vietnam that, although economically poor, provides well-structured primary health care, most cases of severe diarrhoea lead to a consultation of a basic health care institution where the syndrome is recorded. Hence a large if not the largest part of the CDD-surveys that have been conducted were actually superfluous and could have been replaced by "register-based" studies, i.e. sampling from records. The opportunity to compare indicators obtained from a survey with those extracted from the HIS is mostly lost although recently there have been notable exceptions, e.g. the survey from Guatemala on maternal mortality already quoted (Ministerio de Salud Pública y Asistencia Social 2002).

The sample surveys we are discussing are simple cross-sectional studies that concern in principle only the state of affairs at the moment the data are recorded. If, for instance, we are interested in the incidence of an acute disease or the mortality by it as it happens in the framework of EPI, the diagnosis for a case or the cause of a death has to be recorded for a *period of the past*, and can therefore only be determined by asking questions about the past, i.e. by an *a posteriori diagnosis* or an *oral autopsy*, respectively. Sometimes, this may not be very reliable. In any case, the survey should be confronted with the HIS if there is one. In particular, the questionnaire of the survey ought to contain a question about whether the patient had consulted his or her CHC or another health facility or not. Comparing the answers with the entries in the relevant register of consultations would then tell us a lot about the functioning of the HIS and the health system itself.

There is a related problem in the case of indicators defined with respect to *cohorts* that start at birth like infant mortality, child mortality, or vaccination coverage. In their definition, a cohort of children is to be followed from birth on to the age of 1, 5, or 2 years, respectively. They can be estimated directly by a register-based study. By contrast, a sample survey is done at a fixed moment. It either estimates a different indicator that concerns the state of a group of children at this moment as it happens with the usual EPI-coverage surveys, or needs to resort to questions about the past. If the latter strategy is adopted as it is for instance being done within the Demographic Health Surveys (DHSs) when estimating child mortality, care must be taken to analyse possible bias resulting from censuring the 5-year period of the past within which a child was to be followed.

To look at the interplay between sample surveys and register-based studies is also most illuminating when dealing with chronic diseases, especially non-infectious ones. Sample surveys done in Vietnam by an association of cardiologists have shown a recent dramatic increase of the prevalence of hypertension, most of it hitherto hidden. Linking such surveys to the HIS could have provided much useful knowledge.

Sample surveys, like HISs, can play an educative and training role, too, as it happened with the World Fertility Survey that largely relied on local staff. The organizers of a survey who often come from an international organization should always take great care to explain to the local health personnel involved its rationale including both the objectives and the methodology. They do not do it every time, partly because not all of them understand the underlying principles of the methods. They also tend to apply ready-made recipes that do not take into account the local administrative structures. Worse, existing know-how is often not exploited; in some countries certain local personnel is in fact better qualified than the "experts" directing a survey.

For instance, the so-called "30-cluster sampling plan" has been widely used in developing countries (Henderson and Sundaresan 1982). Its first stage is a Madow sampling design (Cochran 1977, p 265). Its second stage is tailor-made for countries that may not have lists of all households nor suitable maps of hamlets or villages. It has been very useful in many situations because it provides a standard method. Although it is not always self-weighting it has been treated as if it were which implies a simple form of the estimators. However, it has also been much applied in contexts where other sampling plans would have been easier and cheaper to implement and also would have been more efficient. This author has seen the Madow design used by a foreign CDD-specialist to select a sample of 30 administrative units from a list of only 32 or 33 such units. The local staff would simply have taken all of these units! Nowadays suitable maps of houses can be cheaply and rapidly drawn by the Geographic Positioning System even for very remote and poor villages.

Another example: in a developing country that operates a high-level research institute for demography and family planning, a baseline survey for a reproductive health programme was conducted by a person from abroad using the above-mentioned World Fertility Survey software although surveys providing a large part of the results had already been done by that institute, and although the institute could very well have done the entire survey itself in a much cheaper and more imaginative manner, profiting at the same time from the training and insights (and money) that go with it.

As said above, baseline surveys of vertical programmes and other surveys are sometimes repeated to monitor changes. To this end, samples are taken repeatedly in an independent fashion. There always exists a splendid opportunity to retain part of the sample and to use it for *longitudinal studies* that are most informative, e.g. household-based ones, but this opportunity is usually missed as it happened in the survey just mentioned.

The need for longitudinal studies was also one of the motivations for creating the concept of a sentinel network. This is a hybrid between a HIS and a sample survey. Since basic health facilities are all too often ill-equipped for making reliable diagnoses, do not have sufficient staff to keep registers and file reports, and cannot rely on good postal or other services to transmit information, the idea arose to select a fixed sample of such institutions, e.g. CHCs. Their capabilities were to be enhanced substantially by furnishing some laboratory equipment, paying additional trained staff, and ensuring better communications. These fixed "sentinels" were to monitor demographic and epidemiologic indicators over time including the impact of interventions. Sentinel networks may, however, give biased information because the measures taken to upgrade the selected sites alter the health situation there. More people might be attracted to use these facilities, better treatment can influence the dynamics of the transmission of infectious diseases, and better health education will reduce the incidence of many ailments including injuries.

Originally, sentinel networks were discussed mainly in the context of single vertical programmes but occasionally also for larger components of primary health care. There was no general scheme and no coordination. More recently, Demographic Surveillance Systems (DDSs) have been installed in various "field sites", i.e. geographically defined populations, in order to monitor their health and demographic status. Let us look at two examples. The first one is the DSS established in the early eighties by an already existing institution, namely the Nouna Health Research Centre in the North-West of Burkina Faso. It covers about 55,000 people (Yé et al. 2002). The second one is a DSS created during the years 1997–1999 in the context of a Vietnamese-Swedish collaborate research project in the district of Ba Vi of the province of Ha Tay in the North of Vietnam which counts around 235,000 inhabitants. It is combined with a field laboratory for epidemiologic research. First results concern among others mortality, death reporting, theory and practice of oral autopsies, knowledge of people about tuberculosis, and cardiovascular diseases (Nguyen et al. 2003).

Starting in 1998, an "International Network of field sites with continuous Demographic Evaluation of Populations and Their Health in developing countries" (INDEPTH) has been built up in order to link existing field sites, and in particular to strengthen them and to enhance their visibility and use (INDEPTH 2002). In 2003 it comprised 31 field sites from 17 countries, among them the DSSs at Nouna and Ba Vi.

6.6   Epidemiologic Studies

We will now take a quick look at how epidemiologic studies, other than register-based studies or straight sample surveys, can satisfy the specific epidemiologic needs of developing countries. We will thus be dealing with studies of the kind treated in the Chaps. I.3, I.5–I.8, and I.12 of this handbook.

The practical problems that a research team might face are summarized in Wawer (2001). Let us look at an example that illustrates one of the worst obstacles, namely loss to follow-up. This study, the Bloemfontein Vitamin A Trial (Chikobvu and Joubert 2003) had in fact a dual purpose: firstly, to investigate the effect of vitamin A on the transmission of HIV from mother to child; secondly, to assess the extent of loss to follow-up in the presence of AIDS with a view to planning and analysis of other cohort studies on HIV/AIDS including clinical trials. A total of 303 HIV positive pregnant women were recruited with 152 randomly allotted to the vitamin A group and 151 to the placebo group, to be followed until their baby was 18 months old. The tracing procedure of these women was precisely defined, the observed loss to follow-up was analyzed in detail, and the kind of bias that may have resulted was discussed. This trial and ten other cohort studies on HIV/AIDS quoted for comparison had losses to follow-up in the order of 10 to 48%. One of the main conclusions was that published studies must adequately discuss the tracing methods used.

Many sample surveys, especially large ones like the World Fertility Surveys or the Demographic Health Surveys, collect data both on risk factors, e.g. social ones, and on outcome variables, for instance morbidity. They can therefore be exploited in the form of cross-sectional studies on the influence of these factors on such outcomes. A good example is the study from Guatemala already quoted (Ministerio de Salud Pública y Asistencia Social 2002). This involves the shortcomings of cross-sectional studies in general which arise from the fact that many variables concern the past or a cohort and not the moment of the survey; we have sketched these problems in the preceding section.

Pure case-control or cohort studies, to be conducted in accordance with a rigid protocol fixed in advance, are relatively rare in developing countries. These countries have been a fertile ground for research in genetic epidemiology, though. For instance studies on thalassemia have a long history in South East Asia. Genetic susceptibility to infectious diseases has been studied intensively. An early example was the evidence for genetic susceptibility to leprosy obtained by a linkage analysis in a closed population, namely on a Caribbean island (Abel et al. 1989). In the realm of parasitic diseases, the role of genetic factors in resistance to malaria had already been established in 1982 (Mims 1982). Recent work done in Sudan concerns schistosomiasis (Dessein et al. 1999) and visceral leishmaniasis (kala-azar) (Bucheton et al. 2003). There have also been *clinical trials*, centring in particular around HIV, e.g. on the prevention of mother-to-child transmission.

Much epidemiologic work in developing countries has the form of *ecological* studies, that are treated in Chap. I.3 of this handbook. Section 4.2.1 of Chap. I.3 gives an example of a large descriptive ecological study in China (Chen et al. 1991). A community-based intervention trial, the Gambia Hepatitis Study, is mentioned in Chap. I.8, and a few other intervention studies of various sorts are quoted in Wawer (2001). Community-based intervention studies are often a useful and feasible type of investigation given the needs and conditions of developing countries, especially in the context of infectious diseases.

However, the most typical, illuminating, and useful type of study looks different in practice. It is more informal, and *prospective*, usually lasting for many years or even decades. Often it starts small, and expands later regarding objectives, study type, and basic population. It may concern anything connected with health: general or reproductive health of a community as time proceeds; nutrition; etiological factors, especially from the environment or social ones; the results of person-based or community-based interventions; and often several of these together. The diseases involved are those already mentioned in the present chapter, but rarely non-infectious ones.

An excellent summary of 34 such surveys plus a detailed presentation of 12 among them was published a few years ago (Das Gupta et al. 1997). It starts with pioneer studies done in China in the early thirties, it is organized by continents: Asia, Latin America, and Africa, and it provides fascinating reading. A good example is the malaria study in the Garki district in Nigeria, a savannah region. It took place from 1969 to 1976, involved 22 villages with a total population of 7423, and has also been the subject of a separate monograph (Molineaux and Gramiccia 1980). The topics studied were manifold: demographic and epidemiologic, in particular intervention evaluation. The epidemiology of malaria included all aspects: immunology, serology, parasitology, entomology, clinical manifestations, and the influence of various factors like weather and nutrition. The interventions consisted in pesticide spraying and mass prophylaxis. Let us quote some of the many results. No significant difference in mortality between mass-treated and untreated villages was found except for infant mortality. Malaria antibodies existed in people in sprayed as well as in unsprayed environments and their level was uncorrelated with that of parasitemia except in infants. The intervention reduced, but did not eliminate, the prevalence of the plasmodia involved, and malaria transmission and vector capacity, which had existed on a high level, persisted.

6.7   Conclusions

Summarizing finally the respective roles of the three sources of epidemiologic knowledge in developing countries we may say that, roughly, HISs have their roots in the daily work of the health workers, especially in their clinical activities; sample surveys are mostly tied to particular projects or programmes and concern mainly the state of affairs at a particular moment; analytic and experimental epidemiologic studies provide the deeper knowledge that is indispensable for all useful planning of health strategies.

The Example India (by A. Kar, A.K. Chakraborty)

The Situation in India

In India, planned intervention in public health is less than sixty years old. In 1947 when the country achieved Independence, health infrastructure was non-existent and infectious diseases periodically swept through the population traumatized by food deprivation. The Report of the Health Survey and Development Committee (1946) stated that the death rate in the year 1937 was 22.4 per 100,000/year while expectancy of life at birth was 27 years (Table 6.1A). Mortality records of British India estimated a maternal mortality rate of 20/1000 live births. Table 6.1B presents a comparison of mortality in infants and children in British India as compared to the United Kingdom and Wales. Cholera, smallpox, and plague accounted for 2.4%, 1.1% and 0.5% of all deaths in the year 1932. Tuberculosis mortality rates in cities ranged between 200–450 per 100,000 population. Only 2% of the population had access to potable water, whilst sanitary facilities were available for only 4.5%

Table 6.1A. Health indicators India

Indicator	1937[1]	1951[2]	1981[2]	2000[2]
Demographic indicators				
LE at birth	26.9(M) 26.5(F)	36.7	54	64.6
Crude birth rate		40.8	33.9 (SRS)	26.1 (1999, SRS)
Crude death rate	22.4/1000	25	12.5 (SRS)	8.7 (1999, SRS)
IMR	162/1000 live births	146	110	70
Epidemiological shifts				
Malaria (cases in million)	100	75	2.7	2.2
Leprosy cases per 10,000 population		38.1	57.3	3.74
Smallpox	69,474 (1.1%)	> 44,887	Eradicated	
Guineaworm (No. of cases)			> 39,792	Eradicated
Polio			29,709	265

(table to be continued)

Table 6.1A. (continued)

Indicator	1937[1]	1951[2]	1981[2]	2000[2]
Infrastructure				
SC/PHC/CHC		725	57,363	163,181
Dispensaries & hospitals (all)		9209	23,555	43,322 (1995–96, CBHI)
Beds (private and public)		111,198	569,495	870,161 (1995–96, CBHI)
Doctors (Allopathy)		61,800	268,700	503,900 (1995–96, MCI)
Nursing personnel		18,054	143,887	737,000 (1999, INC)

[1] Report of Health Survey and Development Committee (1946). In Compendium of Recommendations of Various Committees on Health and Development 1943–1975. Central Bureau of Health Intelligence, Directorate General of Health Services, Ministry of Health and Family Welfare, Government of India. New Delhi
[2] National Health Policy (2002)
SRS = Sample Registration System, CBHI = Central Bureau of Health Intelligence
MCI = Medical Council of India, INC = Indian Nursing Council
LE = Life Expectancy, IMR = Infant Mortality Rate
SC = Subcentre, PHC = Primary Health Centre, CHC = Community Health Centre

Table 6.1B. Deaths at specific age-periods shown as percentages of the total deaths at all ages[1]

	Under one year	1–5 years	5–10 years	Total under 10 years
British India (1935–1939)	24.3	18.7	5.5	48.5
England and Wales (1938)	6.8	2.1	1.1	10.0

[1] Report of Health Survey and Development Committee (1946). In Compendium of Recommendations of Various Committees on Health and Development 1943–1975. Central Bureau of Health Intelligence, Directorate General of Health Services, Ministry of Health and Family Welfare, Government of India. New Delhi

of the populace. Trained health personnel and infrastructure were practically non-existent. This was more pronounced in the rural population, where for example, one institution was available for the 105,626 inhabitants of 224 villages (Report of Health Survey and Development Committee 1946).

After Independence, the country has demonstrated an impressive improvement in health indicators (Table 6.1A/B). Smallpox and guinea worm have been eradi-

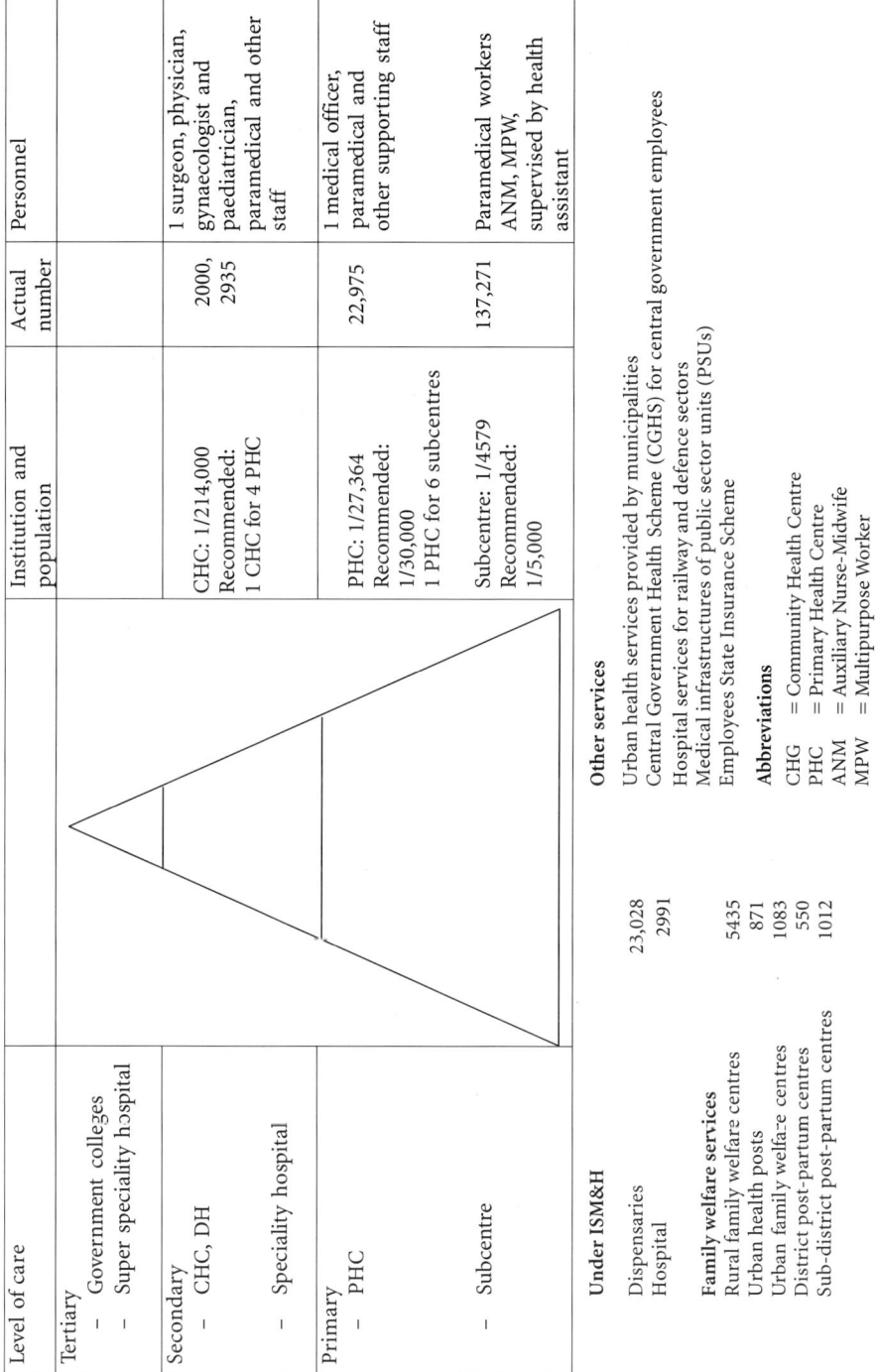

Level of care		Institution and population	Actual number	Personnel

Tertiary
  – Government colleges
  – Super speciality hospital				

Secondary
  – CHC, DH
 	
  – Speciality hospital
		CHC: 1/214,000
		Recommended:
		1 CHC for 4 PHC
			2000,
			2935
				1 surgeon, physician, gynaecologist and paediatrician, paramedical and other staff

Primary – PHC		PHC: 1/27,364 Recommended: 1/30,000 1 PHC for 6 subcentres	22,975	1 medical officer, paramedical and other supporting staff
– Subcentre		Subcentre: 1/4579 Recommended: 1/5,000	137,271	Paramedical workers ANM, MPW, supervised by health assistant

Under ISM&H

Dispensaries   23,028
Hospital   2991

Family welfare services

Rural family welfare centres   5435
Urban health posts   871
Urban family welfare centres   1083
District post-partum centres   550
Sub-district post-partum centres   1012

Other services

Urban health services provided by municipalities
Central Government Health Scheme (CGHS) for central government employees
Hospital services for railway and defence sectors
Medical infrastructures of public sector units (PSUs)
Employees State Insurance Scheme

Abbreviations

CHG   = Community Health Centre
PHC   = Primary Health Centre
ANM   = Auxiliary Nurse-Midwife
MPW   = Multipurpose Worker
ISM&H = Indian Systems of Medicine and Homeopathy

Figure 6.1. Schematic representation of the public health infrastructure

cated and polio is on the verge of extinction (National Polio Surveillance Project; http://www.npspindia.org). There has been a substantial drop in the total fertility rate and infant mortality rate (National Health Policy 2002). Through planned health interventions, India has developed a vast health infrastructure and health manpower (Table 6.1A/B, Fig. 6.1). Unfortunately, the process of expansion of health infrastructure has bypassed the development of systems to manage and document health data. The country does not have a reliable Health Management Information System (HMIS), or a credible disease surveillance system. Demographic data for epidemiological studies are however available. In the first part of this section, we present the sources of population data followed by the sources of health data, as well as the structural organization of the health sector that contributes to the complexity of data management.

In the absence of complete and accurate disease registers, estimating disease incidence and prevalence becomes a major challenge. We illustrate this using the example of tuberculosis, which is the largest cause of infectious morbidity and mortality in the country.

6.9   Sources of Data

Demographic and health statistics in India are collected, compiled and disseminated by the concerned ministries.

6.9.1   Demographic Statistics

Census

The census forms one of the more authentic sources of demographic data in India. The first population census was initiated in various parts of the country between 1865 and 1872, and has subsequently been undertaken uninterruptedly once every ten years. The Census 2001 represents the 14th census of the country.

Detailed description of the methodology for the 2001 Census of India and the checks to ensure data quality are given (Census of India 2001). The task of ensuring data quality becomes apparent from the enormity of the population covered for enumeration (593 districts, 5564 community blocks (*talukas*), 5161 towns and around 640,000 villages). Data collection is supervised by the Union Home Ministry, headed by the Registrar General and Census Commissioner, India. Field offices in thirty States and union territories were responsible for overseeing census work for the Census 2001. The questionnaire for data collection for the 2001 Census was evolved after a data user's conference, followed by a technical review. The census had two questionnaires, the Household List and the Household Schedule (Annex III and IV, Census of India 2001). Table 6.2 lists some of the variables collected in the household schedule of the Census 2001. Enumerators and supervisors were drawn from local school teachers and employees of the Central and State Government. Field work was carried out in two phases after rigorous training of

Table 6.2. Variables of household schedule; Census of India (2001)

A. General and socio-cultural characteristics:
    Number of individuals in the household
    Relationship to head of household
    Age
    Marital status
    Age at marriage
    Religion
    Caste/tribe
    Mother tongue
    Other languages known
    Literacy
    Highest education level
    Disability
B. Characteristics of workers and non-workers
    Employment
    Duration of employment
    Occupation
    Distance from residence to place of work
    Mode of travel to place of work
C. Migration characteristics
    Birth place
    Place of last residence
    Reason for migration
    Duration of stay at place of residence
D. Fertility particulars
    For ever married women
        Number of surviving children
        Total number of children ever born alive
    For currently married women only
        Number of children born alive during last one year

enumerators. In the first phase of field work, house numbering operations were undertaken, followed by the second phase of field work which involved population enumeration through personal interview.

From 1951, post enumeration surveys (PES) form an integral part of the census operation. The objective of PES is to estimate coverage and content error. Error tables for under-coverage of census houses and population are available through periodic publications from the Office of the Registrar General and Census Commissioner. Content error is estimated from a 10% sample of households enumerated in the census, and re-verifying certain specific data in the questionnaire. As is routine for all censuses conducted in the country, enumeration of the houseless population was undertaken for the 2001 Census on the mid-night of the 28th February, 2001. The collection of data at night ensures that the population can be found sleeping on pavements or under trees and thus can be accurately recorded.

The 14th Census introduced a new strategy to ensure long term tracing of a municipal ward or a village. In India, state boundaries are subjected to frequent administrative changes at the district and sub-district level during the inter-censal period. In fact, three months prior to the decadal census, three new States were carved out of three existing States. The 14th Census has assigned an eight digit coding system (termed the permanent location code number, PLCN) that should allow the unique identification of a village or municipality ward irrespective of jurisdictional changes in administrative boundaries. Another much needed innovation of the 2001 Census has been the acknowledgement of the rapid growth of urban slums. For the first time, slum enumeration blocks have been defined, providing a starting point for long-term studies on this population.

The Census Act of 1948 forms the legal basis for conduct of censuses, and it is a legal obligation on the part of the public to cooperate and provide correct information. However, despite quality checks, there remain lacunae in datasets of such magnitude. The most obvious source of error comes from non-sampling error, such as incomplete listing of houses, despite the institution of PES. Illiteracy of the population creates difficulties in terms of ensuring accuracy of social information. For example, data on age, birth intervals, income etc. have to be collected with extreme care due to the illiteracy of the respondents. Long-term utility of the data is also threatened by changing concepts and definitions.

Civil Registration System

The civil registration system for continuous recording of births, deaths and marriages leaves much to be desired in matters of coverage, quality and timeliness of the data. Compulsory registration of births and deaths is required under the Central Births and Deaths Registration Act in 1970. Despite the legislation, there is significant under-registration of vital events, especially in the rural areas. Vital data are collected from the urban and rural registration units and forwarded by the tenth of each month to the data processing unit of each State. In the State of Maharashtra, for example, vital statistics data are obtained from 40,448 villages, 230 municipal councils, 15 corporations, 7 cantonment boards and 4 ordnance factories. It is estimated that in Maharashtra about 80% of births and about 62% of deaths are registered under the civil registration system (Health Status Report Maharashtra 2003).

A number of factors contribute to the poor functioning of the civil registration system in the country. Registration of vital events is an additional responsibility for functionaries, who remain unaware of the importance of registration of vital events. It is worth remembering that many of the functionaries at the grass-root level in rural areas may be barely literate. There is a lack of public awareness about the statutory requirement of registration of vital events, reflecting a lack of demand for birth and death certification in the country. The issue of accessibility to vital registration centres also remains a problem, which is especially true for rural areas. Computerization of vital events is present in only a handful of municipalities in the country. In urban areas, death certificate is compulsory for obtaining permission for cremation or burial. This rule is rendered ineffective in rural areas where regulated cremation areas are often not used.

Sample Registration System

Various attempts have been made to improve the registration of vital events in the country. One of the most reliable estimates of vital rates is obtained from the sample registration system (SRS). The objective of the SRS is to provide reliable annual birth and death rates at the State and national level for urban and rural areas. The SRS is a dual system of registration involving continuous enumeration of births/deaths in sample villages/urban blocks and matching these data with that of a six-monthly retrospective survey. The data obtained through these two sources are verified by matching. Unmatched data are re-verified. This method not only results in unduplicated reporting of events but also has an inbuilt system of quantifying the disparity between the two data sets. Information for vital events is collected from various sources and individuals most likely to be involved in rituals of birth or death, such as the village priest, barber, midwives, socially important persons like the village headman, from nursing homes, maternity homes and from cremation and burial grounds. The half-yearly survey is done by specially trained permanent staff who undertakes house-to-house visit and data collection.

The sample design adopted for SRS uses a simple uni-stage stratified random sample. In rural areas each district within a State has been divided into two strata based on population per village. Villages with a population of greater than 1500 are divided into two segments. Simple random samples of villages and segments have been selected. Urban areas are categorized into five classes based on population size. The sampling unit is a census enumeration block. A simple random sample has been selected from these enumeration blocks from all five classes. The SRS currently has 6671 (4436 rural and 2235 urban) sample blocks covering 6182 million population (4821 million rural and 1361 million urban population) (SRS 2001).

Various studies have been undertaken by the Registrar General and Census Commissioner to evaluate the completeness of the SRS data. The studies have shown that birth registration had improved dramatically over the years. For example, whilst there was a 8% under-registration of births in 1972, the figure had decreased to 1.8% in 1985 (Narasimhan et al. 1997).

Population and Health Data from Surveys

Most recent and accurate scientifically collected baseline data that can be used for epidemiological studies comes from the National Family Health Surveys. The first and second National Family Health Survey (NFHS-1 and 2) were conducted in 1992–1993 and 1998–1999 respectively. The primary purpose of these surveys was to collect data on key indicators for assisting in policy decisions pertaining to the national population policy. In addition to serving as an important demographic database the NFHS provides data on fertility, the practice of family planning, infant and child mortality, maternal and child health and utilization of health services provided to mothers and children. The exhaustive list of variables for which data has been collected is available from periodic publications and from the NFHS (http://www.nfhsindia.org/). The detailed methodology for the NHFS-2 including sample characteristics for States and estimates of sampling errors is available (National Family Health Survey, India 2001). The NFHS-2 sample covered more than 99 percent of India's population living in all 26 States. Over 90,000 women were interviewed. Information has been collected using bilingual questionnaires (English and the regional language of the State). The household questionnaires provide a rich source of demographic data and serve as a source from which eligible respondents for the women's questionnaire were selected. Data on family planning, reproductive health and status of women are available from this questionnaire. A third village questionnaire makes available reliable and accurate baseline data for villages covered under the survey. A post-survey check confirmed the high quality of the data (Singh 1999). The NFHS data is available to researchers for analysis.

6.9.2   Health Data

The Central Bureau of Health Intelligence (CBHI) of the Ministry of Health and Family Welfare and the National Institute of Communicable Diseases are the agencies responsible for the compilation of health information of the country. CBHI is also the nodal agency for implementation of the Health Management Information System (HMIS). Communicable disease data are available from the various national disease control programmes (Table 6.3). The Ministry of Family Welfare collects data on reproductive and child health (RCH), such as immunization and population control measures. Rural health statistics provide data on government health infrastructure and manpower deployment in rural areas. These data have variable accuracy. The biggest lacunae in all these data are that they do not include disease data from the private sector. The country does not have any programmes for non-communicable disease prevention and control. Whilst programmes for prevention and control of diabetes, coronary heart diseases, cancer and mental health are available on paper (Table 6.3), there are no Government services for these ailments and conditions. Thus data are not available with the only exception of cancer, for which data from six population based registries are available (Indian Council of Medical Research 2001).

The Complexity of the Health Sector in India

The health sector in India consists of both public and private health services. The public health sector has a definite organizational structure and is responsible for health promotion, disease prevention and for providing curative services, at no or minimum cost to the Indian population. The private sector consists of individual and corporate private practitioners, and those working from privately owned hospitals and nursing homes. The role of the private sector is to provide

Table 6.3. Major schemes for health and disease control of the Government of India
(http://mohfw.nic.in/MSP-1.pdf)

National AIDS Control Programme
National Leprosy Eradication Programme
Vector Borne Disease Control Programme (malaria, filarial, kala-azar, dengue)
National Tuberculosis Control Programme
National Programme for Control of Blindness
National Cancer Control Programme
Vitamin A Deficiency Programme
Diarrhoeal Disease Control Programme
National Iodine Deficiency Disorders Control Programme
National Surveillance Programme for Communicable Diseases
National Mental Health Programme
Drug-Deaddiction Programme
National Diabetes Control Programme
National Cardiovascular Disease Control Programme
Medical Care for Remote and Marginalized Tribal and Nomadic Communities

curative services for a fee. There are multiple systems of medical practice in India. In addition to allopathic practitioners, licensed practitioners of traditional Indian systems of medicine (e.g. ayurveda, unani, siddha) and homeopathy are widely used by people in all parts of the country. This enormous diversity creates a tremendous complexity, making information management an extremely intimidating task. The public health sector is under bureaucratic control of the government and undergoes periodic review. The private sector, however, is largely unregulated with little control over the quality of services. The number of licensed private practitioners in the country is known from the lists of practitioners graduating from the various medical colleges in the Indian Systems of Medicine and Homeopathy. Updated lists of active practitioners from all systems of medicine are unavailable.

Public Health: Organizational Framework

The blueprint of the public health delivery system originated in 1943 (Report of Health Survey and Development Committee 1946), and was created primarily to serve the under-privileged majority in the country. The utilization of these services, and thus, morbidity data from the public health institutions, is restricted to the under-privileged groups in the Indian society and would not necessarily reflect the health situation of the Indian population in general.

Morbidity data and data on RCH are collected from the rural and urban health infrastructure of the public health system (Fig. 6.1) and forwarded through a series of functionaries to the State level for compilation. The rural infrastructure consists of the primary health care infrastructure, which provides the first level of contact between the population and health care providers. The most peripheral health institution available to the rural population is the subcentre, which is manned by one auxiliary nurse-midwife (ANM) and one multipurpose worker (MPW). These para-medical workers, supervised by a health assistant, have the responsibility to provide basic health care services to the people. These include treatment for minor ailments and injuries, collection of blood smears from all fever (suspected malaria) cases and sending them to the primary health centre (PHC), and to deliver the governmental health developmental programmes to the people. These functionaries are also responsible for referring cases to the PHC. One sub-centre is available to a population of 5000. The PHC is the referral unit for six-subcentres and represent the next level of the health care system. All PHCs have at least one qualified medical officer in charge. A majority of PHCs has four to six in-patient beds. One PHC is available for every 30,000 population. The community health centre (CHC, also termed the First Referral Unit) is a 30 bed hospital that is the first referral unit for four PHCs. One CHC is available for every 200,000 population. The secondary health care infrastructure consists of the district hospitals and other specialty hospitals, while the tertiary health care infrastructure consists of the government medical colleges and super-specialty hospitals. Starting from the sub-centre level, morbidity and health data are collated and forwarded from one level to the next, and ultimately through the district health officers to the Directorate of Health Services of each State.

Unlike rural health services, urban health services do not have the planned and organized primary, secondary, and tertiary services in geographically delineated urban areas. Usually, private practitioners, municipal dispensaries and tertiary care institutions cater to an enormous patient population from both the urban and rural areas. Morbidity data from these institutions are also forwarded through the district health officers to the Directorate of Health Services of each State.

Private and Voluntary Sectors

Although the private health sector is the largest provider of health and medical care to the population, very little information is available on the number of practitioners, available infrastructure or utilization of this sector (Duggal 2000; Report of the Steering Committee on Health for the Xth Five Year Plan, 2002–2007, 2002). Private sector health services range from the services provided by large corporate hospitals, smaller hospitals and nursing homes to dispensaries run by qualified personnel and services provided by unqualified practitioners. The majority of the private sector institutions are single doctor dispensaries with very little infrastructure or paramedical support. Specialty and super-specialty care account for only 1 to 2% of the total number of institutions, while corporate hospitals (i.e. hospitals funded by large business organizations) constitute less than 1% of this infrastructure (Report of the Steering Committee on Health for the Xth Five Year Plan, 2002–2007, 2002). There are no mechanisms for obtaining and analyzing information on disease, infrastructure or manpower from this sector. It is estimated that there are more than 7000 voluntary agencies involved in health related activities, mostly in the rural areas (Report of the Steering Committee on Health for the Xth Five Year Plan, 2002–2007, 2002).

Indian Systems of Medicine and Homeopathy (ISM&H)

There is a vast network of governmental ISM&H institutions. There are 3004 hospitals with 60,666 beds and over 23,000 dispensaries providing primary health care (Report of the Steering Committee on Health for the Xth Five Year Plan, 2002–2007, 2002). Over 16,000 practitioners from 405 colleges qualify every year. There is no estimate of the utilization of this sector, although ISM&H practitioners are extremely popular throughout the country. Inclusion of morbidity data from these practitioners into a disease database would be greatly limited since the rationale for diagnosis and disease classification is entirely different from the allopathic system of medicine.

Utilization of Private and Public Sector Services

The information presented in the preceding sections illustrate the extent of incompleteness of morbidity data in the country. Various surveys have shown that people from all socio-economic strata access the private sector for outpatient services. For inpatient services, 60% of individuals living below the poverty line (26% of the Indian population fall into this category) utilize the public health sector facilities. An equal number of people above the poverty line access the private health sector (National Sample Survey Organization, 1995–1996, 52nd Round 1998). Other surveys have shown that 65% of households go to private hospitals/clinics or doctors for treatment when a family member is ill. Only 29% usually approach the public medical sector. Even among poor households only 34% normally use the public medical sector during illness (NFHS-2 2000). Data of the National Sample Survey Organization (National Sample Survey Organization, 1995–96, 52nd Round 1998) suggest that the majority of physicians in both the modern system of medicine and the ISM&H works in the private sector. There are significant inter-state differences in the distribution of private sector hospitals and beds. Private sector hospitals are present in more prosperous districts and States, while in the poorer districts where health infrastructure is most needed, health services are provided by the public health sector.

Morbidity Statistics

National disease control programmes provide data on reported morbidity for those patients who utilize the public health system. Table 6.3 lists the major disease control programmes and health schemes of the government which were launched at various times after Independence, in order to control and eradicate communicable disease, improve environmental sanitation, raise the standard of nutrition and to implement population control. Under each disease control programme, data are collected from both rural and urban health institutions. For example, in the tuberculosis control programme (termed the Revised National Tuberculosis Control Programme, RNTCP) in the State of Maharashtra data is collected from 29 district tuberculosis centres and 1995 peripheral health institutions in the State. In addition, there are seven tuberculosis hospitals and sanatoria (Health Status Report Maharashtra 2003). The role of each centre is in case finding, treatment, case holding, management, recording and reporting of data. These data represent an obvious under-representation of morbidity, since they do not include data from the private sector.

6.9.3   Epidemiologic Surveillance System

Epidemiologic disease surveillance is an essential prerequisite for the effective control and prevention of communicable diseases, especially in India where environmental conditions are extremely poor. The major national programmes for control of various diseases like malaria, tuberculosis, trachoma, leprosy, cholera, filaria etc. (Table 6.3) have their own vertical surveillance system. Organized efforts to integrate all the ongoing surveillance into a single comprehensive programme for disease surveillance are lacking. Although the private sector provides over 75% of curative care for common illnesses, no attempt has been made to include the data from private health providers into a disease surveillance system. There is a recent endeavour suggested by the Planning Commission of India to compile information pertaining to common epidemic prone diseases or conditions like measles, diarrhoea, diphtheria etc., which are prevalent throughout the country as well as region specific problems such as malaria, filaria and leptospirosis from the endemic areas (Report of the Steering Committee on Health for the Xth Five Year Plan, 2002–2007, 2002). However, since many such programmes have been initiated to no avail, the success of this effort remains to be seen.

Notification System
Usually diseases which are considered to be serious menaces to public health, like measles, whooping cough, diptheria etc. are included in the list of notifiable diseases. In India, there is a conspicuous lack of uniformity in the lists of diseases which are notifiable in different States. Cholera, yellow fever and plague which are internationally quarantinable diseases are notifiable throughout the country as required under international health regulation. Notification of the specific communicable disease is compulsory and non-compliance is punishable by law. However, this provision of the law is very poorly implemented. Moreover, other than the three diseases listed above, most of the important conditions are not uniformly notifiable, resulting in an incomplete picture of morbidity and mortality pattern in India as a whole.

In urban areas, the responsibility for disease notification rests with the municipal health authorities who forward the reports to the district health officer. Private practitioners are by and large not involved in these activities. In rural areas, notification and registration is done traditionally through the village *chowkidar* (watchman), who is often minimally literate, or through the village *panchayat* (village governing body). These functionaries notify the local police station, from where the information is forwarded to the PHC and finally the District Health Officer. It is not surprising therefore, that such a disease reporting system lacks in reliability, promptness and completeness.

Health Information System

Despite several attempts, a Health Management Information System (HMIS) is not in operation in India. Information is collected and compiled in the traditional manner described above. This information is not timely or complete. Thus, decision making is most often ad hoc and not information based.

Tuberculosis Epidemiology   6.10

India is listed first amongst the twenty-two high burden countries that account for 80% of new tuberculosis cases in the world (World Health Organization 2002) The contributions of Indian tuberculosis research to disease control policies have been succinctly reviewed (Chakraborty 1997, Appendix vi; Narayanan et al. 2003). Tuberculosis is a long standing, chronic epidemic which has existed for centuries in the country as seen from descriptions of this disease in ancient ayurvedic texts. The first attempt at estimating disease burden was undertaken shortly after Independence when a national sample survey for tuberculosis was conducted in the country (Indian Council of Medical Research 1959). This survey revealed the prevalence of tuberculosis and identified the requirement of increasing the infrastructure and treatment facilities for tuberculosis. In 1956 the so-called "Madras Study" demonstrated the effectiveness of ambulatory, domiciliary treatment and the fact that such treatment did not increase the risk of tuberculosis amongst family contacts (Tuberculosis Chemotherapy Centre Madras 1959). In 1963 it was demonstrated that most tuberculosis cases approached treatment facilities due to persistence of symptoms, eliminating the need for active case finding for tuberculosis (Bannerji and Andersen 1963). The feasibility of passive case finding using sputum smear microscopy for presence of acid-fast bacilli (AFB) opened the way for establishing tuberculosis diagnosis and treatment facilities in primary health centres throughout the country (Baily et al. 1967). These seminal studies led to the establishment of the National Tuberculosis Programme (NTP) in 1962, having as its core, case detection through sputum microscopy of chest symptomatics attending government health facilities on their own, supplemented by X-ray when needed, and ambulatory treatment of 12 to 18 months duration. The NTP was reviewed in the 1990's and the Revised National Tuberculosis Control Programme (RNTCP) was launched from 1992, having as its guiding principle the DOTS, i.e. directly observed treatment, short course (World Health Organization 1994). Research conducted in 1958 and in the 1980's in India has shown the impact of treatment supervision on improving cure rates, and that intermittent treatment was as efficacious as a daily treatment regimen (Tuberculosis Chemotherapy Centre Madras 1959; Tuberculosis Research Centre Madras and National Tuberculosis Institute Bangalore 1986). Both these findings are integral components of the DOTS strategy. Currently, 50% of the country is covered under the RNTCP (Granich and Chauhan 2003) whilst the NTP is in operation in the rest of the country.

In this part, we restrict the discussion to two major areas viz., estimation of disease burden and investigations to determine the time trends of the tuberculosis epidemic in the country. A more in-depth review is available (Chakraborty 1997; Dye et al. 1999).

6.10.1   Survey Tools for Tuberculosis Infection and Disease

Tuberculin as a Tool for Measuring Tuberculosis Infection

Prevalence of tuberculosis infection in the community is based on the interpretation of tuberculin test results of persons without BCG scar. Tuberculin test results in an induration which is measured between 48 and 96 hours. Size of the induration is plotted in a histogram. It is possible to identify tuberculin reactors from non-reactors, since the induration measures cluster around two modes, separated by an antimode. Four key variables are known to influence comparability between surveys. These are the use of different antigens (i.e. 1TU PPD-RT23 versus 2TU-PPD-RT23) of varying dosages of tuberculin, testing and reading variations, non-specific reactions to tuberculin and BCG immunization (Kumari Indira 2003). The widespread BCG vaccination in the country has been a major confounder in infection measurement since tuberculin reactors are found to be higher in BCG vaccinated populations than in populations that are not vaccinated. However, the problem of BCG induced tuberculin reactions can be eliminated since studies report that the waning pattern of the induration of BCG vaccinated subjects follows a pattern different from true tuberculin reactions (Chanabasavaiah et al. 1993). Another variable influencing infection studies in India is the non-specific reactions due to atypical mycobacteria. Chakraborty et al. (1976) have shown that non-specific infection increases with age, so that the majority of the population above the age group of 15 years is tuberculin positive. Infection surveys are usually carried out in children in the age group of 0–9 years, without BCG scar. Beyond 14 years of age tuberculin testing in India is of no value.

Survey Tools for Determining Disease

Examination of sputum smears for AFB and radiography have been the standard epidemiological survey tools. The specificity of microscopy is high, ranging between 98% and 99%. However, the sensitivity is relatively poor ranging between 50% and 70% or even lower. Repeated sputum examinations are known to improve the sensitivity of microscopy (Nair et al. 1976). For example, when two specimens are studied, case detection improved from 58% to 72%. Only 6% additional cases were detected if eight specimens are examined. However, under field conditions the lack of sensitivity of sputum microscopy becomes a major limitation in identifying cases of tuberculosis. Culture of concentrated bacilli from processed sputum on standard culture medium is more sensitive than microscopy, since culture detects approximately 100 bacilli per millilitre of sample. Expense has been a major limitation in the use of sputum culture in epidemiological studies in India. Transportation of samples from remote areas to the laboratory is another major problem to be addressed during surveys. Radiography has been one of the major tools in epidemiologic investigations. However, X-ray is a non-specific tool since considerable subjectivity exists in the reading of X-radiographs (Gothi et al. 1974). It is generally used in surveys for prior screening of general population groups, selecting eligibles for sputum test, but cost of X-ray is a limitation during a survey.

Survey Strategies

A list of major surveys and their outcomes have been summarized in Chakraborty (1997). Two major methodologies have been used in prevalence studies. In the "X-ray screening" approach, mass miniature radiography (MMR) of the entire population is used to identify individuals with abnormal chest shadows for sputum tests. In the "symptom-screening" method, chest symptomatics in the community have been identified through questioning individuals for the cardinal signs of tuberculosis (i.e. persistent cough, chest pain, low grade fever and hemoptysis). Individuals screened positive by this method are offered sputum examination and chest radiography. Chakraborty et al. (1994) established that estimates of prevalence of disease made by the use of either MMR followed by sputum examination or surveys based on symptom screening yielded identical data. It was subsequently pointed out that the symptom screening method resulted in a significantly higher yield of culture positive cases (Krishnamurthy 2001). One explanation of the higher yield of culture positive cases could be due to improvement in laboratory methods since it is more often found in recent studies.

Defining Disease

Comparability between surveys undertaken at various times in the country have been hampered by lack of a consensus definition of what constitutes a case of tuberculosis. A bacteriological case of tuberculosis is defined as a culture positive individual with or without a radiological abnormality. A second category of tuberculosis case is one that is radiologically positive (i.e. has chest shadows suggestive of pulmonary tuberculosis) but is bacteriologically negative. Survey results that have diagnosed cases on the basis of chest radiography have to be accepted with caution since reader variations in the interpretation of chest abnormalities is a well-known phenomenon. For example, in one study, of the initial 385 persons classified as having sputum negative X-ray active tuberculosis at the first survey, only 22% were subsequently classified as having active tuberculosis, following re-evaluation of the tuberculosis activity status in each through a five-year period of follow-up (Gothi et al. 1974).

Calculating Tuberculosis Burden   6.10.2

As explained in the earlier sections, case notifications from the public health programmes (RNTCP and NTP) cannot be used as a source of data on tuberculosis prevalence and incidence. The extent of incompleteness of the data can be illustrated with the following example. With the implementation of the DOTS strategy, record keeping has improved substantially so that it is possible to get a reliable estimate on case detection and cure rates under the public health programme. However, the discrepancy in the data reported to the World Health Organization is evident from the following data. Detection rates of smear positive cases computed for the period 1993-2000, ranged annually between 25–35 per 100,000 (Chakraborty 2004) as against an expectation of 84 per 100,000 per year, estimated by the World Health Organization for India based on the consensus statement of global rates (Dye et al. 1999). These figures indicate that either these patients are being misdiagnosed or more likely, do not present themselves to the public health system. The tuberculosis control programme has initiated strategies to include private clinicians in tuberculosis control and reporting.

Prevalence estimates of pulmonary tuberculosis have been computed from different surveys that have been conducted from time to time in the country (Chakraborty 1997). The surveys lack in uniformity since the objectives and methodologies have varied. Moreover, the surveys have been conducted in certain specified and restricted areas of the country covering different populations. Thus, the available information is neither uniform in its content nor representative of the country as a whole. The methodology employed for computing prevalence and incidence estimates from different survey results has been extensively discussed (Chakraborty 1997).

A global exercise has been conducted by Dye et al. (1999) directed towards providing an average estimate for the country. The average rates of disease and infection (both prevalence and incidence) as well as death were computed. The sources of data used for estimating prevalence and incidence included survey results, incidence of cases calculated out of the *Annual Risk of Infection* (ARI, explained below) and the likely disease rates computed from notification of cases made to the World Health Organization. The average rates for countries represent the most up to date statement of the burden (Table 6.4). Table 6.5 summarizes the tuberculosis situation in the country.

Disease burden is expressed as an average (including a range) and is used to work out control strategies and estimate the resources that will be required for the control programme. However, such average calculations cannot be used to evaluate changes in the tuberculosis epidemic in the country, for which precise rates, such as those obtained through ARI surveys described below are necessary.

The ARI gives the proportion of the population which will be primarily infected or re-infected with tubercle bacilli in the course of one year (Styblo et al. 1969). It is usually expressed as a percentage or cumulative rate. ARI is estimated through the following formula (Cauthen et al. 1988):

$$\widehat{\text{ARI}} = 1 - (1 - P)^{1/A} \,,$$

where A = average age studied and P = prevalence of infection. The method of calculating average age (A) is described in Cauthen et al. (1988). The estimated ARI is actually demonstrated to be the same as the incidence of infection, worked out by repeat testing of the same population under Indian conditions, and represents the

Table 6.4. Annual risk of tuberculosis infection in various areas in India (modified from Chakraborty 2004)

	Region	Year of survey	ARI (%)
I	*South India*		
	Kerala		
	Trivandrum	1991–1992	0.75
	Karnataka		
	Tumkur Dist	1960–1972	1.66–1.08
	Bangalore rural	1962	1.1
	Bangalore rural	1985	0.61
	Bangalore urban	1996–1999	1.67
	Chingleput rural	1969–1984	1.8–1.9
	Chingleput rural	1991–1996	2.9–3.2
II	*North India*		
	N. India rural	2000–2001	1.62
	N. India urban		2.6
	Uttar Pradesh		
	Rae Bareilly	2000–2001	2.3
	Hardoi		1.9
	Jaunpur		1.5
III	*West India*		
	Rural	2000–2002	1.5 (5.9–9.7)*
	Urban		2.4 (8.3–17.0)*
	Rajasthan	1995	1.44
	Gujarat		
	Junagadh	2000–2002	0.73
	Maharashtra	2000–2002	
	Nagpur rural		1.2 (6.34–6.38)*
	Nagpur urban		1.6 (8.44–8.50)*
	Thane rural		1.6 (8.07–8.10)*
	Thane urban		3.3 (15.75–15.80)*
IV	*East India*		
	Orissa	2000–2002	1.72 (7.5–11.3)*
	Rural		1.62 (7.2–10.3)*
	Urban		2.48 (7.7–19.8)*
	Andaman and Nicobar Island	1986	1.53
	Andaman and Nicobar Island	2002	3.8

* represents 95% confidence interval of prevalence of infection

only observational evidence ever reported (Chakraborty et al. 1992). ARI studies from different parts of India have demonstrated the differences in the tuberculosis situation in different areas in India (Table 6.4). This was also true for prevalence

Table 6.5. Rates and prevalences of tuberculosis in India (average for the country)

Prevalence of infection	38% all ages[*]
	44% all ages[#]
Prevalence of radiologically active abacillary pulmonary tuberculosis	16.0 per thousand[*]
	(3.0; 2.6–4.7)[§]
Prevalence of culture positive cases	4.0 per thousand[*]
	(6.0; 3.0–11.0)[§]
Prevalence of total pulmonary tuberculosis cases	20.0 per thousand[*]
	(9.0; 5.6–15.7)[§]
New culture positive arising annually	1.3 per thousand[*]
Mortality rate (annual)	50–80/100,000[*]
Case fatality rate (annual)	
of untreated culture positive cases[*]	14%
of all tuberculosis cases[#]	24%
Prevalence of all forms of tuberculous disease	5.05 per thousand[#]
Prevalence of smear positive cases	2.27 per thousand[#]
New smear positive arising annually	0.84 per thousand[#]

Total Indian population: 1000 million (850 million older than 5 years of age)

[*] Extrapolating observed rates from population surveys conducted in some areas of India (Chakraborty 1997, 2004).

[§] Numbers in parentheses give mean and range of corrected numbers as per results of correctional surveys carried out in India (Chakraborty 1997)

[#] As per Global Consensus Statement (Dye et al. 1999)

of tuberculosis. Prevalence and incidence of tuberculosis increased by age. Other variables influencing prevalence rates were literacy, economic status, occupation and living standards (Chakraborty 1997, Table 6.5)

6.10.3   Evaluation of Epidemiological Changes Through Time

Longitudinal studies, conducted in a few areas of the country, give an insight into tuberculosis trends. One of the first longitudinal studies was initiated in a rural population residing in 119 randomly selected villages of Bangalore district. Tuberculin surveys were undertaken at intervals of 1.5, 1.5 and 2 years. All persons above 5 years of age were X-rayed, and those with radiological abnormality were bacteriologically investigated. At this time, the tuberculosis control programme was not in operation in this area, and no intervention was available to the population. After a fourth survey, intervention was implemented. A fifth survey was undertaken in a subset of the population after eleven years from the fourth survey (Gothi et al. 1979). A sixth survey was undertaken in the area after 16 years. Twenty-three years after the first survey was initiated, a seventh survey was undertaken in 40 of the original 119 villages (Chakraborty et al. 1982). The results of this study gave one of the first opportunities to observe the time trend of tuberculosis in a rural community in India. The first five years of the study represented the natural history of the disease since there was no intervention. Prevalence and incidence of culture positive and radiologic cases revealed no change during the period of 12 years for which information was available. The mean age of cases was higher at later surveys. ARI had declined from 1.1% to 0.65% in 23 years. Incidence of smear positive cases had declined for the area from about 65 to 23 per 100,000 in the same period, parallel to the falling ARI. The above data was used to estimate future case rates with the help of a mathematical model (Balasangameshwara et al. 1992) which projected that even in 50 years, tuberculosis case rates expressed in terms of prevalence of culture positive cases would come down minimally. It also showed that more energetic and efficient tuberculosis control measures as defined in the model could, however, result in a verifiable change in case rates. Very large population sizes would be required to be surveyed repeatedly to appreciate a change if any.

The epidemic situation in India is probably on a slow downward curve as indicated by the following evidences: declining mortality and case fatality rates due to tuberculosis, decline in meningeal and miliary forms of the disease, relatively high prevalence of cases in higher age with a low rate of positive cases in children, relative concentration of cases in higher ages, higher prevalence of cases in males, especially adult males, and equal prevalence rates across the urban-rural divide. However, even if on a downward trend, the decline could be minimal, as witnessed from high ARI of 1% to 2% and an annual decline of around 0% to 3% reported from the Bangalore rural and Chennai areas (Chakraborty 2004).

Drug Resistance and HIV-TB Co-infection Studies 6.10.4

Two issues that need to be mentioned concern the estimation of drug resistant tuberculosis and HIV-TB co-morbidity in India. Monitoring drug resistance is of utmost importance, not only because drug resistant tuberculosis is more expensive to treat, but also because drug resistance is usually man-made (due to incomplete treatment) and thus indicates a poorly functioning tuberculosis control programme. Drug resistance is of concern in India, where immuno-compromised individuals living in crowded conditions such as those of urban slums would be a potent risk in furthering the transmission of drug resistant disease to the general population. With the exception of few studies, estimates of drug resistance in India have to be viewed with caution (Paramasivan 1998). At the clinical level, reports of drug resistance are often based on lack of improvement in the patient following chemotherapy or a relapse of the symptoms, unconfirmed by laboratory testing of cultures. On the other hand, reports of high incidence of drug resistance in various other studies, are often due to the very small number of patients studied. Primary drug resistance in children was found to range between 5% to 10% for streptomycin and 2% to 11% for isoniazid with nil resistance to rifampicin, suggesting that primary drug resistance is not a cause for alarm in this country. However, acquired drug resistance (i.e. drug resistance in a previously treated case) was much higher, though these data are available from limited studies (Venkataraman and Paramasivan 2003). Studies to verify these observations are ongoing in five cities in the country. Drug-resistance studies are limited by expense and by the absence of qualified laboratories capable of undertaking drug-resistance assays.

The greatest threat to tuberculosis control worldwide comes from the HIV epidemic, since tuberculosis is the only AIDS-related opportunistic infection that can significantly affect the general population. HIV surveillance in India is done by the National AIDS Control Organization (NACO) through 77 sentinel surveillance sites distributed throughout the country (National AIDS Prevention and Control Policy 2002). HIV/AIDS estimates of the country have been fraught with controversy which falls out of the scope of the current discussions (Rao 2003). There is no accurate baseline data for estimating the impact of HIV on the tuberculosis epidemic. Isolated studies have documented increasing HIV seropositivity in tuberculosis patients (Paranjape et al. 1997; Tripathy et al. 2002). Studies on the burden of HIV-TB co-morbidity are urgently required in order to determine the impact on tuberculosis control.

6.11   Conclusions

In this section, we have addressed the issue of availability of denominator and numerator data in India. The key conclusion is that systems to ensure timely, complete and accurate collection of health data have not been a priority in this country. Evidence-based data are of utmost importance in developing countries where interventions have to be implemented on the background of resource limitation. Currently, public health planning in India is based primarily on mortality statistics, supplemented by morbidity data obtained from infrequent surveys for major communicable diseases, nutritional deficiencies or morbidity in women and children. The Planning Commission, the highest authority framing developmental plans for the country, points out the dangers of this approach (Report of the Steering Committee on Health for the Xth Five Year Plan, 2002–2007, 2002). Epidemiological and demographic transition is well under way in the country, and non-communicable diseases will emerge as major public health problems in the near future. Thus, in addition to the emphasis on morbidity data on communicable diseases and health of women and children, systems to document data on chronic illnesses and disabilities need to be put in place. Furthermore, there are wide interstate differences in epidemiological transition (National Human Development Report 2001). Under these conditions it is imperative to develop a system to obtain non-aggregated and reliable data on morbidity and mortality in different States or districts in order to determine appropriate interventions required for health development and reduction in morbidity and mortality. Since in a population of more than a billion, the interventions to ensure healthy living will be many and resources will be limited as compared to the needs, disease surveillance and systems to ensure accurate and reliable morbidity data are urgently required for prioritization of interventions.

We have utilized tuberculosis epidemiology as a case study to illustrate the challenges faced by epidemiologists in deriving prevalence and incidence estimates in the absence of a complete disease reporting system. In lieu of data reporting systems, disease surveys are routinely used for obtaining denominator data. Disease surveys in a populous country like India are extremely expensive, and till now, selecting a sample that is sensitive enough to reflect the characteristics of the billion-plus population have eluded epidemiologists. Whilst discussing tuberculosis case detection, Dye et al. (2003) suggest that infrequent and isolated surveys are not the long-term solution to acquiring denominator data. Rather, the ultimate solution would be the same approach currently used in low incidence countries, namely comprehensive routine disease surveillance. Daunting as the task may appear, it is obvious that strengthening disease surveillance and HMIS systems need to be given a high priority in the country.

Acknowledgement. The authors thank Dr. N.S. Deodhar, Kavita Modi-Parekh and Mugdha Potnis-Lele for comments on the manuscript.

References

References to A

Aaby P (1997) Bandim: an unplanned longitudinal study. In: Das Gupta M, Aaby P, Garenne M, Pison G (eds) Prospective community studies in developing countries. Clarendon Press, Oxford, pp 276–296

Abel L, Demenais F, Baule MS, Blanc M, Muller A, Raffoux C, Millan J, Bois E, Babron MC, Feingold N (1989) Genetic susceptibility to leprosy on a Caribbean island: linkage analysis with fire markers. Int J Leprosy 57:465–471

Bucheton B, Abel L, Sayda El-Safi, Musa M Kheir, Pavek S, Lemainque A, Dessein AJ (2003) A major susceptibility locus on chromosome 22q12 plays a critical role in the control of kala-azar. Am J Hum Genet 73:1052–1060

Chen JS, Campbell TC, Li JY, Peto R (1991) Diet, life-style and mortality in China. A study of the characteristics of 65 Chinese counties. Oxford University Press, Oxford

Cleland J, Scott C (1987) The World Fertility survey, an assessment. Oxford University Press, Oxford

Chikobvu P, Joubert G (2003) Follow-up in longitudinal studies in the presence of HIV/AIDS: The Bloemfontein Vitamin trial, a case study. In: Bull International Statistical Institute 54th Session Proceedings, Invited Paper Meeting 54, ISI, Den Hague

Cochran WG (1977) Sampling techniques. 3rd edn. Wiley, New York

Das Gupta M, Aaby P, Garenne M, Pison G (eds) (1997) Prospective community studies in developing countries. Clarendon Press, Oxford

Dessein AJ, Hillaire D, Nasr Eldin MA Elwali, Marquet S, Qurashi Mohamed-Ali, Mirghani A, Henri S, Ahmed A Abdelhameed, Osman K Saeed, Mubarak MA Magzoub, Abel A (1999) Severe hepatic fibrosis in *schistosoma mansoni* infection is controlled by a major locus that is closely linked to the interferon-g receptor gene

Henderson RH, Sundaresan T (1982) Cluster sampling to assess immunization coverage: a review of experience with a simplified sampling method. Bull World Health Organization 60:253–260

INDEPTH (2002) INDEPTH, health and demography in developing countries, vol 1: Population, health and survival at INDEPTH sites. IDRC, Ottawa

Krickeberg K (1989) Intégration des soins de santé primaires. Lecture at the Faculty of Medicine of Phnom Penh, January 1989. Séminaire de Statistique Médicale, Université de Paris V (1989–90), pp 45–69

Krickeberg K (1994) Health information in developing countries. In: Frontiers in Mathematical Biology, Lecture Notes in Biomathematics 100:550–568

Krickeberg K (1999) The health information system in Vietnam in 1999. Joint Health Systems Development Programme Vietnam-EU (Unpublished report, available from the author: krik@ideenwelt.de)

Krickeberg K (2003) Health information systems in developing countries. Bull International Statistical Institute 54th Session Proceedings, Invited Paper Meeting 54. ISI, Den Hague

Lippeveld T, Sauerborn R, Bodart C (eds) (2000) Design and implementation of health information systems. World Health Organization, Geneva

Mims (1982) Innate immunity to parasitic infections. In: Cohen S, Warren K (eds) Immunology of parasitic infections. Blackwell, Palo Alto, pp 3–27

Ministerio de Salud Pública y Asistencia Social (2002) Línea basal de mortalidad materna para el año 2000. Guatemala

Molineaux L, Gramiccia G (1980) Le projet Garki. Organisation Mondiale de la Santé, Genève

Nguyen Thi Kim Chuc, Diwan V, Dao Lan Huong, Byass P (2003) Public health in Bavi, Vietnam – a collaborative project. Scand J Public Health 31 (Supplement 62)

Wawer MJ (2001) Research collaborations in developing countries. In: Thomas JC, Weber DJ (eds) Epidemiologic methods for the study of infectious diseases. Oxford University Press, Oxford, Chap. 21, pp 431–447

Yé V, Sanou A, Gbangou A, Kouyaté B (2002) The Nouna demographic surveillance system, Burkina Faso. In: INDEPTH, health and demography in developing countries, vol 1: Population, health and survival at INDEPTH sites. IDRC, Ottawa, pp 221–226

References to B

Baily GVJ, Savic D, Gothi GD, Naidu VB, Nair SS (1967) Potential yield of pulmonary tuberculosis cases by direct microscopy of sputum in a district of South India. Bull World Health Organ 37:875–892

Balasangameshwara VH, Chakraborty AK, Chaudhuri K (1992) A mathematical construct of epidemiological time trend in tuberculosis – fifty year study. Ind J Tuber 39:87–98

Bannerji D, Andersen S (1963) A sociological study of awareness of symptoms amongst persons with pulmonary tuberculosis. Bull World Health Organ 29:665–669

Cauthen GM, Pio A, ten Dam HG (1988) Annual risk of tuberculous infection. WHO/TB/88.154, 1–34 World Health Organization, Geneva

Census of India (2001) Provisional population totals – India, Paper 1 of 2001. Registrar General and Census Commissioner of India, Government of India, New Delhi

Chakraborty AK (1997) Prevalence and incidence of TB infection and disease in India: A comprehensive review. WHO/TB/97.231-World Health Organization, Geneva

Chakraborty AK (2004) Current status of the epidemiology of tuberculosis in India: A review in the global context. (in press)

Chakraborty AK, Ganapathy KT, Nair SS, Bhushan K (1976) Prevalence of non-specific sensitivity to tuberculin in a South Indian population. Ind J Med Res 64(57):639–651

Chakraborty AK, Singh H, Srikantan K, Rangawsamy KR, Krishnamurthy MS, Stephen JA (1982) Tuberculosis in a rural population of South India: Report on five surveys. Ind J Tuber 29:153–167

Chakraborty AK, Chaudhury K, Sreenivas TR, Krishnamurthy MS, Shashidhara AN, Channabasavaiah R (1992) Tuberculosis infection in a rural population of South India: 23 year trend. Tubercle and Lung Dis 73:213–218

Chakraborty AK, Channabasavaiah R, Krishnamurthy MS, Shashidhara AN, Krishnamurthy W, Choudhary K (1994) Prevalence of pulmonary tuberculosis in a peri-urban community of Bangalore under various methods of population screening. Ind J Tuber 41:17–27

Chanabasavaiah R, Mohan M, Suryanarayana HV, Krishnamurthry MS, Shashidhara AN (1993) Waning of the BCG scar. Ind J Tuber 40:137–141

Duggal R (2000) The private health sector in India. Nature, trends and a critique. Voluntary Health Association of India, New Delhi

Dye C, Scheele S, Dolin P, Pathania V, Raviglione M (1999) Global burden of tuberculosis. Estimated incidence, prevalence and mortality by country. JAMA 282:677–686

Dye C, Watt CJ, Bleed DM, Williams BG (2003) What is the limit to case detection under the DOTS strategy for tuberculosis control? In: Glimpses. Selected full text articles presented at the 4th World Congress on Tuberculosis. Washington, DCUSA June 3–5, 2002. TB Care, India, pp 14–22

Gothi GD, Chakraborty AK, Banerjee GC (1974) Interpretations of photoflurograms of active pulmonary tuberculosis patients found in epidemiological survey and their five year fate. Ind J Tuber 21:90–97

Gothi GD, Chakraborty AK, Nair SS, Ganapathy KT, Banerjee GC (1979) Prevalence of tuberculosis in a South Indian District twelve years after initial survey. Ind J Tuber 26:121–135

Granich R, Chauhan LS (2003) Status report of the Revised National Tuberculosis Control Programme. J Ind Med Assoc 101(3):150–156

Health Status Report Maharashtra (2003) Public Health Department, Government of Maharashtra, Maharashtra

Indian Council of Medical Research (1959) Tuberculosis in India: A sample survey, 1955–58. Special Report series No. 34, ICMR, New Delhi India, pp 1–121

Indian Council of Medical Research (2001) National cancer registry programme. Consolidated report of the population based cancer registries, 1990–96. ICMR, New Delhi India

Krishnamurthy MS (2001) Problems of estimating the burden of pulmonary tuberculosis in India: a review. Ind J Tuber 48:193–198

Kumari Indira K (2003) Tuberculin survey: An appraisal of its future role in India. Health Admn XV 1–2:175–181

Nair SS, Gothi GD, Naganathan N, Rao KP, Banerjee GC, Rajalakshmi R (1976) Precision of estimates of prevalence of bacteriologically confirmed pulmonary tuberculosis in general population. Ind J Tuber 23:152–159

Narasimhan RL, Retherford RD, Mishra V, Arnold F, Roy TK (1997) Comparison of fertility estimates from India's sample registration system and national family health survey. National Family Health Survey Subject Reports No 4 Mumbai: International Institute for Population Sciences; and Honolulu: East-West Center, USA

Narayanan PR, Garg R, Santha T, Kumaran PP (2003) Shifting the focus of tuberculosis research in India. In: Glimpses. Selected full text articles presented at the 4th World Congress on Tuberculosis Washington, DC USA June 3–5, 2002. TBCare India, pp 58–65

National AIDS Prevention and Control Policy (2002) National AIDS Control Organization Ministry of Health and Family Welfare. New Delhi, India

National Family Health Survey (NFHS-2), 1998–99 (2000) International Institute for Population Sciences Mumbai India, and ORC. Macro Calverton, Maryland, USA (http://www.nfhsindia.org) Accessed May 18, 2004

National Health Policy (2002) Ministry of Health and Family Welfare, Government of India, Nirman Bhavan, New Delhi

National Human Development Report (2001) Planning Commission Government of India March 2002

National Polio Surveillance Project (http://www.npspindia.org) Accessed May 18, 2004

National Sample Survey Organisation (1998) Morbidity and treatment of ailments 52nd Round (July 1995–June 1998). Report No. l, 449, Department of Statistics, New Delhi

Paramasivan CN (1998) An overview of drug resistant tuberculosis in India. Ind J Tuber 45:73–81

Paranjape RS, Tripathy SP, Menon PA (1997) Increasing trend of HIV seroprevalence among pulmonary tuberculosis patients in Pune, India. Ind J Med Res 106:207–211

Rao AS (2003) Can we obtain realistic HIV/AIDS estimates for India? J Biosci 28:367–369

Report of Health Survey and Development Committee (1946) In: Compendium of recommendations of various committees on health and development 1943–1975. Central Bureau of Health Intelligence, Directorate General of Health Services, Ministry of Health and Family Welfare, Government of India, New Delhi

Report of the Steering Committee on Health for the Xth Five Year Plan, 2002–2007 (2002) Government of India, Planning Commission, New Delhi

Sample Registration System (SRS) Bulletin (2001) Volume 35, No. 1 Registrar General and Census Commissioner. India, Vital Statistics Division, New Delhi

Singh P (1999) National family health survey, 1992–93: Post survey check. Economic and Political Weekly 34:3084–3088

Styblo K, Meijer J, Sutherland I (1969) The transmission of tubercle bacilli, its trend in a human population. TSRU report No 1. Bull Int Union Tub XLII:1–104

Tripathy S, Joshi DR, Mehendale SM, Menon P, Joshi AN, Ghorpade SV, Patil U, Paranjape RS (2002) Sentinel surveillance for HIV infection in tuberculosis patients in India. Ind J Tuber 49:17–21

Tuberculosis Chemotherapy Centre, Madras (1959). A concurrent comparison of home and sanatorium treatment of pulmonary tuberculosis in South India. Bull World Health Organ 21:51–144

Tuberculosis Research Centre Madras and National Tuberculosis Institute Bangalore (1986) A controlled clinical trial of 3- and 5-month regimens for the treatment of sputum positive pulmonary tuberculosis in South India. Am Rev Respir Dis 134:27–33

Venkataraman P, Paramasivan CN (2003) Drug resistance in tuberculosis and issues related to multidrug resistance in planning for TB control in India. Health Admin Vol XV, No 1–2:127–136

World Health Organization (1994) Global tuberculosis programme. Framework for effective tuberculosis control. Document WHO/TB/94.179. World Health Organization, Geneva

World Health Organization (2002) Global tuberculosis control – surveillance, planning, financing. Document WHO/CDS/TB/2002.295. World Health Organization, Geneva

Ethical Aspects
of Epidemiological Research

IV.7

Hubert G. Leufkens, Johannes J.M. van Delden

Introduction

> Every UK citizen has the right to medical care, but those rights also involve responsibilities. Better treatments that save more lives come from research into previous patients' experience.
>
> Peto (2001)

> I think you need to give conscious consent to having any data, any personal data used, whether you are identified or not. That's certainly a right. That's your information, it's your medical history. Whether it's identified or not, you should control it.
>
> Patient 14, in Willison et al. (2003)

These two quotes are about values and expectations, about perceived responsibilities, about community benefits and individual rights in medical care and research, and reflect thereby compellingly the tensions, the paradoxes, the different views and ethical aspects concerning biomedical research (Coughlin 2000). Epidemiology is part of the arena of biomedical research and is particularly focussed on determinants of disease occurrences in populations. Ethics is the systematic analysis of values and norms (Weed and Coughlin 1999; Weed and McKeown 2001). Usually ethical reasoning and conduct are not issues that are at the top of a epidemiologist's menu chart (Beauchamp et al. 1991). In previous chapters of this handbook we have seen that most epidemiological methods are non-interventional, e.g. observational by design, meaning that conventional ethical aspects of experiments with human beings (e.g. protocol review, randomisation, placebos, informed consent, etc.) are not applicable as such. Many ethical committees have been struggling with the review of protocols of non-interventional studies because of the rationale and design of the study being directed at not influencing the 'natural' disease course of patients, but at determining statistical inferences between various exposures (e.g. environment, drug treatment, medical practice) and effects in the population in a non-experimental fashion. Observational epidemiology possesses the attractiveness, but also the practical paradox, of scientific investigation with a priori objective of not intervening in the normal course of the study object.

There have been several drivers within and outside the field of epidemiology that have changed the picture of ethical aspects significantly over the last decades. First of all, since the mid-eighties of the last century the development and availability of automated record linkage databases, capturing both exposure and outcome data on an individual level, have raised questions about confidentiality of patient's medical records, authorizing access to person-specific information, and misuse of such databases (Knox 1992). A second driver has been the debate about integrity and conflict of interests related to epidemiological research, in particular in cases of sponsored epidemiological studies and/or when the results of such studies were contradictory and subject of controversy and discourse. Finally, the growing interest of epidemiologists to include molecular variables in their studies (e.g. laboratory data, biomarkers, genetic factors) has fuelled ethical questions and debate about the design, conduct and what to do with the study results of such epidemiological research.

As a consequence, the last decades have shown that concern about the ethical aspects of their research activities has become engaging epidemiologists as much as others who deal with public health, clinical decision making, prioritising and policy making in health care. Ethics guidelines have been prepared and accepted by several epidemiological organizations (Bankowski et al. 1991; IEA 1998) in response to a growing awareness among epidemiologists that ethical conduct is essential to epidemiology. Basic principles of integrity, honesty, truthfulness, fairness and equity, respect for people's autonomy, distributive justice, doing good and not harming have been made explicit. Essentially, the appreciation of these values have their origins in the follow-up of the Nuremberg trials, the UN Declaration on Human Rights, the Declaration of Helsinki, and many later declarations, guidelines and codes of conduct. Basically, these declarations and guidelines reflect a major shift in current society from less priority to collective interests and benefits towards the primacy and protection of the individual (World Medical Association 2000; Coughlin 2000).

Drivers of Awareness of Ethical Aspects in Epidemiology 7.2

Surge of Automated Databases 7.2.1

One of the visionary founders of medical registries has been William Farr who understood already in the nineteenth' century clearly the importance and potential of keeping person-specific records on diagnoses, medical treatments, environmental factors and disease course (Farr 1875). Later various approaches of building and linking datasets for evaluating medical treatments and other determinants of health have been developed. In the early sixties and seventies of the twentieth century, consistent and protocol based medical record keeping became also recognized as an essential tool for clinical practice, and worldwide famous centres of clinical and epidemiological excellence like the Mayo Clinics or the Oxford Radcliff Infirmary earned their appreciation mainly because they were champions in collecting and managing clinically relevant person-specific information in an era when paper charts, pencils and several primitive collecting and retrieving machineries where state of the art technologies (Gostin 1997). The introduction of advanced computer and information technologies changed that picture dramatically in the mid and late eighties of the twentieth century. Storing, assembling and linking clinical information became 'push button' actions and fascinating avenues for epidemiological research capturing data of hundreds of thousands, even millions, of individuals became feasible (Quantin et al. 1998). However, the 'push button' nature and the big numbers involved of these developments gave rise to various ethical questions, in the beginning still vaguely phrased but later in very pronounced way on the table.

The overwhelmingness of the potentials of new information technologies and the speed of the developments have driven the need for a comprehensive balance sheet of all the social, political and ethical aspects involved. Moreover, the owners and stake holders of these automated databases are usually not health care providers or professionals but third party payers, e.g. health insurers, Health Maintenance Organisations, or governmental bodies. These organisations have mostly not their origins in the professional and ethical environment of Hippocratic medicine, and have invested in these data systems with other purposes (e.g. reimbursement of health care providers, cost-containment, risk management) than supporting medical practice (Gostin 1997).

The surge of automated databases has been stirred by the progress in record linkage techniques. Record linkage is the process by which pairs of correctly matched records of person-specific information are brought together in such a fashion that they may be treated as a single record for one individual (Herings et al. 1992). Record linkage provides a powerful tool in epidemiology in order to stratify exposures according to patient outcomes, e.g. bringing data together on food intake and cancer events, or exposure to sleeping pills and hospitalisations for hip fracture. Record linkage has driven the expansion of automated databases and from an ethical point of view there has been at least two major concerns (Herings et al. 1992; Kelman et al. 2002). First of all the operational process of linkage of individual data from a number of sources using a unique person-specific ID (identification) requires patient identification. Researchers in epidemiology have developed for that reason probabilistic approaches of record linkage, using sets of in itself not unique identifiers. However, it is believed by some opponents that this approach of record linkage may also violate data confidentiality rules i.e. each pseudonymised method needs to be validated and then the use of person-specific data (e.g. name or other ID) is essential (Tondel and Axelson 1999). A second concern related to record linkage has always been the fear that (non)medical data (e.g. insurance status, life style, sexual behaviour, socio-economic position) are built-in epidemiological data frames enhancing the feasibility of making unintended and/or undesirable statistical inferences that could cause damage or distress to individuals (Kmietowicz 2001). As a consequence, in the advent of a surge in automated databases, many countries both in North America and Europe have taken comprehensive legal action to assure the protection of personal privacy (Vandenbroucke 1992; UK Parliament Acts 1998; US DHHS 2001; de Vet et al. 2003).

Today's balance sheet of the role of automated databases in epidemiological research looks very positive. Cancer epidemiology, cardiovascular epidemiology, pharmacoepidemiology are branches in epidemiology where such databases are key resources. They all have in common complex multivariate and time-dependent exposure-disease occurrences. Confidentiality of person-specific information is one of the most imperative ethical aspects to consider. We will come back to this later on in this chapter.

Integrity and Conflict of Interest in Epidemiological Research

In the 'ideal' world, basic values of integrity, objectivity, respect and independence should be key to every field of science. Committed to the discovering of the truth, researchers design, conduct and report on study results (Levinski 2002). This notion gives the impression of science being a logical and unbiased human activity. Current society has long relied on scientists' professional commitment to truth and honesty. However, disclosure of for instance a case of fraud by a Dutch neurologist participating in the 'European stroke prevention study 2' (ESPS-2), a multicentre stroke study, scandalized both the medical research community and the public (Hoeksema et al. 2003). The neurologist had committed fraud, in the sense that he had used names and fingered data of existing patients without these patients actually being enrolled in the study. Recently, the University of Connecticut in the US announced clear misconduct by a vaccine expert who had falsified preliminary data in two grant applications (Malakoff 2003). The university removed the expert as head of the research centre and a series of lawsuits between the university and the vaccine researchers took place. We notice here two obvious cases of serious misconduct in biomedical science, e.g. doctoring of data. Other examples of questionable and unethical scientific behaviour include apparent study sponsor induced bias, as well known from research sponsored by the tobacco industry into the association between smoking and lung cancer (Barnes and Bero 1998), and at the very end of the spectrum, fraud and falsification of data. We will come back to industry sponsoring of epidemiological research into drug effects. But there are other more subtle constraints to scientific integrity.

In 2002 Levinski gave a very personal and historical account on how he started as a medical researcher, and reflecting visibly on major ethical questions, e.g. the protection and reimbursement of human research subjects, informed consent, disclosure of financial interests, prestige of the academic institution and personal career building. The account also shows that ethical weighing can vary strongly over time. What we believed as being ethically acceptable in the past, might not be today or vice versa:

In 1963, before the advent of institutional review boards (IRBs), I was a young academic physician studying the regulation of sodium excretion by the kidneys. I paid medical students approximately $50 to serve as subjects for experiments involving only saline infusions and the collection of blood and spontaneously voided urine samples. I do not remember exactly what I told the students about the risks of the experiments but am quite certain that I characterized them as nominal. In one subject, severe phlebitis developed at the site of an intravenous

infusion and required extensive therapy. The research project was funded by the National Institutes of Health. I had no possibility of financial gain from it. My primary motive was academic – the desire to advance knowledge about an important physiological mechanism with a bearing on clinical conditions such as edema. A potent secondary motive was to advance my career by publishing the results of the research and maintaining grant support – academic currency that buys prestige and promotion.
(Levinski 2002).

For epidemiology, conflicts of interest related to research sponsoring are a very contemporary and controversial issue. Thompson has defined conflicts of interests as

a set of conditions in which professional judgment concerning a primary interest (such as a patient's welfare or the validity of research) tends to be unduly influenced by a secondary interest (such as financial gain)
(Thompson 1993).

Financial interests related to the tobacco industry have been subject of intense controversy since decades. This industry has been always active in engaging researchers (as well as public media) for promoting messages contrary to the available epidemiological evidence on health risks of both active and passive smoking. In the field of epidemiology of drug effects two archetypal cases have paved the pathway of debate and controversy on the ethics of research sponsoring, conflict of interest and scientific (mis)conduct:

Cardiovascular Risks of Calcium-Channel Blockers

In 1995 Psaty et al. reported in the JAMA about a population-based case-control study among hypertensive patients in order to assess the association between first myocardial infarction and the use of antihypertensive agents (i.e., beta-blockers, calcium-channel blockers, angiotensin-converting-enzyme inhibitors, diuretics). The main result of the study was that the use of short-acting calcium-channel blockers, especially in high doses, was associated with an increased risk of myocardial infarction (Psaty et al. 1995). An intense controversy on the scientific validity of the study, the consequences for treatment of patients with hypertension, and the financial implications for the companies marketing calcium-channel blockers followed in both the medical literature and the lay press. A surge of commentaries, reviews and additional papers on the topic emerged in the literature. Stelfox et al. (1998) evaluated the obviously visible signatures of the debate in the medical literature and demonstrated a strong association between authors' opinions about the safety of calcium-channel blockers and their financial relationships with those industries having an apparent interest in the hypertension market. Supportive authors had more financial ties with manufacturers of calcium-channel antagonists, while critical authors were much less likely to be involved in industry sponsoring and other financial connections with manufacturers. Although the paper of Stelfox et al. could be criticized for methodological reasons (lack of adjustment for dynamics of actions-reactions of time in the aftermath of the Psaty et al. paper) the overall message remains valid: there is and has been an association between ties with sponsors, choice of study questions and, possibly, study results.

Venous Thrombosis Risk of Oral Contraceptives

In the same year as the calcium-channel blocker controversy emerged 1995, several case-control studies reported on a two-fold increased risk of deep vein thrombosis and pulmonary embolism in females using the so-called third generation oral contraceptives relative to second-generation oral contraceptives (Skegg 2001). These findings engendered a surge of further (for the most part case-control) studies primarily driven by questions on possible confounding by indication (e.g. health user effect meaning preferential prescribing of third generation oral contraceptives to females with more risk factors of cardiovascular disease) and biases related to the method of exposure ascertainment to oral contraceptives.

Many of these studies were sponsored by the pharmaceutical industry and Vandenbroucke observed a contrast between the industry sponsored studies reporting a relative risk of 1.5 or less and the non-funded studies consistently showing an increased risk of about 2.0 (Vandenbroucke 1998) (see also Fig. 7.1).

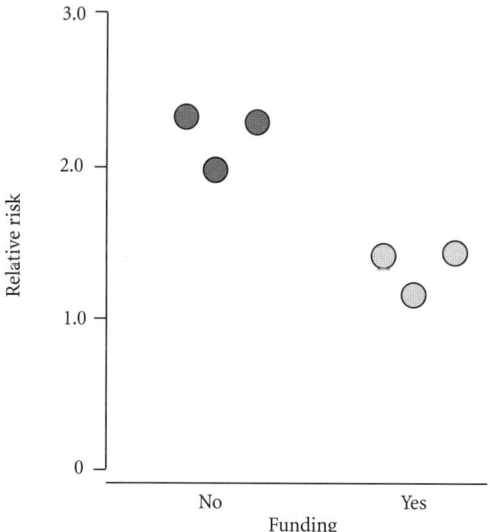

Figure 7.1. Risk of venous thrombosis with third-generation contraceptives stratified for industry sponsoring. From Vandenbroucke (1998)

Answering the question whether this contrast is real, implicating that industry sponsorship is followed by biased research, is much more difficult to answer and is still subject of an ongoing debate. To illustrate the bewildering impression fuelled by the array of conflicting studies captured in Fig. 7.1, Vandenbroucke quotes a pharmacologist involved in early-phase studies for the industry:

> ... this might very well mean that industry-sponsored studies are the better ones
> (Vandenbroucke 1998).

Like in case of the calcium-channel blockers controversy, a surge of commentaries and additional papers on the topic emerged in the literature and the public press. Moreover, as the topic was also subject for several court cases, the legal press covered the issue as well. This controversy has been one of the most striking examples in the last decade of how to find the truth in studying drug exposure-outcome associations, to unravel possible biases and confounding factors, dealing with study sponsor's interests, and at the same time to protect scientific integrity. Researchers are exposed to myriad pressures (e.g. balancing individual and institutional needs, search for professional recognition, and sometimes, even rivalry). The science arena operates as a function of all the influences and pressures. Most progress to untangle the individual impact of all these factors has been made in demanding at least disclosure of all financial interests of the researcher by virtually all scientific journals and scientific communities (Levinski 2002). Epidemiologists need to continue to improve scientific and ethical conduct, to prevent unwanted conflicts of interest and to be aware of the great financial interests of the parties involved (Beauchamp et al. 1991; Coughlin 2000). Various avenues to achieve this goal are either proposed or already in place: (1) codes of ethical conduct are adopted by virtually all professional and scientific societies, (2) the same holds for guidelines for disclosure of possible conflict of interests by authors submitting papers to medical-scientific journals, (3) there is a surge both at the medical and other life science faculties, to include ethics classes in their standard curricula. In addition we think that researchers should submit a declaration of any potential conflicts of interest affecting the study to an institutional review board. These boards should evaluate each study in light of any declared conflicts and ensure that adequate means of mitigation are provided. When appropriate, the board may also require that a potentially conflicting interest be part of the information provided to the respondents. If a potentially serious conflict of interest cannot be adequately mitigated, the committee should not approve the project.

7.2.3   Molecular Epidemiology and Genetics

Molecular epidemiology is a rapidly emerging field and in Chaps. III.6 and III.7 of this handbook we have seen up-to-date accounts on scientific achievements and progress. A growing number of population based molecular epidemiology studies have been set up to explore the roles of molecular factors (e.g. immune response profiling, blood clotting factors, enzymes) and gene mutations and polymorphisms in disease occurrences (Maitland-van der Zee et al. 2000; Nuffield

Council on Bioethics 2003). Issues about participants' consent, confidentiality of information, and the feedback of findings, have been widely addressed. Growing knowledge about molecular pathway-disease associations have led to new opportunities for testing, increasingly important as a guide to prevention, clinical management, and pharmacotherapy. Tests are likely to vary in their predictive value, analytic and clinical validity, clinical utility, and social implications, e.g. access to and affordability of testing, insurance or employment discrimination, stigmatisation, and long-term psychological harms from testing. Molecular epidemiology applying these tests is distinct from most other types of epidemiological research in that such biomarkers or genetic data obtained about an individual also may provide signatures of health about his or her relatives and person-specific future events. For example, concerning the latter, the implications of a positive test for the breast cancer genes BRCA1 or BRCA2 mutation differ considerably for a woman who has not yet had children compared with one who has daughters who might be susceptible as well (Burke et al. 1997).

A pivotal and informative case in identifying and understanding the ethical aspects of these developments is the area of pharmacogenetics (Bolt et al. 2002). The increasing knowledge on the genome has resulted on unprecedented advances in understanding why individuals respond differently to drug therapy (Venter et al. 2001; Roses 2000). Pharmacogenetics focuses on the question of the extent to which genetic variants are responsible for inter-individual variability in drug response among recipients of a specific drug therapy. Few drug therapies are effective for everyone. The ultimate goal of pharmacogenetics is to shape therapy with available medicines in an individualised fashion, e.g. 'tailor-made pharmacotherapy'. Pharmacogenetics integrates epidemiology, pharmacology and genetics and is focussed on an understanding of the genetic determinants of individual variability in drug therapy (Maitland-van der Zee et al. 2000). This research parallels the surge in discoveries of genes and protein expression patterns affecting the susceptibility to disease. There is evidence that certain disease susceptibility genes are also determining drug action, and thereby therapy response.

The Nuffield Council on Bioethics (2003) has identified a number of ethical issues specifically raised by pharmacogenetics: (1) consent, privacy and confidentiality (2) management of information about response to therapy likelihood (3) implications of differentiating individuals into groups based on response to therapy likelihood. The key question in pharmacogenetics is unravelling the genetic traits of efficacy and/or safety of medicines. When that information is available it can guide prescribers to select specific drugs or dosage schemes. Recently, it has been shown that on the one hand male carriers of the Apolipoprotein-E 44 variant are more prone to discontinue therapy with anticholesterol lowering agents (Maitland-van der Zee et al. 2003). Although the precise mechanism underlying this association is still not known, prescribers, pharmacists, and patients can improve therapy knowing this risk-factor of non persistence by enhancing compliance with the regimen, tailor-made counselling and the like. On the other hand, we know that Apolipoprotein-E is also associated with various cardiovascular and neurological risks (e.g. Alzheimer disease). The level of evidence of the mentioned

Apolipoprotein-E associations is still subject of ongoing research and all the three ethical issues mentioned by the Nuffield Council on Bioethics are visibly present in this case. This is particularly true in an area where we don't know today what kind of new genetic traits are discovered tomorrow and what kind of implications that has for already collected biological material (e.g. DNA samples). We see a surge in post-hoc genotyping in both clinical and epidemiological research. This is feasible as individual genetics do not change over time and when biological samples (blood, urine or buccal cells) are still available, a major ethical question is whether the informed consent (maybe completed decades ago!) still holds for the current new situation. And what about the ethical questions provoked by genotyping cases and controls in for instance a case-control study revealing that certain study subjects carry serious susceptibility genes (e.g. BRCA1 or BRCA2 mutations)? Genotyping of the cases may be well covered by informed consent in the protocol, but this may be not valid for the controls sampled from the study base anonymously. And what about the 'right not to know' of both the study subjects and their inherited relatives?

The application of pharmacogenetics information to drug development also fuels ethical questions. Preferential inclusion of tested full responders into clinical trials increases the efficiency of such programs. However, such an approach would hide important information about the actions of the drug in other patients. In case the group of responders would be (too) small to develop the compound to an economically feasible medicine, the industry might decide to discontinue the project. The latter picture has led to the illustrious quote 'Will all drugs become orphans?' (Maitland-van der Zee et al. 2000)

7.3 Ethical Principles: Weighing Ethical 'Benefits' and 'Costs'

On the background of all the developments addressed so far, ethical principles are highly prevalent, but in many cases badly defined, virtually invisible or denied. Weighing of ethical 'benefits' and 'costs' is becoming an essential, additional perspective in designing and conducting sound epidemiological research (Nilstun and Westrin 1994). In the late eighties of the last century the Americans Beauchamp and Childress proposed four ethical principles in order to provide a more or less neutral, analytical framework to help doctors, researchers and all others who are engaged in medical decision and policy making, when reflecting on moral issues that arise at work: respect for autonomy, beneficence, non-maleficence, and justice (Beauchamp and Childress 1989). Despite rapid and thought-provoking changes in medical technology and the practice of medicine, we believe that these four principles, plus attention to their scope of application, may encompass most of the moral issues that arise in today's health care and public health arena (Gillon 1994, 2003).

Autonomy

Autonomy is a widely discussed principle in bioethics and the word has several meanings. By and large, however, two focusses can be discerned: on the one hand autonomy can be perceived as a right to self-determination, and on the other as an ideal of deliberated self rule. The first is about sovereignty, the second about authenticity. With respect to research ethics, autonomy is most visible in the practice of informed consent. Autonomy may be infringed if individuals are denied the right to choose whether or not to be enrolled in clinical or epidemiological research. Respecting people's autonomy requires consulting patients or other study subjects and obtaining their agreement before inclusion in a study. Medical confidentiality is an instrument to protect privacy, which in itself is based on the respect for a patient's autonomy.

Privacy refers to freedom of the person to choose for himself or herself the time and circumstances under which and, most importantly, the extent to which, his or her attitudes, beliefs, behaviour, and opinions are to be shared with or withheld from others. Confidentiality refers to managing private information; when a subject shares private information with (confides in) an investigator, the investigator is expected to refrain from sharing this information with others without the subject's authorisation or some other justification. Without confidentiality patients will be also far less open about all their personal concerns, symptoms and other pieces of highly private information. Such information is very often critical to assign diagnoses and treatment scenarios to individual patients. This will have implications for clinical practice, but also for research. Study subjects should have more than enough reasons to trust researchers. Respecting autonomy also means not abusing this trust.

Beneficence and Non-maleficence

The principle of beneficence means that health-care professionals and investigators have a responsibility to do good for those whom they treat. The traditional Hippocratic moral obligation of medicine is to provide net medical benefit to patients with minimal harm. Therefore, beneficence and non-maleficence are viewed as basic components of a balance sheet aiming at producing net benefit over harm. For epidemiology this means that a research project should add to the existing knowledge base on exposure-disease occurrences in order to treat populations of patients effectively and to prevent health hazards or even mortality in the community. In epidemiology the interests, and thereby the benefits, for the individual patient are less obvious, since often no treatment is offered. However, part of the benefit that communities, groups and individuals may reasonably expect from participating in studies is that they will be told of findings that pertain to their health. Where findings could be applied in public health measures to improve community health, they should be communicated to the health authorities. In informing individuals of the findings and their pertinence to health, their level of literacy and comprehension must be considered. Research protocols should include provision for communicating such information to communities and individuals (Bankowski et al. 1991).

The principle of non-maleficence applied to epidemiology reflects the moral obligation not to do harm to study subjects. In many cases of research it is still uncertain what the benefits are of a specific intervention (as this is part of the study question). The principle of non-maleficence teaches that at least participating in the study should do no harm and should involve only minimal risks. Likewise, epidemiological investigators studying activities that pose risks to the well-being of subjects are ethically obligated to propose to subjects with whom they interact any feasible steps that can be taken to minimise their exposure to risk. Furthermore, harm may occur, for instance, when scarce health personnel are diverted from their routine duties to serve the needs of a study, or when, unknown to a community, its health-care priorities are changed. It is wrong to regard members of communities as only impersonal material for study, even if they are not harmed. Ethical review must always assess the risk of subjects or groups suffering stigmatization, prejudice, loss of prestige or self-esteem, or economic loss as a result of taking part in a study.

7.3.3   Justice

This principle underpins the moral obligation of a fair distribution of burdens and benefits between people. One way of looking at justice is treating those with equal need equally. Justice can also be described as the requirement to act on the basis of fair settlement between competing claims or demands. Equity is at the heart of justice, and since centuries people have argued about the morally relevant criteria for regarding and treating people as equals and those for regarding and treating them as unequals. This principle has become prominent in an era of cost-containment and rationing of health care resources. Allocation of resources may conflict between several common moral concerns (e.g. individual access to and affordability of resources, fair distribution of scarcity, autonomy of professionals to make the best decisions for their patients). All concerns may be morally justified but not all can be fully met simultaneously. Epidemiology is the science of land-scaping and explaining differences (in health, socio-economic status, resources, risk factors) within populations and is thereby a critical 'monitor' of (in)equity (Weed and McKeown 2001).

7.3.4   Balancing the Four Principles

Although, all the four principles together are seen as a comprehensive frame for moral reflection in medicine and epidemiology, we can observe a shift in emphasis and a greater prominence of autonomy as the leading manual for ethical conduct. This shift of putting the individual first is welcomed with mixed feelings and has made balancing individual rights with those of the whole society to become a key issue in contemporary Western society:

Autonomy is, then, de facto given a place of honour because the trust of individualism, whether from the egalitarian left or the market oriented right, is to give people maximum liberty in devising their own lives and values. (Callahan 2003).

Nilstun and Westrin have proposed a model to cross the four ethical principles with the perspectives of each of the parties involved, and then to assess and weigh the ethical 'benefits' and 'costs' for each individual party in the event the study is or is not conducted (Nilstun and Westrin 1994). Earlier in this chapter we have addressed the scientific and political debate about the risk of deep vein thrombosis and pulmonary embolism in females using the so-called third generation oral contraceptives relative to second-generation agents. In 1999 Herings et al. published a follow-up study on this topic using anonymous exposure data related to females using one of these oral contraceptives and anonymous, but person-specific, outcomes data on hospitalizations for either deep vein thrombosis or pulmonary embolism (Herings et al. 1999). The study confirmed the differential risk between the two categories of oral contraceptives and showed that the highest risk was in young females, newly starting with this contraceptive method. We use the study accessible through this paper to illustrate the model of Nilstun and Westrin.

The analysis starts with identifying the relevant parties (females using OC, society at large, industry, prescribers). In Table 7.1 possible outcomes of an analysis of the most relevant 'benefits' and 'costs' are listed concerning the two dimensions of ethical principles and parties involved in the event that the study will be conducted. If the study is done, there are possible 'benefits' for society at large, for prescribers, for (other) women using oral contraceptives. For the industry the conduct of the study results in an ambiguous picture. Manufactures of the second generation oral contraceptives considered the study as 'good news', for manufactures of the third generation the results of the study were less favourable. For industry as a whole one may argue that every piece of science that contributes to the benefit-risk balance is advantageous, although this is not perceived like this in real life. Although this is reasonably understandable, it marks also the complexity and paradoxal nature of such multi-interest cases. Because the study confirmed earlier findings that most of the risk is concentrated in the very young users, the paper provided important guidance to decision makers and young females in choosing the most suitable oral contraceptive.

With respect to the potential 'costs', respect for autonomy (violating privacy, absence of individual informed consent) of the females and (possibly) the prescribers involved in the study is critical. Data used in the study were anonymous but person-specific, meaning that the investigator could not link the research data to any individual women. The linkage procedure of the Dutch Pharmaco-Morbidity (PHARMO) record linkage database has been internationally acknowledged (PHARMO data have been used in more than 100 studies) and brings community pharmacy and hospital data within established hospital catchments regions, together on the basis of patients' birth date, gender, and general practitioner (GP) code (yielding a sensitivity and specificity of linking person-specific data from two separate databases of over 98% each, which means that 98% are correctly linked) (Herings et al. 1992). PHARMO has been linked also to primary care data, population surveys, laboratory data, cancer and accident registries, and other outcomes data using the same linkage model. Individual informed consent from all females involved in this study was not obtained and there are certain autonomy advocates who argue that this should be accomplished. Practical and methodological (those who refuse are mostly most relevant to the research) constraints would make individual informed consent virtually unfeasible. Instead, general informed consent in order to use the data for research purposes is obtained at the time a person enters the PHARMO area. The same holds for the participating physicians. PHARMO assures to them that all analyses are doctor-anonymous in order to prevent personalized auditing or other ways of influencing prescribing practice. Looking at the principle of 'beneficence', participating females have contributed (although not in conscious fashion) to the research and have taken their share in the solidarity of bringing together relevant data for solving an important public health problem.

Table 7.1. Most important possible 'benefits' and 'costs' when the study is done

	Autonomy	Beneficence non-maleficence	Justice
Study subjects	Costs	Benefit	Mixed
Physicians	Costs	Benefit	
Industry		Mixed	
Society at large		Benefit	Benefit

Whatever the outcomes of such an exercise are they provide a systematic frame for reflection and identification 'where things can go wrong'. The latter is a pivotal role of ethics in epidemiology (Coughlin 2000). Each preliminary idea of a study protocol should be accompanied with such an 'ethical scan'. Not only for the purpose of moral justification of the research but also for reasons of improving the quality of the research. Experiences in coping with requirements to assure data privacy have been dominated mainly by technical (e.g. probabilistic linking, de-identification, introduction of random error on an individual level, but not on a population level, etc.) or procedural (e.g. standard operating procedures, good practice standards, security, etc.) dimensions (Roos and Nicol 1999). From a pragmatic view these dimensions may fully satisfy. However, ethical weighing of 'benefits' and 'costs' also includes critical reflection of the aims, deliverables and consequences for the stakeholders (e.g. patients, physicians, etc.) involved. The latter goes beyond finding 'smart tricks' to deal with privacy regulations or clinical trial directives.

As stated before, the ability to link person-specific clinical, exposure and disease course data is a critical objective of epidemiology. Of all ethical issues and considerations, respecting autonomy by protecting privacy and confidentiality are the most crucial ones. Virtually all current legal systems in the Western world acknowledge the basic right of the patient to be assured that all his medical and personal data are confidential. Only in case of few well-defined exceptions disclosure of person-specific information is allowed, e.g. prevention of serious risk to public health, order by a court of law in a crime case, and under certain safeguards, scientific research. The tension between assuring personal privacy and access to medical data for epidemiological research has drawn ample attention from various stakeholders (individual patients, the public, politicians, health professionals, and the research community). In Table 7.1 possible violations of personal privacy related to either study subjects or physicians are classified as 'costs'.

The scientific community of epidemiologists struggles with these two concepts and tries to convince politicians and policy-makers of the importance of collective benefit to society from research with medical data and that we cannot rule out significant adverse effects to public health when epidemiological research has been made virtually impossible. Others take the pragmatic route using methodology that includes contemporary computer and statistical technology in order to build, within the framework of existing privacy legislation, aggregated, de-identified but person-specific, information. Court cases in several parts of Europe have concluded that the use of fully anonymous, de-identified patient data for the purpose of scientific epidemiological or clinical research is permissible under current law. In cases where it is not feasible to use primary data (collected directly from clinical practice for a specific, well-defined, purpose) in an anonymous fashion, informed consent should always be obtained. Epidemiological researchers may rely on access to non-anonymous medical records but access to patient records for a research purpose requires individual patient informed consent.

The effect on research quality will be determined by the proportion of individuals who refuse consent, or in the case of large automated databases, who are simply not contactable. Researchers, cautioned by privacy advocates, very often overestimate participation rates in consent procedures. There is growing evidence available that patients are willing to allow personal information to be used for research purposes. Several studies have shown that refusal to comply with consent procedures are most often not higher than in about one out of ten. A recent study form Canada suggests however, that study subjects want to be actively consulted before the start of an epidemiological study where personal information is collected, whenever this is practically feasible (Willison et al. 2003). Secondary use of data (use of existing data for purposes other than those for which they were originally obtained) remains controversial as some interpreters of the law feel that secondary data use is prohibited because of the requirement for data to be used only for purposes compatible with those for which it was originally collected. In practice we see that this requirement is solved by obtaining general informed consent, although many researchers have sought exemption from the consent requirements in order to minimise selection bias, logistical obstacles, time consumption and costs. Record linkage provides a powerful tool for the study of the natural history of diseases, the aetiology of rare diseases, or the study of drug-effect associations with a (long) induction period between exposure and outcome (Herings et al. 1992). The process of linkage of individual data from a number of sources, such as primary care records, secondary care records, prescribing and mortality data, requires patient identification and in many countries is not permitted because this is believed to breach data protection laws. In order to comply with confidentiality rules, researchers very often rely on medical staff providing them with a list of patients' names and addresses to be used as a sampling frame. Although no medical details are given, the provision of names and addresses is clearly not anonymous and this is likely to be in breach of European and US legislation (UK Parliament Acts 1998; US DHHS 2001). Experiences so far in record linkage represent a patchwork of various approaches to link individual sets of drug exposure and clinical data. In absence of a (national) unique identifier, researchers have to rely on other approaches for bringing separate datasets together to a patient-specific linked set.

7.4 Ethical Issues Specific to Epidemiology

7.4.1 Unethical Quality of Research

This brings us to another ethical angle of epidemiological research, namely poorly conducted research. That kind of research will for sure not benefit patients or society, but may cause harm when it leads to unsubstantiated and wrong decision making in clinical practice or policy making in public health. Taubes (1995) has addressed this issue in his thoughtful paper on the limits of epidemiology where he accuses the field for producing repeatedly exposure-outcome associations that do not hold very long because subsequent studies either contradict the findings or are unable to reproduce the main study results. Although scientific controversies are essential to progress and evolution in science, conflicting data and secondary turmoil in epidemiology do most often more harm than good (Vandenbroucke 1998; Skegg 2001). This means the 'Good Epidemiology Practices' with the purpose to prevent or adjust a priori poorly designed studies, are as important for quality assurance as for ethical reasons (IEA 1998).

7.4.2 Global Bioethics and Inequity

A remaining, but not less important ethical challenge for future epidemiological research is the gigantic inequity in global health. Large differences in disease burden, variable access to efficacious and safe medical technology, gaps in pharmaceuticals and health services are an enormous concern (World Medical Association 2000). Fighting against inequity in global health as a feature of modern medical and epidemiological ethics goes beyond the application of the Hippocratic oath. It is about prioritising, about creating affordability and access, and epidemiology is and will be the pivotal science of fuelling policy making and strategic action with quantitative evidence for managing this global problem (Reich 2000; World Health Organization 2003). The triangle global inequity, epidemiology and ethics contrasts extremely with the ethics of individual 'autonomy' of for instance a patient objecting against participating in a database study in the US or Europe. So far, ethicists have been struggling with 'prioritising' ethical issues. Questions whether a disease burden of an orphan disease with a prevalence of less than 1 : 10,000 in the EU is, or should be, as equally important as the burden of a tropical disease affecting millions and millions of people are still difficult to address. The future will teach us how far we can go with the 'equal' approach. We will face important challenges for epidemiologists and ethicists involved in these 'contrasting' areas. Some criteria, however, have been developed already. Both the declaration of Helsinki in its fifth amendment (2000) and the CIOMS guidelines for biomedical research state that research undertaken in populations with limited resources should be responsive to the health needs of the population. Moreover sponsors and investigators must ensure that products or knowledge generated by the research will be made reasonably available for the benefit of the population.

Epidemiological Determinism and Preventive Medicine   7.4.3

In the late nineties of the last century, James Le Fanu, a UK based general practitioner, wrote a reflecting and alluring book titled the 'Rise and fall of modern medicine' (Le Fanu 1999). In his book, the author is very critical about numerous features of contemporary medicine and health care, in particular about the role of epidemiology in medical education, knowledge building and clinical practice. Many of his arguments are close to the ethical questions arising from the determinism of epidemiology resulting in stratifying populations in categories of disease susceptibility, consequently leading to screening, 'healthy' behaviour and preventive medicine. The promise of genomics and other molecular strategies for improving the practice of medicine must be pursued taking into account the fundamental ethical principles of autonomy, beneficence, non-maleficence and justice. Because genetics are linked to family ties the 'right of not to know' for instance goes beyond the individual judgement and decision making of the persons involved in the study themselves.

Precautionary Principle and Scientific Evidence   7.4.4

Closely related to the former issue of epidemiological determinism is the question how strong the evidence of the relationship between a hypothesised cause (i.e. environmental factor, medical intervention, drug treatment) and the effect should be before implementation and public health action is justified (Rogers 2003). This is at the heart of the science of epidemiology, as we have seen in previous chapters, and there are many cases of 'established' exposure-outcome associations which had to be revoked afterwards because new studies and data became available, e.g. reserpine and breast cancer or fenoterol and asthma death (Fraser 1996; Spitzer et al. 1992). According to the precautionary principle, a principle widely embraced nowadays by politicians and consumer advocates, particularly in the area of assessing environmental risks, it is uncertainty that justifies and requires pro-active measures and regulations, and a reversal of the burden of proof. A manufacturer intending the marketing of a new product or a government planning to build a new power plant have the obligation to provide solid evidence on efficacy and safety of the innovation before authorisation is granted. The pharmaceutical market knows this system already since the early sixties of the last century, but also other areas of medical technology anticipate more pro-active assessment of the benefits and risks. The application of the precautionary principle is controversial because, according to its opponents, it drives behaviour of counterproductive risk-avoidance and defensive strategies in balancing risks and benefits of innovation. Assessment and prediction of health effects of any intervention depend on a synthesis of all available epidemiological and mechanistic evidence to produce a valid estimate of the likely effect. Epidemiology is an important scientific resource to fuel the precautionary principle. From that perspective the adverse effects of this principle in terms of, for instance, exclusion of susceptible patients from certain medical technologies because proof of safety is still lacking (e.g. pregnant women, children), or neglecting and discontinuing research and development in specific risky areas, call for ethical reasoning.

7.4.5   Medical Ethics and Epidemiology

Singer and colleagues (2001) have identified a number of important drivers in medical ethics:

— New ethical challenges posed by advances in biotechnology
— Maturation of clinical ethics by strengthening the research base and developing graduate programmes and fellowships
— Emphasising the intersection between clinical ethics and health policy, including a focus on ethics of health care institutions and health systems
— Increasing public education and involvement
— Developing the conceptual foundations of bioethics
— Changes in the doctor-patient relationship.

Epidemiology is very close to clinical medicine, as epidemiologists provide scientific underpinnings of (1) the diagnosis, (2) aetiology of the disease, and (3) the prognosis (and determinants of disease) in populations, both healthy and diseased. We anticipate that all major developments in medical genetics will have consequences for epidemiology ethics as well, directly or indirectly. But because epidemiology is frequently directed at the healthy part of the population, meaning those who are not (yet) ill, the field carries specific ethical responsibilities with respect to predictive competences, e.g. identifying risk factors and preventive medicine. Moreover, as stated before, there are not many scenarios in epidemiological research where study subjects individually can benefit directly from the study and/or the research results. Partly this is a consequence of the historical nature of for instance retrospective case-control or many cohort studies, the anonymity of the data, and the large numbers involved, making person-specific implementation of the study results to study subjects hardly feasible. These features contrast with clinical research with more options for direct patient benefit. Direct patient benefit (or harm) is also an important driver of the discussion on the ethics of placebo-controlled clinical trials in case there is an efficacious therapy available and not treating might harm the patient for sure, e.g. by severe worsening of the disease or mortality in oncology research, or suicide risk in evaluating antidepressive therapies (Storosum et al. 2001; Michels and Rothman 2003). In general it is accepted that placebo controlled trials are only morally acceptable in the absence of proven effective therapy.

Conclusions

7.5

Among many other factors, innovation in automated databases, the surge in molecular and genetic knowledge, and controversies about scientific integrity, conflict of interest and related issues, have increased apprehension of the importance of ethical aspects in epidemiology. In the beginning, concern about loss of privacy has been a key driver of ethical questioning in epidemiology and various techniques have been developed to cope with the confidentiality issue. The creation of unbiased person-specific histories (including both data on various exposure and outcomes) is a crucial requirement in epidemiology. Ethical weighing of 'benefits' and 'costs' can play an additional and relevant role as a vehicle for thoughtful reasoning (Beauchamp et al. 1991). Indeed, there have been expressed concerns about the various ways of misusing such data. In particular in the era of genetics and the increased interests of health insurers to reduce their business risks, there is a great need for prudence, protection and careful weighing (Bolt et al. 2002; Nuffield Council on Bioethics 2003). Discovery of genes determining the response to drugs is an emerging area of genomic research as well and will produce new and intriguing ethical questions.

When considering the four ethical principles of beneficence, non-maleficence, autonomy and justice on a scale of individual versus society as a whole, it is apparent that most of the 'benefits' of epidemiological research can be attributed to the collective level (community, society), and that most of the 'costs' fall down on the individual level. That makes epidemiology vulnerable for controversies where the individual-collective dimension is sensitive. The two examples of calcium-channel blockers and the users of oral contraceptives exemplified that participating study subjects themselves are virtually not benefiting from the study results. Current or future users of both drug categories however are in a much better position after the research has been done than before.

It is not a rare occurrence that epidemiological researchers perceive ethics as cumbersome, conservative and anti-scientific. Although these feelings may be justifiable in some cases, the ultimate balance sheet of more ethical weighing and reasoning will be positive. Ethical reasoning helps also to be concise in defining the research question, the design and conduct of the study. Ethics and the linked formal and legal frameworks (e.g. scientific conduct guidelines, privacy protocols, ethical review board, etc.) undoubtedly have delivered in terms of quality push, critical reflection and scientific enlightenment, and will continue to do so in the future. The research community, clinical medicine and patients, all are major stakeholders in searching for and achieving mutual benefit from integrating ethics into epidemiological science (Gillon 2003).

References

Bankowski Z, Bryant JH, Last JM (eds) (1991). Ethics and epidemiology: International Guidelines. CIOMS, Geneva

Barnes DA, Bero LA (1998) Why review articles on the health effects of passive smoking reach different conclusions. JAMA 279:1566–1570

Beauchamp TL, Childress JF (1989) Principles of biomedical ethics, 3rd edn. Oxford University Press, New York

Beauchamp TL, Cook RL, Fayerweather WE, Raabe GK, Thar WE, Cowles SR, Spivey GH (1991) Ethical guidelines for epidemiologists. J Clin Epidemiol 44(Suppl 1):151S–169S

Bolt LLE, Delden JJM van, Kalis A, Derijks HJ, Leufkens HGM (2002) Tailor-made pharmacotherapy: future developments and ethical challenges in the field of pharmacogenomics. Center for Bioethics and Health Law (CBG), Utrecht

Burke W, Daly M, Garber J, Botkin J, Kahn MJ, Lynch P, McTiernan A, Offit K, Perlman J, Petersen G, Thomson E, Varricchio C (1997) Recommendations for follow-up care of individuals with an inherited predisposition to cancer. II. BRCA1 and BRCA2. Cancer Genetics Studies Consortium. JAMA 277:997–1003

Callahan D (2003) Principlism and communitarianism. J Med Ethics 29(5):287–291

Coughlin SS (2000) Ethics in epidemiology at the end of the 20th century: ethics, values, and mission statements. Epidemiol Rev 22:169–175

De Vet HCW, Dekker JM, van Veen EB, Olsen J (2003) Access to data from European registries for epidemiological research: results from a survey by the International Epidemiological Association European Federation. Int J Epidemiol 32:1114–1115

Farr W (1875) Supplement to the 35th annual report of the registrar general for the years 1861–70. HMSO, London

Fraser HS (1996) Reserpine: a tragic victim of myths, marketing, and fashionable prescribing. Clin Pharmacol Ther 60:368–373

Gillon R (1994) Medical ethics: four principles plus attention to scope. Br Med J 309:184–188

Gillon R (2003) Ethics needs principles – four can encompass the rest – and respect for autonomy should be first among equals. J Med Ethics 29:307–312

Gostin L (1997) Health care information and the protection of personal privacy: ethical and legal considerations. Ann Intern Med 127:683–690

Herings RMC, Stricker BHCh, Nap G, Bakker A (1992) Pharmaco-morbidity linkage: a feasibility study comparing morbidity in two pharmacy-based exposure cohorts. J Epid Comm Health 46:136–140

Herings RM, Urquhart J, Leufkens HGM (1999) Venous thromboembolism among new users of different oral contraceptives. Lancet 354(9173):127–128

Hoeksema HL, Troost J, Grobbee DE, Wiersinga WM, van Wijmen FC, Klasen EC (2003) A case of fraud in a neurological pharmaceutical clinical trial. Ned Tijdschr Geneeskd 147(28):1372–1327

IEA (International Epidemiological Association) (1998) Good Epidemiological Practice. Proper conduct in epidemiologic research. Prepared by the European Epidemiology Group

Kelman CW, Bass AJ, Holman CD (2002). Research use of linked health data – a best practice protocol. Aust NZ J Public Health 26:251–255

Kmietowicz Z (2001) Registries will have to apply for right to collect patients' data without consent. Br Med J 322:1199

Knox EG (1992) Confidential medical records and epidemiologic research. Br Med J 304:727–728

Le Fanu J (1999) The rise and fall of modern medicine. Little Brown, London

Levinski NG (2002) Nonfinancial conflicts of interest in research. New Eng J Med 347:759–761

Maitland-van der Zee AH, de Boer A, Leufkens HGM (2000) The interface between pharmacoepidemiology and pharmacogenetics. Eur J Pharmacol 410:121–130

Maitland-van der Zee AH, Stricker BH, Klungel OH, Mantel-Teeuwisse AK, Kastelein JJ, Hofman A, Leufkens HGM, van Duijn CM, de Boer A (2003) Adherence to and dosing of beta-hydroxy-beta-methylglutaryl coenzyme A reductase inhibitors in the general population differs according to apolipoprotein E-genotypes. Pharmacogenetics 13:219–223

Malakoff D (2003) The multiple repercussions of a fudged grant application. Science 300:40

Michels KB, Rothman KJ (2003) Update on unethical use of placebos in randomised trials. Bioethics 17(2):188–204

Nilstun T, Westrin CG (1994) Analysing ethics. Health Care Analysis 2:43–46

Nuffield Council on Bioethics (2003) Pharmacogenetics: ethical issues http://www.nuffieldfoundation.org/bioethics/

Peto R (2001) Newsnight, BBC2, 18 May; Today Programme, Radio 4, 19 May

Psaty BM, Heckbert SR, Koepsell TD, Siscovick DS, Raghunathan TE, Weiss NS, Rosendaal FR, Lemaitre RN, Smith NL, Wahl PW, Wagner EH, Furberg CD (1995) The risk of myocardial infarction associated with antihypertensive drug therapies. JAMA 274:620–625

Quantin C, Bouzelat H, Allaert FA, Benhamiche AM, Faivre J, Dusserre L (1998) Automatic record hash coding and linkage for epidemiological follow-up data confidentiality. Methods Inf Med 37:271–277

Reich MR (2000) The global drug gap. Science 287:1979–1981

Rogers MD (2003) Risk analysis under uncertainty, the precautionary principle, and the new EU chemicals strategy. Regulatory Toxicol Pharmacol 37(3):370–381

Roos LL, Nicol JP (1999) A research registry: uses, development, and accuracy. J Clin Epidemiol 52:39–47

Roses AD (2000) Pharmacogenetics and the practice of medicine. Nature 405:857–865

Skegg DCG (2001) Evaluating the safety of medicines, with particular reference to contraception. Stat Med 20:3557–3569

Singer PA, Pellegrino ED, Siegler M (2001). Clinical ethics revisited. BMC Med Ethics 2(1):1

Spitzer WO, Suissa S, Ernst P, Horwitz RI, Habbick B, Cockcroft D, Boivin JF, McNutt M, Buist AS, Rebuck AS (1992) The use of beta-agonists and the risk of death and near death from asthma. N Engl J Med 326:501–506

Stelfox HT, Chua G, O'Rourke K, Detsky AS (1998). Conflict of interest in the debate over calcium-channel antagonists. New Eng J Med 338:101–106

Storosum JG, van Zwieten BJ, van den Brink W, Gersons BP, Broekmans AW (2001) Suicide risk in placebo-controlled studies of major depression. Am J Psychiatry 158(8):1271–1275

Taubes G (1995) Epidemiology faces its limits. Science 269 (5221):164–169

Thompson DF (1993) Understanding financial conflicts of interest. N Engl J Med 329:573–576

Tondel M, Axelson O (1999) Concerns about privacy in research may be exaggerated. Br Med J 319:706–707

UK Parliament Acts. European Data Protection Act (1998) http://www.hmso.gov.uk/acts1998/19980029.htm

US Department of Health and Human Services (2001) National Standards to Protect Patients' Personal Medical Records http://www.hhs.gov/

Vandenbroucke JP (1992) Privacy, confidentiality and epidemiology: the Dutch ordeal. Int J Epidemiol 21:825–826

Vandenbroucke JP (1998) Medical journals and the shaping of medical knowledge. Lancet 352:2001–2006

Venter JC, Adams MD, Myers EW, et al (2001) The sequence of the human genome. Science 291:1304–1351

Weed DL, Coughlin SS (1999) New ethics guidelines for epidemiology: background and rationale. Annals Epidemiol 9(5):277–280

Weed DL, McKeown RE (2001) Ethics in epidemiology and public health, [I] technical terms, [II] applied terms. J Epidemiol Public Health 55:855–857 [I], 56:739–741 [II]

Willison DJ, Keshavjee K, Nair K, Goldsmith C, Holbrook AM (2003) Patients' consent preferences for research uses of information in electronic medical records: interview and survey data. Br Med J 326:373–378

World Health Organization (2003). World Health Report 2003. Shaping the future. World Health Organization, Geneva

World Medical Association (2000) The Revised Declaration of Helsinki. Interpreting and Implementing Ethical Principles in Biomedical Research. Edinburgh: 52nd WMA General Assembly. JAMA 284:3043–3045 http://www.wma.net/e/policy/17e.html

List of Contributors

Wolfgang Ahrens
Division of
Epidemiological Methods
and Ethiologic Research
Bremen Institute
for Prevention Research
and Social Medicine (BIPS)
Linzer Str. 8–10
28359 Bremen
Germany

Karin Bammann
Devision of Biometry
and Data Management
Bremen Institute
for Prevention Research
and Social Medicine (BIPS)
Linzer Str. 8–10
28359 Bremen
Germany

Olga Basso
The Department
of Epidemiology
and Social Medicine
University of Aarhus
Vennelyst Boulevard 6
8000 Aarhus C
Denmark

Heiko Becher
Department
of Tropical Hygiene
and Public Health
Ruprecht Karls University

Im Neuenheimer Feld 324
69120 Heidelberg
Germany

Jacques Benichou
University of Rouen
Medical School
and Rouen University
Hospital
Department of Biostatistics
CHU de Rouen
1, rue de Germont
76031 Rouen Cedex
France

Marianne Berwick
Department
of Epidemiology
and Biostatistics
Memorial Sloan-Kettering
Cancer Center
1275 York Avenue
New York, 10021
USA

Caroline Beunckens
Biostatistics
Centre for Statistics
Limburg University Centrum
Universitaire Campus
Building D
3590 Diepenbeek
Belgium

Heike Bickeböller
Department
of Genetic Epidemiology
University of Göttingen
Medical School
Humboldtallee 32
37073 Göttingen
Germany

John F. Bithell
Department of Statistics
University of Oxford
1 South Parks Road
Oxford OX1 3TG
UK

Maria Blettner
Johannes Gutenberg
University
Institute for Medical
Biometry,
Epidemiology
and Informatics
Obere Zahlbacher Str. 69
55131 Mainz
Germany

Paolo Boffetta
Gene Environment
Epidemiology Group
IARC
150, Cours Albert-Thomas
69372 Lyon Cedex 08
France

Freddie I. Bray
Descriptive
Epidemiology Group
IARC
150, cours Albert Thomas
69372 Lyon Cedex 08
France

Norman E. Breslow
Department of Biostatistics
University of Washington
Box 357232
Seattle, WA 98195-7232
USA

Reinhard Busse
Institut of Health Sciences
Berlin University
of Technology
EB2 – Straße des 17. Juni 145
10623 Berlin
Germany

Jeffrey S. Buzas
Department of Mathematics
and Statistics
University of Vermont
16 Colchester Ave
Burlington, Vermont 05401

Asit Kumar Chakraborty
Bikalpa
557, 4th Block
8th Main
Koramangala
Bangalore 560 034
India

Tarani Chandola
Dept. of Epidemiology
and Public Health
University College London
1-19 Torrington Place
London WC1E 6BT
UK

Sylvaine Cordier
INSERM U435
Université de Rennes I
Campus de Beaulieu
35042 Rennes Cedex
France

Johannes J.M. van Delden
Centre for Bioethics
and Health Law
Utrecht University
Heidelberglaan 2
3584 CS Utrecht
Netherlands

Janet D. Elashoff
Research Institute
Atrium Annex Room 101
Cedars-Sinai Medical Center
8700 Beverly Boulevard
Los Angeles, CA 90048
USA

John W. Farquhar
Stanford Prevention
Research Center
Stanford University
School of Medicine
Hoover Pavilion, Room 229
221 Quarry Road
Stanford, CA 94305-5705
USA

Arlène Fink
Public Health –
Health Services/
Med-GIM&HSR
mail code: 173617
911 Broxton Plz/1562 Casale
Pacific Palisades CA 90272
USA

Stephen P. Fortmann
Stanford Prevention
Research Center
Stanford University
School of Medicine
Hoover Pavilion, Room N229
211 Quarry Road
Stanford, CA 94305-5705
USA

Silvia Franceschi
Infection and Cancer
Epidemiology Group
IARC
150, Cours Albert-Thomas
69372 Lyon Cedex 08
France

Edeltraut Garbe
Institute for Clinical
Pharmacology
Charité-University
Medicine Berlin
Schumannstr. 20/21
10117 Berlin
Germany

Christian A. Gericke
Institute of Health Sciences
Berlin University
of Technology
EB2 – Straße des 17. Juni 145
10623 Berlin
Germany

David C. Goff Jr.
Public Health Sciences
and Internal Medicine
Wake Forest University
School of Medicine
Medical Center Boulevard
Winston Salem
NC 27157-1063
USA

Ellen B. Gold
Devision of Epidemiology
Department
of Public Health Sciences
University of California
One Shields Avenue
Davis, CA 95616-8638
USA

Sander Greenland
Department of Epidemiology
UCLA School of Public Health
and
Department of Statistics
UCLA College of
Letters and Science
Los Angeles,
CA 90095-1772
USA

Gordon H. Guyatt
Departments of Medicine
and Clinical Epidemiology &
Biostatistics
McMaster University
Health Sciences Centre,
Room 2C12
Hamilton, Ontario, L8N 3Z5
Canada

Timo Hakulinen
Finnish Cancer Registry
Institute for Statistical
and Epidemiological
Cancer Research
Liisankatu 21B
00170 Helsinki
Finland

Ivy Jansen
Biostatistics
Centre for Statistics
Limburg University Centrum
Universitaire Campus
Building D
3590 Diepenbeek
Belgium

Anita Kar
Reader in Health Sciences
School of Health Sciences
University of Pune
Pune 411007
India

Philip H. Kass
Department of Population
Health and Reproduction
1018B Haring Hall
School of Veterinary Medicine
University of California
One Shields Avenue
Davis, CA 95616
USA
    and
Department of Epidemiology
and Preventive Medicine
School of Medicine
University of California
Davis, CA
USA

Michael G. Kenward
London School of Hygiene &
Tropical Medicine
Medical Statistics Unit
Keppel Street
London WC1E 7HT
UK

Lothar Kreienbrock
Department for Biometry,
Epidemiology and
Information Processing
Hannover School
of Veterinary Medicine
Bünteweg 2
30559 Hannover
Germany

Klaus Krickeberg
Le Châtelet
63270 Manglieu
France
    or
Großer Kamp 4
33619 Bielefeld
Germany

Darwin R. Labarthe
Division of Adult
and Community Health,
National Centre for
Chronic Disease Prevention
and Health Promotion
4770 Buford Highway NE
Mailstop K-30
Atlanta, GA 30341
USA

John M. Last
University of Ottawa
451 Smyth Road
Ottawa K1H 8M5
Canada

Stanley Lemeshow
School of Public Health,
Centre for Biostatistics
The Ohio State University
M161 Starling-Loving Hall
320 West 10th Avenue
Columbus, OH 43210-1240
USA

Hubert G. Leufkens
Department
of Pharmacoepidemiology
and Pharmacotherapy
Utrecht Institute
for Pharmaceutical Sciences
PO Box 80082
3508 TB Utrecht
Netherlands

Dorothy Mackerras
Menzies School
of Health Research,
Northern Territory
PO Box 41096
Casuarina NT 0811
Australia

Barrie M. Margetts
Public Health Nutrition
Institute of Human Nutrition
University of Southampton
Southampton
General Hospital
Southampton SO16 6YD
UK

Michael Marmot
Department of Epidemiology
and Public Health
University College London
1-19 Torrington Place
London WC1E 6BT
UK

Giuseppe Matullo
Department
of Genetic Biology
and Biochemistry
University of Torino
Via Santena 19
10126 Torino
Italy

Franco Merletti
Unit of Cancer Epidemiology
and Centre
for Oncologic Prevention
University of Torino
Via Santena, 7
10126 Torino
Italy

Anthony B. Miller
Department
of Public Health Sciences
Faculty of Medicine
University of Toronto
Toronto, Ontario, MSS 1A8
Canada

Dario Mirabelli
Unit of Cancer Epidemiology
and Centre
for Oncologic Prevention
University of Torino
Via Santena, 7
10126 Torino
Italy

Geert Molenberghs
Biostatistics
Centre for Statistics
Limburg University Centrum
Universitaire Campus
Building D
3590 Diepenbeek
Belgium

Jørn Olsen
The Danish Epidemiology
Science Centre
University of Aarhus
Vennelyst Boulevard 6
Building 260
8000 Aarhus C
Danmark

Mari Palta
Departments of
Population Health Sciences,
and Biostatistics
and Medical Informatics
University of Wisconsin
610 Walnut St.
Madison, WI 53726
USA

D. Maxwell Parkin
Descriptive Epidemiology
Group
International Agency for
Research on Cancer (IARC)
150, cours Albert Thomas
69372 Lyon Cedex 08
France

Neil Pearce
Centre for Public
Health Research
Research School
of Public Health
Massey University
Wellington Campus
Private Box 756
Wellington
New Zealand

Iris Pigeot
Division of Biometry
and Data Management
Bremen Institute
for Prevention Research
and Social Medicine (BIPS)
Linzer Str. 8–10
28359 Bremen
Germany

Martyn Plummer
Infection and Cancer
Epidmiology Group
IARC
150, Cours Albert-Thomas
69372 Lyon Cedex 08
France

Preetha Rajaraman
Division of Cancer
Epidemiology and Genetics
National Cancer Institute
6120 Executive Boulevard
MSC 7242 Bethesda,
Maryland 20892-7335
USA

Raoult Ratard
Louisiana Department
of Health and Hospitals
Office of Public Health
Infectious Disease
Epidemiology Section
325 Loyola Ave, Room 615
New Orleans, LA 70112
USA

Lorenzo Richiardi
Unit of Cancer Epidemiology
and Centre
for Oncologic Prevention

University of Torino
Via Santena, 7
10126 Torino
Italy

Hilkka Riihimäki
Department of Epidemiology
and Biostatistics
Finnish Institute
of Occupational Health
(FIOH)
Topeliuksenkatu 41 a A
00250 Helsinki
Finland

Måns Rosén
Centre for Epidemiology
The National Board of Health
and Welfare
106 30 Stockholm
Sweden

Kenneth J. Rothman
Department
of Epidemiology
and Department
of Medicine
Boston University
Medical Centre
715 Albany Street
Boston, MA 02118
USA

Jonathan M. Samet
Department of Epidemiology
Bloomberg School
of Public Health
The Johns Hopkins University
615 N. Wolfe Street
Suite W6041
Baltimore, MD 21205
USA

Peter D. Sasieni
Cancer Research UK
Department of Epidemiology,
Mathematics & Statistics
Cancer Research UK
Clinical Centre at Barts
  and
The London Wolfson Institute
of Preventive Medicine
Charterhouse Square
London EC1M 6BQ
UK

Thomas Schäfer
University of Applied Sciences
Gelsenkirchen
Fachbereich Wirtschaft
Bocholt
Statistik und
Wirtschaftsmathematik
Münsterstraße 265
46397 Bocholt
Germany

Peter Schlattmann
Institut für Medizinische
Informatik, Biometrie
und Epidemiologie
Charité –
Universitätsmedizin Berlin
Campus Benjamin Franklin
Hindenburgdamm 30
12200 Berlin
Germany

Holger J. Schünemann
Departments
of Medicine and Social &
Preventive Medicine
School of Medicine
and Biomedical Sciences
University at Buffalo
270 Farber Hall
3435 Main St
Buffalo, NY 14214
USA
  and

Department
of Clinical Epidemiology
and Biostatistics
McMaster University
Hamilton, Ontario
Canada

Leonard A. Stefanski
Department of Statistics
North Carolina
State University
Room 201-B,
Patterson Hall
2501 Founders Drive
Raleigh, NC 27695
USA

Patricia A. Stewart
Department of Health
and Human Services
National Institutes of Health
National Cancer Institute
Rockville, MD 20892
USA

Susanne Straif-Bourgeois
Louisiana Department of
Health and Hospitals
Office of Public Health
Infectious Disease
Epidemiology Section
325 Loyola Ave, Room 615
New Orleans, LA 70112
USA

Samy Suissa
Departments
of Epidemiology
and Biostatistics
McGill University
687 Av. des Pins Ouest
Ross 4.29
Montréal, Québec H3A 1A1
Canada

Herbert Thijs
Biostatistics
Centre for Statistics

Limburg University Centrum
Universitaire Campus
Building D
3590 Diepenbeek
Belgium

Tor D. Tosteson
Dartmouth Medical School
Rubin 7927
One Medical Center Drive
Lebanon, NH 03756
USA

Geert Verbeke
Biostatistics
Centre for Statistics
Limburg University Centrum
Universitaire Campus
Building D
3590 Diepenbeek
Belgium

Paolo Vineis
Dipartimento
di Scienze Biomediche
e Oncologia Umana
University of Torino
Via Santena, 7
10126 Torino
Italy
  and
Environmental Epidemiology
Department of Epidemiology
and Public Health
Imperial College London,
St Mary's Campus
Norfolk Place W2 1PG London
UK

Pascal Wild
INRS
Département Epidémiologie
en Entreprises
Avenue de Bourgogne
BP 27
54501 Vandoeuvre Cédex
France

Printing: Saladruck, Berlin
Binding: Stein+Lehmann, Berlin